Teaching Atlas of Spine Imaging

Teaching Atlas
of Spine Imaging

Ruth G. Ramsey
Professor of Radiology
Head, Section of Neuroradiology
The University of Chicago
Chicago, Illinois

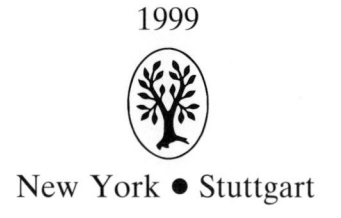

1999

New York • Stuttgart

Thieme New York
333 Seventh Avenue
New York, NY 10001

Executive Editor: Jane E. Pennington, Ph.D.
Editorial Assistant: Jinnie Kim
Editorial Director: Avé McCracken
Developmental Editor: Kathleen P. Lyons
Director, Production & Manufacturing: Maxine Langweil
Production Editor: Michele Mulligan
Marketing Director: Phyllis Gold
Sales Manager: David Bertelsen
Chief Financial Officer: Seth S. Fishman
President: Brian D. Scanlan
Cover Designer: Kevin Kall
Compositor: Bi-Comp, Inc.
Printer: Courier, Inc.

Library of Congress Cataloging-in-Publication Data

Ramsey, Ruth G.
   Teaching atlas of spine imaging / Ruth G. Ramsey.
     p. cm.
   Includes bibliographical references and index.
   ISBN 0-86577-778-0.—ISBN 3-13-115791-7
   1. Spine—Imaging—Atlases. 2. Spine—Imaging—Case studies.
I. Title.
   [DNLM: 1. Spinal Diseases—diagnosis atlases. 2. Spinal Diseases—
diagnosis case studies. 3. Spine—pathology atlases. 4. Magnetic
Resonance Imaging atlases. WE 18R183t 1998]
RD768.R36 1998
617.5′60754—dc21
DNLM/DLC
for Library of Congress   98-27857
                                                                                          CIP

Copyright © 1999 by Thieme Medical Publishers, Inc. This book, including all parts thereof, is legally protected by copyright. Any use, exploitation or commercialization outside the narrow limits set by copyright legislation, without the publisher's consent, is illegal and liable to prosecution. This applies in particular to photostat reproduction, copying, mimeographing or duplication of any kind, translating, preparation of microfilm, and electronic data processing and storage.

Important note: Medical knowledge is ever-changing. As new research and clinical experience broaden our knowledge, changes in treatment and drug therapy may be required. The authors and editors of the material herein have consulted sources believed to be reliable in their efforts to provide information that is complete and in accord with the standards accepted at the time of publication. However, in view of the possiblity of human error by the authors, editors, or publisher of the work herein, or changes in medical knowledge, neither the authors, editors, publisher, nor any other party who has been involved in the preparation of this work, warrants that the information contained herein is in every respect accurate or complete, and they are not responsible for any errors or omissions or for the results obtained from use of such information. Readers are encouraged to confirm the information contained herein with other sources. For example, readers are advised to check the product information sheet included in the package of each drug they plan to administer to be certain that the informaiton contained in this publication is accurate and that changes have not been made in the recommended dose or in the contraindications for administration. This recommendation is of particular importance in connection with new or infrequently used drugs.

Some of the product names, patents, and registered designs referred to in this book are in fact registered trademarks or proprietary names even though specific reference to this fact is not always made in the text. Therefore, the appearance of a name without designation as proprietary is not to be construed as a representation by the publisher that it is in the public domain.

Printed in the United States of America

5 4 3 2

TNY ISBN 0-86577-778-0
GTV ISBN 3-13-115791-7

For Michael, Thomas, and Timothy—

thanks for all your understanding

Contents

Preface xv
Acknowledgments xvii

I. Normal Anatomy

    A. Cervical spine
        Example 1. Sagittal 5
        Example 2. Midsagittal 9
    B. Thoracic spine
        Example 1. Sagittal short TR image 20
        Example 2. Sagittal long TR image 22
        Example 3. Sagittal short TR image in a pediatric patient 24
        Example 4. Sagittal long TR image in a pediatric patient 25
    C. Lumbar spine
        Example 1. Midsagittal short TR images 30
        Example 2. Midsagittal short TR images 34
        Example 3. Coronal short TR images 35
        Example 4. Parasagittal short TR images 37
        Example 5. Normal pediatric lumbar spine 40
        Example 6. Sagittal short TR images 42
        Example 7. Axial short TR images 45
        Example 8. Preinfusion and postinfusion axial short TR images . 51
        Example 9. Long TR images 52
        Example 10. Axial long TR images 54
        Example 11. Axial computed tomography images 56
        Example 12. Multiple Tarlov cysts 58

II. Congenital

    Case 1. Chiari I malformation with focal syrinx cavity 67
    Case 2. Chiari I malformation with lower cervical and thoracic syrinx cavity 71
    Case 3. Chiari I malformation and thoracic syrinx 74
    Case 4. Chiari type II malformation with a large meningomyelocele, sacral agenesis 77
    Case 5. Chiari II malformation with meningomyelocele, dysraphic spine, cerebellar tonsillar
        herniation, tethered cord, deformed vertebrae, and expanded foramen magnum . . 80
    Case 6. Chiari I malformation with syrinx cavity, postoperative changes with shunt
        tube placement 83
    Case 7. Chiari type III malformation 86
    Case 8. Anterior sacral myelomeningocele 88
    Case 9. Tethered cord, meningomyelocele, and coccygeal agenesis 90
    Case 10. Sacral agenesis with filum terminale lipoma and lower-than-normal spinal cord . . 93
    Case 11. Caudal regression syndrome with tethered cord and multiple vertebral anomalies . . 97
    Case 12. Partial sacral and coccygeal agenesis, sinus tract, spinal dysraphism, tethered
        spinal cord 100
    Case 13. Tethered cord, sacral agenesis, horseshoe, pelvic kidney 102
    Case 14. Tethered cord with filum terminale lipoma, syrinx of the distal cord, expanded
        lumbar vertebral canal 104
    Case 15. Tethered cord, sinus tract 107
    Case 16. Tethered cord, lipoma, myelomeningocele 109

Case 17. Klipple-Feil anomaly associated with the Chiari I malformation, tethered cord, lipoma, sacral agenesis 112
Case 18. Diastematomyelia, scoliosis, vertebral body 115
Case 19. Diastematomyelia 119
Case 20. Diastematomyelia with atrophic spinal cord with two slightly asymmetric hemicords and an associated syrinx cavity, *forme fruste* of a Chiari I malformation with deformity of the posterior fossa 122
Case 21. Neurofibromatosis type 1, multiple neurofibromata along the spine, a large plexiform neurofibroma along the course of the brachial plexus on the right arm 125
Case 22. Neurofibromatosis type 2, with multiple schwannomas, postoperative changes, spinal cord tethering 128
Case 23. Bilateral acoustic schwannomas and multiple spinal schwannomas; small right internal auditory canal lipoma 130
Case 24. Down's syndrome with C1-2 dislocation, congenital heart disease with atrial septal defect 133

III. Spinal Cord Tumors

A. Intramedullary
   Case 1. Ependymoma 137
   Case 2. Astrocytomas; neurofibromas of the dorsal root ganglion bilaterally 141
   Case 3. Pilocytic astrocytoma 145
   Case 4. Glioma of the cervical spinal cord and cerebellum, confirmed at surgery 149
   Case 5. Spinal cord lesion, a metastasis from the patient's known leiomyosarcoma, confirmed at surgery 151
   Case 6. Pilocytic astrocytoma, confirmed at surgery 154
   Case 7. Postoperative changes in a patient who had previous surgical removal of a spinal cord ependymoma 161
   Case 8. Pilocytic astrocytoma, confirmed by biopsy 164
   Case 9. Astrocytoma, confirmed at surgery; tumor arose from within the spinal cord and grew in an exophytic fashion; soft tissue schwannomas 167

B. Intradural
   Case 1. Schwannoma 175
   Case 2. Isolated schwannoma 178
   Case 3. Schwannoma; multiple myeloma 180
   Case 4. Schwannoma at L3; osteoporosis; postoperative changes 182
   Case 5. Meningioma, confirmed at surgery 184
   Case 6. Meningioma 186
   Case 7. Myxopapillary ependymoma 189
   Case 8. Myxopapillary ependymoma with areas of hemorrhage 192
   Case 9. Ependymoma; dilated Virchow-Robin spaces in the brain of unknown significance 195
   Case 10. Drop metastasis from recurrent posterior fossa ependymoma 198
   Case 11. Metastatic colon carcinoma 201

C. Neurofibromatosis
   Case 1. Neurofibromatosis type 1 with multiple plexiform neurofibromas 211
   Case 2. Neurofibromatosis type 1 with multiple plexiform and dumbbell-shaped tumors . . 217
   Case 3. Neurofibromatosis type 1 with multiple plexiform neurofibromas at all levels on the spine 225
   Case 4. Neurofibromatosis type 2 with plexiform neurofibromas in the intervertebral foramina, deep to the sternocleidomastoid muscle, and in the intradural space in the cervical and thoracic region 230
   Case 5. Probable nonenhancing low grade astrocytoma of the distal spinal cord 233
   Case 6. Neurofibromatosis type 2 with multiple spinal schwannomas, meningiomas, and ependymomas, as well as cerebral meningiomas and acoustic schwannomas 235
   Case 7. Neurofibromatosis with bilateral acoustic schwannomas, meningiomas, and spinal cord ependymomas 241

CONTENTS

    D. Miscellaneous
        Case 1. Chordoma, with postoperative changes 249
        Case 2. Metastatic chordomas: postsurgical changes 253
        Case 3. Chordoma within the vertebral body of L3, confirmed at biopsy 256
        Case 4. Multiple hemangioblastomas in a patient with von Hippel-Lindau disease 258
        Case 5. Sacral teratoma 260
        Case 6. Dermoid tumor, low spinal cord (proved at surgery) 263

IV. Trauma
        Case 1. Traumatic compression fracture with spinal cord edema 269
        Case 2. Compression fracture of L1 and distraction of the interfacet joints at the
                L1-2 level 272
        Case 3. Fracture dislocation of T6-7 with cord contusion and paraspinal hematoma
                formation 276
        Case 4. Flexion injury with fracture dislocation of the L1-2 spinous processes with tear in the
                dura and leakage of cerebrospinal fluid and blood into the soft tissue and muscles of
                the back 282
        Case 5. Compression fracture of L1 with spinal cord hematoma 284
        Case 6. Traumatic anterolisthesis of C4 on C5 with a traumatically herniated disc on the left
                side at the C4-5 level 286
        Case 7. Probably old fracture dislocation of C4 on C5 associated with a scoliosis and
                formation of a posttraumatic syrinx cavity at C4; presumed child abuse 289
        Case 8. Fracture dislocation of C2 on C3 in a "hangman's" type of fracture with a
                traumatically herniated disc at the C2-3 level 292
        Case 9. Old odontoid fracture; type 2 odontoid fracture 298
        Case 10. Bilateral perched facets 300
        Case 11. Anterior dislocation of C5 on C6 with disruption of the nucal ligament and
                traumatic herniation of the intervertebral disc at the C5-6 level 302
        Case 12. Small epidural hematoma 306
        Case 13. Epidural hematoma; blood in the thecal sac; air in the vertebral canal in the lower
                thoracic region 308
        Case 14. Spontaneous epidural hematoma 313
        Case 15. Spontaneous epidural hematoma in the midthoracic region secondary to
                coumadin treatment 317
        Case 16. Benign compression fractures of T4 and T12 secondary to osteoporosis 320
        Case 17. Multiple compression fractures 322
        Case 18. Multiple benign compression fractures secondary to osteoporosis 324

V. Metastases
        Case 1. Isolated metastatic breast carcinoma to the L3 vertebral body, proved at biopsy . . 331
        Case 2. Postradiation changes 338
        Case 3. Metastatic osteoblastic prostate cancer within the bone marrow; multiple para-aortic
                lymph nodes also show signs of metastatic disease 340
        Case 4. Postsurgical changes with placement of a metallic plate and multiple screws in the
                vertebral bodies at C5, 6, and 7; diffuse metastases to multiple vertebral bodies and
                spinous processes 344
        Case 5. Vertebral metastases and multiple pathologically enlarged lymph nodes secondary to
                non-Hodgkin's lymphoma 347
        Case 6. Diffuse metastases secondary to innumerable osteoblastic lesions related to the
                prostate cancer 350
        Case 7. Metastatic adenocarcinoma with bone destruction and spinal cord compression . . 353
        Case 8. Metastatic breast cancer with vertebral body involvement and
                pathologic adenopathy 357
        Case 9. Metastatic breast cancer involving multiple vertebral bodies and the brachial plexus 360
        Case 10. Metastatic lung cancer, biopsy proved; multiple additional lung nodules were present
                on the chest CT scan 362

Case 11.	Metastatic colon carcinoma to T12 with bone expansion and cord compression	367
Case 12.	Metastatic Ewing's sarcoma with cord compression at the T2 level	369
Case 13.	Metastatic renal cell cancer to the right lung and the vertebrae in the thoracic and lumbar region and involving the paratracheal lymph nodes	371
Case 14.	Chloroma, secondary to acute myelogenous leukemia	377
Case 15.	Metastatic renal cell carcinoma involving the C3 vertebral body with cord compression	380
Case 16.	Breast cancer, metastatic to the C2 vertebral body with cord compression	383
Case 17.	Metastatic lung cancer with bony and epidural metastases and cord compression	386
Case 18.	Multiple myeloma with involvement of the spine and bony calvarium	389
Case 19.	Multiple myeloma with diffuse marrow involvement and multiple pathologic compression fractures	392
Case 20.	Multiple myeloma	395
Case 21.	Diffuse metastases involving multiple vertebral bodies with a pathologic fracture at T6	397
Case 22.	Multiple myeloma with rapid progression	399
Case 23.	Multiple myeloma involving the bony structures and forming a soft tissue mass dorsal to the spinal cord resulting in cord compression	402
Case 24.	Multiple myeloma with diffuse infiltration of the bone marrow of the vertebral bodies and with a soft tissue mass	404
Case 25.	Multiple myeloma; multilevel epidural hematoma predominantly posteriorly, but also present anteriorly; bilateral bloody pleural effusions	407
Case 26.	Metastatic breast cancer with diffuse osteoblastic metastases	410
Case 27.	Breast cancer with osteoblastic metastases with soft tissue epidural component and spinal cord compression	412
Case 28.	Metastatic osteoblastic prostate carcinoma	414
Case 29.	Diffuse osteoblastic metastatic disease with mild soft tissue component in the lower cervical region and multiple pathologic fractures	417
Case 30.	Diffuse osteoblastic metastases from the patient's known primary osteogenic sarcoma	421

VI. Carcinomatosis

Case 1.	Spinal and cerebral meningeal carcinomatosis secondary to breast cancer, with involvement of the leptomeninges (pia and arachnoid) of the spine and brain; presumed metastatic deposit in the inferior end plate of the L4 vertebrae	429
Case 2.	Recurrent cerebral glioblastoma multiforme with drop metastases and resulting meningeal carcinomatosis	433
Case 3.	Diffuse bone metastases and spinal meningeal carcinomatosis	439
Case 4.	Diffuse leukemic infiltrate throughout the visualized marrow, resulting in diffuse decreased signal within the marrow of the vertebral bodies; minimal pathologic fracture of the L1 vertebral body; metastases in the distal end of the thecal sac; meningeal carcinomatosis; polycystic disease of the kidney (incidental finding)	443
Case 5.	Metastatic colon cancer in the subarachnoid space	447
Case 6.	Recurrent posterior fossa medulloblastoma with multiple drop metastases from medulloblastoma	449
Case 7.	Germinoma with drop metastases and resulting spinal meningeal carcinomatosis	451
Case 8.	Leukemic infiltrate in the marrow of the vertebral bodies and meningeal carcinomatosis with enhancement of the nerve roots of the cauda equina	455
Case 9.	Metastatic breast cancer to the vertebral body marrow and the spinal epidural space	458
Case 10.	Diffuse osteoblastic and osteolytic metastatic deposits throughout the bony structures; cerebral meningeal carcinomatosis	461

VII. Inflammatory

Case 1.	Discitis with soft tissue component and destruction of the vertebral body end plate	467

Case 2. Discitis, following trauma with an unusual organism as the etiologic agent; bilateral psoas abscesses and an abscess surrounding the abdominal aorta 470
Case 3. Discitis, involving the intervertebral disc with paraspinal extension; enhancement of the vertebral body reflects the presence of vertebral osteomyelitis 477
Case 4. Postoperative wound infection with draining sinus tract and postoperative disc infection; inflammatory process extends into the soft tissues of the back and into the intervertebral foramenae bilaterally 480
Case 5. Discitis and epidural and paraspinal abscess secondary to *Mycobacterium tuberculosis* 483
Case 6. Discitis, vertebral osteomyelitis; bilateral psoas abscesses; epidural abscess extending from the lumbar region through the thoracic spine; thick-rimmed thoracic paraspinal muscle abscess 487
Case 7. Multilevel anterior and posterior epidural abscess, meningitis and multiple dorsal and paraspinal, and psoas muscle abscesses 491
Case 8. Loculated, multilevel anterior and posterior epidural abscess secondary to retropharyngeal abscess; etiologic organism was not cultured 498
Case 9. Chemical meningitis with arachnoid adhesions 503
Case 10. Probably pneumonitis and meningitis with *Mycobacterium tuberculosis* 507
Case 11. *Mycobacterium tuberculosis* without evidence of sarcoidosis 509
Case 12. *Mycobacterium tuberculosis* in the interfacet joints of the thoracic and lumbar regions 512
Case 13. Cervical spinal cord involvement with sarcoidosis 516
Case 14. Cytomegalovirus radiculitis 519

VIII. Cervical Spine

Case 1. Large herniated disc at the C5-6 level on the right side 527
Case 2. Right-sided herniated intervertebral disc at the C5-6 level 532
Case 3. Left lateral herniated disc at the C4-5 level 535
Case 4. Herniated midline and left paracentral cervical disc at the C4-5 level 538
Case 5. Degenerative changes with osteophyte formation and trauma resulting in myelomalacia 540
Case 6. Rheumatoid arthritis with C1-2 dislocation; herniated disc at the C3-4 and C4-5 levels 544
Case 7. Atlantoaxial fusion; Klippel-Feil anomaly; right-sided herniated disc at the C4-5 level 549
Case 8. Herniated disc at C3-4 level; posterior longitudinal ligament ossification 553
Case 9. Posterior longitudinal ligament calcification/ossification 557
Case 10. Recent surgery for disc removal at the C4-5 and C5-6 levels with bony fusion plugs in place 561
Case 11. Large midline herniated disc at C3-4; postoperative changes with fusion at the C5-6 and C6-7 levels 563
Case 12. Postoperative changes with fusion at C4-5; bony osteophyte at the C4-5 level with compromise of the subarachnoid space; area of myelomalacia at the C4-5 level . . 567
Case 13. Degenerative change in the cervical spine with subsequent postoperative changes . . 570
Case 14. Right-sided herniated nucleus pulposus at C5-6 and resulting myelomalacia 574
Case 15. Postoperative changes; cervical spinal cord syrinx 579
Case 16. Diffuse idiopathic skeletal hyperostosis 581

IX. Thoracic Spine

Case 1. Herniated intervertebral disc at the T6-7 level 587
Case 2. Calcified, herniated intervertebral disc at the T6-7 level 591
Case 3. Herniated, calcified intervertebral disc at the T8-9 level 593
Case 4. Calcified, herniated intervertebral disc at the T6-7 level with compromise of the vertebral canal in the midline and on the left side 595
Case 5. von Hippel-Lindau disease with multiple cerebellar hemangioblastomas and spinal cord hemangioblastomas 599

TEACHING ATLAS OF SPINE IMAGING

Case 6.	Thoracic spinal cord ischemia and presumed infarction	602
Case 7.	Probable spinal cord ischemia with areas of enhancement	607
Case 8.	Spinal cord arteriovenous malformation with subarachnoid hemorrhage and spinal cord ischemia	610

X. Lumbar Disc

Case 1.	Large herniated disc at the L4-5 level; degenerated discs at the L3-4 and L5-S1 levels	619
Case 2.	Herniated, extruded disc	622
Case 3.	Laterally herniated disc at the L5-S1 level	625
Case 4.	Large left paracentral herniated disc at the L5-S1 and a moderately sized disc at the L4-5 level	629
Case 5.	Herniated, sequestered disc with nerve root enhancement	632
Case 6.	Large recurrent herniated disc fragment with peripheral enhancement	637
Case 7.	Recurrent herniated disc which has migrated behind the L5 vertebral body	640
Case 8.	Herniated disc, probably arising from the L2-3 level; surgically proved	645
Case 9.	Left laterally herniated disc at the L4-5 level with encroachment on the intervertebral foramen	647
Case 10.	Midline herniated disc at the L2-3 level; large extruded herniated disc with a sequestered fragment at the L4-5	651
Case 11.	Grade 1 spondylolisthesis secondary to bilateral spondylolysis at the L4-5 level	655
Case 12.	Bilateral spondylolysis and grade 1 spondylolisthesis	659
Case 13.	Grade 4 spondylolisthesis	662
Case 14.	Synovial cyst	666
Case 15.	Synovial cyst arising from the left interfacet joint at the L3-4 level	670
Case 16.	Spinal stenosis at the L3-4 level secondary to hypertrophy of the ligamentum flavum and encroachment upon the dorsal aspect of the vertebral canal; incidental Paget's disease of the lumbar spine at the L5, S1, and S2 levels, as well as the sacral alae and the iliac crests	673
Case 17.	Diffusely bulging disc, largest on the left side; lateral recess stenosis on the right side	677
Case 18.	Spinal stenosis with vacuum degenerative changes of the intervertebral disc	679
Case 19.	Spinal stenosis at the L4-5 and L3-4 levels with bulging discs at L3-4, L4-5, and L5-S1	681

XI. Miscellaneous

Case 1.	Multiple sclerosis of the brain and spinal cord	689
Case 2.	Multiple sclerosis of the brain and spinal cord	694
Case 3.	Probable multiple sclerosis	699
Case 4.	Multiple sclerosis of the spinal cord	703
Case 5.	Multiple sclerosis of the spinal cord	707
Case 6.	Transverse myelitis of unknown cause	709
Case 7.	Postimmunization transverse myelopathy (myelitis)	712
Case 8.	Postvaccination encephalomyelopathy (acute disseminated encephalomyelopathy) secondary to vaccination	716
Case 9.	Transverse myelitis, most likely secondary to multiple sclerosis	719
Case 10.	Transverse myelitis, cause unknown	722
Case 11.	Postradiation changes in the spinal cord and the vertebral bodies	725
Case 12.	Postradiation change with enhancement of the spinal cord	728
Case 13.	Postradiation change	731
Case 14.	Retained pantopaque; herniated disc at L4-5	733
Case 15.	Extensive postoperative changes with scarring and adhesions of the nerve roots of the cauda equina	736
Case 16.	Postoperative adhesive arachnoiditis	739
Case 17.	Epidural hematoma	742
Case 18.	Multilevel epidural hematoma in the lumbar region	744

Case 19.	Spinal cord lipoma	747
Case 20.	Epidural lipomatosis	750
Case 21.	Extramedullary hematopoiesis	752
Case 22.	Sickle cell anemia with multiple bone infarcts	756
Case 23.	Amyloidosis secondary to chronic renal failure with β_2 microgloblinemia	758
Case 24.	Scoliosis with dorsal encroachment secondary to degenerative changes, no tumor; secondary to poliomyelitis; postpolio syndrome	760
Case 25.	Postpolio syndrome	766
Case 26.	Postoperative change with focal atrophy of the spinal cord and anterior tethering of the cord to the posterior margin of the vertebral body	768
Case 27.	Multiple endplate herniations of the intervertebral discs called Schmorl's node deformities	771
Case 28.	Cavernous angioma of the spinal cord with hemorrhage	773

XII. Unknown Cases

Case 1.	Discitis with vertebral osteomyelitis at the L3-4 level and severe spinal stenosis	781
Case 2.	Epidural and prevertebral abscess	785
Case 3.	Multiple sclerosis of the brain and spinal cord	790
Case 4.	Neurofibromatosis type 2 with multiple schwannomas	793
Case 5.	Diffuse osteolytic and osteoblastic metastases involving all the visualized bony structures	795
Case 6.	Epidural hematoma, cause unknown	799
Case 7.	Diffuse osteoblastic and osteolytic metastases from prostate cancer	802
Case 8.	Multiple schwannomas and postoperative changes with laminectomy and tethering of the spinal cord posteriorly at the T12-L1 level	804
Case 9.	Desmoid tumor (unrelated to the recent trauma)	806
Case 10.	Chiari I malformation, postoperative changes in the posterior fossa; syrinx cavity	810
Case 11.	Neurofibromatosis type 1 with plexiform neurofibromata at all levels in the cervical spine	813
Case 12.	Lipoma at the L2 level with tethered spinal cord and diastematomyelia	818
Case 13.	C1-2 subluxation in association with Down syndrome	823
Case 14.	Large far laterally herniated disc at the L3-4 level; small midline herniated disc at the L4-5 level	826
Case 15.	Chordoma of the distal lumbar spine, iliac crest, sacrum, and coccyx	831
Case 16.	Cavernous angioma of the spinal cord	834
Case 17.	Metallic fusion plate and fixating screws	838
Case 18.	Diffuse bony metastases with pathologic fractures of T10, L1, and L2 and a metastatic deposit in the right lobe of the liver	842
Case 19.	Metastatic cancer involving the T11 and L4 vertebral bodies with epidural metastases	845
Case 20.	Spinal cord ependymoma with an associated syrinx cavity	849
Case 21.	Leukemic infiltrate of the bone marrow; leptomeningeal carcinomatosis	853
Case 22.	von Hippel-Lindau disease with multiple spinal and cerebral hemangioblastomas	857
Case 23.	Diffuse leukemic infiltrate of the marrow of the vertebral column; granulocytic sarcoma (chloroma) of the soft tissues of the neck; dural based meningeal metastases; bony calvarium metastases (?) chloroma	861

Index . . . 871

Preface

Teaching Atlas of Spine Imaging, a collection of both classic and challenging cases, is formatted to reflect "real-life" presentations. These cases, the emphasis of which is not rare and unusual cases, but those seen in a busy practice regardless of the clinical setting, begin with a brief clinical presentation, followed by a series of images, and a section entitled Radiologic Findings. The large format of the volume allows life-size presentation of the images to simulate the clinical setting at the time of interpretation. Armed with the clinical presentation, the images, and the radiologic findings, the reader should be able to make a diagnosis, which is subsequently provided, along with the differential diagnosis and a brief discussion of the abnormality. The need for clinical correlation and relevance is repeatedly emphasized. The clinical information, often not included on the consultation request, is frequently the key to diagnosis. In cases in which it is not possible to arrive at a diagnosis at the time of initial imaging evaluation, follow-up images are provided as well. Practical guidelines to diagnosis and imaging, called pearls and pitfalls, are highlighted in the margins.

Because the ability to evaluate abnormal anatomy requires an understanding of normal anatomy, the first section of the book evaluates the normal spine. The next nine sections—Congenital, Spinal Cord Tumors, Trauma, Metastases, Carcinomatosis, Inflammatory, Cervical Spine, Thoracic Spine, Lumbar Disc, and Miscellaneous Cases—address a wide variety of abnormalities that affect the vertebral column and the spinal cord. An up-to-date bibliography is included with each section. The final section is devoted to unknown cases. The reader may use these cases for self-assessment by either using the given clinical data or by using the images alone. These typical clinical cases cover a wide variety of clinical entities.

Evaluation of the vertebral column and spinal cord has evolved from plain film evaluation to the use of computed tomography (CT), to CT in conjunction with myelography, and most recently to magnetic resonance (MR) imaging in conjunction with a variety of basic and sophisticated techniques. At present, MR imaging has essentially replaced other imaging methods for evaluation of the vertebral spinal column and spinal cord. Although these news modalities are better for diagnosing spine abnormalities, this technology requires a keen eye and solid understanding of how the various abnormalities are imaged. It is my hope that this volume, developed as a response for an easy to use imaging guide for a variety of abnormalities of the spine will be used by both new and experienced practitioners alike to diagnose these special patients.

Acknowledgments

The vast majority of the photography was performed by Mr. Harold Tyler, without whose help this book would have been very difficult. Special thanks to the Neuroradiology fellows as well, especially Rajiv Shah who always watched for interesting teaching cases, Donna Bower Kim, Robert Wankmuller, Vivek Sehgal, and Sundeep Nayak. Thanks to Sharon Byrd for many of the pediatric cases. Thanks to the residents whose questions allowed me insight into what is complicated and difficult for them to understand about spine imaging. Thanks also to my clinical colleagues who suffered through all the teaching files that were made during the course of this project.

Thanks to Anne Healy, who always provided the necessary technical assistance and support, Margaret Caldwell my secretary, as well as the entire secretarial staff who pitched in when needed: Charlene Sheridan, Leslie Cleveland, Debbie Cop, and Evelyn Ruzik. The entire technology staff, who made certain that excellent images were obtained on all our patients. The film library staff also deserve special thanks for helping me to find the cases.

I would certainly be remiss if I did not mention the staff at Thieme Medical Publishers, including Hilary Evans, who encouraged me to start this project; Jane Pennington for her excellent advice; Michele Mulligan for her patience and perseverance; Kathy Lyons, who listened to all the phone calls and shepherded all the images through the process; and their colleagues in the New York office.

Thanks to Martin J. Lipton, Chairman of the Department of Radiology, for his help and encouragement.

Section I

Normal Anatomy

A. Cervical Spine

NORMAL ANATOMY

Cervical Spine

Evaluation of the normal cervical spine includes sagittal short and long TR images. Intermediate TR images in the sagittal plane may also be obtained. Axial images are obtained through any areas of interest using short TR sequences or sequences that result in increased signal intensity cerebrospinal fluid.

Contrast material is used in any patient who has had previous surgery. Contrast material should also be used in patients who are being evaluated for a possible tumor in the cervical region, an inflammatory process or a process such as meningeal carcinomatosis, or demyelinating disease such as multiple sclerosis.

The standard imaging sequences and planes may be modified in a variety of ways depending upon the clinical presentation and anatomic area and level of interest.

For various diseases, the following sequences are suggested:

1. Disc disease
   - Sagittal short and long TR images: fast spin-echo sequences may be used.
   - Axial short TR images or axial gradient-echo images: axial images should be obtained through all abnormal levels.

2. Intramedullary tumor
   - Sagittal short and long TR images.
   - Sagittal short TR images postcontrast.
   - Axial short TR images precontrast and postcontrast.

3. Cervical spinal cord multiple sclerosis
   - Sagittal short and long TR images.
   - Sagittal short TR images postcontrast.
   - Axial short TR images precontrast and postcontrast.
   - Axial long TR images or gradient echo images.

4. Cervical spine tumor
   - Sagittal short and long TR images.
   - Sagittal short TR images postcontrast.
   - Axial short TR images precontrast and postcontrast.

5. Cervical spine syrinx cavity with and without Chiari malformation
   - Sagittal short and long TR images including the skull base.
   - Axial short TR images.
   - Sagittal and axial images should include the entire length of the syrinx cavity.
   - The thoracic spinal cord should also be evaluated to determine the entire extent of the syrinx cavity.

6. Cervical spine congenital malformation
   - Sagittal short and long TR images.
   - Axial short TR images.
   - Axial images with increased signal intensity cerebrospinal fluid.
   - Additional images as needed for evaluation of the abnormality.
   - Short TR images post contrast material as needed.

Additional imaging sequences, such as fat-saturated images in any plane, should be used as necessary. Many cases need to be evaluated on a case-by-case basis. In complicated cases, it is necessary to monitor the imaging and alter the sequences and the planes of imaging as necessary for complete and accurate evaluation.

NORMAL ANATOMY

Example 1

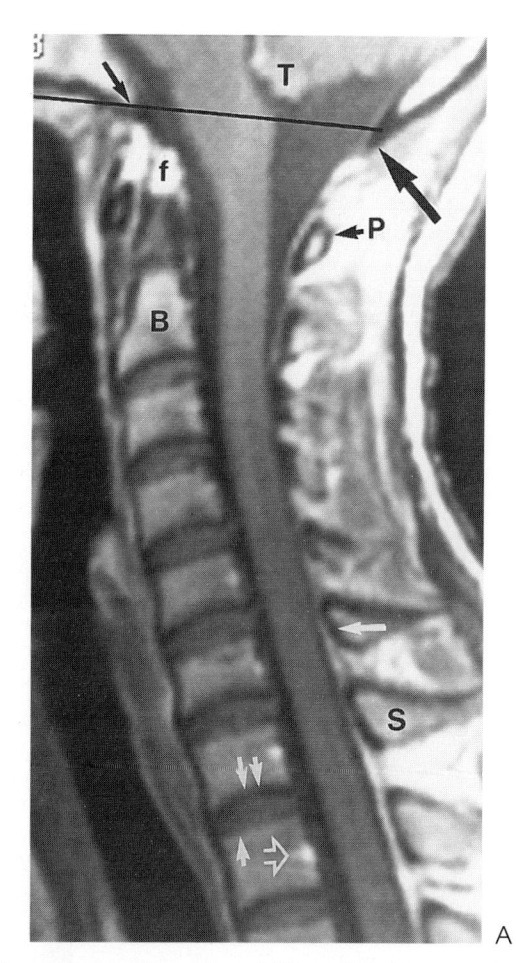

(Fig. A) Normal cervical spine short TR sagittal image. The outer table and the inner table of the bony calvaria both appear as linear areas of decreased signal intensity. The diploe of the calvaria is filled with fat and therefore appears as increased signal intensity. The point where the outer and inner table meet marks the posterior margin of the foramen magnum. Chamberlain's line is a line connecting the posterior margin of the foramen magnum with the posterior margin of the hard palate; basilar impression is present if half or more of the odontoid process projects above this line. The foramen magnum is defined as a line from the posterior margin of the hard palate to the posterior margin of the foramen magnum; in this patient, it is superimposed upon Chamberlain's line.

The posterior arch of C1 appears as an oval area of decreased signal intensity which represents the cortical bone margin with a central area of high signal intensity secondary to the normal marrow. The spinal laminar line is a low signal intensity line that is formed at the point that the laminae of the vertebral bodies join together and are viewed tangentially.

The inferior end plates of the vertebral bodies appear thicker and more decreased signal intensity than the superior end plates of the vertebral bodies. This appearance is secondary to chemical shift artifact. *T*, cerebellar tonsil; *long black arrow*, posterior margin of the foramen magnum; *short black arrow*, caudal end of the clivus; *f*, normal fat at the bottom of the clivus; *B*, body of the C2 vertebral body; *P-arrow*, posterior arch of C1; *long white arrow*, spinal laminar line; *short double white arrows*, inferior end plate of C7; *short single white arrow*, superior end plate of T1; *S*, spinous process; *long black line*, Chamberlain's line; *open arrow*, entrance point of venous plexus.

TEACHING ATLAS OF SPINE IMAGING

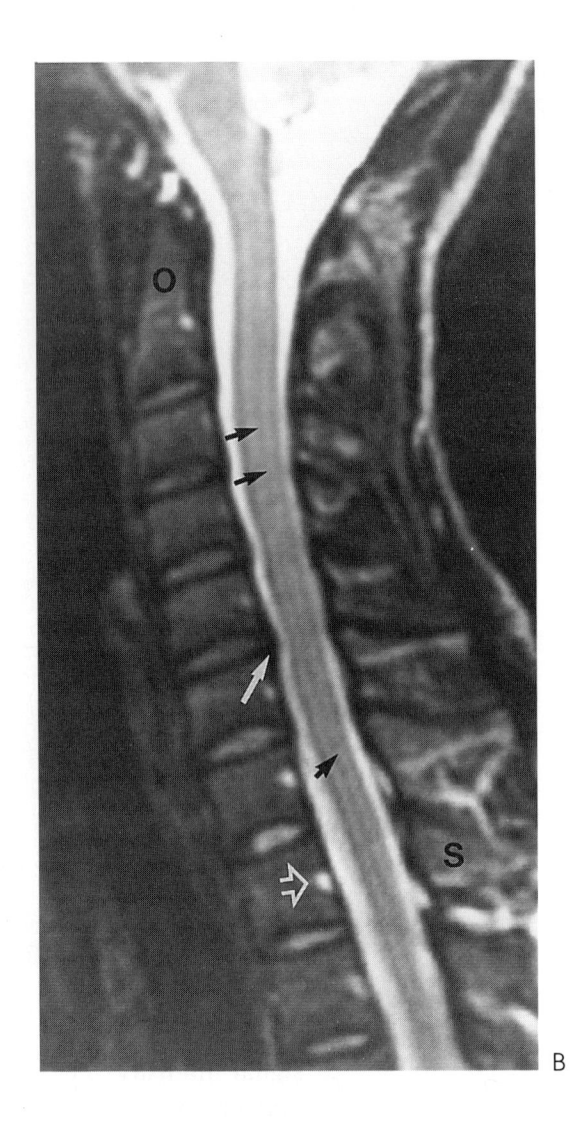

(Fig. B) Normal long TR sagittal image. *O*, odontoid process; *S*, spinous process; *white arrow*, small prominence of the C5-6 intervertebral disc; *black arrows*, longitudinal lines of increased and decreased signal intensity within the spinal cord secondary to truncation artifact; *open arrow*, basivertebral venous plexus.

NORMAL ANATOMY

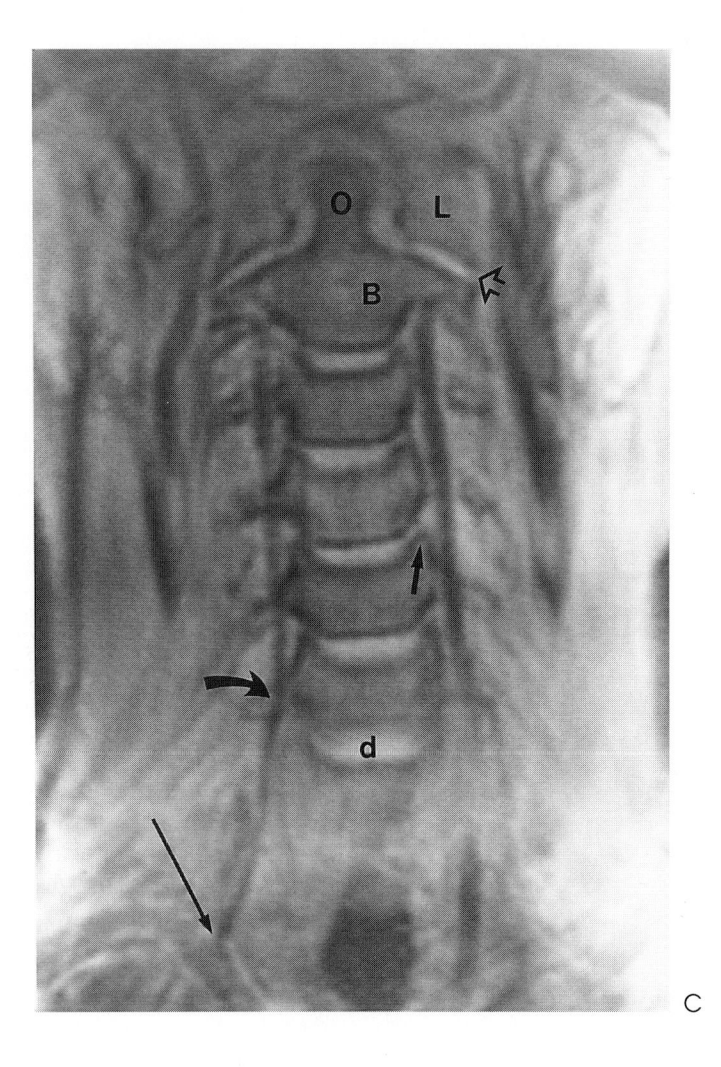

(Fig. C) Normal long TR coronal image of the cervical spine. The right and left vertebral arteries appear as areas of flow void within the foramena transversarium bilaterally. The left vertebral artery is larger than the right vertebral artery, a normal anatomic variant. The uncinate process is a small protuberance of bone that is beveled such that the vertebral body above is held in place by these bony processes. Degenerative changes frequently occur around these uncinate processes. *O*, odontoid process; *B*, body of the C2 vertebral body; *L*, lateral mass of the C1 vertebral body; *d*, intervertebral disc; *open arrow*, joint space between the lateral masses of C1 and C2; *short black arrow*, uncinate process; *long black arrow*, origin of the vertebral artery; *curved arrow*, entrance of the right vertebral artery into the foramen transversarium at the C6-7 level.

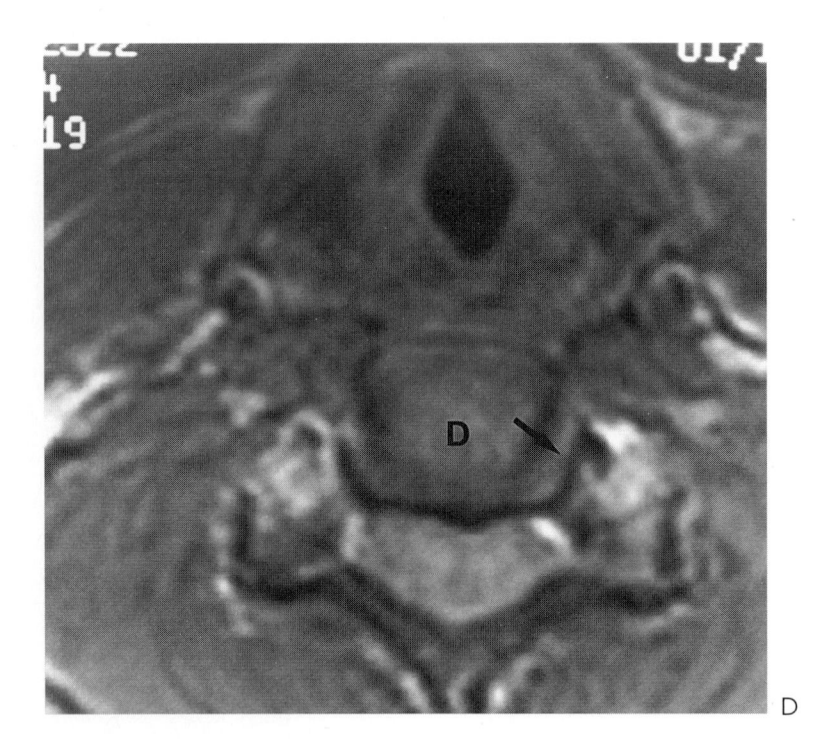

(Fig. D) Normal axial short TR image at the level of C4. The uncinate process defines the lateral margin of the vertebral body. *D*, intervertebral disc; *arrow,* marrow-filled uncinate process.

Example 2

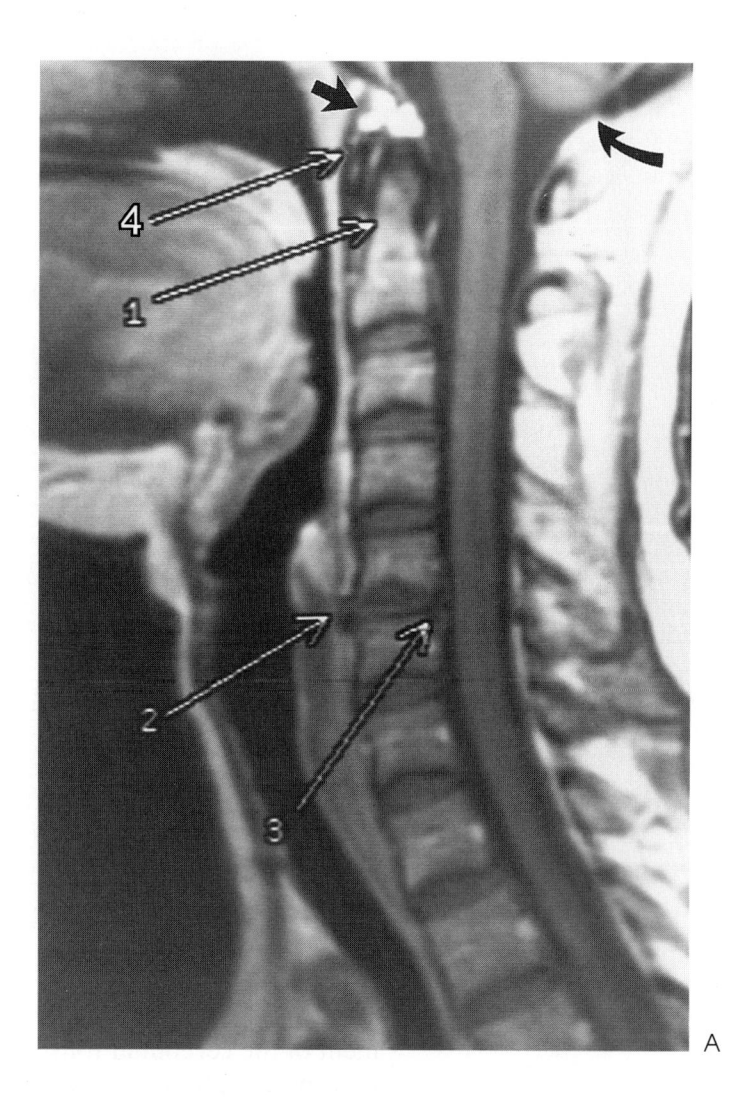

(Fig. A) Midsagittal short TR image of the cervical spine. *1*, odontoid process; *2*, small osteophytes on the anterior-inferior aspects of the end plate of C5 and the anterior-superior aspects of the end plate of C6; *3*, small posterior osteophyte on the posterior-superior aspects of the end plate of C6; *4*, anterior arch of the C1 vertebral body; *straight black arrow,* normal, irregularly marginated, high signal intensity area of fat that identifies the bottom of the clivus and projects just above the odontoid process. The high signal intensity of the fat is helpful in identifying the anterior margin of the foramen magnum. *curved black arrow,* normal posterior margin of the foramen magnum.

TEACHING ATLAS OF SPINE IMAGING

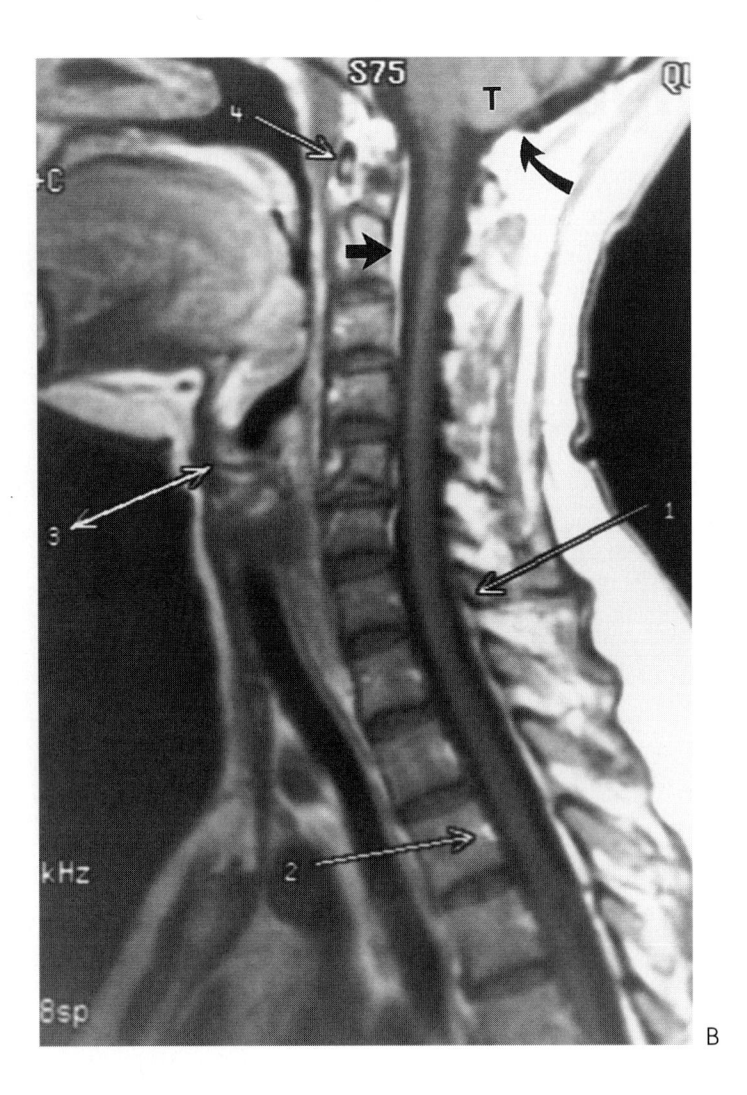

(Fig. B) Sagittal short TR image. Tonsillar "ectopia" is downward displacement of the cerebellar tonsils below the foramen magnum and is considered a normal anatomic variant. *1*, base of the spinous process; *2*, entrance of the venous plexus into the vertebral body; *3*, laryngeal ventricle; *4, black arrow,* behind the C2 vertebral body and extending to the level of the inferior end plate of C3, there is a streak of increased signal intensity that is the contrast-enhanced normal epidural venous plexus; *curved arrow,* posterior margin of the foramen magnum.

The Chiari I malformation is defined as: 1) downward displacement of one cerebellar tonsil at least 5 mm below the foramen magnum; 2) both cerebellar tonsils 3 to 5 mm below the foramen magnum into the upper cervical canal; 3) no history of myelomeningocele or radiologic evidence of a Chiari II malformation; 4) no prior cranial or cervical spinal surgery; 5) no mass causing the herniation.

NORMAL ANATOMY

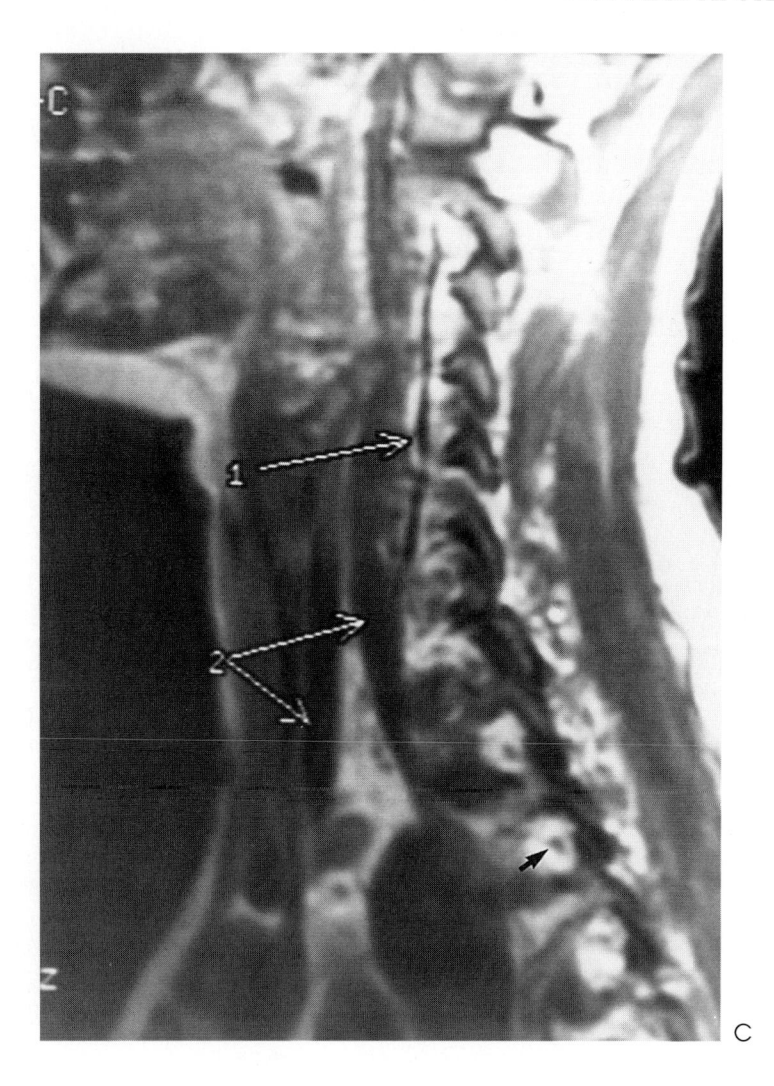

(Fig. C) Parasagittal short TR image at the level of the foramina transversaria. The vertebral artery enters into the foramen transversarium between the C6 and C7 vertebral bodies. *1*, vertebral artery in the foramen transversarium; *2*, anterior and middle scalenus muscles; *black arrow,* the nerve in the intervertebral foramen surrounded by normal high signal intensity fat.

TEACHING ATLAS OF SPINE IMAGING

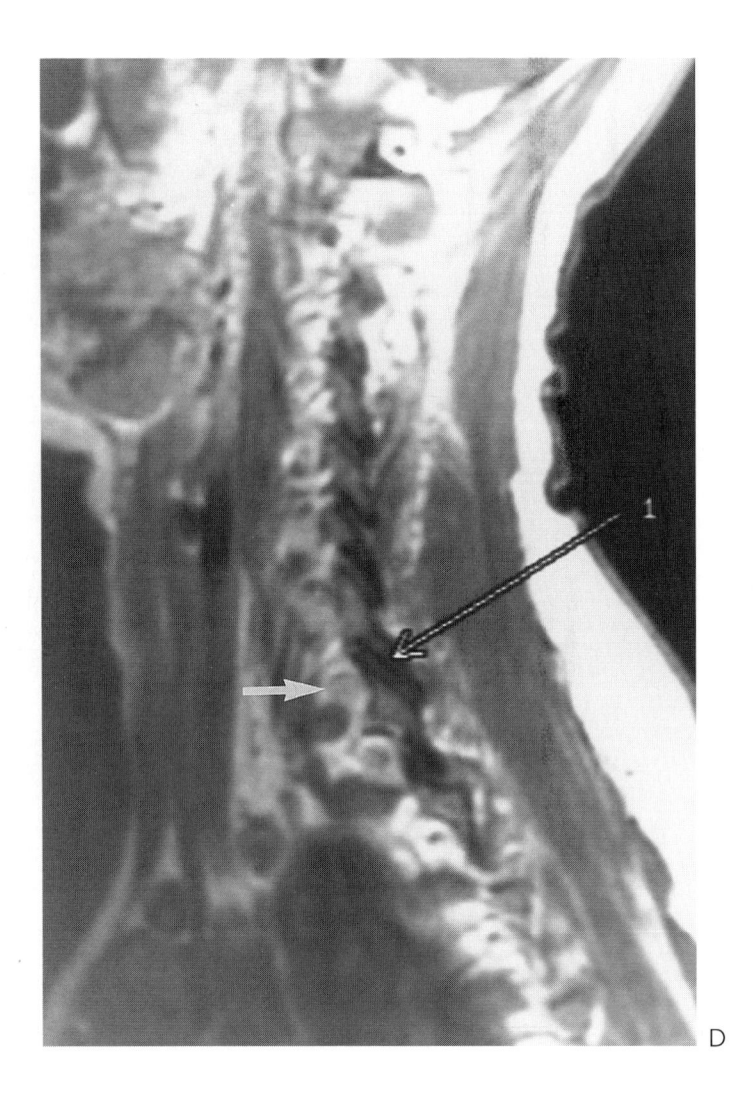

(Fig. D) Parasagittal short TR image at the level of the interfacet joint. *1*, normal interfacet joint; *white arrow,* normal dorsal root ganglion.

NORMAL ANATOMY

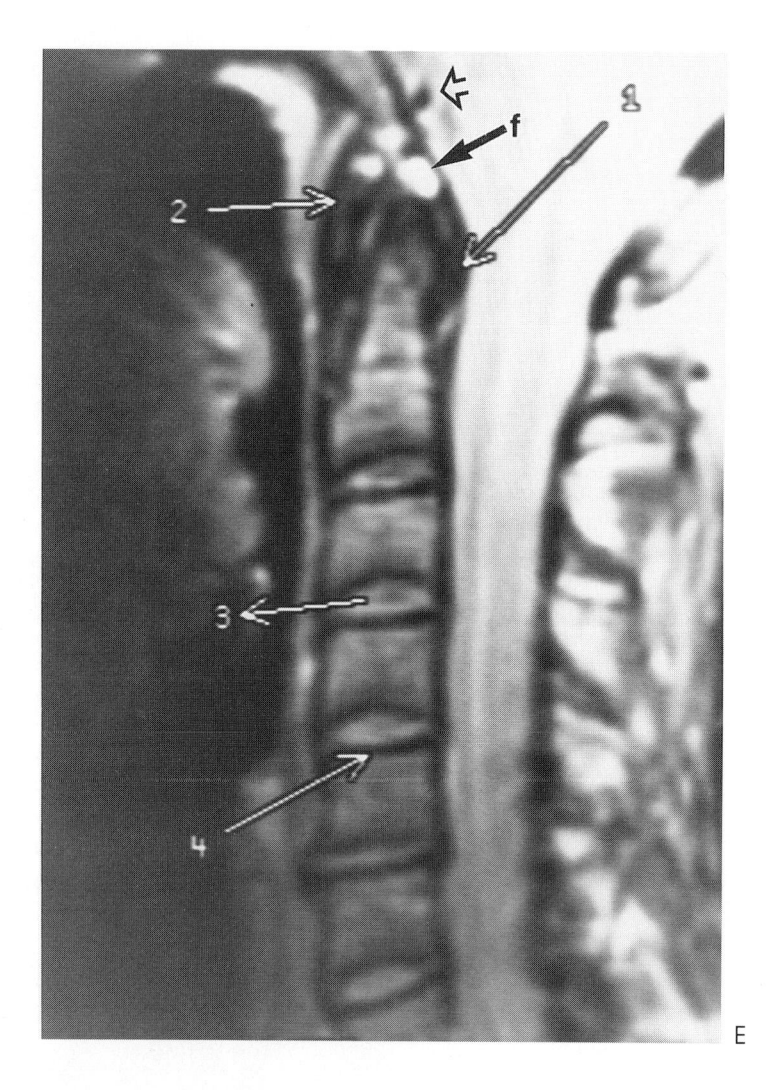

(Fig. E) Sagittal long TR image. *1*, normal low signal intensity of the transverse and cruciate ligaments; *2*, anterior arch of C1; *3*, normal intervertebral disc; *4*, normal decreased signal intensity of the superior end plate of the vertebral body; *f-arrow,* identifies the fat at the inferior end of the clivus and marks the anterior margin of the foramen magnum; *open arrow,* flow void of the vertebral body.

TEACHING ATLAS OF SPINE IMAGING

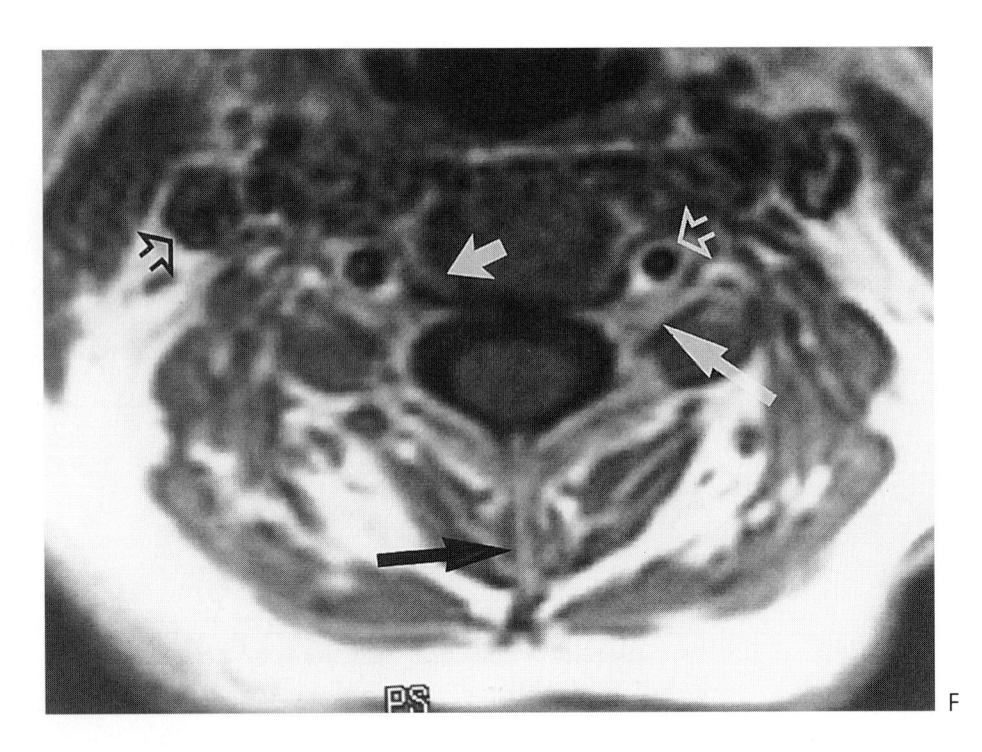

(Fig. F) Normal short TR image postinfusion. *Open black arrow*, jugular vein; *open white arrow*, flow void of the left vertebral artery; *short solid white arrow*, uncinate process; *long solid white arrow*, enhancing dorsal root ganglion; *long solid black arrow*, spinous process.

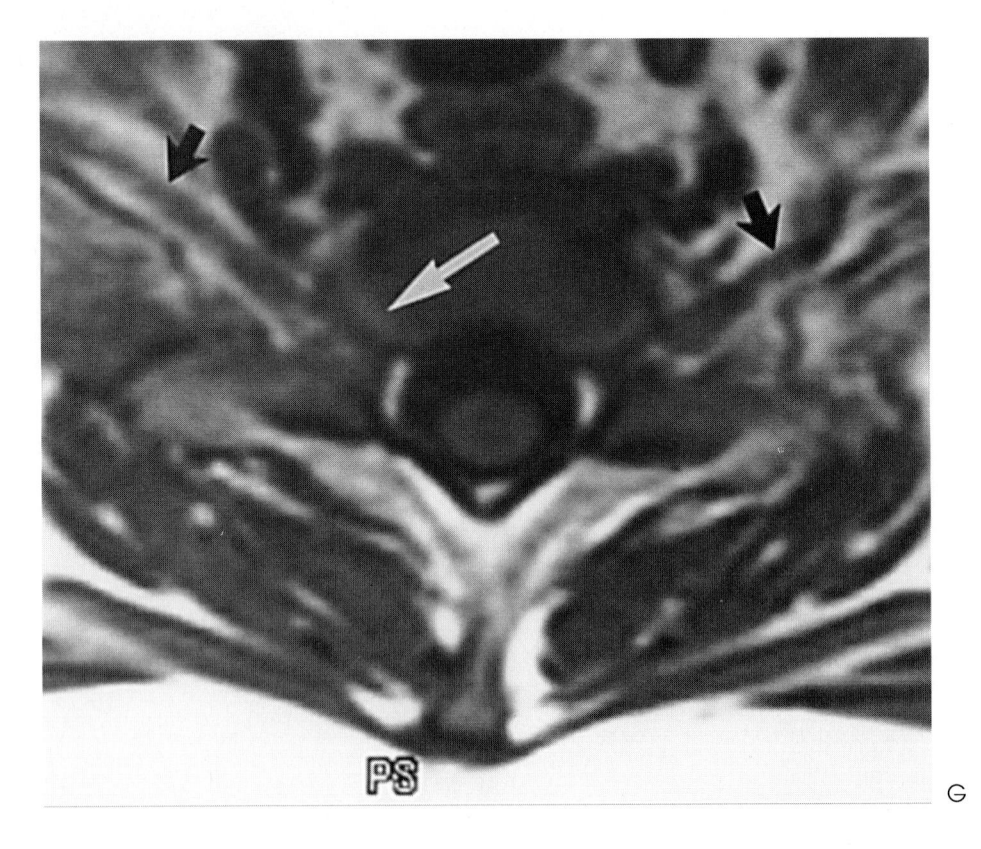

(Fig. G) Axial short TR image in the lower cervical region. *Black arrows*, nerves of the brachial plexus surrounded by high signal intensity fat; *white arrow*, the curvilinear high signal intensity of the marrow-filled uncinate process.

NORMAL ANATOMY

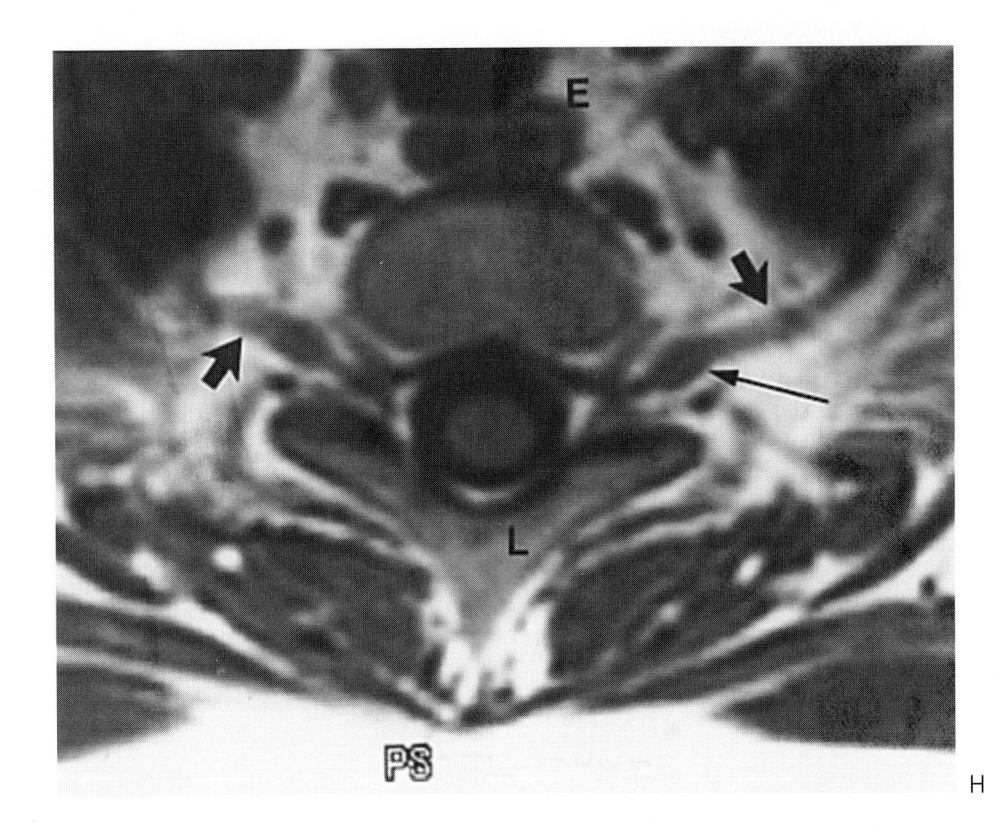

(Fig. H) Axial short TR image in the lower cervical region. Just lateral to the spine, the nerves of the brachial plexus are positioned between the anterior and middle scalenus muscles. *Short black arrows,* nerve roots of the brachial plexus; *long arrow,* dorsal root ganglion; *L,* lamina of the vertebral; *E,* esophagus

Section I
Normal Anatomy
B. Thoracic Spine

Thoracic Spine

Imaging of the normal thoracic spine includes sagittal short and long TR images as well as axial short TR images through any areas of interest or demonstrated abnormality.

Contrast material is generally not used for the evaluation of thoracic disc disease. However, contrast material is mandatory if the patient has had previous surgery, for the evaluation of a spinal cord tumor, for evaluation of a tumor in the thoracic vertebral canal, for the evaluation of meningeal carcinomatosis, or for the evaluation of a vascular malformation.

Axial images may also be obtained with a variety of other imaging sequences that result in increased signal intensity cerebrospinal fluid.

Images should be annotated such that they include the skull base or the distal end of the lumbar vertebral column so that the exact level of any abnormality can be identified in the lumbar spine.

Example 1

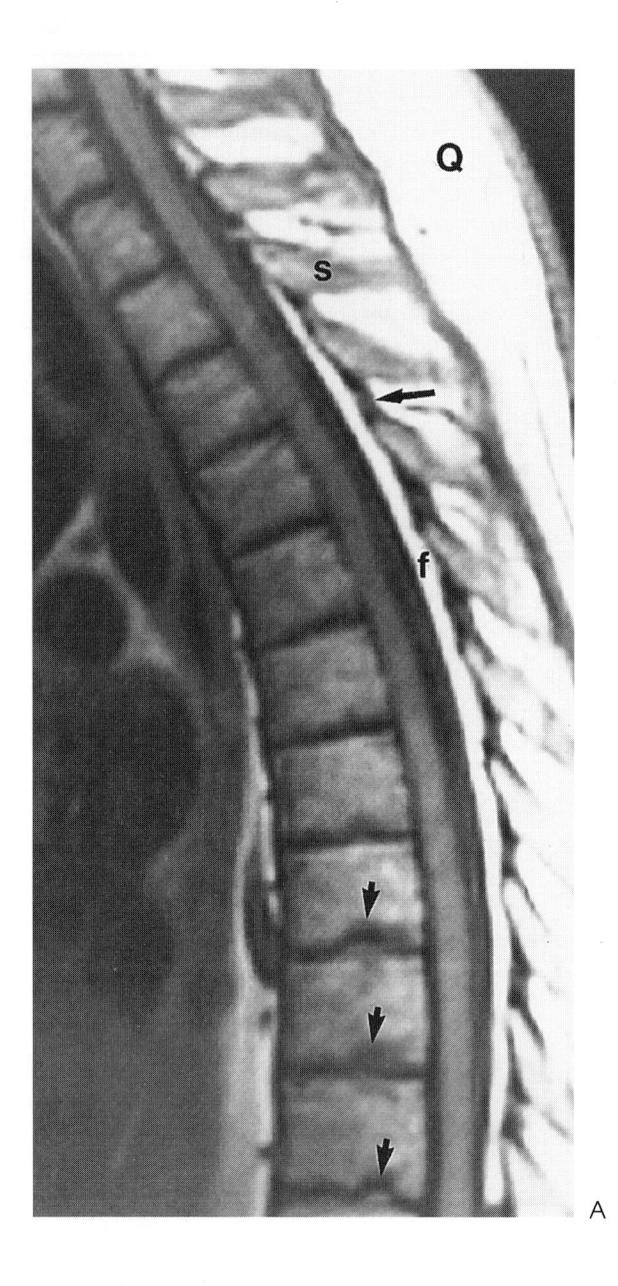

(Fig. A) Normal short TR image of the thoracic spine. The spinal cord follows a normal curvilinear path along the posterior margin of the vertebral column. There is a normal thoracic kyphosis. The spinal cord appears as intermediate signal intensity surrounded by the decreased signal intensity of the normal cerebrospinal fluid. *Q*, high signal intensity subcutaneous fat; *S*, spinous process; *F*, normal high signal intensity epidural fat; *black arrows,* small Schmorl's node deformities in the inferior end plates of three lower thoracic vertebral bodies.

NORMAL ANATOMY

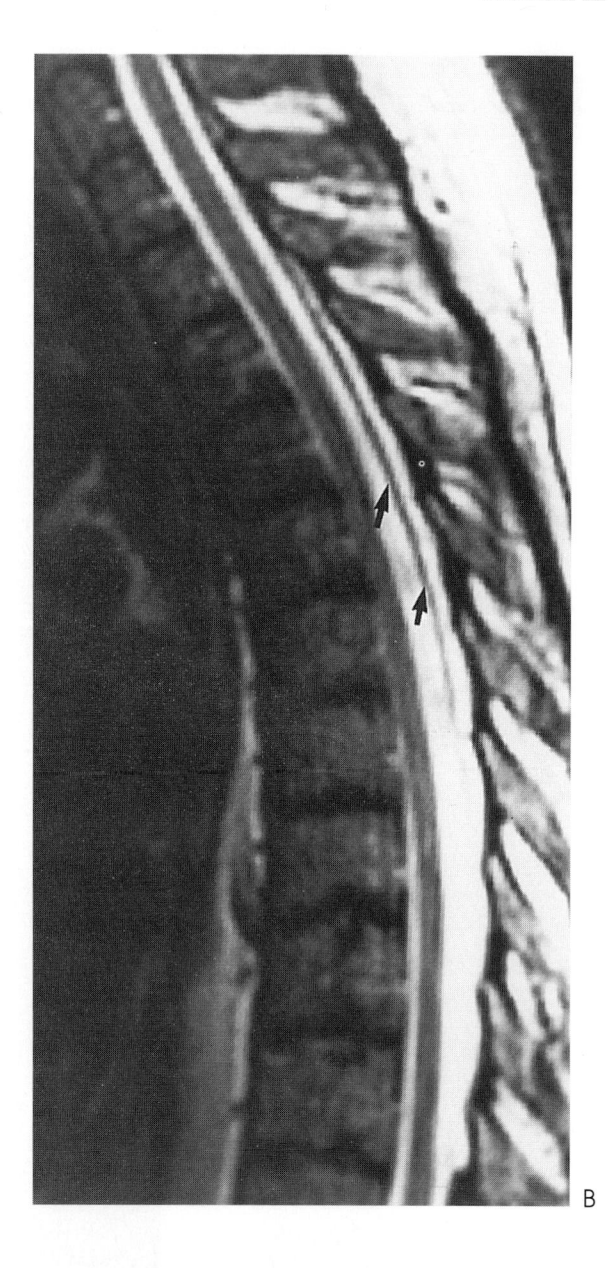

(Fig. B) Normal sagittal long TR image. The black arrows identify a curvilinear area of decreased signal intensity which is an area of flow-related enhancement secondary to movement of the cerebrospinal fluid dorsal to the thoracic spinal cord. The spinal cord appears as decreased signal intensity surrounded by the high signal intensity of the cerebrospinal fluid.

TEACHING ATLAS OF SPINE IMAGING

Example 2

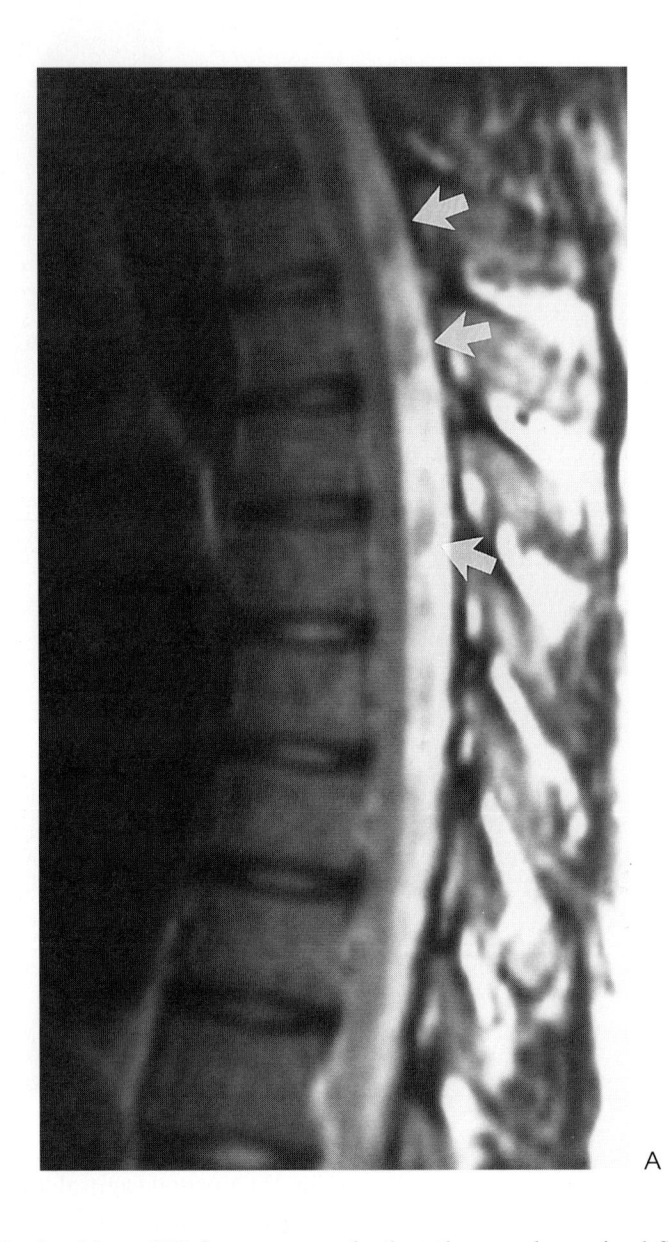

(Fig. A) Sagittal long TR image reveals that the cerebrospinal fluid appears as increased signal intensity. Within the cerebrospinal fluid and dorsal to the spinal cord (*arrows*), there are areas of decreased signal intensity secondary to flow-related enhancement of cerebrospinal fluid.

NORMAL ANATOMY

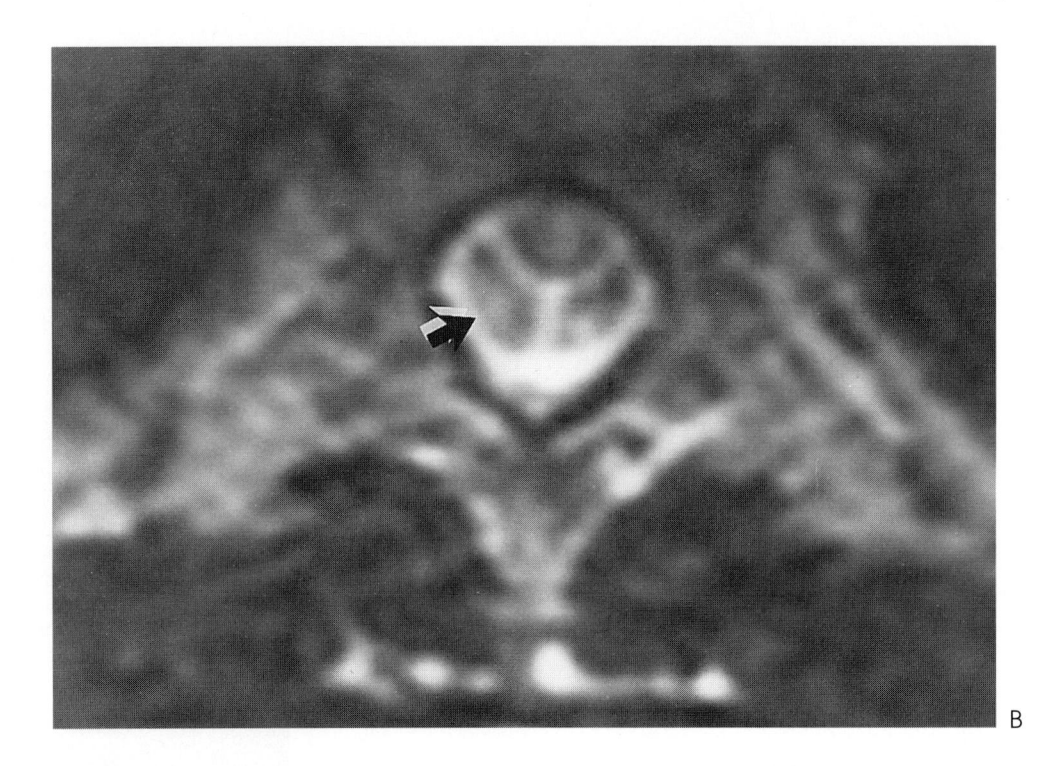

(Fig. B) Axial long TR image also reveals the areas of decreased signal intensity dorsal to the spinal cord secondary to flow-related enhancement of the cerebrospinal fluid (*arrow*).

Be aware that this type of flow-related enhancement may occur. This finding of flow-related enhancement does not indicate the presence of a spinal cord arteriovenous malformation.

TEACHING ATLAS OF SPINE IMAGING

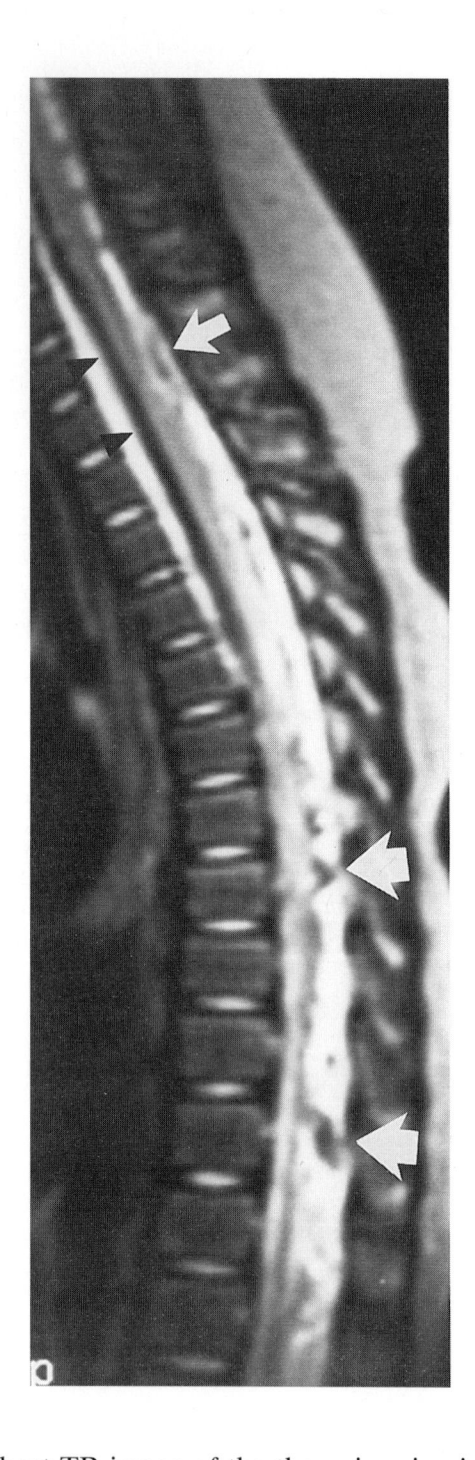

Example 3

(Fig. A) Sagittal short TR image of the thoracic spine in a pediatric spine. The intervertebral disc (disk) and adjacent cartilagenous end plates of the adjacent vertebral bodies appear as increased signal intensity (*white arrows*). The vertebral body appears as decreased signal intensity as compared to the intervertebral disc; this is the reverse of the appearance seen in adults. The thoracic spinal cord enlarges slightly in its distal portion and ends at the level of L1 intervertebral disc (*O*); this is slightly higher than the normal level.

NORMAL ANATOMY

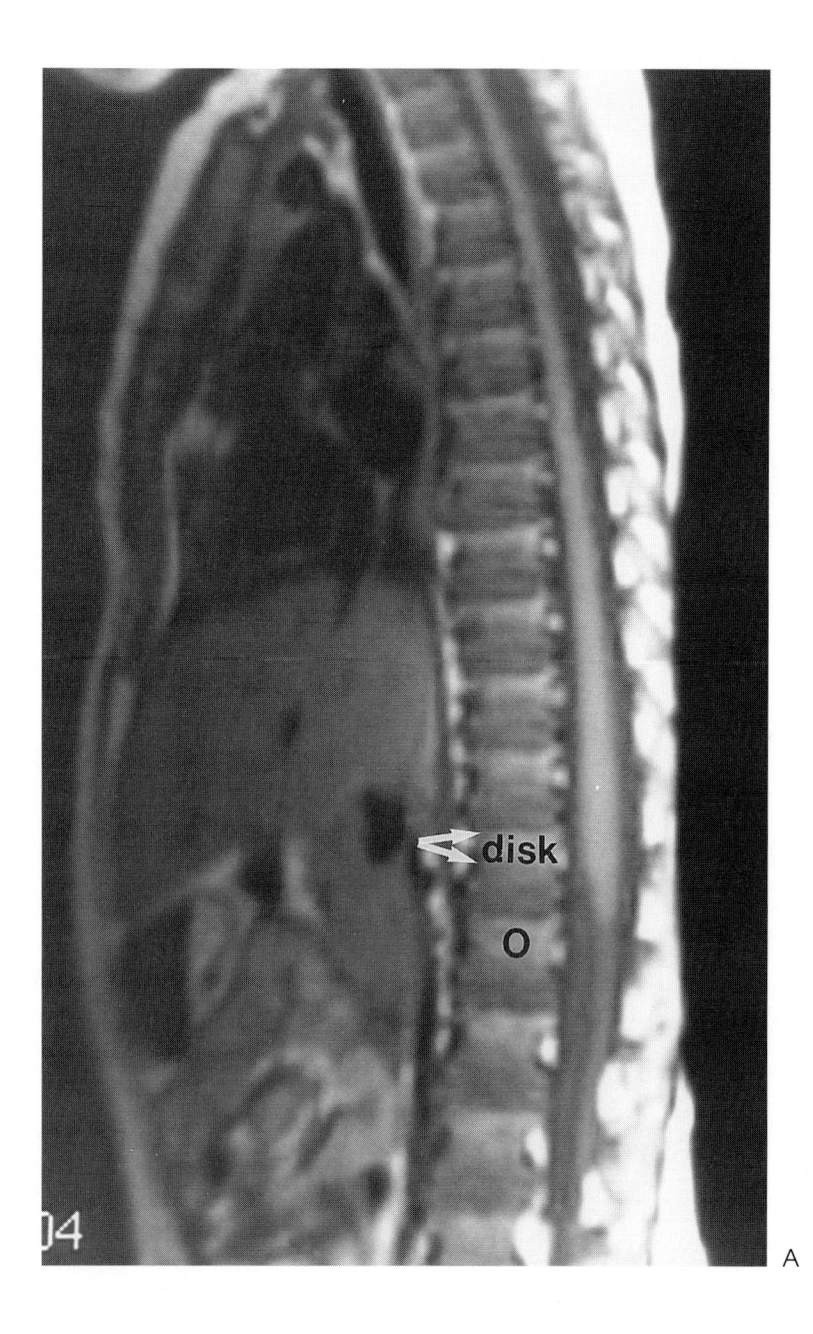

Example 4

(Fig. A) Pediatric thoracic spine. Sagittal long TR image of the thoracic spine reveals curvilinear areas of decreased signal intensity dorsal to the spinal cord (*white arrows*) and a long thin area of decreased signal intensity ventral to the spinal cord (*black arrowheads*). These areas represent turbulent flow dorsal to the spinal cord and smooth linear flow ventral to the spinal cord. The normal intervertebral discs appear as increased signal intensity.

Section I

Normal Anatomy

C. Lumbar Spine

Lumbar Spine

Magnetic resonance imaging is an excellent method for evaluating the entire vertebral column. The normal high signal intensity adipose tissue surrounding the various neural structures provides an excellent contrast material. The spine can be imaged using a wide variety of imaging sequences. Each of these sequences has advantages and disadvantages. Normal examination of the spine includes sagittal short and long TR images that extend from one side to the opposite side of the vertebral column. Axial images are also obtained using either short TR images or images with increased signal intensity cerebrospinal fluid such as long TR images or gradient-echo images. The axial images include parallel-stacked slices through the lowest three lumbar intervertebral discs and additional stacked images angled through and parallel to the intervertebral discs. Ideally, the axial images include parallel slices as well as angled slices. At a minimum, the axial images should extend from the level of the vertebral pedicle of one vertebral body to the level of the pedicle of the adjacent vertebral body. In the evaluation of disc disease, long TR images should be obtained so that any decrease in signal intensity, which reflects the presence of degenerative change, can be identified.

Indications for Contrast Enhancement

Evaluation for disc disease does not require the use of contrast material unless the patient has had previous surgery. Contrast material should be used in all patients who have had previous surgery.

Contrast material should be used in all patients who are being evaluated for meningeal carcinomatosis or spinal cord or vertebral canal tumor. Contrast material is generally not necessary for the evaluation of bony metastases unless there is a soft tissue component.

TEACHING ATLAS OF SPINE IMAGING

Example 1

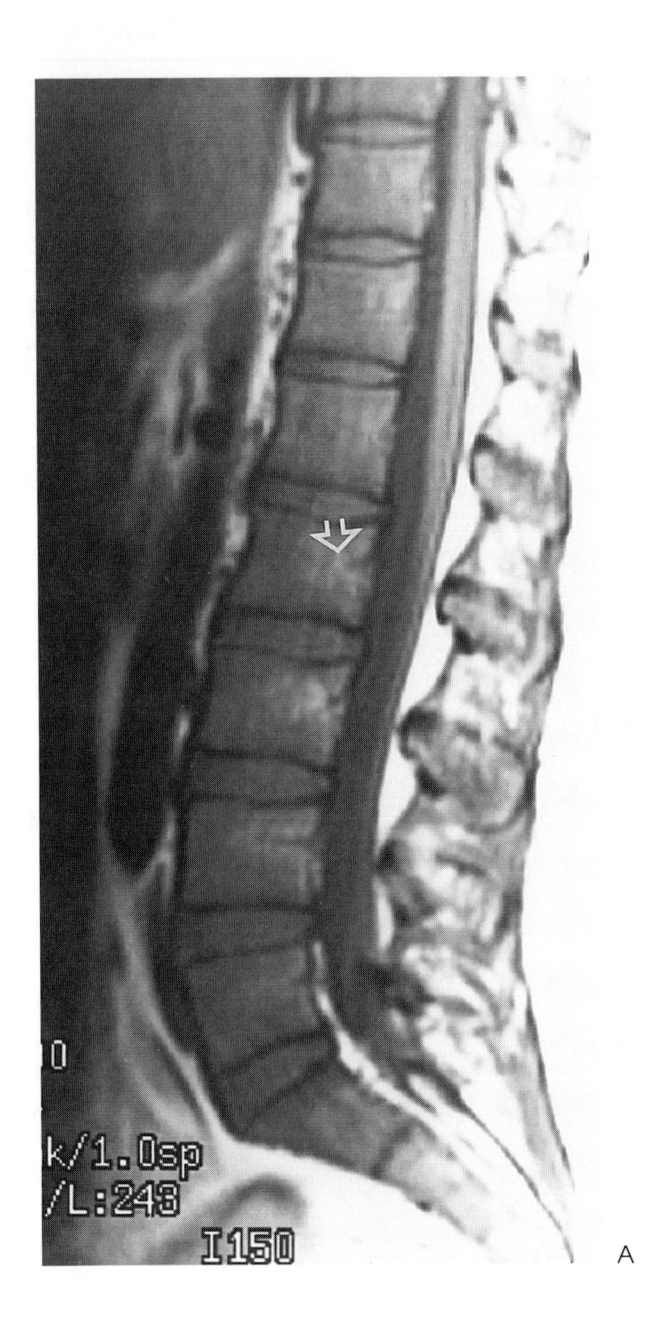

(Fig. A) Midsagittal short TR image. The vertebral body height and intervertebral disc height are normal at all levels. The point of entrance of the normal basivertebral venous plexus is seen in the posterior margin of the vertebral body (*open arrow*). The normal spinal cord ends at the level of the inferior end plate of the L1 vertebral body. The normal epidural fat appears as increased signal intensity dorsal to the thecal sac. The normal dorsal epidural fat is triangular in configuration and is outlined by the base of the spinous processes of the vertebral bodies. The first sacral segment is positioned at an angle to the L5 vertebral body and tapers inferiorly.

NORMAL ANATOMY

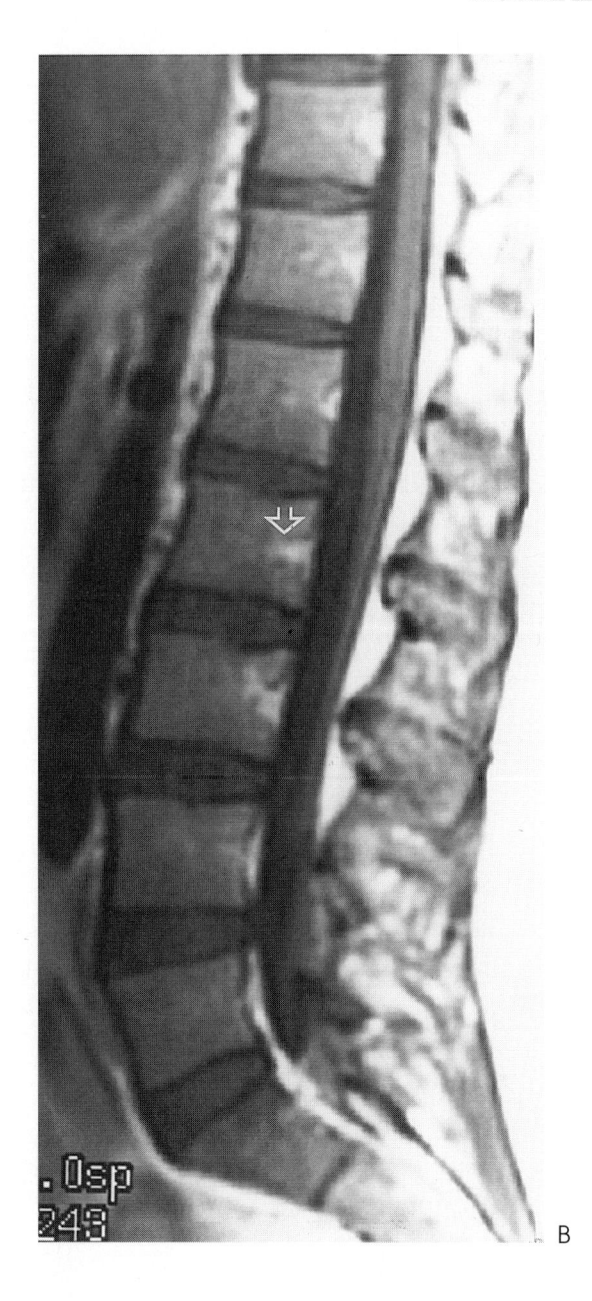

(Fig. B) Midsagittal short TR image postcontrast. The normal intravertebral basivertebral venous plexus enhances (*open arrow*). There is enhancement of the normal epidural venous plexus behind the L4 and L5 vertebral bodies.

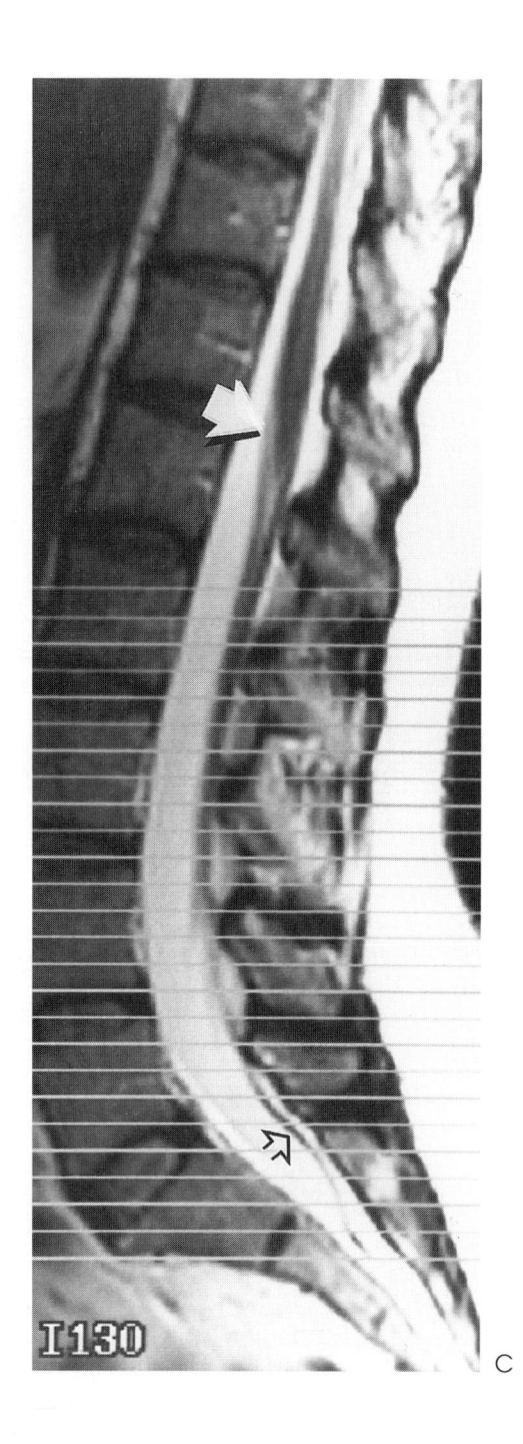

(Fig. C) Midsagittal long TR image demonstrates the tapered distal end of the thoracic spinal cord (*solid arrow*) as it ends at the level of the L1 vertebral body. The filum terminale is seen as a linear area of decreased signal intensity in the distal end of the thecal sac (*open arrow*). Multiple superimposed lines represent the lines of the levels that are scanned in a routine magnetic resonance study of the lumbar spine. The study utilizes a fast spin-echo technique, so the normal high signal intensity fat remains high signal intensity. When using the standard spin-echo technique, the normally high signal intensity fat would appear as slightly decreased signal intensity.

NORMAL ANATOMY

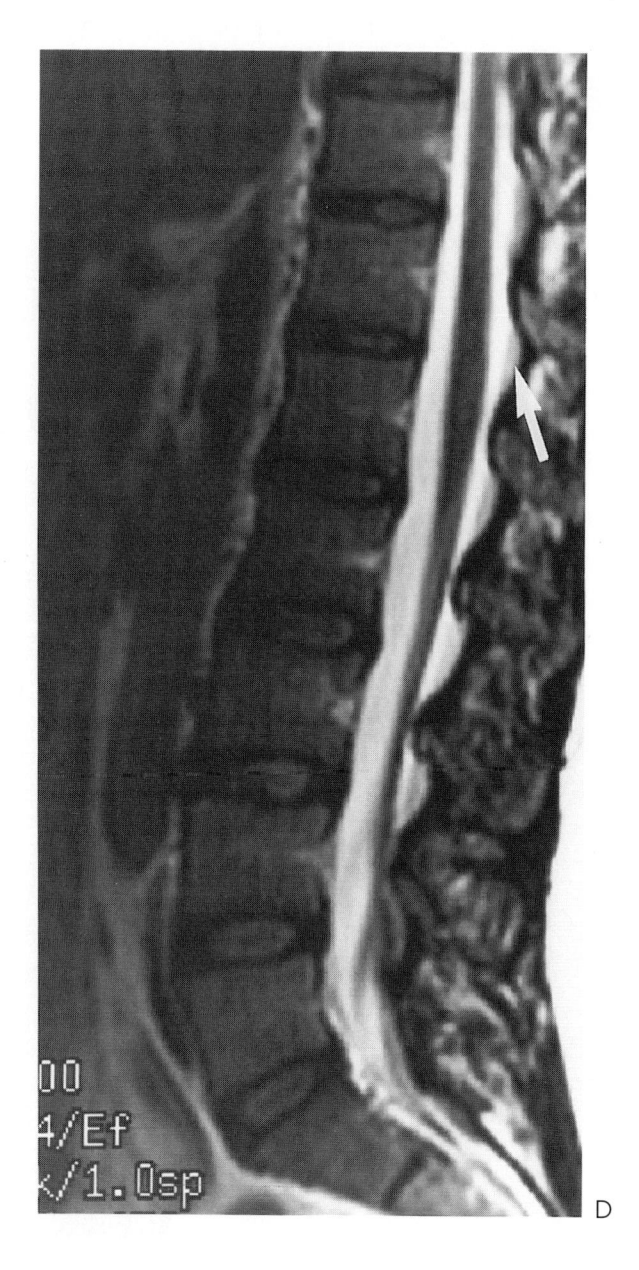

(Fig. D) Midsagittal long TR image using standard spin-echo technique reveals the decreased signal intensity spinal cord surrounded by increased signal intensity cerebrospinal fluid. The intervertebral disc appears as increased signal intensity. The epidural fat appears as decreased signal intensity (*arrow*).

TEACHING ATLAS OF SPINE IMAGING

Example 2

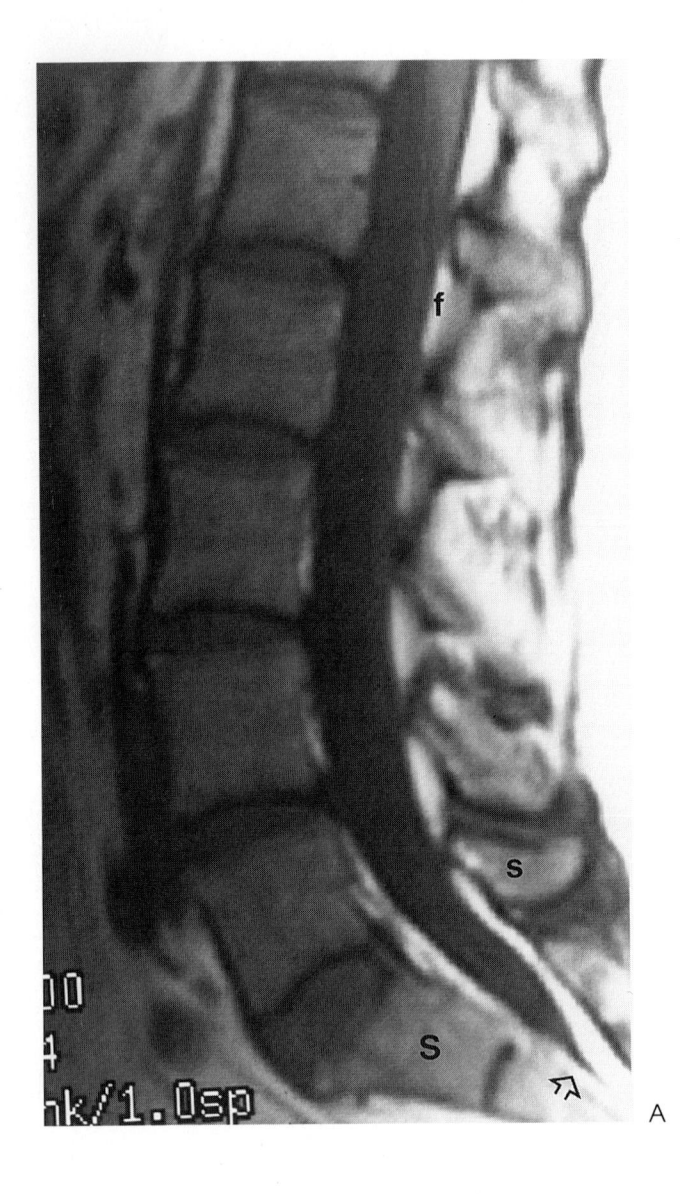

(Fig. A) Midsagittal short TR image of the lumbar spine. *f*, normal high signal intensity fat in the epidural space; *S*, normal first sacral segment; *s*, spinous process of L5; *open arrow,* normal termination of the distal end of the thecal sac at the level of the midbody of the second sacral segment.

NORMAL ANATOMY

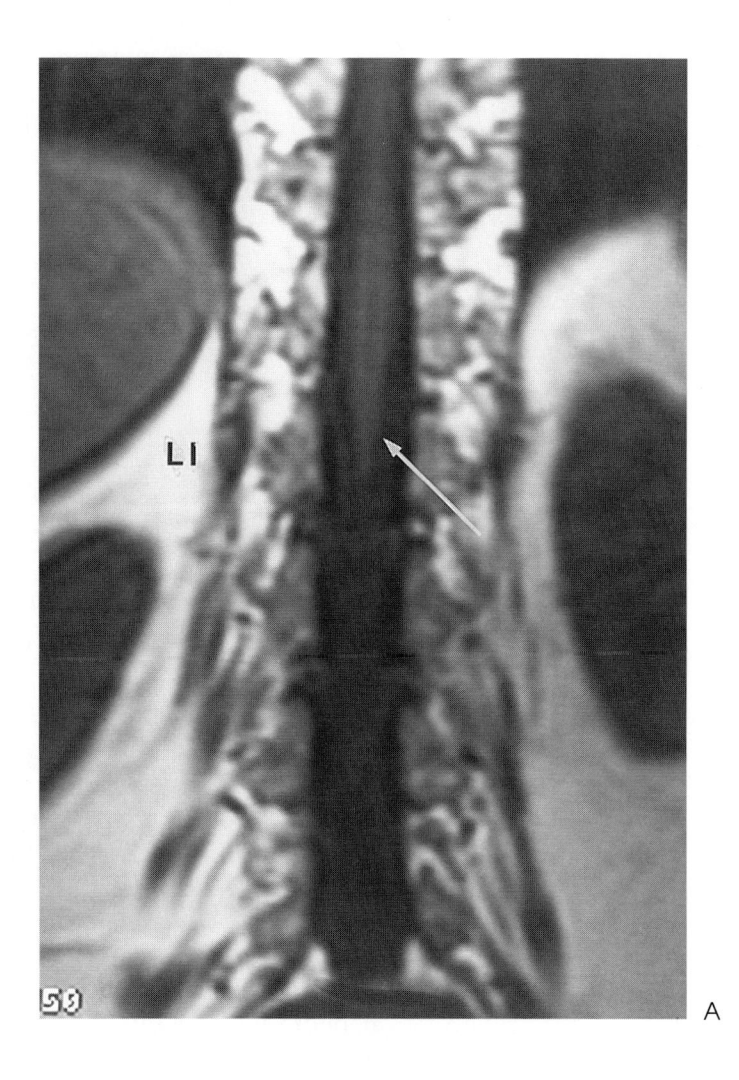

Example 3

(Fig. A) Coronal short TR image at the level of L1 (*L1*). *arrow,* the termination of the distal end of the spinal cord at the level of the L1 vertebral body.

35

TEACHING ATLAS OF SPINE IMAGING

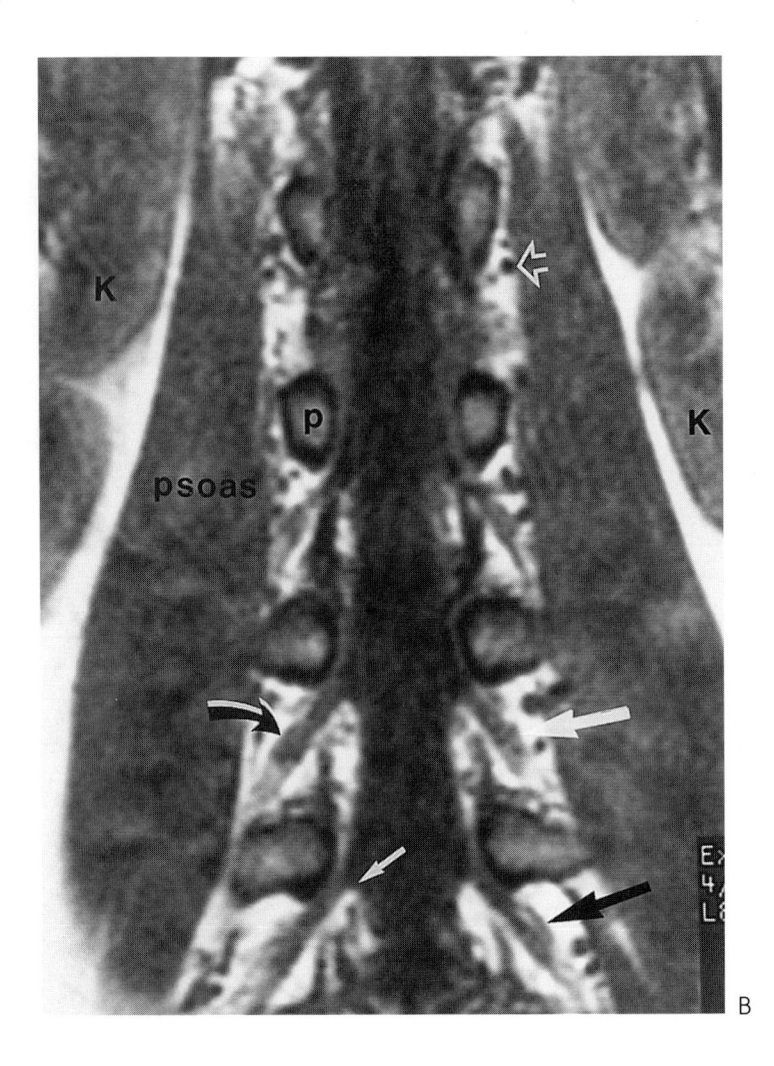

(Fig. B) Normal short TR coronal image. *K,* kidney; *psoas,* psoas muscle; *p,* pedicle; *long white arrow,* normal nerve; *long black arrow,* normal nerve; *curved black and white arrow,* dorsal root ganglion; *short white arrow,* "axilla" of the normal root sleeve; *open arrow,* flow void of one of the vessels of the venous plexus.

NORMAL ANATOMY

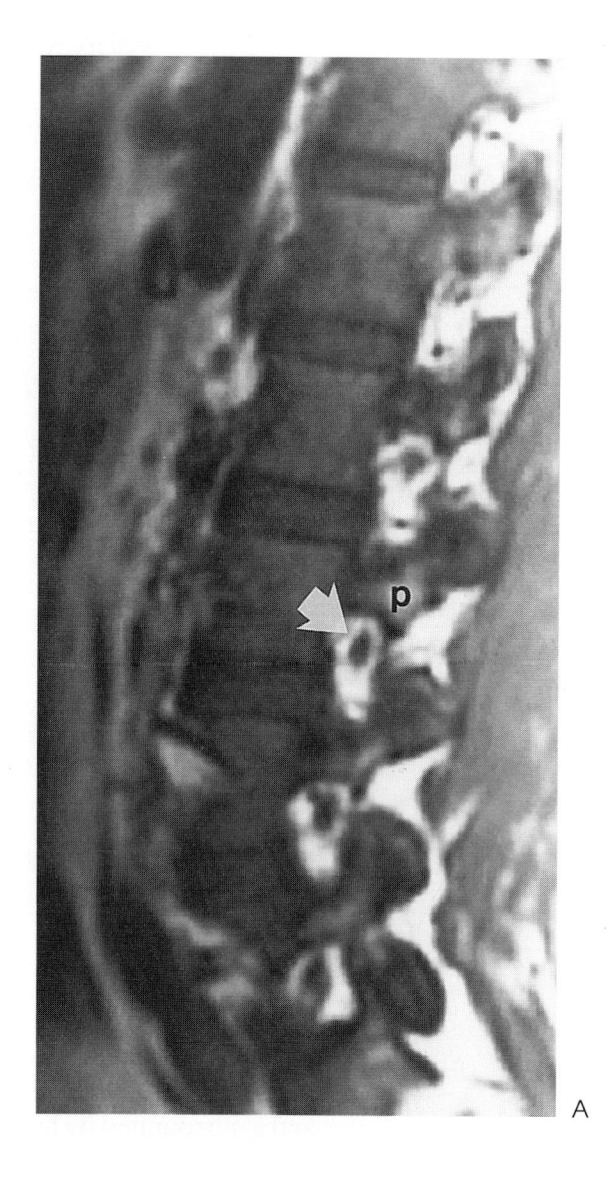

Example 4

(Fig. A) Parasagittal short TR image at the level of the intervertebral foramina. *P*, pedicle; *white arrow,* dorsal root ganglion.

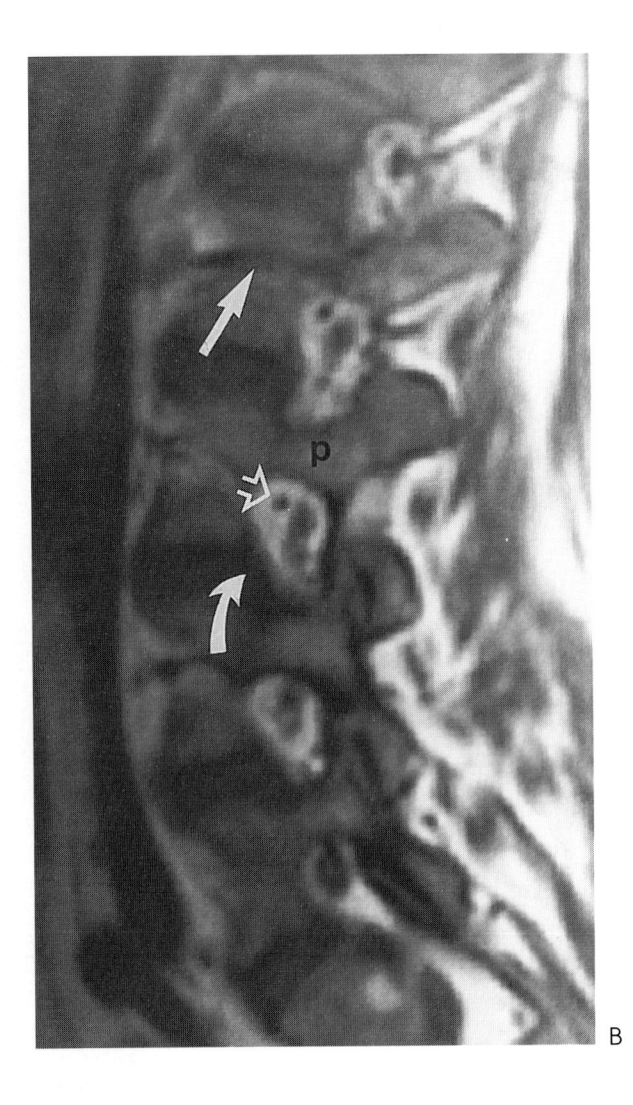

(Fig. B) Parasagittal short TR image at the level of the intervertebral foramen. The dorsal root ganglion is anatomically positioned immediately below the level of the vertebral body pedicle. It is intermediate signal intensity and is surrounded by high signal intensity fat. The intervertebral disc projects into the lower portion of the intervertebral foramen. Thus, a herniated disc will encroach upon the nerve as it exits via the intervertebral foramen. *p*, pedicle; *open arrow*, flow void of the vessels of the basivertebral venous plexus; *straight arrow*, flow void of one of the vessels of the basivertebral venous plexus; *curved arrow*, intervertebral disc.

NORMAL ANATOMY

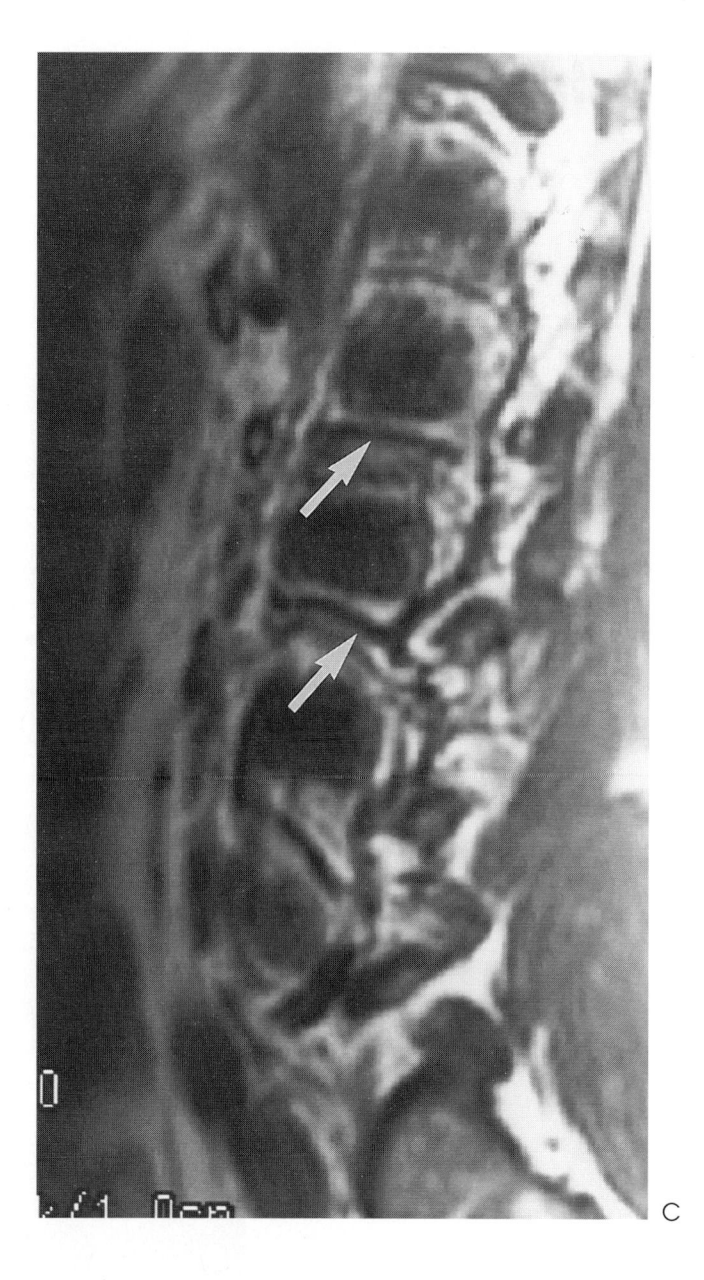

(Fig. C) Parasagittal short TR image at the level of the lateral margin of the vertebral body. *Arrows,* flow voids of the basivertebral venous plexus as they surround the vertebral body.

TEACHING ATLAS OF SPINE IMAGING

Example 5

Normal pediatric lumbar spine.

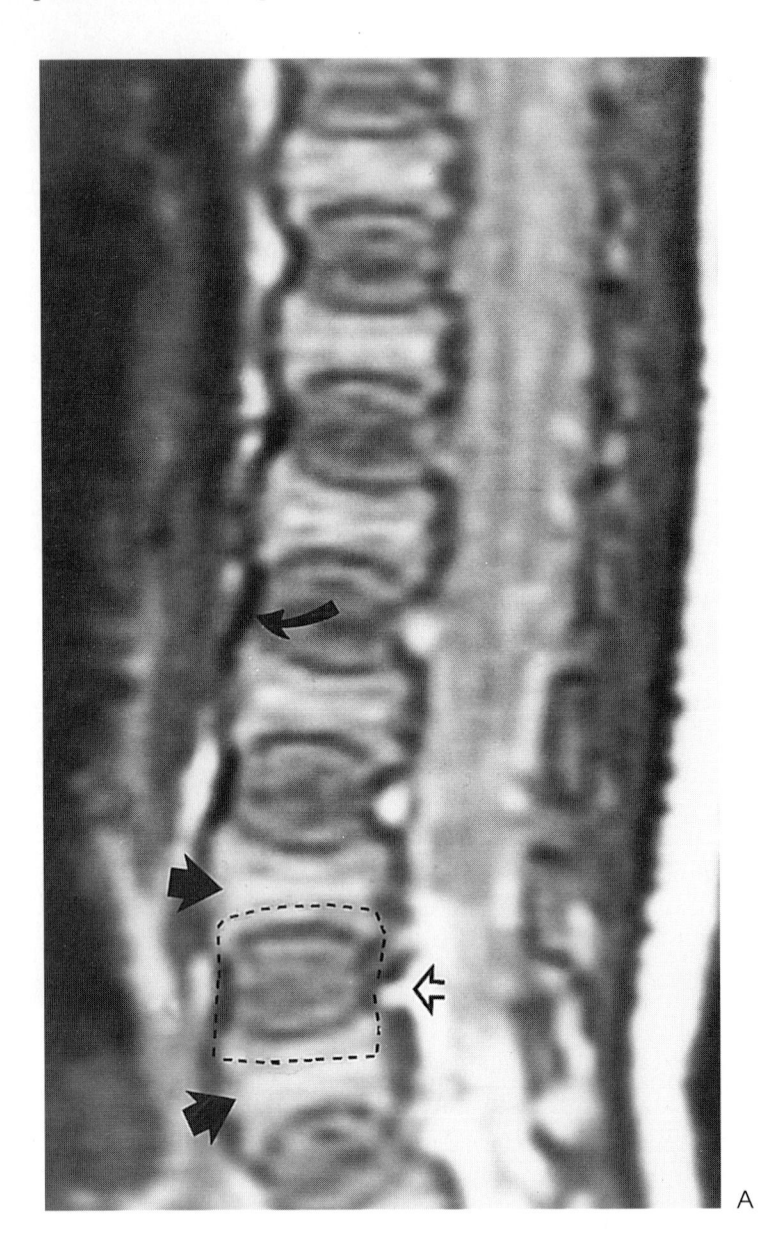

(Fig. A) Sagittal short TR image. *Wide arrows,* intervertebral discs; *open arrow,* entrance of basivertebral venous plexus; *curved arrow,* low signal intensity of the anterior margin of the vertebral body.

NORMAL ANATOMY

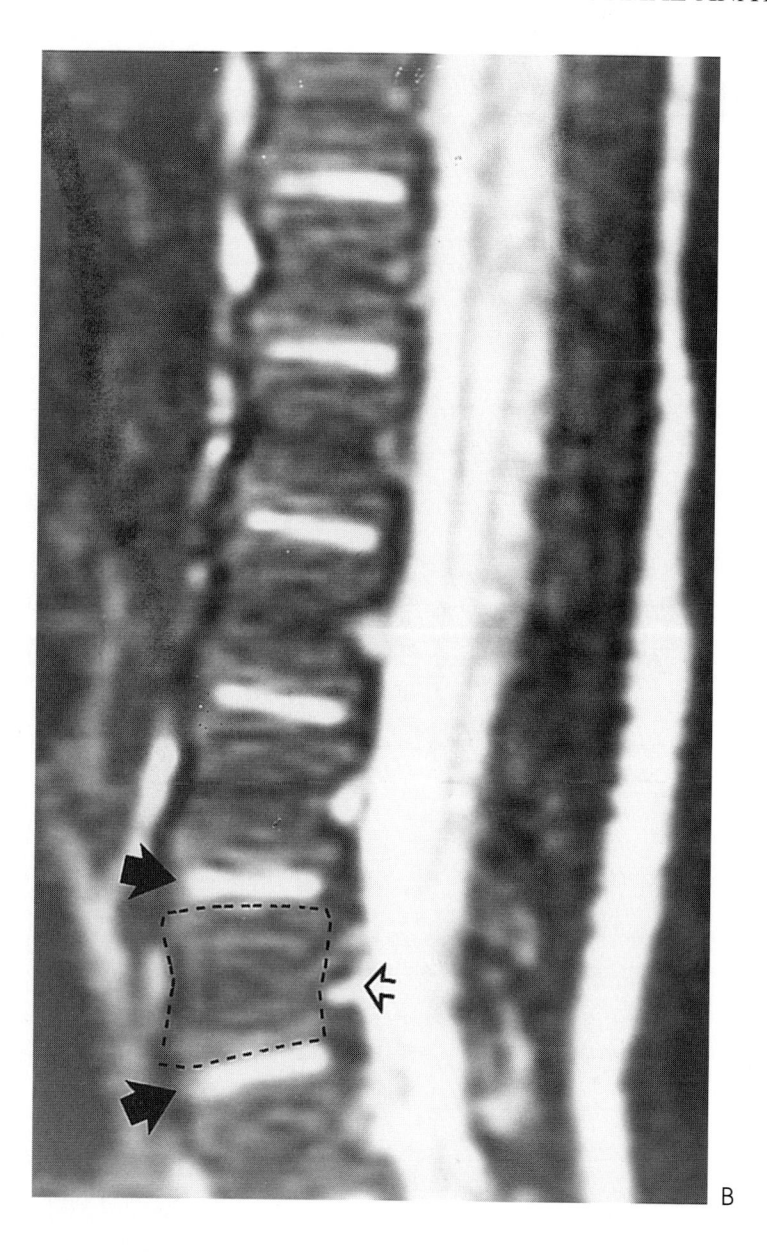

(Fig. B) Sagittal long TR image. The dotted lines on both images outline the vertebral body. On the short TR images, the cartilagenous end plates of the vertebral bodies appear as increased signal intensity, while the cartilage appears as decreased signal intensity on the long TR images. In general, the intervertebral disc appears as increased signal intensity on all imaging sequences, but this appearance is much more marked with the longer TR or more T2-weighted images. *solid arrows,* intervertebral disc; *open arrow,* entrance of basivertebral venous plexus.

41

TEACHING ATLAS OF SPINE IMAGING

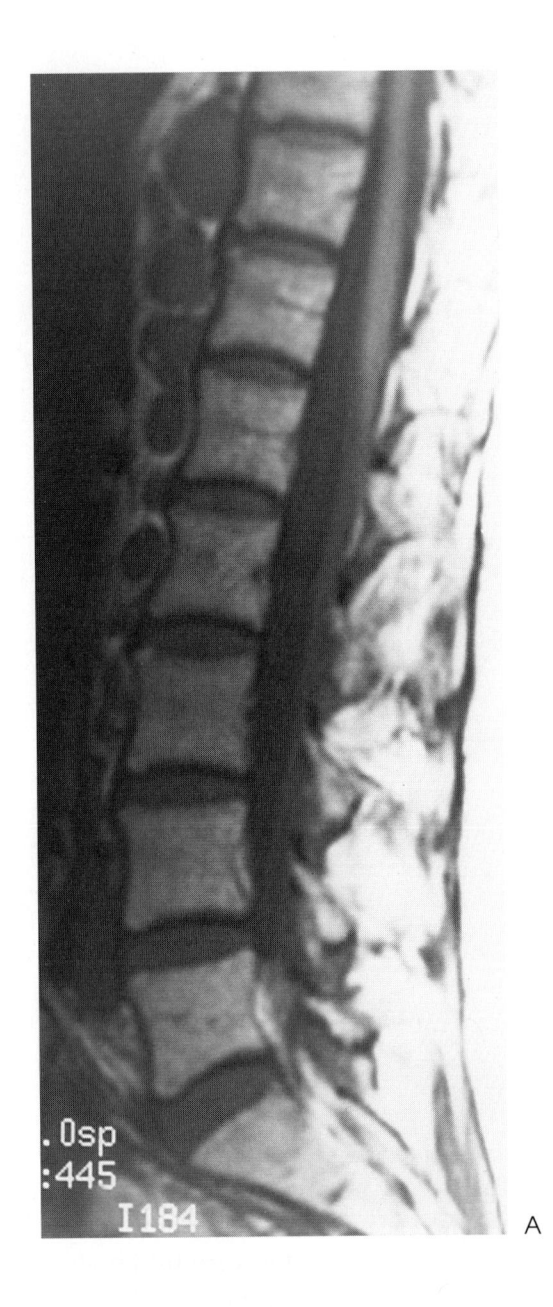

Example 6

(Fig. A) Sagittal short TR image of the lumbar spine. The vertebral body height and intervertebral disc height is normal. The spinal cord is normal in position. However, there are multiple enlarged lymph nodes in the prevertebral space. The patient has acquired immunodeficiency syndrome (AIDS) and systemic lymphoma.

NORMAL ANATOMY

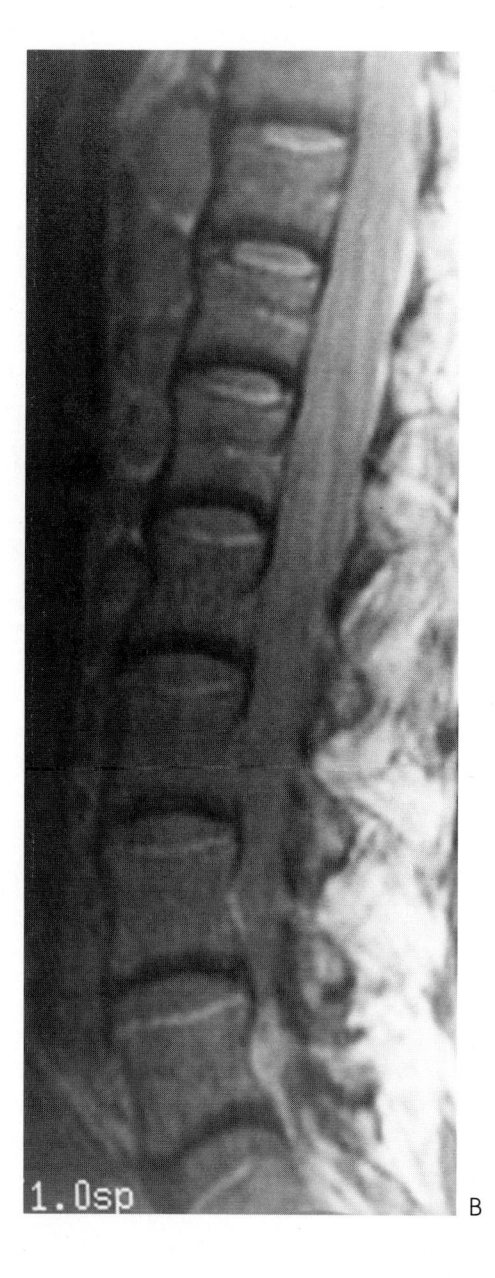

(Fig. B) Sagittal intermediate signal intensity image reveals chemical shift artifact with the inferior end plates of the vertebral bodies appearing as decreased signal intensity while the superior end plates appear as intermediate signal intensity with an adjacent increased signal intensity parallel line.

TEACHING ATLAS OF SPINE IMAGING

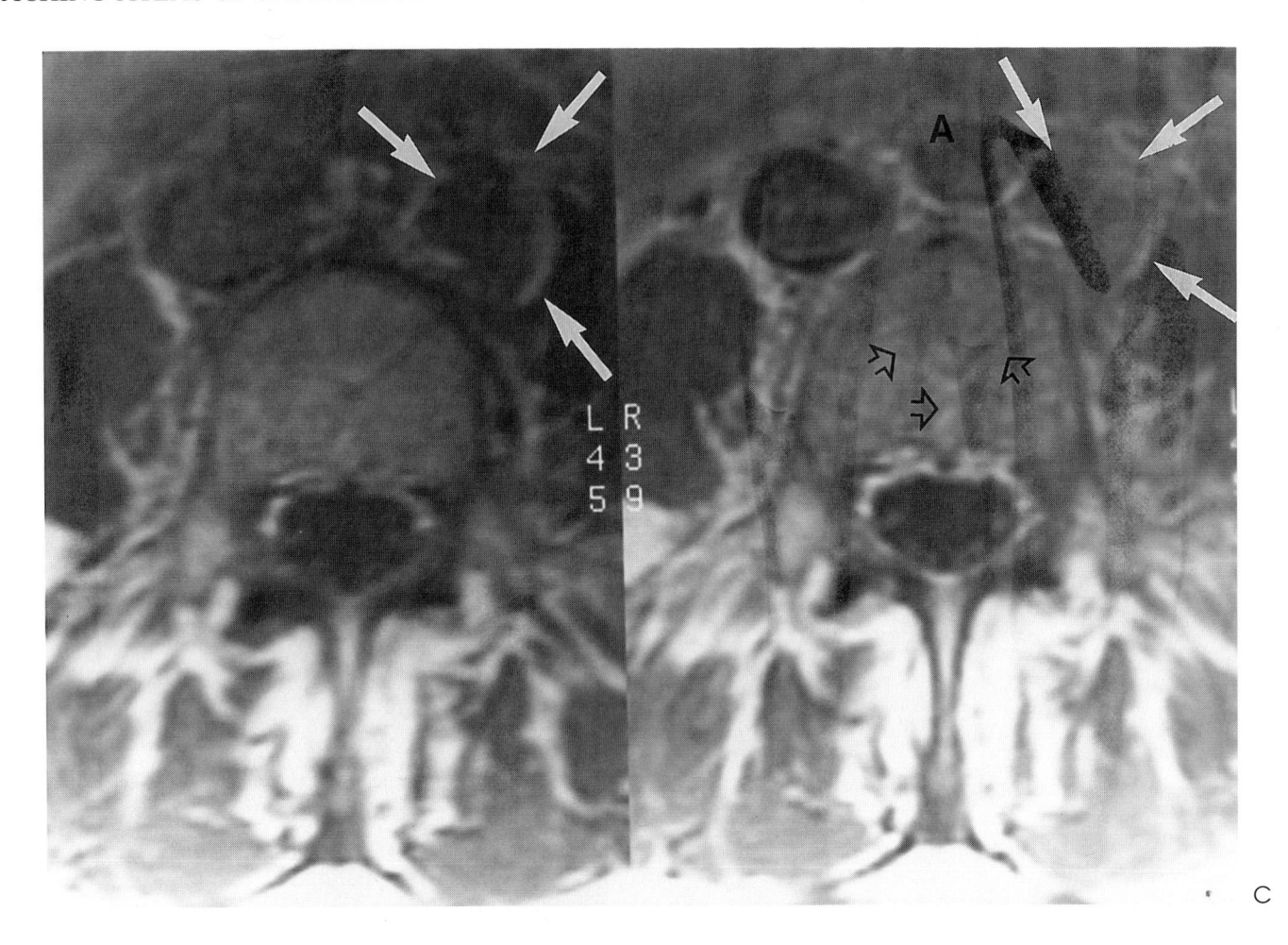

(Fig. C) Precontrast (*left*) and postcontrast (*right*) axial short TR images reveal multiple prevertebral lymph nodes (*white arrows*) which project to the left of the flow void of the abdominal aorta (*A*). The intravertebral portion of the basivertebral venous plexus is also seen (*open arrows*).

NORMAL ANATOMY

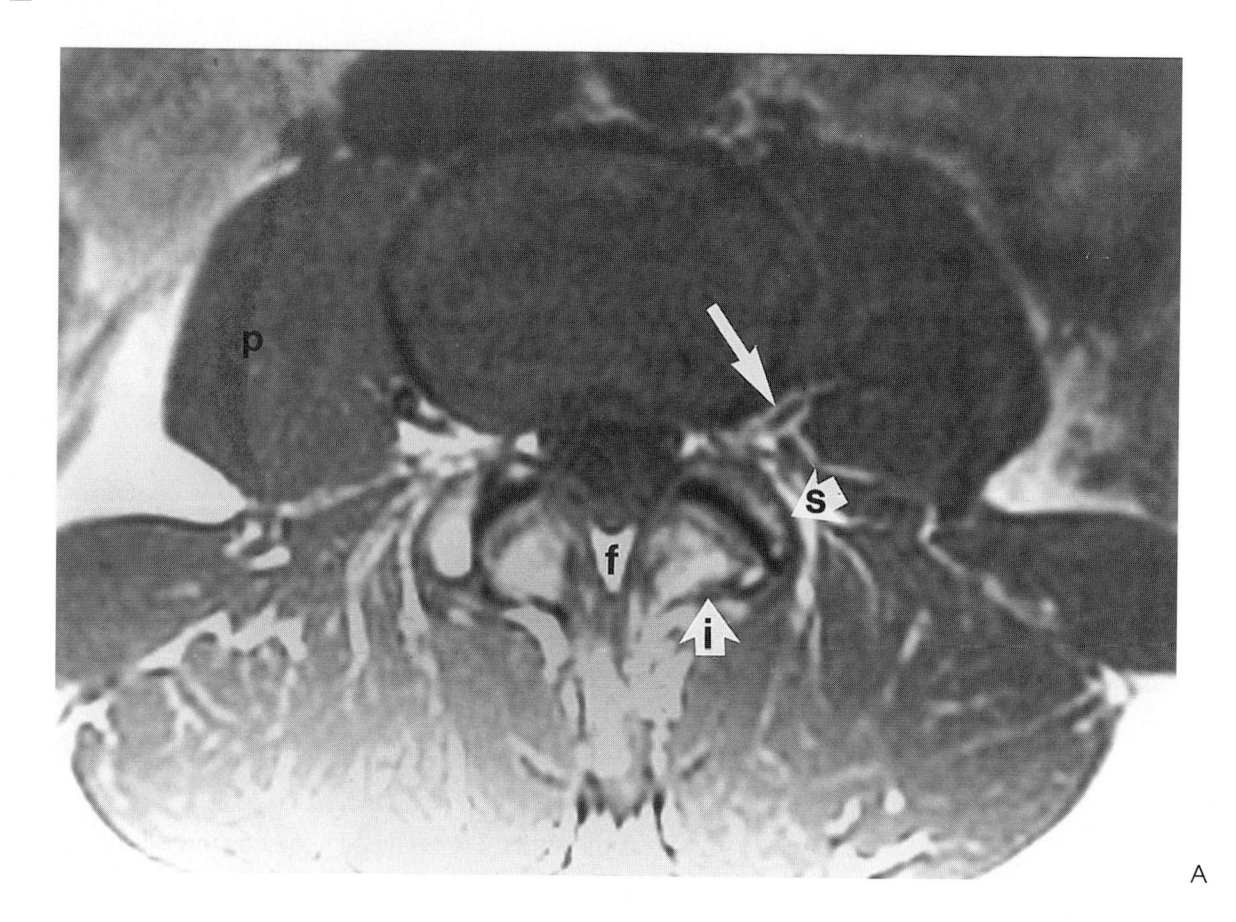

Example 7

(Fig. A) Axial short TR image at the level of the intervertebral disc. *Long white arrow,* normal nerve surrounded by high signal intensity fat; *s/arrow,* superior articulating facet; *i/arrow,* inferior articulating facet; *f,* normal epidural fat between the laminae of the vertebral bodies at the base of the spinous process; *p,* psoas muscle.

TEACHING ATLAS OF SPINE IMAGING

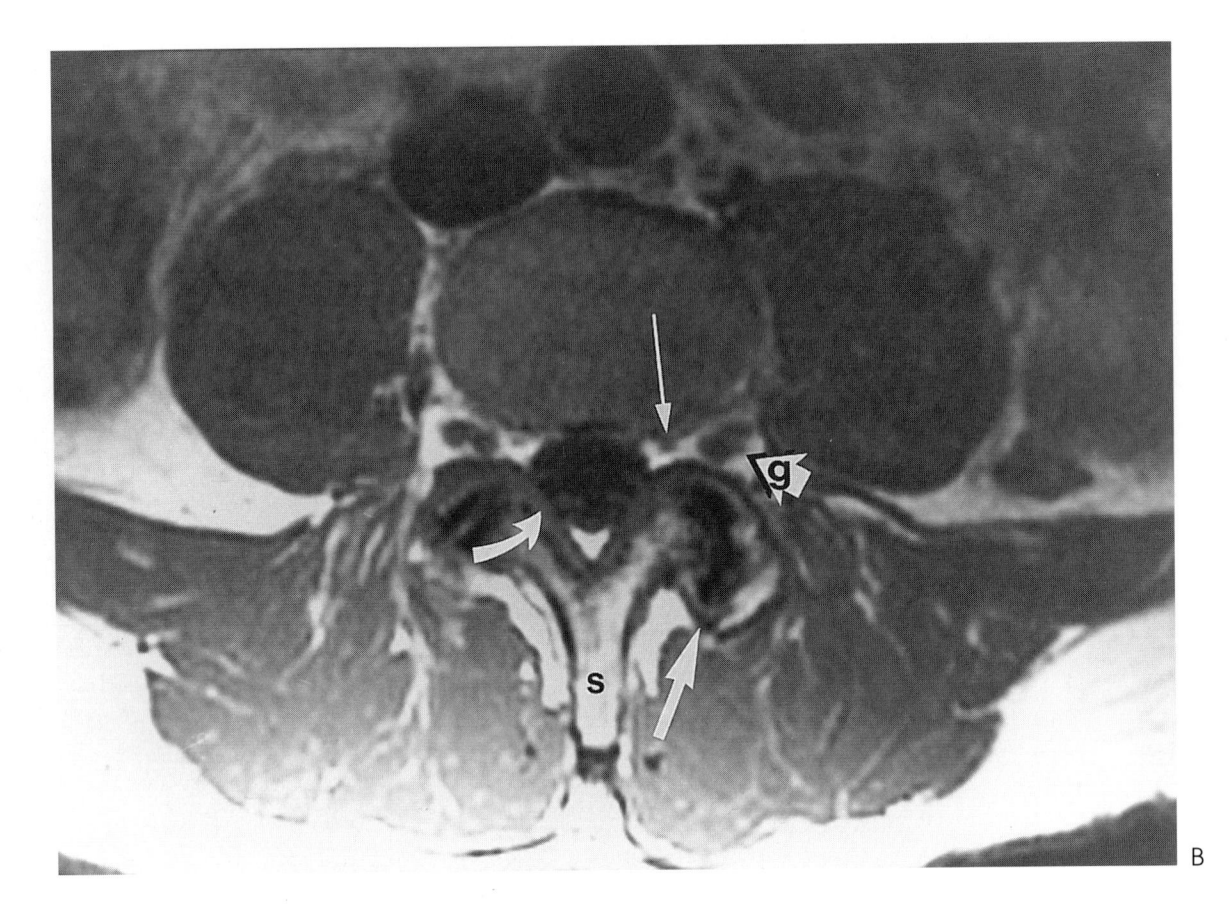

(Fig. B) Axial short TR image. The psoas muscle projects on either side of the vertebral body. The aorta is an area of flow void anterior to the vertebral body and just to the left of the midline, while the inferior vena cava is an oval-shaped area of flow void just to the right of the midline. *s*, spinous process; *g/arrow*, normal dorsal root ganglion; *long thin white arrow*, anterior epidural vein; *curved arrow*, ligamentum flavum; *long thick white arrow*, interfacet joint with degenerative changes with cupping of the superior articulating facet around the inferior articulating facet.

NORMAL ANATOMY

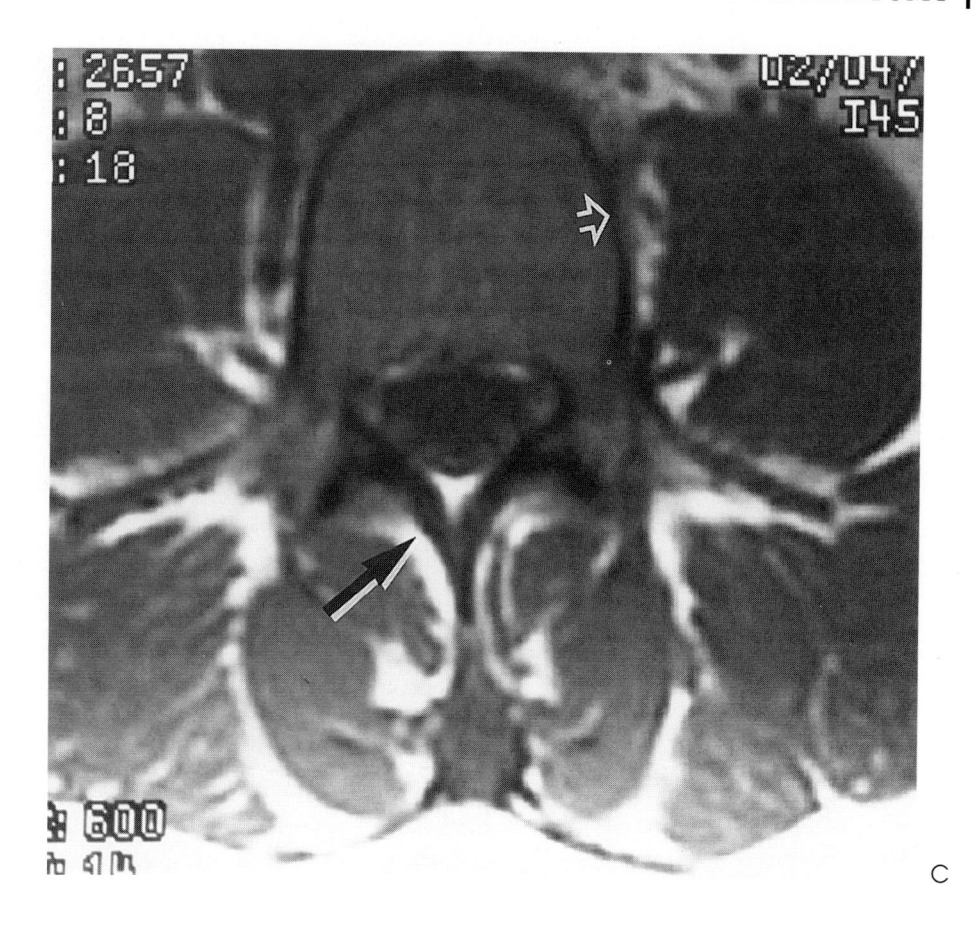

(Fig. C) Axial short TR image at the level of the vertebral pedicle. *Open arrow,* decreased signal intensity of the cortical margin of the vertebral body; *black-and-white arrow,* decreased signal intensity of the cortical margin of the lamina of the vertebral body.

TEACHING ATLAS OF SPINE IMAGING

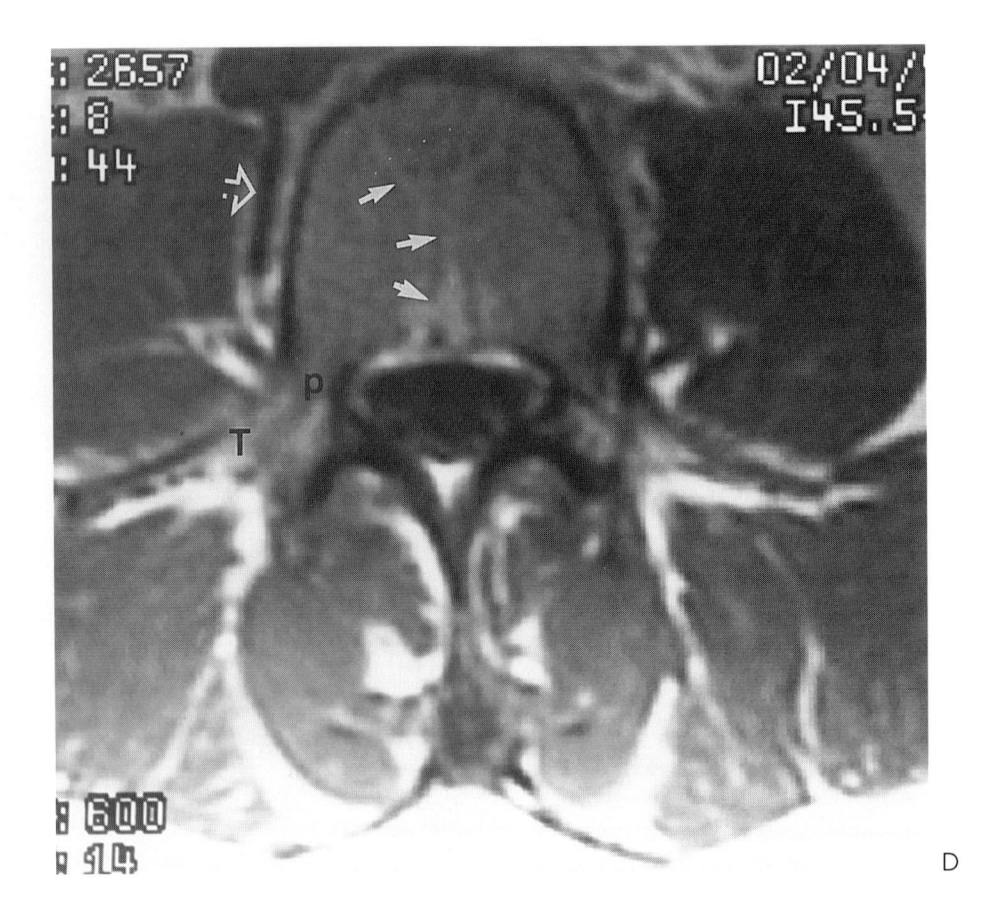

(Fig. D) Axial short TR image at the same level as Figure C, postcontrast. The basivertebral venous plexus typically forms a Y-shaped area within the vertebral body. *Open arrow,* flow void of the vessel of the basivertebral venous plexus; *p,* pedicle; *T,* transverse process; *solid arrows,* enhancing intravertebral portion of the basivertebral venous plexus; *open arrow,* flow void of vein of basivertebral venous plexus.

NORMAL ANATOMY

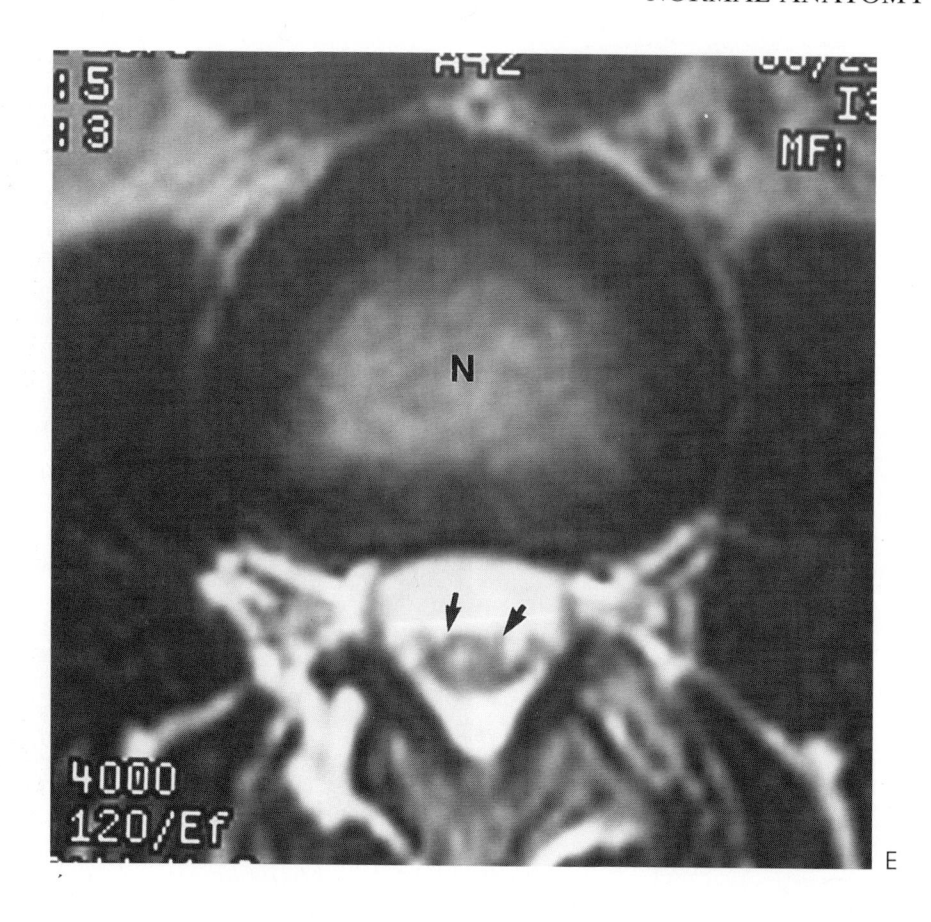

(Fig. E) Axial long TR image at the level of the intervertebral disc. The normal nerves of the cauda equina appear as small rounded areas of intermediate signal intensity within the thecal sac (*arrows*). The annulus fibrosus appears decreased signal intensity and surrounds the nucleus pulposus. The normal nucleus pulposus is identified with N.

TEACHING ATLAS OF SPINE IMAGING

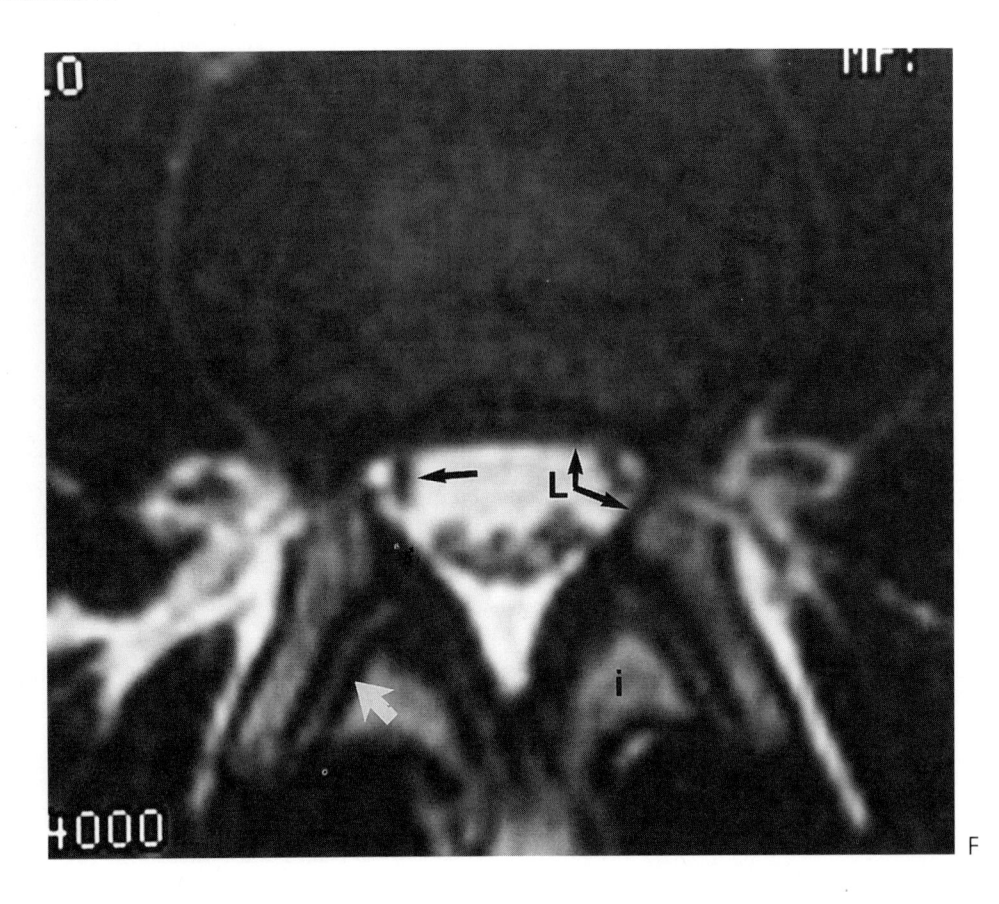

(Fig. F) Axial long TR image. The lateral recess is formed by the superior articulating facet and the posterior margin of the vertebral body. The distance between these structures should not be less than 5 mm. *White arrow*, the normal low signal intensity of the cortical bone of the inferior articulating facet adjacent to the intermediate signal intensity of the interfacet joint; *L-arrows*, the normal lateral recess; *black arrow*, nerve root as it passes through the lateral recess; *i*, inferior articulating facet.

Example 8

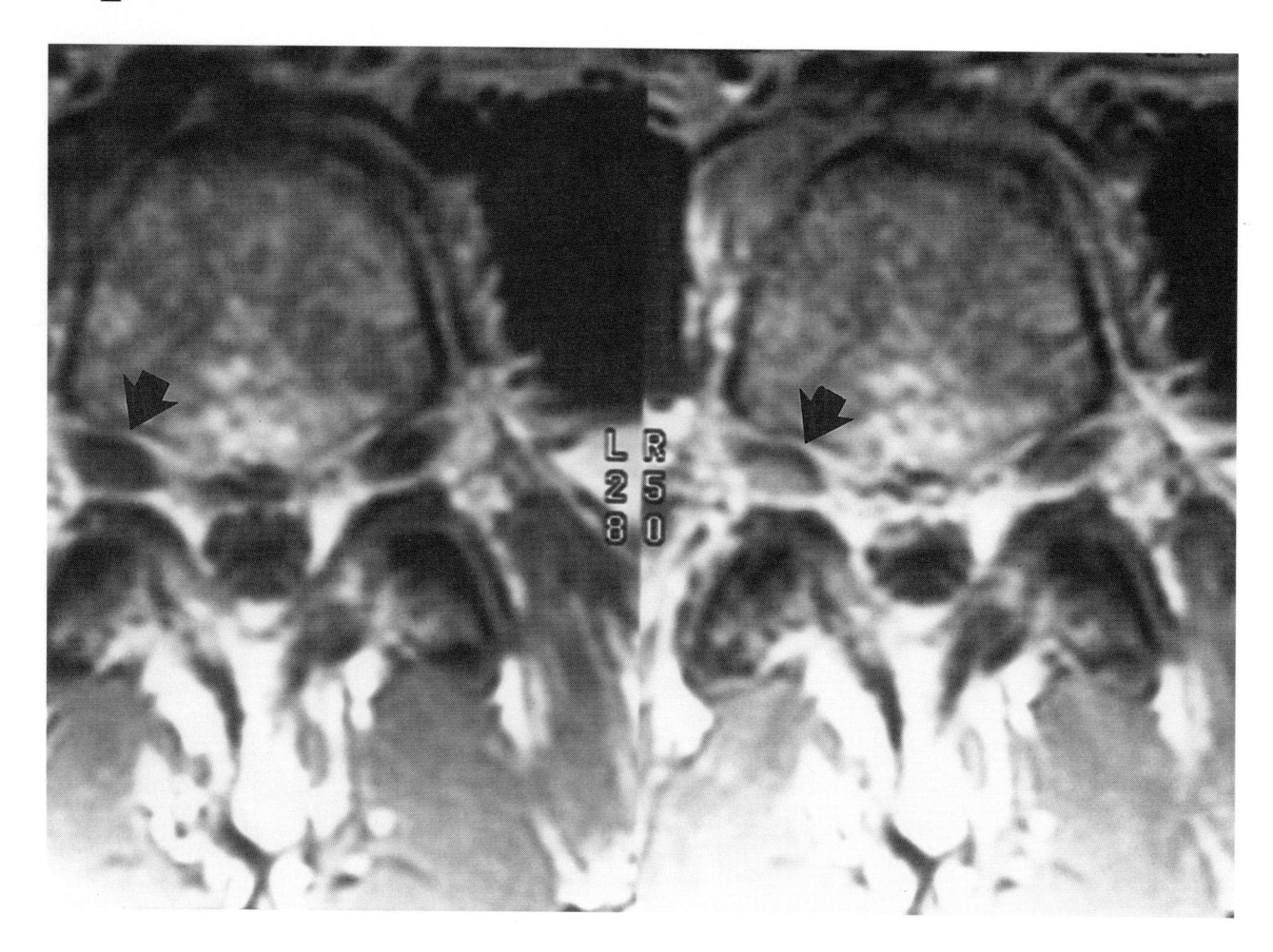

NORMAL ANATOMY

(Fig. A) Preinfusion (*left*) and postinfusion (*right*) axial short TR images at the level of the dorsal root ganglion. The normal dorsal root ganglion is seen bilaterally (*black arrows* point to the right dorsal root ganglion) which enhances postinfusion (*right*). This normal enhancement should not be mistaken for a schwannoma.

TEACHING ATLAS OF SPINE IMAGING

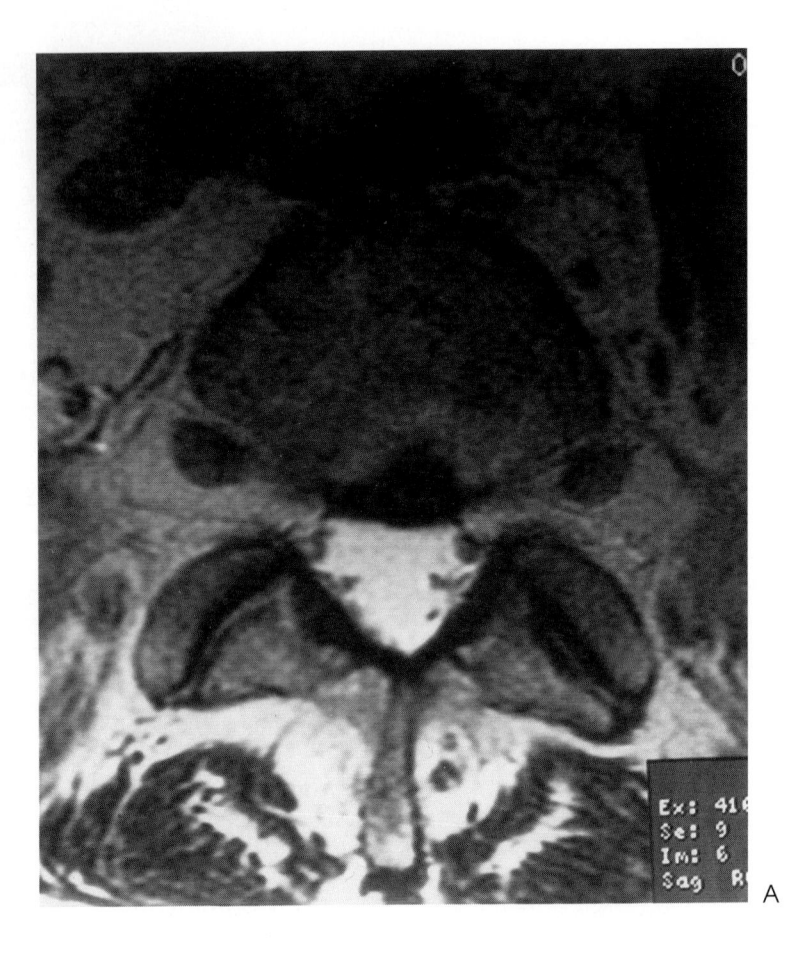

Example 9

(Fig. A) Long TR image at the level of the nerve root ganglion of the L5 vertebral body. The vertebral body is lemon shaped at the L5 level. The dorsal root ganglion appears as an area of intermediate signal intensity surrounded by normal high signal intensity fat. The cerebrospinal fluid appears as increased signal intensity, and the nerve roots of the cauda equina appear as dotlike areas of intermediate signal intensity within the thecal sac.

NORMAL ANATOMY

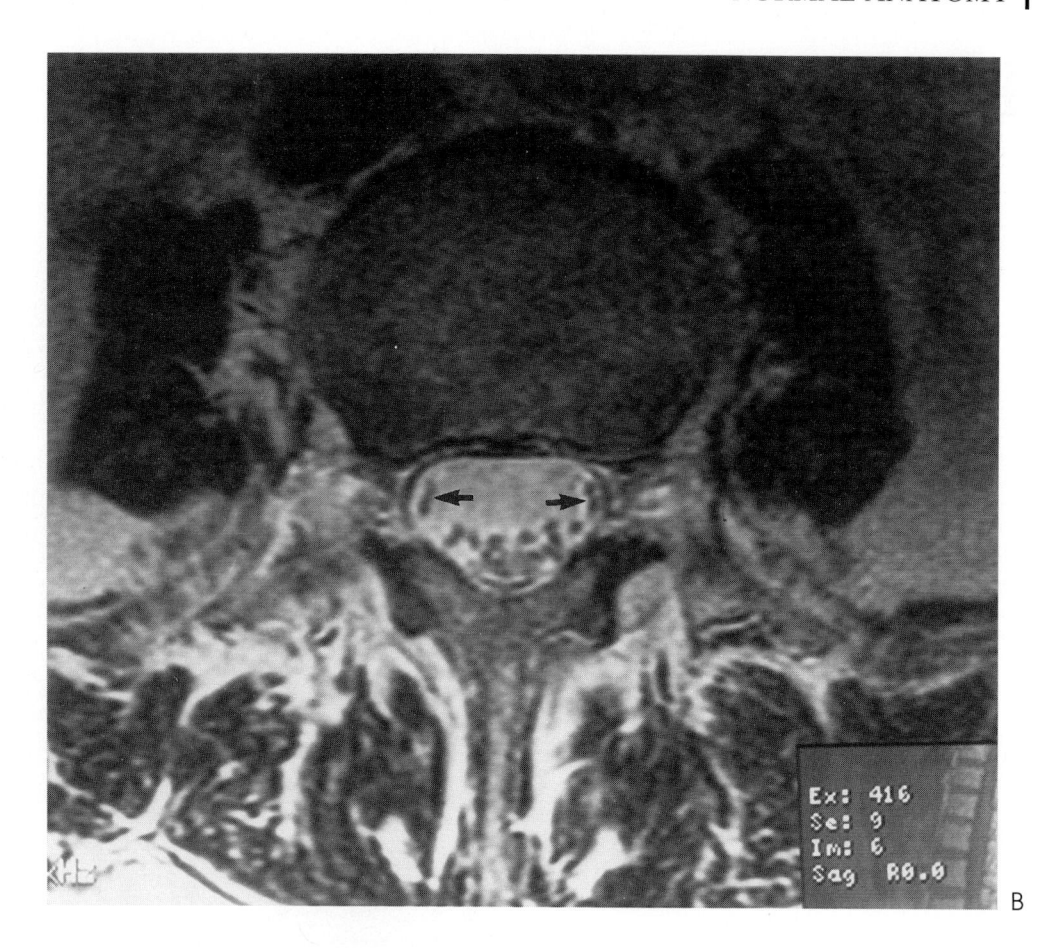

(Fig. B) Long TR image at the level of the L3-4 intervertebral disc. The disc has a normal concave margin which follows the posterior margin of the vertebral body. The intermediate signal intensity of the normal nerve roots are surrounded by high signal intensity cerebrospinal fluid. The nerve roots that are positioned laterally will soon exit from the thecal sac (*arrows*).

TEACHING ATLAS OF SPINE IMAGING

Example 10

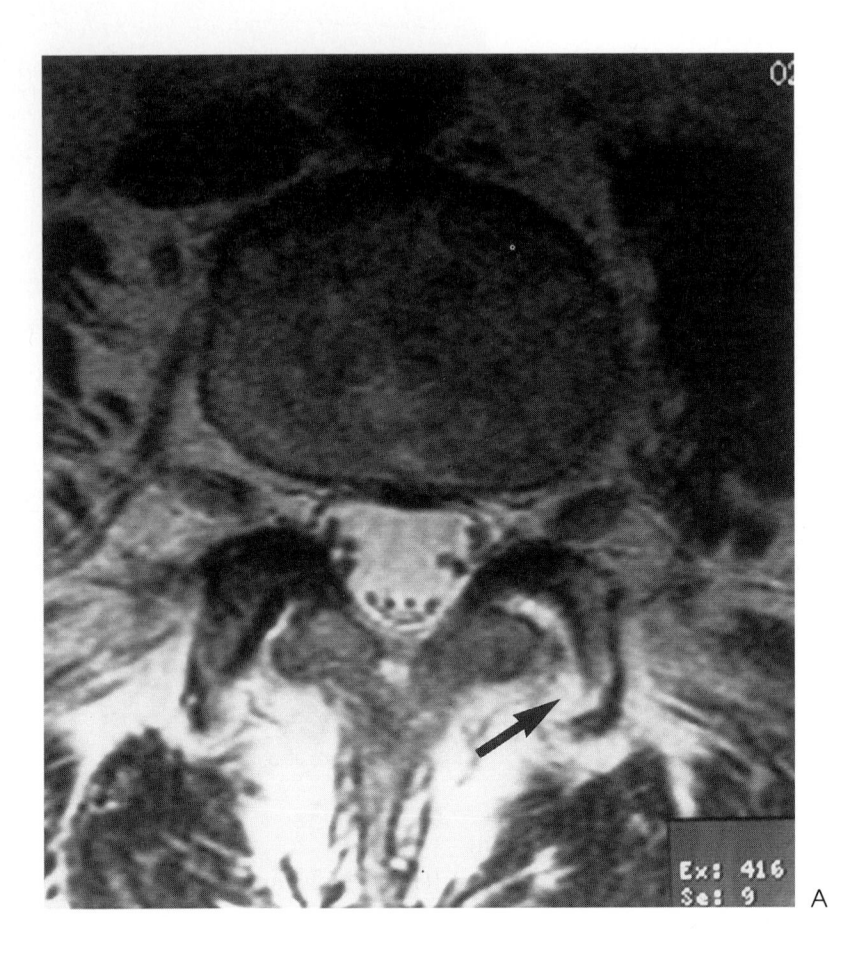

(Fig. A) Axial long TR image at the level of the dorsal nerve root ganglion. There are degenerative changes involving the interfacet joints bilaterally with cupping of the superior articulating facet around the inferior articulating facet. There is also widening of the interfacet joint on the left side (*arrow*).

NORMAL ANATOMY

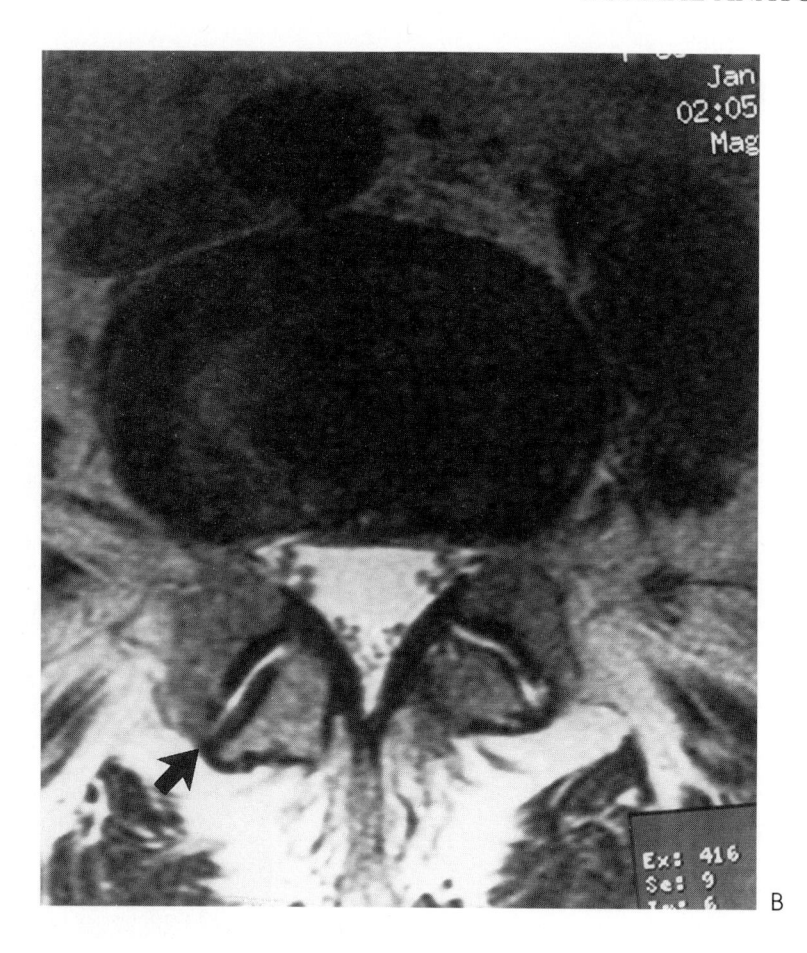

(Fig. B) Axial long TR image at the level of the intervertebral disc reveals diffuse expansion or bulging of the disc. The fluid within the interfacet joint appears as increased signal intensity (*arrow*). The nerve roots of the cauda equina appear as small rounded areas of intermediate signal intensity within the thecal sac.

TEACHING ATLAS OF SPINE IMAGING

Example 11

A

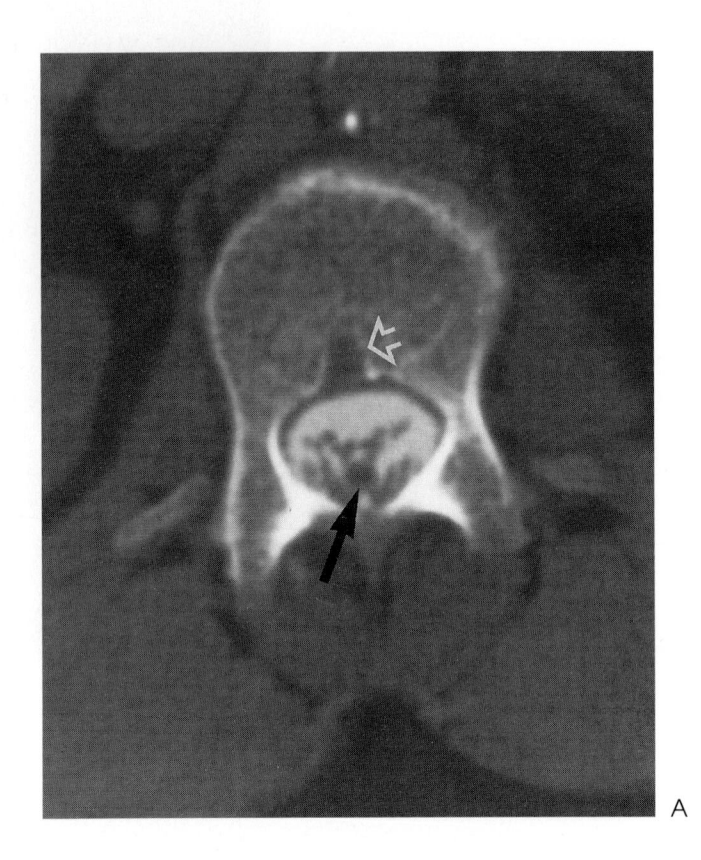

(Fig. A) Axial computed tomographic (CT) image postmyelogram at the level of the vertebral pedicle reveals the point of entrance of the basivertebral venous plexus into the posterior aspect of the vertebral body (*open arrow*). The nerve roots of the cauda equina appear as rounded areas of intermediate density within the contrast-filled thecal sac. The filum terminale at the very distal end of the spinal cord appears as a slightly larger rounded area of intermediate density (*solid arrow*). Below this level, the normal filum terminale cannot be differentiated from the nerve roots of the cauda equina.

CONGENITAL

Case 2

Clinical Presentation

The patient is a 6-year-old male unable to keep up with his class mates in gym class.

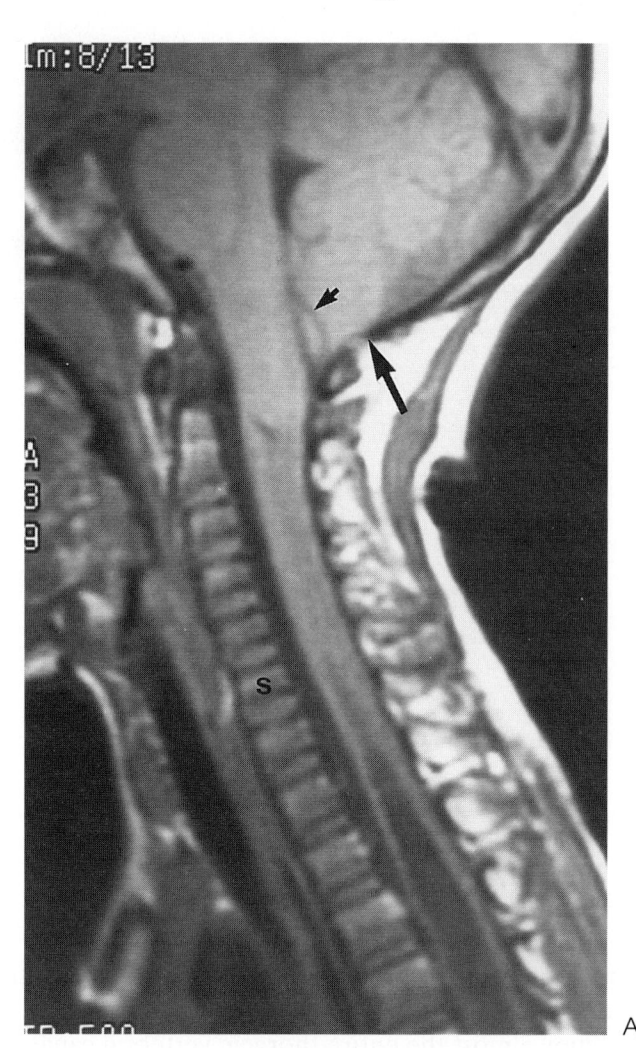

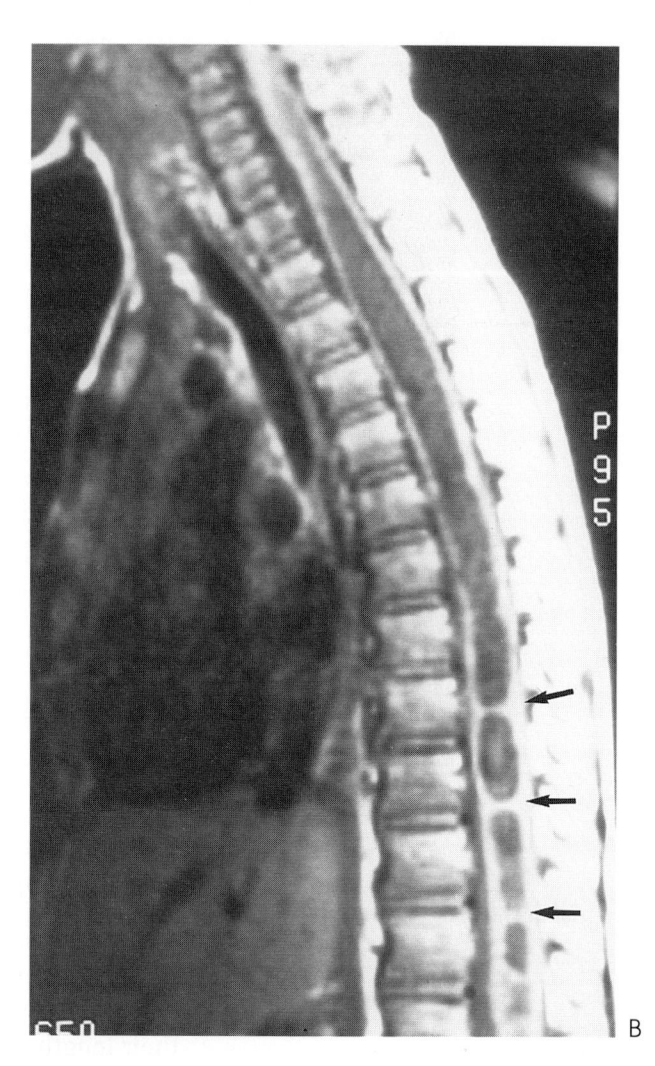

Radiologic Findings

Sagittal short TR image (Fig. A) reveals the posterior margin of the foramen magnum (*long arrow*). This bone is thinned secondary to long-standing pressure from the downward displacement of the inferior cerebellum and the cerebellar tonsils. The cerebellar tonsils are displaced below the level of the foramen magnum and appear pointed. The posterior inferior cerebellar artery appears as a curvilinear area of flow void (*short arrow*). The tapered upper end of a centrally placed cavity can be seen at the level of C6 (*s*). The cavity extends inferiorly into the thoracic spine region.

Sagittal short TR image (Fig. B) reveals the syrinx cavity with multiple internal septae (*arrows*).

TEACHING ATLAS OF SPINE IMAGING

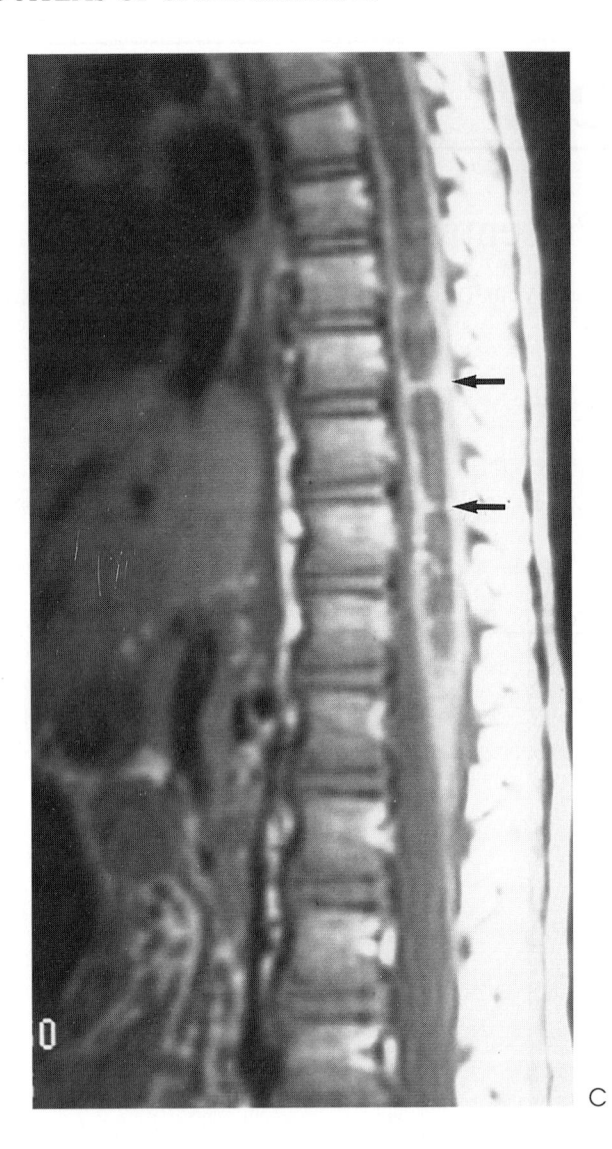

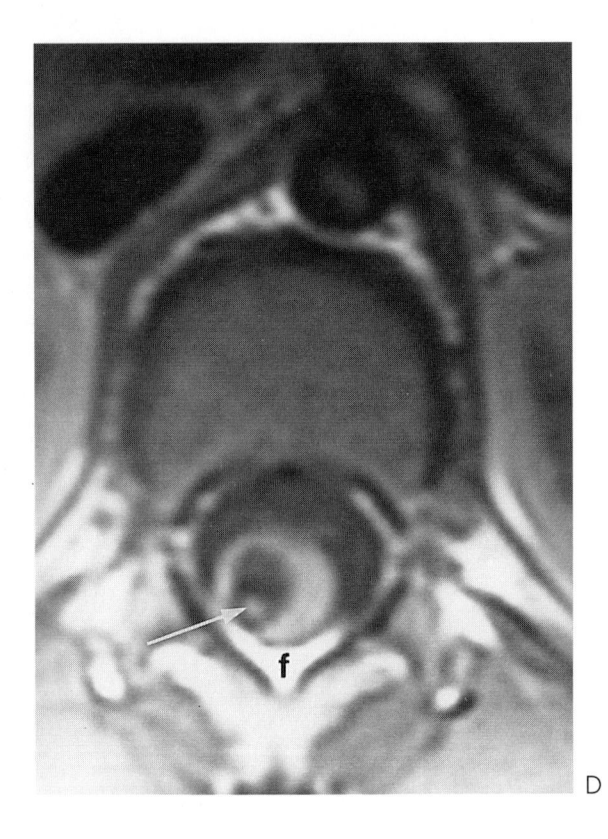

C

D

Radiologic Findings (continued)

Sagittal short TR image including the distal spinal cord (Fig. C) reveals the multiple internal septations (*arrows*) extending to the distal end of the spinal cord. The lower cervical and thoracic spinal cord are expanded throughout their length and occupy almost the entire thoracic vertebral canal, resulting in obliteration of the surrounding subarachnoid space. The vertebral canal is enlarged throughout its length, which reflects the long-standing nature of this process.

Axial short TR image in the distal thoracic region (Fig. D) reveals the low signal intensity cavity, which is slightly eccentrically placed within the spinal cord. There is a small rounded area of increased signal intensity within the dorsal aspect of the cavity (*arrow*). The normal epidural fat appears as increased signal intensity (*f*).

PEARLS

- In the patient with a Chiari I malformation, the entire spinal cord should be evaluated to determine the exact extent of the cavity.

- The small rounded area of increased signal intensity within the syrinx cavity is secondary to an area of flow related enhancement.

PITFALL

- At the time of surgery, the multiple internal septae may make shunting of the syrinx cavity difficult because these septae may interfere with free communication between the various compartments.

Diagnosis

Chiari I malformation with lower cervical and thoracic syrinx cavity.

Differential Diagnosis

- Chiari I malformation with lower cervical and thoracic syrinx cavity

Discussion

Although Chiari I malformation is one of the more common congenital anomalies of the central nervous system that exhibits typical findings on imaging, there are frequently minor variations on the theme of these deformities. There are often variations in the appearance of the low lying tonsils, a highly variable difference in the size of the syrinx cavity, and a variety of clinical presentations. Typical surgical treatment of this anomaly includes removal of the inferior aspect of the occipital bone to allow free flow of cerebrospinal fluid around the region of the foramen magnum.

For a definition of Chiari I malformation, see Case 1.

TEACHING ATLAS OF SPINE IMAGING

Case 3

Clinical Presentation

The patient is an 8-year-old male with progressive lower extremity weakness.

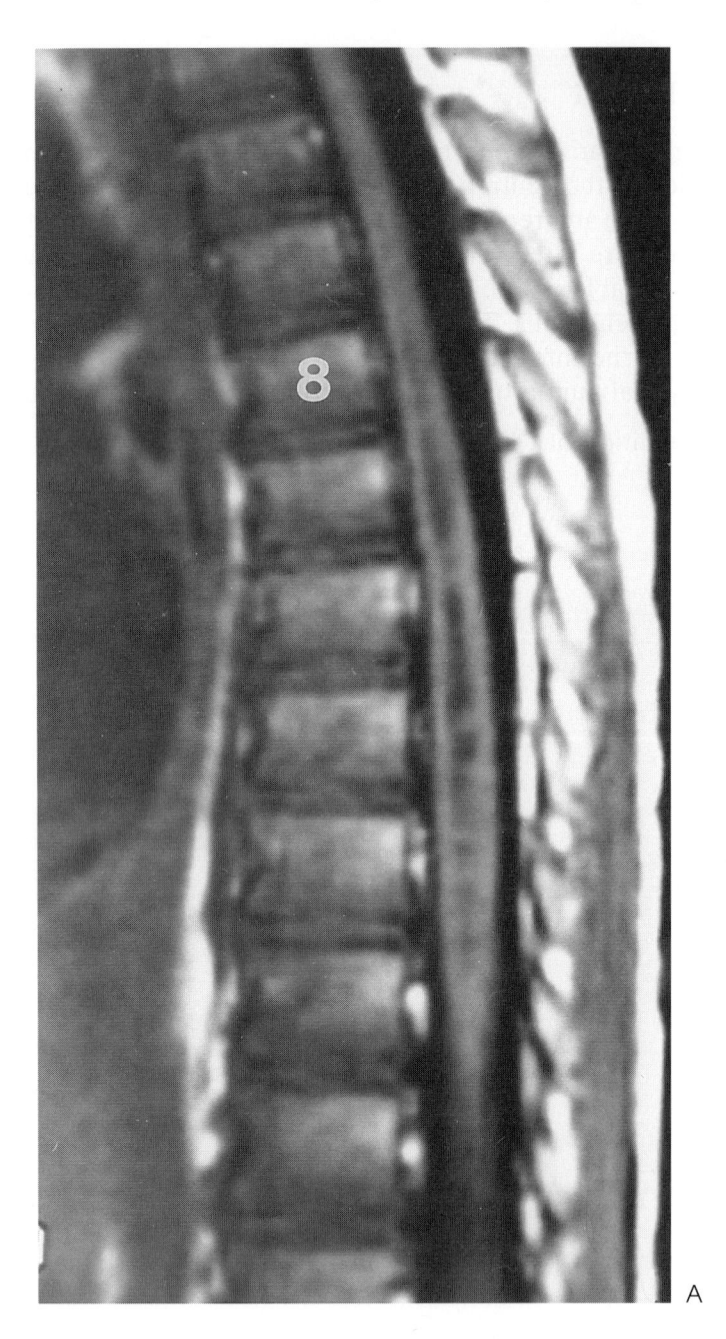

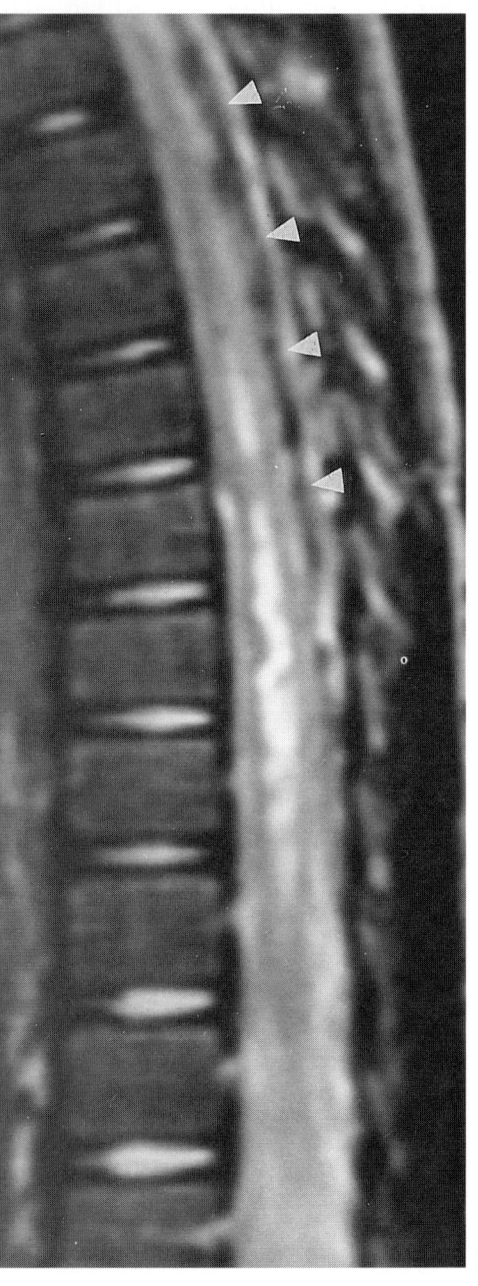

CONGENITAL

C

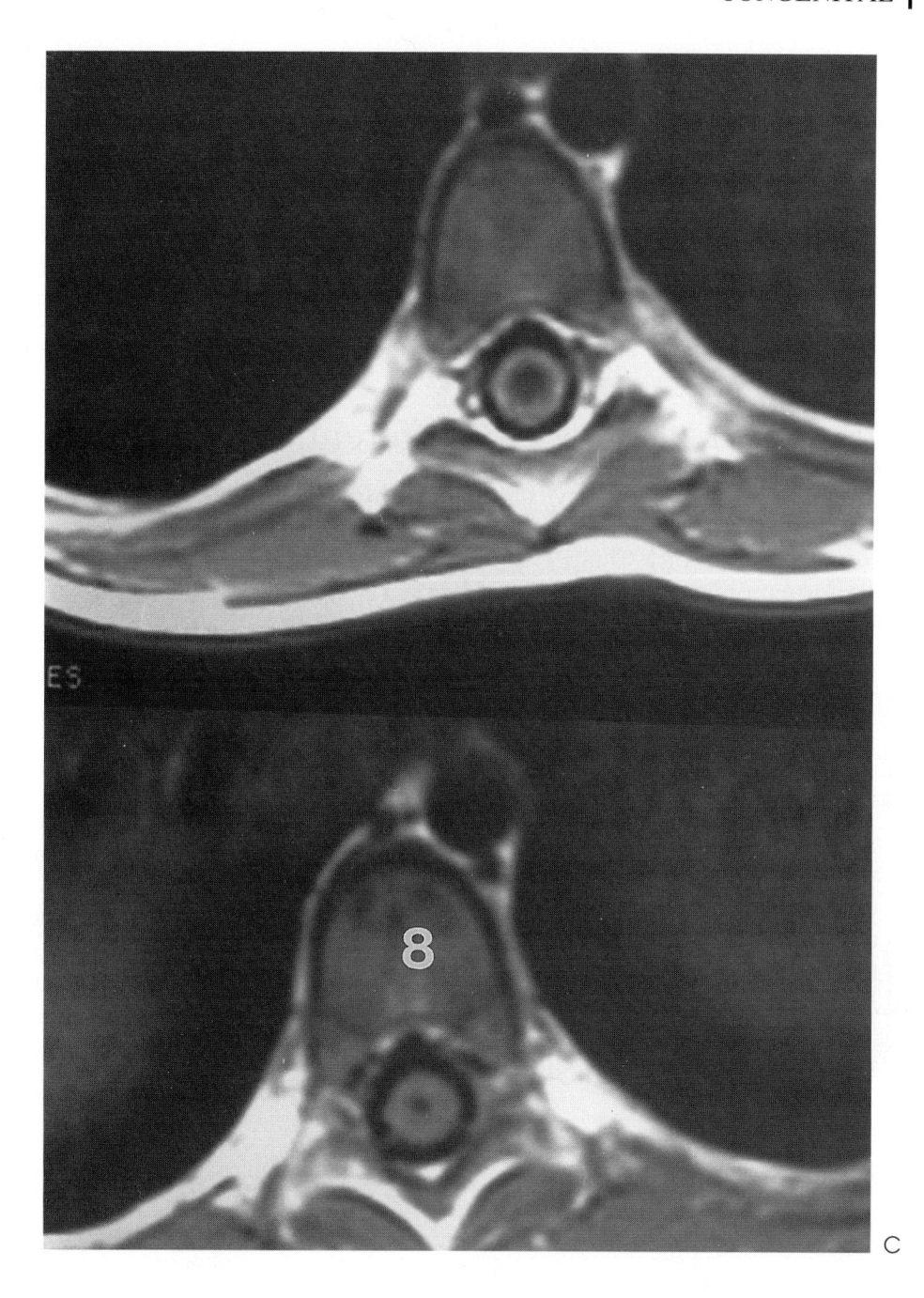

Radiologic Findings

Sagittal short TR image (Fig. A) reveals a small, multisegment, loculated syrinx cavity in the mid and distal thoracic spinal cord. The cerebrospinal fluid (CSF) containing cavity begins at the level of the inferior endplate of T7 and extends to the level of the midbody of L1. There is slight expansion of the spinal cord throughout the spinal cord at the area of the syrinx cavity. 8 = T8 vertebral body.

Sagittal long TR image (Fig. B) reveals that the fluid within the syrinx cavity exhibits marked increased signal intensity. Note the areas of decreased signal intensity dorsal to the spinal cord superior to the syrinx cavity (*arrowheads*). These represent areas of flow void in the CSF secondary to transmitted heart beat and respiration.

TEACHING ATLAS OF SPINE IMAGING

Axial short TR images (Fig. C) reveal the central area of decreased signal intensity within the spinal cord secondary to the syrinx cavity. In the midportion of the thoracic spine, at the level of T8 (*8*), the cavity is smaller, whereas at the more distal end of the spinal cord the cavity is larger in size (*upper image*).

Diagnosis

Chiari I malformation and thoracic syrinx.

Differential Diagnosis

- Chiari I malformation and thoracic syrinx

Discussion

There was downward displacement of the cerebellar tonsils below the level of the foramen magnum in this patient consistent with a Chiari I malformation (not illustrated). There was no syrinx cavity present in the cervical spinal cord. The location of the syrinx cavity in the thoracic region is uncommon, but otherwise typical of Chiari I malformation.

The size and location of the syrinx cavity in patients with Chiari I malformation is highly variable. In some patients these cavities are small, whereas in others they are large. There is also variation in the number of internal septations that may be seen. CSF flow may be evaluated by magnetic resonance imaging with directional annotation so that caudal flow has increased signal intensity while cepahalad flow exhibits decreased signal intensity. The flow may also be quantitative and therefore, changes that may occur following any corrective surgical procedure can be evaluated.

For a definition of Chiari I malformation, see Case 1.

PEARLS

- The cervical spinal cord also should be evaluated to rule out the presence of a syrinx cavity.

- In the presence of a Chiari I malformation and a cervical spinal cord syrinx cavity, the entire length of the spinal cord should be evaluated.

PITFALL

- The multiple areas of decreased signal intensity dorsal to the thoracic spinal cord represent areas of flow void secondary to transmitted heart beat and respiration and should not be mistaken for the flow void of an arteriovenous malformation.

CONGENITAL

Case 4

Clinical Presentation

The patient is a newborn male with a large soft tissue mass arising in the lower dorsal region of the lumbar spine.

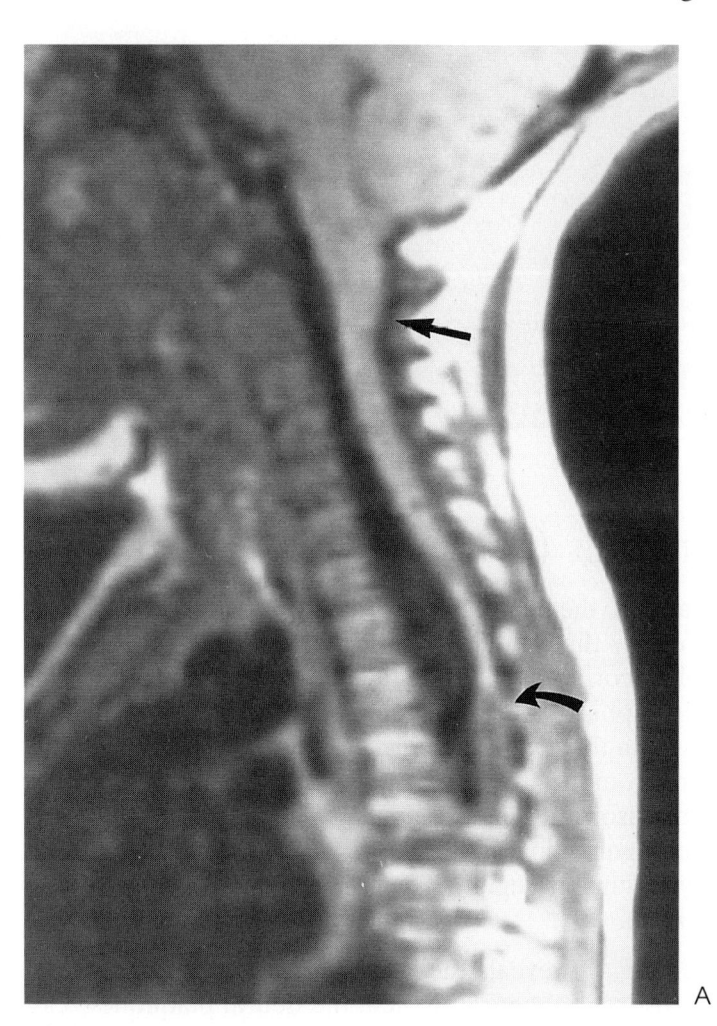

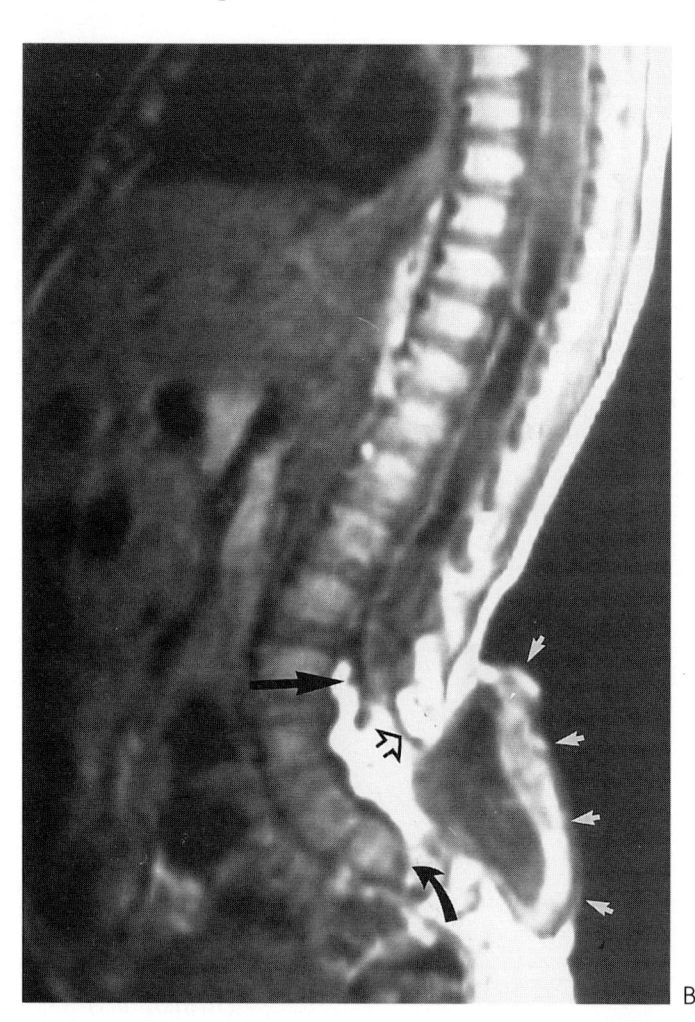

Radiologic Findings

Sagittal short TR image at the level of the cervical spine (Fig. A) reveals cerebellar tonsillar herniation (*straight arrow*). The cervical spinal cord is displaced posteriorly into the lower cervical region and the upper portion of a syrinx cavity is seen in the upper thoracic region (*curved arrow*). The cervical vertebral canal is expanded. Incidentally, there is platybasia of the skull base, with absence of the normal curvilinear angulation between the brain stem, medulla, and upper spinal cord.

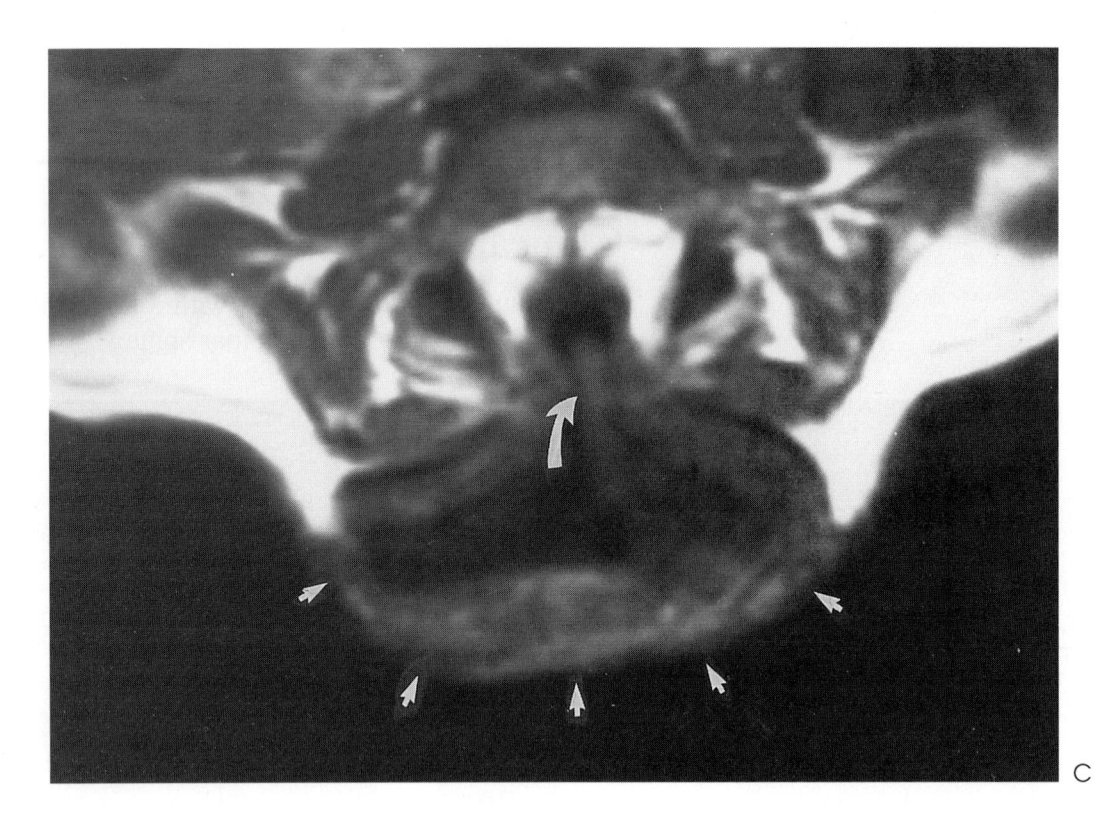

Radiologic Findings (continued)

Sagittal short TR image of the lumbar vertebral canal (Fig. B) reveals a multiloculated syrinx cavity that extends from the thoracic region into the lumbar region. The spinal cord is tethered distally at the level of L3 (*straight black arrow*). Spinal dysraphism and a heart-shaped, thick-walled meningomyelocele (*white arrows*) in the lower lumbar region are visible. The meningocele extends outward from the dysraphic lumbar vertebral canal into the subcutaneous area. The disordered neural tissue (*open arrow*) can be seen extending into the meningomyelocele. There is an increase in the normal epidural fat in the lower lumbar region. The sacrum is missing below the level of S1 (*curved arrow*).

Axial short TR image (Fig. C) reveals the thick-walled meningomyelocele (*straight arrows*). The disordered neural tissue—the neural plaquode—can be seen extending into the vertebral canal (*curved arrow*). Spinal dysraphism is visible. There is an increase in the epidural fat in the widened vertebral canal and an increase in the amount of adipose tissue in the subcutaneous tissue adjacent to the meningocele.

PEARLS

- The entire spinal cord should be visualized to evaluate for tethering of the spinal cord and the presence and extent of syringohydromyelia. Magnetic resonance imaging accurately reflects the anatomic findings and surgery can be based on these findings.

- This patient also has sacral agenesis with an increase in the amount of subcutaneous fat. In 30% of cases, infants with sacral agenesis have a diabetic mother.

- The dorsal displacement of the upper portion of the thoracic spinal cord is probably secondary to dorsal tethering of the spinal cord at this level. The normal basal angle, formed by a line connecting the nasion to the tuberculum sellae to the anterior margin of the foramen magnum is 125 to 143 degrees.

PITFALL

- Vertebral anomalies may also be seen in patients with the Chiari malformations.

Diagnosis

Chiari type II malformation with a large meningomyelocele, sacral agenesis.

Differential Diagnosis

- Chiari type II malformation with a large meningomyelocele, sacral agenesis

Discussion

In the Chiari II malformation, the cerebellar tonsils are downwardly displaced and a meningocele or meningomyelocele is found in the lumbar region. There may be an associated syrinx cavity within the spinal cord, or an associated aqueduct stenosis and therefore an associated hydrocephalus. Other abnormalities of the brain that may be seen in association with the Chiari II malformation include enlarged massa intermedia, downward pointed floors of the lateral ventricles, towering vermis of the cerebellum, scalloping of the posterior margin of the petrous bones, kinking of the brainstem, colpocephaly, absent septum pellicidum, absence of the corpus callosum, enlarged foramen magnum, and tectal beaking.

This patient exhibits a large constellation of findings that may be seen in patients with congenital anomalies of the spine. As with congenital anomalies of the brain, when one anomaly is present, there are frequently additional anomalies. It also may be helpful or even necessary to evaluate the intracranial contents in these patients to fully evaluate the extent of abnormalities.

TEACHING ATLAS OF SPINE IMAGING

Case 5

Clinical Presentation

The patient is a 1-year-old male with a history meningomyelocele repair at birth.

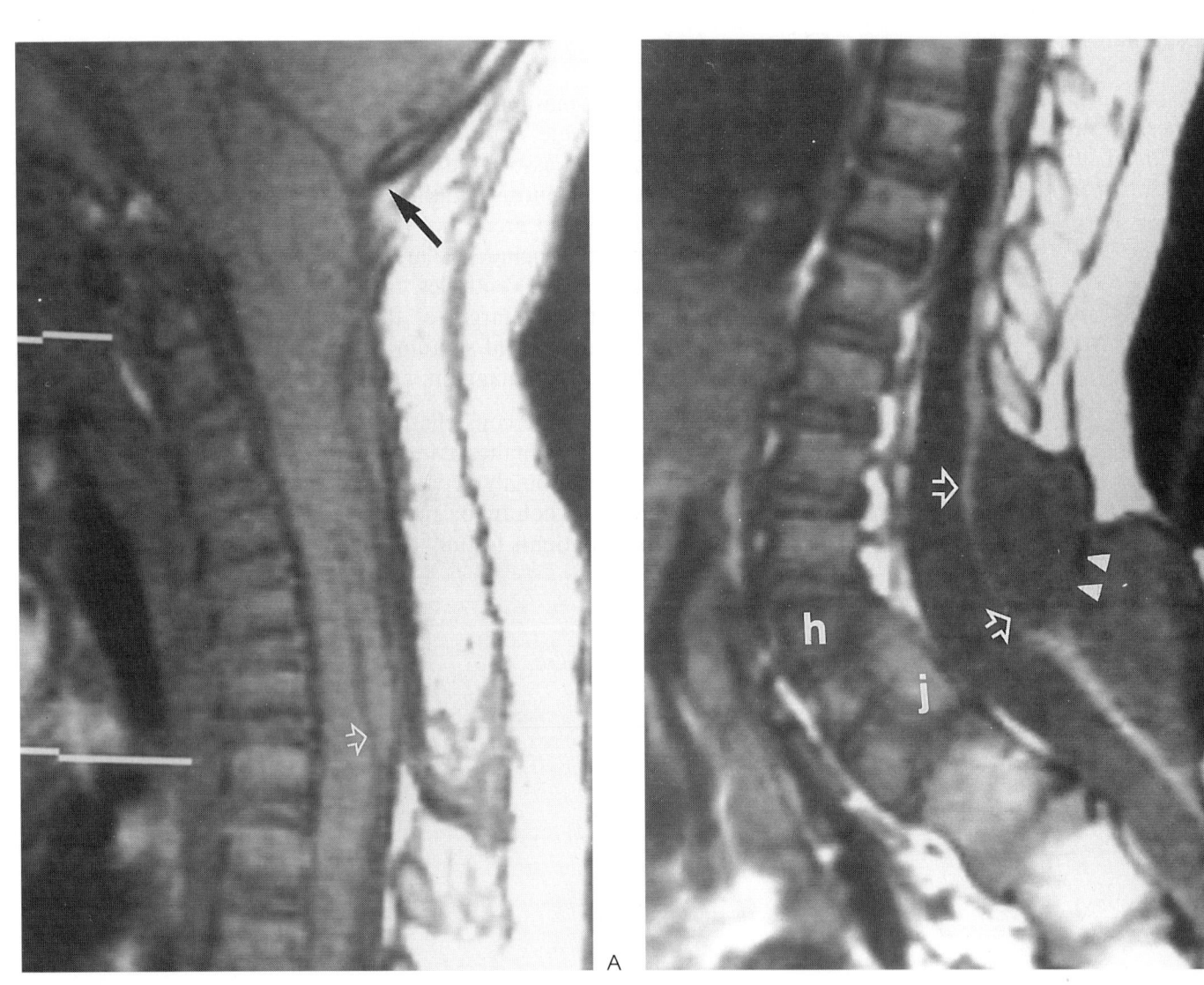

Radiologic Findings

Sagittal short TR image (Fig. A) reveals extraordinarily marked downward displacement of the cerebellar tonsils (*solid arrow*). The tonsils are elongated and pointed and extend down to the T1 level (*open arrow*).

Diagnosis

Chiari type III malformation.

Differential Diagnosis

- Chiari type III malformation

Discussion

The Chiari III malformation includes the presence of an occipital meningocele or meningoencephalocele. There may also be an associated cervical spinal cord syrinx cavity. In this patient, there is an occipital meningoencephalocele, cerebellar tonsillar herniation, agenesis of the corpus callosum, kinking of the brainstem, syringohydromyelia of the cervical spinal cord, and a small posterior fossa. This constellation of findings is seen in the patient with the Chiari III malformation. It is important to determine the contents of the soft tissue mass. If the mass contains only meninges without cerebellar tissue, it can be removed surgically with impunity. However, if the sac also contains cerebral tissue, then the surgical implications are much greater, and surgery cannot be attempted without danger to the patient. MR imaging is the procedure of choice for evaluation.

PEARL
- The physical findings in this patient are obvious to the clinician; therefore, the clinical diagnosis is obvious. There are typical findings which are seen in a patient with this diagnosis, and these changes should be looked for when evaluating the images.

PITFALL
- If one is unaware of the typical findings, the various subtleties of the case may not be appreciated.

TEACHING ATLAS OF SPINE IMAGING

Case 8

Clinical Presentation

The patient is a 2-year-old female with lower extremity paralysis and bowel and bladder incontinence; a pelvic mass was identified on ultrasound.

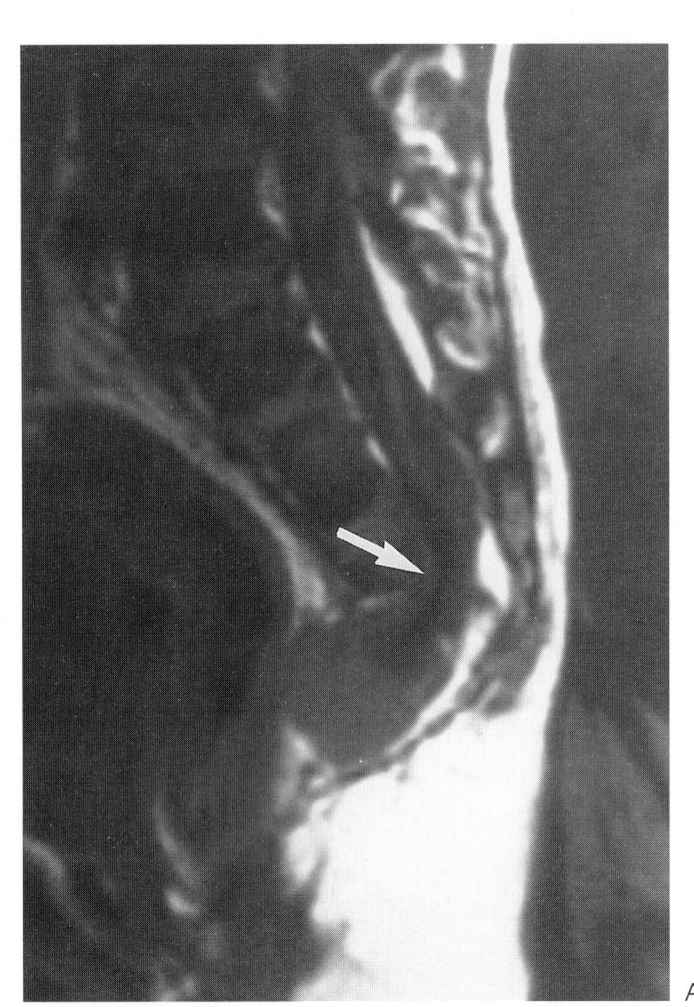

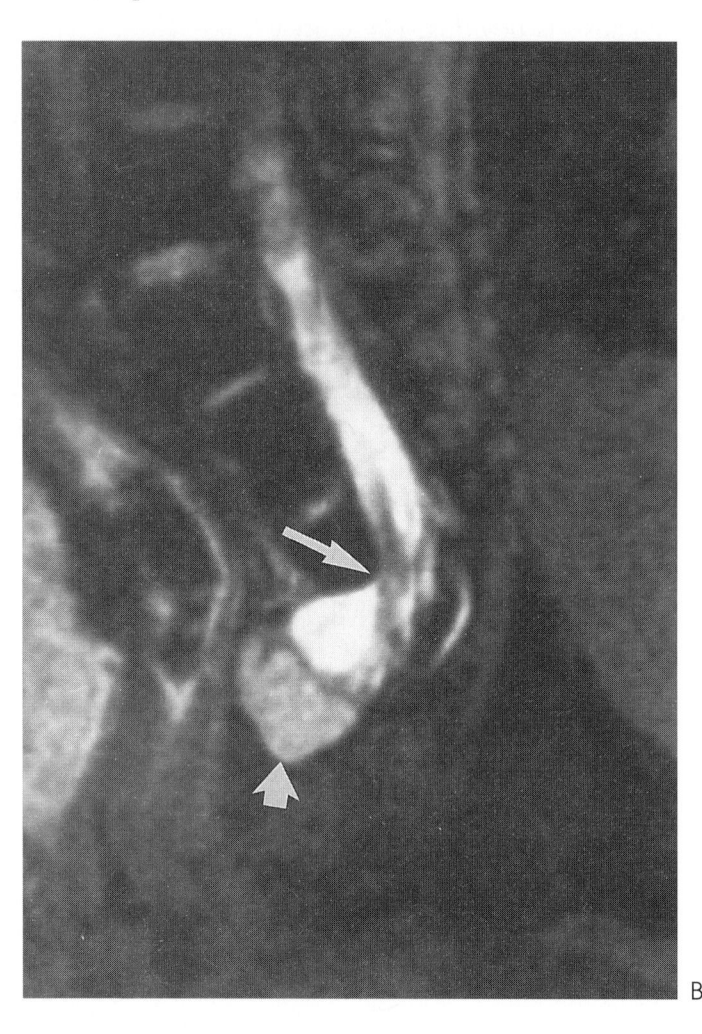

Radiologic Findings

Sagittal short TR image in the lower lumbar region (Fig. A) reveals extension of the thecal sac into the pelvis anterior to the sacrum. The thecal sac is expanded, with a large component extending anteriorly into the pelvis (*arrow*). The material within the sac is a combination of cerebrospinal fluid (CSF) and the deformed neural tissue; therefore, the signal intensity within the sac is variable and is secondary to this wide variety of soft tissue structures. The bowel and bladder are both dilated.

Sagittal long TR image (Fig. B) reveals the nerve roots of the cauda equina extending into the sacral meningocele. The sac contains CSF and neural tissue (*short arrow*). The distal end of the sacrum is absent (*long arrow*), as is the coccyx.

CONGENITAL

Diagnosis

Anterior sacral myelomeningocele.

Differential Diagnosis

- retrorectal cyst-hamartoma (tailgut cyst)
- dermoid cyst
- duplication cyst of rectum
- neurenteric cyst
- rectal leiomyosarcoma
- chordoma
- sacral teratoma

Discussion

Prior to the development of magnetic resonance (MR) imaging, evaluation of sacral meningocele was performed with myelography. Following the injection of iodinated contrast material into the subarachnoid space, radiopaque contrast material would accumulate in the meningocele. The myelogram would typically be followed by a computed tomography (CT) scan, which would then evaluate the amount of neural tissue elements and CSF within the sac. This was a much more invasive and less accurate examination than MR imaging. In general, surgery may be planned in these patients based solely on the MR findings.

PEARLS

- There also is caudal regression with absence of a portion of the sacrum and the coccyx, and tethering of the spinal cord.

- CT scanning also may be helpful to better evaluate the bony abnormalities.

- The remainder of the spine should be evaluated for the possibility of a syrinx cavity within the spinal cord.

- A sacral teratoma could have a similar appearance but would not communicate with the thecal sac.

PITFALL

- Communication may occur with the gastrointestinal tract, resulting in central nervous system infections.

Case 9

Clinical Presentation

The patient is a 3-month-old female with a small dimple on the lower back.

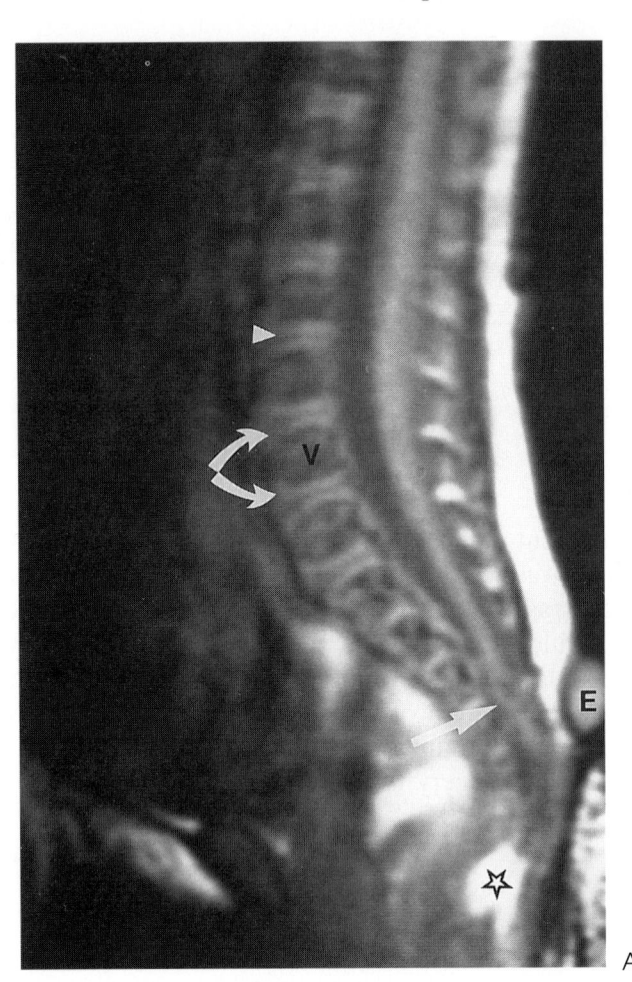

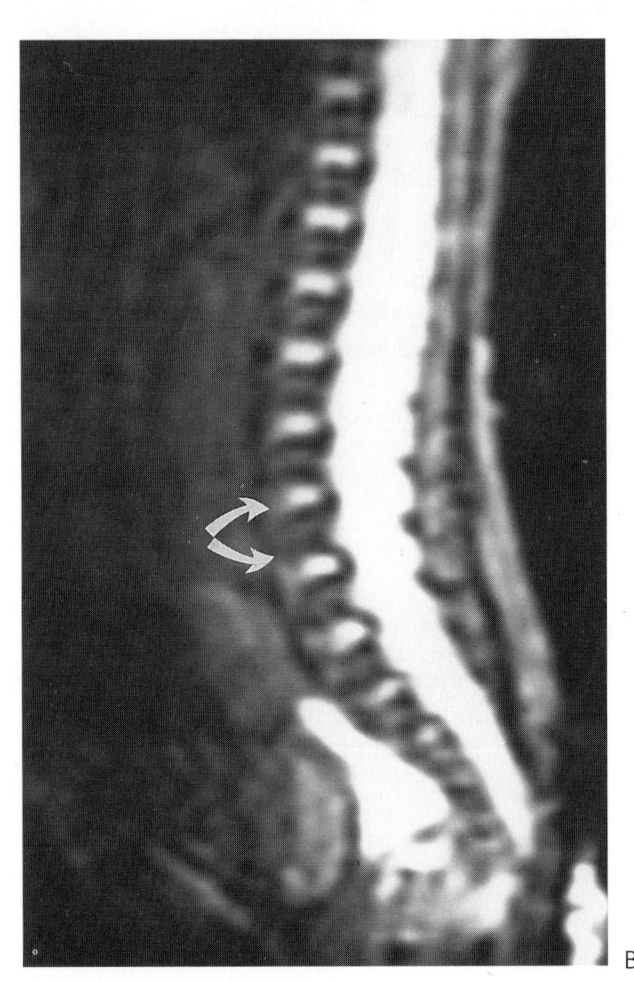

Radiologic Findings

Sagittal short TR image of the lumbar spine (Fig. A) does not demonstrate the true conus. The spinal cord is a solid structure down to the level of the junction between the sacrum and the coccyx (*long arrow*). A vitamin E capsule (*E*) identifies the skin abnormality. There is absence of the coccyx and a small irregularly marginated accumulation of fat (*) marks the distal end of the vertebral column. The vertebral bodies and intervertebral discs demonstrate their immature form. The vertebral body is identified with a *V* and the superior and inferior cartilaginous end plates are marked with curved arrows. The intervertebral disc is identified with an *arrowhead*.

CONGENITAL

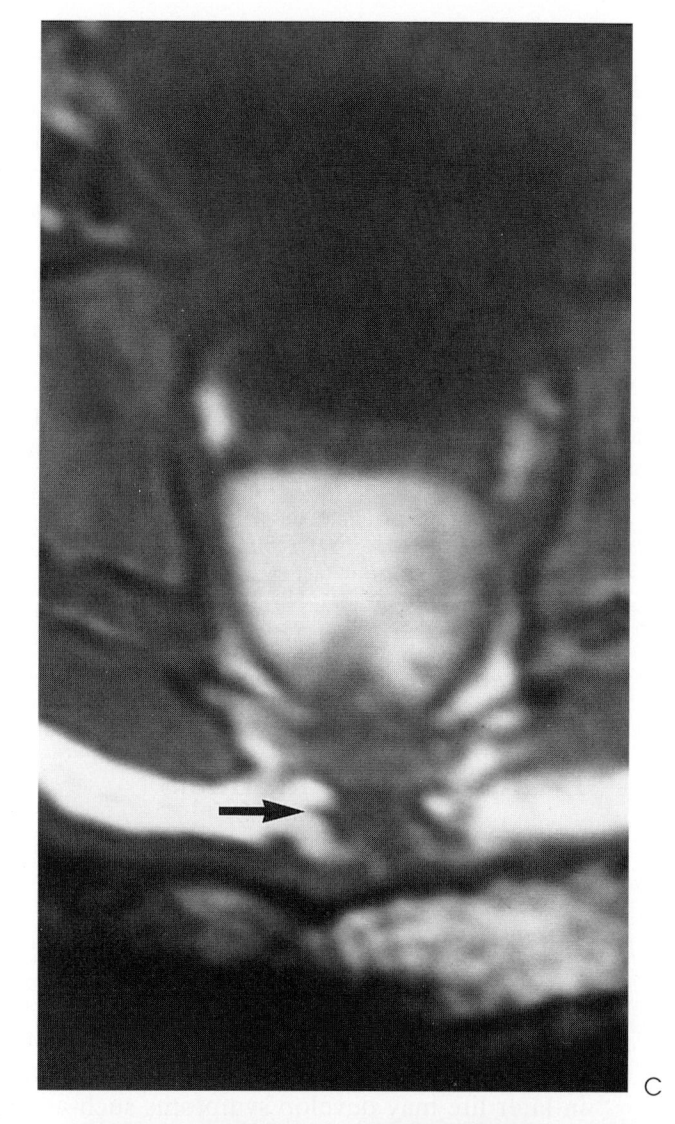

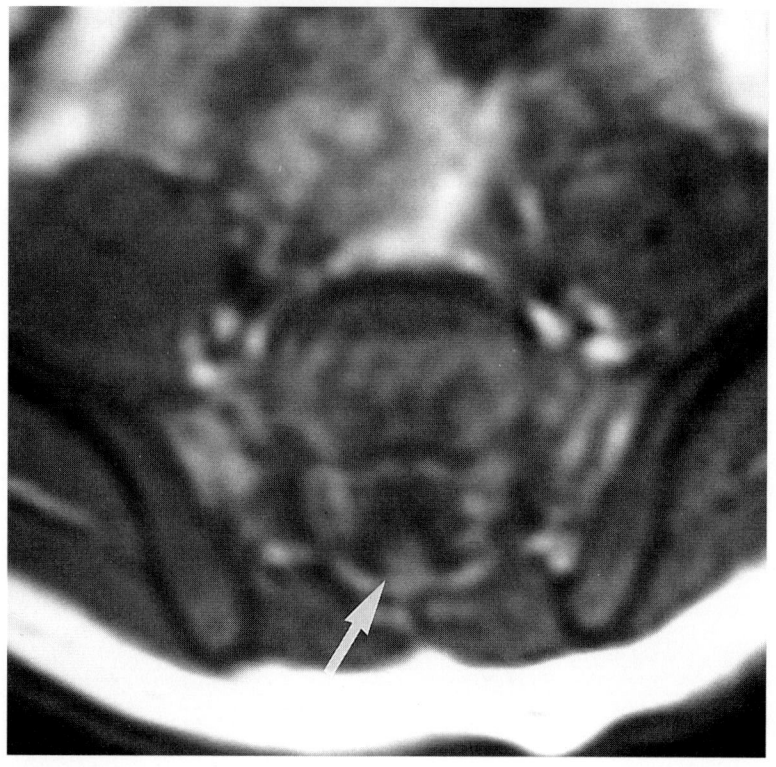

91

Radiologic Findings (continued)

On the long TR image (Fig. B) the cartilaginous endplates of the vertebral bodies appear markedly decreased in signal intensity (*arrows*), whereas the intervertebral disc appears bright. The lumbar vertebral canal is enlarged throughout. The dilated vertebral canal appears as increased signal intensity; the spinal cord is not seen.

The axial short TR image in the lower lumbar region (Fig. C) reveals a dysraphic spine and the soft tissue density material replacing the subcutaneous fat (*arrow*).

Axial short TR image in the sacral region (Fig. D) reveals a dysraphic spine and the tethered spinal cord positioned posteriorly in the thecal sac (*arrow*). There is no lipoma of the distal cord; however, the neural tissue is abnormally located outside of the vertebral canal.

> **PEARL**
> - Evaluation of the craniovertebral junction may reveal the presence of low lying cerebellar tonsils.

Diagnosis

Tethered cord, meningomyelocele, and coccygeal agenesis.

Differential Diagnosis

- tethered cord, meningomyelocele, and coccygeal agenesis

> **PITFALL**
> - The entire sacrum and coccyx should be visualized so that anomalies can be identified.

Discussion

The presence of a low lumbar skin dimple may herald the presence of a tethered cord or other anomaly. Magnetic resonance imaging is the best method for evaluation. Patients may be asymptomatic in younger life, but in later life may develop symptoms such as urinary retention. If there is a sinus tract associated with the skin dimple and resulting communication with the spinal subarachnoid space, repeated central nervous system (CNS) infections such as meningitis may occur. A sinus tract should not be probed for fear of introducing infection into the CNS.

CONGENITAL

Case 10

Clinical Presentation
Newborn male with imperforate anus.

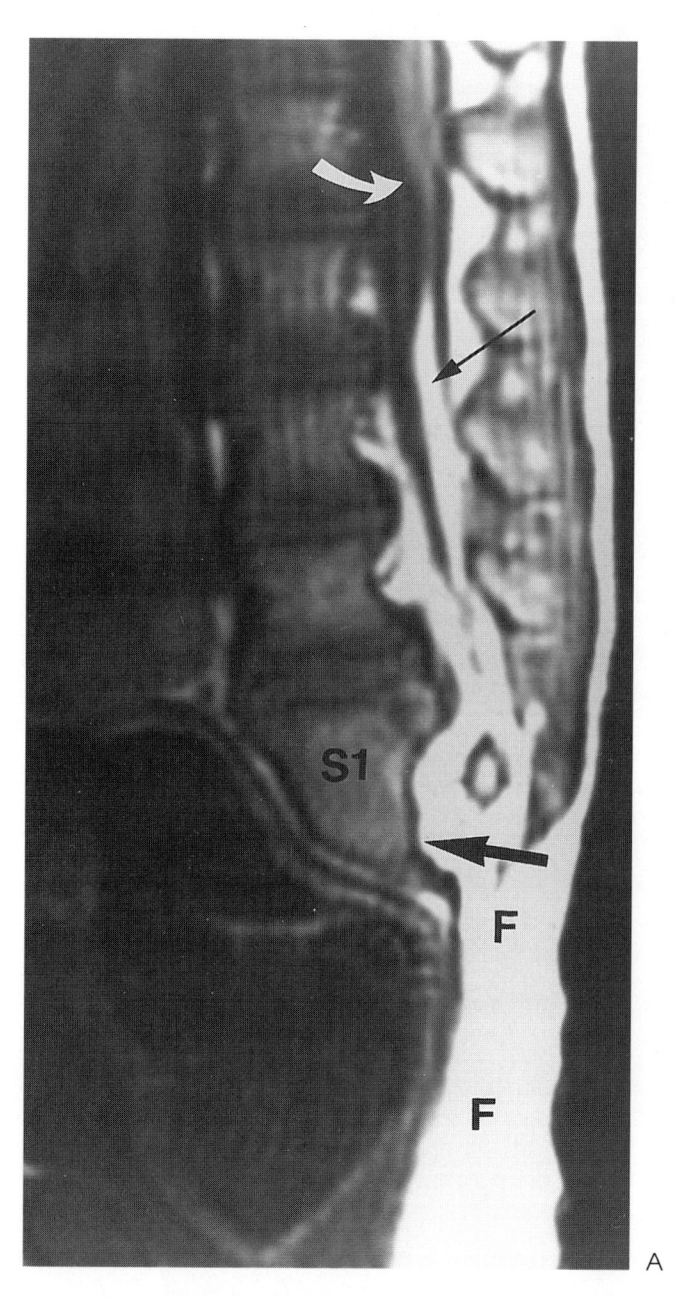

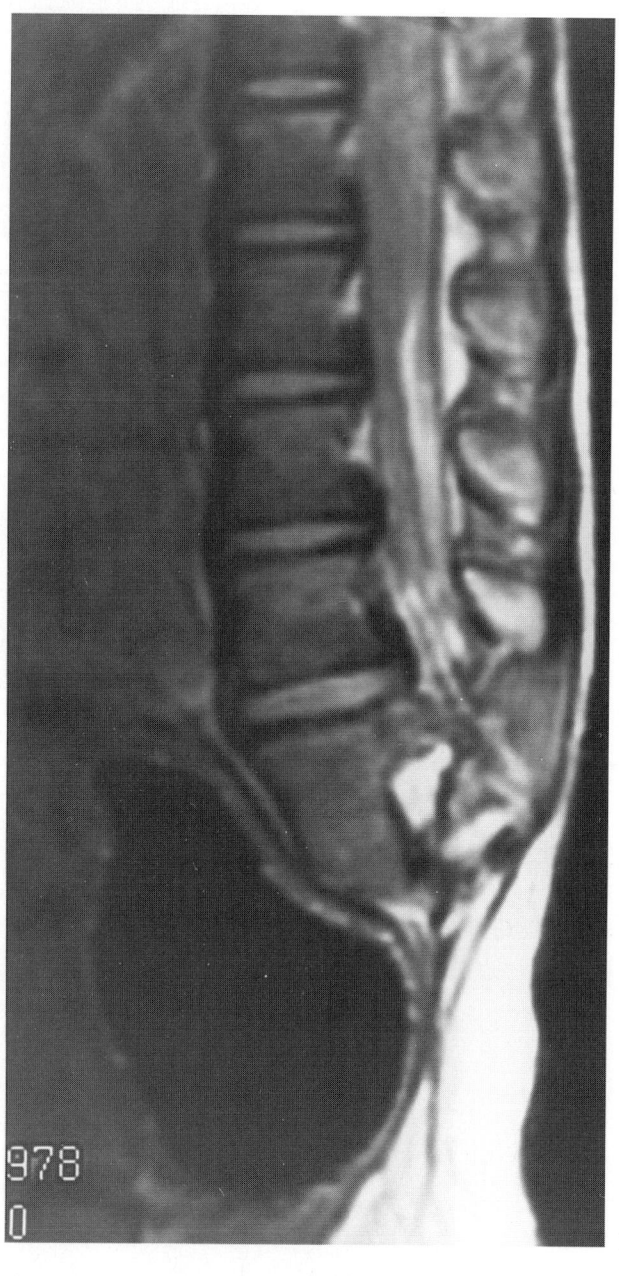

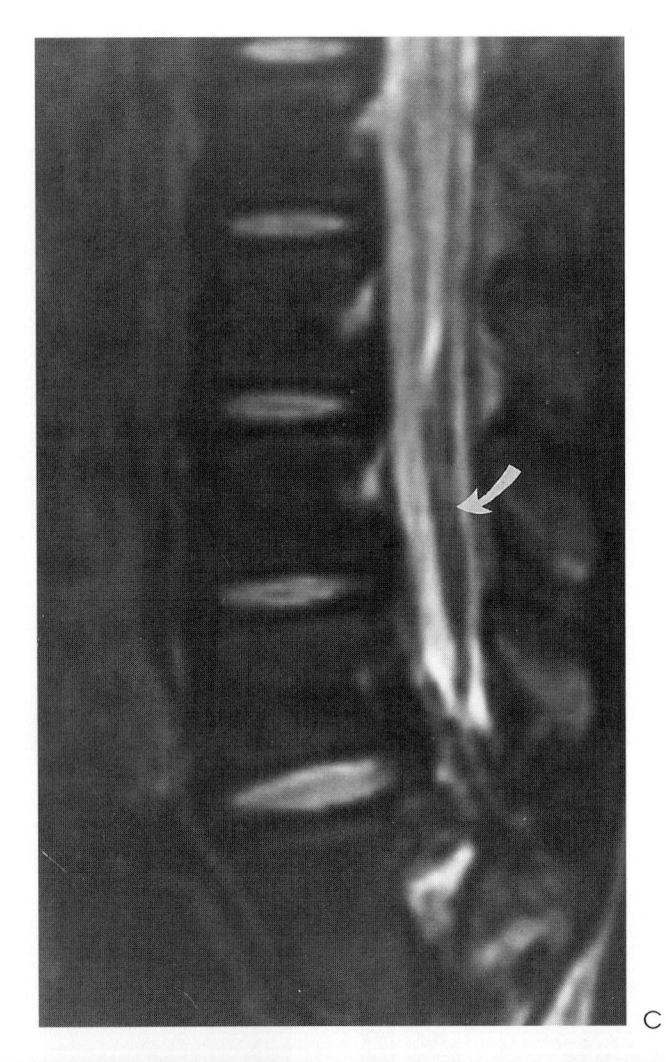

TEACHING ATLAS OF SPINE IMAGING

C

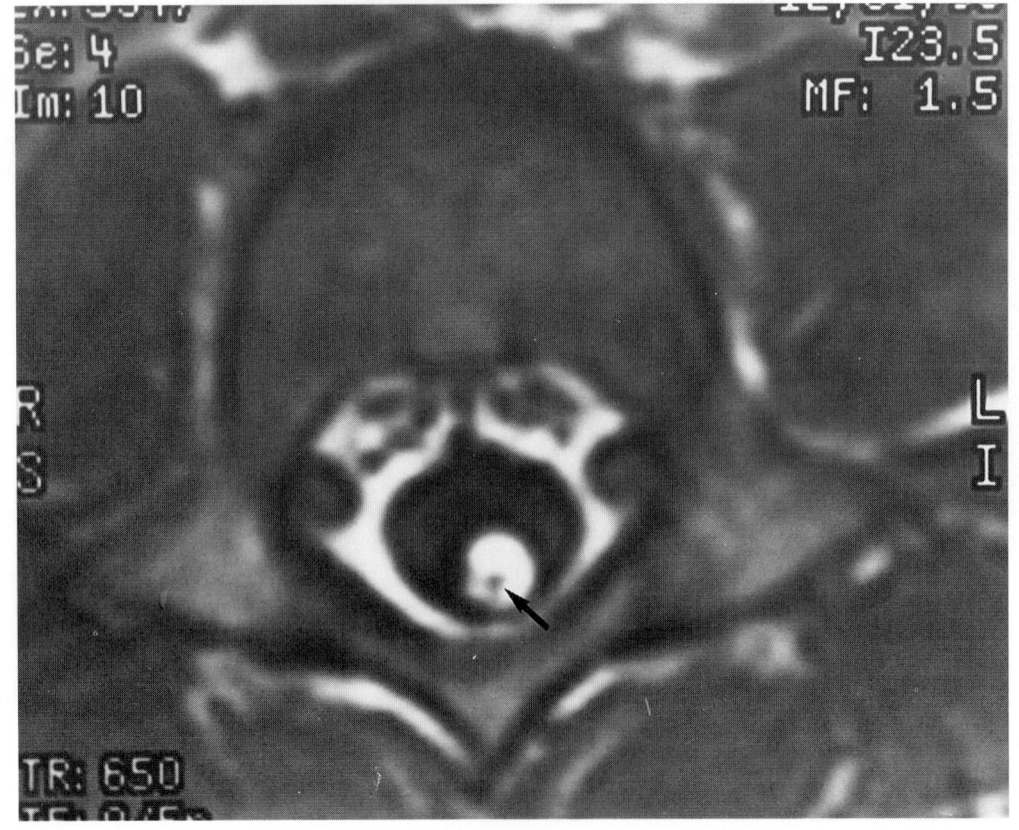

D

CONGENITAL

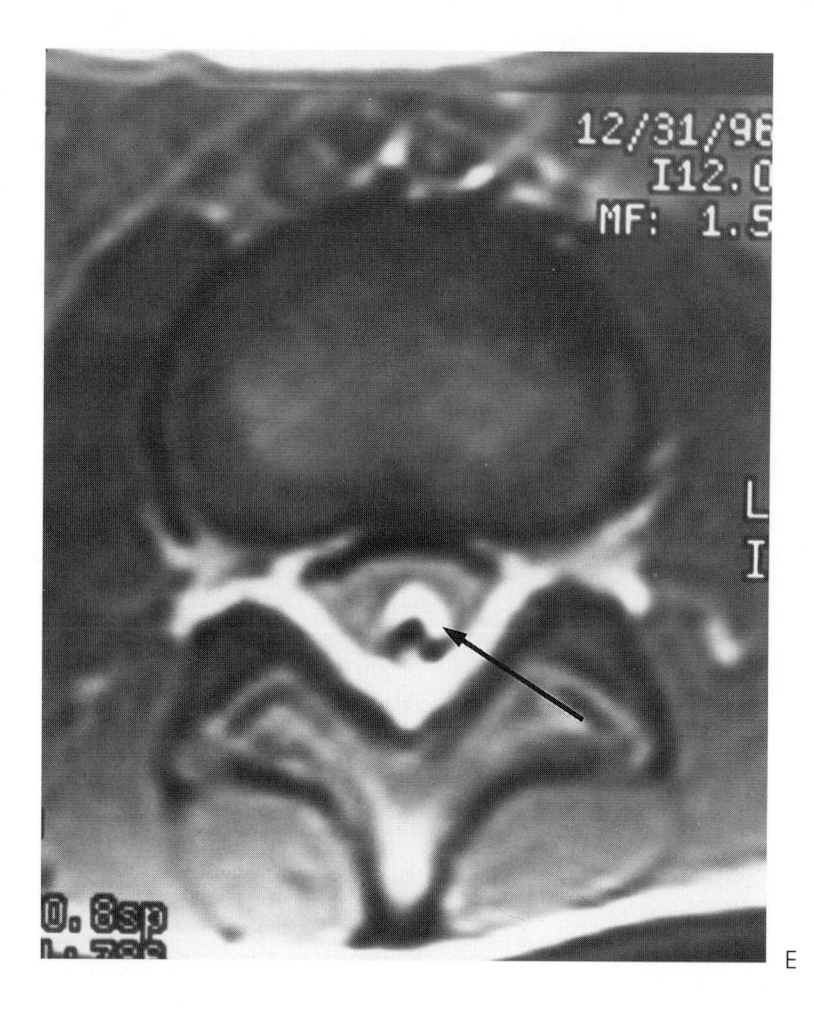

Radiologic Findings

Sagittal short TR image (Fig. A) reveals that the spinal cord ends at the level of the inferior endplate of L2 (*curved arrow*). There is an increased signal intensity elongated soft tissue mass that begins at the level of the midbody of L3 and extends inferiorly to mid-L5 (*thin black arrow*). The S1 vertebral body (*S1*) is deformed (*thick black arrow*), and there is an increase in the amount of fat in the subcutaneous area in the anticipated position of the sacrum and coccyx (*F*). The rectum and distal bowel are greatly dilated. Sagittal intermediate TR image (Fig. B) reveals that the cerebrospinal fluid now appears as intermediate signal intensity; the soft tissue mass appears as increased signal intensity.

Long TR image (Fig. C) reveals that the soft tissue mass now appears decreased signal intensity (*arrow*).

Axial short TR image at the level of L4 (Fig. D) reveals that the filum terminale (*arrow*) appears as an area of rounded decreased signal intensity within the increased signal intensity mass seen in Figures A through C.

Short TR image at the level of the intervertebral disc of L4-5 (Fig. E) reveals chemical shift artifact (*arrow*) associated with the increased signal intensity mass.

PEARL

- It is reported that 30% of infants with caudal regression syndrome are born to mothers with diabetes mellitus.

PITFALLS

- The entire sacrum and coccyx should be included at the time of imaging.

- Plain film evaluation may be necessary.

- CT scanning may better demonstrate the bony abnormalities.

Diagnosis

Sacral agenesis with filum terminale lipoma and lower-than-normal spinal cord.

Differential Diagnosis

- an area of subacute hemorrhage could mimic the appearance of lipoma

- sacral teratoma (unlikely)

Discussion

Other anomalies such as kidney lesions also may be seen in patients with sacral agenesis. Magnetic resonance imaging is the procedure of choice for diagnosis. The entire vertebral column should be evaluated for the presence of various anomalies and the possibility of a syrinx cavity in the spinal cord. Abdominal imaging with CT and/or ultrasound and in the evaluation of related organsystem anomalies.

CONGENITAL

Case 11

Clinical Presentation

The patient is a 6-month-old male with lower extremity weakness.

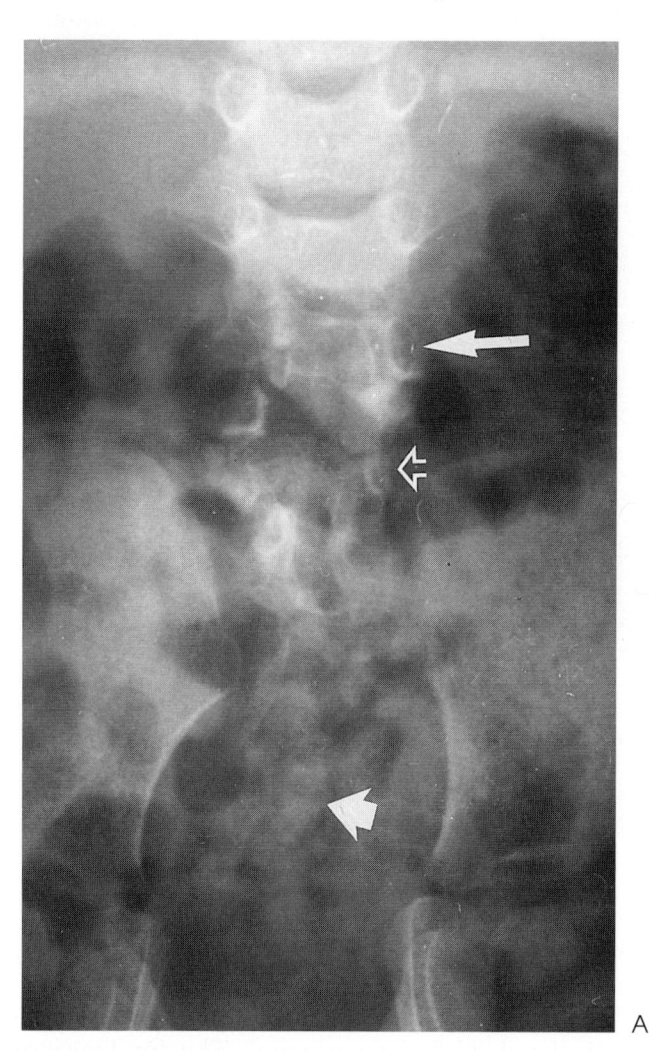

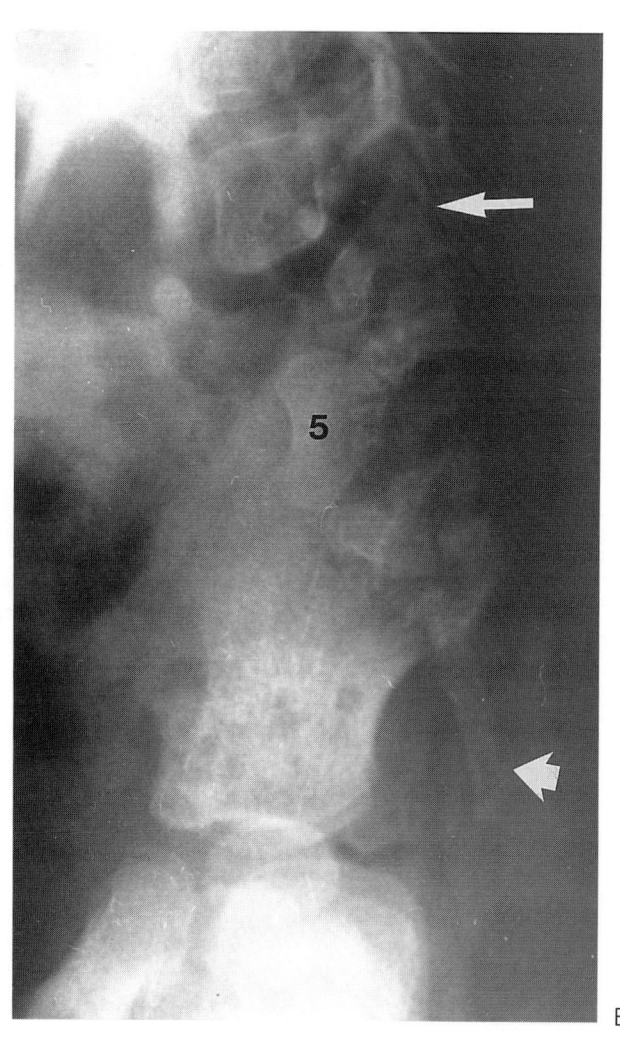

Radiologic Findings

Anteroposterior (Fig. A) and lateral (Fig. B) views of the abdomen reveal that there is incomplete development of the sacrum and coccyx. Only a small rod-like bone appears in the anticipated position of the sacrum and coccyx (*short arrow*, Figs. A and B). L3 is a small rounded malformed piece of bone. L4 (*long arrow*, Figs. A and B) is a hemivertebrae with a deformed pedicle on the right side. L5 (*5*, Fig. B) appears to be incompletely formed with a hemivertebrae on the left side (*open arrow*, Fig. A).

TEACHING ATLAS OF SPINE IMAGING

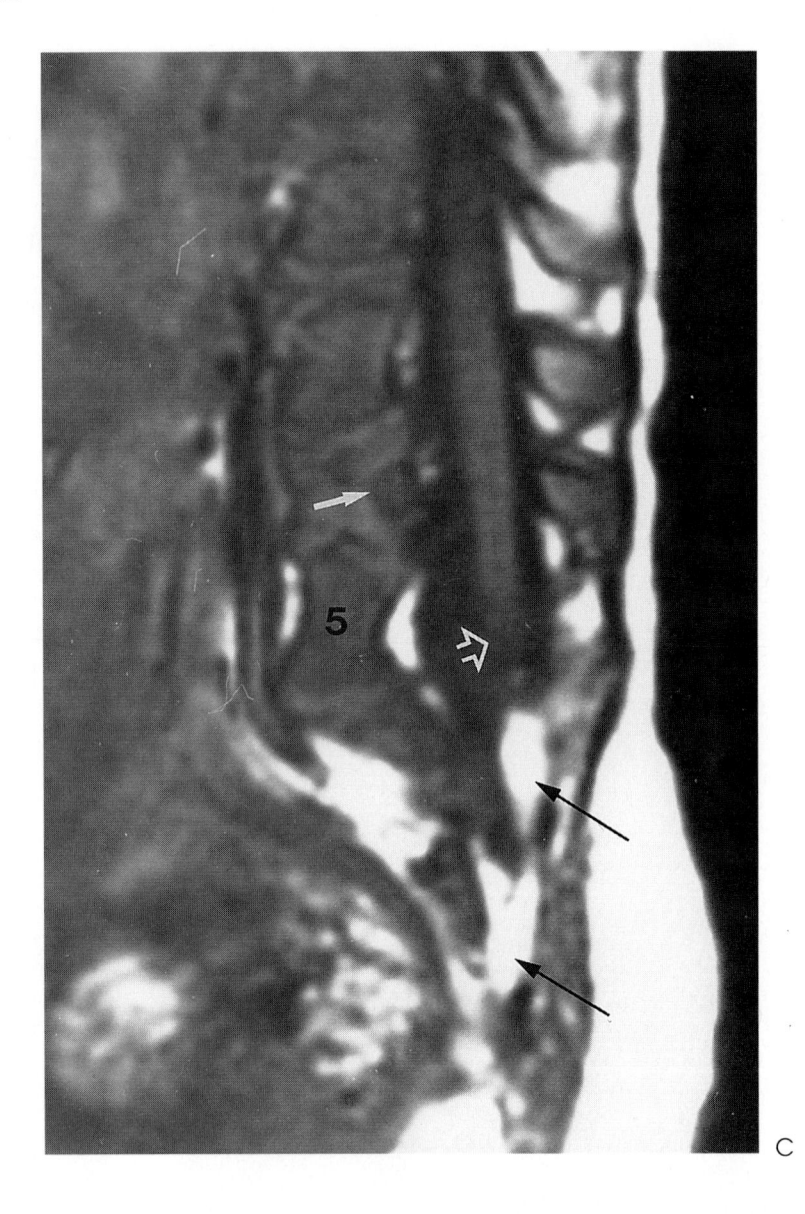

Radiologic Findings (continued)

Sagittal short TR image (Fig. C) reveals that the spinal cord is tethered and extends caudally to the level of L5 (5; *open arrow*). The dural sac is expanding into the lumbar region. L3 can be seen as a small rounded segment of bone (*white arrow*). L4 and L5 appear similar in appearance to the plain spine films. The rod-like structure of the sacrum and coccyx are seen surrounded by high signal intensity fat (*black arrows*).

CONGENITAL

PEARLS
- 30% of infants with caudal regression syndrome have diabetic mothers.

- Magnetic resonance imaging is the ideal method of evaluating congenital abnormalities of the spine.

PITFALLS
- If a myelogram is attempted in a patient with a tethered spinal cord, the needle should be placed eccentrically in the outer thirds of the thecal sac such that the needle will not injure the tethered spinal cord.

- Tethered cord may potentially be associated with low cerebellar tonsils (as if the tethered spinal cord "pulls" the cerebellar tonsils inferiorly). Therefore, if a cervical spinal tap is attempted the cerebellar tonsils could potentially be at risk for injury.

Diagnosis

Caudal regression syndrome with tethered cord and multiple vertebral anomalies.

Differential Diagnosis

- sacral teratoma
- dermoid
- lipoma

Discussion

The bulbous, frequently squared off appearance of the distal spinal cord is typical of the caudal regression syndrome. However, other anomalies such as spinal cord lipomas may also be seen in association with this anomaly.

TEACHING ATLAS OF SPINE IMAGING

Case 12

Clinical Presentation

The patient is a 2-day-old female with spinal dysraphism with hypoplasia of the lowest two lumbar and first sacral vertebral body segments on plain film examination. The opening of a dermal defect is visible in the lower lumbar region on direct physical examination.

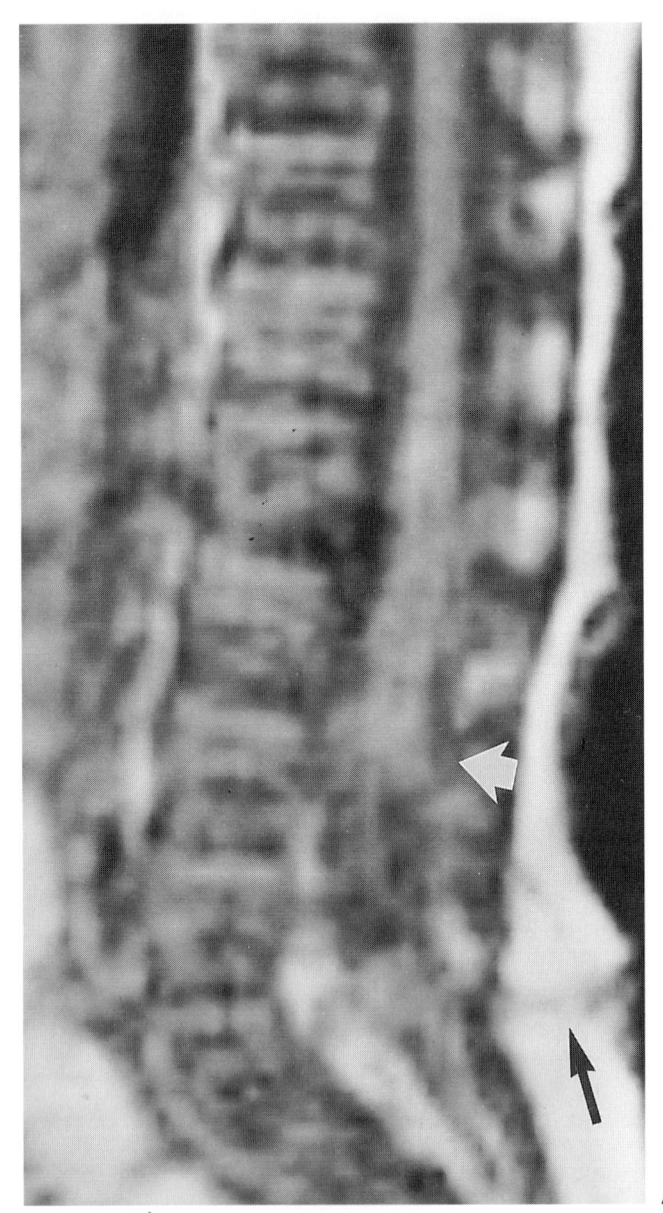

A

PEARL

- The intermediate signal intensity linear structure represents the sinus tract. In some patients the sinus tract may be very small in size and only faintly or not at all visible on MR imaging. Therefore, a vitamin E capsule taped to the patient's skin is useful to mark the position of the opening of the sinus tract and to aid in the identification and characterization of the abnormality by MR imaging.

PITFALL

- The sinus tract should *not* be probed for fear of introducing infection.

Radiologic Findings

Sagittal short TR image (Fig. A) reveals a faint intermediate signal intensity linear structure extending from the skin defect to the level of the lumbar thecal sac (*black arrow*). The distal end of the spinal cord is blunted, bulbous, and distorted (*white arrow*). There is increased fat in the anterior epidural space from L5 through the sacrum.

Diagnosis

Partial sacral and coccygeal agenesis, sinus tract, spinal dysraphism, tethered spinal cord.

Discussion

The full extent of the sinus tract may not be visible on magnetic resonance (MR) examination; however, its location can be identified by scanning, and the sinus tract may then be followed to its termination at the time of surgery. Multiple anomalies are common in patients with caudal regression, therefore when one anomalie is identified, evaluation should be made for additional anomalies. These additional anomalies may be within the central nervous system and/or in other organ systems.

TEACHING ATLAS OF SPINE IMAGING

Case 13

Clinical Presentation

Newborn male with flaccid anal sphincter.

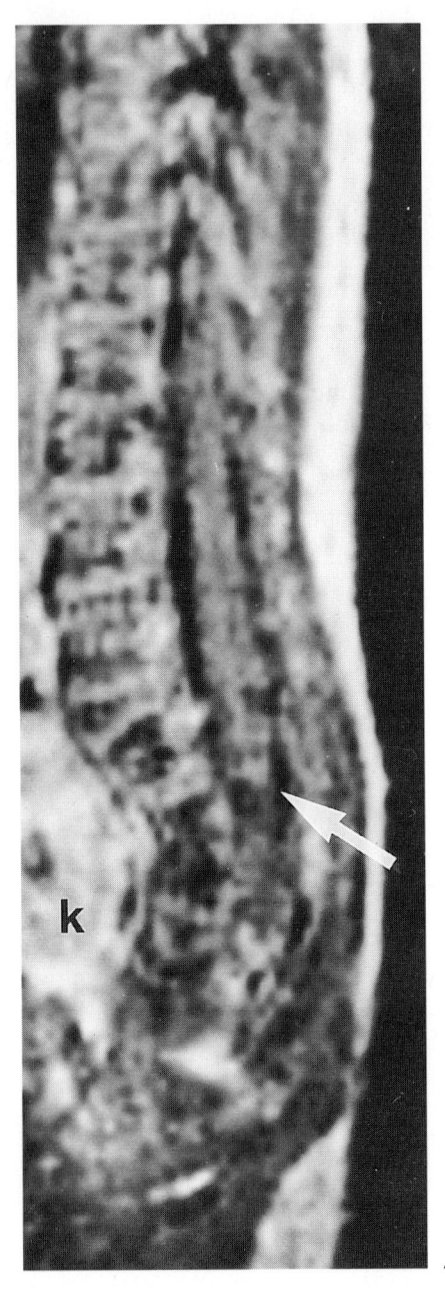

A

CONGENITAL

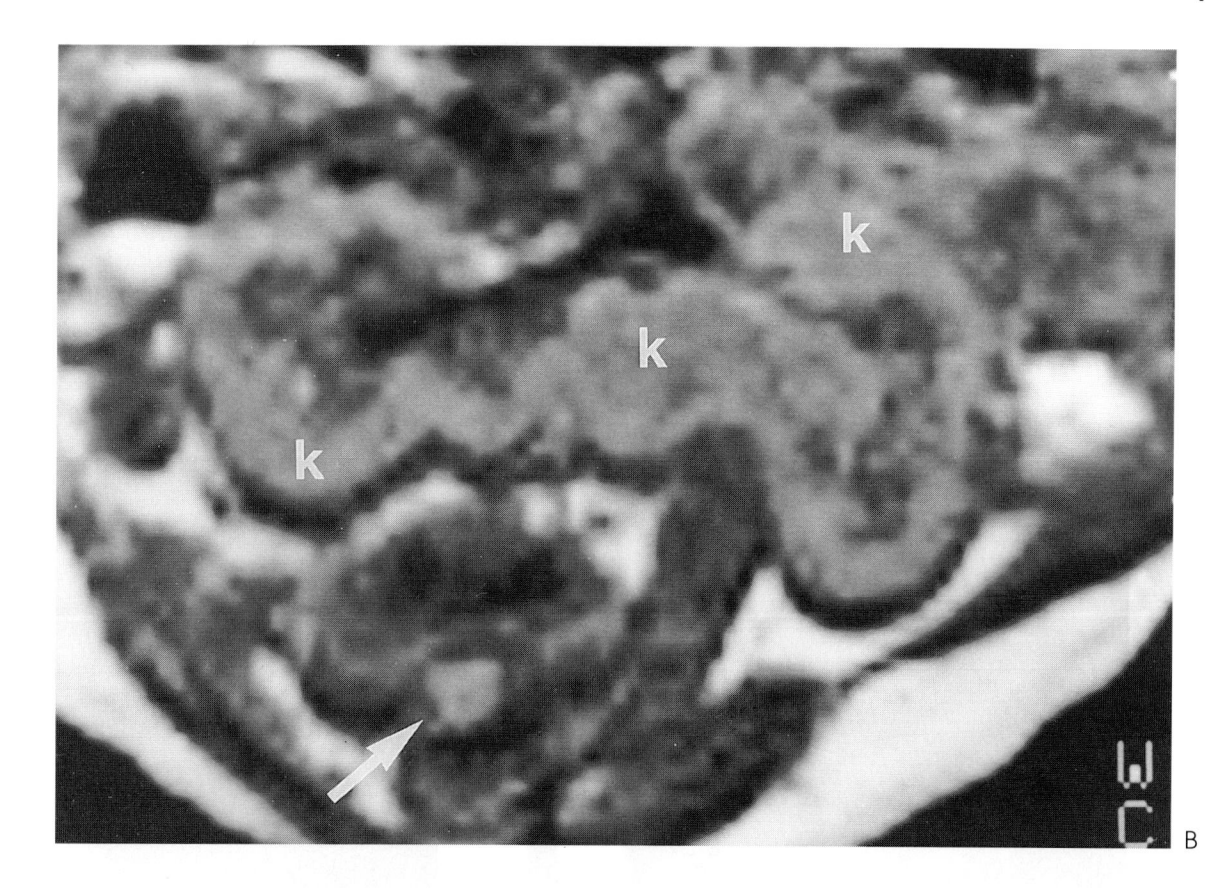

Radiologic Findings

Sagittal short TR image (Fig. A) reveals that the spinal cord appears as a large solid structure that extends down to the level of S1 (*arrow*). The sacrum was absent below the level of S2. A pelvic kidney (*k*) projects anterior to the sacrum.

Sagittal short TR image at the level of the lower lumbar spine (Fig. B) reveals tethered cord in the vertebral canal (*white arrow*), and a horseshoe kidney (*k*) at the level of the lumbosacral function.

PEARL
- The newborn is difficult to image because of its very small size. It may be advantageous to image such a small child in a small coil such as the knee coil.

Diagnosis

Tethered cord, sacral agenesis, horseshoe, pelvic kidney.

Differential Diagnosis

- tethered cord, sacral agenesis, horseshoe, pelvic kidney

Discussion

Multiple anomalies are common in patients with caudal regression, so when one anomaly is identified, evaluation should be made for additional anomalies both within the central nervous system and other organ systems.

TEACHING ATLAS OF SPINE IMAGING

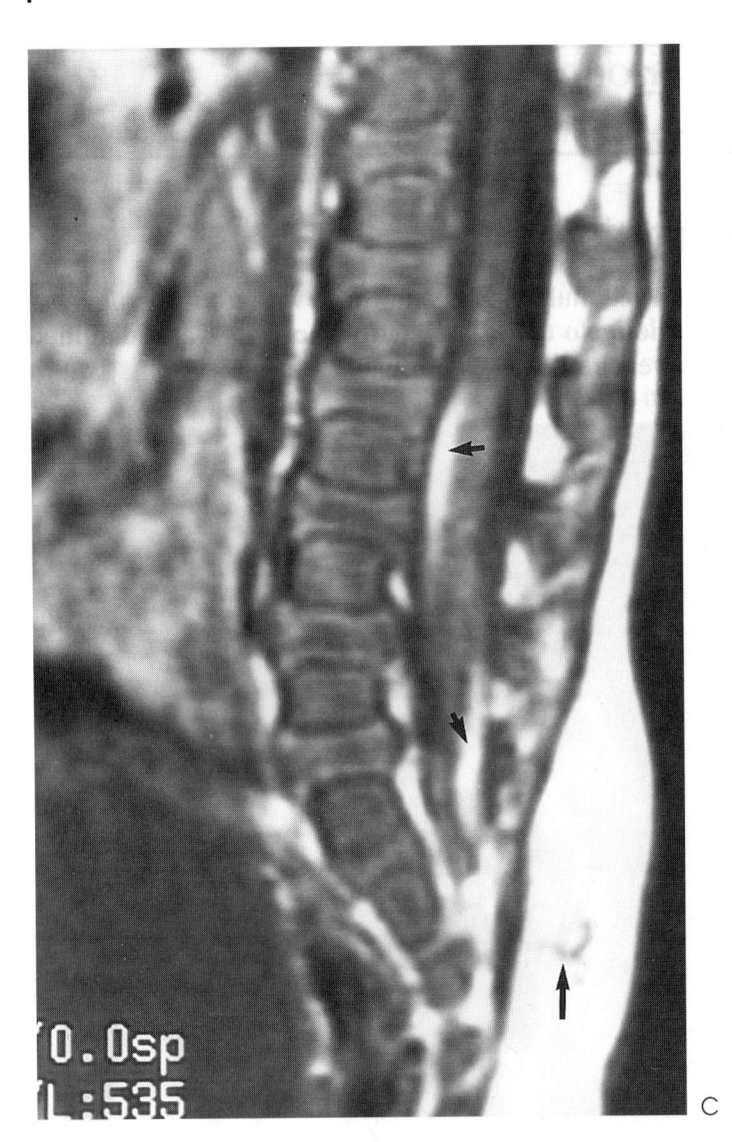

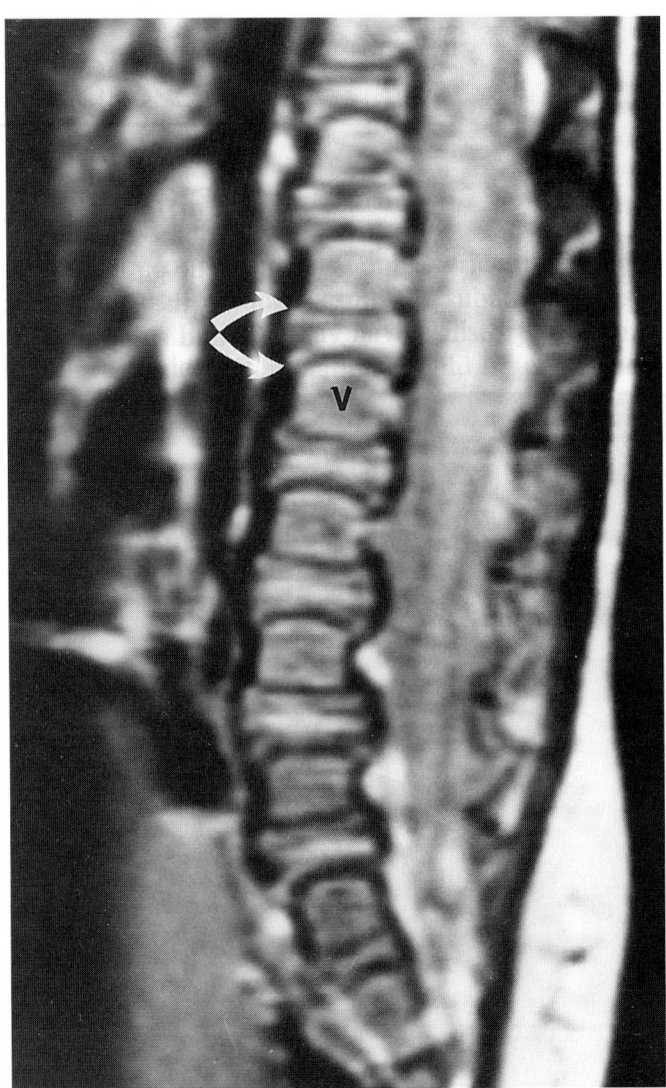

C

D

Radiologic Findings

Sagittal short TR midline image (Fig. A) reveals that the spinal cord is a solid structure that extends down to the level of L4. An irregularly marginated increased signal intensity mass is present in the distal end of the thecal sac (*L*). The vertebrae and intervertebrae exhibit their infantile appearance. The vertebral body (*V*) appears relatively decreased in signal intensity compared with the intervertebral disc. The disc appears higher in signal intensity than the vertebral body and contains a decreased signal intensity line the nuclear cleft (*curved arrow*). The endplates of the vertebral bodies are cartilagenous (*straight arrow*).

Parasagittal image on the right side (Fig. B) reveals that the increased signal intensity mass (*L*) extends superiorly along the lateral margin of the thecal sac to the level of L2. No dorsal elements are visible at the level of S2. Increased signal intensity tissue containing internal areas of decreased signal intensity tissue (*arrow*) extend outside of the vertebral canal and into the clinically noted prominent subcutaneous fat in the lower lumbar and upper sacral region.

Parasagittal image on the left side (Fig. C) reveals two small, linear areas of increased signal intensity tissue that extend along the lateral margin of the thecal sac (*short arrows*). An area of intermediate signal intensity deformed and disordered tissue is seen in the dorsal subcutaneous fat (*long arrow*).

Sagittal intermediate signal intensity image (Fig. D) reveals that the vertebral body (*V*) appears as slightly increased signal intensity. The cartilagenous endplates of the vertebral body appear as decreased signal intensity (*arrows*). The disc itself appears as increased signal intensity.

Diagnosis

Tethered cord, lipoma, myelomeningocele.

Discussion

The increased signal intensity tissue is a lipoma and the internal areas of curvilinear intermediate signal intensity are the disordered neural tissue. These deformed nerve roots can be seen as areas of intermediate signal intensity that extend into the subcutaneous fat/lipoma of the lower back. Patients with tethered cord may become symptomatic as they grow older because the vertebral column continues to grow and the spinal cord is "pulled" up into the vertebral canal. Because it is tethered in the lumbar region, a scoliosis may develop.

In the very young infant, the disc may be mistaken for the vertebral body. However, on the long TR images the intervertebral disc appears as increased signal intensity and the vertebral body as decreased signal intensity. Therefore, the differentiation between the two is more easily appreciated.

PEARL

- Magnetic resonance (MR) imaging is the procedure of choice for evaluation of any patient suspected of having a meningocele.

PITFALLS

- Plain films must be evaluated carefully: Although the plain films for this patient were reported as normal, a dysraphic spine was noted on the MR scan.

- The lower lumbar and sacral region may be difficult to evaluate in the very young patient because of overlying bowel gas.

TEACHING ATLAS OF SPINE IMAGING

Case 17

Clinical Presentation

The patient is a 19-year-old female with lower extremity weakness.

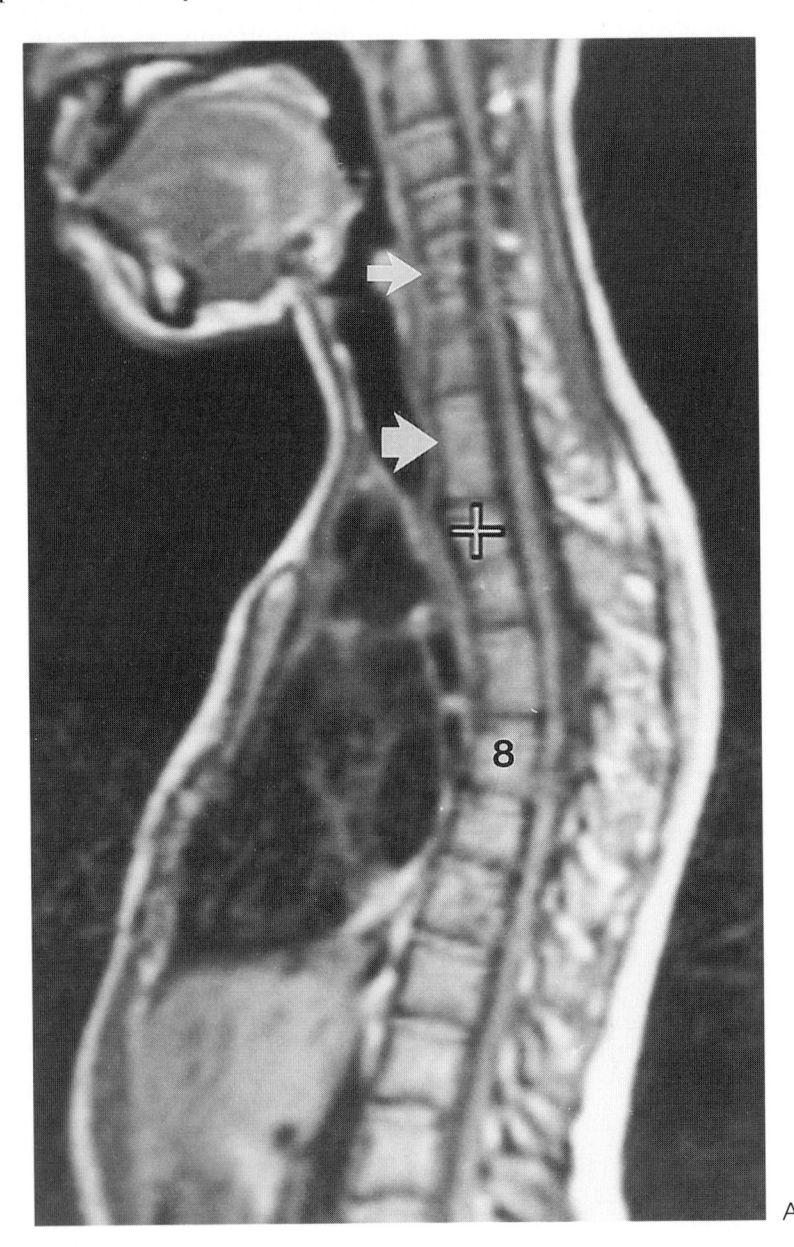

Radiologic Findings

Sagittal short TR image (Fig. A) reveals fusion of multiple cervical vertebral body segments (*upper arrow*). T1 and T2 are also fused (*lower arrow*), as are T6 and T7.

CONGENITAL

Radiologic Findings

Sagittal short TR images (Fig. A) reveal a cystic area of cerebrospinal fluid signal intensity in the distal thoracic spinal cord (*white arrow*). The spinal cord appears as a solid structure down to the level of L3 where there is a lobulated, elongated area of increased signal intensity that extends from the lower margin of L3 through the distal end of the thecal sac. The thecal sac is diffusely enlarged. There is a lobulated area of soft tissue signal intensity dorsal to the spinal cord extending from T12 to L2 (*black arrowheads*).

Coronal short TR images (Fig. B) reveal a rounded area of increased signal intensity in the midportion of the lower thoracic vertebral canal (*curved arrow*). The spinal cord below this level is divided into two separate cords. The area of increased signal intensity projects just to the right of the distal end of the hemicords, which join together at this level. There is a deformed, butterfly type vertebral body at the level of the curved arrow.

Axial short TR image in the lumbar region (Fig. C) reveals two hemicords in the dilated spinal vertebral canal. The vertebral body is deformed in a curvilinear pattern. The dorsal elements of the vertebral body are absent at this level.

Midsagittal short TR image of the brain (Fig. D) reveals thinning of the anterior portion of the corpus callosum (*open arrow*). The genu of the corpus callosum is hypoplastic. There is an area of pachygyria in the frontal region (*black arrowheads*). There is downward displacement of the cerebellar tonsils into the foramen magnum.

Diagnosis

Diastematomyelia

Differential Diagnosis

- vertebral anomalies

Discussion

Vertebral anomalies with diastematomyelic spur, syringomyelia, deformed neural plaquode of tissue (black arrowheads), tethered cord, two hemicords, lipoma, and spinal dysraphism? Associated cerebral anomalies include parital agenesis of the corpus callosum, pachygyria, and low cerebellar tonsils.

> **PEARL**
> - There are frequently multiple congenital abnormalities present. Imaging should be performed of the entire vertebral column and evaluation should also be performed of the brain.

> **PITFALL**
> - If a spinal tap is necessary, care must be taken to avoid those areas of the vertebral canal that contain neural tissue.

TEACHING ATLAS OF SPINE IMAGING

Case 20

Clinical Presentation

The patient is a 10-year-old female with unsteady gate and progressive scoliosis.

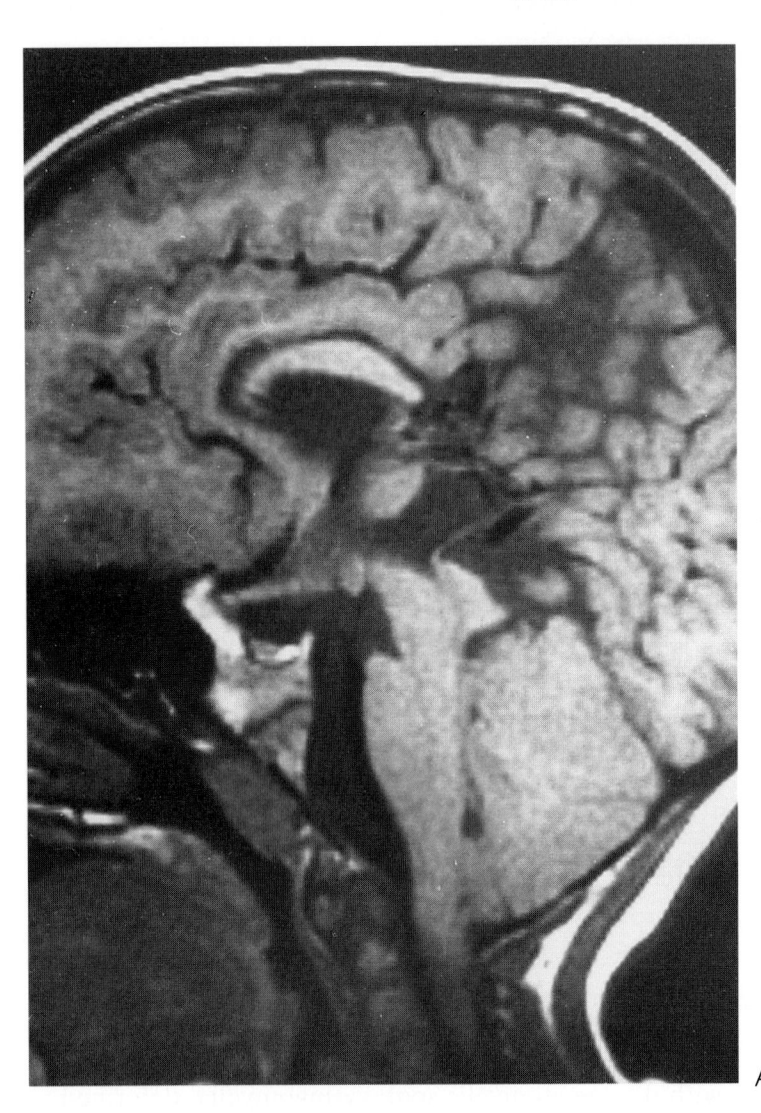

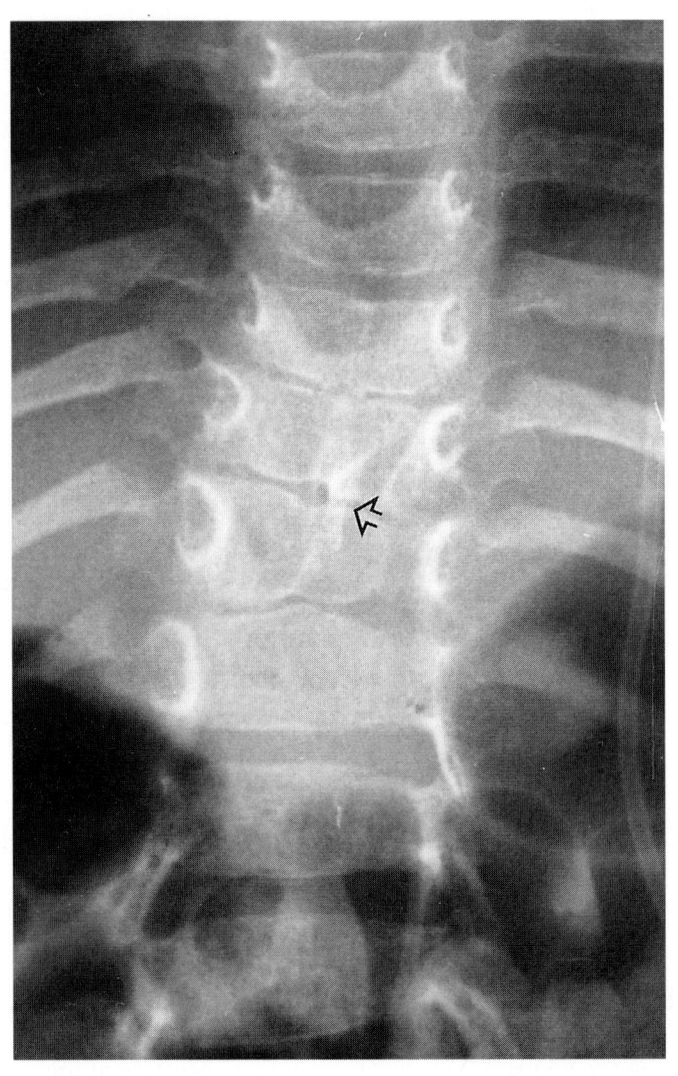

A

B

Radiologic Findings

Sagittal short TR image (Fig. A) reveals a small posterior fossa. The quadrigeminal plate is deformed and pointed. The fourth ventricle is elongated, inferiorly displaced, and small. The cerebellar tonsils are deformed and pointed. There is basilar kyphosis with a very small basal angle of the calvarium and partial agenesis of the corpus callosum.

CONGENITAL

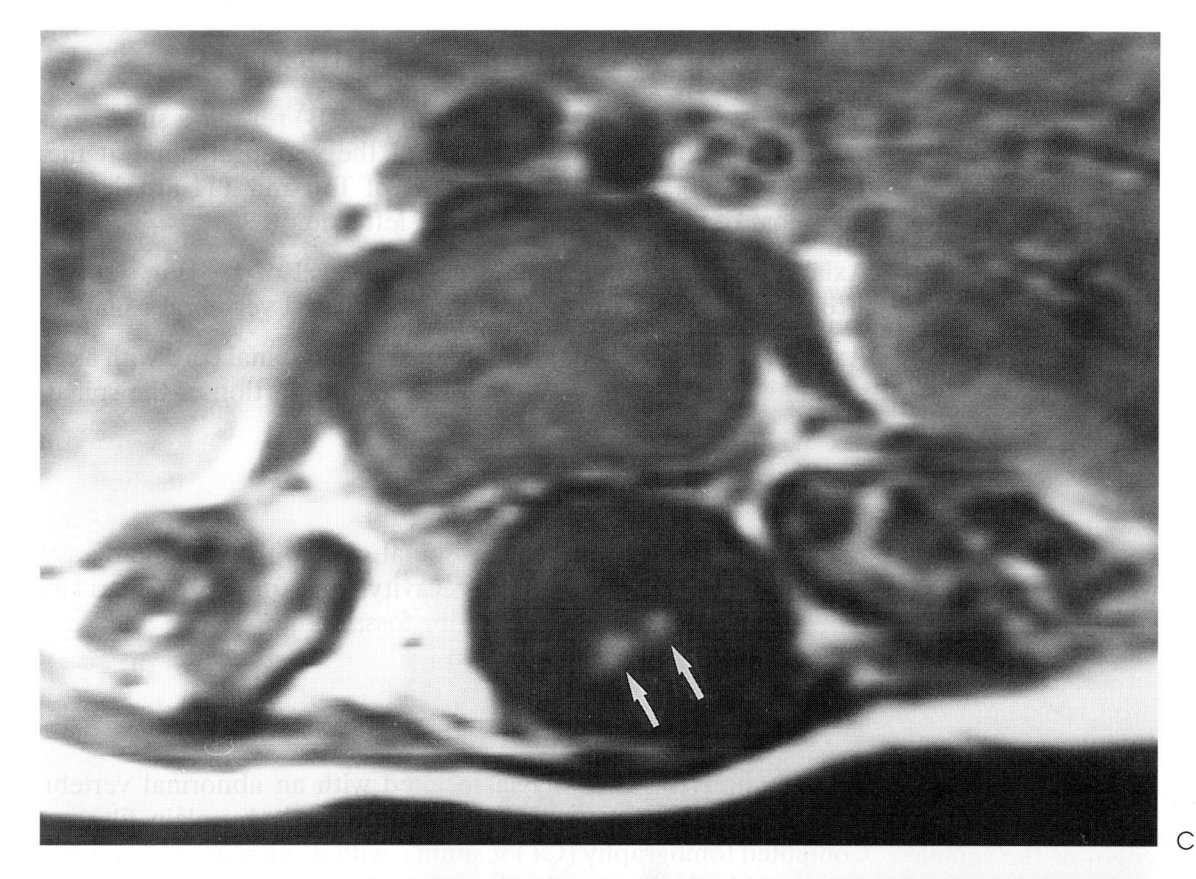

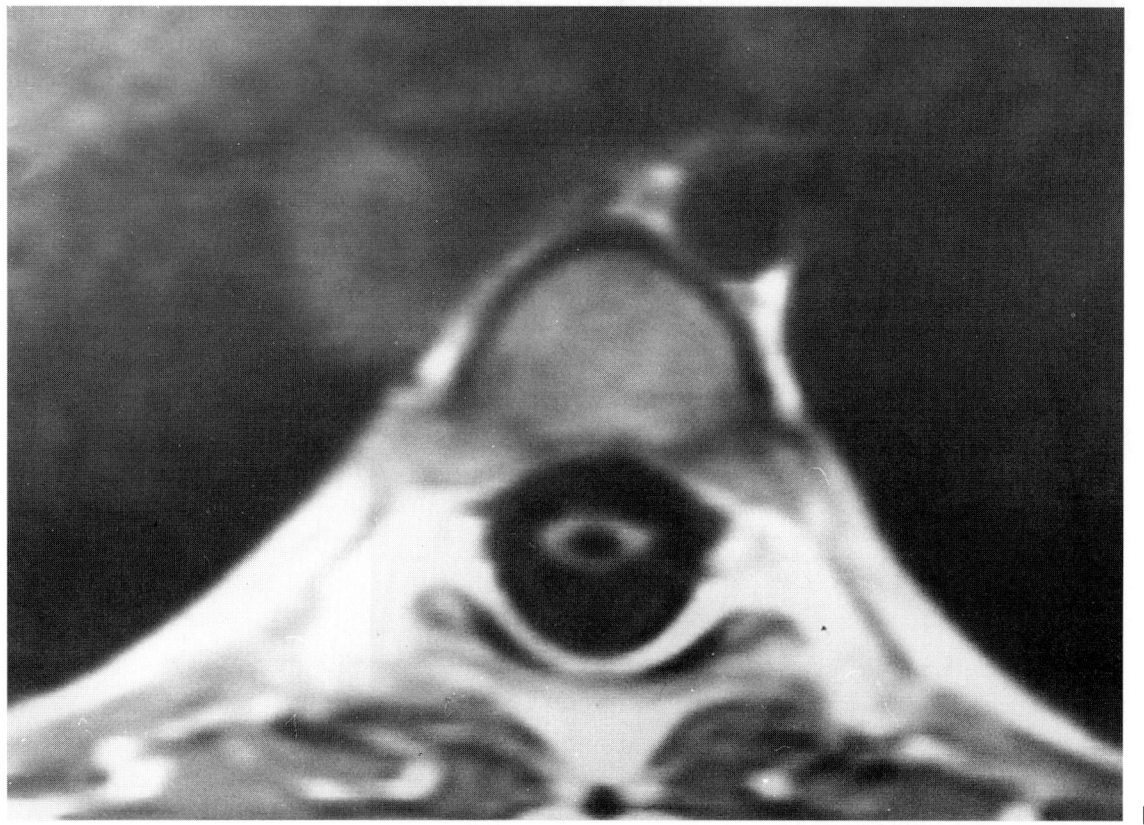

C

D

TEACHING ATLAS OF SPINE IMAGING

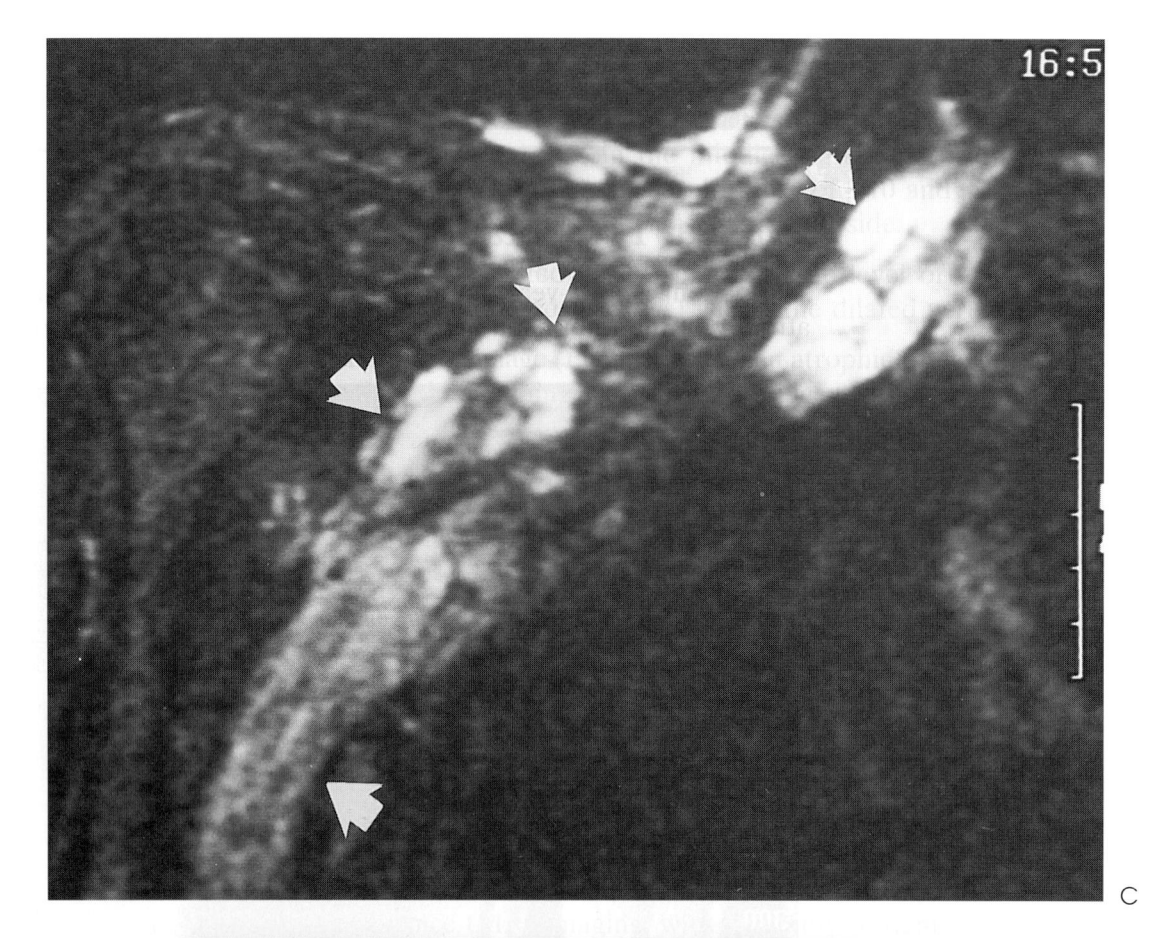

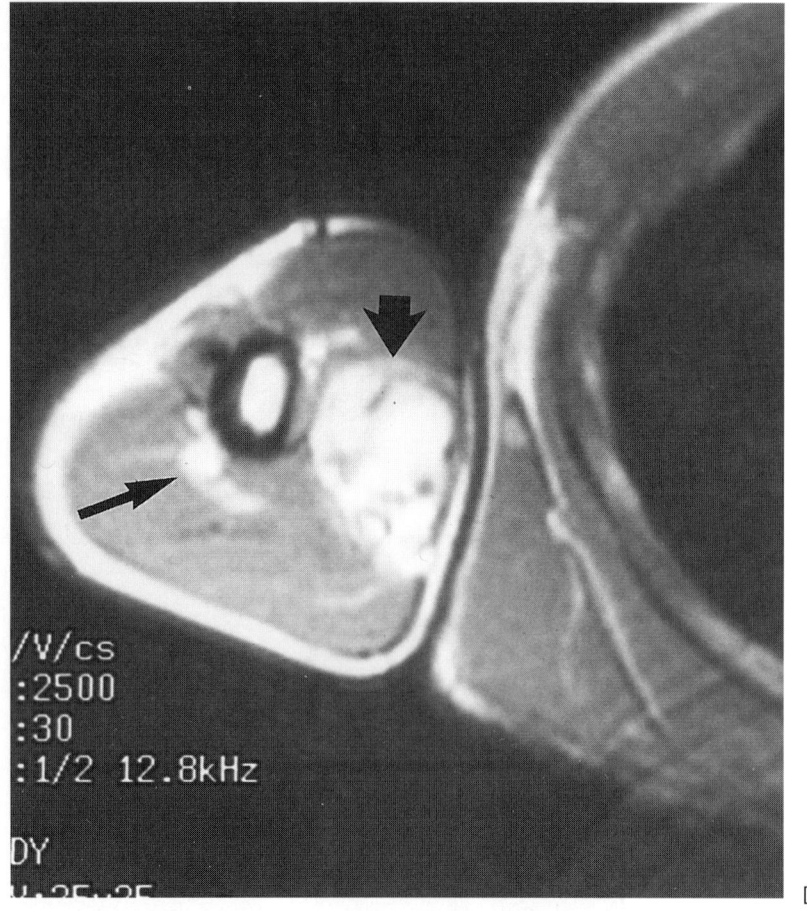

CONGENITAL

Radiologic Findings

Coronal short TR image of the chest and thoracic spine (Fig. A) reveal multiple paraspinal intermediate signal intensity masses on the left side. There is scoliosis of the thoracic and lumbar spine with a soft tissue mass on the left side of the spine in the lower thoracic region (*arrow*).

Short TR image of the right supraclavicular region (Fig. B) reveals diffuse enlargement of the nerves of the brachial plexus (*black arrows*) just distal to their point of origin from the cervical vertebral canal. The flow void of the vertebral artery can be seen where it arises from the subclavian artery (*white arrow, v*). The subclavian and axillary arteries can be seen projecting below the level of the mass.

The long TR image (Fig. C) reveals that the masses, which extend into the axilla, all exhibit increased signal intensity (*arrows*).

Axial postcontrast image at the level of the midhumerus (Fig. D) reveals that the mass appears as increased signal intensity (*thick arrow*). Additional nerves in the arm are also increased signal intensity (*thin arrow*).

Diagnosis

Neurofibromatosis type 1 (NF1), multiple neurofibromata along the spine, a large plexiform neurofibroma along the course of the brachial plexus on the right arm.

Discussion

Identification of plexiform neurofibromata is important because NF1 is autosomal dominant, with an abnormality of chromosome 17 with variable penetrance. Because the disease is inherited, genetic counseling is in order. In this case, the patient's brother also had NF1.

NF1 is also known as the peripheral form of neurofibromatosis. It is associated with plexiform neurofibromas and may result in "dumbbell" type of tumors that involve the vertebral canal and paraspinal area. Magnetic resonance (MR) imaging is the best method of evaluating these abnormalities.

PEARLS
- These plexiform neurofibromas of the spine may extend into the vertebral canal at one or multiple levels.

- MR without and with the infusion of contrast material and multiplanar imaging is the best method of evaluation.

PITFALL
- Surgical management of these multilevel lesions is difficult.

TEACHING ATLAS OF SPINE IMAGING

Case 22

Clinical Presentation

The patient is a 24-year-old male who underwent previous surgery to remove a thoracolumbar schwannoma.

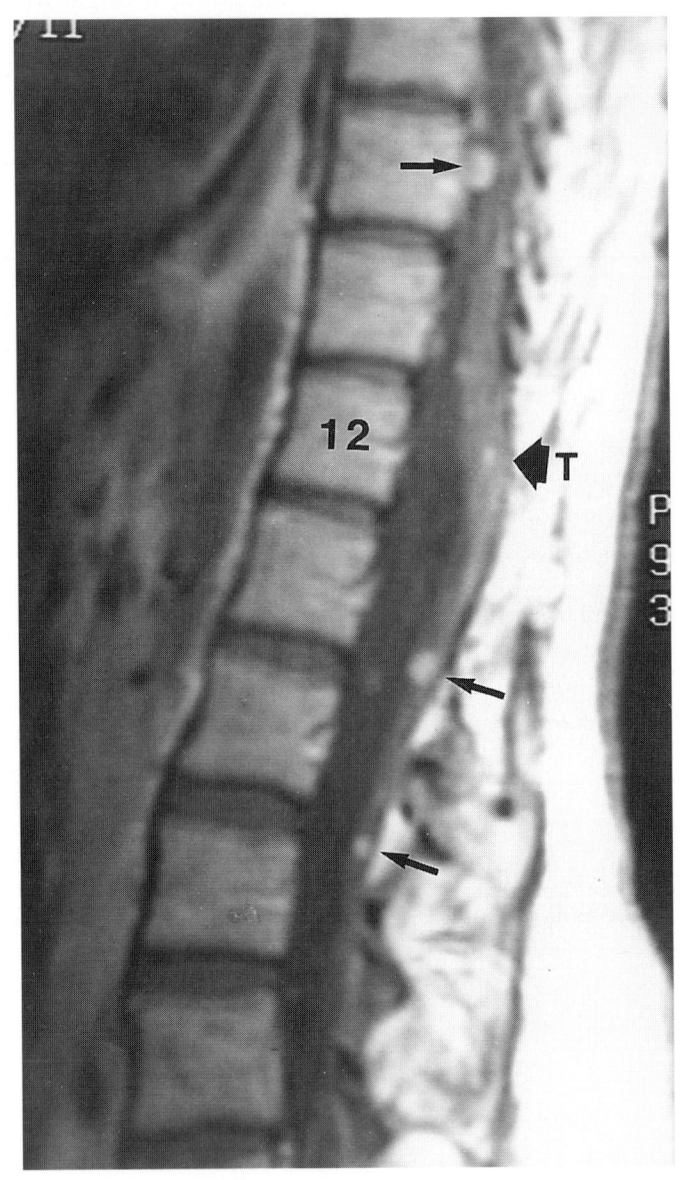

A

PEARLS

- Tethering of the spinal cord at the surgical site is not an indication of a surgical complication, but rather occurs not infrequently at the point where the dura is opened at the time of surgery. Patients' symptoms may improve following surgical removal of a tumor, only to recur when there is secondary tethering of the spinal cord because of scar formation at the surgical site.

- Magnetic resonance imaging is the procedure of choice for evaluation.

PITFALL

- Clinical history is very helpful in the evaluation of these patients, particularly to rule out metastases versus multiple schwannomas.

Radiologic Findings

Sagittal short TR postcontrast MR image (Fig. A) reveals multiple rounded areas of enhancement scattered throughout the lower thoracic and upper lumbar thecal sac. The larger of these masses are highlighted (*small arrows*). Multiple additional smaller masses are also present. Postlaminectomy changes are noted in the lower thoracic and upper lumbar region with absence of the spinous processes of the vertebrae at multiple levels. The spinal cord is tethered posteriorly in the lower thoracic/upper lumbar region at the level of the previous surgery (*thick arrow*). The central portion of the tethered cord is at the level of T12.

Diagnosis

Neurofibromatosis type 2 (NF2) with multiple schwannomas, postoperative changes, spinal cord tethering.

Differential Diagnosis

- drop metastases (unlikely)

Discussion

NF is an autosomal dominant hereditary disease with a defect on chromosome 22 with variable penetrance. It is also known as the central form of NF and is typically associated with bilateral acoustic schwannomas. Spinal cord ependymomas are the typical tumor that is seen in these patients. This disease may be remembered with the mnemonic MISME: *m*ultiple *i*nherited *s*chwannomas, *m*eningiomas, and *e*pendymomas. The meningiomas typically involve the cerebral meningies whereas the ependymomas typically affect the spinal cord.

TEACHING ATLAS OF SPINE IMAGING

Case 23

Clinical Presentation

The patient is a 48-year-old male with known neurofibromatosis type 2 (NF2), with bilateral deafness who now presents with low back pain.

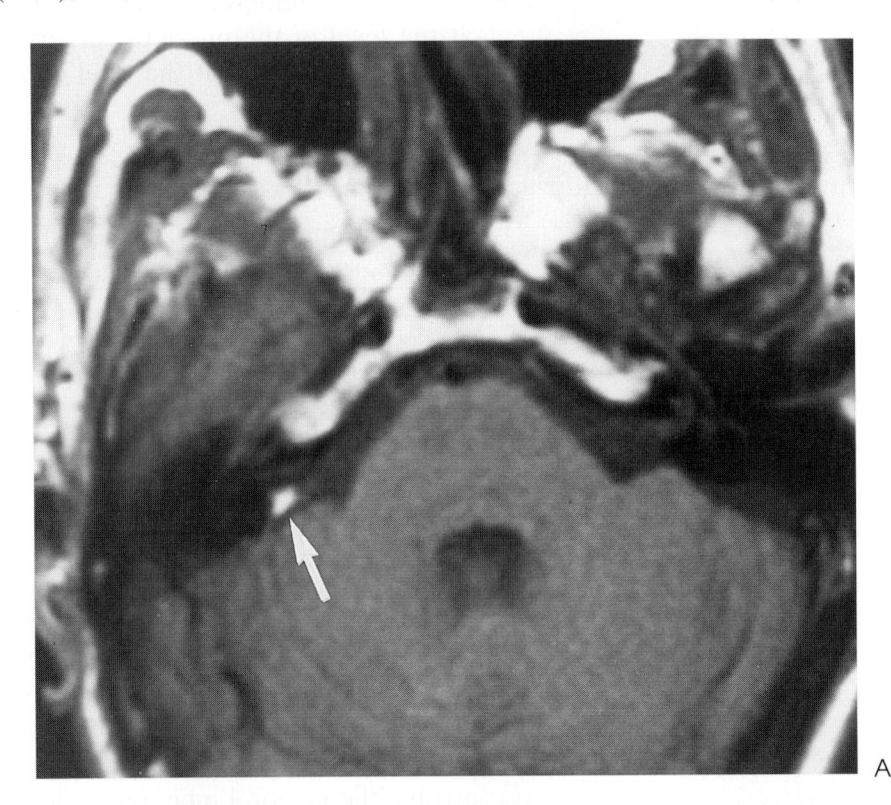

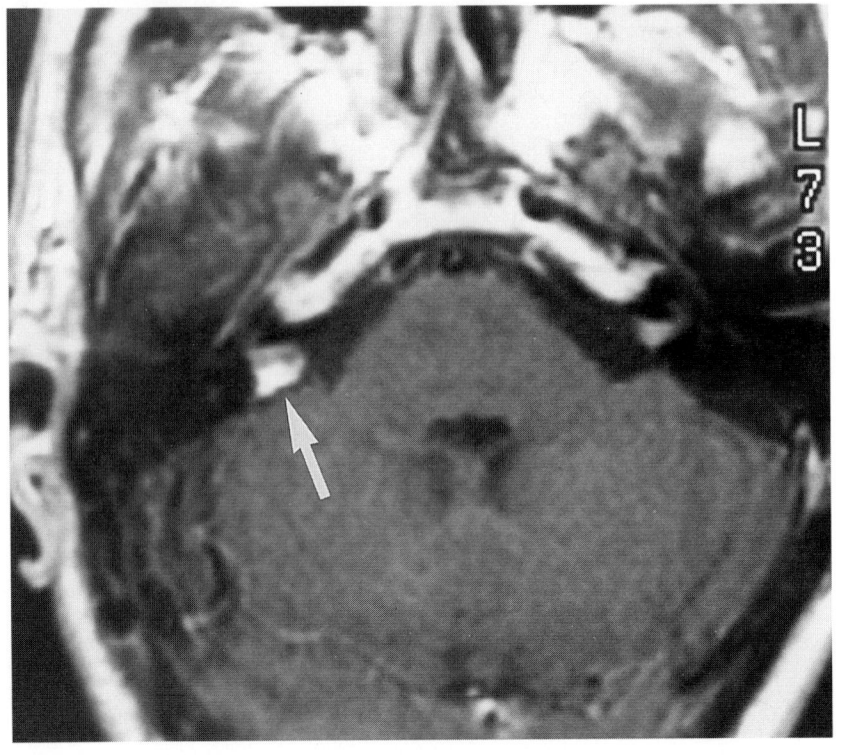

A

B

130

CONGENITAL

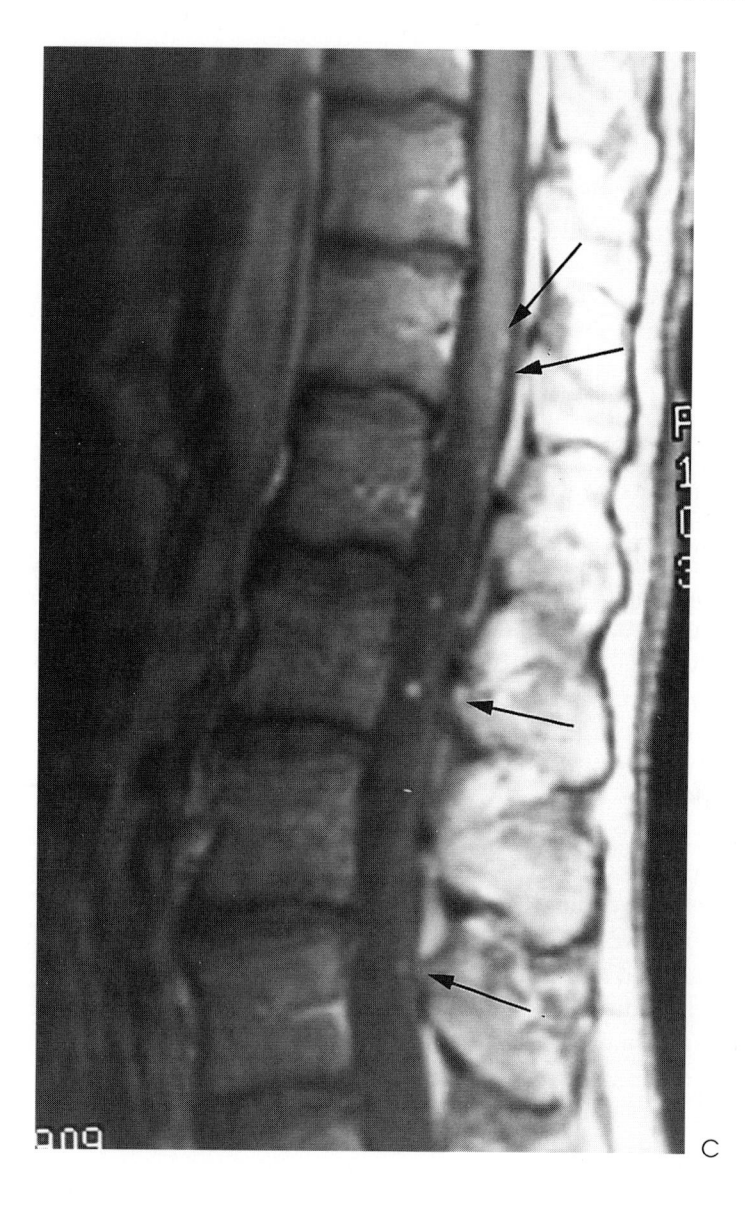

Radiologic Findings

Precontrast axial short TR image (Fig. A) reveals a small, high signal intensity soft tissue mass in the right internal auditory canal (*arrow*).

Postcontrast axial short TR image (Fig. B) reveals enhancement of bilateral acoustic masses (right larger than left). The right-sided acoustic mass extends slightly into the cerebellopontine angle (*arrow*); the left acoustic mass is intracanalicular.

Postcontrast sagittal short TR of the lumbar spine (Fig. C) reveals multiple small (1–2 mm) rounded areas of enhancement along the dorsal aspect of the distal thoracic spinal cord and the nerve roots of the cauda equina (*arrows*).

PEARL

- The mnemonic of MISME (*m*ultiple *i*nherited, *s*chwannomas, *m*eningiomas, and *e*pendymomas) helps one to remember the lesions that are seen in the patient with NF2.

PITFALL

- Because lipomas of the internal auditory canal may exist without schwannomas, and because their increased signal intensity could be mistaken for an enhancing lesion if only a postinfusion study is performed, all studies of the internal auditory canals should be performed prior to and following the infusion of contrast material and should not be performed postinfusion only. A very rare entity such as hemorrhage into the nerves in the internal auditory canal may also appear as increased signal intensity on the precontrast images.

Diagnosis

- Bilateral acoustic schwannomas and multiple spinal schwannomas
- Small right internal auditory canal lipoma

Differential Diagnosis

- hemorrhagic infarct of right eighth cranial nerve

Discussion

Neurofibromatosis type 2 is known as central neurofibromatosis. These patients may appear clinically normal and do not have the external stigmata seen in patients with NF type 1. NF type 2 is characterized by bilateral acoustic schwannomas, spinal ependymomas, and meningomas. Symptoms tend to present at a younger age than in patients with NF1.

CONGENITAL

Case 24

Clinical Presentation

The patients is an 18-year-old female with polycythemia due to cyanotic congenital heart disease, visual disturbance, head shaking, and poor responsiveness lasting a few minutes.

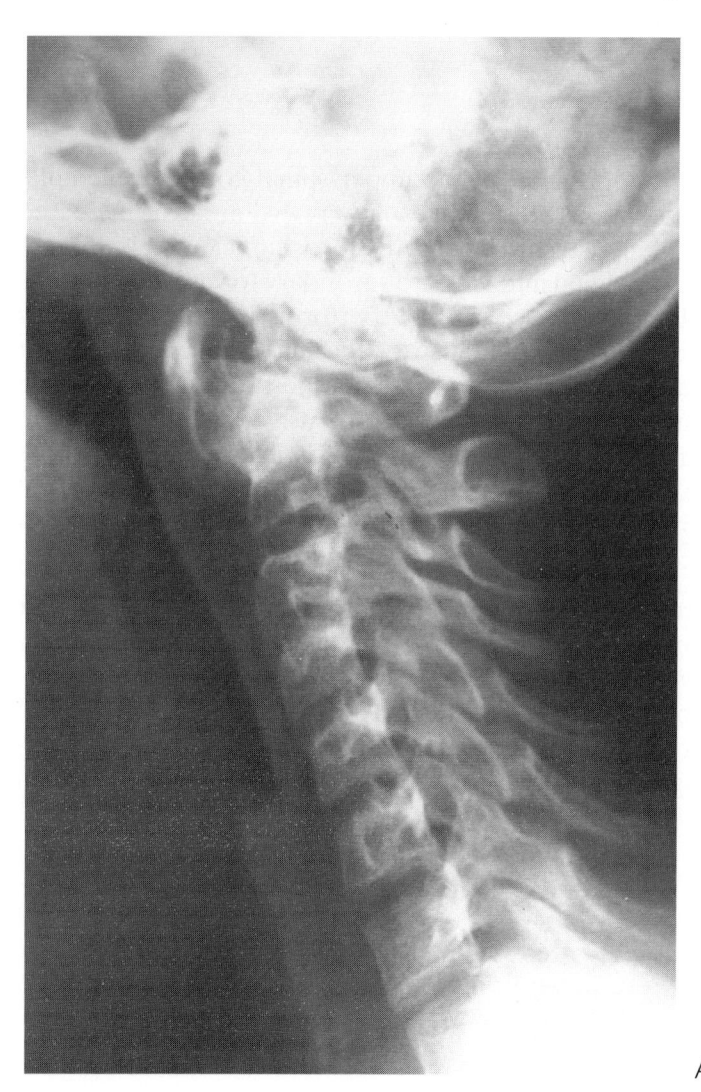

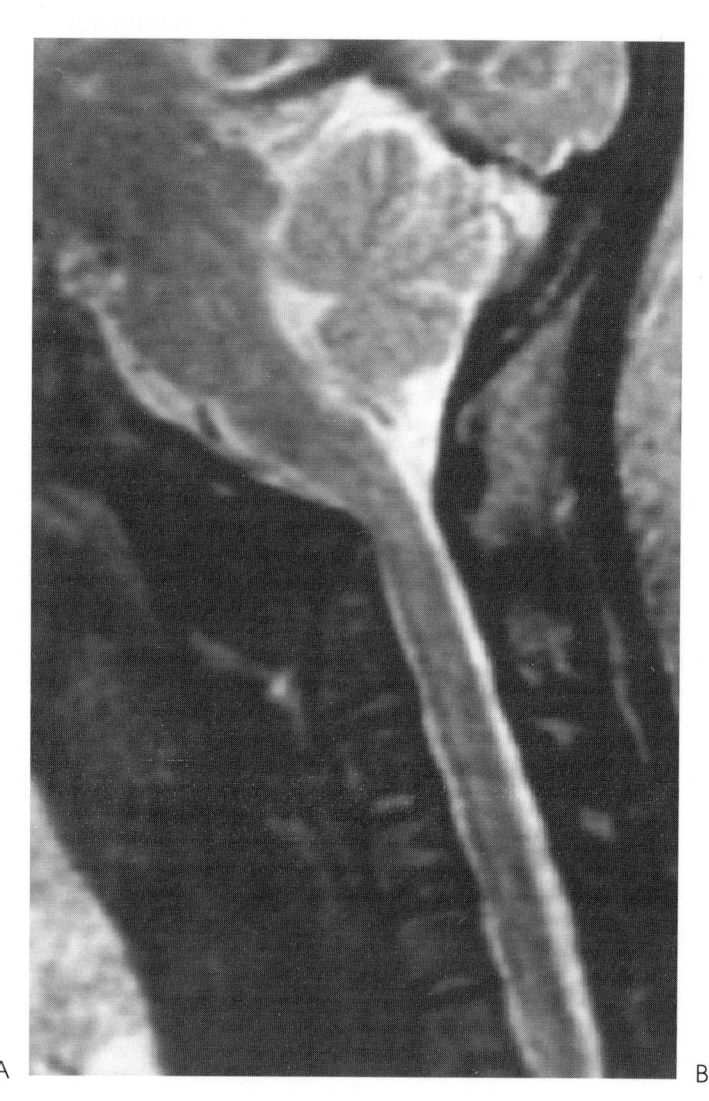

Radiologic Findings

Lateral view of the cervical spine (Fig. A) reveals posterior subluxation of the odontoid process relative to the anterior arch of C1.

Sagittal short TR image (Fig. B) reveals posterior dislocation of the odontoid process relative to the anterior arch of C1 and widening of the space between C1 and C2. There is posterior curvilinear displacement of the spinal cord. There is compromise of the subarachnoid space at the level of C1-2 and the foramen magnum.

PEARL
- Because C1-2 subluxation may be present in Down's syndrome patients, MR imaging may be used for evaluation prior to allowing these patients to participate in athletic competition.

PITFALL
- MR imaging evaluation may include short TR images in the sagittal plane with the patient in the neutral, flexed, and extended positions.

Diagnosis

Down's syndrome with C1-2 dislocation, congenital heart disease with atrial septal defect.

Differential Diagnosis

- rheumatoid arthritis with C1-2 dislocation
- posttraumatic dislocation

Discussion

Subluxation results in compression of the upper spinal cord and medulla. Long TR magnetic resonance (MR) images may reveal areas of increased signal intensity within the spinal cord if compression is sufficient. It is thought that the areas of increased signal intensity are secondary to vascular compromise. Sagittal short TR images also may be performed with the patient's neck flexed and extended to better demonstrate the amount of encroachment upon the vertebral canal and spinal cord in these positions. Care must be used when manipulating the neck in these patients. Because there is an increase in the amount of space surrounding the cervical spinal cord in the upper cervical region compared with the remainder of the spine, the spinal cord frequently follows a curvilinear course around the posteriorly positioned odontoid process.

A similar type of increased mobility of the odontoid process also may occur in patients with rheumatoid arthritis. In these cases the increase in mobility is secondary to laxity of the transverse and cruciate ligaments, which normally hold the odontoid process against the anterior arch of the C1 vertebral body. Rheumatoid arthritis is seen in older patients and is generally associated with other changes in the bony structures.

Section III

Spinal Cord Tumors

A. Intramedullary

SPINAL CORD TUMORS

Case 1

Clinical Presentation

The patient is a 49-year-old male with progressive upper extremity weakness, right arm greater than left.

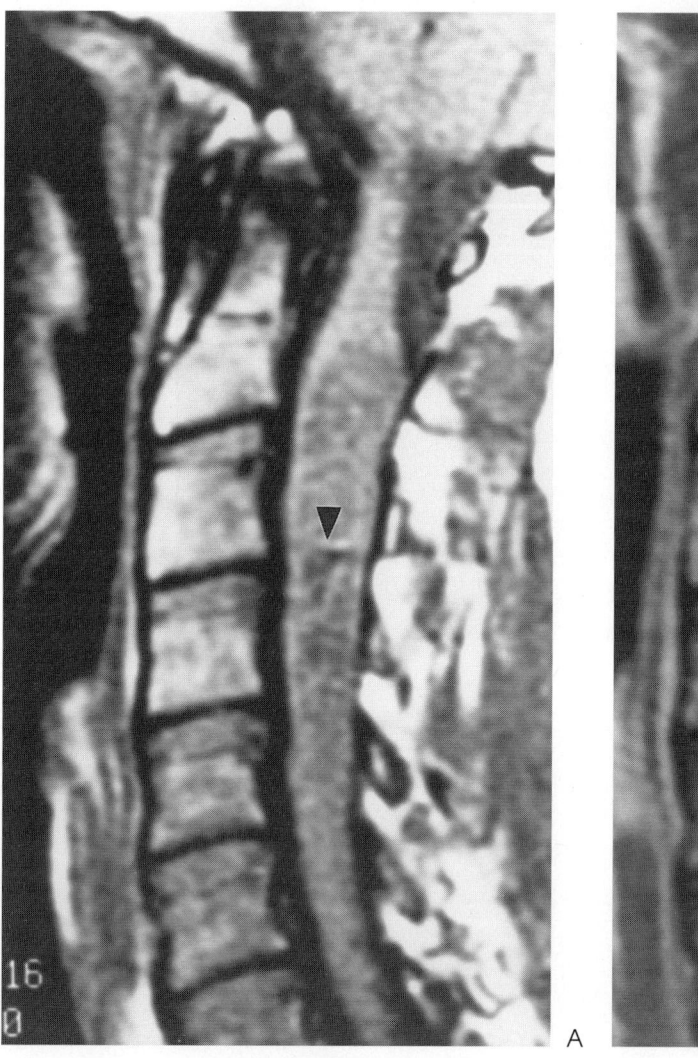

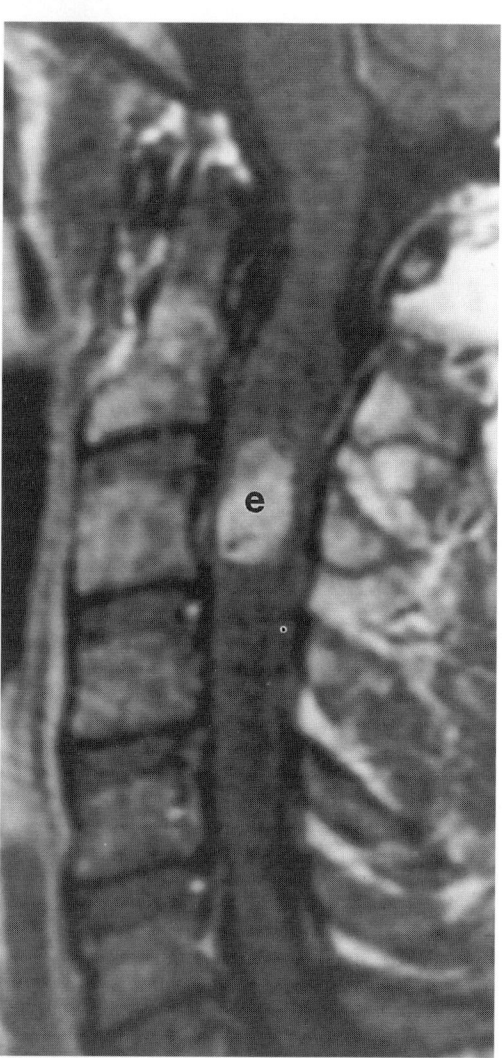

Radiologic Findings

Sagittal short TR image (Fig. A) reveals expansion of the cervical spinal cord beginning at the level of the midbody of C2 and extending to the level of C5. There is compromise of the subarachnoid space from the level of C2 inferiorly to approximately C5. At the level of C3, there is an amorphous streaklike area of decreased signal intensity (*arrowhead*).

TEACHING ATLAS OF SPINE IMAGING

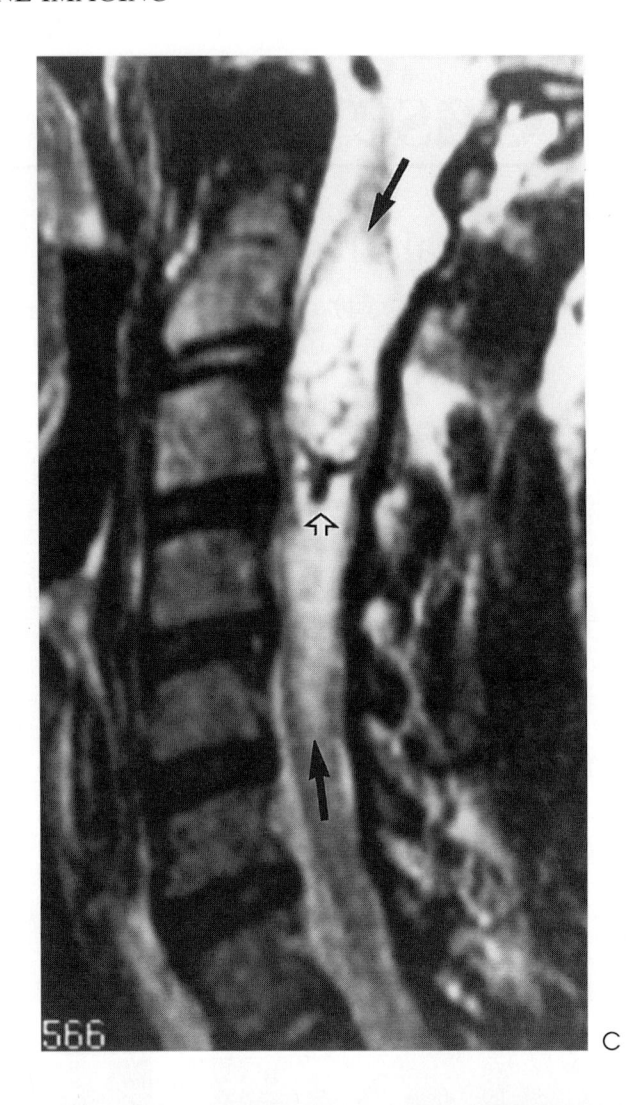

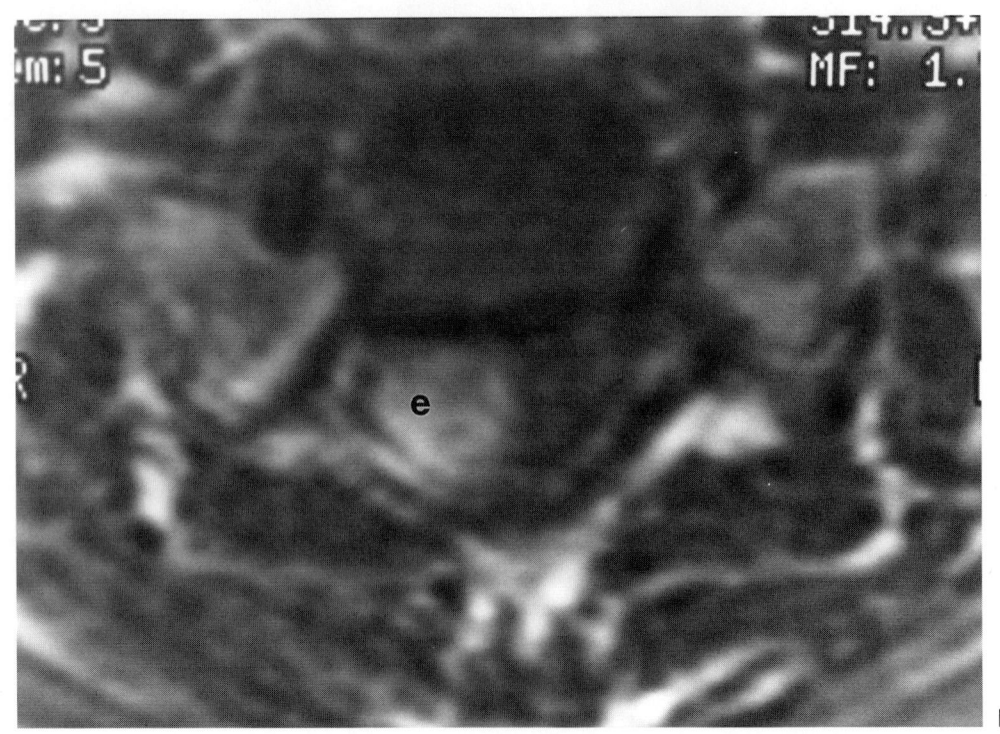

SPINAL CORD TUMORS

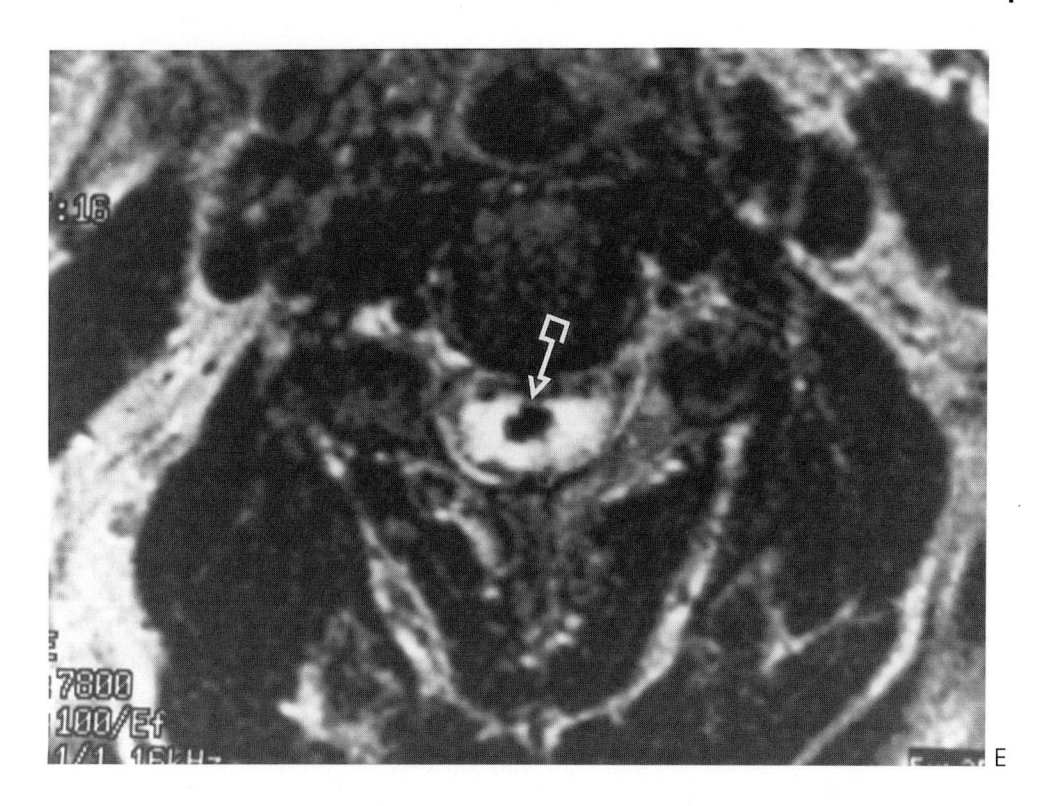

Radiologic Findings (continued)

Sagittal short TR image postcontrast (Fig. B) reveals a nodule of enhancement (e) in the anterior two thirds of the spinal cord beginning at the level of the C2-3 intervertebral disc and extending to the inferior end plate of C3. The area of decreased signal intensity in Figure A is visible in the inferior portion of the enhancing nodule.

Sagittal long TR image (Fig. C) reveals that there is an oval-shaped area of increased signal intensity extending from the base of the odontoid process (*top black arrow*) to the inferior end plate of C5 (*lower black arrow*). There are several patchy and curvilinear areas of persistent decreased signal intensity within the area of increased signal intensity at the level of C3 (*open arrow*).

Axial short TR image at C3 after the infusion of contrast (Fig. D) reveals the enhancing nodule (e) in the right side of the cervical spinal cord. The right side of the spinal cord is expanded at this level.

Axial long TR image (Fig. E) reveals the central area of decreased signal intensity (*arrow*) surrounded by increased signal intensity within the expanded spinal cord.

TEACHING ATLAS OF SPINE IMAGING

PEARLS
- The tumor nodule is the enhancing nodule at the C3 level with edema extending above and below this level.

- Enhancement is the rule with spinal cord tumors, although rarely no enhancement may be seen. The enhancement pattern may also be effected by the administration of steroids, which decrease the amount of enhancement.

PITFALLS
- The areas of persistent decreased signal intensity may also be seen with areas of calcification.

- Computed tomographic (CT) scanning is more accurate than magnetic resonance scanning for the evaluation of the presence of calcification. However, as treatment will probably not be altered whether calcification is present or not, the need for CT is not urgent.

Diagnosis
Ependymoma.

Differential Diagnosis
- spinal cord astrocytoma
- spinal cord metastases

Discussion

Ependymomas may exhibit areas of hemorrhage that appear as areas of decreased signal intensity secondary to magnetic susceptibility artifact, as seen in this case. A spinal cord astrocytoma could have a similar appearance, but the area of hemorrhage with hemosiderin makes this diagnosis less likely. Spinal cord metastases may also have a similar appearance; however, spinal cord metastases are uncommon. Intramedullary metastases may develop from such primary tumors as medulloblastoma, breast and lung cancer, and various sarcomas.

Other tumors that may exhibit areas of decreased signal intensity are vascular tumors such as occult vascular malformations or cavernous angiomas. Cavernous angiomas are more common in the brain but may also be seen in the spinal cord. The cavernous malformation tends to have a typical appearance of a central area of increased signal intensity on the short TR images with a surrounding, slightly irregularly margined, peripheral rim of decreased signal intensity. This decreased signal intensity is thought to be secondary to episodes of hemorrhage, with leaking of blood into the tissues surrounding the cavernous angioma.

SPINAL CORD TUMORS

Case 2

Clinical Presentation

The patient is a 37-year-old female with neurofibromatosis type 1 with upper extremity weakness.

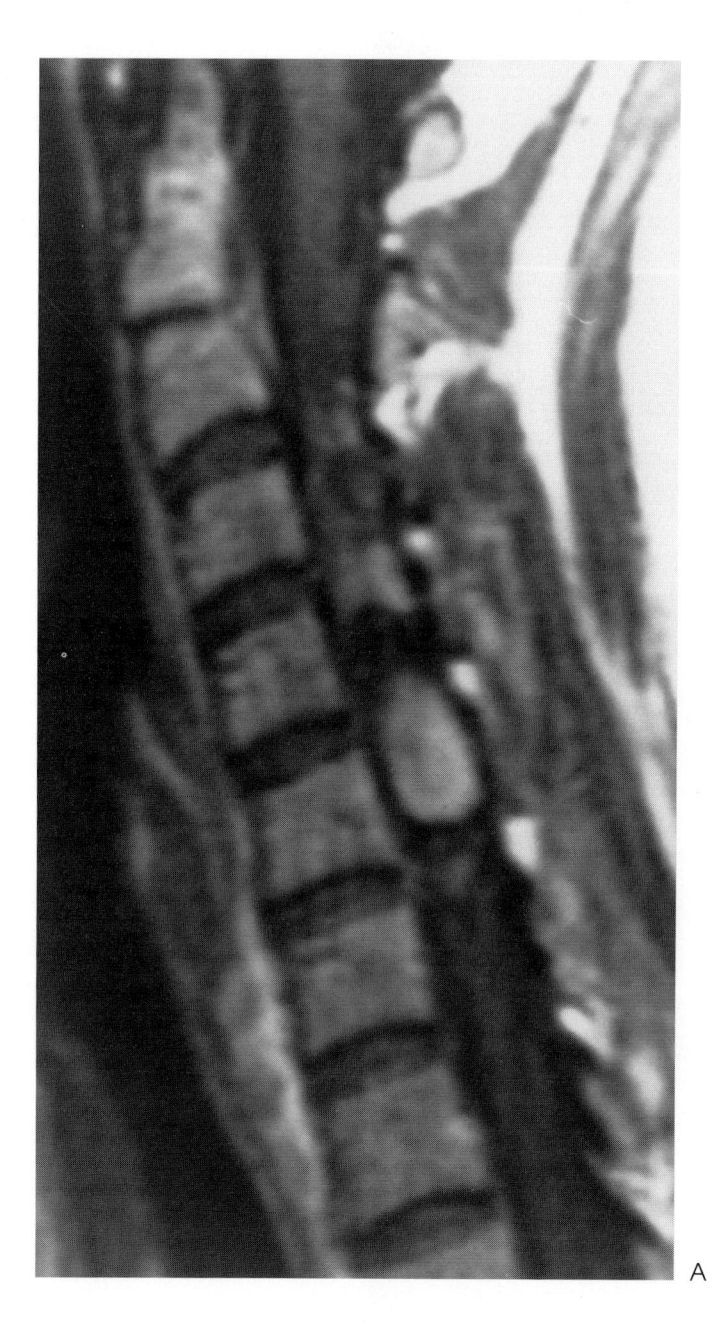

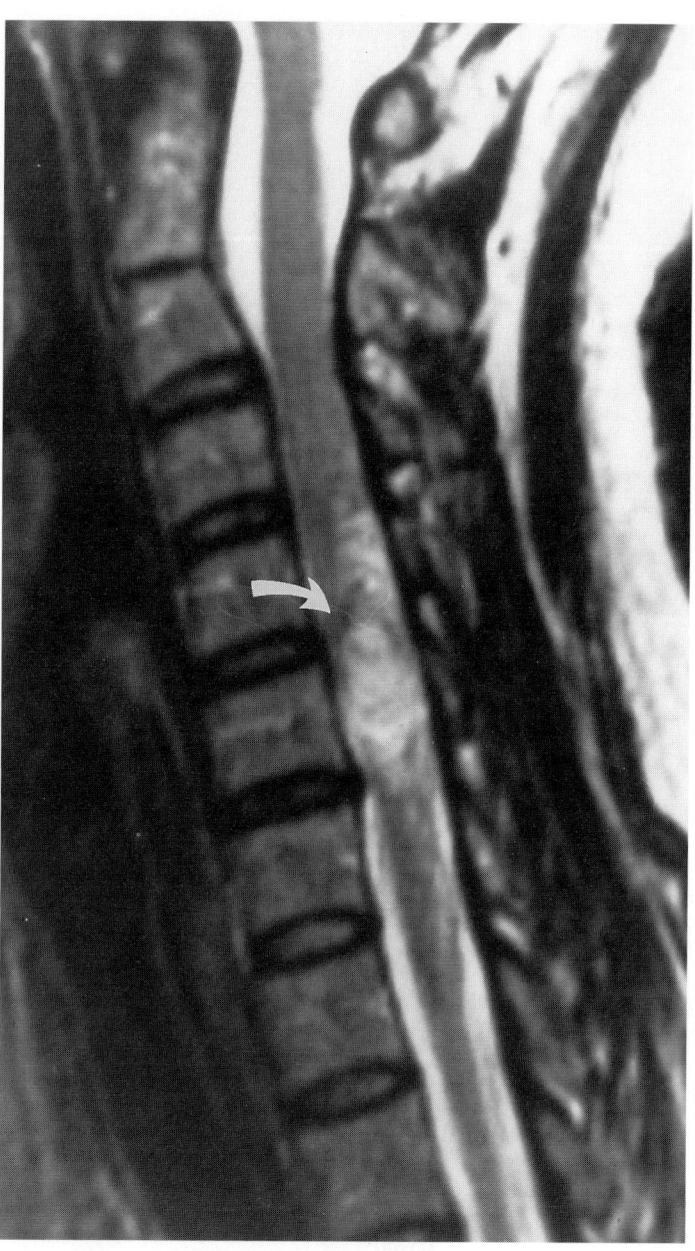

A

B

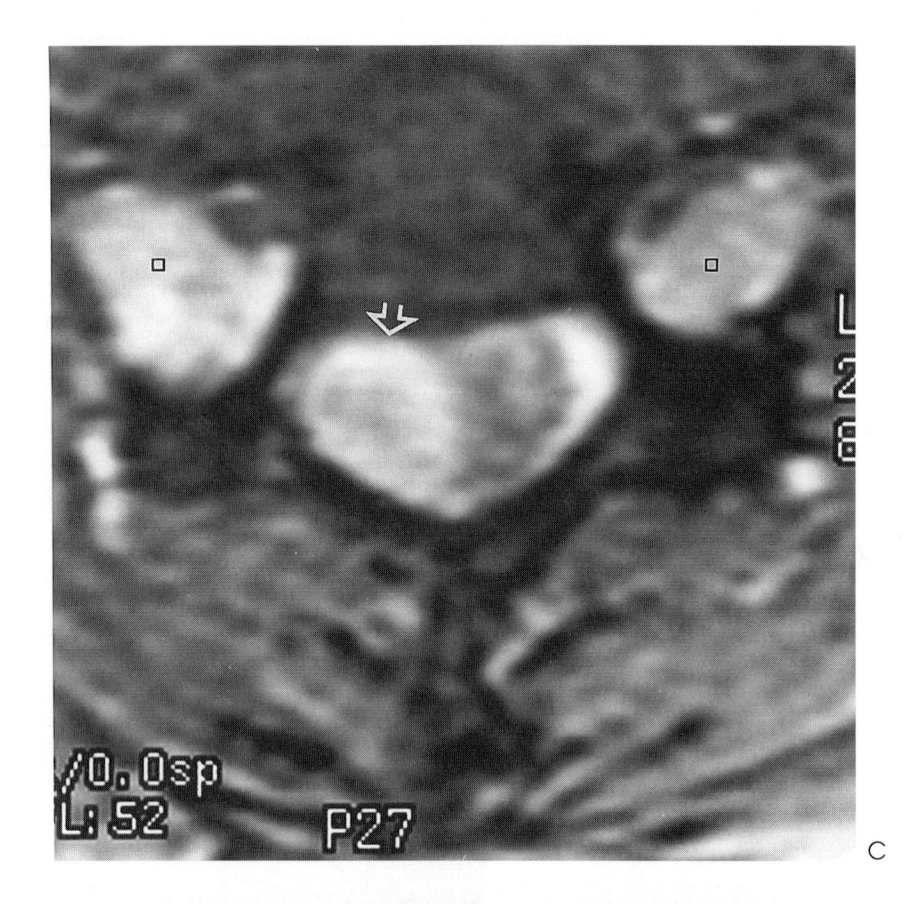

TEACHING ATLAS OF SPINE IMAGING

C

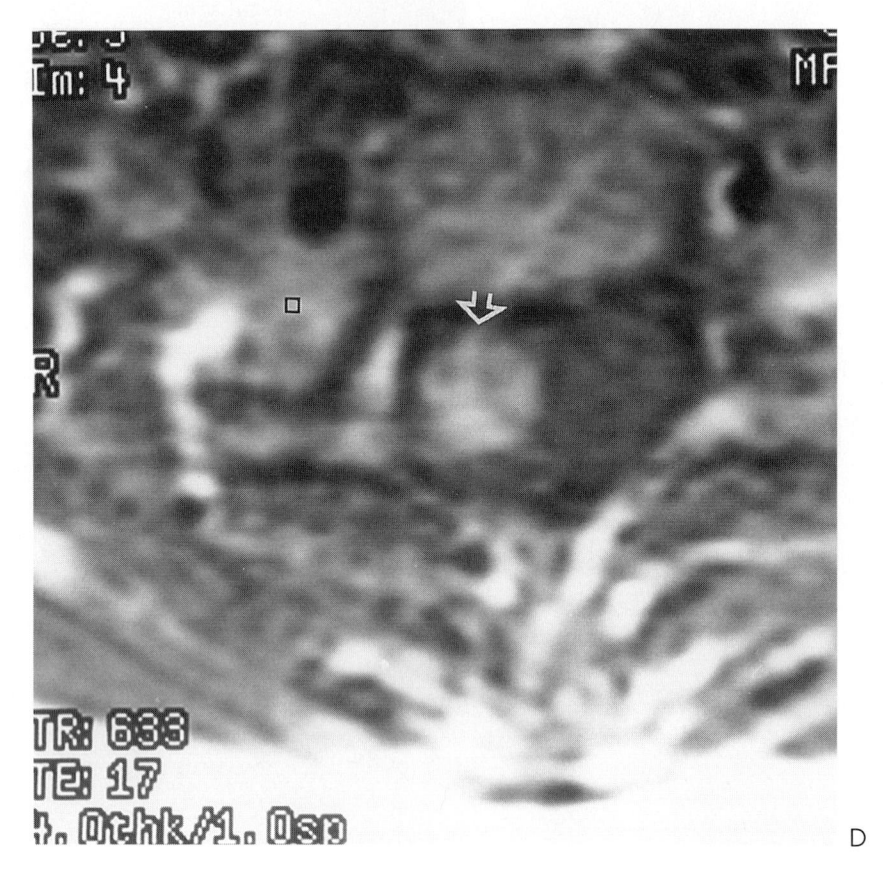

D

142

SPINAL CORD TUMORS

Radiologic Findings

Sagittal short TR image postcontrast (Fig. A) reveals a 1.2-cm oval area of enhancement at the C6 level that extends to the level of the intervertebral disc at C5-6. There are also smaller less well-defined areas of enhancement above and below this level. There is reversal of the curve of the spine and expansion of the spinal cord. Note the incidental finding of congenital fusion between the C2 and C3 vertebral bodies.

Sagittal long TR image (Fig. B) reveals expansion of the spinal cord from C3-4 through approximately C7. There are areas of increased signal intensity within the central portion of the spinal cord from the C4-5 level through the C7 level. The increased signal has faint concentric rings of increased signal intensity with a few internal curvilinear areas of decreased signal intensity (*curved arrow*).

Axial long TR image (Fig. C) reveals a thick-walled ring of increased signal intensity in the right side of the spinal cord (*arrow*). There are oval-shaped areas of increased signal intensity in the region of the dorsal root ganglia bilaterally (*squares*).

Axial short TR image postcontrast (Fig. D) reveals a rounded area of enhancement in the right side of the cervical spinal cord (*arrow*). The mass in the region of the right dorsal root ganglion is also seen to enhance (*square*).

PEARL
- Because these tumors may metastasize, the entire spinal column should be evaluated.

PITFALL
- The areas of decreased signal intensity could represent areas of hemosiderin deposition, making ependymoma a diagnostic consideration.

Diagnosis

Astrocytoma; neurofibromas of the dorsal root ganglion bilaterally.

Differential Diagnosis

- astrocytoma
- ependymoma

Discussion

Astrocytomas of the cervical spinal cord are less common than those in the brain. In the spinal cord, both the astrocytoma and the ependymoma arise from the glial cells of the spinal cord. Astrocytomas are the most common primary tumor in the spinal cord, particularly in the pediatric age group, but they may be seen in any age group. These tumors may be focal or extend over multiple vertebral body segments. Exophytic growth may also occur. The pattern of enhancement generally reveals a dense area of enhancement in the cervical cord, which is localized to a one or two segment region.

There may be associated cysts within the tumor, and there may also be an associated syrinx cavity. Typically, spinal cord astrocytomas exhibit enhancement on the postcontrast study, although very rarely enhancement will not be seen. If there is an associated syrinx cavity, the wall of the syrinx typically does not enhance. Although attempts have been made to differentiate astrocytoma from ependymoma based on the anatomic location within the spinal cord, this is usually not possible. The pattern of enhancement in astrocytoma generally reveals a dense area of enhancement in the cervical cord that is localized to a one or two segment region. The axial images usually reveal that the tumor is not in the midline, but rather is off center. It does not appear that this is a reliable imaging method. Mixed cell type tumors may also be seen.

Treatment is surgical with resection of as much of the tumor as possible.

A specific histologic type of astrocytoma is the pilocytic astrocytoma. This tumor derives its name of "pilocytic" because the cells that make up the tumor are long, thin, and "hair like" (i.e., pilocytes). These may occasionally be metachronous lesions or may represent metastatic lesions.

The differential diagnosis would include ependymoma, although astrocytoma would be more common in the setting of a patient with neurofibromatosis type 1. It is said that astrocytomas tend to involve multiple segments while ependymomas are less extensive. The presence of areas of decreased signal intensity within the tumor is more consistent with the diagnosis of ependymoma. It is impossible to differentiate between the diagnosis of ependymoma and astrocytoma by imaging appearances alone.

SPINAL CORD TUMORS

Case 3

Clinical Presentation

The patient is a 39-year-old female with difficulty signing her name.

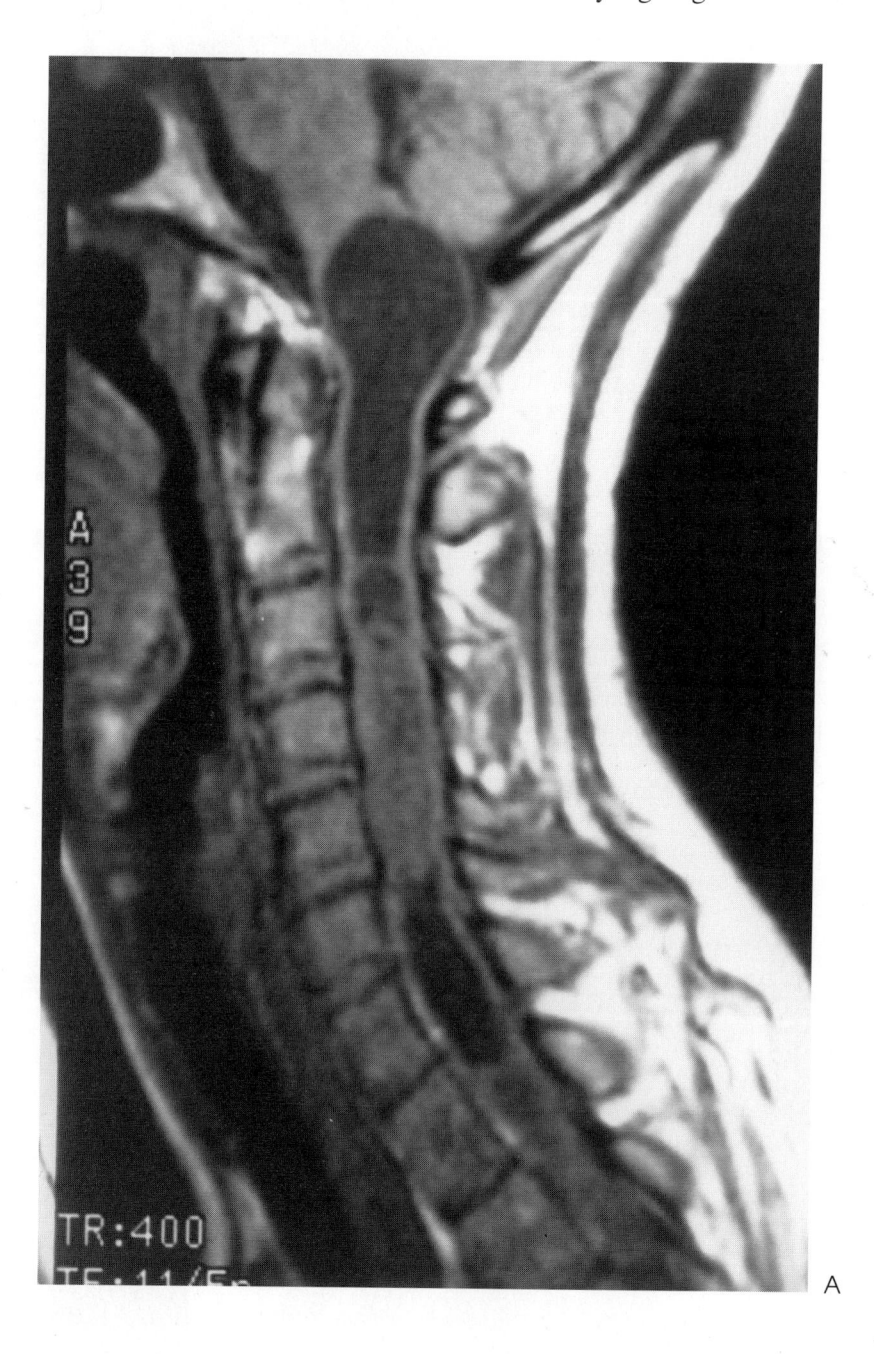

A

TEACHING ATLAS OF SPINE IMAGING

B

C

D

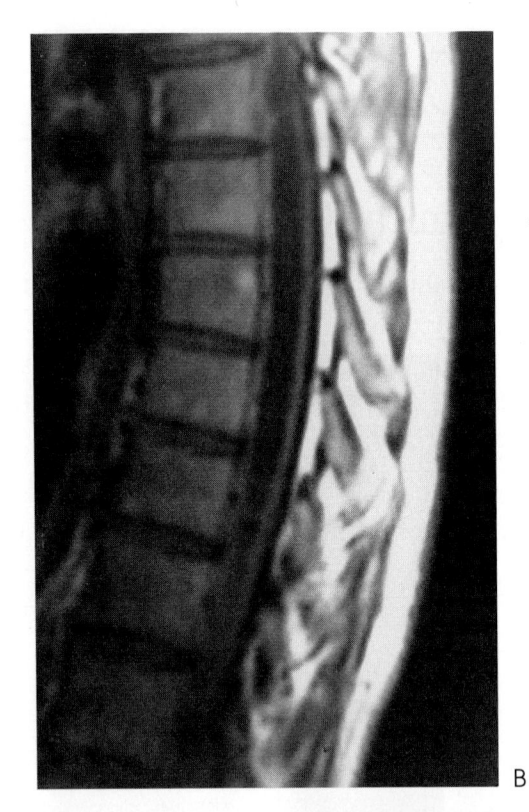

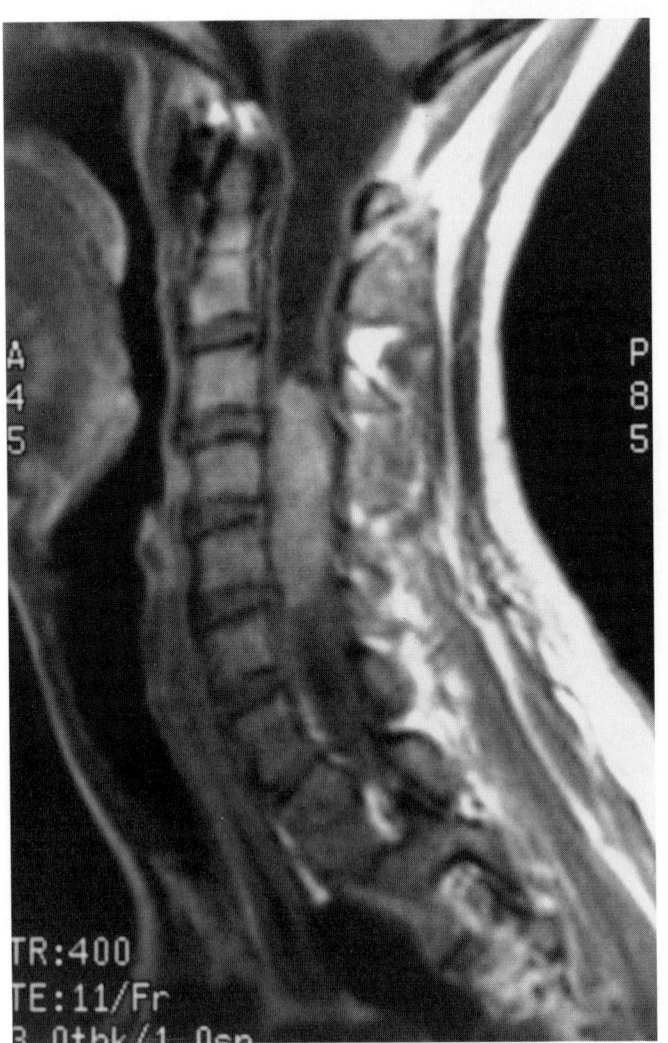

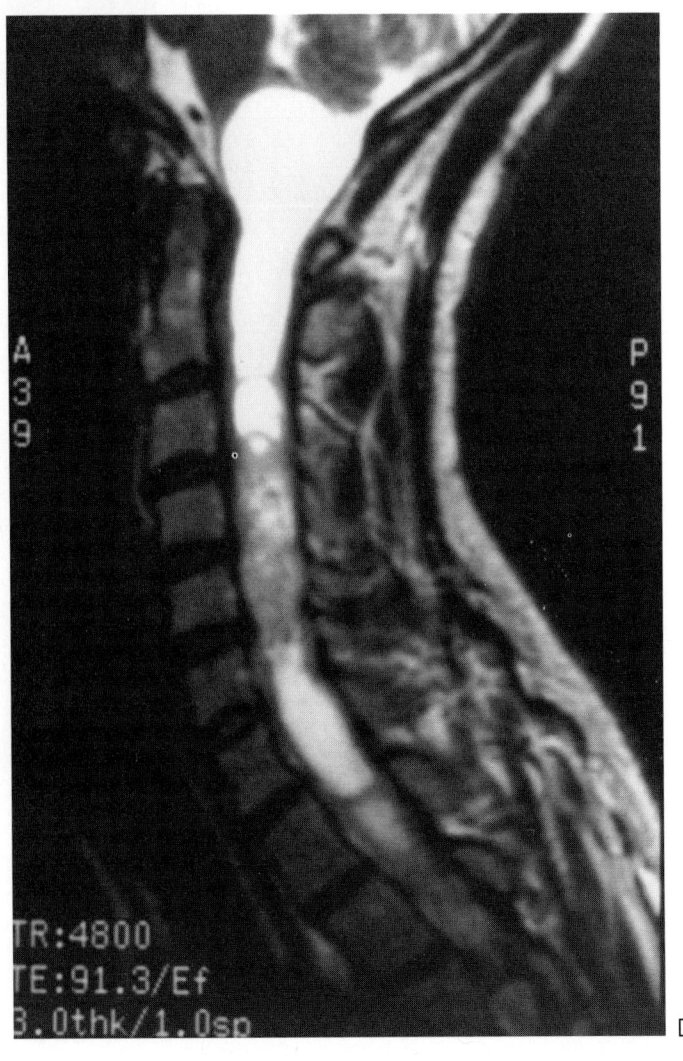

146

SPINAL CORD TUMORS

Radiologic Findings

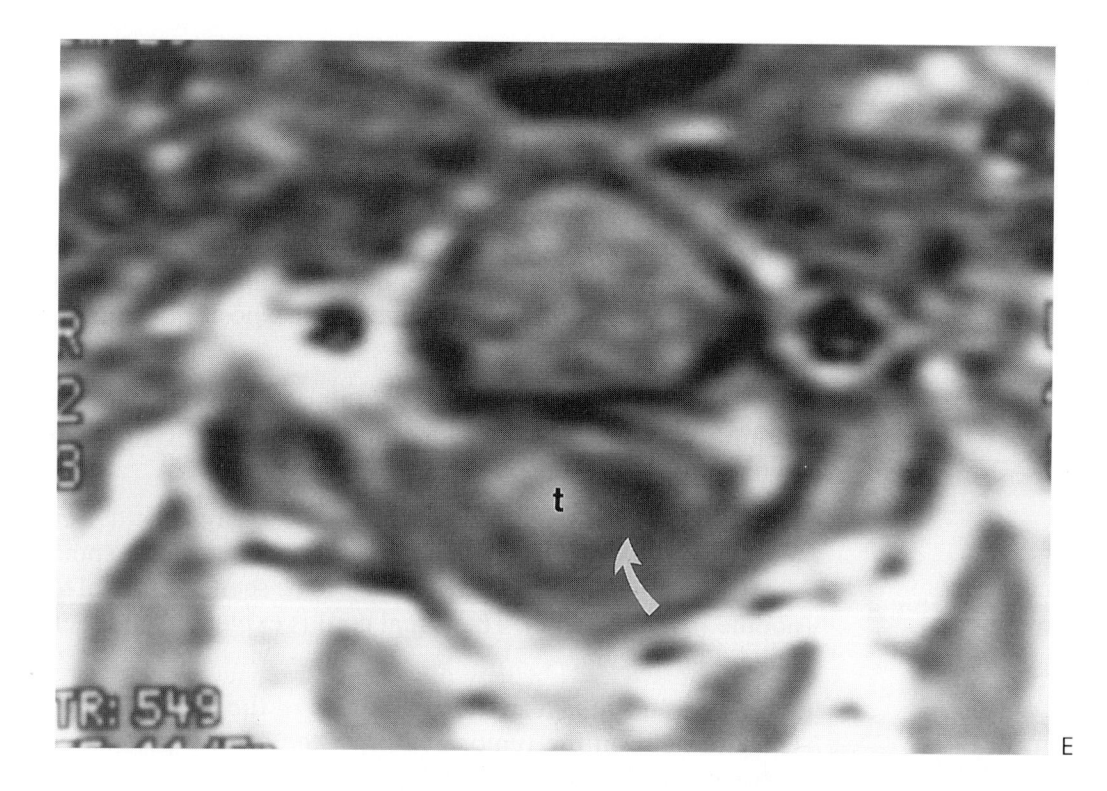

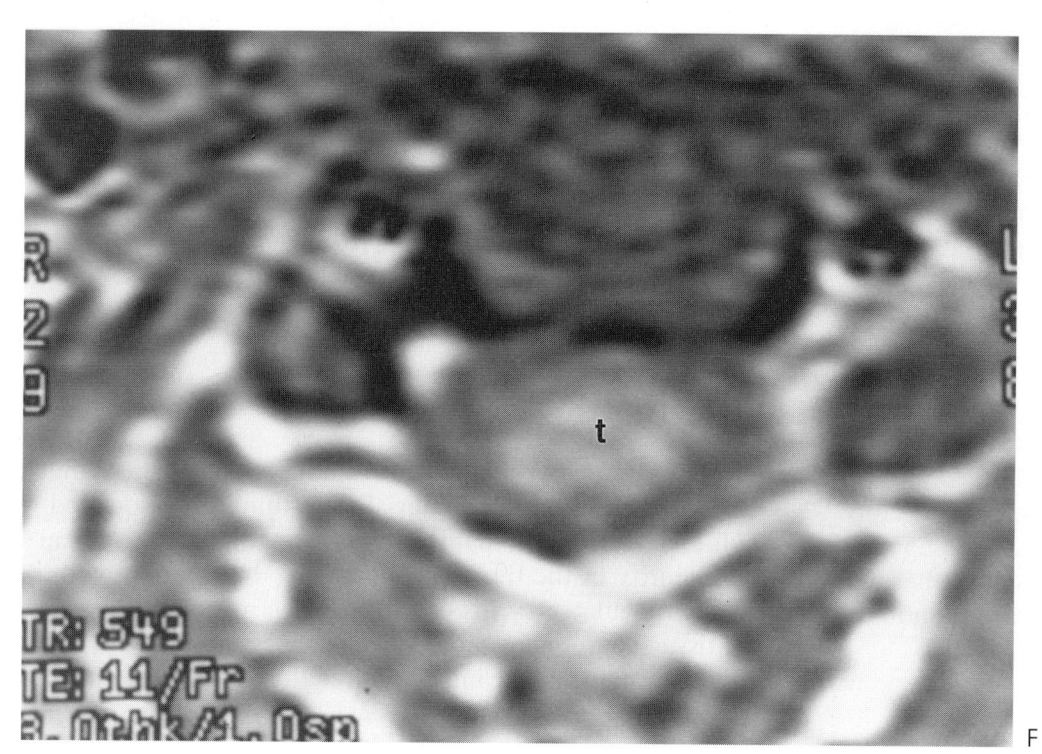

Sagittal short TR image of the cervical spine (Fig. A) reveals a multiloculated cyst that extends from the intracranial medulla throughout the entire visualized spinal cord. There is an isointense soft tissue mass that begins at the level of the midbody of C3 and extends through the level of the intervertebral disc at C5-6.

147

TEACHING ATLAS OF SPINE IMAGING

Radiologic Findings (continued)

Sagittal short TR image in the midthoracic level (Fig. B) reveals a syrinx cavity extending into the lower thoracic region. There are faint internal septations.

Sagittal short TR image postcontrast (Fig. C) reveals dense, slightly inhomogeneous enhancement of the nodule of tumor. There is a slightly lobulated peripheral margin that corresponds to the posterior margins of the vertebral bodies.

Sagittal long TR image (Fig. D) reveals persistent decreased signal intensity within the tumor nodule. The cystic areas become markedly increased in signal intensity.

Axial short TR image postcontrast (Fig. E) reveals a 1-cm eccentrically placed nodule of enhancement in the right side of the spinal cord (t). The decreased signal intensity cavity can also be seen just lateral to the enhancing nodule (*curved arrow*). The spinal cord is expanded and there is only a thin remaining margin.

Axial short TR image in the midportion of the tumor (Fig. F) reveals dense enhancement on the tumor nodule in the central portion of the expanded cervical spinal cord (t).

Diagnosis

Pilocytic astrocytoma.

Differential Diagnosis

- ependymoma

Discussion

The neoplastic portion of the tumor is the portion that enhances after the infusion of contrast material. The tumor is associated with a "benign" multiloculated syrinx that involves the medulla, the cervical spinal cord, and the majority of the thoracic spinal cord. In a patient with a smaller tumor, the multiloculated syrinx cavity could be mistaken for a benign syrinx. The soft tissue component should be closely evaluated with a contrast-enhanced study and multiplanar imaging after the infusion of contrast material.

PEARL

- The entire spinal cord should be evaluated because other areas of enhancement secondary to the presence of tumor may be seen. The study should be performed with the infusion of contrast to identify those portions of the tumor that enhance. The nonenhancing areas presumably represent edema without the presence of tumor.

PITFALL

- This tumor cannot be differentiated from a spinal cord ependymoma. Ependymomas may develop metastases with seeding of the subarachnoid space; therefore, the entire thecal sac should be imaged.

SPINAL CORD TUMORS

Case 4

Clinical Presentation

The patient is a 10-year-old with ataxia and upper and lower extremity weakness.

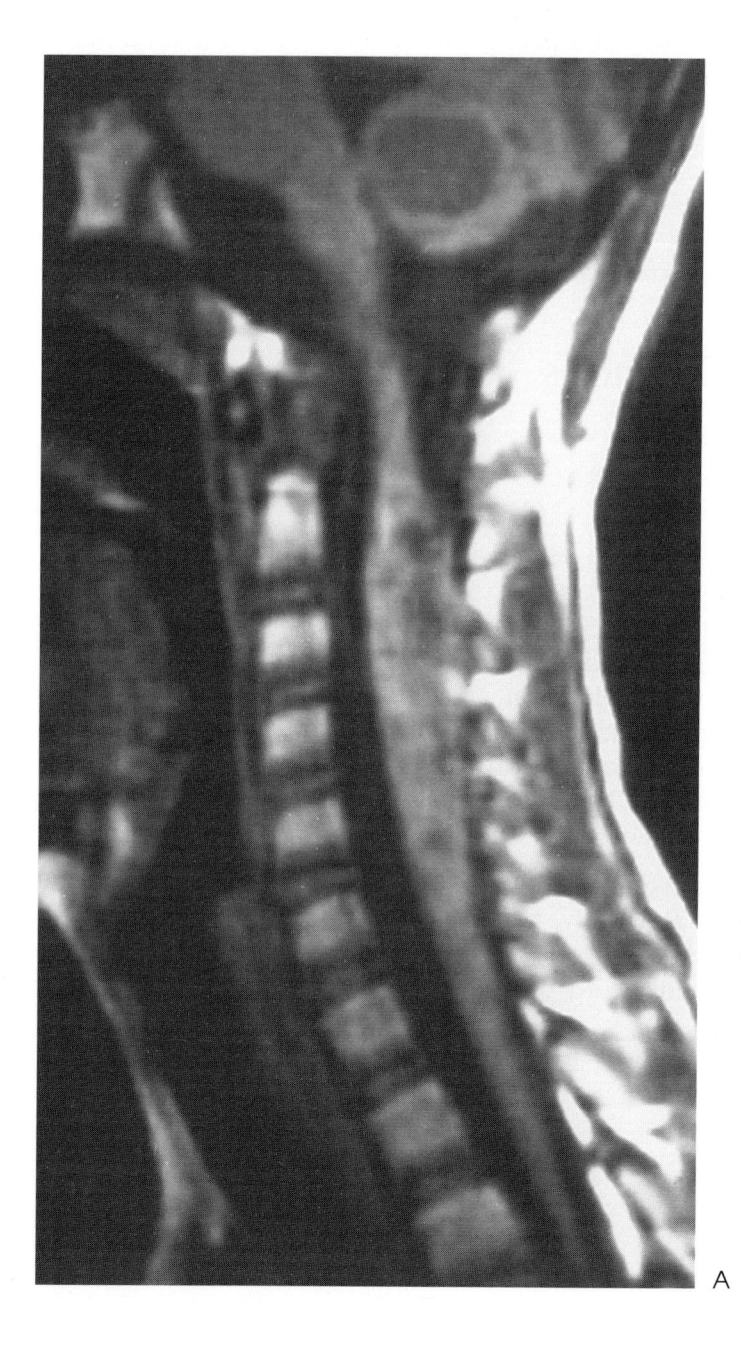

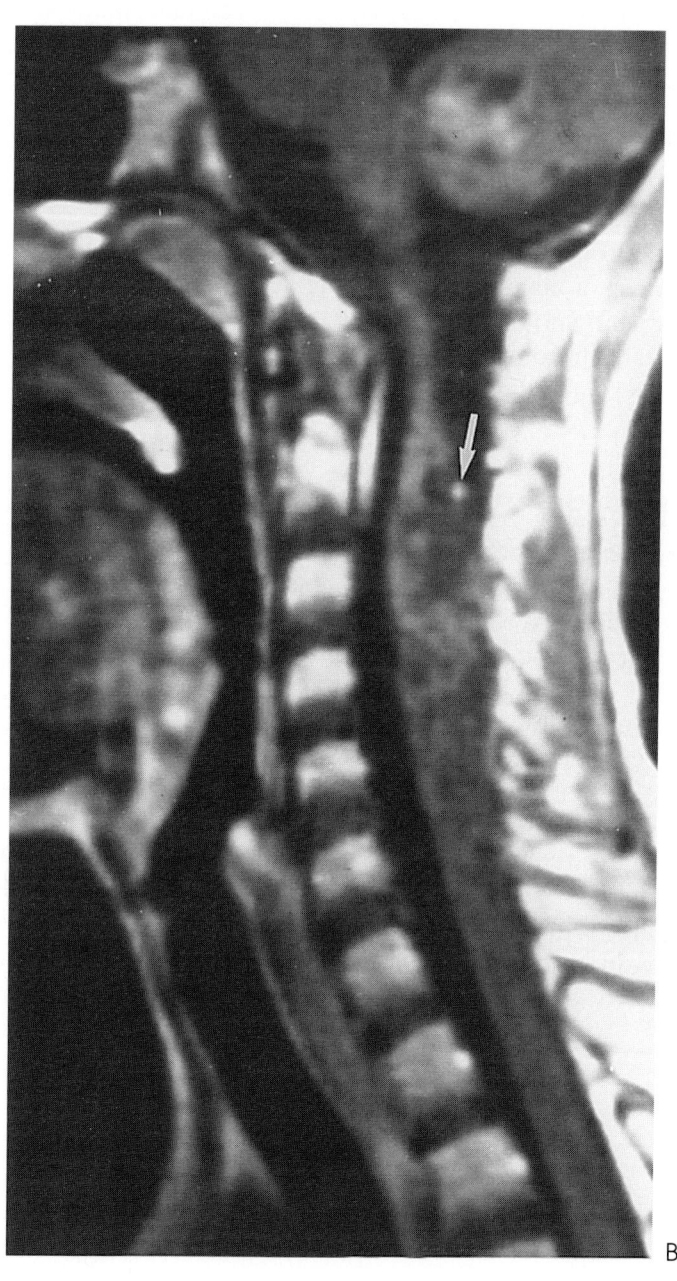

TEACHING ATLAS OF SPINE IMAGING

Radiologic Findings

Sagittal T1W image (Fig. A) reveals widening of the cervical spinal cord from C2 through C6. There are mottled areas of both increased and decreased signal intensity within the spinal cord. There is essentially complete obliteration of the subarachnoid space dorsal to the spinal cord. Also note the approximately 1.5- to 2.0-cm cystic appearing mass in the inferior part of the cerebellum in the midline.

Sagittal T1W image postcontrast (Fig. B) reveals only a very small dot of enhancement along the dorsal aspect of the spinal cord at the level of C2 (*arrow*). An area of irregular enhancement within the cystic mass is visible in the posterior fossa.

PEARL
- Clinical correlation with a possible history of neurofibromatosis type 2 would favor a diagnosis of multiple ependymomas. No history of neurofibromatosis type 2 was present in this patient.

Diagnosis

Glioma of the cervical spinal cord and cerebellum, confirmed at surgery.

Differential Diagnosis

- pilocytic astrocytoma
- ependymoma

PITFALLS
- Although unlikely, cerebellar and spinal cord metastases could have a similar appearance.
- Areas of hemorrhage within the cervical spinal cord could have a similar appearance with either decreased or increased signal intensity or both. The areas of decreased signal intensity could also represent areas of flow void in a vascular tumor.

Discussion

Calcification was identified within the cervical spinal cord tumor on the patient's computed tomographic scan, and presumably the areas of mottled signal intensity represent the areas of calcification. Areas of calcification sometimes present with the paradoxical appearance of increased signal intensity on the T1W images. The area of enhancement seen on Figure B is consistent with a vessel such as an artery or vein.

Differential diagnosis would include pilocytic astrocytoma of the spinal cord and cerebellum. Remotely, hemangioblastoma could have a similar appearance, but would be unlikely. Ependymoma primary in the cerebellum with spread to the spinal cord or vice versa could also be a diagnostic consideration.

SPINAL CORD TUMORS

Case 5

Clinical Presentation

The patient is a one-year-old female with a history of leukemia and new onset of right-sided numbness.

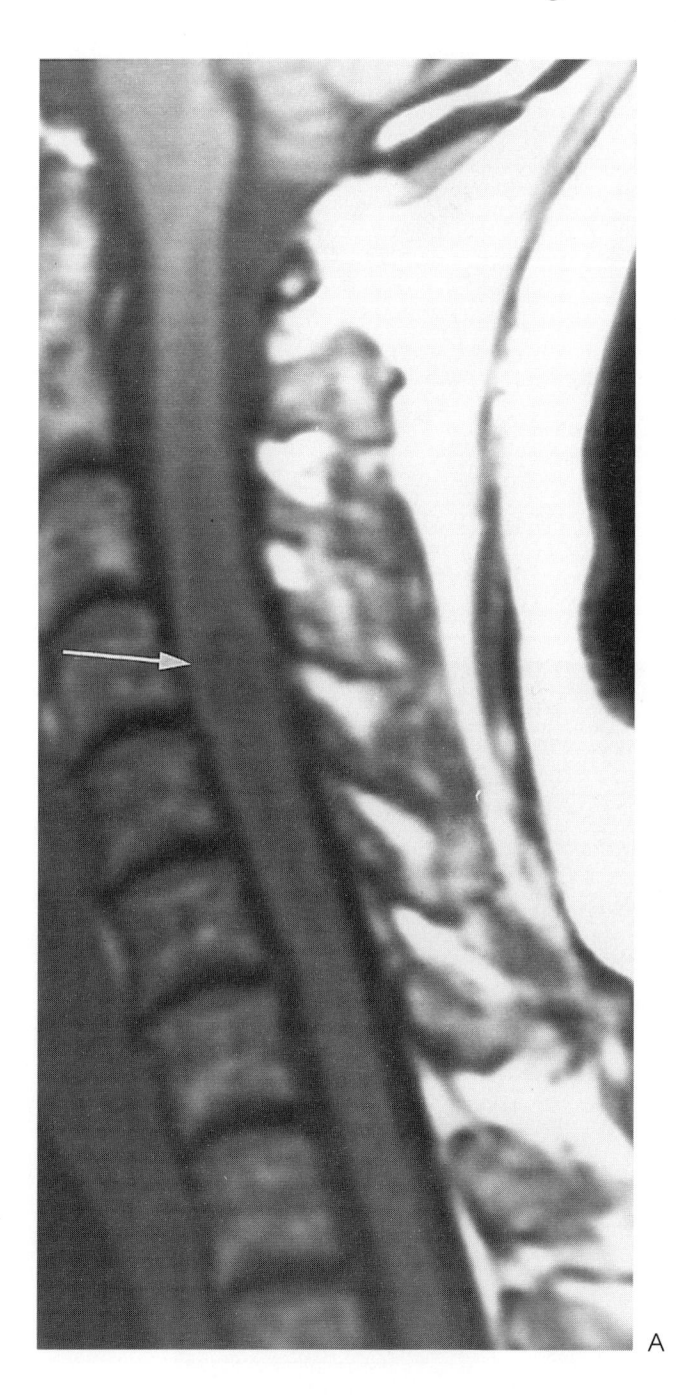

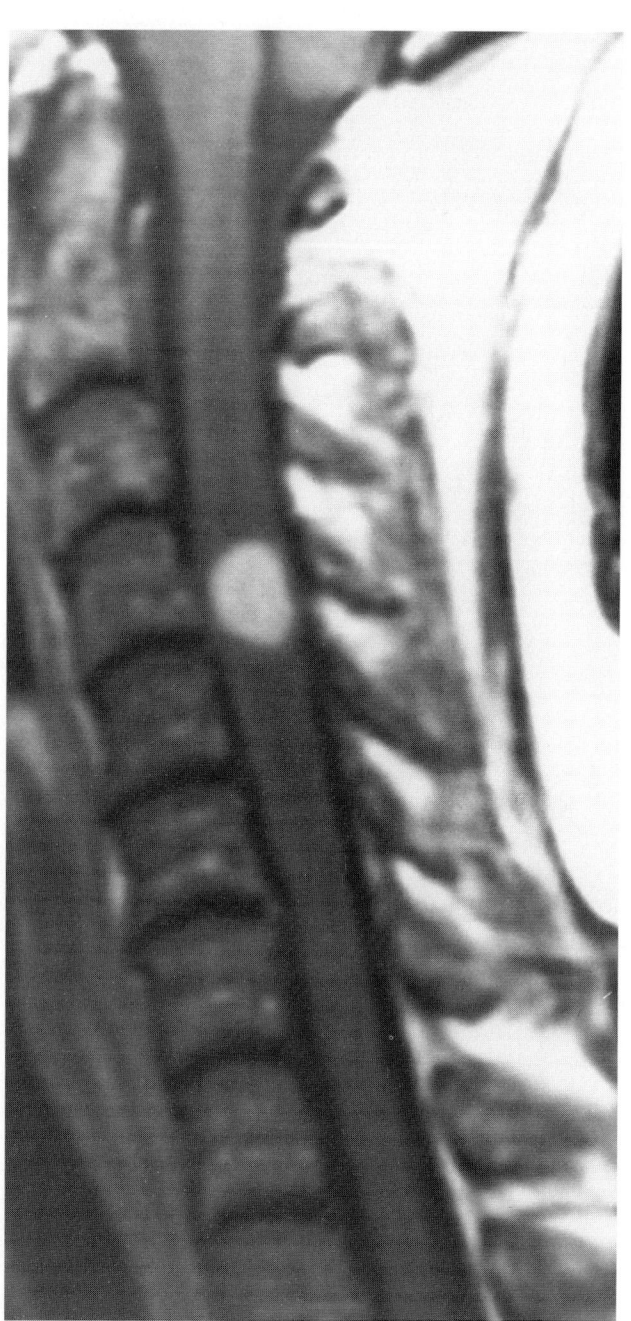

A

B

151

TEACHING ATLAS OF SPINE IMAGING

C

D

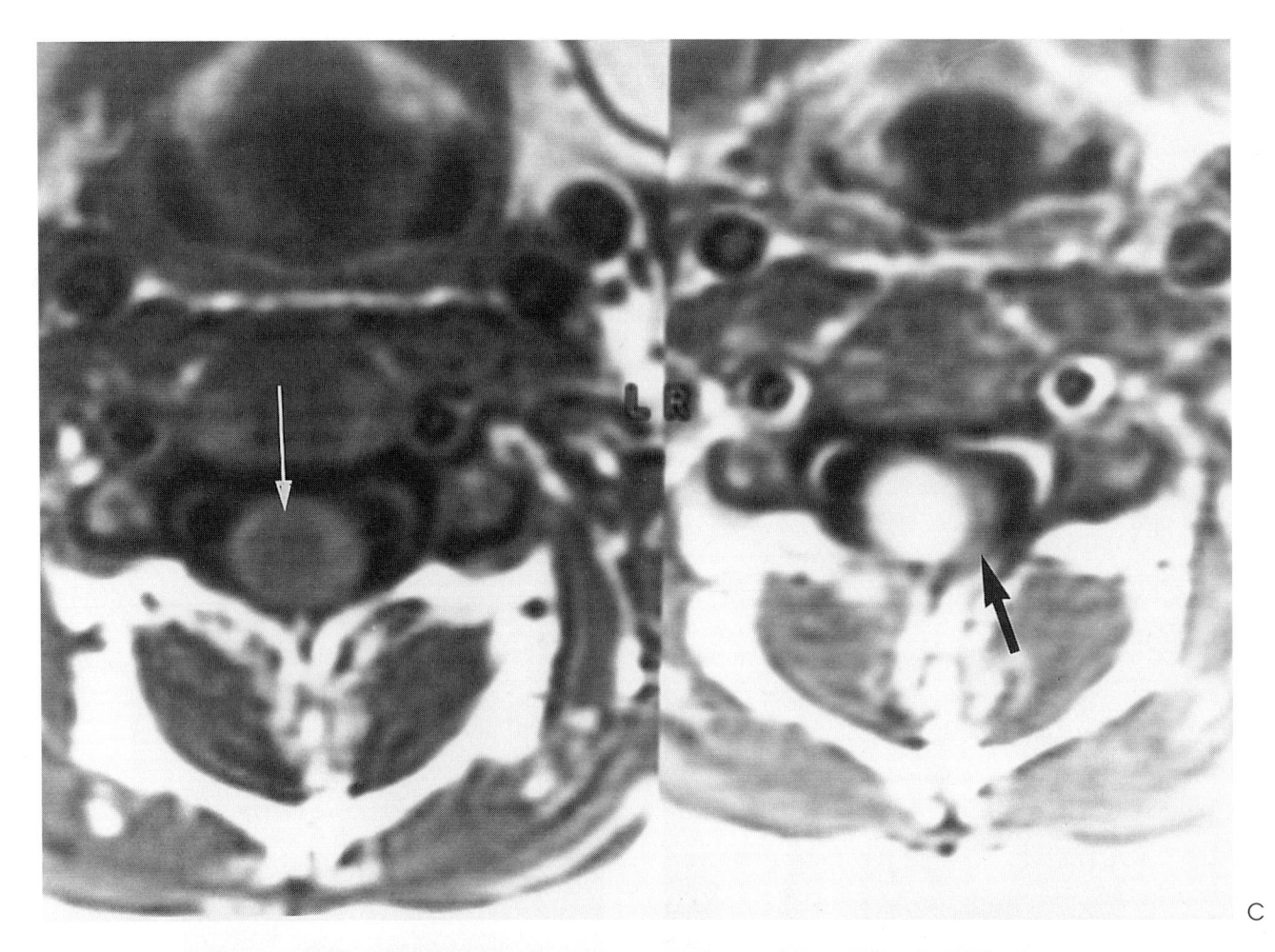

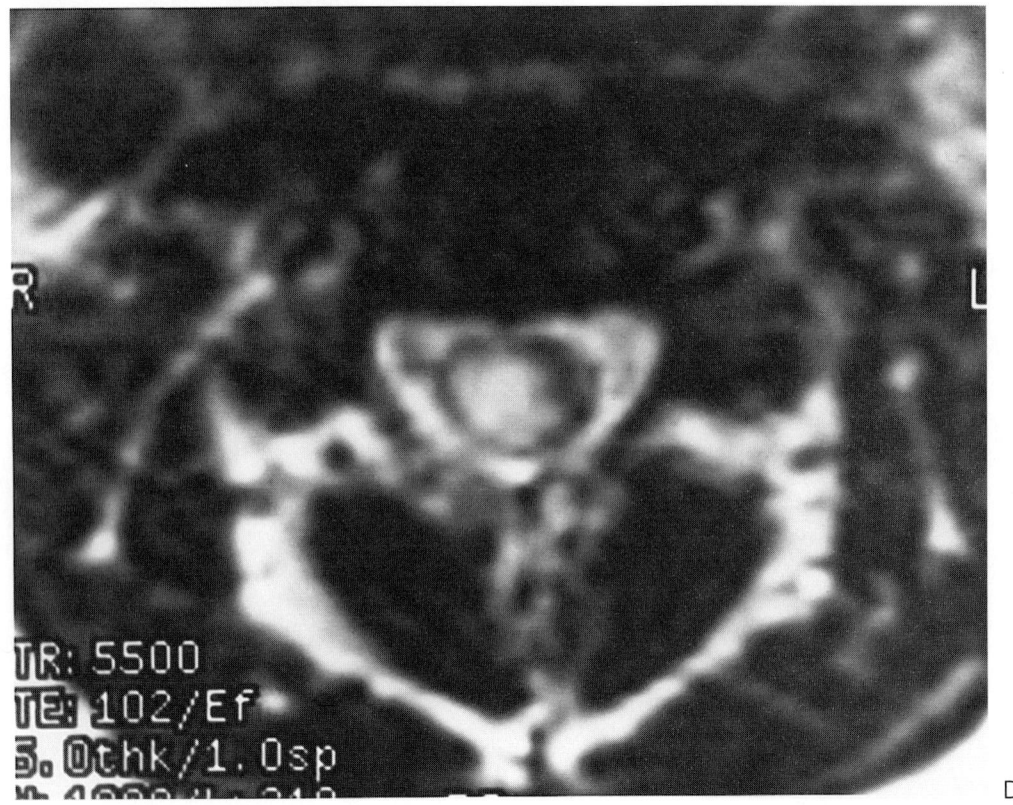

152

SPINAL CORD TUMORS

Radiologic Findings

Sagittal short TR image (Fig. A) reveals fusiform swelling of the cervical spinal cord, which is most marked at the C4 level. At this level, a faint rounded area of slightly lower signal intensity with a slightly increased signal intensity rim can be seen (*arrow*).

Sagittal short TR image postcontrast (Fig. B) reveals dense enhancement of a rounded soft tissue mass in the spinal cord at the C4 level.

Pre- (Fig. C, *left*) and postcontrast (Fig. C, *right*) axial short TR images. The precontrast study reveals a rounded area of decreased signal intensity within the spinal cord, slightly eccentrically displaced toward the right side (*left, white arrow*). After the infusion of contrast material (*right*), there is dense homogeneous enhancement of this soft tissue mass. The normal spinal cord is displaced toward the left side in a crescentic fashion (*black arrow*).

Axial long TR image (Fig. D) reveals that the soft tissue mass exhibits increased signal intensity. There is a slightly irregular peripheral margin.

Additional history reveals that the patient is known to have a primary leiomyosarcoma with secondary leukemia.

Diagnosis

Spinal cord lesion, a metastasis from the patient's known leiomyosarcoma, confirmed at surgery.

Differential Diagnosis

- ependymoma
- astrocytoma

Discussion

The differential diagnosis in this patient would include a primary spinal cord tumor such as an ependymoma or astrocytoma; these diagnoses would be much more likely than a metastasis to the spinal cord. In addition to this spinal cord lesion, the patient had widespread metastatic disease to the lungs and skeletal system.

PEARLS

- The clinical history is very important in this patient to allow an accurate diagnosis.
- Surgery was justified by the fact that this patient was becoming paraplegic; this reversed following surgical removal of the tumor.

PITFALL

- The entire spinal cord and spinal subarachnoid space should be screened for additional lesions, as the presence of multiple lesions may dictate a different approach to management. Multiple lesions would favor treatment with radiation therapy rather than surgery.

TEACHING ATLAS OF SPINE IMAGING

Case 6

Clinical Presentation

The patient is a 26-year-old female with spasticity in the lower extremities, right greater than left. There is flaccidity in the right upper extremity and paresis in the left upper extremity.

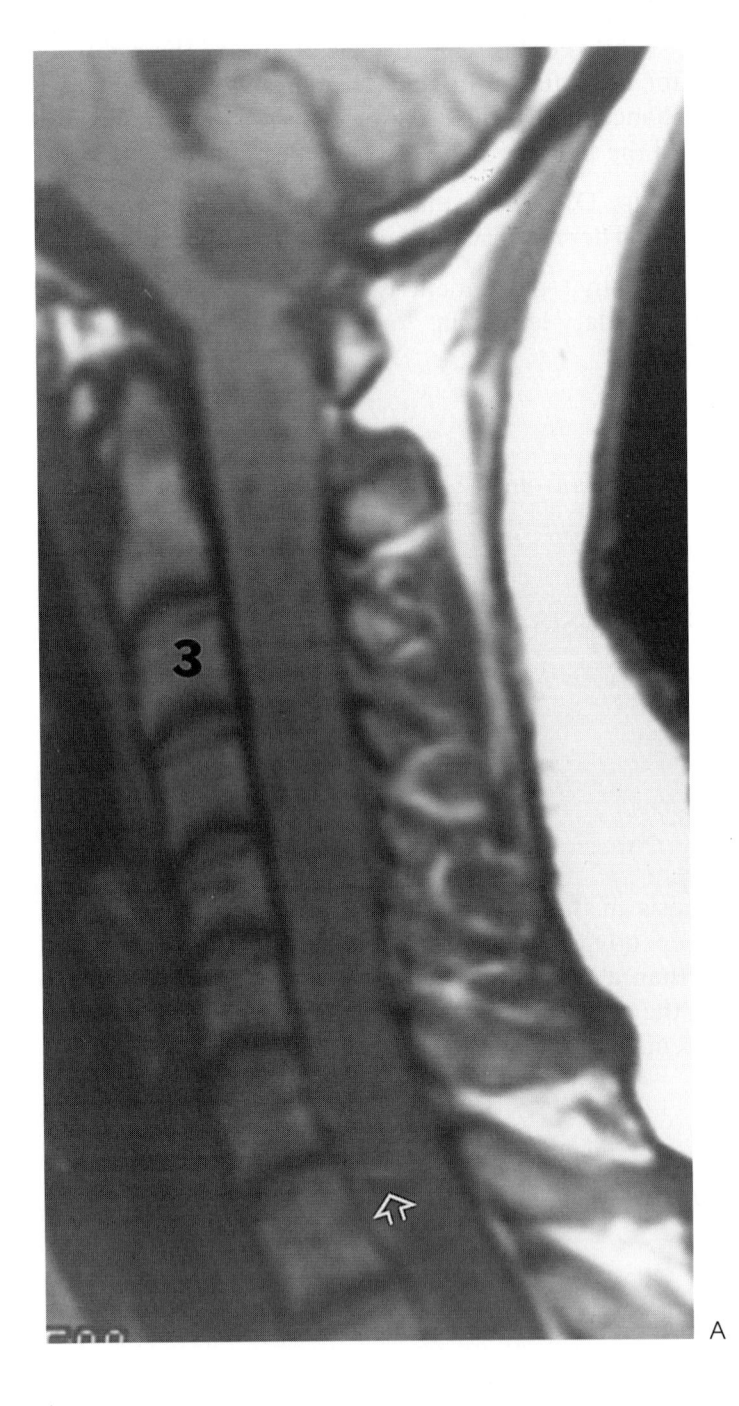

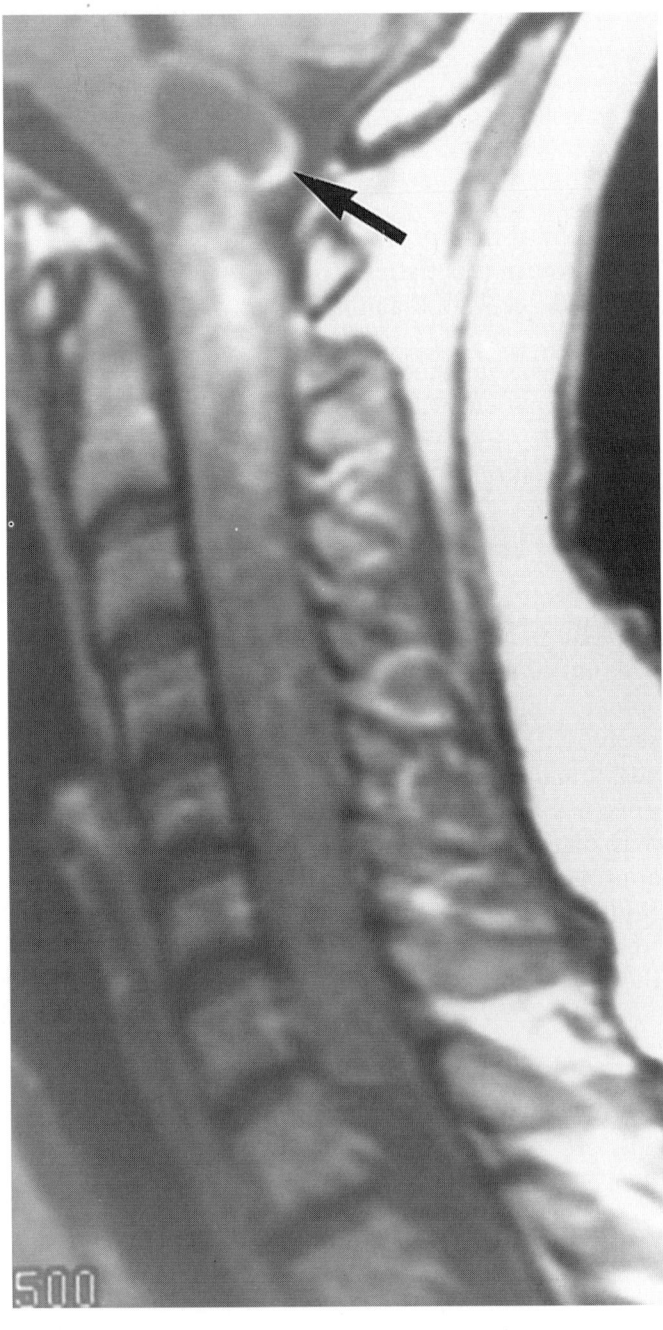

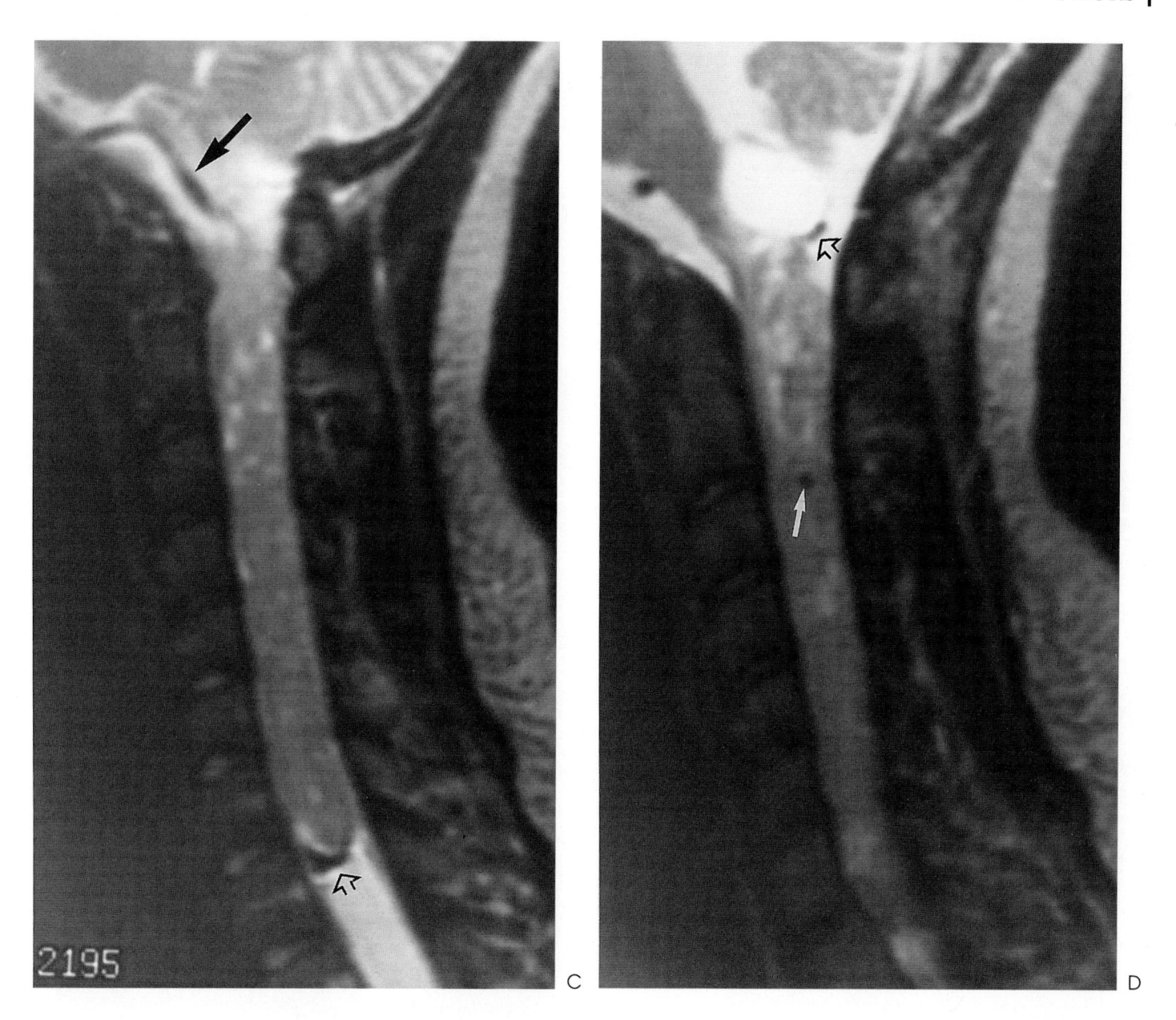

SPINAL CORD TUMORS

155

TEACHING ATLAS OF SPINE IMAGING

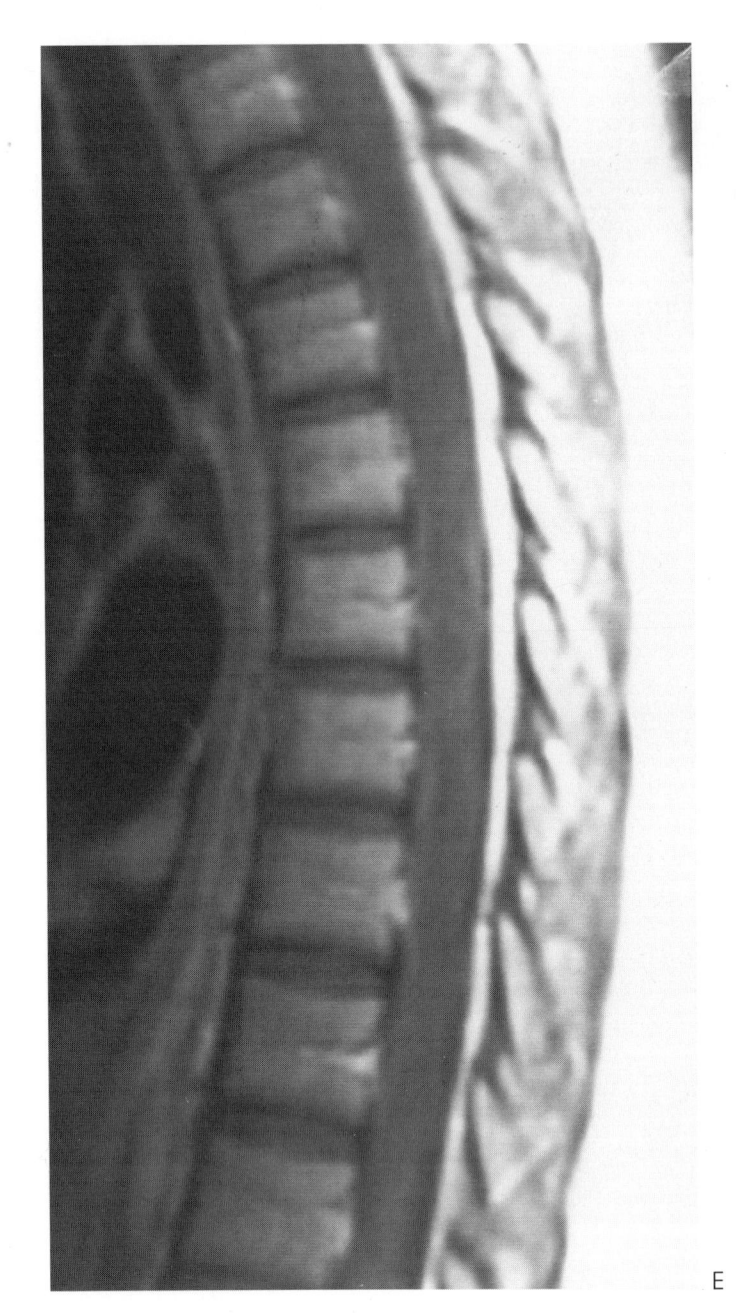

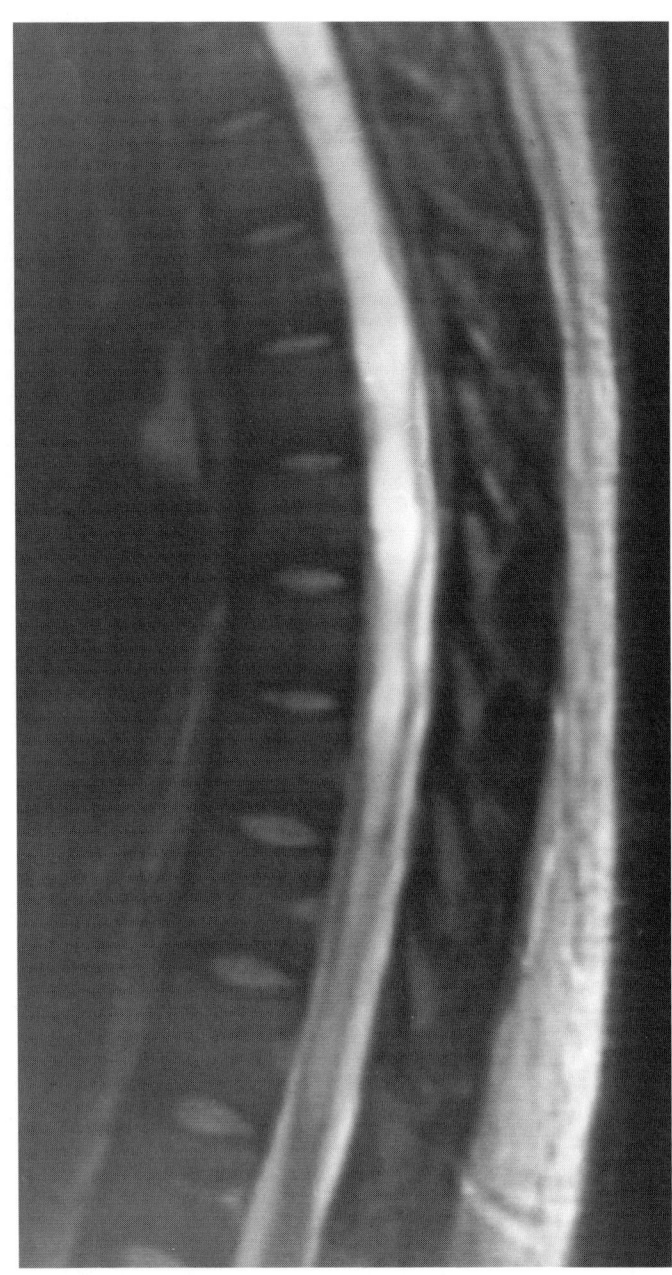

SPINAL CORD TUMORS

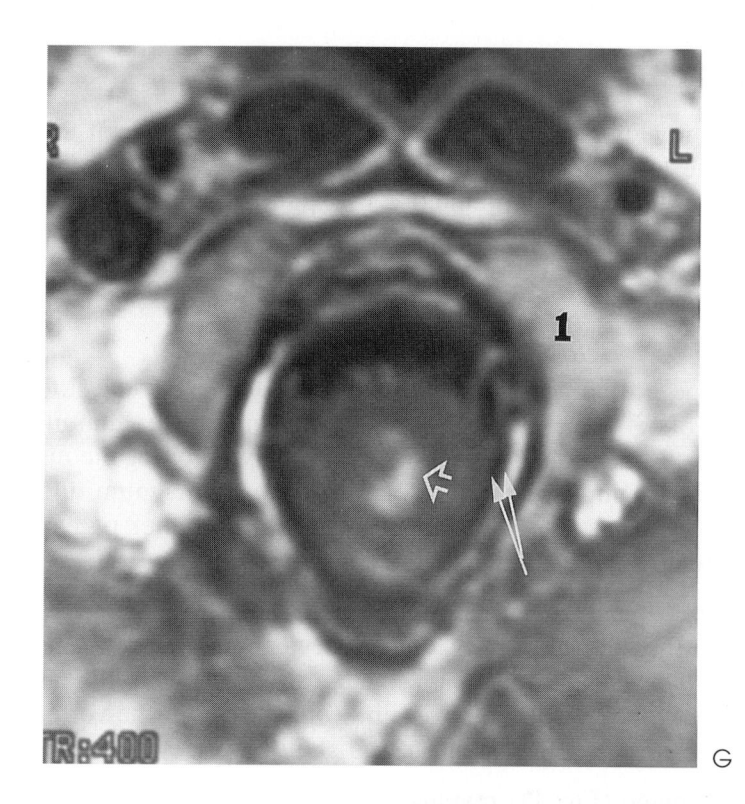

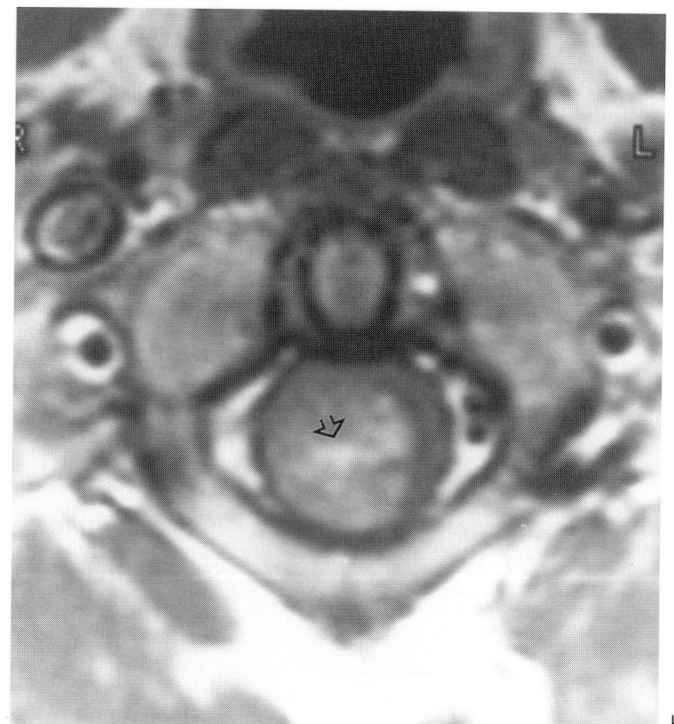

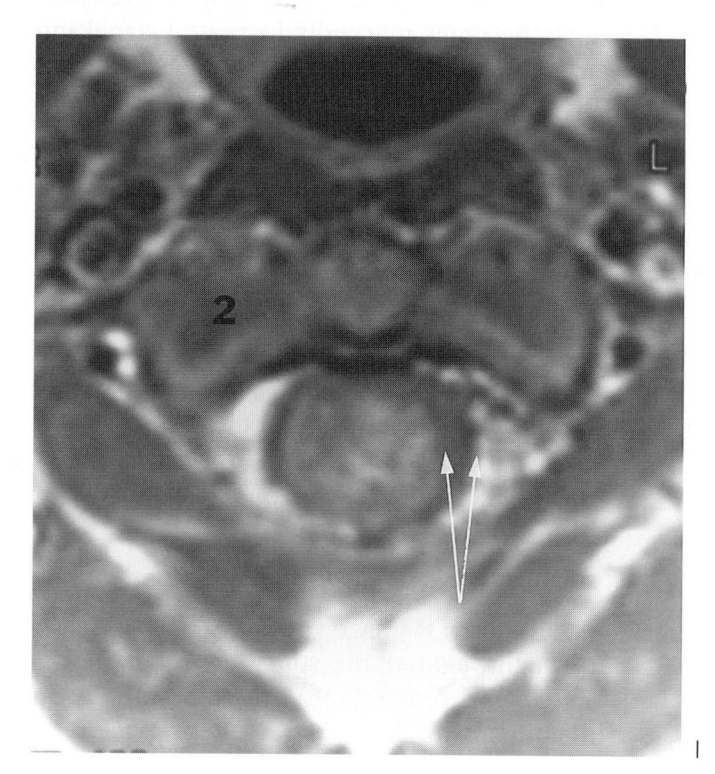

Radiologic Findings

Sagittal short TR image (Fig. A) reveals a 1 × 1.5-cm cystic lesion in the medulla just below the level of the foramen of Magendie and just above the foramen magnum. The cervical spinal cord is expanded from the level of the foramen magnum through the length of the visualized spinal cord. There are curvilinear areas of both decreased and increased signal intensity at the level of the first thoracic vertebrae (*open arrow*). The C3 vertebral body is identified with 3.

Sagittal short TR image postcontrast (Fig. B) reveals that the cystic lesion has a peripheral rim of enhancement along its posterior inferior margin (*arrow*). An area of moderate enhancement in a relatively inhomogeneous pattern can be seen beginning at the level of the foramen magnum and extending through the C2-3 level. There are also multiple smaller patchy areas of enhancement throughout the visualized cervical spinal cord.

Sagittal long TR image (Fig. C) reveals a large area of persistent decreased signal intensity within the central portion of the cervical spinal cord. This extends from the C1 level through the T1 level. There is a small curvilinear area of decreased signal intensity at the lower end (*open arrow*). The vertebral artery appears as an area of flow void at the skull base (*solid arrow*).

Parasagittal long TR image (Fig. D) reveals that the cyst in the posterior fossa becomes markedly increased signal intensity (open arrow). There is a small rounded area of decreased signal intensity within the spinal cord at the C3 level (*solid arrow*).

Sagittal short TR image in the thoracic spine (Fig. E) reveals diffuse enlargement of the spinal cord. There is almost complete obliteration of the subarachnoid space.

Sagittal long TR image (Fig. F) reveals an elongated, scalloped marginated segment of variable increased signal intensity throughout the length of the spinal cord.

Axial short TR image postcontrast at the level of C1 (Fig. G) reveals a curvilinear area of enhancement in the left side of the spinal cord (*open arrow*). The two long white arrows identify the compromised subarachnoid space. The lateral mass of C1 is identified with 1.

Axial short TR image at the tip of the odontoid (Fig. H) reveals multiple small irregular areas of enhancement within the spinal cord (*open arrow*).

Axial short TR image at C2 (Fig. I) reveals a speckled area of faint enhancement throughout the spinal cord. There is only a thin semilunar area of spinal cord remaining on the left side (*arrows*). The lateral mass of C2 is identified with 2.

SPINAL CORD TUMORS

PEARLS

- It is not possible to differentiate a pilocytic astrocytoma from an ependymoma by imaging alone. Magnetic resonance imaging is the ideal method for diagnosis as well as follow-up in these patients.

- The presence of a cystic component is in favor of the diagnosis of pilocytic astrocytoma. Because these tumors are relatively benign and patients tend to do well following surgical removal, careful evaluation for the presence of a cystic component should be performed.

Diagnosis

Pilocytic astrocytoma, confirmed at surgery.

Differential Diagnosis

- astrocytoma

Discussion

The multilevel segment of involvement seen in this case is typical of astrocytoma. The cystic portion of the tumor seen here in the cerebellum would be typical of a pilocytic astrocytoma. The internal areas of decreased signal intensity represent areas of hemorrhage or calcification. The increased signal intensity in the thoracic spinal cord is secondary to formation of a syrinx cavity as well as edema extending down the spinal cord.

At surgery the tumor was totally removed and the patient improved significantly. Follow-up postoperative scans revealed the following:

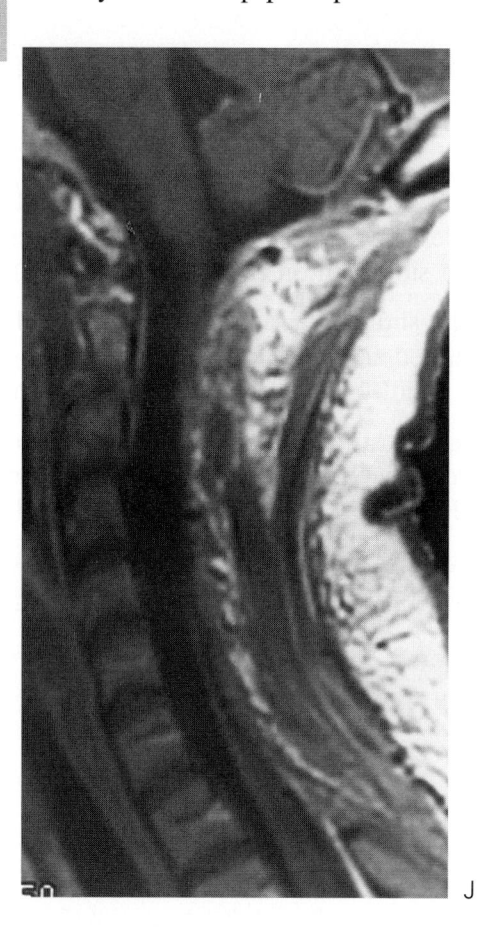

Sagittal short TR image postcontrast (Fig. J) reveals that the cervical spinal cord is markedly thinned and displaced posteriorly in the vertebral canal.

Sagittal long TR image (Fig. K) reveals that the cervical spinal cord cannot be demonstrated with certainty from the level of the foramen magnum to the level of C5. A shunt tubing device can be seen with the tip at the level of C4 (*open arrow*). Several rounded areas of decreased signal intensity are seen in the tube in the thoracic region (*white arrows*).

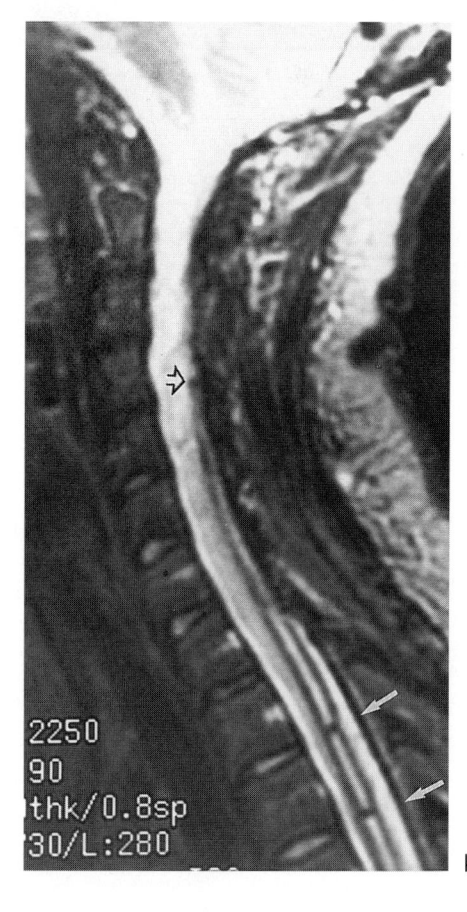

PITFALL

- Because these tumors may spread, the entire vertebral canal should be evaluated for the presence of additional lesions.

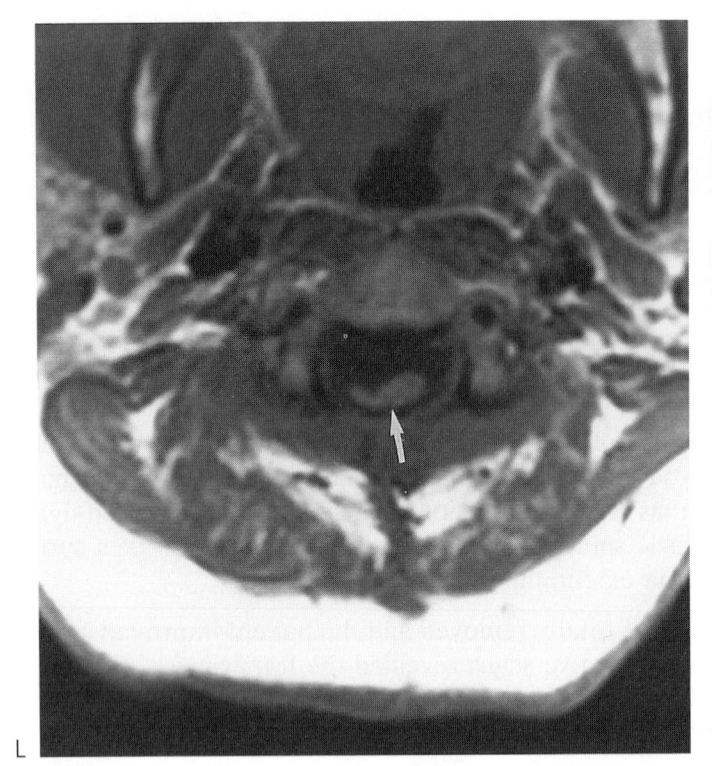

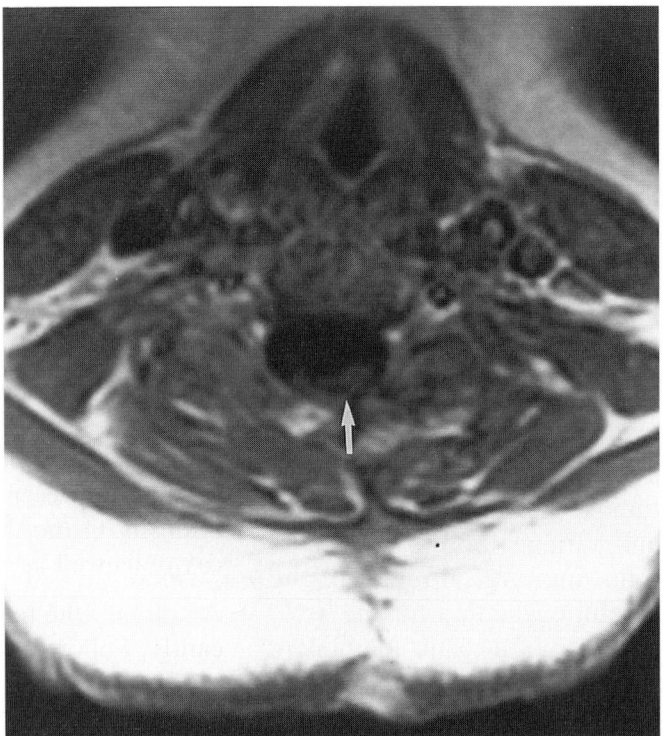

Axial short TR image (Fig. L) reveals the cervical spinal cord displaced posteriorly in the vertebral canal. The spinal cord is flattened, more on the right side than on the left side (*arrow*).

Axial short TR image (Fig. M) reveals the flattened spinal cord. A small rounded area of decreased signal intensity within the spinal cord represents the shunt tube in place within the spinal cord (*arrow*).

These postoperative changes are the result of total removal of the spinal cord pilocytic astrocytoma. The posterior displacement of the spinal cord is due in part to adhesions tethering the cord posteriorly.

SPINAL CORD TUMORS

Case 7

Clinical Presentation

The patient is a 53-year-old male who presents for follow-up.

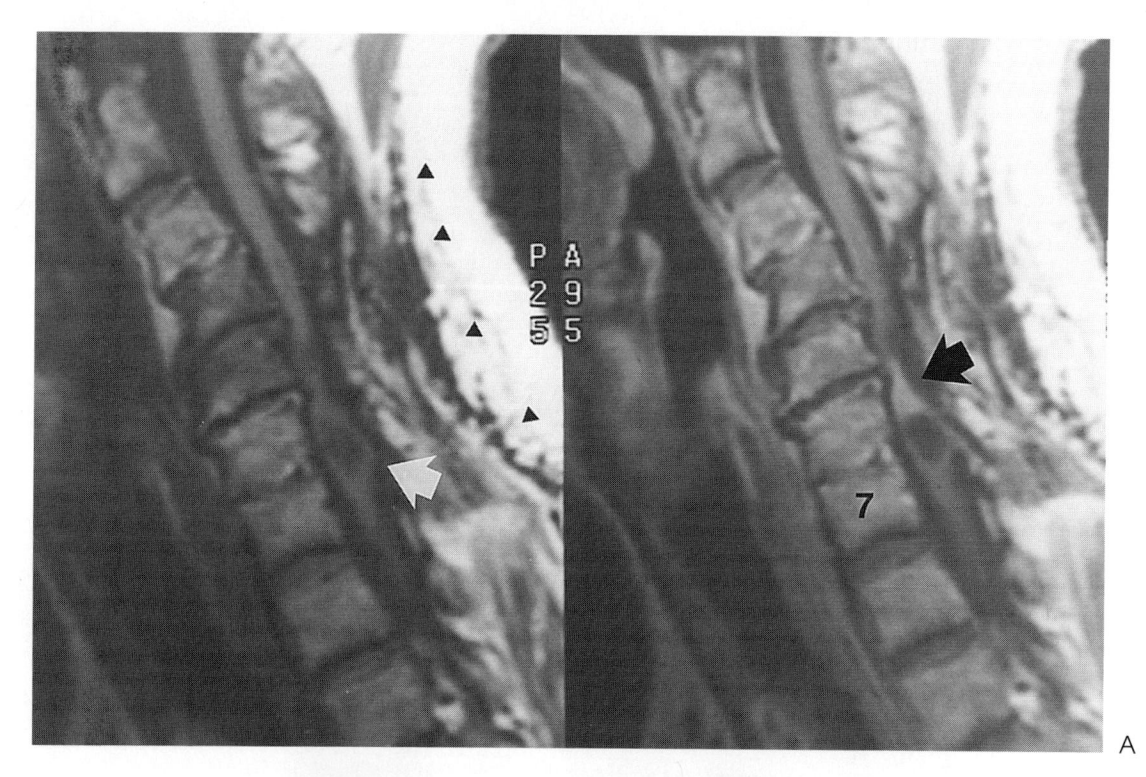

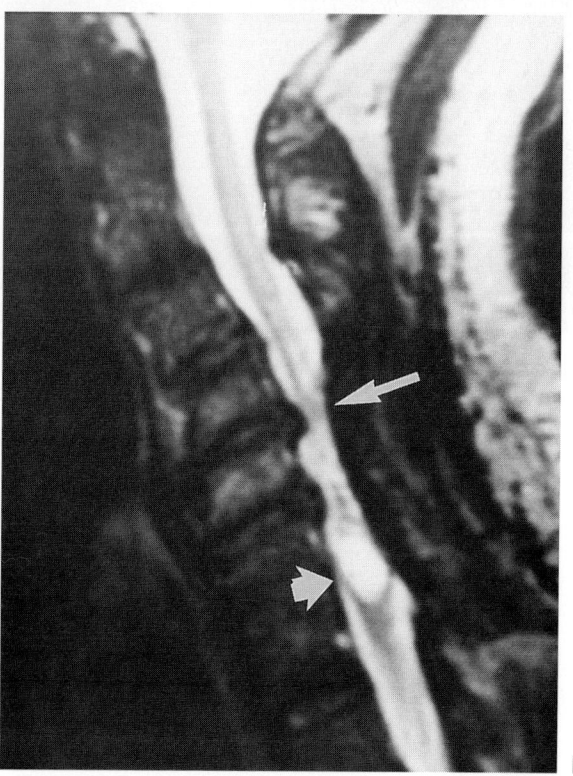

TEACHING ATLAS OF SPINE IMAGING

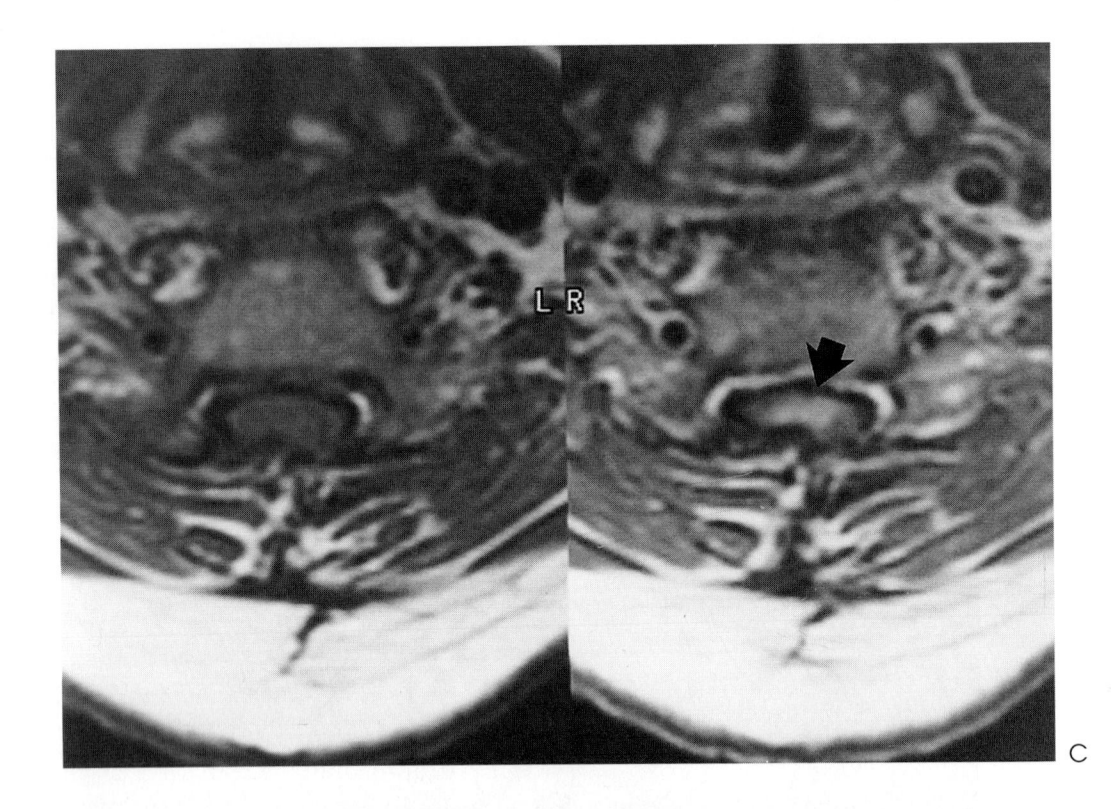

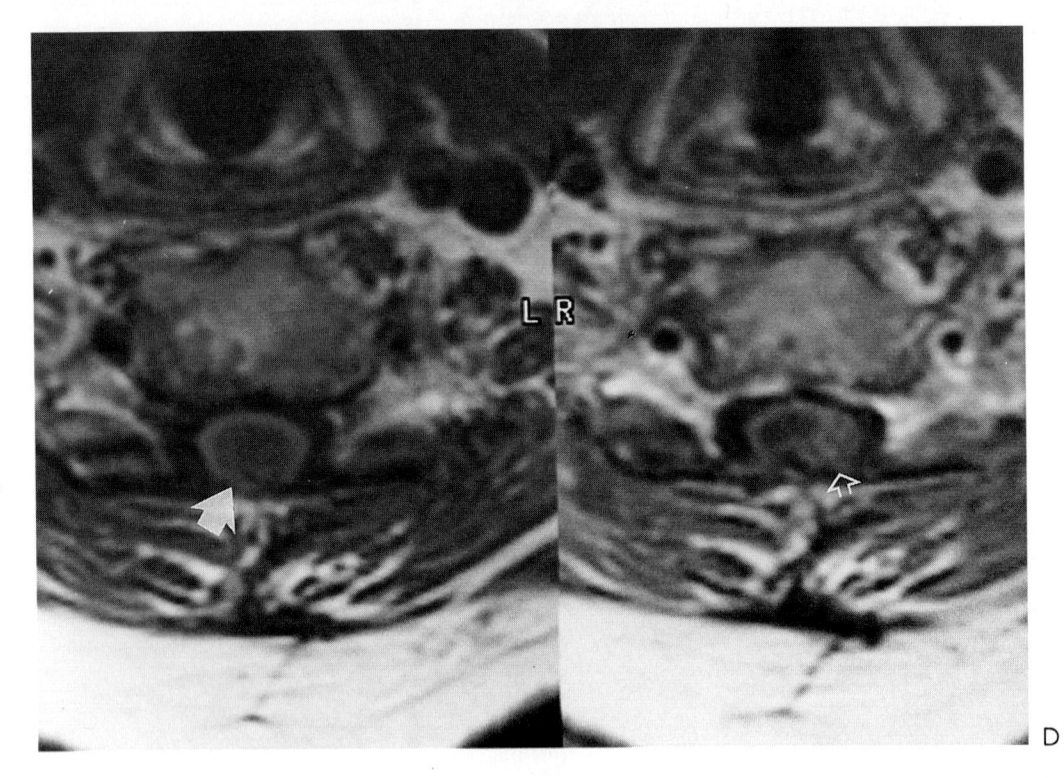

SPINAL CORD TUMORS

Radiologic Findings

Pre- (Fig. A, *left*) and postcontrast (Fig. A, *right*) sagittal short TR images in the cervical spine reveal that the patient has undergone a laminectomy with removal of the cervical spinous processes (left, arrowheads). There is an 8-mm cystic area within the central portion of the cervical spinal cord at the C6 level (*left, white arrow*). Postcontrast (*right*) there is a triangular shaped area of enhancement just above the level of the cyst (*black arrow*). The spinal cord is markedly thinned above the level of the cyst. There are extensive degenerative changes with anterior and posterior osteophytes at multiple levels. These are encroaching on the subarachnoid space and displacing the spinal cord posteriorly. The 7th vertebral body is identified by 7.

The cystic area (Fig. B) appears as increased signal intensity (*short arrow*) on sagittal long TR image. There is also a decreased signal intensity area dorsally, which results in a multisegment encroachment on the subarachnoid space (*long arrow*).

Pre- (Fig. C, *left*) and postcontrast (Fig. C, *right*) axial short TR images reveal the area of enhancement (*right, arrow*).

Pre- (Fig. D, *left*) and postcontrast (Fig. D, *right*) axial short TR images below the level of the cyst reveal the wall of the cyst (*left, solid arrow*) with enhancement of a portion of the spinal cord along the left side (*right, open arrow*).

PEARL
- The most helpful approach for evaluation in this patient is additional follow-up magnetic resonance (MR) scans.

PITFALLS
- The area of enhancement may simply be normal postoperative enhancement and does not necessarily imply remaining or recurrent tumor.
- In addition to remaining tumor, scarring and tethering of the spinal cord to the dura may occur at the level of the laminectomy. MR imaging is the ideal method for evaluating these changes.

Diagnosis

Postoperative changes in a patient who has had previous surgical removal of a spinal cord ependymoma.

Differential Diagnosis

- posttraumatic syrinx cavity
- Wallerian degeneration
- ependymoma

Discussion

It is not possible to determine if the small triangular area of enhancement is or is not remaining tumor. There are extensive postoperative changes with straightening of the spine, postlaminectomy changes, and dorsal encroachment on the subarachnoid space secondary to scar formation. In the appropriate clinical setting, a posttraumatic syrinx cavity could have a similar appearance. Wallerian degeneration may also be associated with surgery or be seen following spinal cord trauma. This type of degeneration may result in areas of increased signal intensity.

Ependymomas may develop metastases with seeding of the subarachnoid space. This spread of tumor may be very extensive; therefore, the entire spinal subarachnoid space should be evaluated to determine the extent of the disease.

TEACHING ATLAS OF SPINE IMAGING

Case 8

Clinical Presentation

The patient is a 15-year-old female with a clinical history of progressive upper and lower extremity weakness.

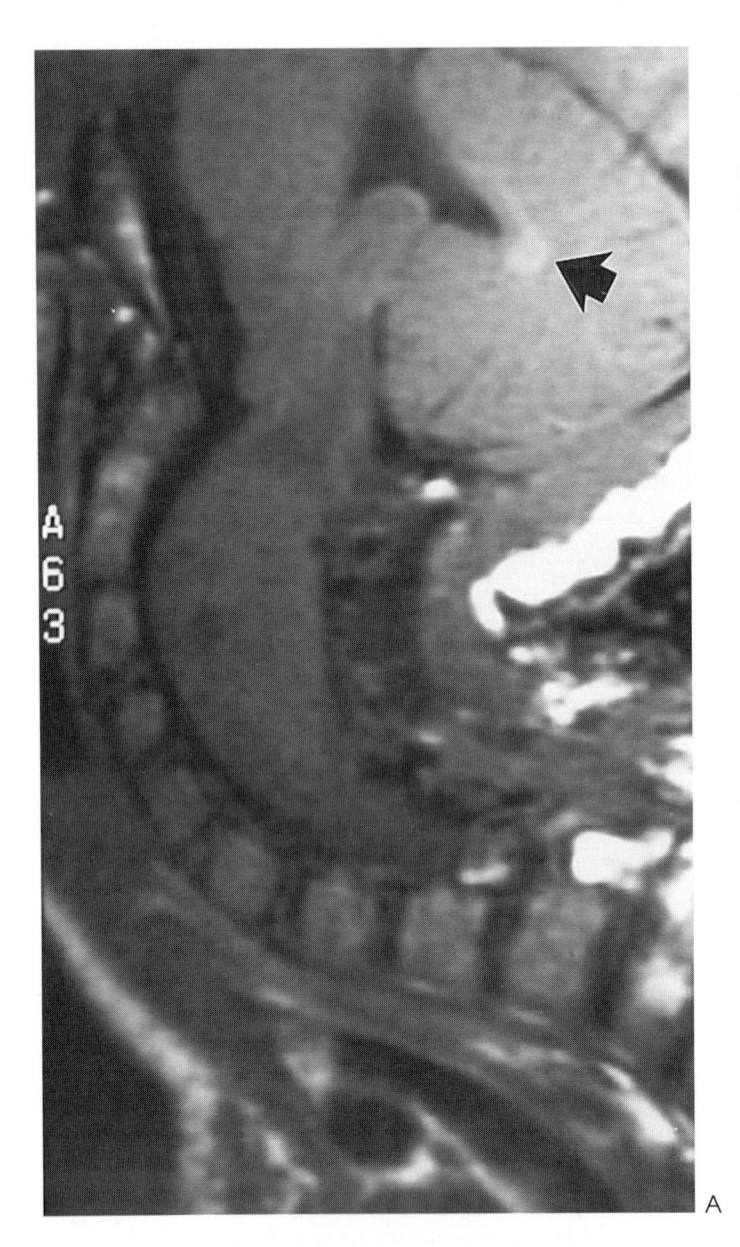

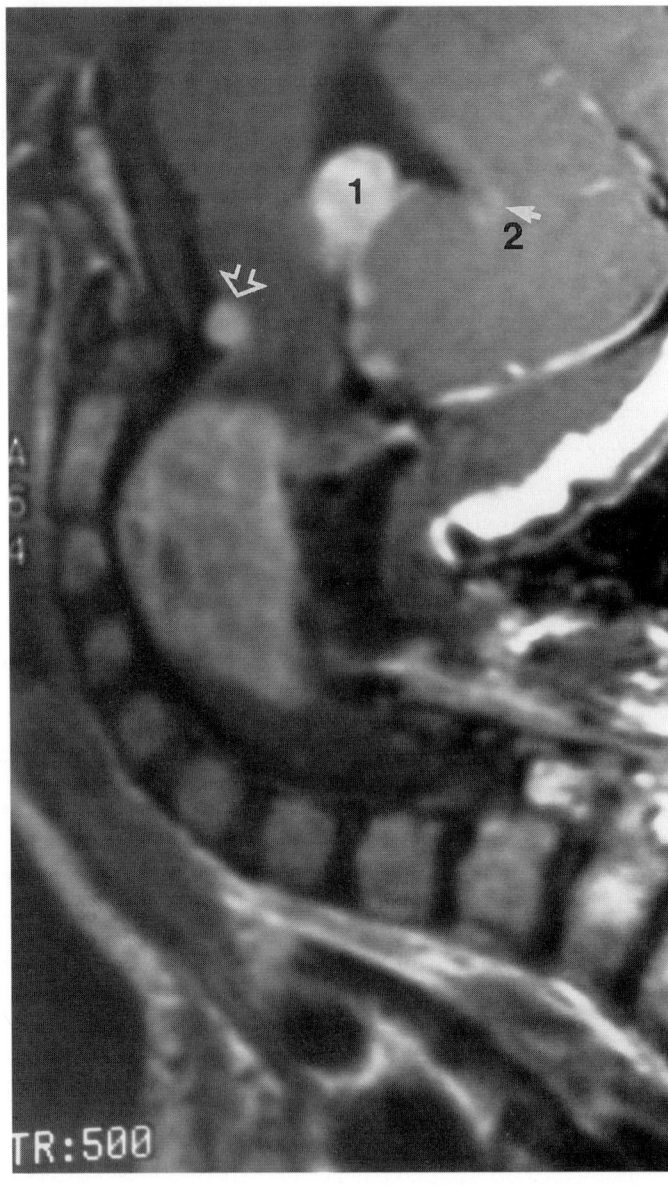

SPINAL CORD TUMORS

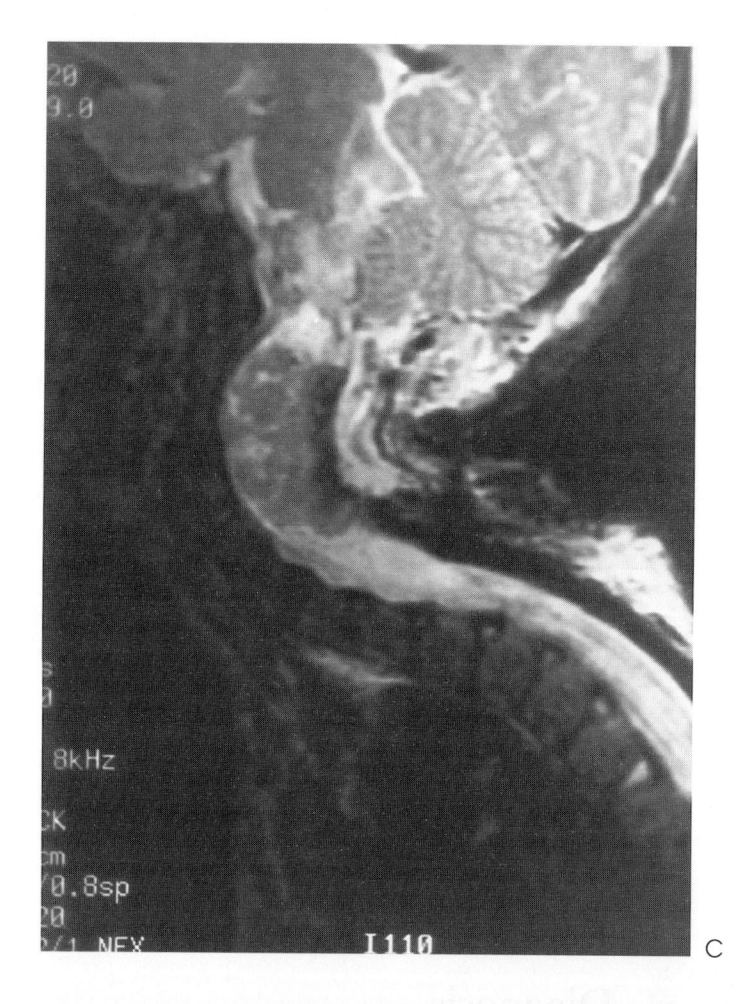

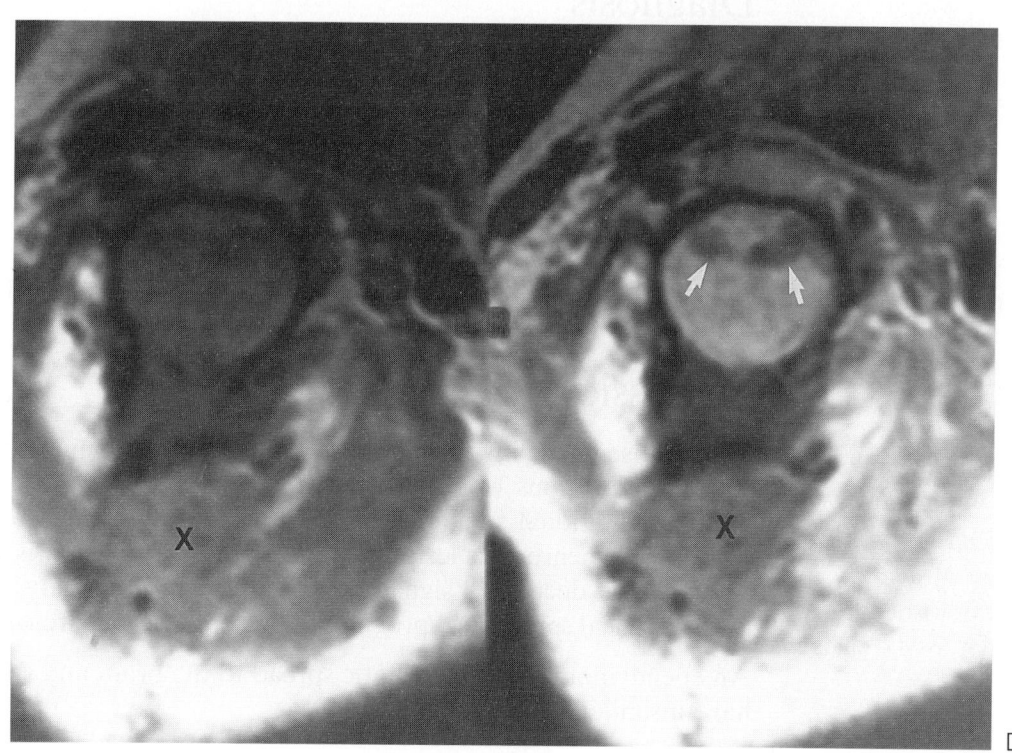

165

Radiologic Findings

Sagittal short TR image (Fig. A) reveals marked expansion of the cervical spinal cord. The medulla is also greatly expanded. There is also an approximately 5 mm area of increased signal intensity at the apex of the fourth ventricle (*arrow*). Also visible are marked expansion of the vertebral canal in the cervical region and marked accentuation of the cervical spine lordosis.

Sagittal short TR image postcontrast (Fig. B) reveals dense, slightly inhomogeneous enhancement of the soft tissue mass in the cervical spinal cord. There are also additional rounded areas of enhancement in the bottom of the fourth ventricle (*1*), at the ventral aspect of the cervicomedullary junction (*open arrow*), and at the apex of the fourth ventricle (*2*). There are several smaller nodules of enhancement in the region of the foramen of Magendie and along the bottom of the cerebellar tonsils.

Sagittal long TR image (Fig. C) reveals a multilobulated decreased signal intensity soft tissue mass within the cervical spinal cord. There are a few internal areas of increased signal intensity, and a variable pattern of areas of increased and decreased signal intensity in the medulla and bottom of the fourth ventricle.

Pre- (Fig. D, *left*) and postcontrast (Fig. D, *right*) axial short TR images reveal the markedly expanded cervical spinal cord. There is dense enhancement postcontrast (*right*). There are several internal areas of smoothly marginated decreased signal intensity anteriorly within the spinal cord (*right, arrows*). Postoperative changes are noted in the dorsal aspect of the neck (*X*).

Diagnosis

Pilocytic astrocytoma, confirmed by biopsy.

Differential Diagnosis

- astrocytoma
- ependymoma

Discussion

The multisegment involvement seen in this case is typical of astrocytoma. The cystic portions would be consistent with a pilocytic astrocytoma. The multiple additional smaller lesions represent either metastatic deposits or additional synchronous lesions. In this patient, the legion is very extensive. The areas of decreased signal intensity seen on the axial short TR images of the cervical spinal cord probably represent internal areas of calcification.

An ependymoma with metastatic spread to the brain and spinal cord could have a similar appearance.

PEARL
- The entire vertebral canal and intracranial contents should also be evaluated. Magnetic resonance represents the method of choice for follow-up in a patient such as this.

PITFALLS
- Total surgical removal of a tumor such as this is generally not possible.

- These patients may have only minor symptoms relative to the size of the lesion. Surgery may be attempted, primarily for diagnosis of cell type and to dictate treatment. However, surgery is unlikely to be curative with such an extensive lesion.

SPINAL CORD TUMORS

Case 9

Clinical Presentation

The patient is a 34-year-old male with neurofibromatosis type 2 who now presents with upper extremity weakness.

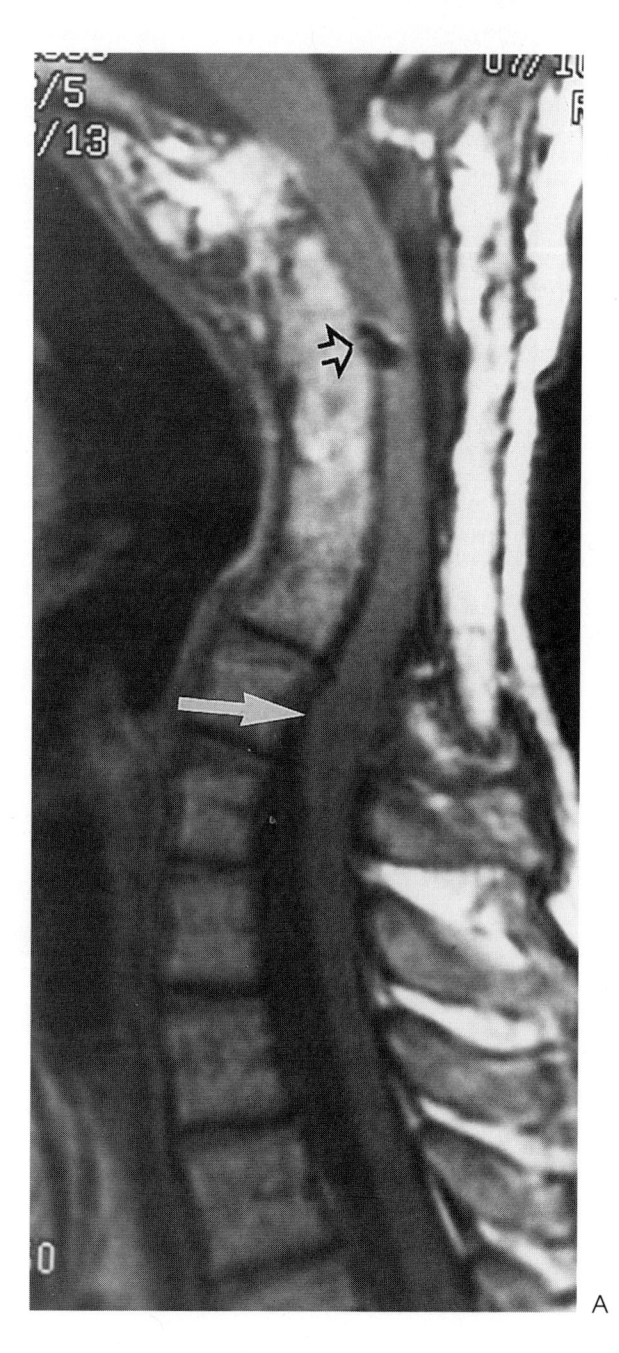

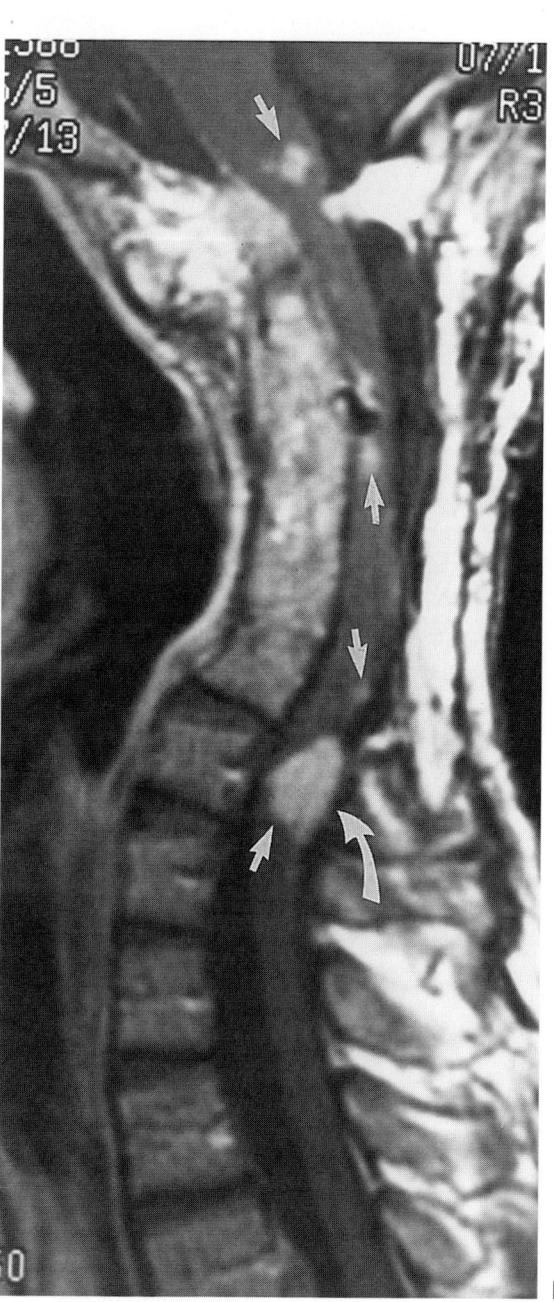

TEACHING ATLAS OF SPINE IMAGING

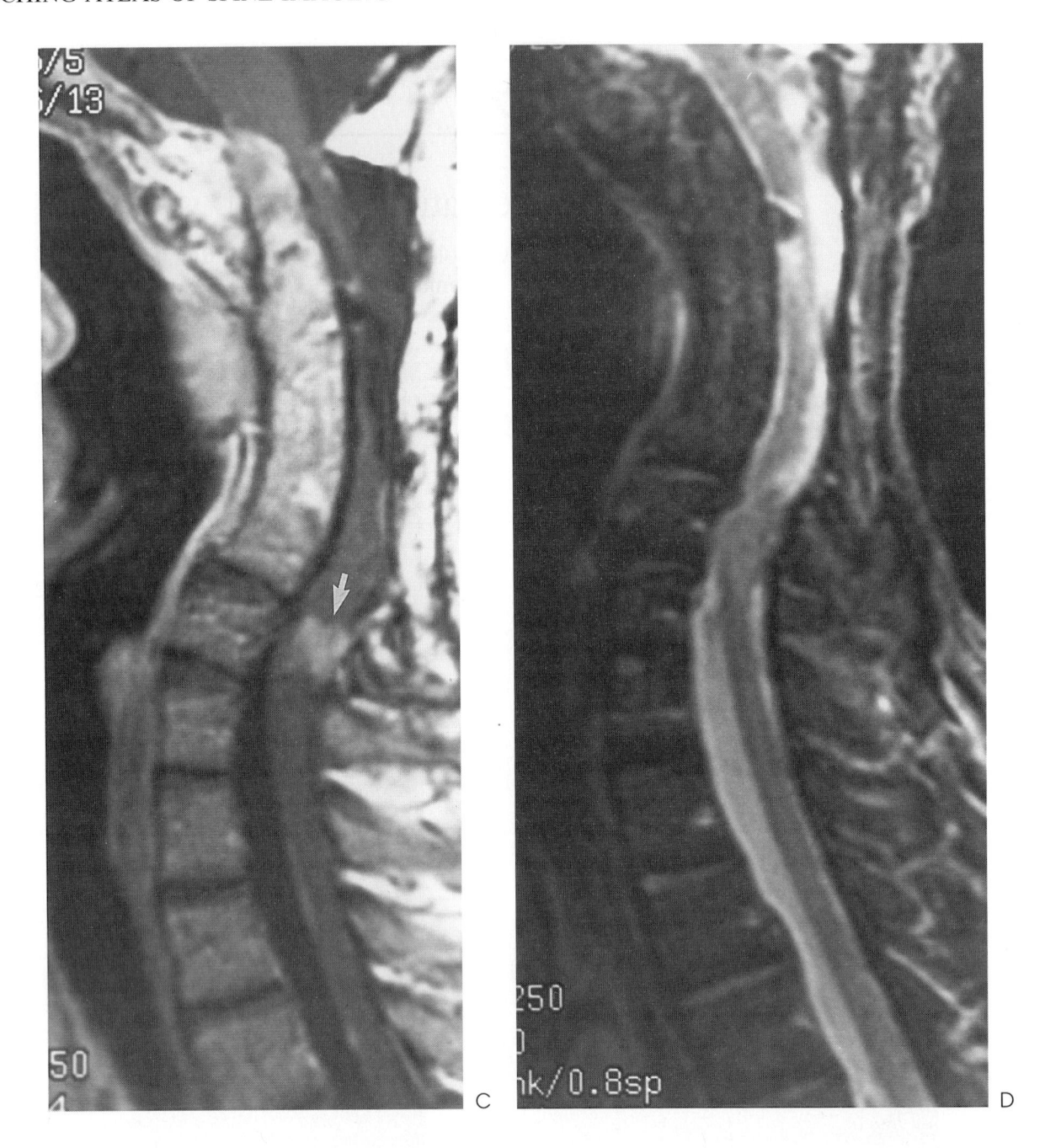

168

SPINAL CORD TUMORS

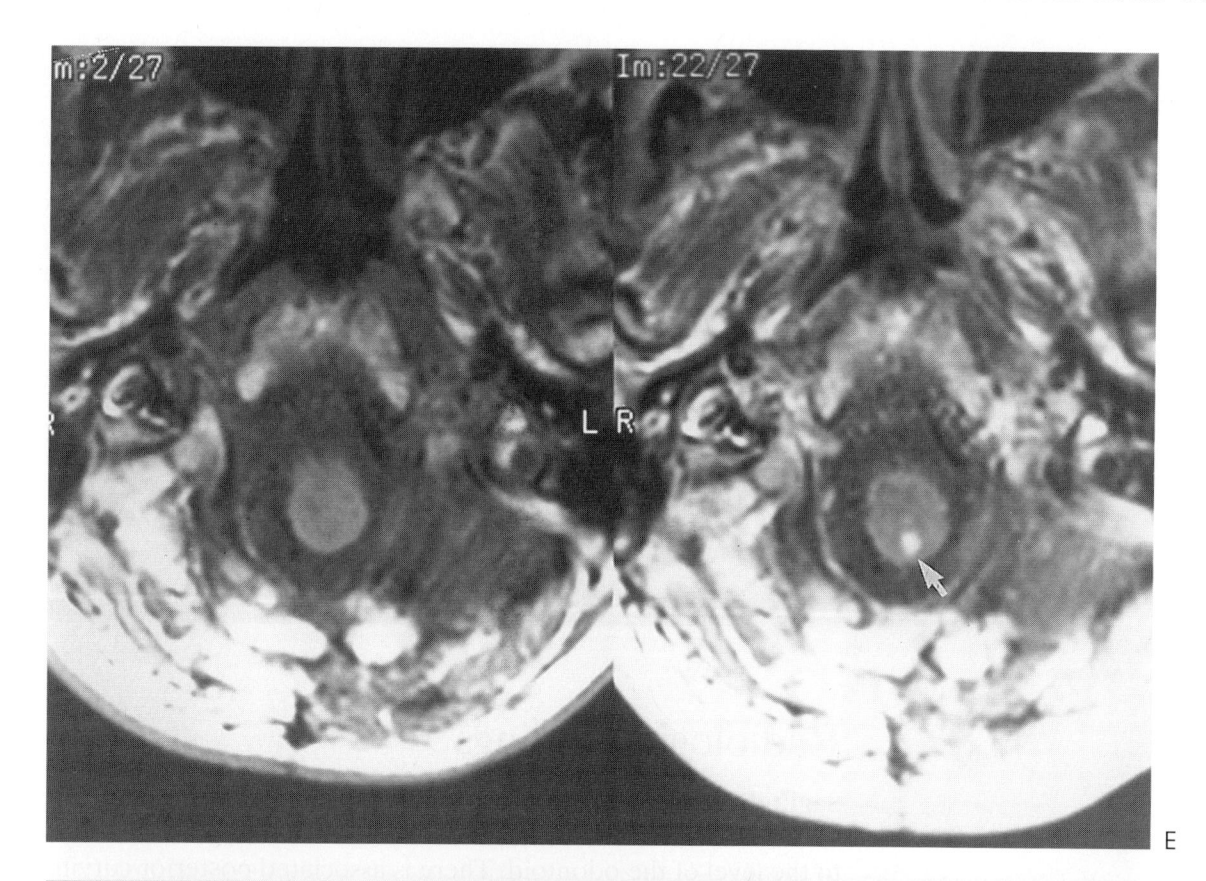

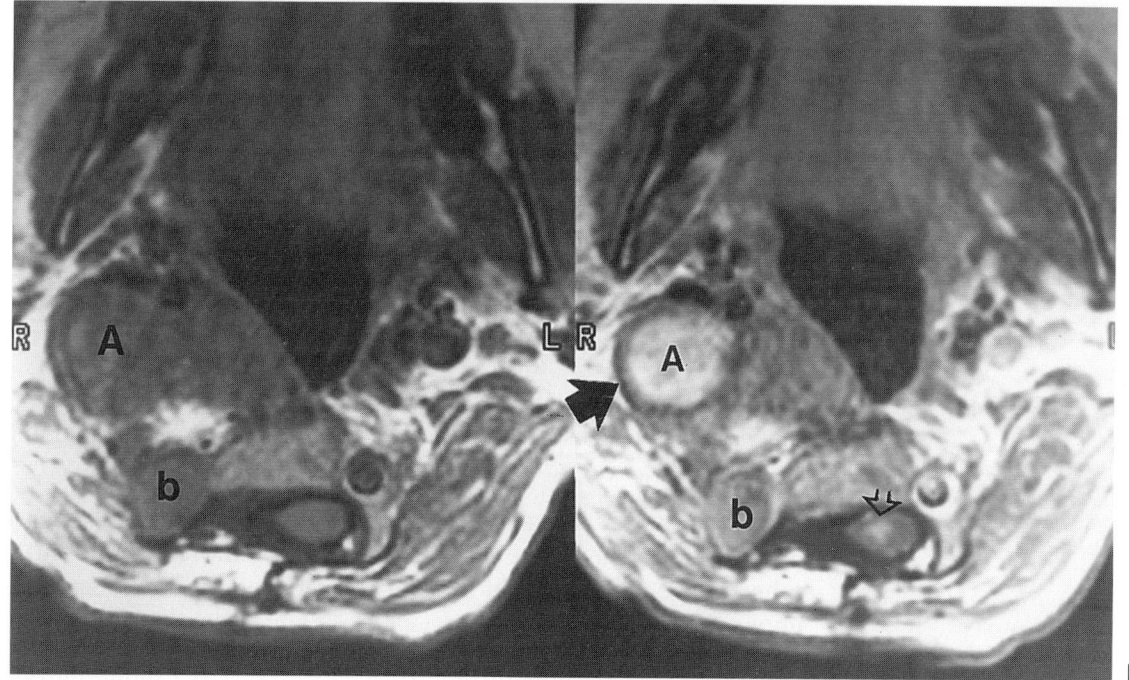

TEACHING ATLAS OF SPINE IMAGING

G

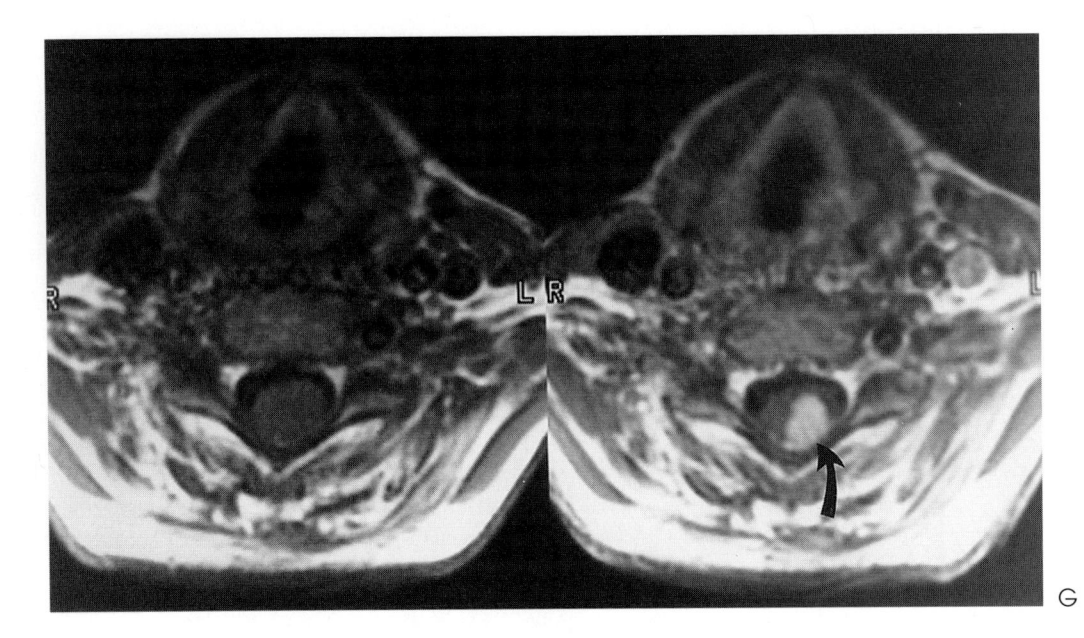

Radiologic Findings

Sagittal short TR image (Fig. A) reveals surgical fusion of multiple cervical vertebral bodies with reversal of the normal cervical lordosis extending up to the level of the odontoid. There is associated posterior curvilinear distortion of the cervical spinal cord. There is a small oval area of decreased signal intensity in the upper cervical region (*open arrow*). There is a focal area of widening of the cervical spinal cord in the upper thoracic region that appears slightly decreased in signal intensity (*solid arrow*). The spinous processes are surgically absent in the cervical region.

Sagittal short TR image postcontrast (Fig. B) reveals enhancement of multiple lesions within the medulla and spinal cord (*straight arrows*). In the lower cervical region, the lesion exhibits an intradural rather than an intramedullary appearance. The mass appears to arise from the dura dorsally (*curved arrow*).

Sagittal short TR image postcontrast (Fig. C) reveals an area of enhancement that appears to arise from the dura posteriorly and to invaginate into the spinal cord (*arrow*).

Sagittal long TR image (Fig. D) reveals that the area of decreased signal intensity anterior to the spinal cord appears more prominent than on the other images. There is an area of focal widening of the spinal cord in the upper thoracic area.

Pre- (Fig. E, *left*) and postcontrast (Fig. E, *right*) axial short TR images reveal a densely enhancing approximately 3-mm nodule within the dorsal portion of the cervical spinal cord (*right, arrow*).

Pre- (Fig. F, *left*) and postcontrast (Fig. F, *right*) axial short TR images reveal a small irregular area of enhancement within the spinal cord (*right, open arrow*). There are also two enhancing soft tissue masses in the neck on the right side (*A, b*). The more anterior lesion (*A*) enhances densely in its central portion and has a decreased signal intensity rim (*right, solid*

SPINAL CORD TUMORS

arrow). There is effacement of the oral pharynx at the level of this mass. The second lesion (*b*) is smaller and arises at the level of the intervertebral foramen.

Pre- (Fig. G, *left*) and postcontrast (Fig. G, *right*) axial short TR images reveal that the spinal cord is enlarged. There is a dense area of enhancement on the postinfusion portion of the study. This area has a slightly irregular peripheral margin and extends to the dorsal surface of the spinal cord adjacent to the dura (*right, curved arrow*).

Diagnosis

Astrocytoma; confirmed at surgery. The tumor arose from within the spinal cord and grew in an exophytic fashion soft tissue schwannomas.

Differential Diagnosis

- ependymoma

Discussion

There is an increased incidence of all types of brain and spinal cord tumors in patients with neurofibromatosis; although the diagnosis was astrocytoma in this patient, ependymoma would be a more likely diagnosis. The exophytic nature of this tumor is unusual. The appearance also suggests that this could be an intradural mass that invaginates into the spinal cord rather than an exophytic tumor growing out of the spinal cord. The decreased signal intensity areas seen in both the short and long TR images anterior to the spinal cord is magnetic susceptibility artifact secondary to the surgical clips from the patient's previous surgery.

The patient also had a history of surgical removal of multiple soft tissue schwannomas and acoustic neuromas. This history of multiple meningiomas and schwannomas is typical for patients with neurofibromatosis type 2; however, a diagnosis of spinal cord ependymoma would be more likely than astrocytoma.

PEARLS

- The preinfusion scans on these patients may be normal, and the enhancing lesions are only visible after the infusion of contrast material.

- Multiplanar imaging with thin slices may be helpful to define the extent of the lesion as well as the anatomic compartment of origin.

PITFALL

- The exophytic portion of the tumor compressed against the dorsal aspect of the vertebral canal, giving the appearance of an intradural mass invaginating into the cervical spinal cord.

- Spinal cord ependymomas in patients with neurofibromatosis may have multiple lesions at various levels, so the entire spinal cord should be evaluated.

- Because seeding may also occur into the spinal subarachnoid space, the entire thecal sac should be evaluated.

Section III

Spinal Cord Tumors

B. Intradural

SPINAL CORD TUMORS

Case 1

Clinical Presentation

The patient is a 29-year-old female with a one-year history of right-sided low back pain.

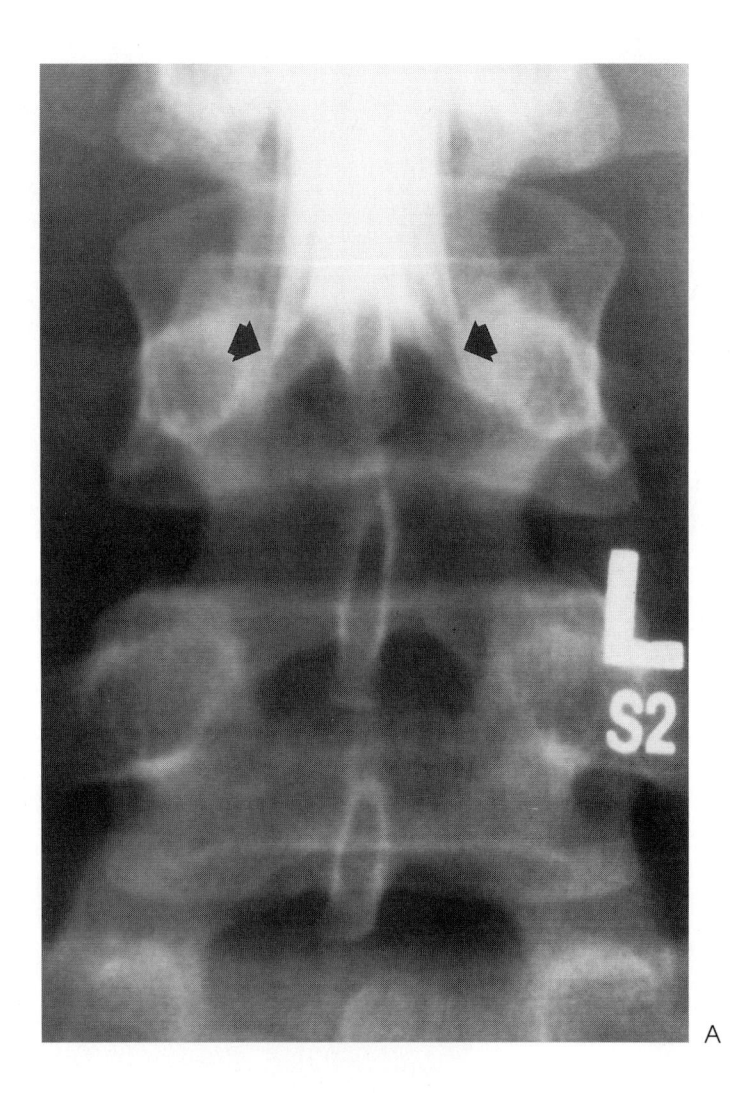

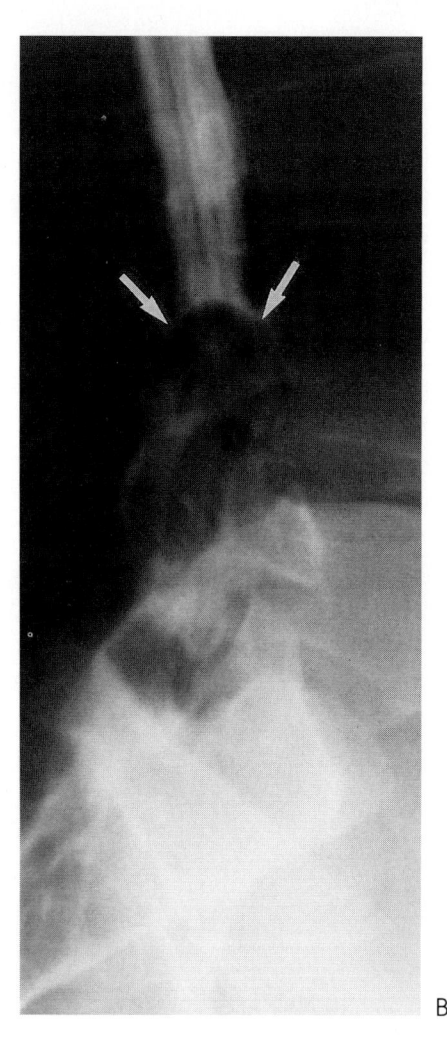

Radiologic Findings

Anteroposterior view of a lumbar myelogram (Fig. A) reveals a complete block to the flow of contrast material at the level of the midbody of L4. There is flaring of the contrast column at this level (*arrows*).

Lateral view of the myelogram (Fig. B) reveals a complete block to the flow of contrast material. There is a upwardly convex soft tissue mass that forms acute angles with the contrast column anteriorly and posteriorly (*arrows*).

TEACHING ATLAS OF SPINE IMAGING

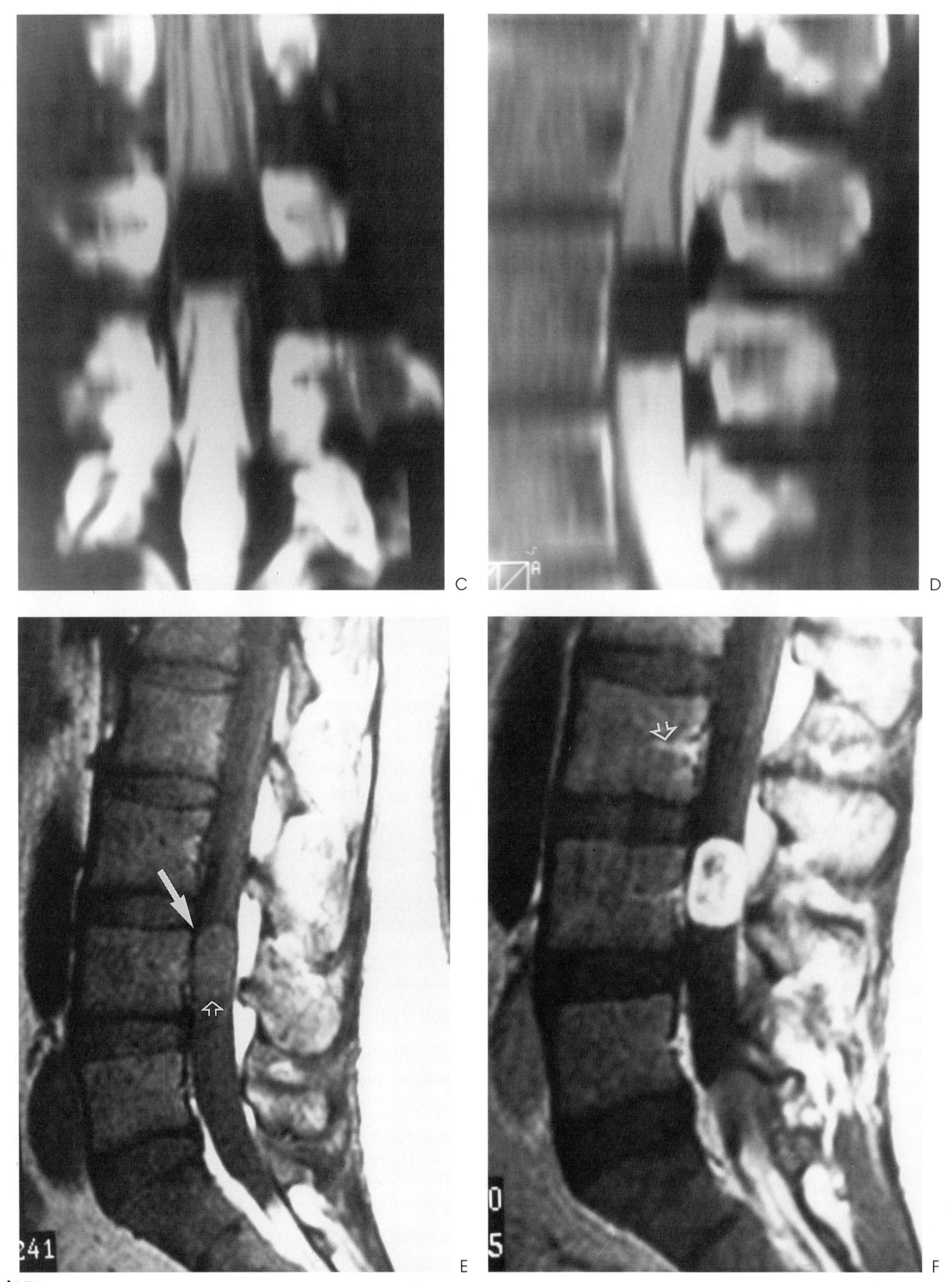

SPINAL CORD TUMORS

Radiologic Findings (continued)

Coronal reconstruction view of the postmyelogram computed tomographic (CT) scan (Fig. C) reveals a filling defect in the contrast column at the L4 level. The nerve roots of the cauda equina are displaced laterally.

Sagittal reconstruction view of the postmyelogram CT (Fig. D) reveals a filling defect in the contrast column at the L4 level. The nerve roots of the cauda equina are displaced dorsally.

Sagittal short TR image (Fig. E) reveals an oval-shaped mass of slightly higher signal intensity than cerebrospinal fluid. The mass exhibits an acute angle with the subarachnoid space at the level of the superior end plate of L4 (*solid arrow*), and the inferior margin is seen at the level of the lower portion of the L4 vertebral body (*open arrow*).

The sagittal short TR image postcontrast enhancement (Fig. F) reveals dense slightly inhomogeneous enhancement of the schwannoma. The normal basivertebral plexus also enhances and is well demonstrated at the L3 level (*arrow*).

Diagnosis

Schwannoma

Differential Diagnosis

- schwannoma
- neurofibroma
- myxopapillary ependymoma
- drop metastasis

Discussion

Schwannomas may be cystic or may reveal central area of necrosis that appear as areas of internal decreased signal intensity as seen in this example. Schwannomas may occur at any level of the spinal cord, but are most common in the lumbar region. They are seen as isolated tumors or in association with neurofibromatosis. They are slightly more common than neurofibromas. Schwannomas, if sufficiently large, could mimic the appearance of a myxopapillary ependymoma. In this case, the differential diagnosis would include schwannoma, solitary neurofibroma, myxopapillary ependymoma, or remotely, a drop metastasis from a central nervous system primary or other metastatic tumor.

PEARLS

- Schwannomas may hemorrhage and therefore may appear increased signal intensity on the preinfusion scan. If hemorrhage is present, a variety of signal intensities with various magnetic resonance image sequences may result.

- The patient with neurofibromatosis type 2 may have multiple schwannomas.

PITFALLS

- A hemorrhagic schwannoma could be mistaken for a hematoma. However, in the patient with a hematoma, one would anticipate a history of recent spinal tap, spinal anesthesia, or other type of spinal trauma.

- In some cases, the soft tissue mass may be very subtle on the precontrast images, and it is possible to overlook the presence of such a mass. Therefore, careful evaluation should be performed when necessary.

TEACHING ATLAS OF SPINE IMAGING

Case 2

Clinical Presentation

The patient is a 47-year-old female school teacher with a history of Hodgkin's disease who has had increasing lower extremity weakness.

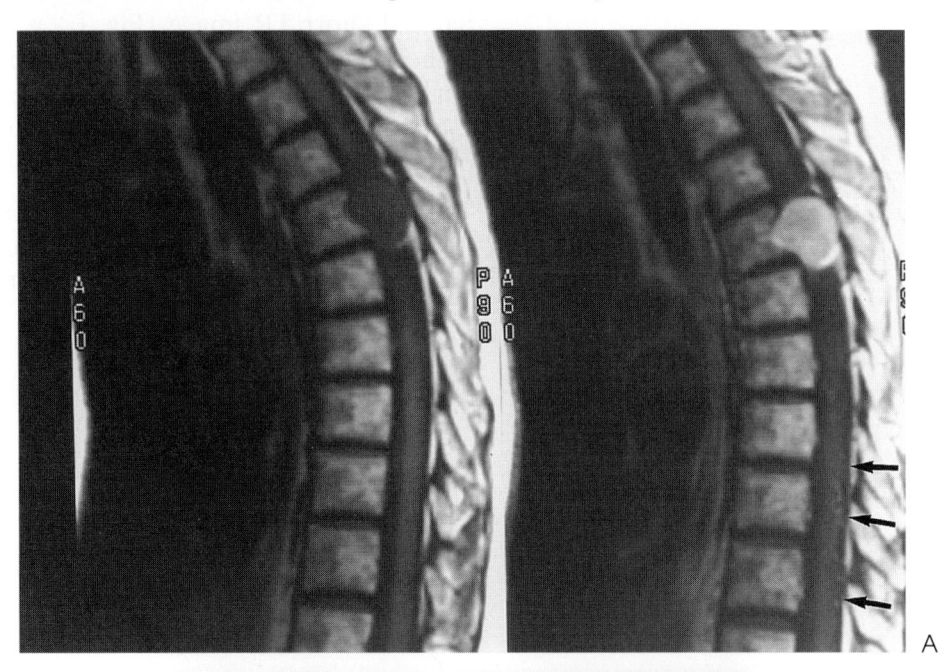

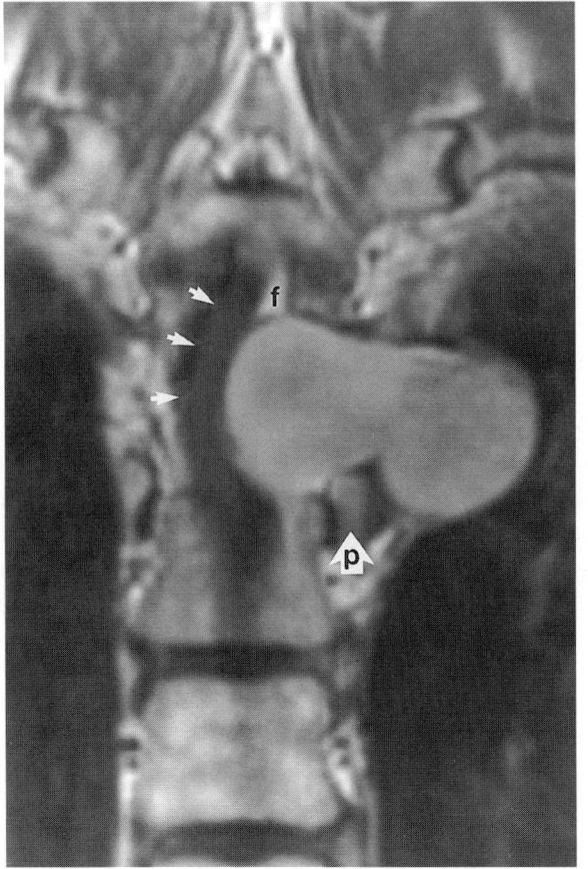

SPINAL CORD TUMORS

Radiologic Findings

Pre- (Fig. A, *left*) and postcontrast (Fig. A, *right*) sagittal short TR images reveal a slightly lobulated area of soft tissue signal intensity at the T6 level. There is curvilinear erosion of the posterior margin of the vertebral body at this level. Neither the spinal cord nor the dorsal epidural fat can be seen at this level. The postcontrast study reveals dense homogeneous enhancement of the mass. There are small curvilinear and dot like areas of enhancement below the level of the mass (*right, arrows*).

Coronal short TR image postcontrast (Fig. B) reveals enhancement of the bilobed mass. The spinal cord is displaced to the right (*small arrows*). Epidural fat (*f*) is seen above the level of the mass. The pedicle projects below the mass on the left side (*p/arrow*).

Diagnosis

Isolated schwannoma

Differential Diagnosis

- neurofibroma

Discussion

The tumor appears bilobed at the point where it extends through the intervertebral foramen, forming a typical dumbbell appearance. The mass is both intradural and extradural. The epidural fat is widened on the side of the lesion because the dura is displaced away from the lateral aspect of the vertebral canal. The faint curvilinear areas of enhancement seen below the mass represent dilated vessels on the dorsal aspect of the spinal cord.

A neurofibroma could also have this appearance. Neurofibromas are typically multiple and are seen in the clinical setting of neurofibromatosis type 1.

PEARLS

- Schwannomas may be solitary or multiple. Solitary neurofibromas are rare.

- A meningioma could rarely have this appearance, but it is very unlikely because typically meningiomas do not have an extradural component or the "dumbbell" appearance seen in this case.

PITFALL

- Because neurofibromas are rarely solitary, the entire length of the vertebral canal should be evaluated.

TEACHING ATLAS OF SPINE IMAGING

Case 3

Clinical Presentation

The patient is an 86-year-old male with known multiple myeloma and new complaints of gradual onset of progressive low back pain.

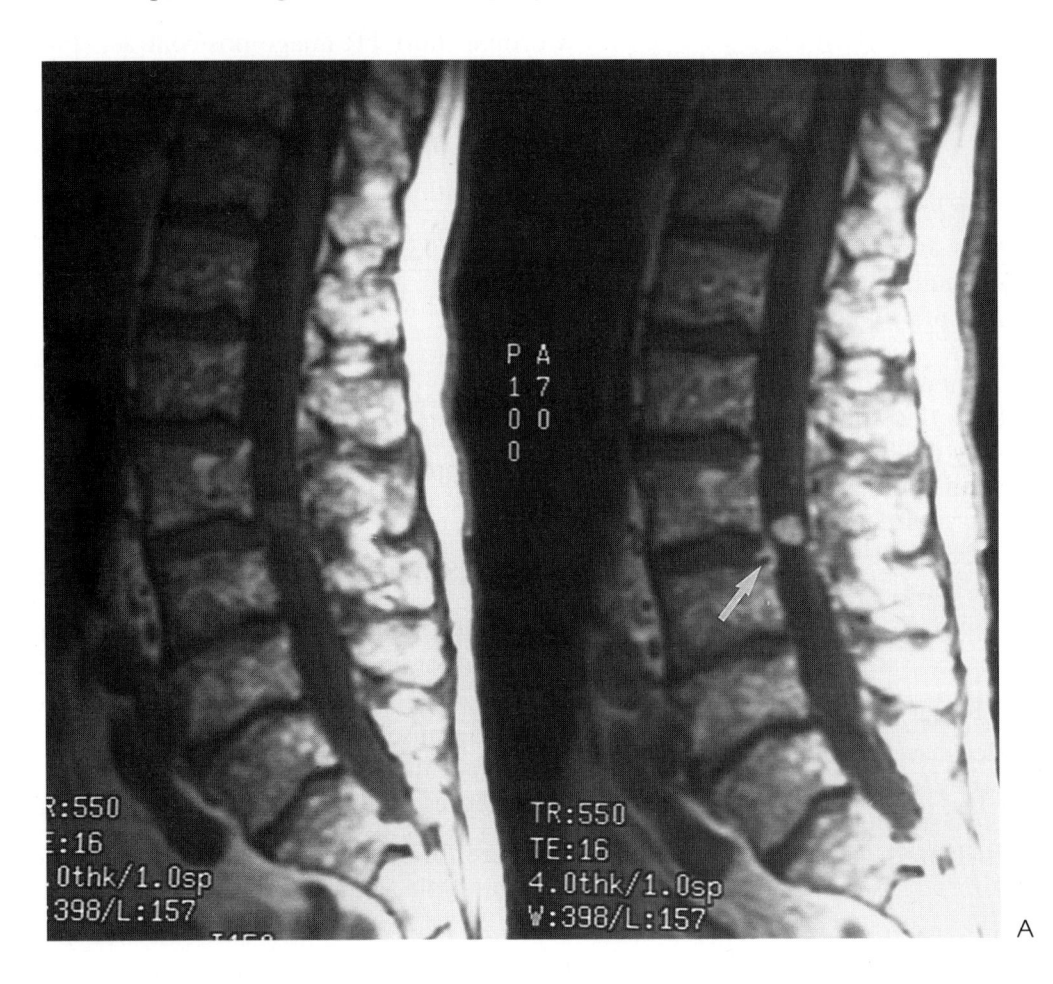

Radiologic Findings

Pre- (Fig. A, *left*) and postcontrast (Fig. A, *right*) sagittal short TR images in the lumbar region. There is a faint rounded area, approximately 8 mm at its greatest diameter, at the L2-3 level in the middle of the vertebral canal. After the infusion of contrast material, there is dense enhancement of the slightly irregularly marginated mass. The marrow within the vertebral bodies and spinous processes exhibits diffuse mottled signal intensity.

SPINAL CORD TUMORS

PEARLS

- Multiple myeloma is occasionally better seen by computed tomographic (CT) scanning than magnetic resonance (MR) imaging because CT may demonstrate the areas of cortical bone destruction that cannot be appreciated by MR scanning.

- The back pain in this patient was probably due to the schwannoma, although multiple myeloma may also cause low back pain.

- If there is question or concern regarding the clinical condition in this patient, a follow-up MR study with contrast enhancement is an excellent, noninvasive method of follow-up.

PITFALLS

- The mottled pattern of decreased signal intensity could be mistaken for the mottled increased signal intensity of osteoporosis.

- A solitary neurofibroma could have a similar appearance but would be unlikely in this patient.

Diagnosis

Schwannoma; multiple myeloma.

Differential Diagnosis

- schwannoma

- metastatic disease

Discussion

The rounded dense pattern of enhancement is typical of schwannoma. The clinical history of multiple myeloma in this patient is helpful to arrive at a correct diagnosis. The densely enhancing lesion is independent of the diagnosis of multiple myeloma. The entire vertebral column should be evaluated to search for additional lesions and pathologic fractures and to rule out cord compression.

In this patient, there are also areas of degenerative change. There is a slight anterior spondylolisthesis of L2 on L3 and slight enhancement of the disc posteriorly at the L2-3 level (*right, arrow*). There is disc space narrowing at the L3-4 through L5-S1 levels secondary to degenerative disc disease.

Differential diagnosis in this patient would include metastatic prostate carcinoma. Small diffuse metastases from any primary tumor could have a similar appearance.

Case 4

Clinical Presentation

The patient is a 76-year-old female with a 10-year history of back pain that was recently exacerbated.

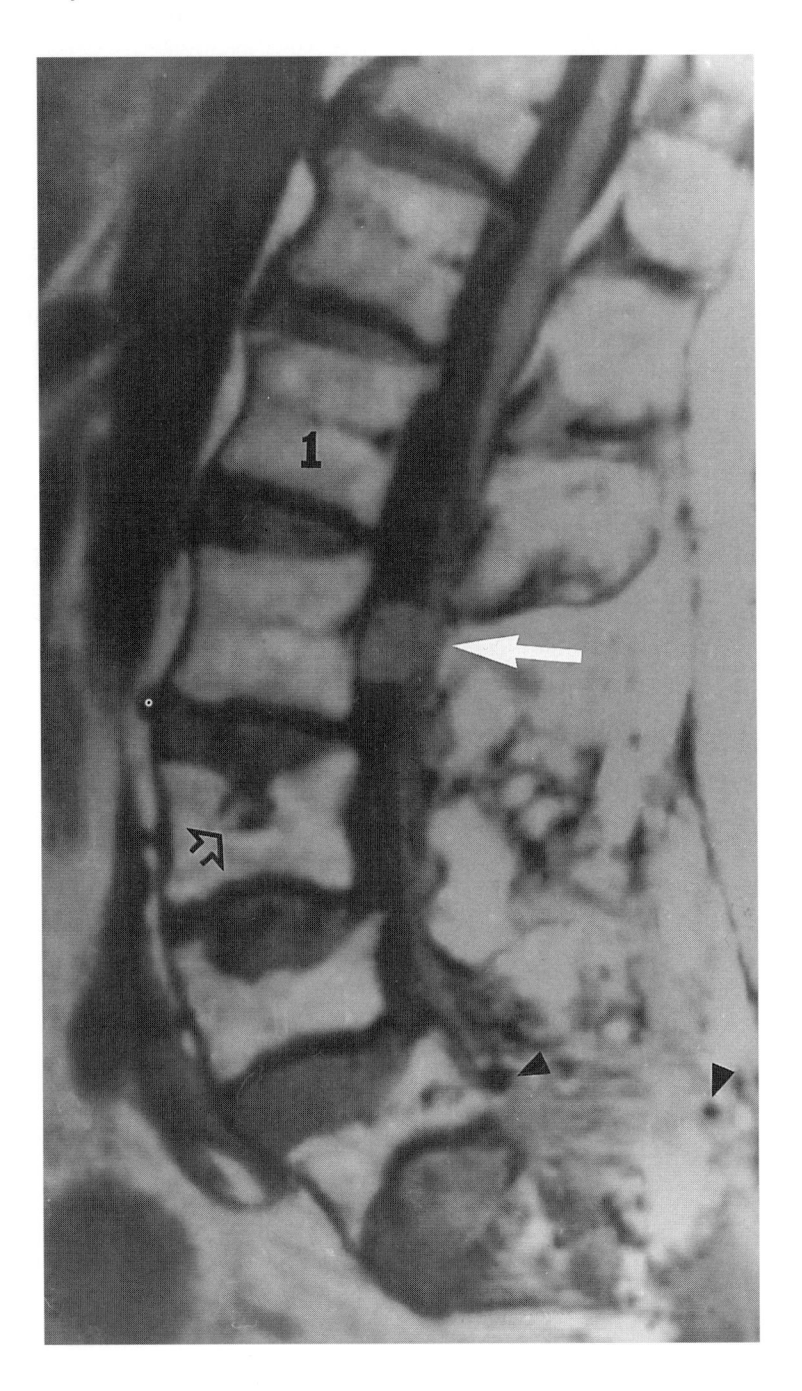

SPINAL CORD TUMORS

Radiologic Findings

Sagittal short TR image without contrast material (Fig. A) reveals an approximately 9-mm oval soft tissue mass in the midportion of the vertebral canal at the L2 level (*white arrow*). A polypoid defect is visible in the superior end plate of the L3 vertebral body (*open arrow*). There is diffuse increase in signal intensity in the marrow of all the visualized vertebral bodies. Compression fractures of the L3, L4, and L5 vertebral bodies can be seen. There is anterior spondylolisthesis with forward displacement of L4 on L5; this is secondary to interfacet degenerative changes. In addition, there are small rounded areas of decreased signal intensity in the soft tissues of the back at the L5-S1 level (*arrowheads*). The L1 vertebral body is identified with 1.

Diagnosis

Schwannoma at L3; osteoporosis; postoperative changes.

Differential Diagnosis

- schwannoma
- drop metastasis
- epidermoid

Discussion

This patient has an isolated schwannoma. The nerve roots of the cauda equina are displaced posteriorly in the vertebral canal. There is a Schmorl's node deformity in the superior end plate of the L3 vertebral body. This occurred because the end plate was weak, the nucleus pulposus fractured the end plate, and it herniated into the vertebral body. There are benign compression fractures of the lowest three lumbar vertebral bodies.

The postoperative changes in the lower lumbar region are secondary to laminectomy. The very low signal intensity rounded areas are secondary to magnetic susceptibility artifact because of the previous surgery. These changes may be seen even if no metallic clips are visible on plain film evaluation.

Osteoporosis results in an increase in the amount of adipose tissue within the vertebral body. Fat is high signal intensity on short TR images, so all the vertebrae appear as increased signal intensity. The vertebrae are weaker when there is osteoporosis, so benign compression fractures may occur.

This appearance is typical of a schwannoma, and it is the most likely diagnosis. However, a drop metastasis from a primary tumor such as breast or lung carcinoma could have a similar appearance, as could metastatic melanoma. An epidermoid secondary to previous spinal tap might also have a similar appearance.

PEARLS

- Multiplanar imaging should be performed to identify the laterality of the lesion so that a surgical approach can be performed appropriately.

PITFALLS

- This schwannoma could potentially have been present at the time of the patient's previous surgery.

- When evaluating a patient for low back pain, the imaging should include up to the T10 vertebral body because a mass as high as T10 may cause symptoms that mimic the low back pain of lumbar disc disease.

- This evaluation may be performed with magnetic resonance imaging and should also be performed in the patient who has had a myelogram.

TEACHING ATLAS OF SPINE IMAGING

Case 5

Clinical Presentation

The patient is a 33-year-old female with clinical myelopathy presenting with lower extremity weakness. The imaging study was performed to rule out demyelinating disease.

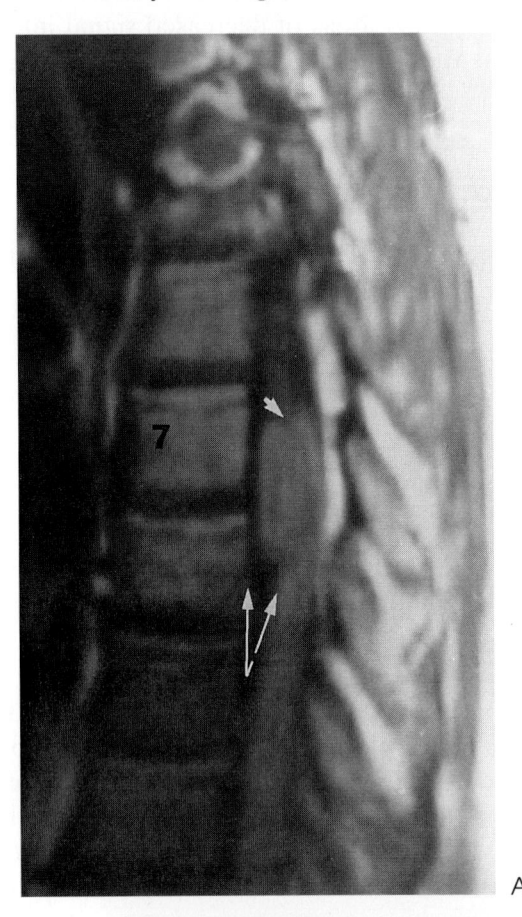

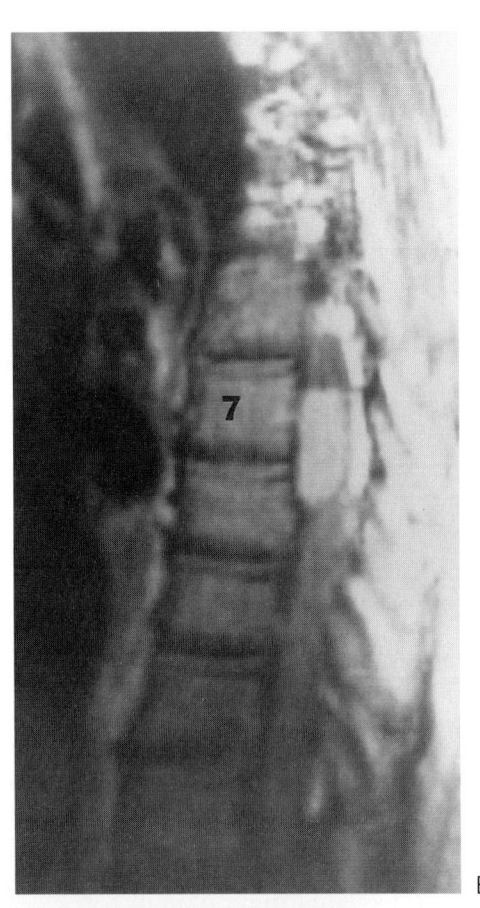

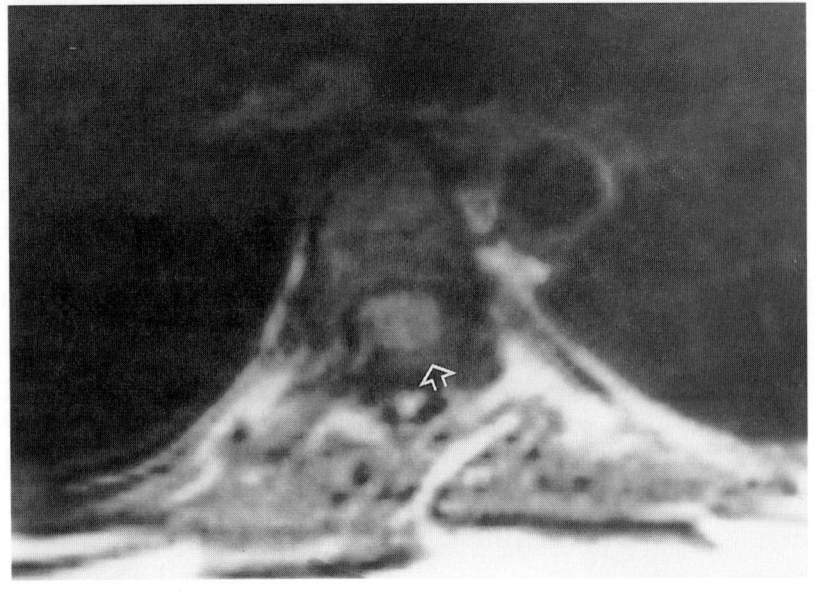

A

B

C

SPINAL CORD TUMORS

PEARLS
- The convex "meniscus" sign is typical for an intradural lesion.

- Myelography may be performed; however, in a case such as this, the myelogram would need to be performed via both a lumbar and a cervical spinal tap with instillation of contrast material. Magnetic resonance scanning is the better method of evaluation and is essentially noninvasive.

PITFALLS
- Note that in one plane the spinal cord will appear displaced away from the mass and compressed by the mass, while in the opposite plane the spinal cord will appear widened because it is compressed and flattened. Therefore, it is vital to obtain orthogonal views to prove that the mass is arising outside of the spinal cord and not from within the spinal cord.

- Meningiomas may calcify, and areas of calcification may be identified by computed tomographic scanning, rarely by plain film evaluation.

Radiologic Findings

Sagittal short TR image (Fig. A) reveals an oval-shaped soft tissue mass in the midthoracic area that displaces the spinal cord posteriorly. The mass forms an acute angle with the spinal cord anteriorly (*short arrow*). There is widening of the subarachnoid space (*double arrow*) on top of the mass. Similar changes are also present below the mass. The T7 vertebral body is identified with 7.

Sagittal short TR image after the infusion of contrast material (Fig. B) reveals dense homogeneous enhancement of the mass. The mass is at the level of the T7 vertebral body (7).

Axial short TR image postcontrast (Fig. C) reveals dense enhancement of the mass, which is anterior to the spinal cord. The spinal cord is an intermediate signal intensity structure that is compressed into a crescentic shaped dorsal to the mass (*arrow*).

Diagnosis

Meningioma, confirmed at surgery.

Differential Diagnosis

- meningioma
- schwannoma

Discussion

The thoracic region is the typical location of these spinal cord meningiomas, 80% of which are found in women. The appearance is typical of an intradural mass. These masses arise from the dura and displace the spinal cord away from the site of origin. The cerebrospinal fluid space is widened on the side of the tumor, and the spinal cord is compressed and displaced by the tumor. A schwannoma could have this appearance, but is less likely.

Spinal meningiomas may exhibit a dual tail sign similar to that seen with cerebral meningiomas.

TEACHING ATLAS OF SPINE IMAGING

Case 6

Clinical Presentation

The patient is a 57-year-old female with a history of progressive lower extremity weakness and unsteady gait.

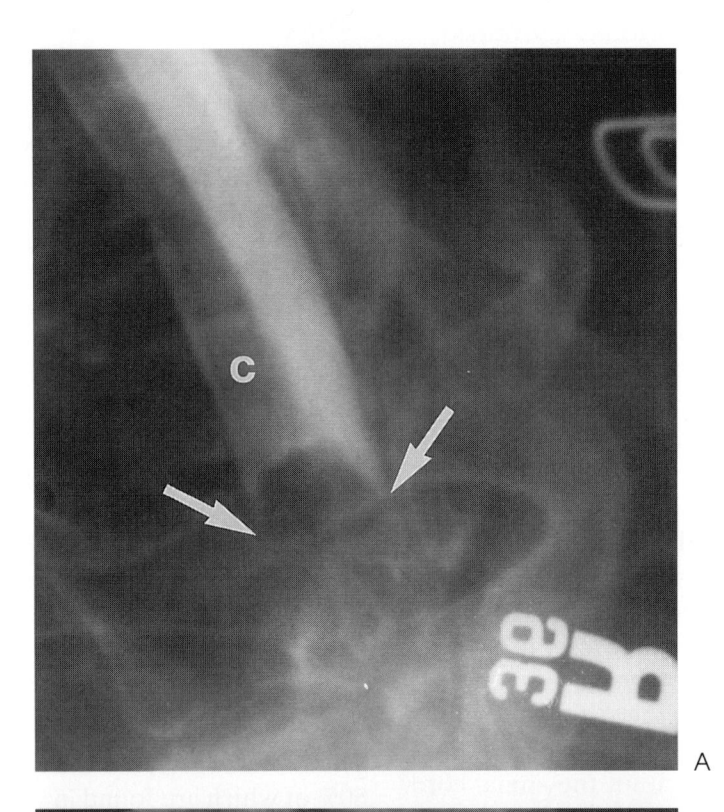

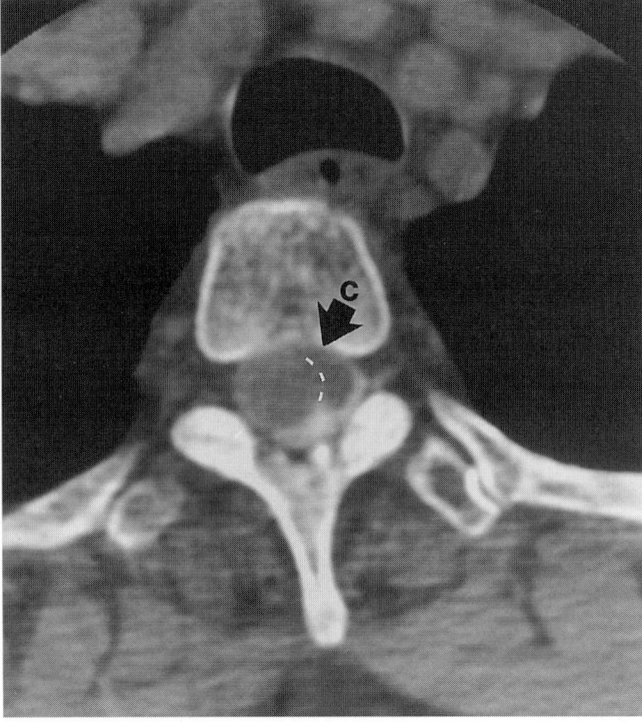

SPINAL CORD TUMORS

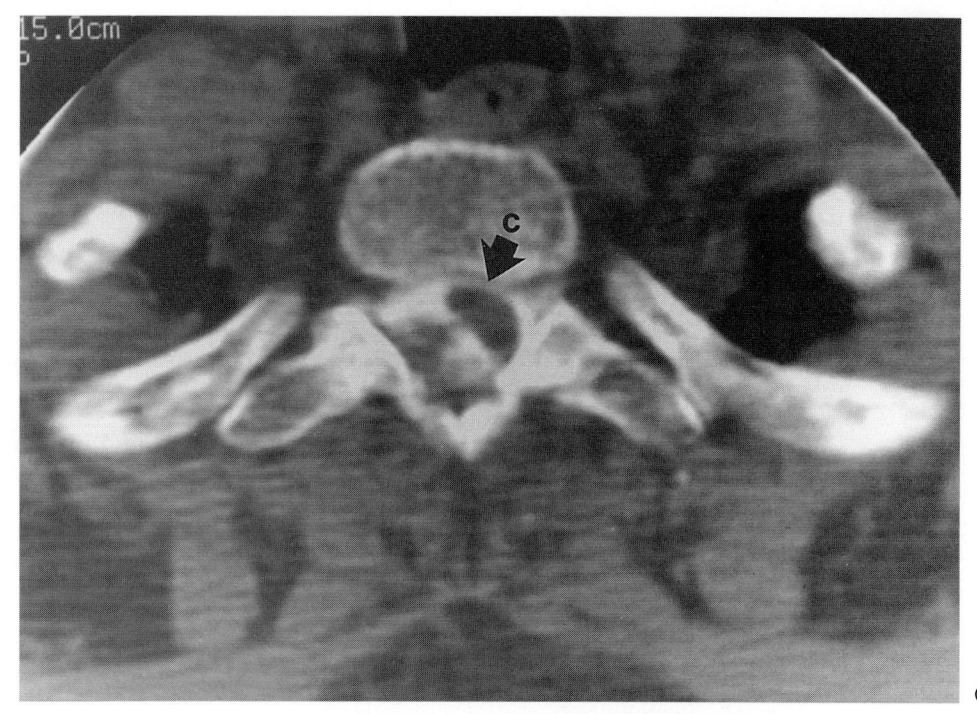

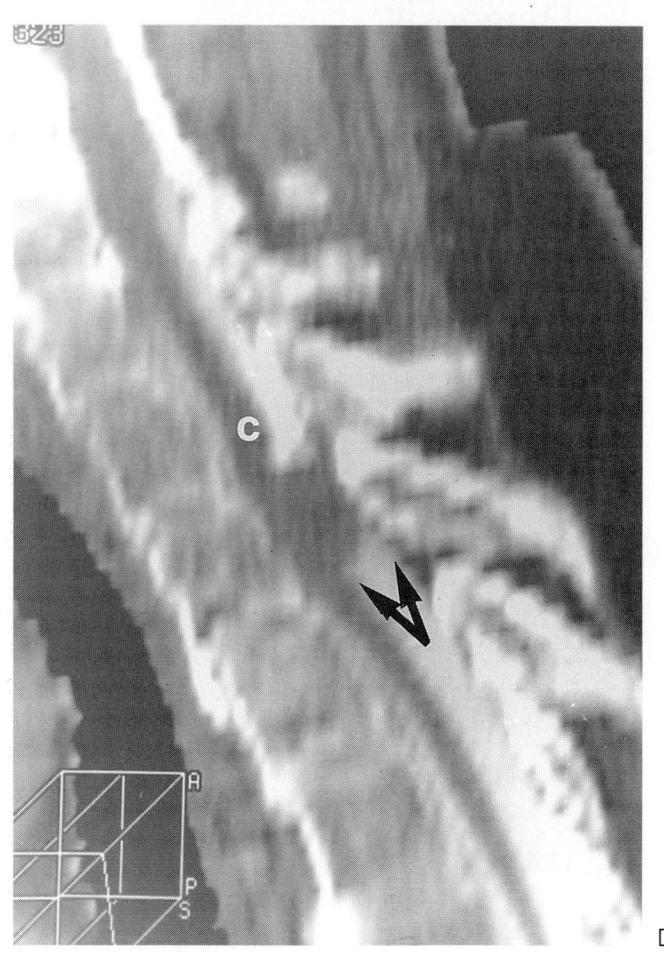

Radiologic Findings

Lateral view of a myelogram performed via cervical tap (Fig. A) reveals a mass with an upwardly convex border that forms an acute angle with the margins of the dura anteriorly and posteriorly (*arrows*). The spinal cord (*c*) is displaced anteriorly. The contrast-filled subarachnoid space is widened dorsally.

Axial computed tomographic (CT) scan at the level of the mass (Fig. B) reveals the spinal cord (*c-arrow*) displaced toward the left side. The dotted line marks the interface between the mass and the spinal cord.

Axial postmyelogram CT scan just above the level of the mass (Fig. C) reveals the spinal cord (*c-arrow*), which is flattened into an oval shape and displaced to the left. The top of the mass is visible in the subarachnoid space on the right side.

Sagittal reconstruction view of the postmyelogram CT scan again (Fig. D) reveals the spinal cord displaced anteriorly (*c*) and the widening of the contrast-filled subarachnoid space posteriorly (*arrows*).

Diagnosis

Meningioma.

Differential Diagnosis

- meningioma
- schwannoma
- drop metastasis

Discussion

The age and gender of the patient as well as the location of the mass make the diagnosis of meningioma the most likely diagnosis. A schwannoma could also have this appearance. A drop metastasis could also have a similar appearance, but the latter two diagnoses are less likely than meningioma.

The appearance of this meningioma visualized by myelography is very similar to the patient illustrated in case 5.

PEARLS

- The appearance is typical for a meningioma.

- Magnetic resonance imaging with contrast enhancement with multiplanar imaging is the procedure of choice for diagnosis and evaluation of a patient with any type of spine or spinal cord tumor.

PITFALLS

- The postmyelogram CT scan helps to define both the upper and lower margins of the mass so that surgery can be planned appropriately.

- If a myelogram is performed via lumbar spinal tap, care should be taken to remove only a very small amount of contrast material. If there is complete block to flow of contrast material, removal of a large amount of contrast may make the patient's condition worse because of the creation of a vacuum below the level of the block.

SPINAL CORD TUMORS

Case 7

Clinical Presentation

The patient is a 20-year-old male with urinary retention, back pain, and impotence.

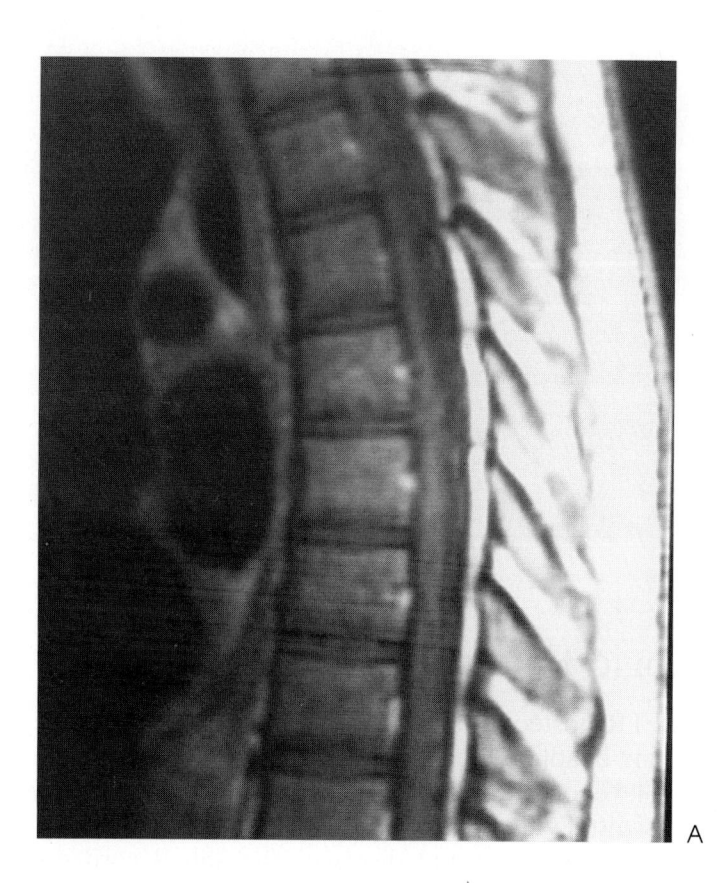

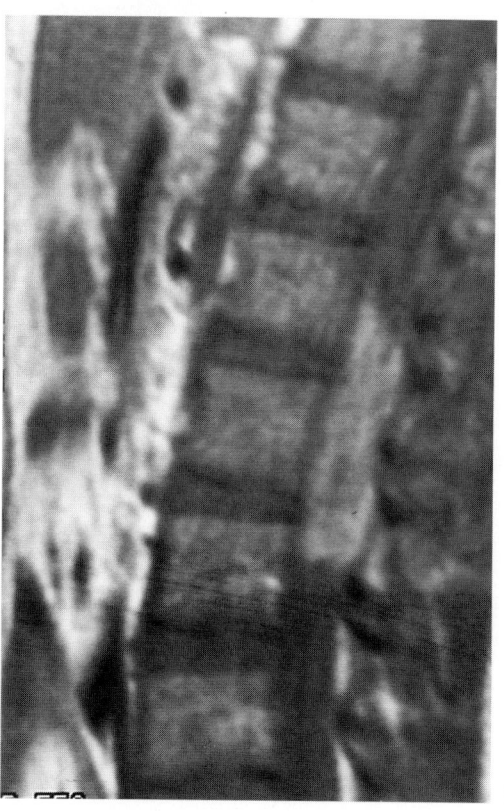

Radiologic Findings

Sagittal short TR postcontrast image (Fig. A) reveals a normal appearing upper and midthoracic spinal cord. There are multiple small rounded, bead-like areas of enhancement along the dorsal aspect of the spinal cord in the lower thoracic region (*thin arrow*). In the very low thoracic spine region, there is an intradural slightly irregularly enhancing mass anterior to the spinal cord in the low thoracic/upper lumbar region (*thick arrow*). The spinal cord is displaced posteriorly and compressed. The subarachnoid space is widened anterior to the spinal cord and the spinal cord is compressed.

Sagittal short TR image postcontrast (Fig. B) reveals dense homogeneous enhancement of the mass, which extends from the level of the midbody of L1 through the midbody of L3.

TEACHING ATLAS OF SPINE IMAGING

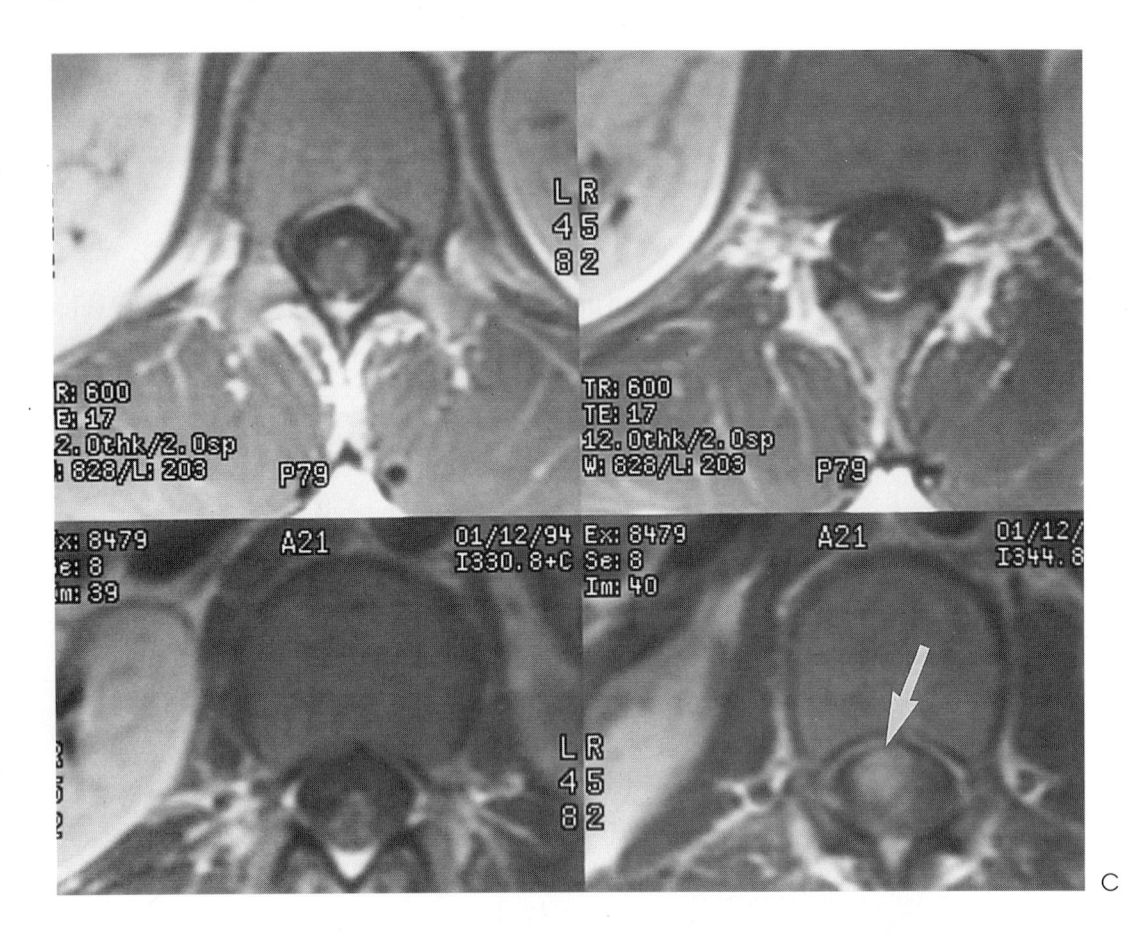

Radiologic Findings (continued)

Axial short TR postcontrast images in the lower thoracic region (Fig. C) reveal the tiny beadlike areas of enhancement on the surface of the spinal cord. At the level of T12-L1, the enhancing mass (*lower right, arrow*) visualized on the sagittal view is also seen on the axial view. The mass is approximately 1 cm in diameter and displaces the spinal cord posteriorly. The cerebrospinal fluid-filled subarachnoid space is almost completely obliterated.

SPINAL CORD TUMORS

PEARL
- The location and enhancing characteristics are typical for a myxopapillary ependymoma.

PITFALL
- Care must be taken to evaluate the entire visualized length of the spinal cord and spinal subarachnoid space. In this example, the abnormality was initially visualized only at the very inferior margin of the image.

Diagnosis

Myxopapillary ependymoma.

Differential Diagnosis

- myxopapillary ependymoma
- drop metastasis

Discussion

This appearance is typical of myxopapillary ependymoma. These ependymomas may also contain areas of hemorrhage and so may appear as decreased signal intensity on both the short and long TR images. A drop metastasis from a primary central nervous system tumor such as medulloblastoma, ependymoma, or pinealoma could also have a similar appearance.

TEACHING ATLAS OF SPINE IMAGING

Case 8

Clinical Presentation

The patient is a 35-year-old male with a history of low back pain and impotence.

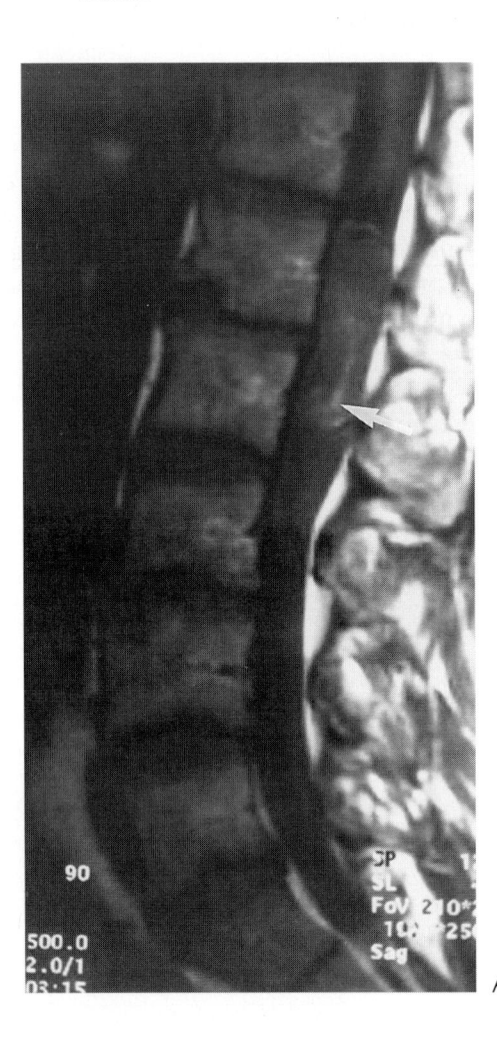

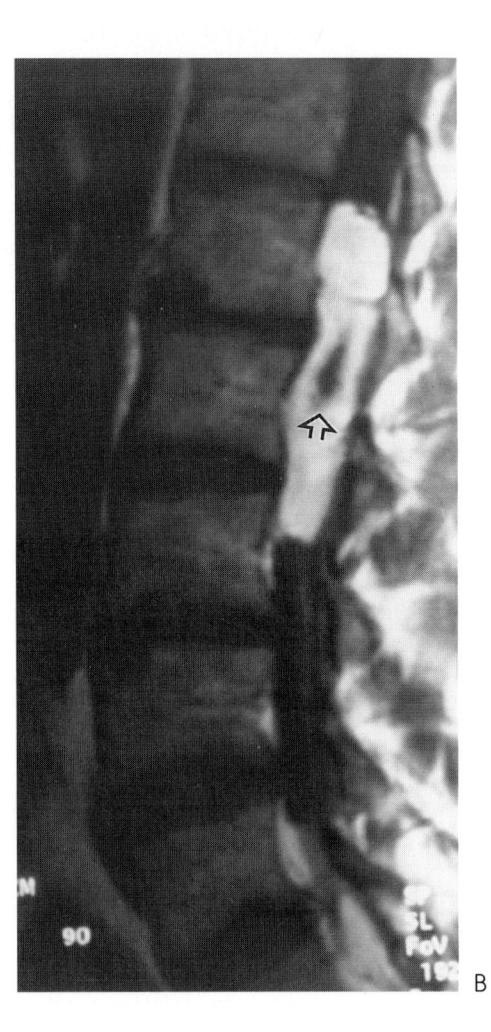

Radiologic Findings

Sagittal short TR image in the lumbar region (Fig. A) reveals a mottled area of slight increased and decreased signal intensity that begins at the level of the superior end plate of L1 and extends to the midbody of L2. Areas of increased signal intensity are seen in the lower portion of the mass (*arrow*).

Sagittal short TR image postcontrast (Fig. B) reveals dense enhancement of the mass. There is a remaining area of persistent decreased signal intensity within the central portion of the mass (*arrow*).

SPINAL CORD TUMORS

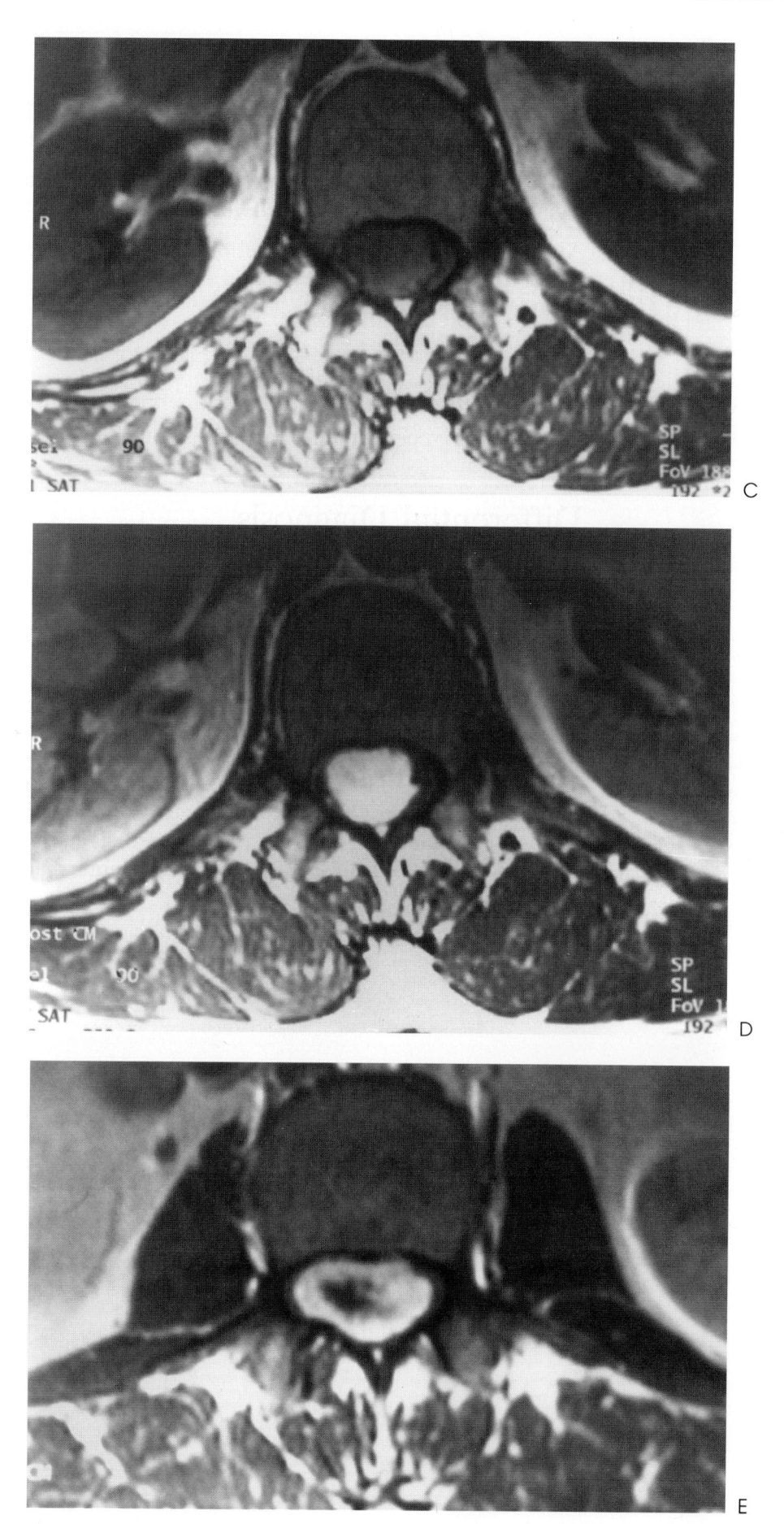

C

D

E

193

TEACHING ATLAS OF SPINE IMAGING

Radiologic Findings (continued)

Axial short TR image preinfusion (Fig. C) reveals a slightly inhomogeneous mass that is located in the right side of the vertebral canal.

Axial short TR image postcontrast (Fig. D) reveals dense homogeneous enhancement of the mass, which fills the entire vertebral canal.

Axial short TR image at the level of the midportion of this mass (Fig. E) reveals the central area of decreased signal intensity. This area has a slightly irregular peripheral margin.

Diagnosis

Myxopapillary ependymoma with areas of hemorrhage.

Differential Diagnosis

- myxopapillary ependymoma

Discussion

The age and appearance of the mass are typical of the diagnosis of myxopapillary ependymoma. The elongated appearance is because the mass takes on the configuration of the lumbar vertebral canal. Metastases from these tumors may occur and can be quite extensive, occupying the entire spinal subarachnoid space. Therefore, the length of the spinal subarachnoid space should be evaluated. The areas of increased signal intensity on the short TR images are presumably related to areas of hemorrhage with methemoglobin formation.

PEARL
- The area of decreased signal intensity is consistent with an area of hemorrhage, and the presence of this type of hemorrhage is very typical of ependymoma in the lumbar region.

PITFALL
- Calcification could also give the appearance of decreased signal intensity within the mass, but would be much less likely than hemorrhage. Areas of calcification may also exhibit areas of increased signal intensity on short TR images secondary to the paradoxical effect related to the chemical composition of the areas of calcification.

SPINAL CORD TUMORS

Case 9

Clinical Presentation

The patient is an 18-year-old male with low back pain and urinary retention.

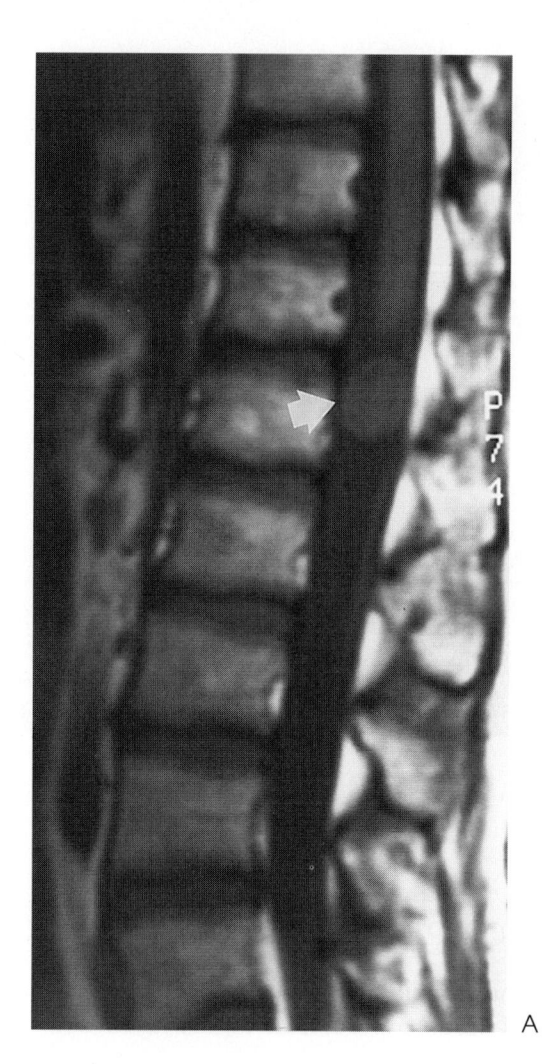

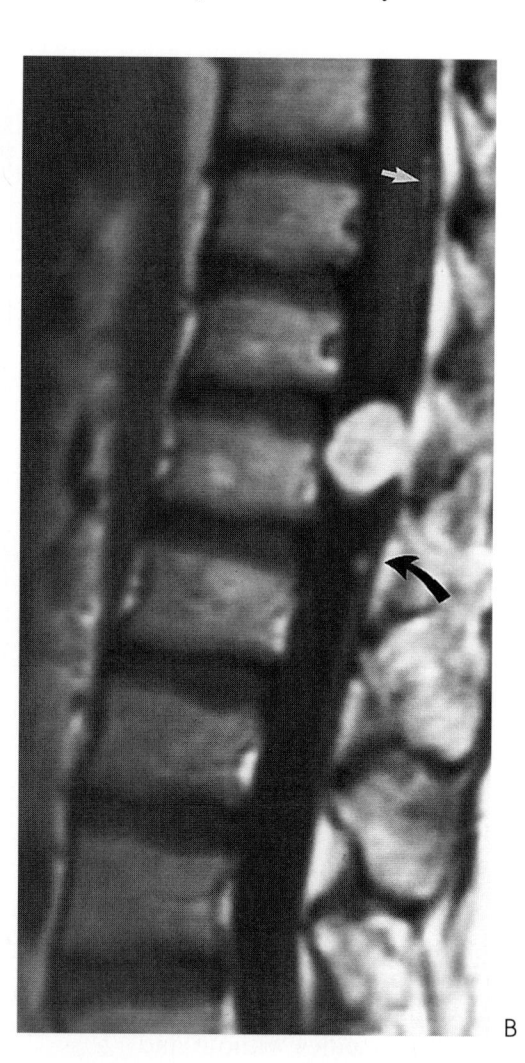

Radiologic Findings

Sagittal short TR image (Fig. A) reveals an isointense, slightly elongated rounded soft tissue mass in the vertebral canal at the level of L1 (*arrow*).

Sagittal short TR image postcontrast (Fig. B) reveals dense, slightly inhomogeneous enhancement of the soft tissue mass. Above the level of the mass, there is a streaklike area of enhancement along the dorsal aspect of the distal spinal cord (*white arrow*). Below the mass, there is a second rounded area of enhancement (*black curved arrow*).

TEACHING ATLAS OF SPINE IMAGING

C

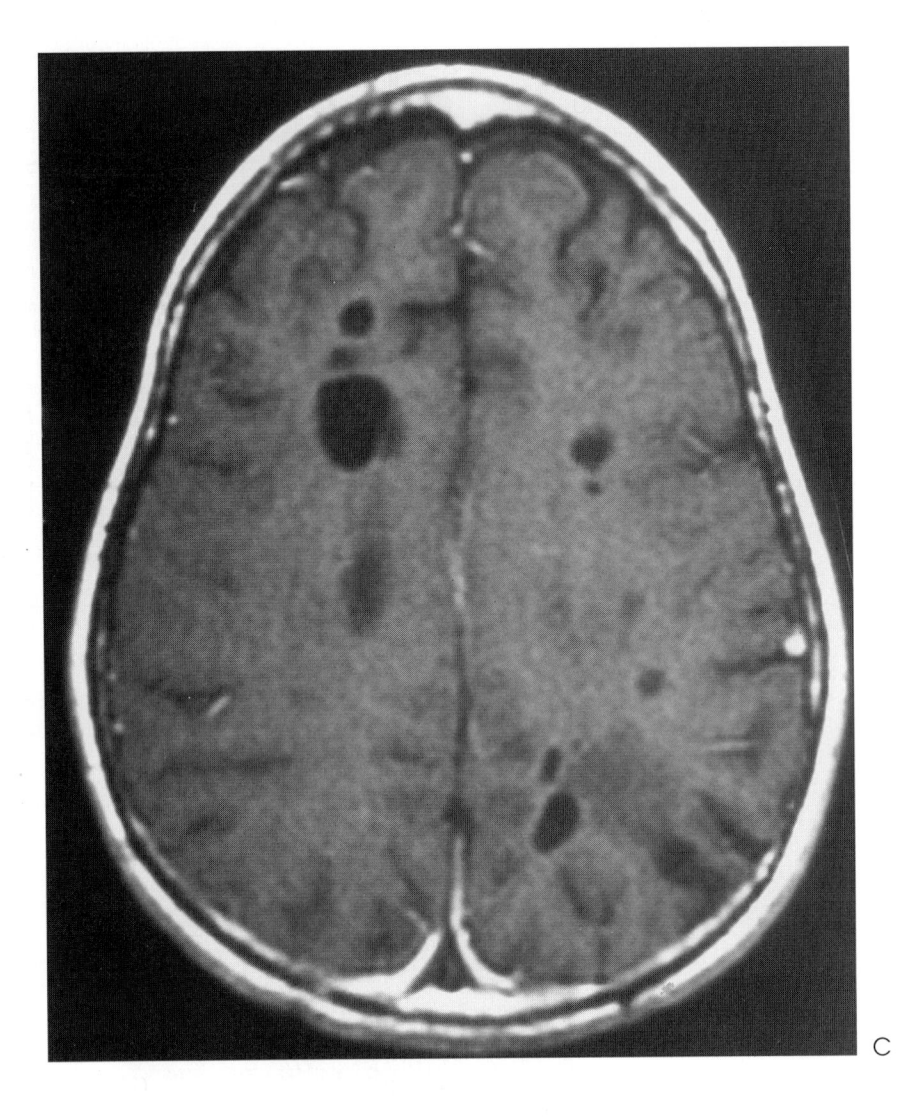

PEARLS

- Because ependymoma may lead to metastatic deposits, the entire length of the vertebral canal should be evaluated. Evaluation of the spine should include studies without and with the infusion of contrast material.

- Tumors that are primary in the brain may also metastasize to the spinal subarachnoid space. If this is a diagnostic consideration, magnetic resonance (MR) imaging of the brain without and with contrast should be performed.

Radiologic Findings (continued)

Axial short TR image of the brain (Fig. C) reveals multiple bilateral rounded areas of cerebrospinal fluid signal intensity.

Diagnosis

Ependymoma; dilated Virchow-Robin spaces in the brain of unknown significance.

Differential Diagnosis

- ependymoma

- metastasis

SPINAL CORD TUMORS

PITFALLS
- The MR appearance of the spinal cord lesion is also typical of schwannoma, and schwannoma would be the most likely diagnosis in this patient in the absence of a history of previous ependymoma.

- Metastatic spread from a primary tumor outside of the central nervous system may also have a similar appearance.

Discussion

This patient had a history of previous resection for a spinal cord ependymoma. The internal areas of decreased signal intensity are probably related to areas of hemorrhage. The areas of enhancement above and below the mass are dilated vessels in the subarachnoid space. Dilated vessels are occasionally seen above the level of a mass that is causing a complete block to the flow of contrast material. In an older patient, a metastasis from a primary tumor such as melanoma could have a similar appearance.

TEACHING ATLAS OF SPINE IMAGING

Case 10

Clinical Presentation

The patient is a 5-year-old female with recurrent ependymoma of the spine who is status postcranial and spinal radiation and now presents with lower extremity weakness.

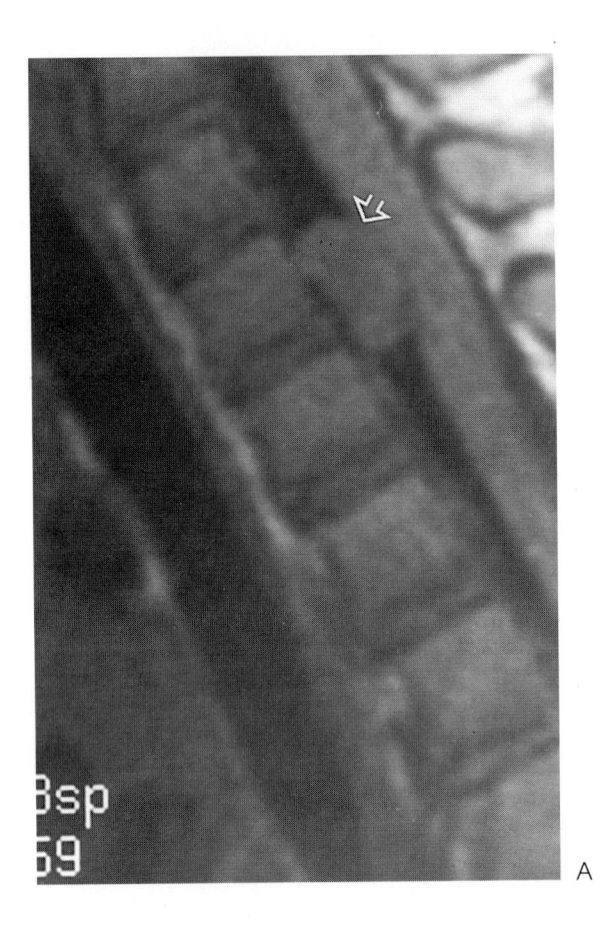

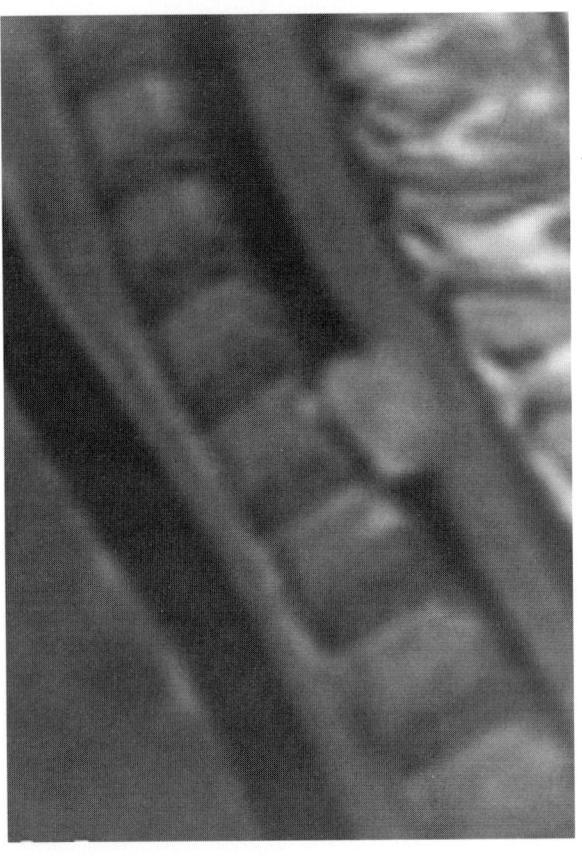

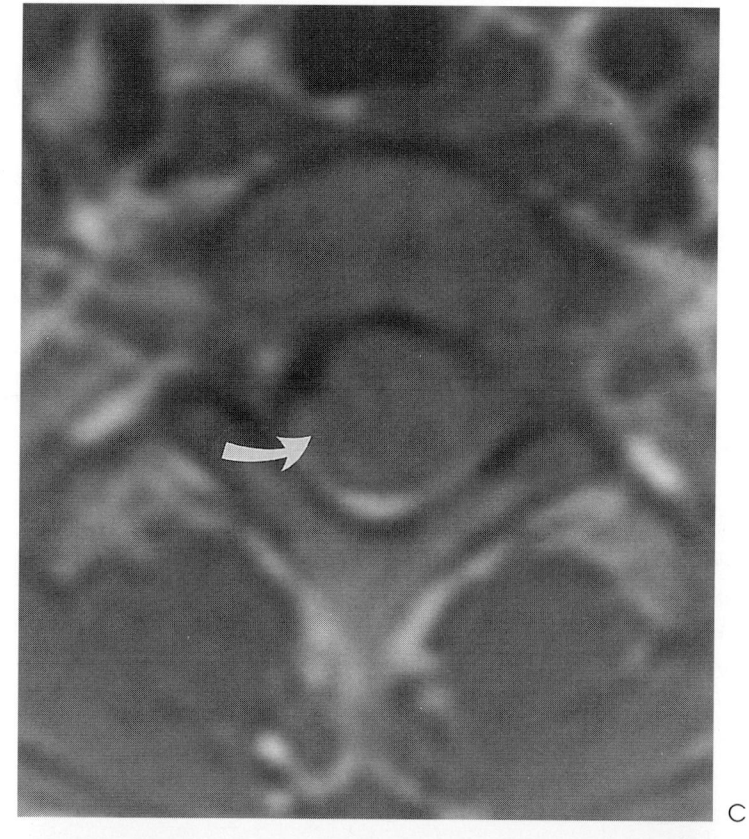

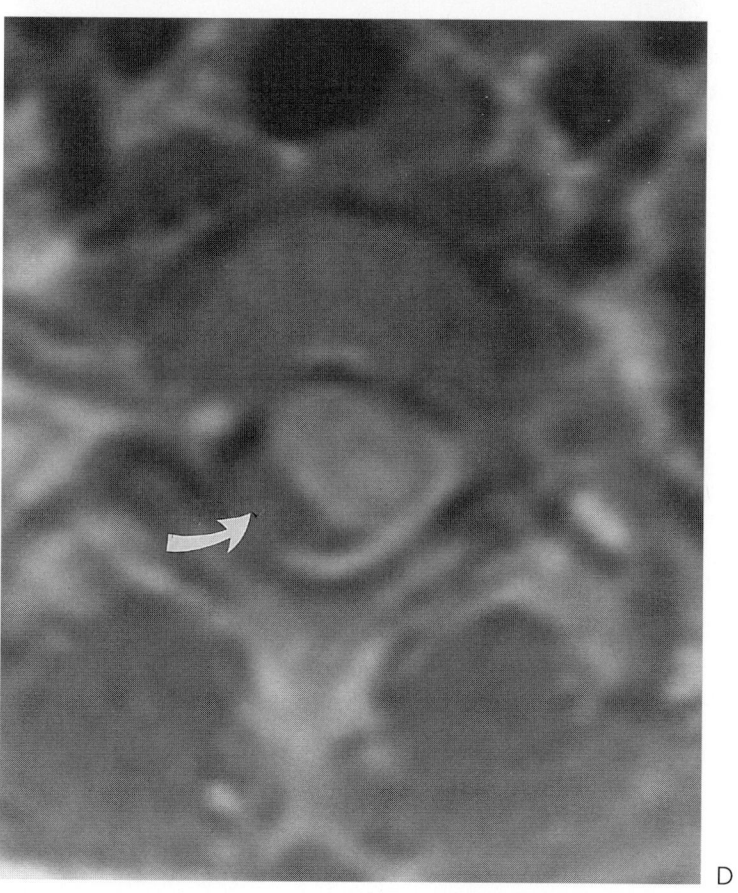

SPINAL CORD TUMORS

C

D

Radiologic Findings

Sagittal short TR image in the cervical region (Fig. A) reveals a slightly lobulated mass arising anterior to the spinal cord at the level of T1 (*arrow*).

Sagittal short TR image postcontrast (Fig. B) reveals dense enhancement of the mass.

Axial short TR image precontrast (Fig. C) reveals that the spinal cord is displaced far posteriorly and compressed into a crescentic shape (*arrow*).

Axial short TR image postcontrast (Fig. D) reveals dense homogeneous enhancement of the mass anteriorly and on the left side displacing the spinal cord posteriorly and to the right (*arrow*).

Diagnosis

Drop metastasis from recurrent posterior fossa ependymoma.

Differential Diagnosis

- drop metastasis
- schwannoma
- neurofibroma

Discussion

The magnetic resonance evaluation of the posterior fossa reveals postsurgical change as well as an enhancing lesion consistent with recurrent tumor. Analysis of the cerebrospinal fluid also revealed cells compatible with recurrent ependymoma. The appearance is consistent with a drop metastasis from a primary ependymoma. A drop metastasis from a disease process such as medulloblastoma could also have this appearance. A schwannoma or neurofibroma could also have this appearance.

PEARL
- The clinical history is important here for the correct diagnosis. The entire spinal axis should be evaluated for complete evaluation in this patient.

PITFALL
- In a patient with a tumor known to metastasize to the craniospinal axis, evaluation of the entire system should be obtained at the time of initial diagnosis as well as at the time of follow-up.

SPINAL CORD TUMORS

Case 11

Clinical Presentation

The patient is a 49-year-old female with evidence of cord compression with progressive inability to walk.

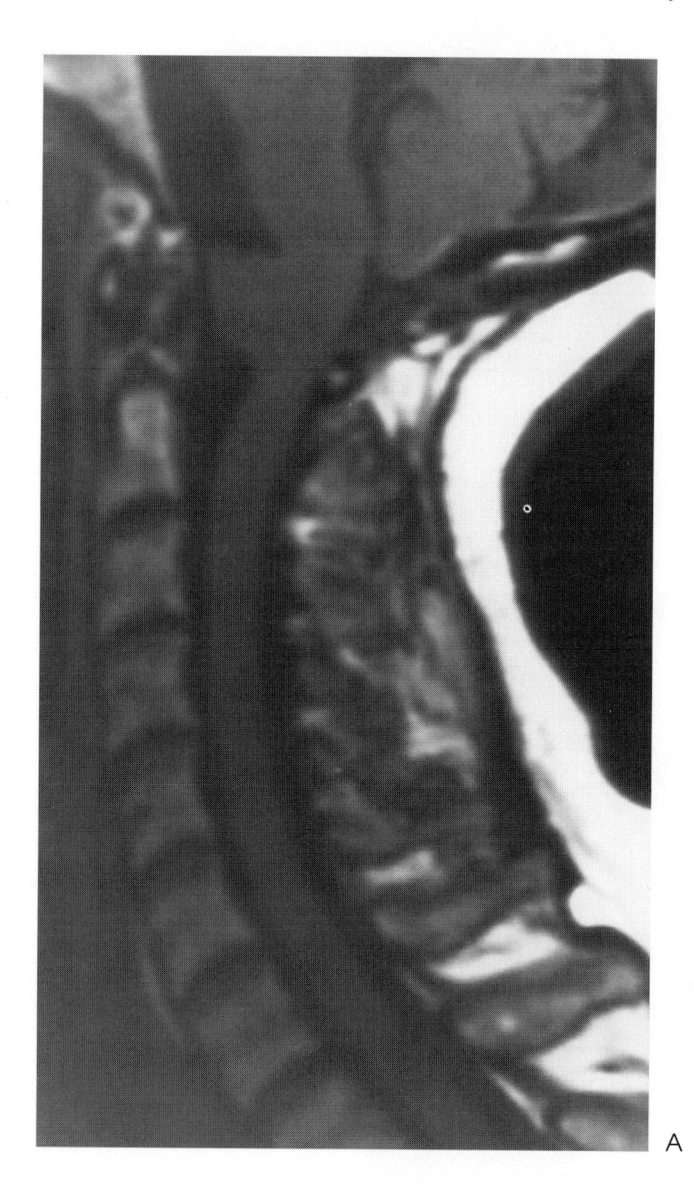

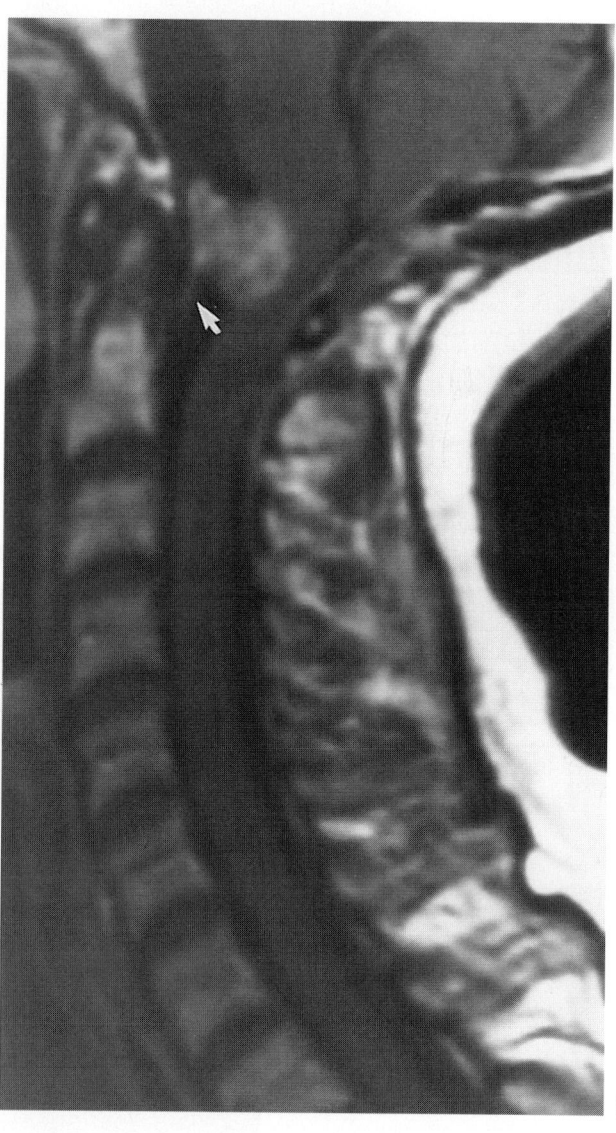

TEACHING ATLAS OF SPINE IMAGING

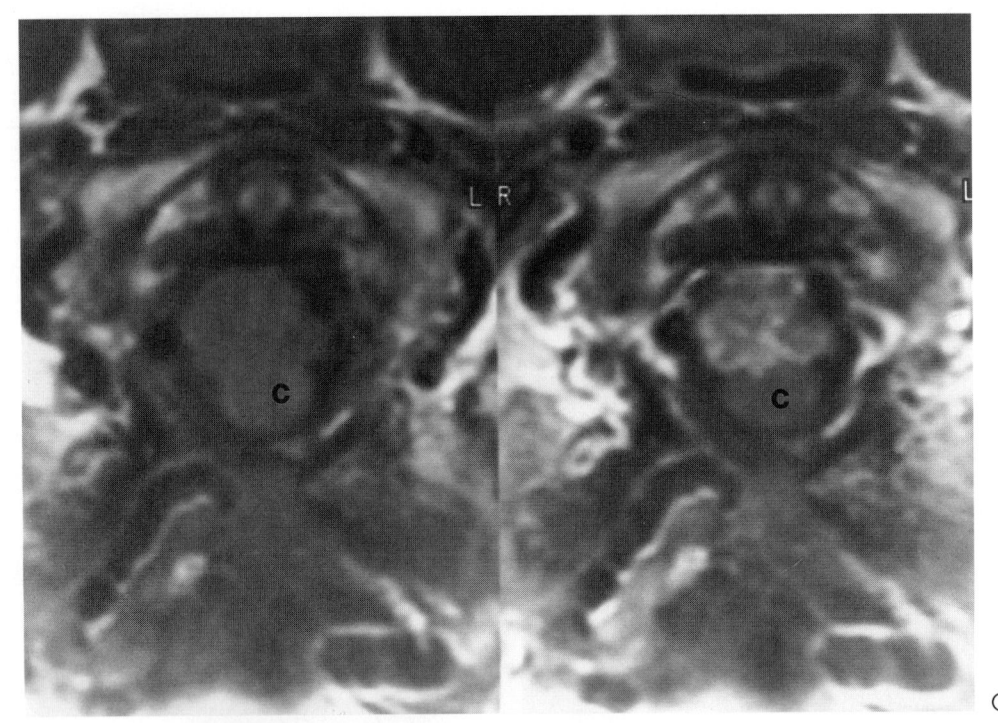

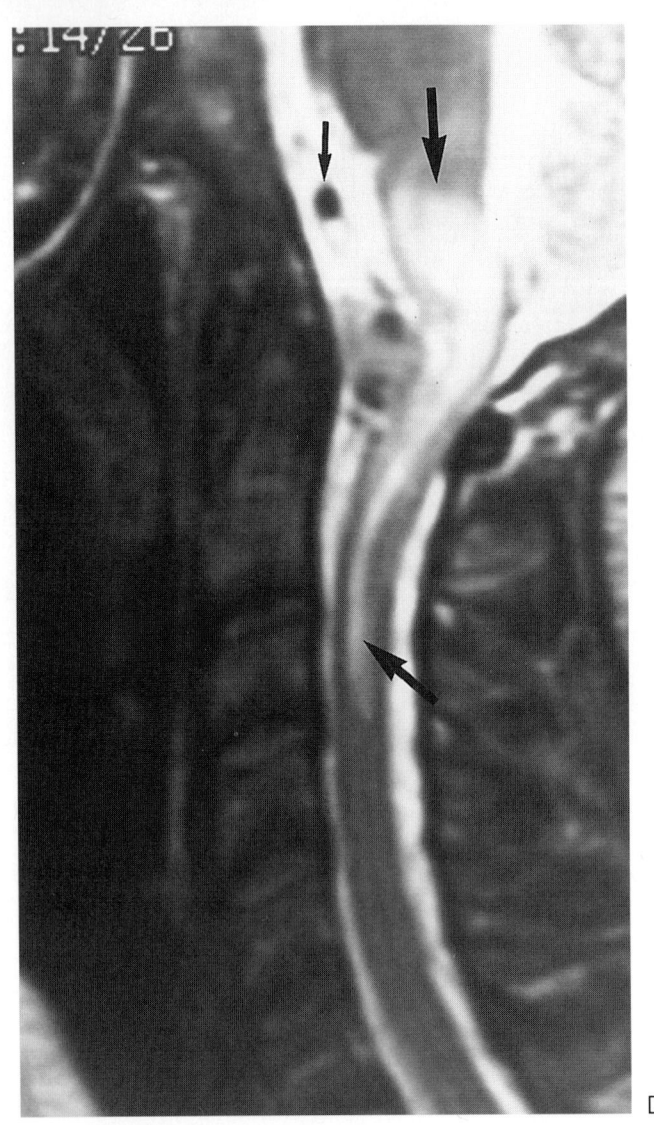

202

SPINAL CORD TUMORS

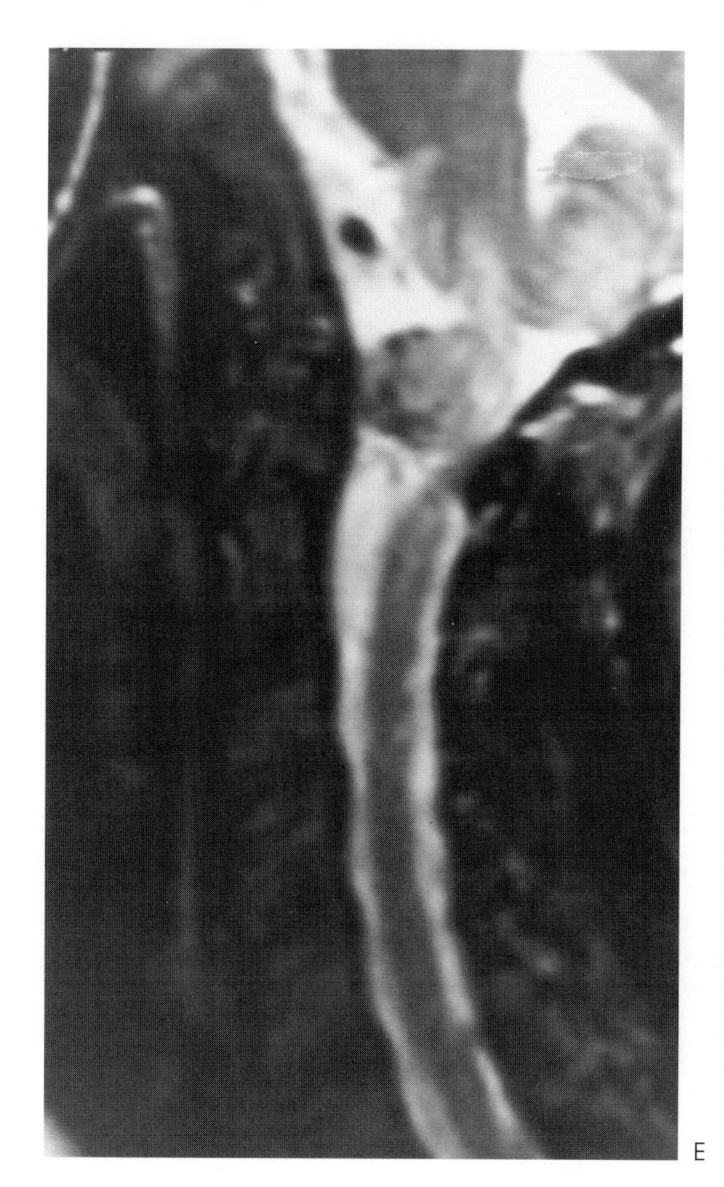

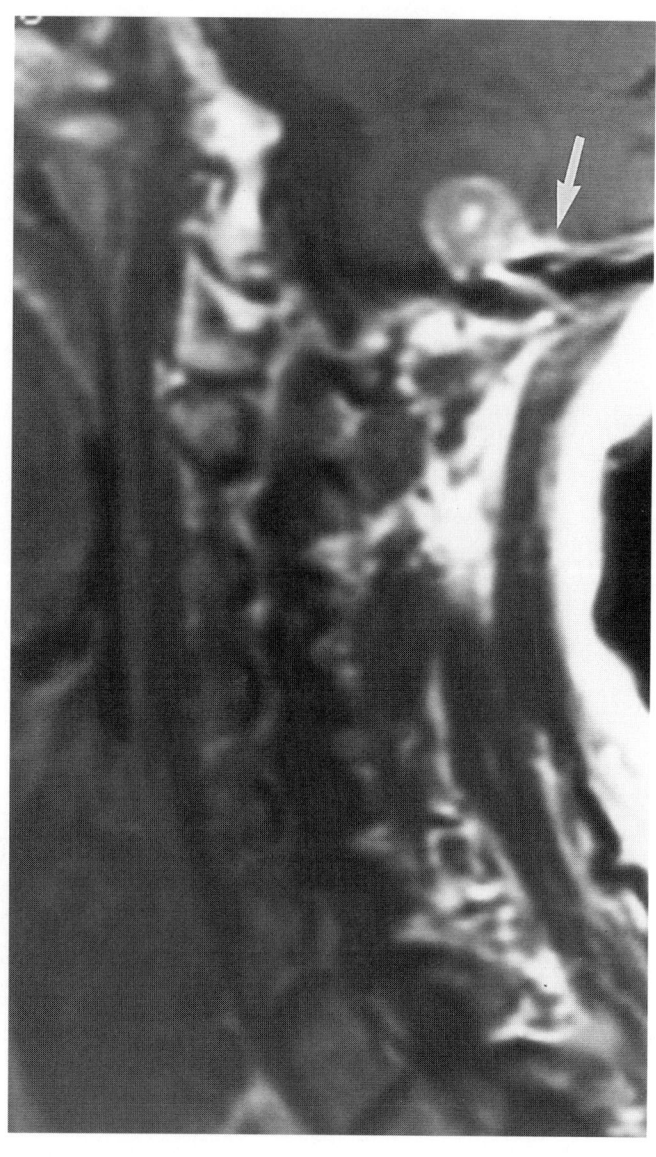

TEACHING ATLAS OF SPINE IMAGING

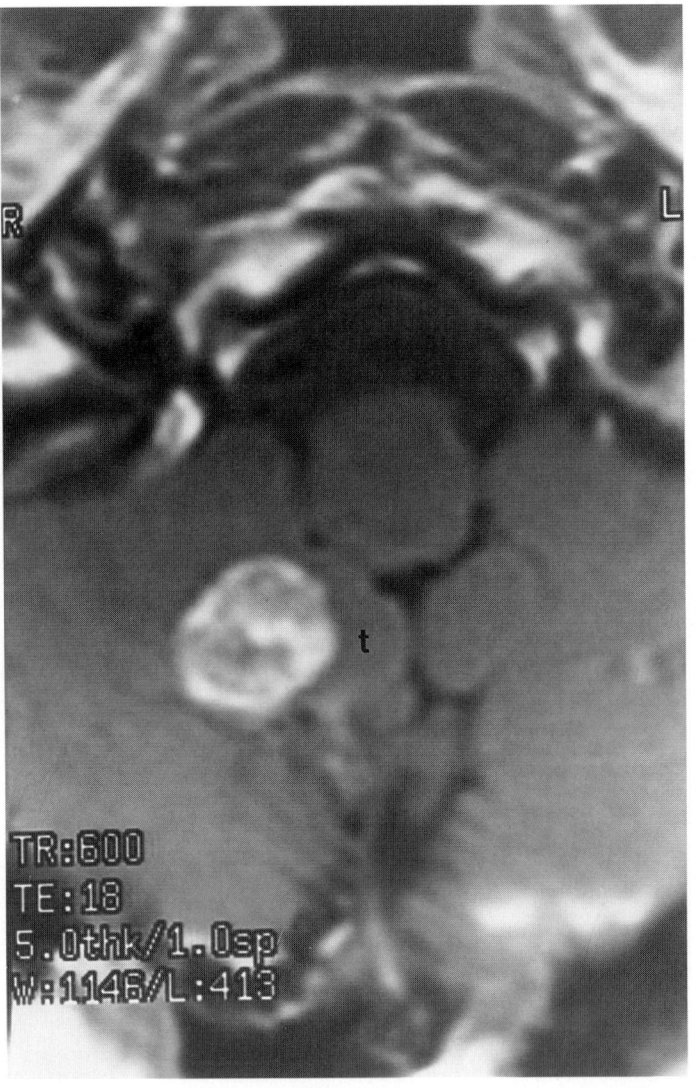

Radiologic Findings

Sagittal short TR image in the cervical region (Fig. A) reveals a slightly irregularly marginated mass behind the odontoid process of C2. The spinal cord and lower medulla are displaced posteriorly.

Sagittal short TR image postcontrast (Fig. B) reveals dense enhancement of the soft tissue mass. There is a short extension of these areas of enhancement along the dura anteriorly (*white arrow*).

Pre- (Fig. C, left) and postcontrast (Fig. C, right) axial short TR images reveal that the spinal cord (*c*) is displaced posteriorly by the soft tissue mass. On the postcontrast study (*right*), the mass exhibits inhomogeneous enhancement and has an irregular peripheral margin.

Sagittal long TR image (Fig. D) reveals that the mass exhibits increased signal intensity with two rounded areas of decreased signal intensity. The medulla and upper cervical spinal cord reveal marked increased signal intensity (*large arrows*). There is a rounded area of low density anterior to the medulla behind the clivus (*small arrow*).

SPINAL CORD TUMORS

Parasagittal long TR image (Fig. E) reveals that the mass appears as variable signal intensity and contains large areas of decreased signal intensity.

Parasagittal short TR image postcontrast (Fig. F) reveals a second area of variable enhancement arising from the dura in the floor of the posterior fossa. This mass appears to have a small extension along the dura (*arrow*).

Axial short TR image postcontrast (Fig. G) reveals irregular enhancement of the mass, which projects up into the right cerebellar hemisphere. The cerebellar tonsil (*t*) is displaced medially.

> **PEARL**
> - Findings must be correlated with clinical history. In a patient with a clinical history of neurofibromatosis type 2, these lesions could represent either meningiomas or schwannomas.

> **PITFALL**
> - While meningiomas may exhibit a "dural tail sign," other tumors may also have a dural tail, as in this case of metastatic colon cancer. Meningiomas typically have a more rounded peripheral margin.

Diagnosis

Metastatic colon carcinoma.

Differential Diagnosis

- metastatic disease
- meningioma

Discussion

The patient was known to have widespread colon cancer. The metastases had even involved the subcutaneous tissues of the patient's forearms. Metastatic colon cancer may be mucin producing and so may appear as variable signal intensity on various magnetic resonance imaging sequences. The "dural tails" with extension along the dura suggest that multiple meningiomas could be a diagnosis in this patient.

Contrast enhancement with multiplanar imaging is very helpful for complete evaluation, and evaluation should include imaging of the entire brain and spine in this patient. Work up should also include evaluation of other organ systems.

The rounded area of low density anterior to the medulla behind the clivus is the flow void of the vertebral artery.

Metastatic disease from a primary tumor such as breast cancer, lung cancer, or melanoma could also have a similar appearance. Melanoma may also be hemorrhagic and so exhibit variable signal intensity on a variety of pulse sequences; melanoma may also develop skin metastases.

Suggested Readings

Berenguer J, Bargalló N, Sanchez M, et al. Magnetic resonance imaging of paraganglioma of the cauda equina. *Canad Assoc Radiol J.* 1995;46:37–39.

Berger RK, Williams AL, Daniels DL, et al. Contrast enhancement in spinal MR imaging. *AJR.* 1989;153:387–391.

Breslau J, Eskridge JM. Preoperative embolization of spinal tumors. *JVIR.* 1995;6:871–875.

Cheng TJ, Wu TT, Hsu JD. Dumbbell spinal lipoma presenting as a neck mass: CT and MR demonstration. *Pediatr Radiol.* 1995;25:570–571.

Cummings TM, Johnson MH. Neurofibroma manifested by spinal subarachnoid hemorrhage. *AJR.* 1994;162:959–960.

De Bruine FT, Kroon HM. Spinal chordoma: radiologic features in 14 cases. *AJR.* 1988;150:861–863.

Debray MP, Ricolfi F, Brugières P, et al. Epidermoid cyst of the conus medullaris: atypical MRI and angiographic features. *Neuroradiol.* 1996;38:526–528.

Demachi H, Takashima T, Kadoya M, et al. MR imaging of spinal neurinomas with pathological correlation. *JCAT.* 1990;14:250–254.

Di Chiro G, Doppman JL, Awyer AJ, et al. Tumors and arteriovenous malformations of the spinal cord: assessment using MR. *Radiology.* 1985;156:689–697.

Dillon WP, Norman D, Newton TH, Bolla K, Mark A. Intradural spinal cord lesions: Gd-DPTA-enhanced MR imaging. *Radiology.* 1989;170:229–238.

Do D-D, Rovira MJ, Ho VB, et al. Childhood onset of myxopapillary ependymomatosis: MR features. *AJNR.* 1995;16:835–839.

Duong JH, Tampieri D, Melancon D, et al. Intramedullary schwannoma. *Canad Assoc Radiol J.* 1995;46:179.

Egelhoff JC, Bates DJ, Ross JS, Rothner AD, Cohen BH. Spinal MR findings in neurofibromatosis types 1 and 2. *AJNR.* 1992;13:1071–1077.

Enzmann DR, Rubin JB. Cervical spine: MR imaging with a partial flip angle, gradient-refocused pulse sequence. II. Spinal cord disease. *Radiology.* 1988;166:473–478.

Fine MJ, Kricheff II, Freed D, Epstein FJ. Spinal cord ependymomas: MR imaging features. *Radiology.* 1995;197:655–658.

Friedman DP, Tartaglino LM, Fisher AR, et al. MR imaging in the diagnosis of intramedullary spinal cord diseases that involve specific neural pathways or vascular territories. *AJR.* 1995;165:515–524.

Friedman DP, Tartaglino LM, Flanders AE. Intradural schwannomas of the spine: MR findings with emphasis on contrast-enhancement characteristics. *AJR.* 1992;158:1347–1350.

Goy AMC, Pinto RS, Raghavendra BN, et al. Intramedullary spinal cord tumors: MR imaging, with emphasis on associated cysts. *Radiology.* 1986;161:381–386.

Horton WA, Wong V, Eldridge R. Von Hippel-Lindau disease: clinical and pathological manifestations in nine families with 50 affected members. *Arch Intern Med.* 1976;136:769–777.

Hosoi K. Intradural teratoid tumors of the spinal cord. *Arch Pathol.* 1931;11:875–883.

Ishii N, Matsuzawa H, Houkin K, et al. An evaluation of 70 spinal schwannomas using conventional computed tomography and magnetic resonance imaging. *Neuroradiol.* 1991;33:542.

Isoda H, Takahashi M, Mochizuki T, et al. MRI of dumbbell-shaped spinal tumors. *JCAT.* 1996;20:573.

Kahan H, Sklar EML, Donovan MJ, et al. MR characteristics of histopathologic subtypes of spinal ependymoma. *AJNR.* 1996;17:143–150.

Katz D, Quencer R. Hamartomatous spinal cord lesion in neurofibromatosis. *AJNR.* 1989;10:101.

Klatte E, Franken E, Smith J. The radiographic spectrum in neurofibromatosis. *Semin Roentgenol.* 1976;9:17–33.

Lewis T, Kingsley D. Magnetic resonance imaging of multiple spinal neurofibromata: neurofibromatosis. *Neuroradiol.* 1987;29:562–564.

Li MH, Holt AS. MR imaging of spinal neurofibromatosis. *Acta Radiol.* 1991;32:279–285.

Li MH, Holtås S, Larsson E-M. MR imaging of intradural extramedullary tumors. *Acta Radiol.* 1992;33:207–212.

Marty R, Minckler DS. Radiation myelitis simulating tumor. *Atch Neurol.* 1973;29:352–354.

Mascalchi M, Dal Pozzo G, Bartolozzi C. Effectiveness of the short T1 inversion recovery (STIR) sequence in MR imaging of intramedullary spinal lesions. *Magn Reson Imaging.* 1993;11:17–25.

Mautner VF, Tatagiba M, Lindenau M, et al. Spinal tumors in patients with neurofibromatosis type 2: MR imaging study of frequency, multiplicity, and variety. *AJR.* 1995;165:951–955.

Meyer JE, Lepke RA, Lindfors KK, et al. Chordomas: their CT appearance in the cervical thoracic and lumbar spine. *Radiology.* 1984;153:683–696.

Mulvhill JJ (moderator). Neurofibromatosis 1 (Recklinghausen disease) and neurofibromatosis 2 (bilateral acoustic neurofibromatosis): an update. *Ann Intern Med.* 1990;113:39–52.

Murphey MD, Andrews CL, Flemming DJ, Temple HT, Smith WS, Smirniotopoulos JG. From the archives of the AFIP: primary tumor of the spine: radiologic-pathologic correlation. *RadioGraphics.* 1996;16:1131–1158.

Neumann HPH, Eggert HR, Weigel K, et al. Hemangioblastomas of the central nervous system: a 10-year study with special reference to von Hippel-Lindau syndrome. *J Neurosurg.* 1989;70:24–30.

Parizel PM, Baleriaux D, Rodesch G, et al. Gd-DPTA-enhanced MR imaging of spinal tumors. *AJNR.* 1989;10:249–258.

Pont MS, Elster AD. Lesions of skin and brain: modern imaging of the neurocutaneous syndromes. *AJR.* 1992.

Provenzale JM, McLendon RE. Spinal angiolipomas: MR features. *AJNR.* 1996;17:713.

Quekel LGBA, Versteege CWM. "Dural tail sign" in MRI of spinal meningiomas. *JCAT.* 1995;19:890–892.

Quencer RM, El Gammal T, Cohen G. Syringomyelia associated with intradural extramedullary masses of the spinal canal. *AJNR.* 1986;7:143–148.

Roeder MB, Bazan C, Jinkins JR. Ruptured spinal dermoid cyst with chemical arachnoiditis and disseminated intracranial lipid droplets. *Neuroradiol.* 1995;37:146–147.

Roeder MB, Jinkins JR, Bazan C III. Subependymoma of filum terminale: MR appearance. *JCAT.* 1994;18:129.

Russo CP, Katz DS, Corona RJ Jr, et al. Gangliocytoma of the cervicothoracic spinal cord. *AJNR.* 1995;16:889–891.

Shiono T, Yoshikawa K, Iwasaki N. Huge lumbar spinal cystic neurinomas with unusual MR findings. *AJNR.* 1995;16:881–882.

Shrier DA, Rubio A, Numaguchi Y, et al. Infarcted spinal schwannoma: unusual MR finding. *AJNR.* 1996;17:1566–1568.

Sibilla L, Martelli A, Farina L, et al. Ganglioneuroblastoma of the spinal cord. *AJNR.* 1995;16:875–877.

Sze G. Gadolinium-DPTA in spinal disease. In Lee H, Zimmerman A, eds. *The Radiology Clinic of North America. Imaging in Neuroradiology.* Vol 5, Philadelphia, PA: WB Saunders, 1988; 1009–1024.

Sze G, Abramson A, Krol G, et al. Gd-DPTA in evaluation of intradural extramedullary spinal diseases. *AJNR.* 1988;9:153–163.

Sze G, Abramson A, Krol G, et al. Gadolinium-DPTA in evaluation of intradural extramedullary spinal diseases. *AJR.* 1988;150:911–921.

Sze G, Bravo S, Krol G. Spinal lesions: quantitative and qualitative temporal evolution of gadopentetate dimeglumine enhancement in MR imaging. *Radiology.* 1989;170:849–856.

Varma DGK, Moulopoulos A, Sara AS, et al. MR imaging of extracranial nerve sheath tumors. *JCAT.* 1992;16:448–453.

Wertelecki W, Rouleau G, Superneau D, et al. Neurofibromatosis 2: clinical and DNA linkage studies of a large kindred. *N Engl J Med.* 1988;319:278–283.

Williams AL, Haughton VM, Pojunas KW. Differentiation of intramedullary neoplasms and cysts by MR. *AJR.* 1987;149:159–164.

Windisch TR, Naul LG, Bauserman SC. Intramedullary gliofibroma: MR, ultrasound, and pathologic correlation. *JCAT.* 1995;19:646–648.

Wippold FJ, 2nd, Smirniotopoulos JG, Pilgram TK. Lesions of the cauda equina: a clinical and pathology review from the Armed Forces Institute of Pathology. *Clinical Neurology and Neurosurgery.* 1997;99:229–234.

Section III

Spinal Cord Tumors

C. Neurofibromatosis

CONGENITAL

Case 1

Clinical Presentation

The patient is a 15-year-old male with recent difficulty voiding who is being evaluated to rule out cord compression.

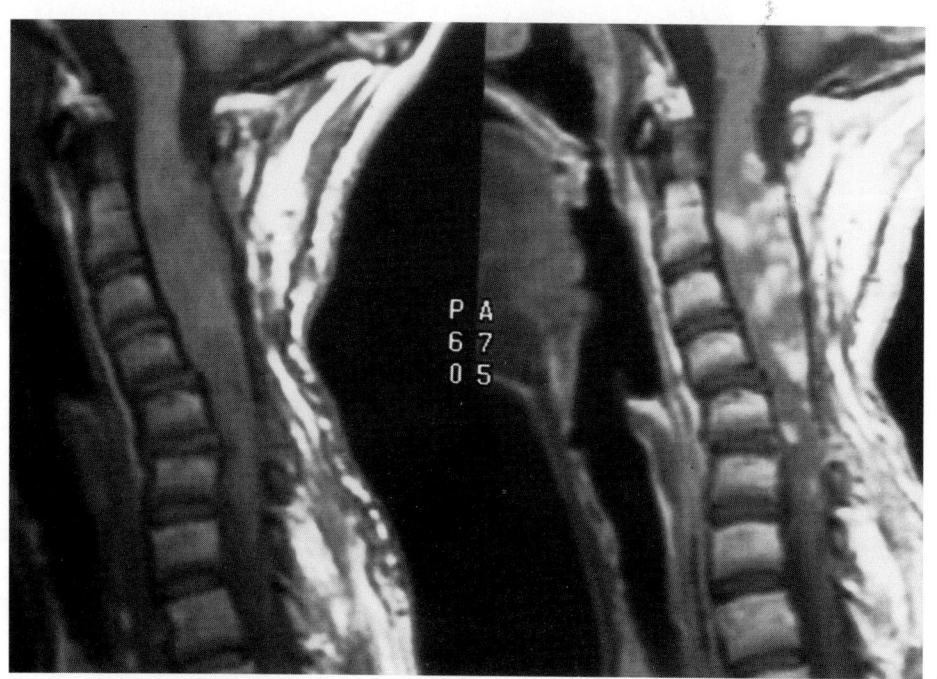

A

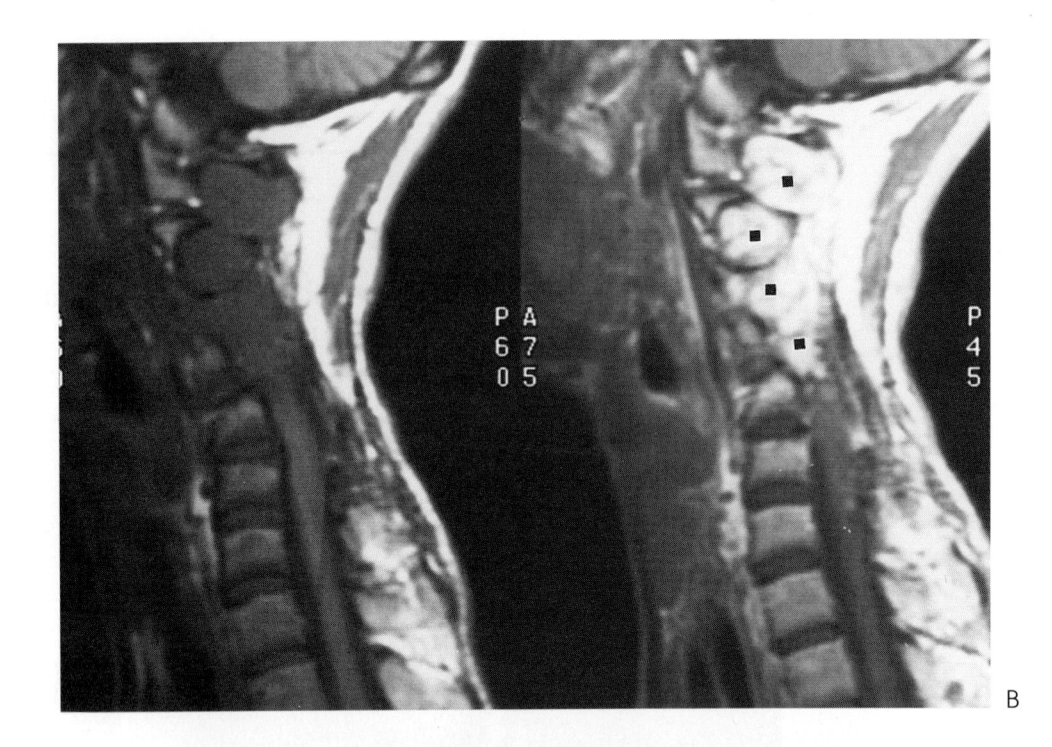

TEACHING ATLAS OF SPINE IMAGING

B

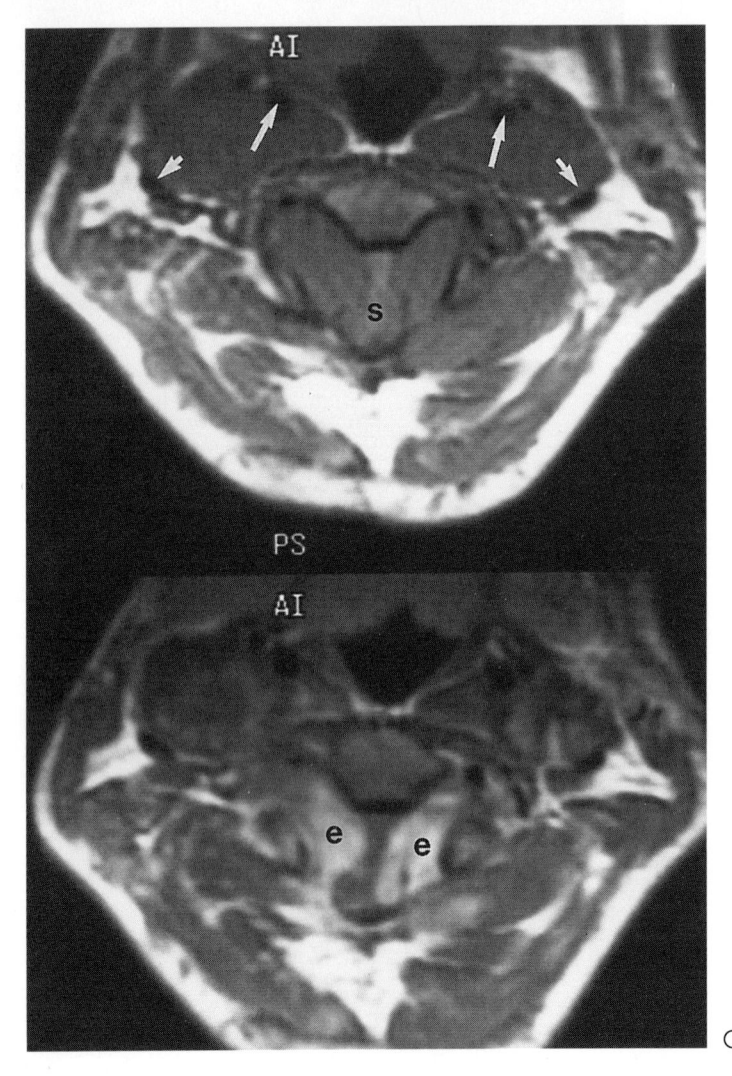

C

SPINAL CORD TUMORS

D

E

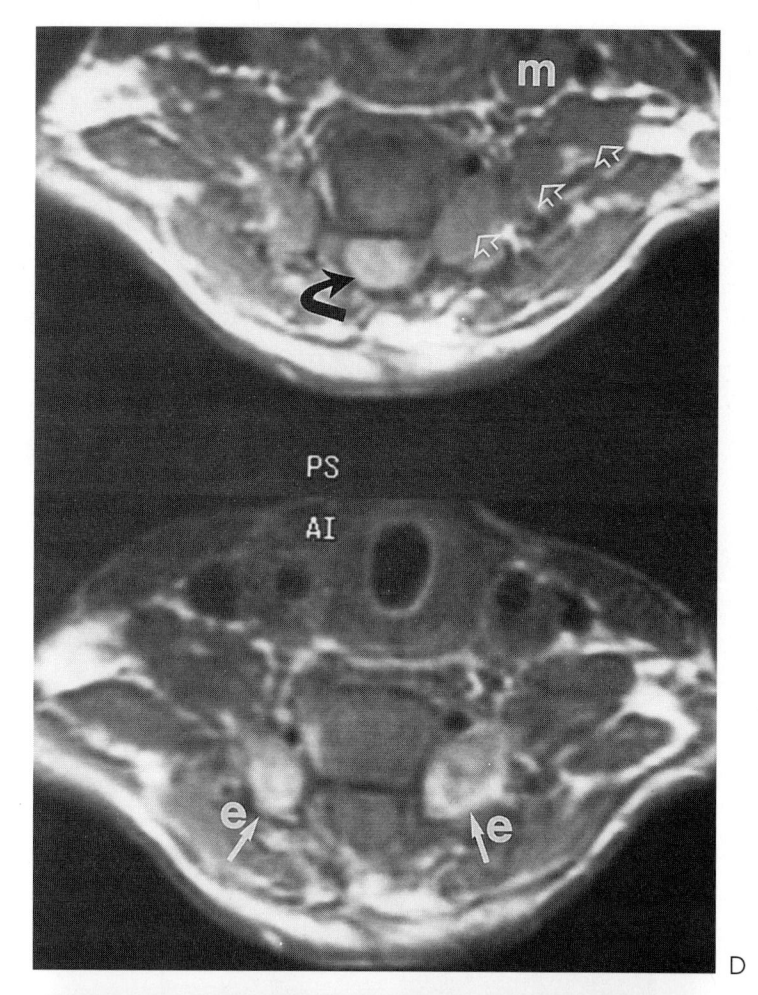

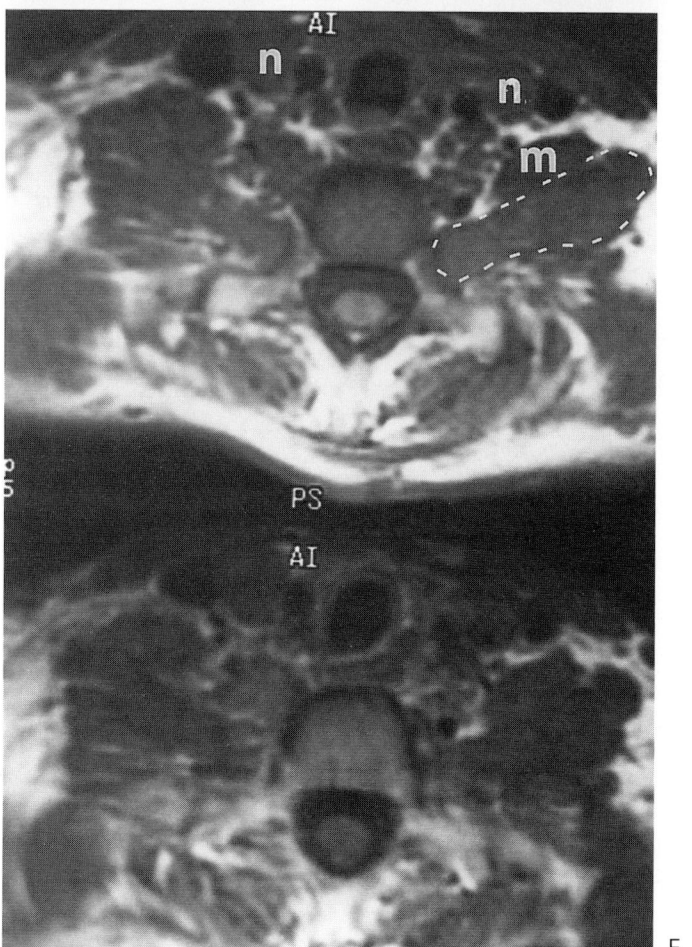

213

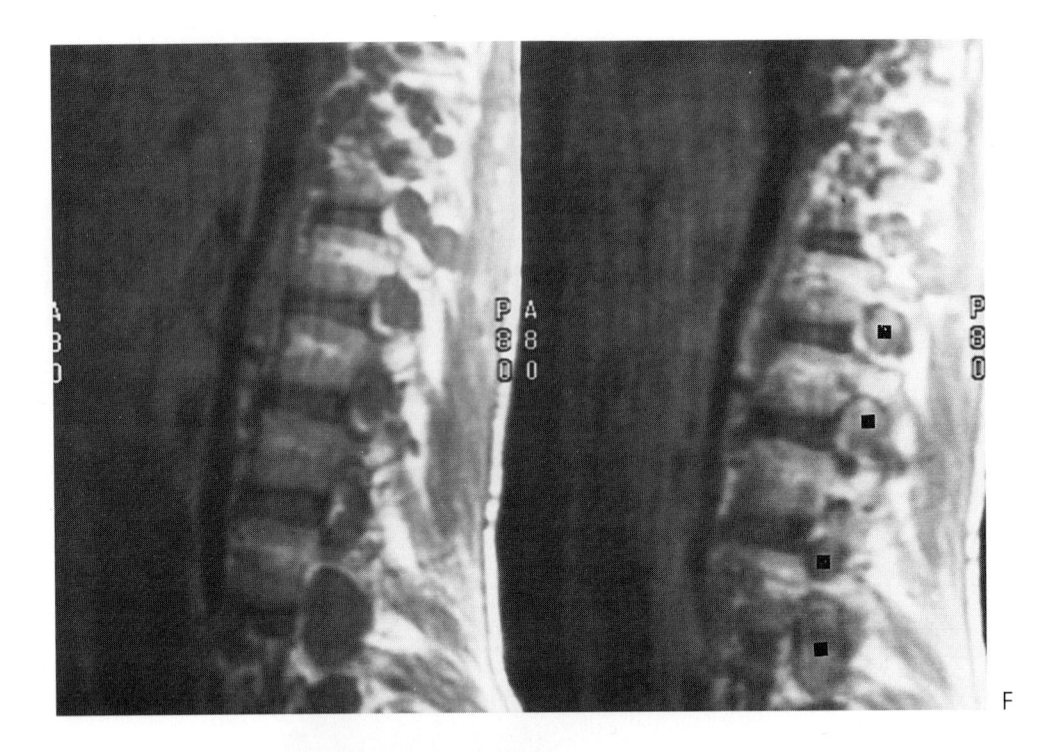

TEACHING ATLAS OF SPINE IMAGING

F

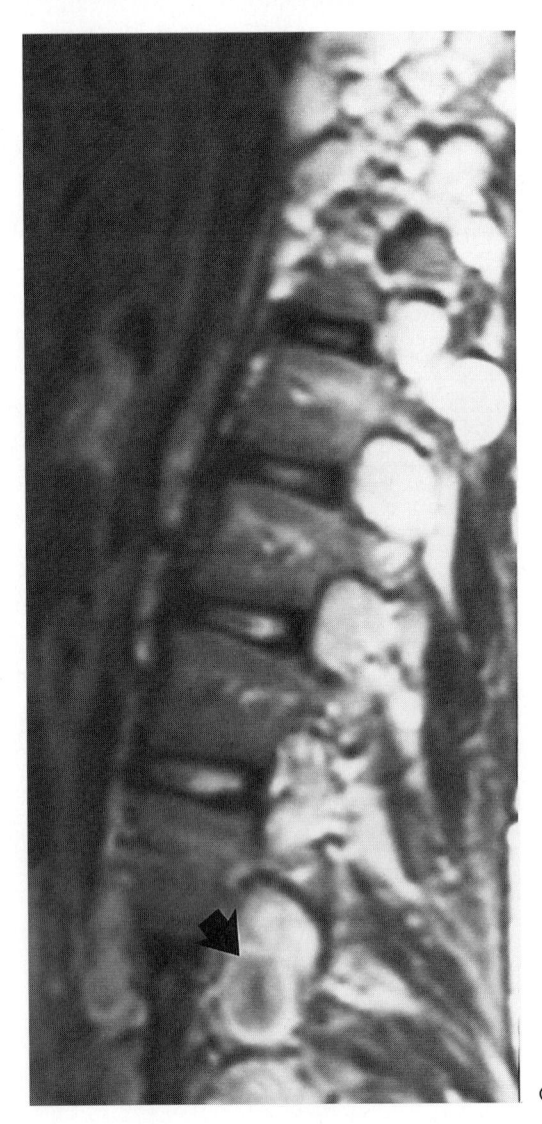

G

SPINAL CORD TUMORS

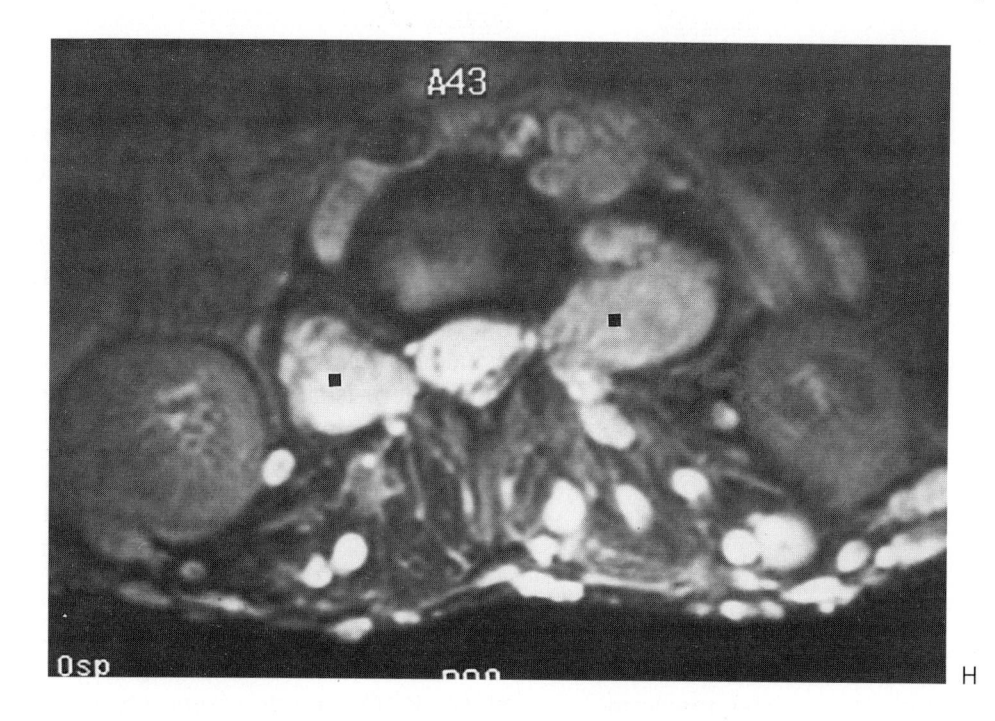

Radiologic Findings

Pre- (Fig. A, *left*) and postcontrast (Fig. A, *right*) sagittal short TR images in the cervical region reveal diffuse widening of the cervical spinal cord from the level of C2 through the level of C5-6. There is reversal of the lordotic curve of the cervical spine. The postcontrast study reveals multiple flocculent areas of enhancement extending from the C2 through the C6 levels.

Pre- (Fig. B, *left*) and postcontrast (Fig. B, *right*) parasagittal short TR images reveal diffuse enlargement of the intervertebral foramen at all levels in the cervical region by multiple, soft tissue, intermediate signal intensity masses. There is dense enhancement on the postinfusion study (*squares*).

Pre- (Fig. C, *top*) and postcontrast (Fig. C, *bottom*) axial short TR images reveal bilateral soft tissue signal intensity masses in the region of the intervertebral foramen. There is dense, slightly inhomogeneous enhancement of these soft tissue lesions (*bottom, e*) that extend into the vertebral canal via the intervertebral foramen and compress the spinal cord into an elongated oval shape (*top, s*). Soft tissue masses displace the flow void of the carotid artery anteriorly (*top, long arrows*); the jugular vein is compressed and displaced posterior and laterally (*short arrows*).

Pre- (Fig. D, *top*) and postcontrast (Fig. D, *bottom*) axial short TR images at the level of C4 reveal bilateral soft tissue signal intensity masses in the region of the intervertebral foramen. On the left side, there are several contiguous soft tissue masses which extend along the course of the brachial plexus (*top, open arrows*). There is another mass between the flow voids of the carotid artery and jugular vein (*m, top*); a similar smaller mass is seen on the opposite side. Within the vertebral canal, there is a rounded area of enhancement that obliterates the vertebral canal (*curved arrow*). The spinal cord cannot be identified with certainty. There is dense, slightly inhomogeneous enhancement of these soft tissue lesions on the postinfusion study (*bottom, e-arrows*).

Precontrast axial short TR images in the lower cervical region at the C5-6 level (Fig. E) reveal a slightly lobulated mass that follows the course of the brachial plexus on the left side (*top, dotted line*). The anterior scalenus muscle projects anterior to this mass (*top, m*). There are soft tissue masses between the internal carotid artery and jugular vein (*top, n*).

Pre- (Fig. F, *left*) and postcontrast (Fig. F, *right*) parasagittal short TR images reveal enlargement of the intervertebral foramina at all levels of the lumbar spine. There is slightly inhomogeneous enhancement of all the soft tissue masses in the intervertebral foramina (*right, squares*).

Parasagittal long TR image (Fig. G) reveals diffuse increased signal intensity within all of the soft tissue masses in the intervertebral foramina. There is a central area that does not exhibit increased signal in the lower lumbar region (*arrow*).

Axial long TR image at the level of L1 (Fig. H) reveals multiple rounded and oval areas of increased signal intensity. These are in the region of the intervertebral foramen (*squares*), in the para-aortic region, and in the muscles of the paraspinal region.

Diagnosis

Neurofibromatosis type 1 with multiple plexiform neurofibromas.

Differential Diagnosis

Intramedullary enhancing lesions

Discussion

The sagittal pre- and postcontrast images in the cervical region reveal dense enhancement of the multiple plexiform neurofibromas. These plexiform tumors extend into the cervical vertebral canal at multiple levels and markedly compress the cervical spinal cord medially, widening the spinal cord. This gives the false impression that there are multiple intramedullary enhancing lesions. However, the axial image confirms the fact that these lesions are actually intradural and extradural rather than intramedullary. The axial image also reveals that there is a soft tissue neurofibroma of the vagus nerve in the vascular bundle in the neck on the right side that displaces the carotid artery anteriorly and the jugular vein posteriorly as seen in Figure C.

Neurofibromatosis type 1 is an hereditary disease that is autosomal dominant with involvement of chromosome number 17.

PEARLS
- This is the typical appearance of extensive plexiform neurofibroma in the patient with neurofibromatosis type 1.

- The entire vertebral column should be evaluated for accurate determination of the extent of the disease because symptoms may actually be minimal even when the lesions are quite extensive.

PITFALLS
- Without multiplanar imaging, the appearance suggests that these are really intramedullary rather than intradural masses.

- Patients with neurofibromatosis type 2 may have multiple intramedullary tumors, such as ependymomas, even when there are minimal or no clinical symptoms.

SPINAL CORD TUMORS

Case 2

Clinical Presentation

The patient is a 22-year-old female with minimal lower extremity weakness.

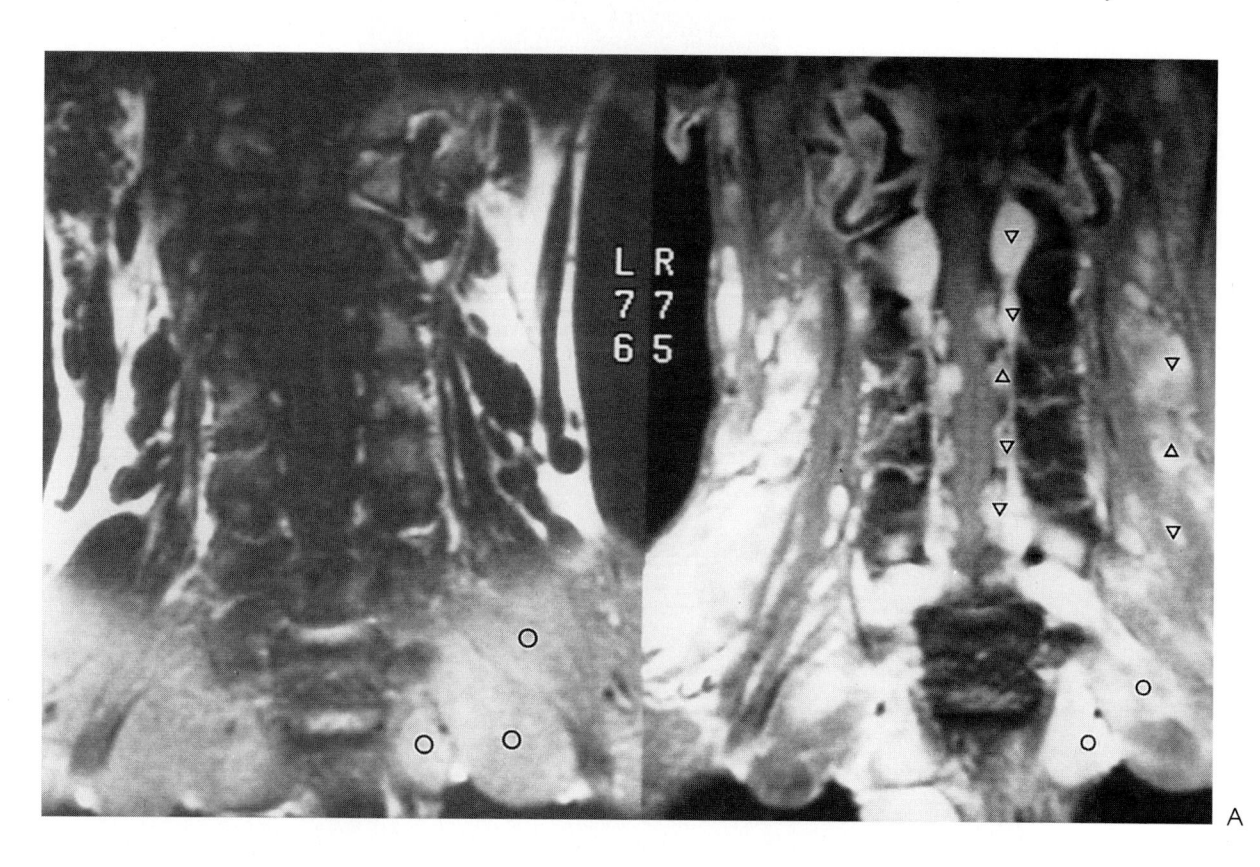

A

TEACHING ATLAS OF SPINE IMAGING

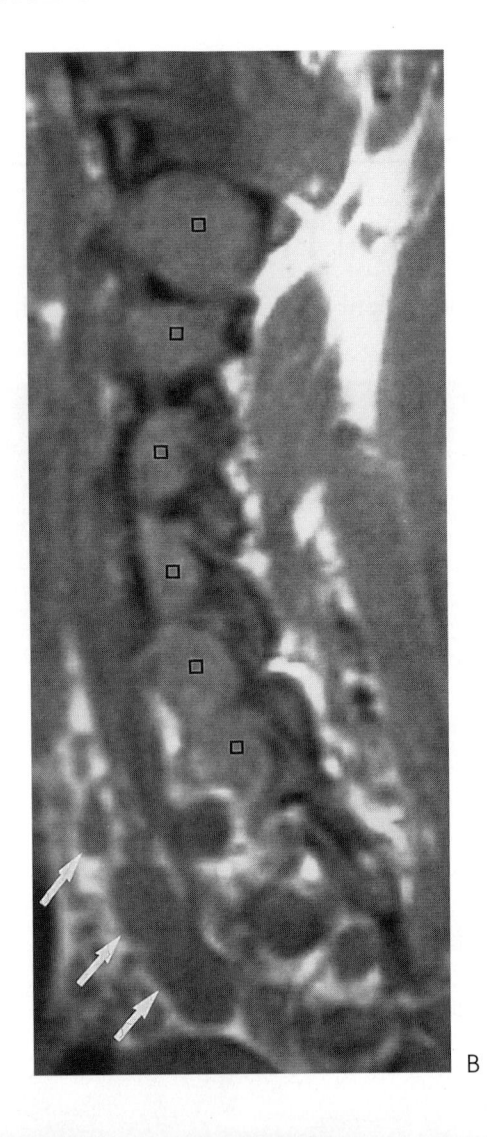

B

C

SPINAL CORD TUMORS

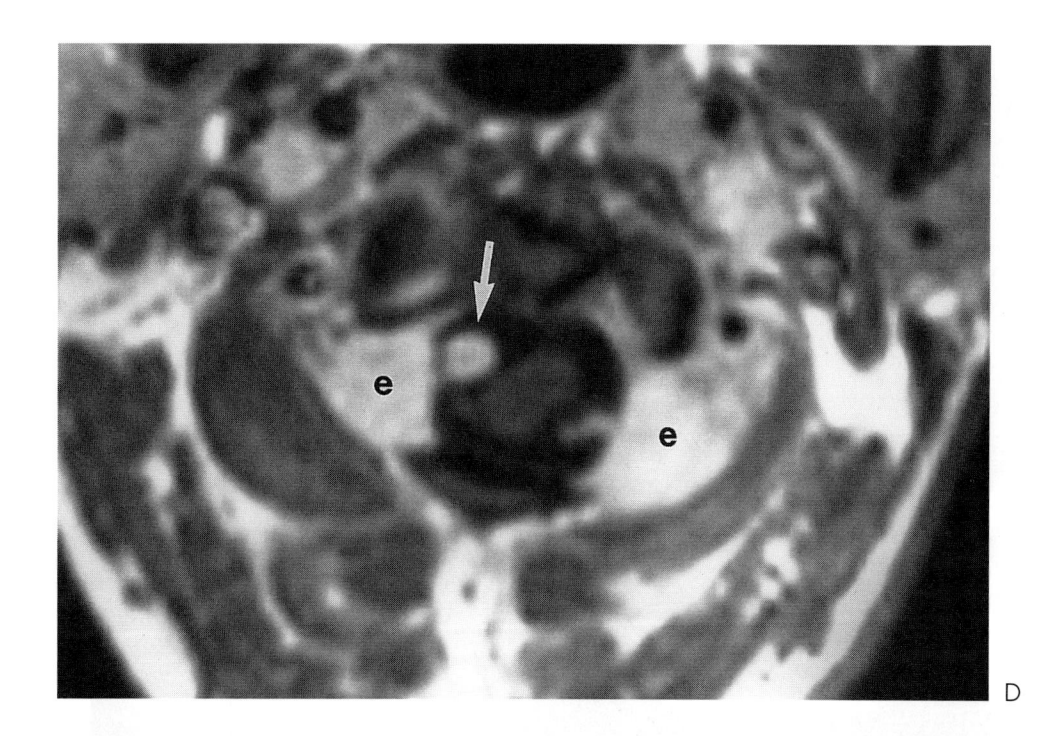

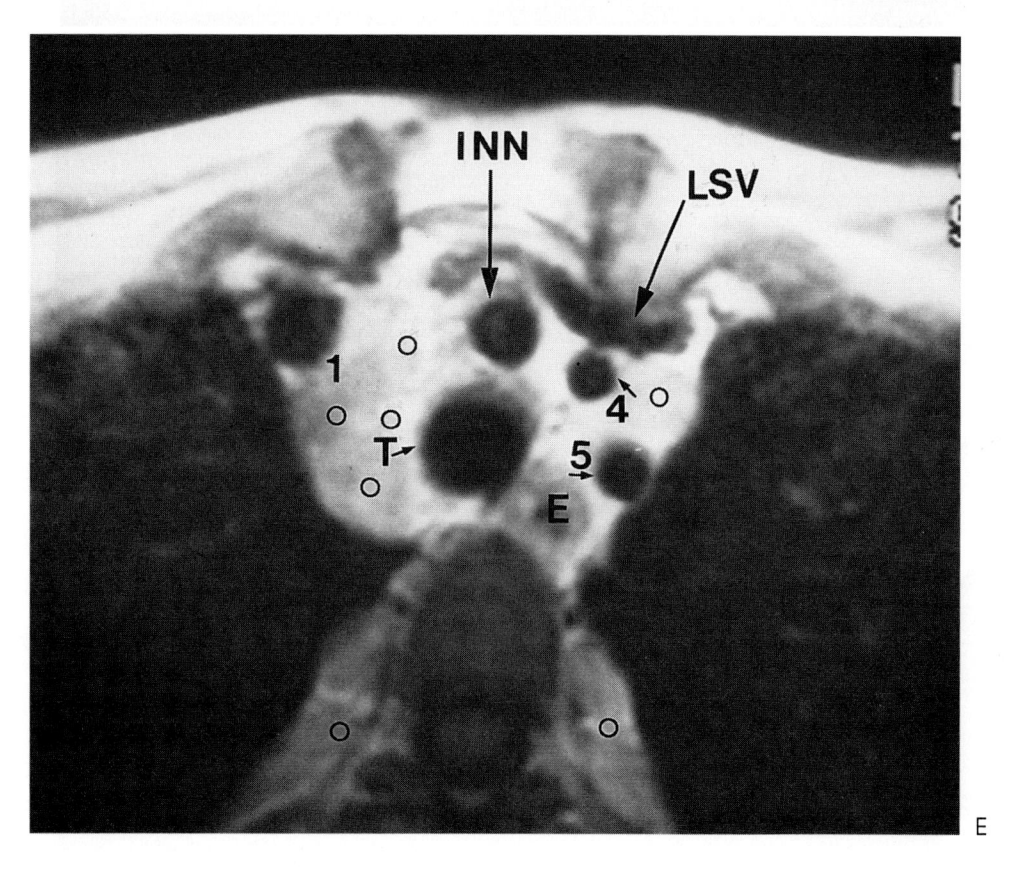

TEACHING ATLAS OF SPINE IMAGING

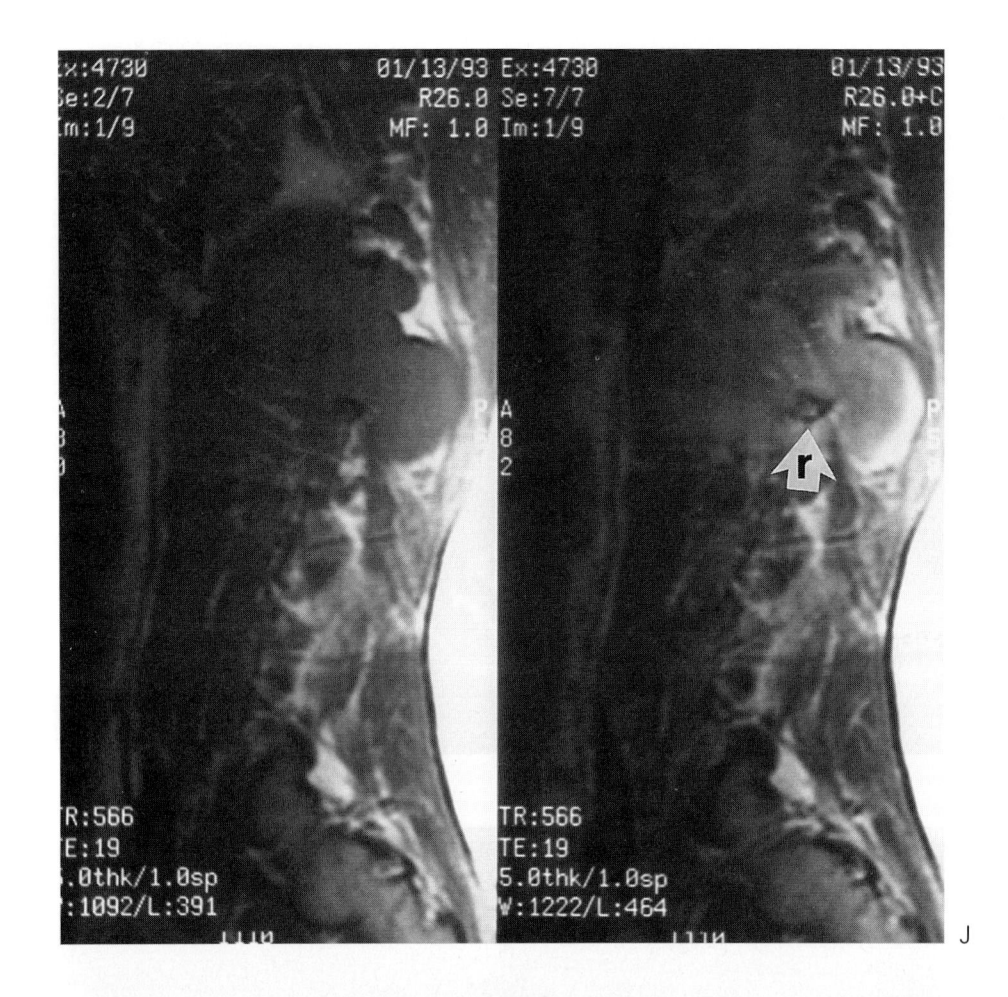

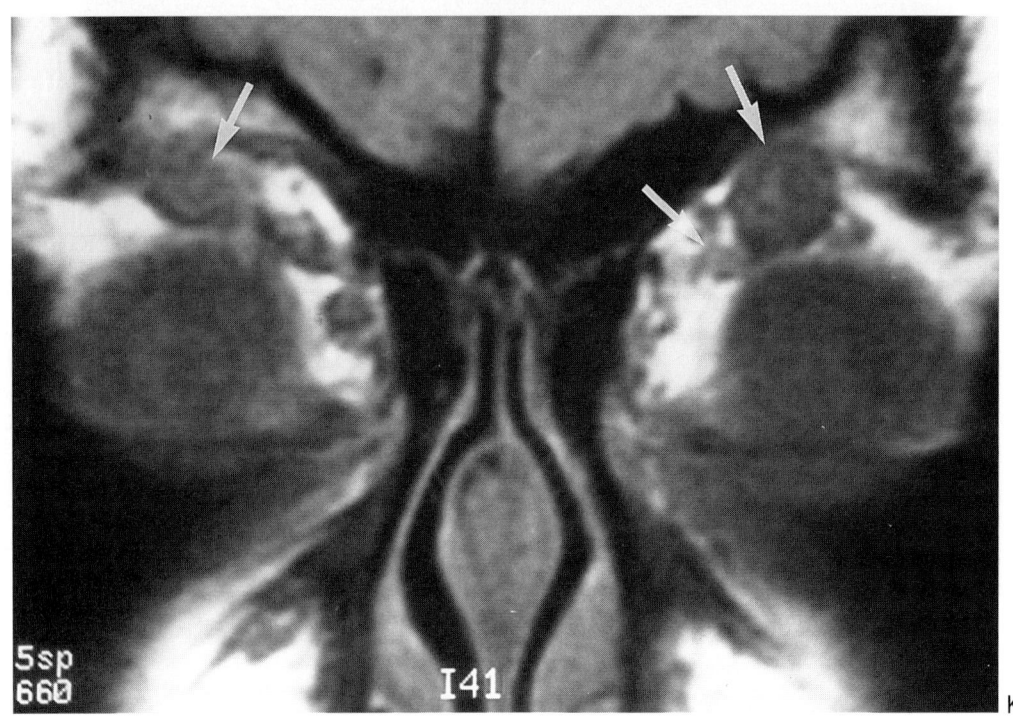

Radiologic Findings

Precontrast (Fig. A, *left*) coronal short TR image reveals multiple soft tissue density masses in the supraclavicular regions bilaterally (*circles*). The postcontrast (Fig. A, *right*) coronal short TR image shows dense enhancement of multiple areas within the vertebral canal (*medial triangles*), along the anterior margin of the middle scalenus muscle (*triangles*), and in the supraclavicular region (*circles*).

Parasagittal short TR image at the level of the intervertebral foramen (Fig. B) reveals that the normal increased signal intensity fat is replaced by soft tissue signal intensity masses at all levels of the intervertebral foramina (*squares*). The intervertebral foramina are enlarged. There are also multiple small soft tissue density masses along the course of the anterior scalenus muscle (*arrows*).

Pre- (Fig. C, *left*) and postcontrast (Fig. C, *right*) axial short TR images at the level of C5 reveal separation of the anterior (*a*) and middle (*m*) scalenus muscles by soft tissue density masses (*dotted line*). These masses exhibit dense enhancement postinfusion (*right, circles*). The anterior scalenus muscle is displaced anteriorly and flattened.

Axial short TR image at the level of C2 (Fig. D) reveals enhancing soft tissue masses in the intervertebral foramina bilaterally (*e*). There is a small enhancing mass that extends into the vertebral canal on the right side (*arrow*).

Axial short TR image after the infusion of contrast material (Fig. E) reveals multiple enhancing soft tissue density masses that surround the flow void of the vessels at the level of the thoracic inlet (*circles*). The vessels that are seen include: right subclavian vein (1), left subclavian vein (LSV), innominate artery (INN), left carotid artery (4), and left subclavian artery (5), trachea (T).

Axial short TR image at the level of L2 (Fig. F) reveals a lobulated soft tissue mass on the right side that extends into the vertebral canal via the intervertebral foramen (*long white arrow*). Multiple additional rounded soft tissue masses in the left paraspinal region and in the paraspinal muscles are also visible (*short white arrows*). There is a rounded soft tissue mass in the paraspinal muscles of the back (*black arrow*).

Axial long TR image at the same level as Figure E (Fig. G) reveals that the spinal cord is displaced to the left (*open arrow*). A large lobulated mass is noted on the right side. A portion of the tumor extends posteriorly (*r/arrow*). There are also multiple areas of increased signal intensity in the paraspinal regions and within the paraspinal muscles.

Axial short TR image slightly below the levels of Figures F and G (Fig. H) reveals marked expansion of the intervertebral foramen. The spinal cord is displaced far to the left (*arrow*). The kidney is seen on the left side.

Axial long TR image (Fig. I) reveals the lobulated soft tissue mass that appears as increased signal intensity. The spinal cord is compressed and displaced to the left (*arrow*). There are multiple smaller areas of increased signal intensity in the paraspinal muscles of the back.

Pre- (Fig. J, *left*) and postcontrast (Fig. J, *right*) parasagittal short TR images reveal enhancement of a lobulated mass. A portion of this mass herniates over the rib (*r/arrow*) into the soft tissues of the back. This is the same mass seen in Figure G.

Coronal short TR image of the orbit (Fig. K) reveals bilateral soft tissue masses that project above the globes of the orbit (*arrows*).

Diagnosis

Neurofibromatosis type 1 with multiple plexiform and dumbbell-shaped tumors.

Differential Diagnosis

- Neurofibromatosis type 1.

Discussion

The appearance is typical of patients with neurofibromatosis type 1. In the cervical region, there is enlargement of all of the intervertebral foramina because of neurofibromas at all levels of the cervical spine. These neurofibromas appear as increased signal intensity on the long TR images. There is pressure erosion of the bony structures at the level of the intervertebral foramen because of the longstanding nature of these lesions.

In the lumbar region, the spinal cord is displaced toward the left side. The spinal cord is also compressed into a triangular shape. The posterior lobulation of the mass seen in Figure G on the right side is secondary to herniation of a small portion of the mass through the ribs into the paraspinal muscles of the back. Symptoms may be minor because the neurofibromas are very slow growing and the spinal cord is able to accommodate compression when it occurs over a long period of time.

PEARL
- In patients with neurofibromatosis, large masses may be seen even in the patient with minimal or mild symptoms. Because the slow growth of these lesions may allow them to reach a relatively large size, imaging with magnetic resonance using intravenous contrast material will allow an accurate determination of the extent of the disease and also provide a baseline for future comparison at the time of follow-up.

PITFALL
- The entire canal should be evaluated because neurofibromas may be present even when there are no symptoms.

SPINAL CORD TUMORS

Case 3

Clinical Presentation

The patient is a 16-year-old male with progressive scoliosis, increasing lower left leg pain, and bowel and bladder incontinence.

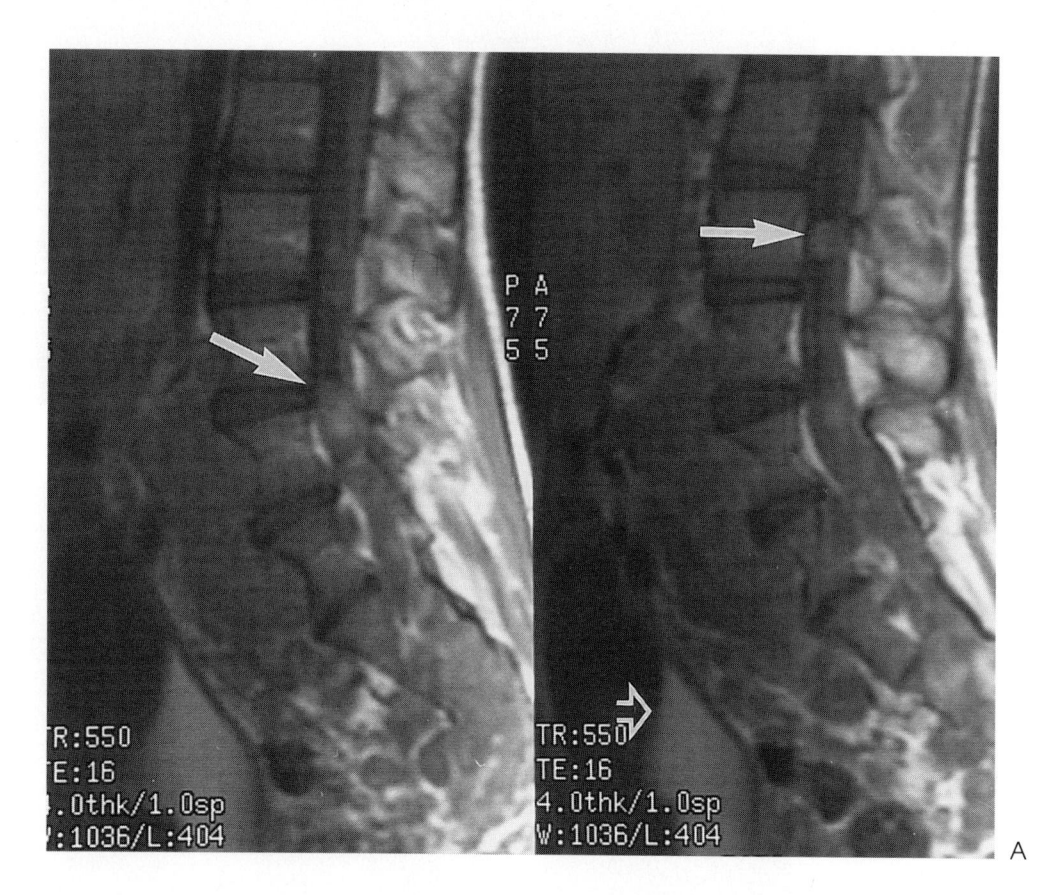

TEACHING ATLAS OF SPINE IMAGING

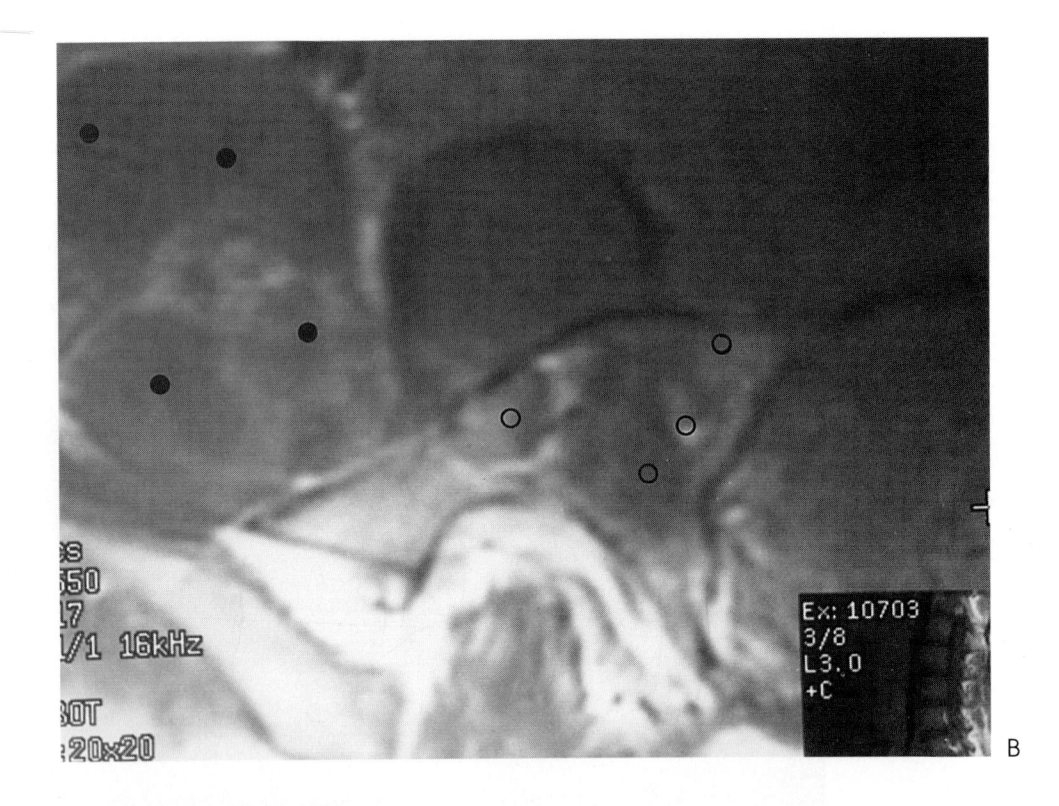

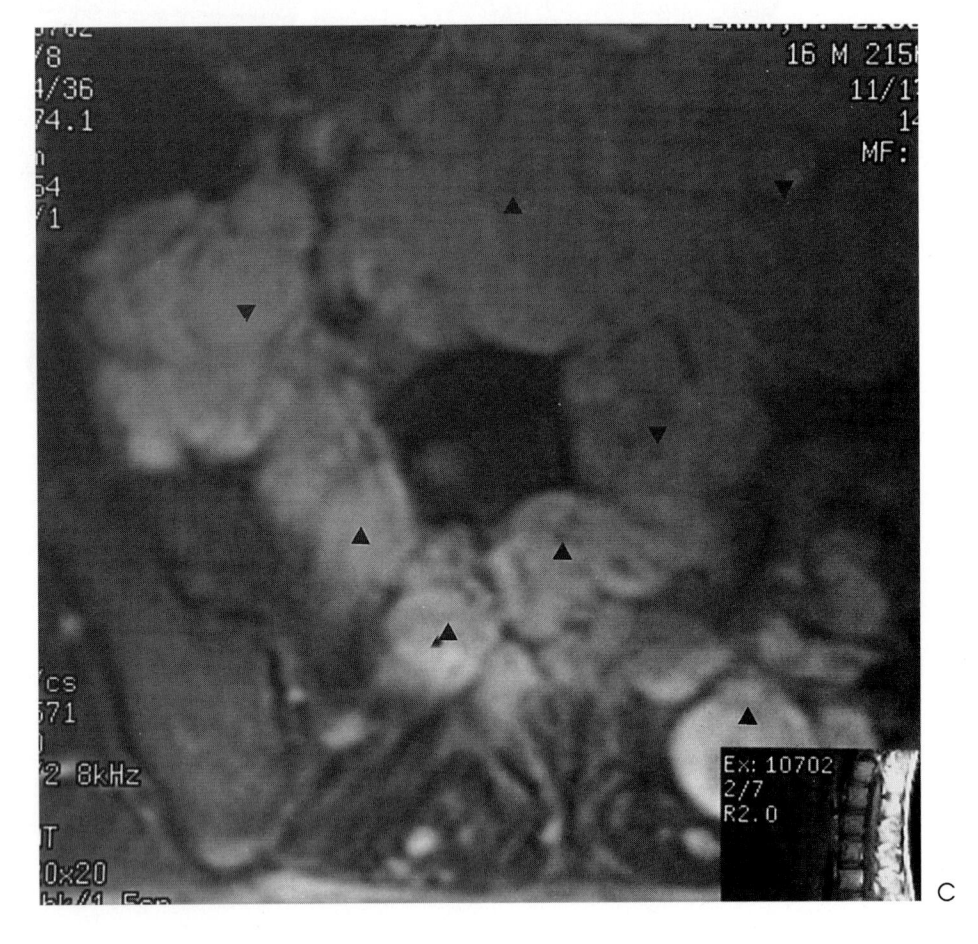

SPINAL CORD TUMORS

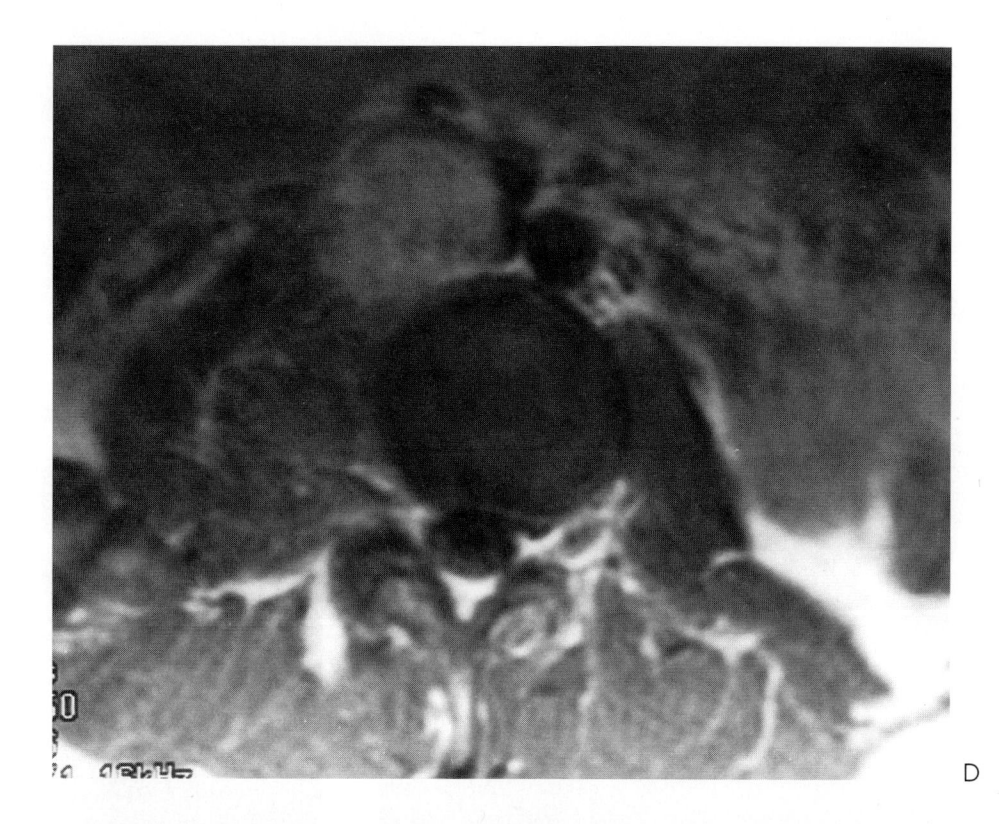

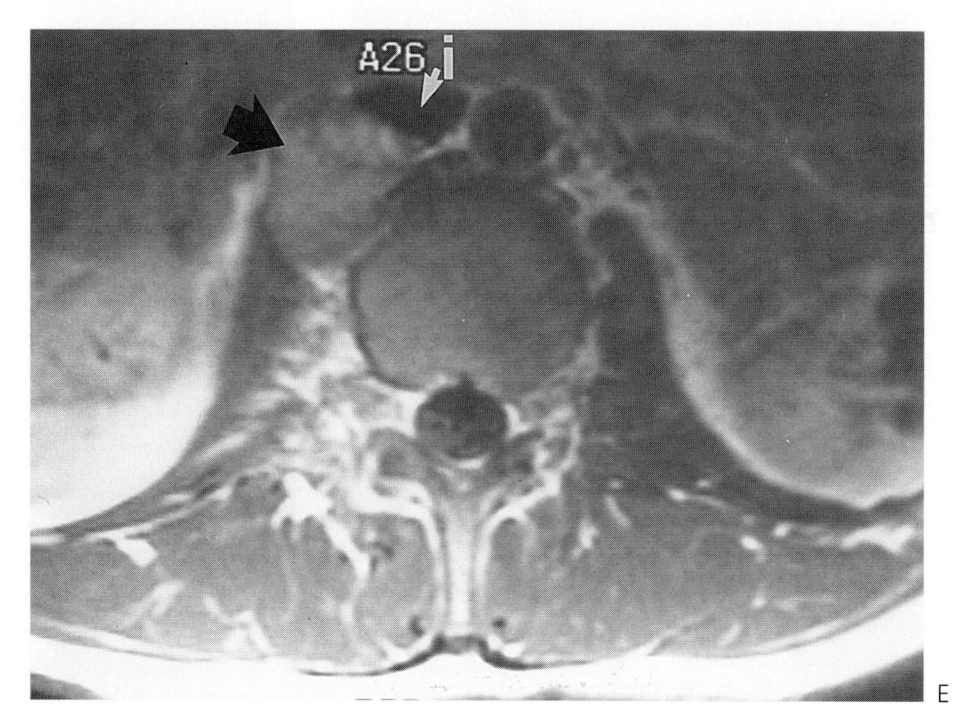

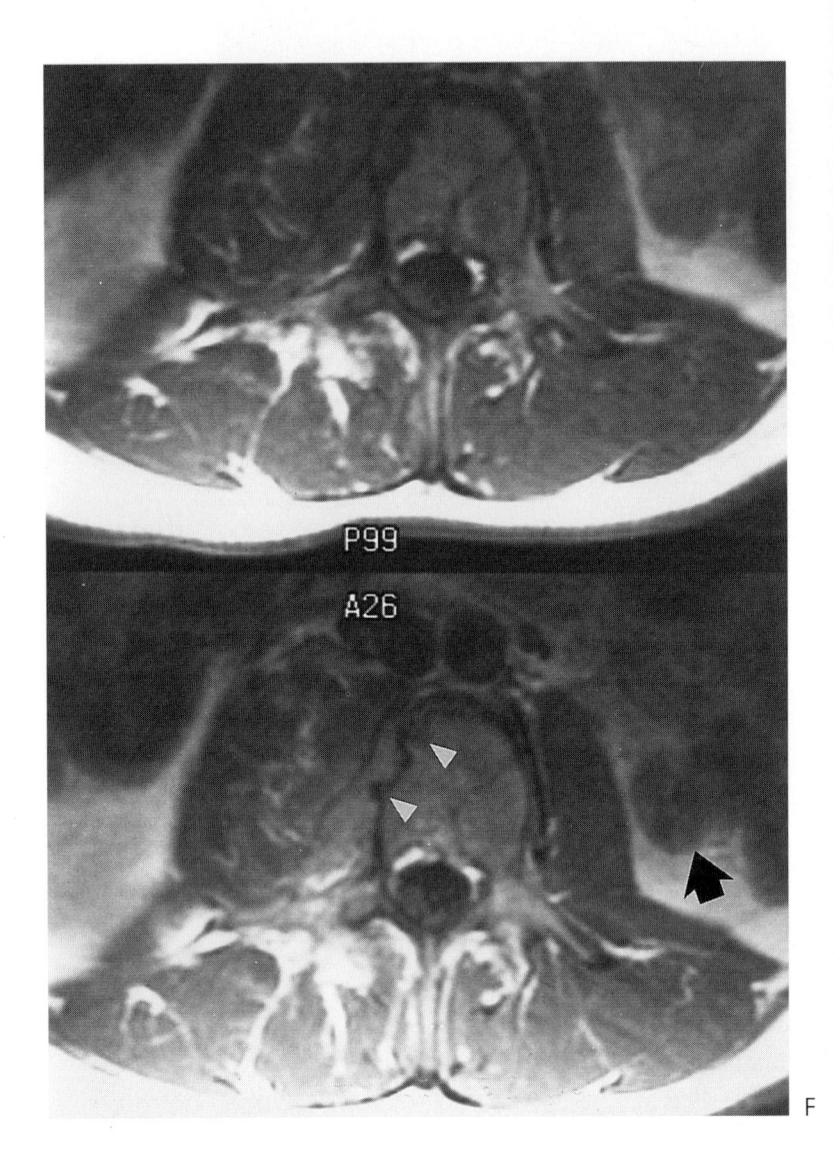

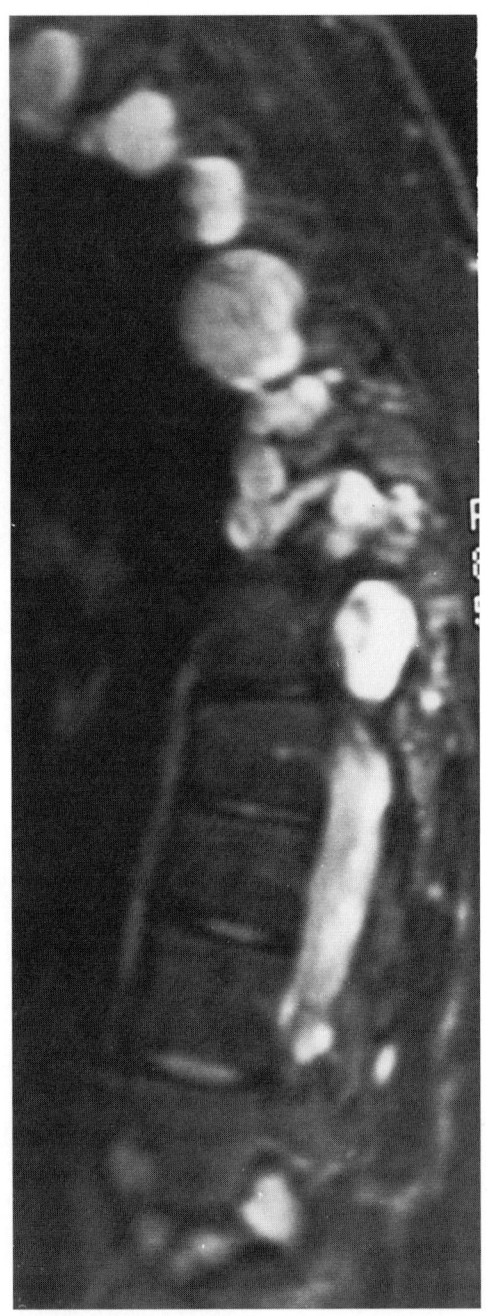

Radiologic Findings

Pre- (Fig. A, *left*) and postcontrast (Fig. A, *right*) sagittal short TR images reveal multiple soft tissue masses in the prevertebral region, within the spinal canal (*solid arrows*), and in the pelvis. Note fluid/fluid level in the bladder with accumulation of gadolinium in the dependent portion of the bladder (*right, open arrow*).

Axial short TR image postcontrast at the level of L5 (Fig. B) reveals multiple soft tissue masses within the vertebral canal (*open circles*), in the left prevertebral area, and in the paraspinal region (*solid circles*).

SPINAL CORD TUMORS

Radiologic Findings (continued)

Axial long TR image in the pelvis (Fig. C) reveals multiple confluent rounded areas of increased signal intensity that surround the distal colon and rectum (*arrowheads*).

Axial short TR image postcontrast at the level of L3 (Fig. D) reveals multiple rounded areas of enhancement adjacent to the inferior vena cava and in the paraspinal region within the psoas muscles.

Axial postcontrast image in the upper lumbar region (Fig. E) reveals a rounded, enhancing mass (*black arrow*) which displaces the inferior vena cava anteriorly (*i, white arrow*).

Axial short TR image postcontrast (Fig. F) reveals the pressure erosion of the lateral margin of the vertebral body (*white arrowheads*), with an associated soft tissue mass in the paraspinal area. There is a rounded, enhancing, soft tissue mass on the left side also (*black arrow*).

Parasagittal long TR image in the thoracic region (Fig. G) reveals that all the intervertebral foramina are enlarged by soft tissue masses that appear as increased signal intensity on the long TR images.

Diagnosis

Neurofibromatosis type 1 with multiple plexiform neurofibromas at all levels on the spine.

Differential Diagnosis

- Neurofibromatosis type 1 with multiple plexiform neurofibromas.

Discussion

There is extension of the multiple plexiform neurofibromas into the expanded distal vertebral canal. In addition, there are multiple, intradural enhancing lesions in the distal lumbar vertebral canal and para-aortic neurofibromas. Pressure erosion of the lateral margin of the vertebral body secondary to the neurofibromas is also visible. These findings are typical of patients with neurofibromatosis type 1 with multiple plexiform neurofibromas. Surgery is frequently impossible in these patients because the extensive nature of these tumors makes surgical removal impossible.

PEARL
- Magnetic resonance imaging (MRI) with contrast enhancement is the most sensitive method of evaluation of these patients. The study should be performed with multiplanar imaging.

PITFALLS
- Spinal tap may be very difficult in a patient such as this case because the multiple intradural and extradural masses obliterate the subarachnoid space.

- Previously myelography was used for evaluation of these patients. However, since the availability of MR, this newer technique has replaced the use of myelography and postmyelography computed tomography for evaluation

- These patients are difficult to manage because of the presence of multiple lesions.

TEACHING ATLAS OF SPINE IMAGING

Case 4

Clinical Presentation

The patient is an 11-year-old male with left arm pain after stretching. Physical exam revealed brisk deep tendon reflexes and positive Babinski's sign.

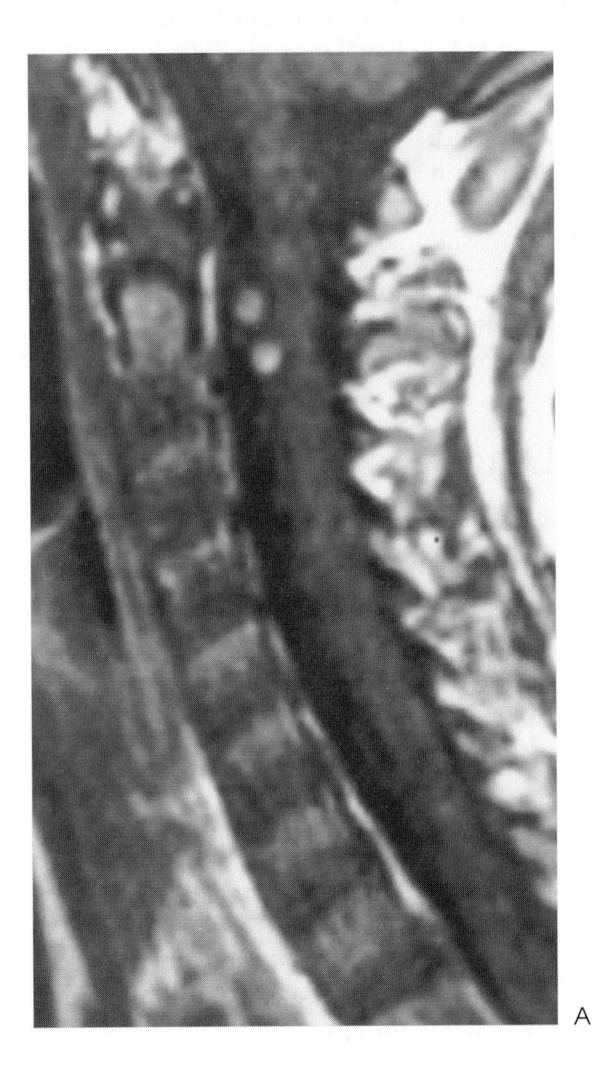

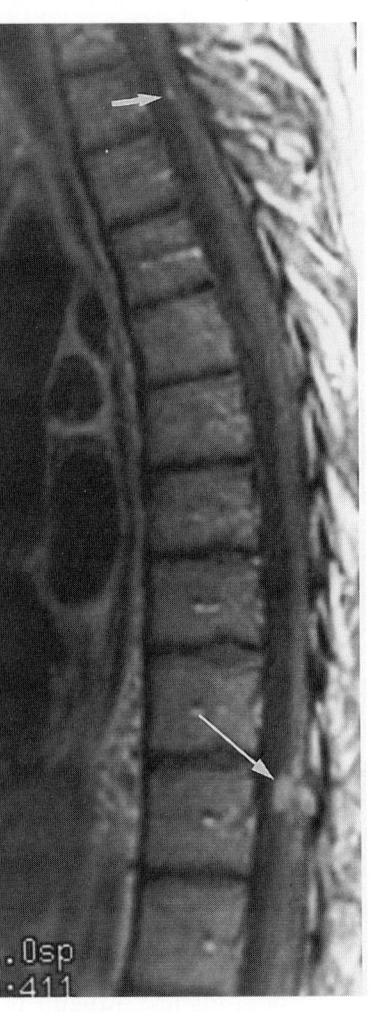

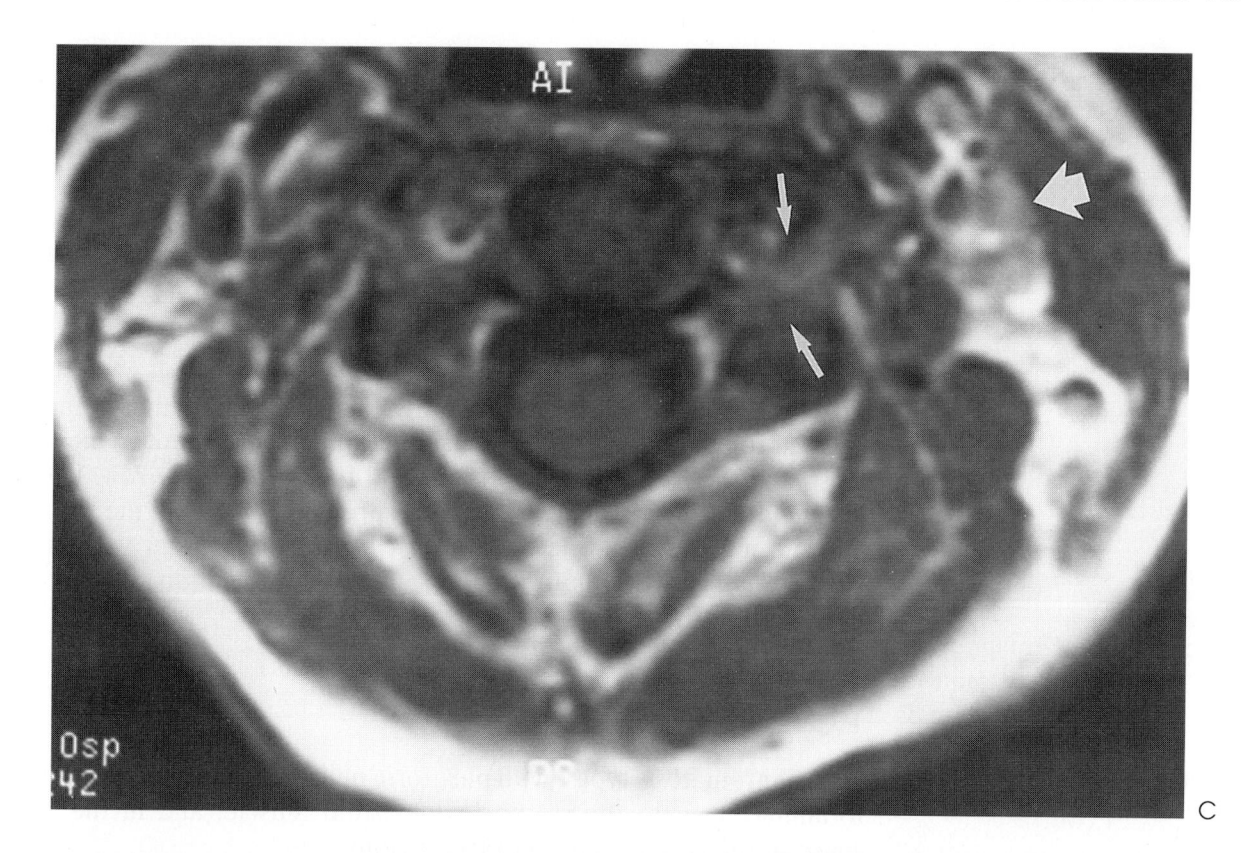

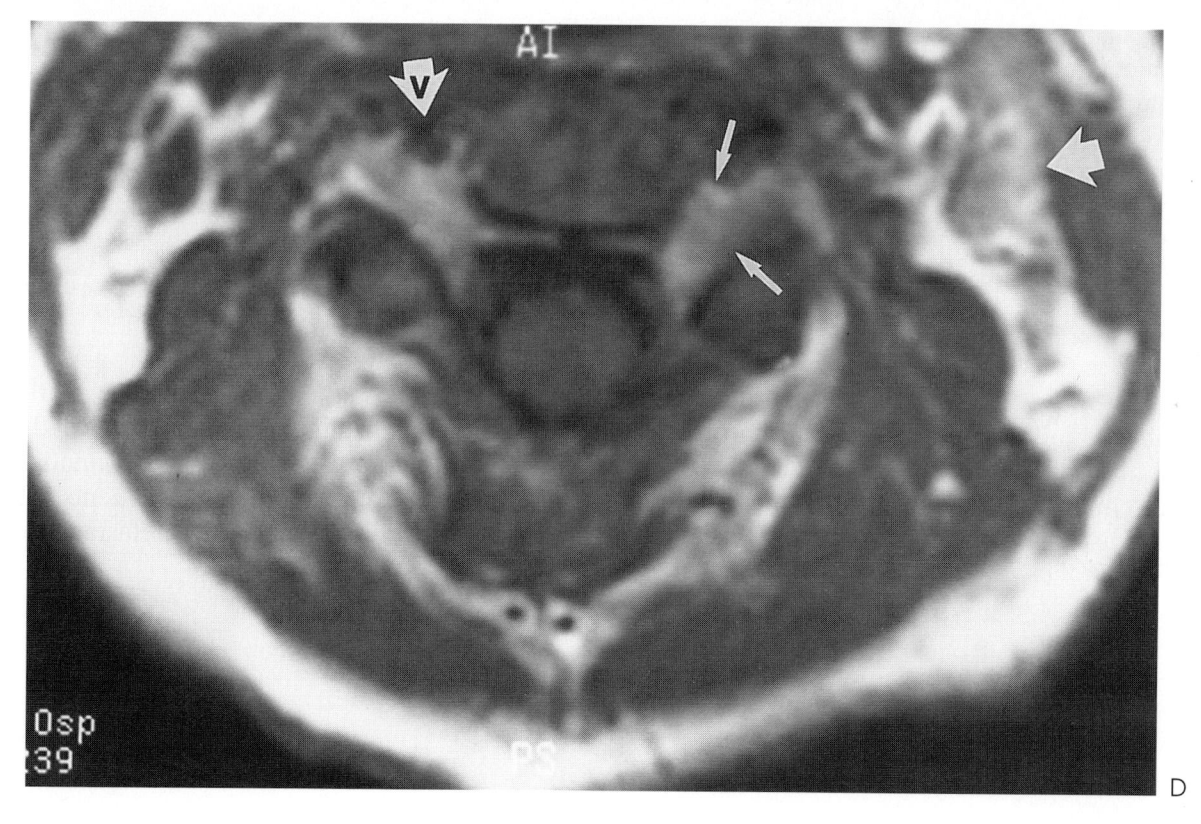

SPINAL CORD TUMORS

TEACHING ATLAS OF SPINE IMAGING

Radiologic Findings

Sagittal short TR image after the infusion of contrast (Fig. A) reveals two small rounded areas of enhancement projecting anterior to the spinal cord at the C2 level.

Sagittal short TR image postcontrast (Fig. B) reveals three small oval-shaped areas of enhancement in the distal thoracic region (*long arrow*). There is also a very small rounded area of enhancement anterior to the spinal cord in the upper thoracic region (*short arrow*).

Pre- (Fig. C) and postcontrast (Fig. D) axial short TR images through the cervical spine at the C5 level reveal bilateral enhancement of the soft tissue masses at the level of the intervertebral foramen (*thin arrows*). There are also multiple soft tissue density masses projecting beneath the sternocleidomastoid muscle on the left side (*thick arrows*). The right vertebral artery (Fig. D, *v/arrow*) is abutted along its posterior margin by an enhancing lesion in the right intervertebral foramen.

Diagnosis

Neurofibromatosis type 1 with plexiform neurofibromas in the intervertebral foramina, deep to the sternocleidomastoid muscle, and in the intradural space in the cervical and thoracic region.

Differential Diagnosis

- Schwannomas
- Metastatic deposits

Discussion

The process is less extensive in this patient than in many patients with neurofibromatosis. The relatively small number of lesions seen in this patient would raise the possibility that these represent multiple schwannomas rather than neurofibromas. Schwannomas may also be seen in patients with neurofibromatosis. In addition, the possibility of multiple metastatic deposits is also a clinical consideration.

PEARLS

- Magnetic resonance imaging is the ideal method for evaluation of the multiple lesions that may be seen in patients with this disease. The study should be performed with contrast enhancement.

- It is not uncommon that the patient may palpate these neurofibromas, which are more superficial in location, particularly those that are beneath the sternocleidomastoid muscle.

PITFALL

- It is possible to fail to appreciate those neurofibromas which are remote from the spinal or paraspinal area.

SPINAL CORD TUMORS

Case 5

Clinical Presentation

The patient is a 13-year-old male with lower extremity weakness.

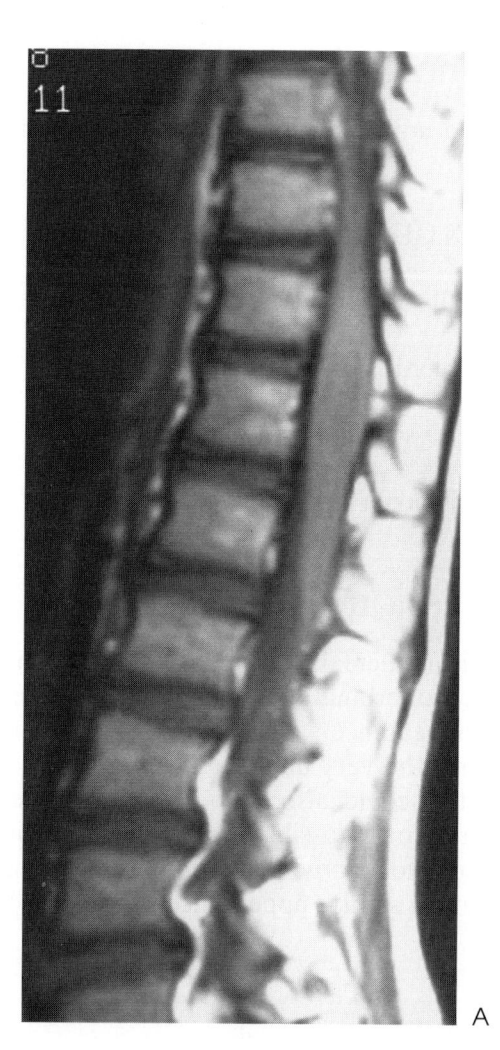

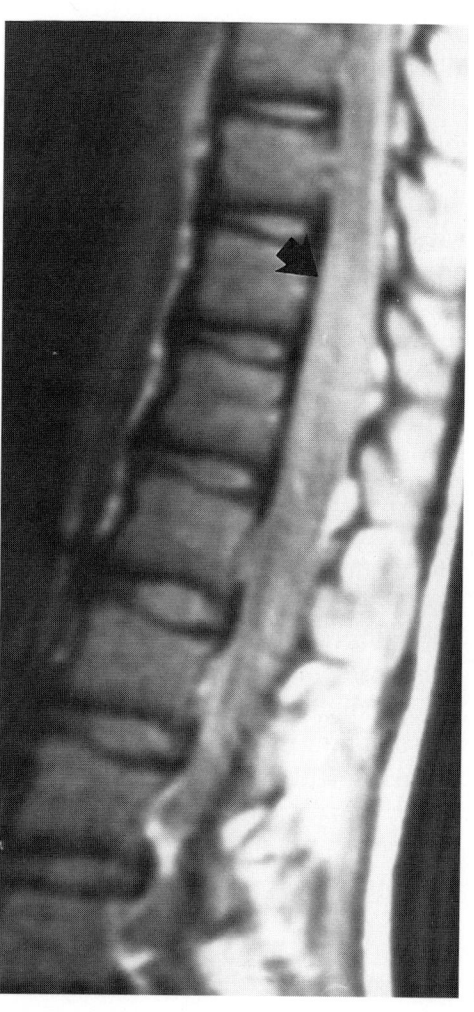

TEACHING ATLAS OF SPINE IMAGING

Radiologic Findings

Sagittal short TR image at the level of the conus medullaris (Fig. A) reveals focal widening of the distal end of the spinal cord. There is a central area of decreased density within the spinal cord.

Sagittal intermediate TR image (Fig. B) reveals increased signal intensity within the distal end of the spinal cord (*arrow*).

Diagnosis

Probable nonenhancing low grade astrocytoma of the distal spinal cord.

Differential Diagnosis

- Neurofibromatosis type 1
- Spinal cord infarct
- Acute disseminated encephalomyelitis (ADEM)
- Ependymoma

Discussion

There is an increased incidence of brain and spinal cord tumors in patients with neurofibromatosis type 1. In an older patient, this magnetic resonance (MR) appearance would be consistent with a spinal cord infarct. However, this would be very unlikely in a 13-year-old patient. An area of transverse "myelitis" could also have a similar appearance. The patient should be evaluated for a possible recent viral infection and a resulting ADEM. Another histologic type of spinal cord tumor such as an ependymoma would also have a similar appearance.

PEARLS
- Watchful waiting may be the best course of action in this patient. MR provides the ideal method of follow-up.
- Most spinal cord tumors exhibit enhancement postcontrast, so the lack of enhancement in this patient is not in favor of a neoplasm.

PITFALL
- Subtle changes in the appearance of the spinal cord may not be appreciated, particularly if there is no enhancement of the lesion. Knowledge of the clinical presentation is very helpful when interpreting images in which there are only subtle changes.

SPINAL CORD TUMORS

Case 6

Clinical Presentation

The patient is a 14-year-old female with deafness and headaches.

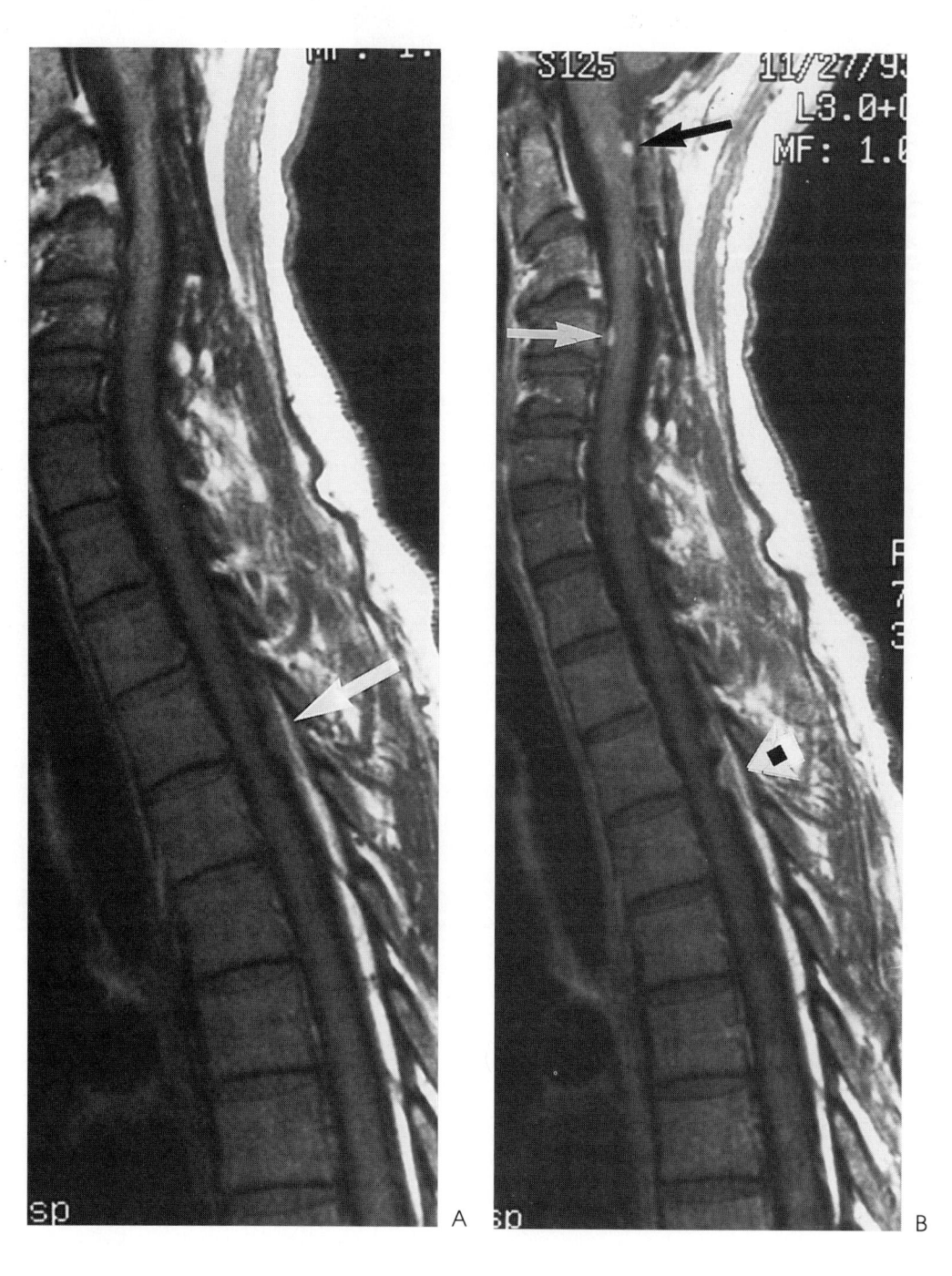

235

TEACHING ATLAS OF SPINE IMAGING

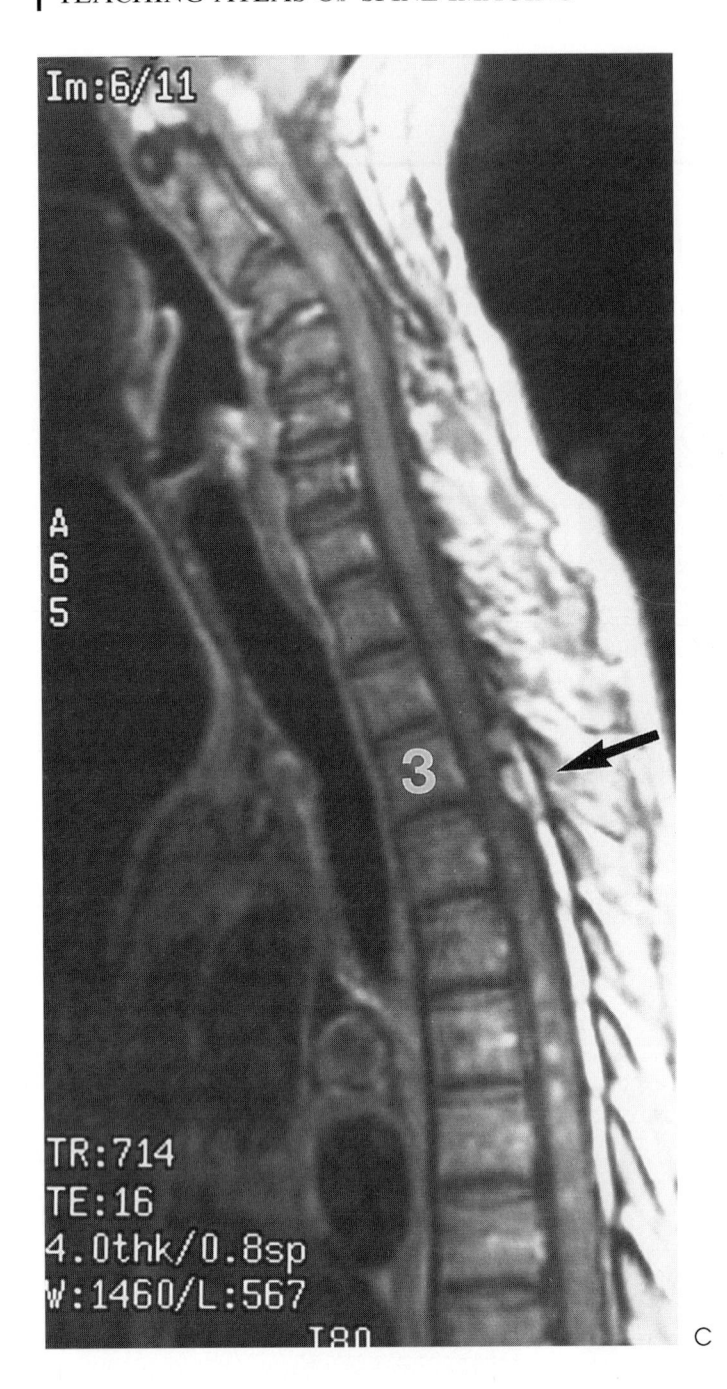

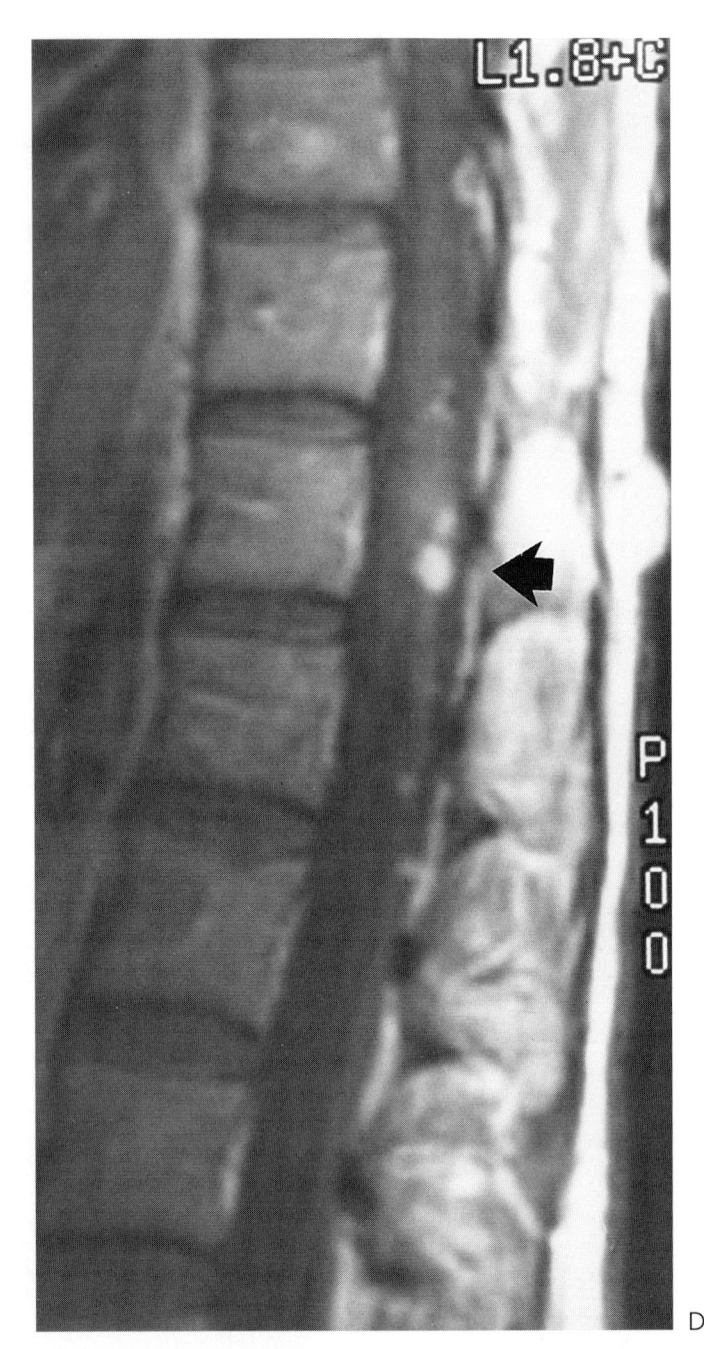

SPINAL CORD TUMORS

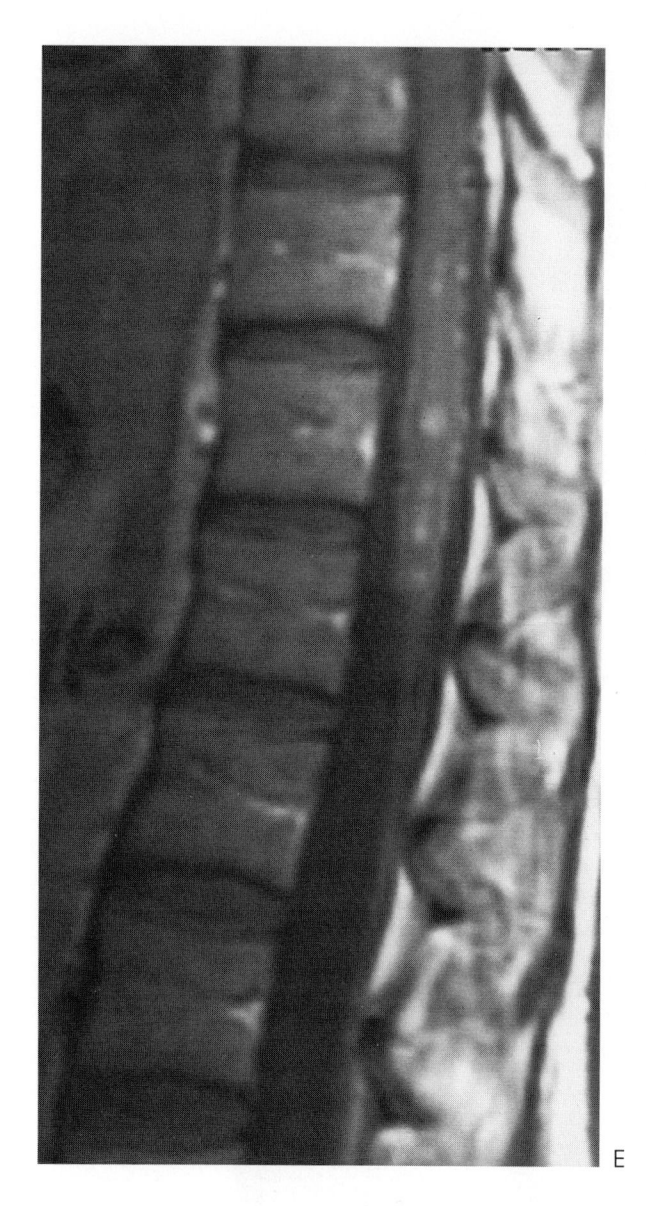

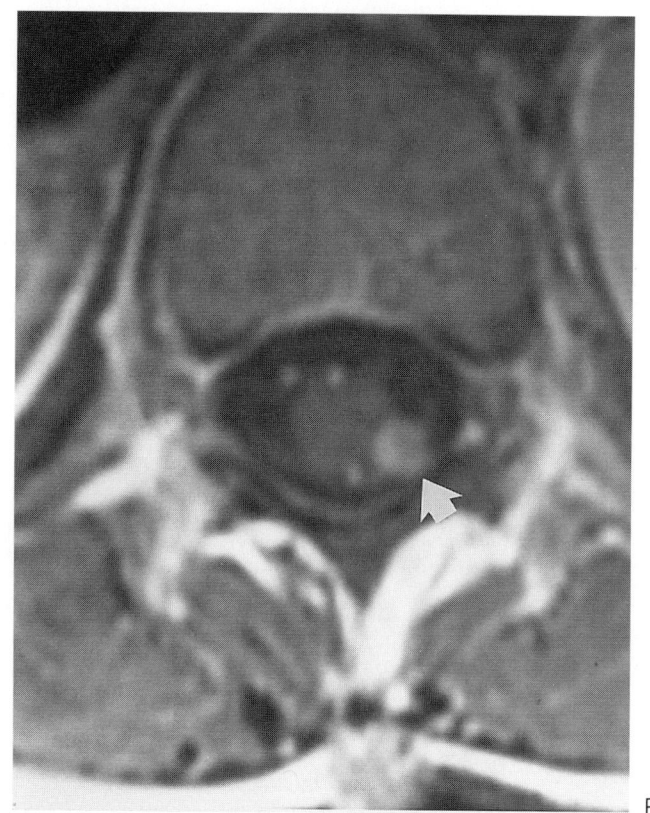

E

F

237

TEACHING ATLAS OF SPINE IMAGING

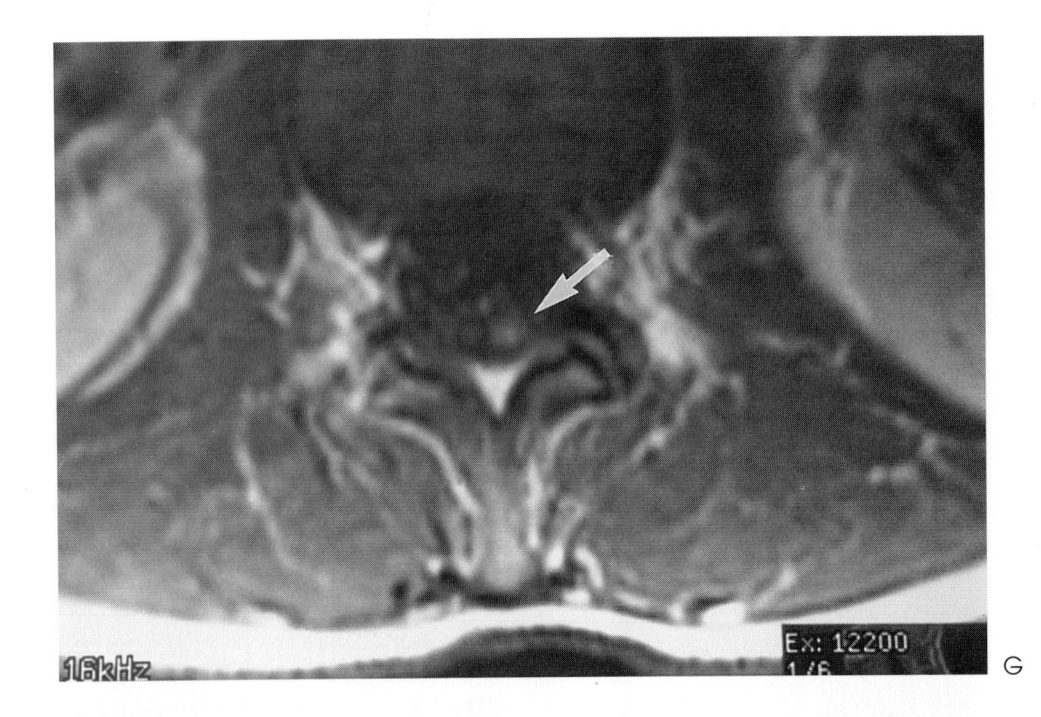

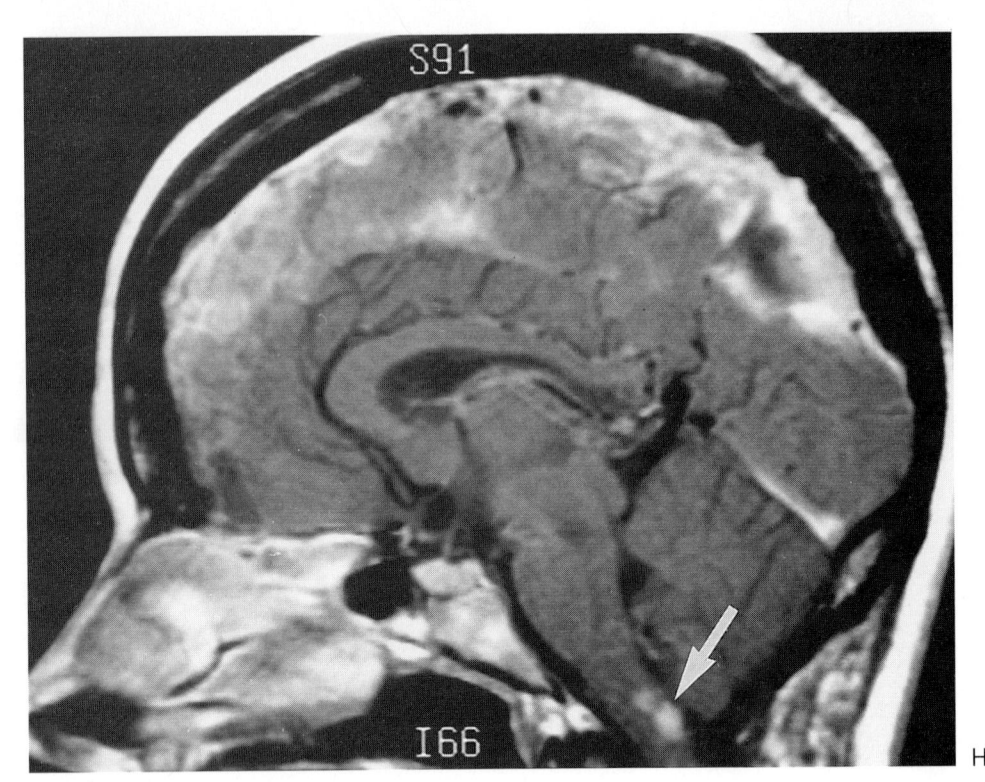

SPINAL CORD TUMORS

Radiologic Findings

Sagittal T1-weighted image of the cervical and thoracic spine (Fig. A) reveals reversal of the normal lordotic curve of the cervical spine. The spinal cord appears normal in size throughout. There is a broad-based approximately 8 mm soft tissue mass dorsal to the spinal cord at the T3 level (*arrow*).

Sagittal T1-weighted image postcontrast (Fig. B) reveals dense enhancement of a 2 to 3 mm schwannoma dorsal to the cord at the C2 level (*black arrow*). There are multiple additional smaller areas of enhancement at the level of C2 and C4 (*white arrow*). A broad-based, enhancing mass that can be seen at T3 (*white arrow with black square*). There is also a second, smaller broad-based mass just superior to this large mass, which is also faintly seen on the preinfusion study in Figure A.

Follow-up 1 year later. Sagittal T1-weighted image postcontrast again (Fig. C) reveals the new enhancing lesions at the level of T3-4 (*arrow*). On this image, there are also multiple enhancing intramedullary lesions that begin at the level of the lower medulla and are visible in the cervical region and then again in the midthoracic spinal cord down to the level of T8. The T3 thoracic level is identified with 3.

Sagittal T1-weighted images postcontrast (Figs. D and E) reveal multiple small areas of enhancement scattered throughout the lower thoracic and upper lumbar subarachnoid space. The largest of these (Fig. D, *arrow*) is also seen in Figure G.

Axial T1-weighted image at the level of T12 (Fig. F) reveals the densely enhancing mass seen in Figure D (*white arrow*). There are also multiple, additional rounded areas of enhancement.

Axial T1-weighted image postcontrast in the region of the cauda equina (Fig. G) reveals multiple small areas of enhancement, the largest of which is highlighted by the white arrow.

Sagittal T1-weighted image postcontrast (Fig. H) reveals dense enhancement of the falx cerebri. There are also multiple focal areas of increased enhancement. The intramedullary spinal cord enhancing lesion is again seen (*arrow*); this lesion is consistent with an ependymoma. The patient also had bilateral masses in the internal auditory canals.

Diagnosis

Neurofibromatosis type 2 with multiple spinal schwannomas, meningiomas, and ependymomas, as well as cerebral meningiomas and acoustic schwannomas.

Differential Diagnosis

- Meningioma

- Intramedullary ependymomas

PEARLS

- The appearance of the constellation of findings in this patient is really pathognomonic of neurofibromatosis type 2. This disease is autosomal dominant and is associated with a defect on chromosome number 22. This disease is also typically associated with bilateral acoustic schwannomas, which are thought to be diagnostic.

- Although many of these tumors are relatively benign and if surgically removed will result in a cure, their location may preclude removal. Additionally, the number of lesions may make satisfactory treatment very difficult.

- The mnemonic of M-I-S-M-E—*m*ultiple, *i*nherited *s*chwannomas, *m*eningiomas, and *e*pendymomas—is very helpful for recalling the lesions associated with neurofibromatosis type 2.

- Neurofibromatosis type 2 has been called "central" neurofibromatosis, while neurofibromatosis type 1 has been called "peripheral" neurofibromatosis. These names reflect the anatomic locations of the abnormalities and are a practical, if not scientific method, of differentiating between the two diseases.

TEACHING ATLAS OF SPINE IMAGING

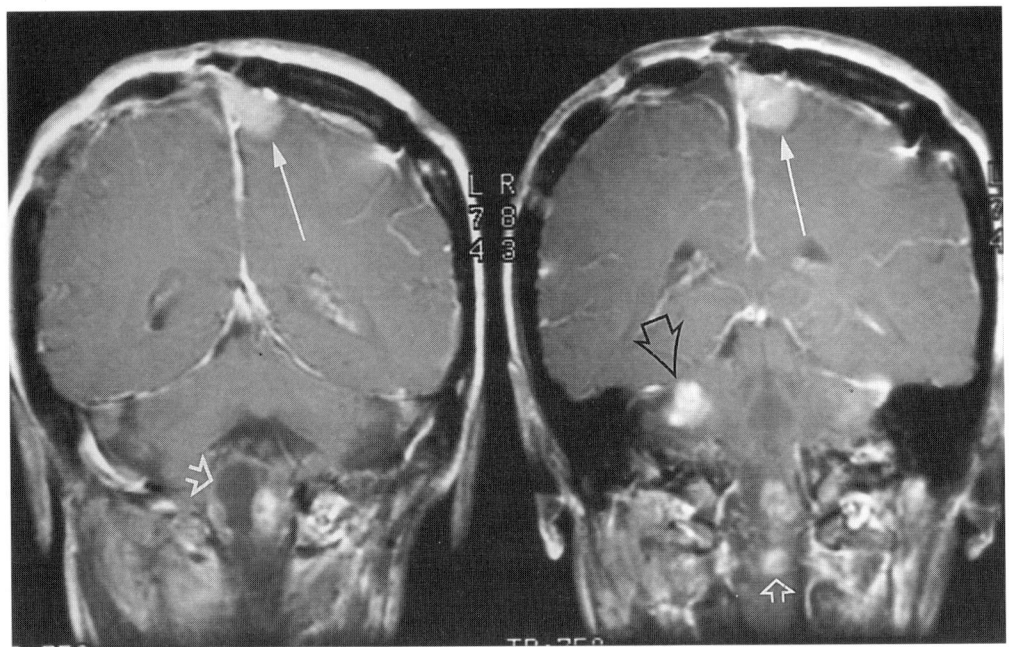

F

Radiologic Findings

Sagittal T1-weighted images. The preinfusion image (Fig. A, *left*) reveals a cystic lesion in the region of the cerebellar tonsils. The spinal cord at the level of the cervicomedullary junction is enlarged. There is a rounded signal intensity mass located slightly higher than spinal cord within the spinal cord at the C2 level (*arrowhead*). Postinfusion (Fig. A, *right*) there is a rounded area of enhancement at this level (*arrowhead*). On the postinfusion study, there is also enhancement of a lobulated mass in the cervical spinal cord above the level of the midbody of the C2 vertebral body extending to the level of the bottom of the fourth ventricle. Magnetic susceptibility artifact, noticeable on both images (*g*), marks the location of metallic sutures from previous surgery. There is also a small broad-based mass that projects behind the intervertebral disc at the C5-6 level (*left, arrow*).

Sagittal long TR image (Fig. B). The cystic lesion in the floor of the posterior fossa is increased in signal intensity. The spinal cord tumor appears as an area of decreased signal intensity in the upper spinal cord (*arrow*).

Axial short TR image postcontrast (Fig. C) reveals bilateral enhancing acoustic schwannomas. There is a small cyst that projects behind the right acoustic tumor (*arrow*).

A slightly higher image slice (Fig. D) reveals the bilateral internal auditory canal and densely enhancing masses, including a mass along the anterior margin of the petrous bone on the left side (*arrow*).

Parasagittal postcontrast short TR image (Fig. E) reveals the enhancing mass in the right internal auditory canal with the cystic component projecting posteriorly (*arrow*).

Coronal short TR images postcontrast (Fig. F) reveal the cystic mass in the posterior fossa (*open white arrow, left*) at the level of the foramen magnum. There is a densely enhancing left parietal, parasagittal mass (*long white arrow, left and right*); slightly more anteriorly the right-sided acoustic neu-

SPINAL CORD TUMORS

PEARLS
- The finding of bilateral acoustic schwannomas is typical of the diagnosis of neurofibromatosis type 2.

- Intramedullary ependymomas are found in patients with neurofibromatosis type 2; however, because patients may be asymptomatic, it is advised that these tumors be observed rather than operated.

PITFALLS
- If a postcontrast study is not performed, the intramedullary ependymomas may not be appreciated.

- While the multiplicity of lesions could suggest the diagnosis of metastases, the distribution of the lesions and their pattern of occurrence is not in favor of metastatic disease.

roma is again seen (*open black arrow, right*). Two enhancing lesions are seen in the upper spinal cord (*open white arrow, right*). There are surgical defects in the bony calvaria bilaterally from previous craniectomies for removal of convexity tumors.

Diagnosis

Neurofibromatosis, with bilateral acoustic schwannomas, meningiomas, and spinal cord ependymomas.

Differential Diagnosis

- Neurofibromatosis

Discussion

Clinical history is very helpful in the diagnosis of this abnormality. Neurofibromatosis is described by using the helpful mnemonic of MISME (*m*ultiple, *i*nherited *s*chwannomas, *m*eningiomas, and *e*pendymomas). Using this mnemonic is very helpful because it aids in the identification of these various abnormalities. The previous surgery was for removal of cerebral meningiomas.

Section III

Spinal Cord Tumors

D. Miscellaneous

SPINAL CORD TUMORS

Case 1

Clinical Presentation

The patient is a 53-year-old male with a history of neck pain and upper and lower extremity weakness.

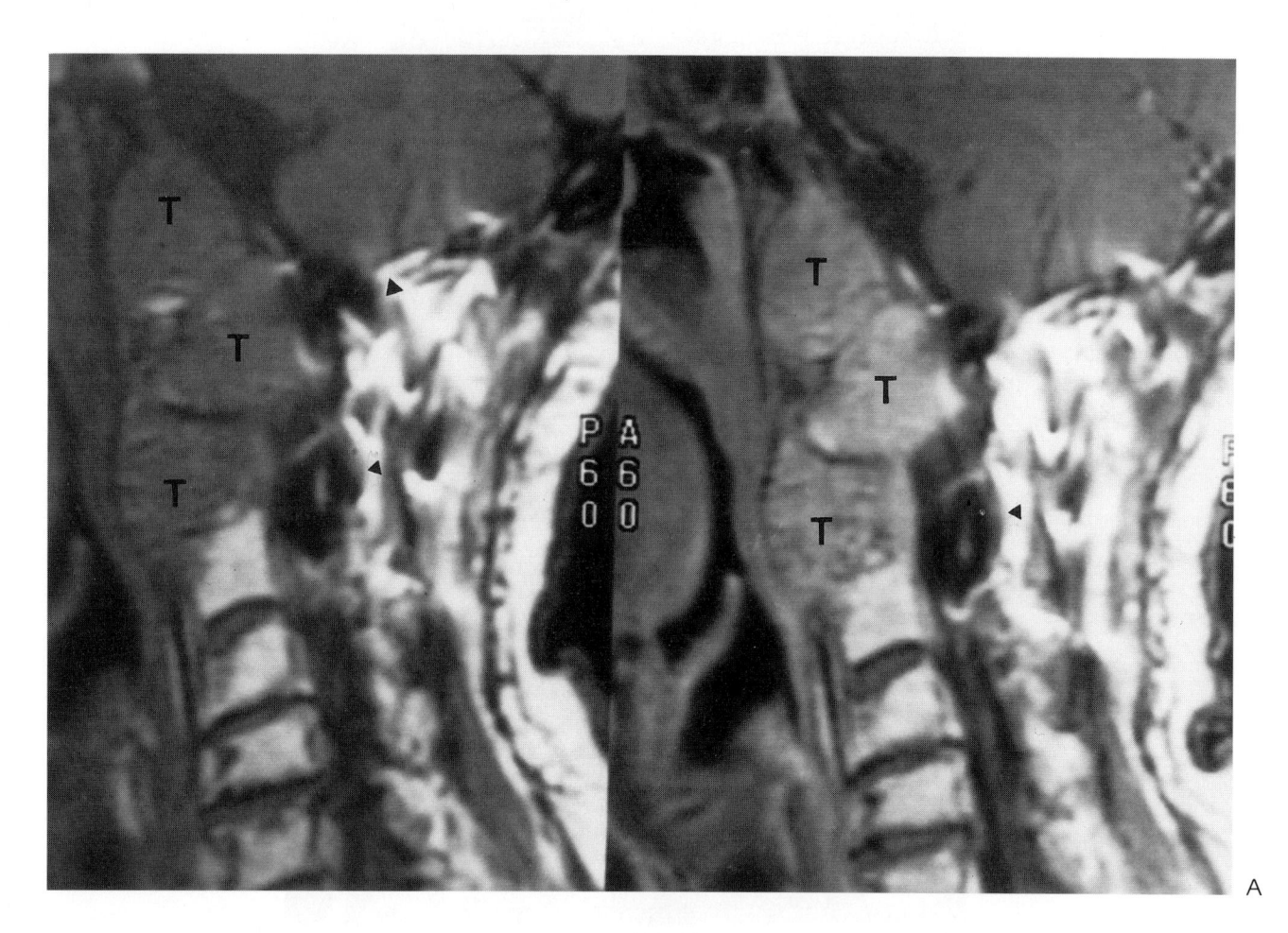

TEACHING ATLAS OF SPINE IMAGING

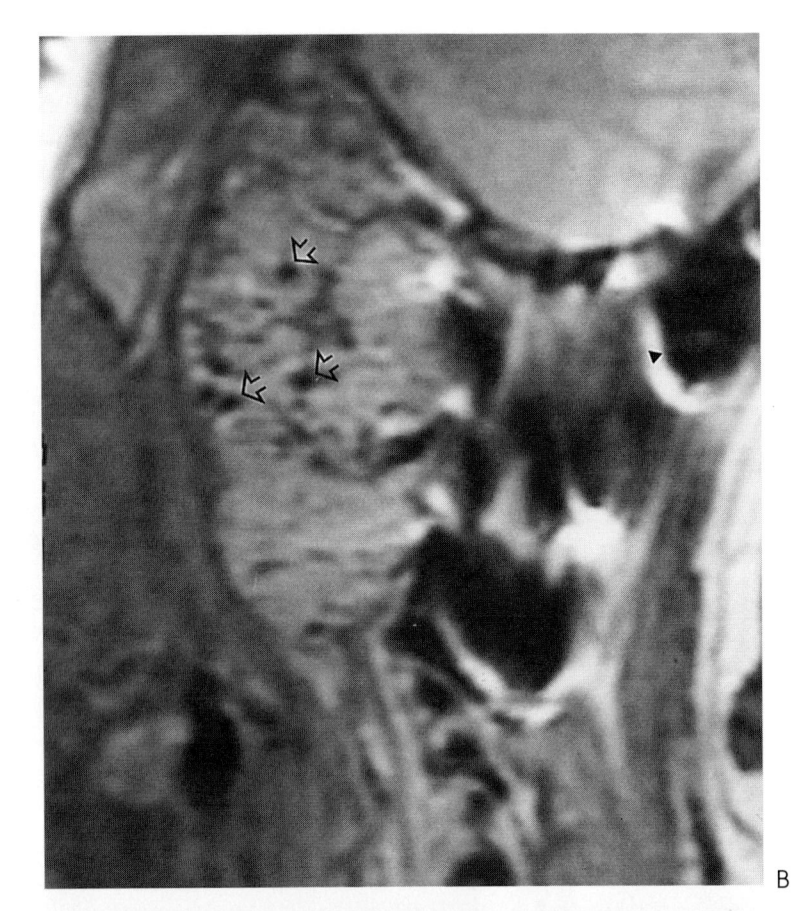

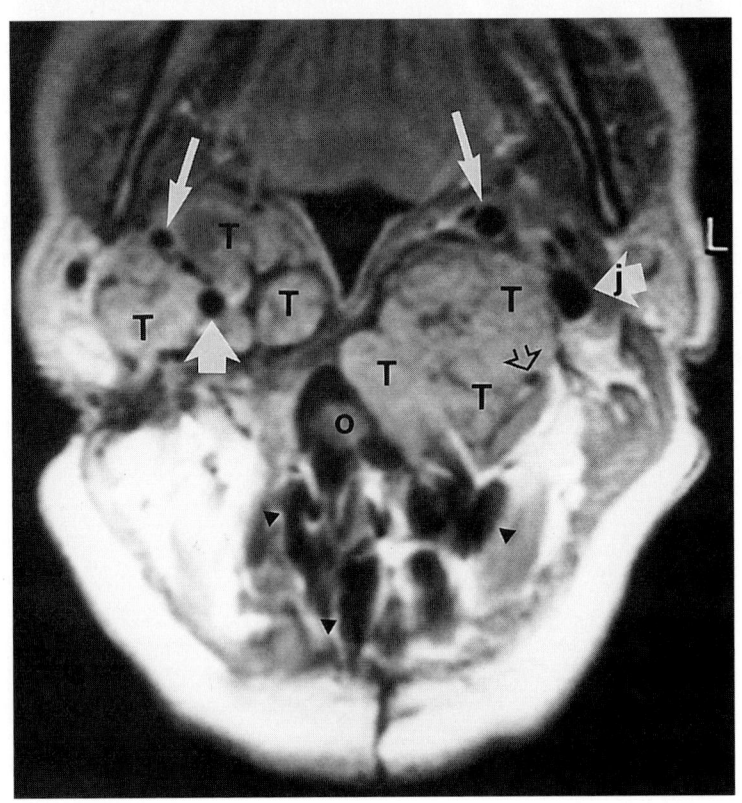

B

C

SPINAL CORD TUMORS

Radiologic Findings

Pre- (Fig. A, *left*) and postcontrast (Fig. A, *right*) sagittal short TR images at the level of the skull base and upper cervical spine reveal a lobulated soft tissue mass (*T*), which has destroyed the inferior margin of the clivus, the odontoid process, and the C3 vertebral body. The remaining cervical vertebral bodies appear diffusely increased in signal intense. Mild degenerative changes are also noted with osteophyte formation. The masses all exhibit dense enhancement on the postinfusion study (*right*). There are multiple rounded and oval areas of decreased signal intensity, which exhibit thin increased signal intensity rims (*arrowheads*).

Sagittal intermediate TR image (Fig. B) reveals multiple small rounded areas of decreased signal intensity within the mass (*open arrows*). In the suboccipital region, there are multiple rounded areas of decreased signal with thin increased rounded rims, the highest of which is identified by an arrowhead.

Axial short TR image postcontrast (Fig. C) reveals multiple varying sized masses (*T*) in the prevertebral, paraspinal, and lateral neck region. The jugular vein is seen on the left side as an area of flow void (*j/arrow*). The carotid artery is surrounded by the masses on the right side (*wide white arrow*). The flow void of the external carotid arteries are seen anteriorly (*long white arrows*). The spinal cord is identified (*circle*), and the surrounding subarachnoid space is effaced along the left lateral and anterior margins. There are multiple oval and rounded areas of decreased signal intensity with the increased signal intensity rims again identified (*arrowheads*). A thin decreased signal intensity line in the midline dorsally in the subcutaneous fat indicates a previous laminectomy.

Diagnosis

Chordoma, with postoperative changes.

Differential Diagnosis

- Chordoma
- Metastatic deposits
- Rheumatoid arthritis

Discussion

Chordomas occur from remnants of the primitive notocord of the spine. They typically occur at the far upper end of the spinal cord in the region of the clivus or at the very distal end of the notochord in the region of the sacrum. However, chordomas may occur at any point along the vertebral column. Metastatic deposits might be a consideration in this case; however, metastases tend to be more permeative in nature. In Figure B, the small internal areas of flow void are secondary to multiple enlarged arteries and

Pearls
- Clinical history is very important in this patient. Chordomas frequently recur following surgery, and total removal is almost impossible. Multiplanar imaging, as in this case, will frequently allow demonstration of the spinal cord in at least one plane, even in the presence of extensive metallic fixating wires, screws, or plates.
- Magnetic resonance is the ideal method for diagnosis and follow up.

Pitfall
- If the metallic artifact from previous surgery is sufficiently extensive and the spinal cord and its relationship to the surrounding structures cannot be demonstrated, it may be necessary to perform a myelogram and postmyelogram computed tomographic scan.

draining veins. Rheumatoid arthritis, with pannus formation, would not result in such extensive changes.

Magnetic susceptibility artifact is visible because of multiple metallic wires that hold the spine in place. The artifact results in the multiple areas of decreased signal intensity. The increased signal intensity is secondary to previous radiation therapy and a relative increase in the amount of adipose tissue within the marrow of the vertebral bodies.

SPINAL CORD TUMORS

Case 2

Case Presentation

The patient is a 35-year-old male with a history of previous surgery for a tumor arising from the clivus. The patient now presents with progressive lower extremity weakness and difficulty breathing.

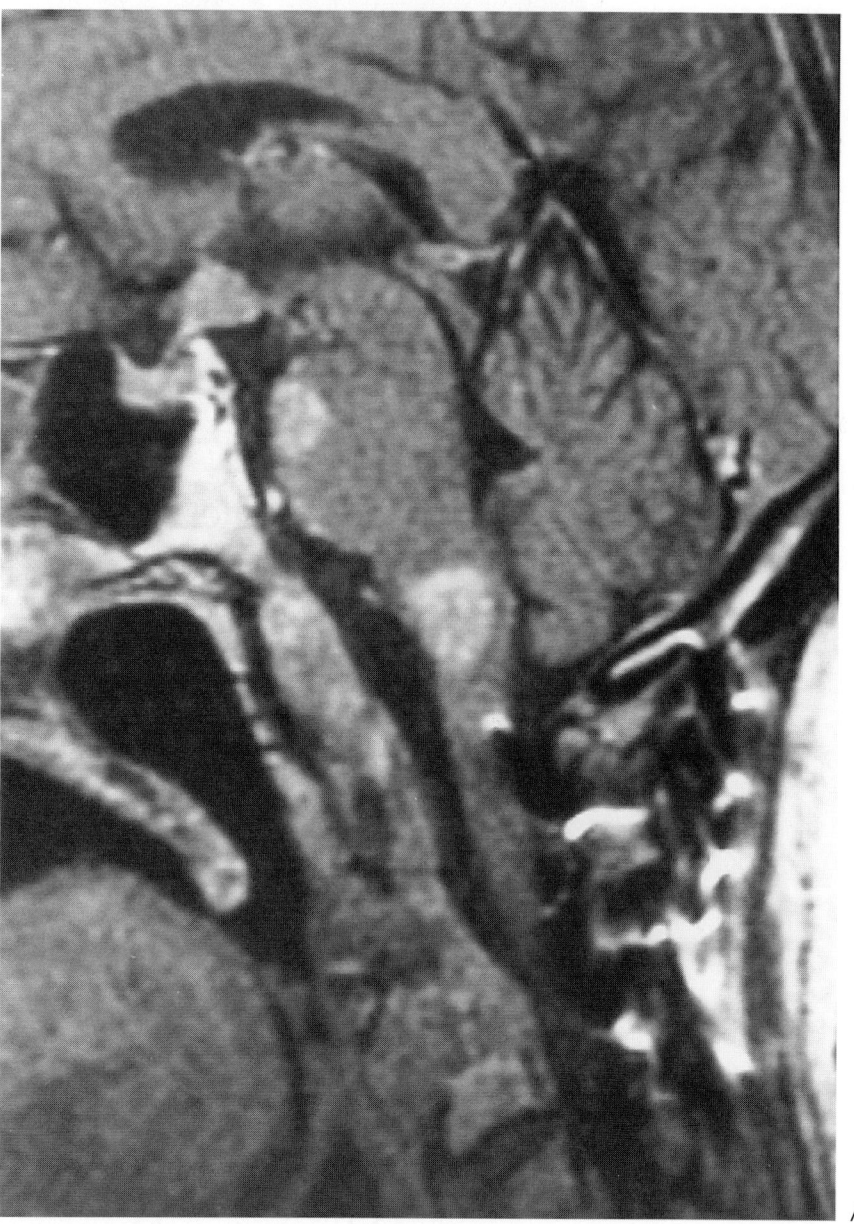

A

TEACHING ATLAS OF SPINE IMAGING

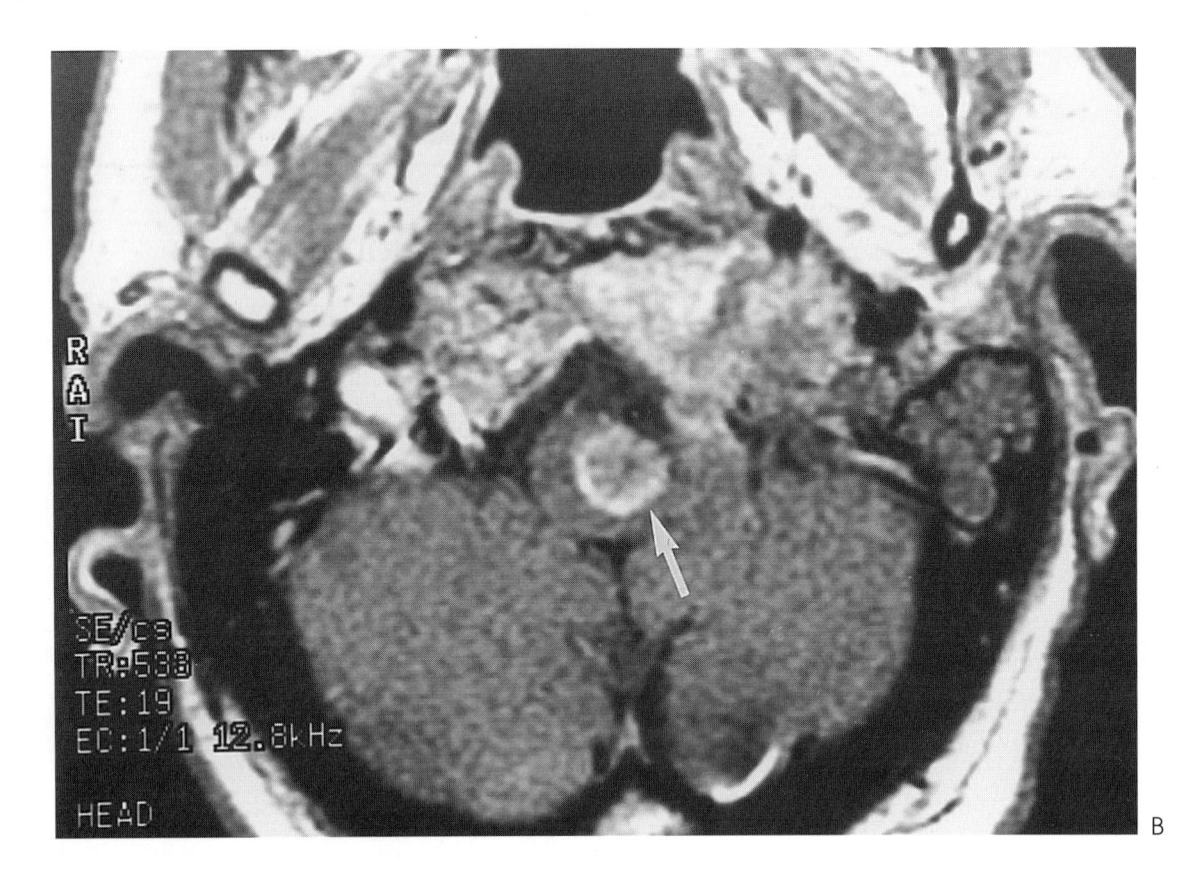

Radiologic Findings

Sagittal short TR image after the infusion of contrast material (Fig. A) reveals postoperative changes in the upper cervical region with fusion between the lower end of the clivus, the odontoid process, and the body of C2 and the anterior arch of C1. There are two irregularly marginated areas of bone graft in place at the C1 and C2 levels. There are multiple rounded areas of enhancement noted. These are in the suprasellar cistern, in the upper anterior margin of the pons, and in the medulla. Multiple rounded and oval areas of decreased signal intensity with increased signal intensity peripheral rims appear in the suboccipital region and extend down the spinous processes in the upper cervical region dorsally.

Axial short TR image (Fig. B) reveals the rounded area of enhancement in the medulla, which is on the left side and extends to the midline (*arrow*).

Diagnosis

Metastatic chordomas; postsurgical changes.

Differential Diagnosis

- Metastatic tumor
- Metastatic chordoma

SPINAL CORD TUMORS

Pearls
- The entire vertebral column and intracranial contents should be evaluated in a patient such as this.

- Because these tumors are often slow growing, patients may survive multiple surgical resections.

- Magnetic resonance is the ideal method of diagnosis and follow-up.

Pitfall
- Total surgical removal of chordomas is almost impossible.

Discussion

The patient's initial surgery was for removal of a clivus chordoma. Although unusual, metastatic deposits from an aggressive chordoma may occur. More typically, chordomas recur with local extension in and around the bed of the original tumor. Other metastatic tumors could have a similar appearance; however, the previous history in this patient makes metastatic chordoma the likely diagnosis.

Chordomas frequently appear as variable signal intensity because of areas of calcification and because of the variable internal histologic make-up. The multiple areas of decreased signal intensity with increased signal intensity peripheral margins are magnetic susceptibility artifacts from metallic wires at the skull base and extending into the upper cervical region.

Section IV

Trauma

TRAUMA

Case 1

Clinical Presentation

The patient is a 45-year-old female who developed severe back pain after falling from a sitting position when the boat in which she was a passenger hit a large wave.

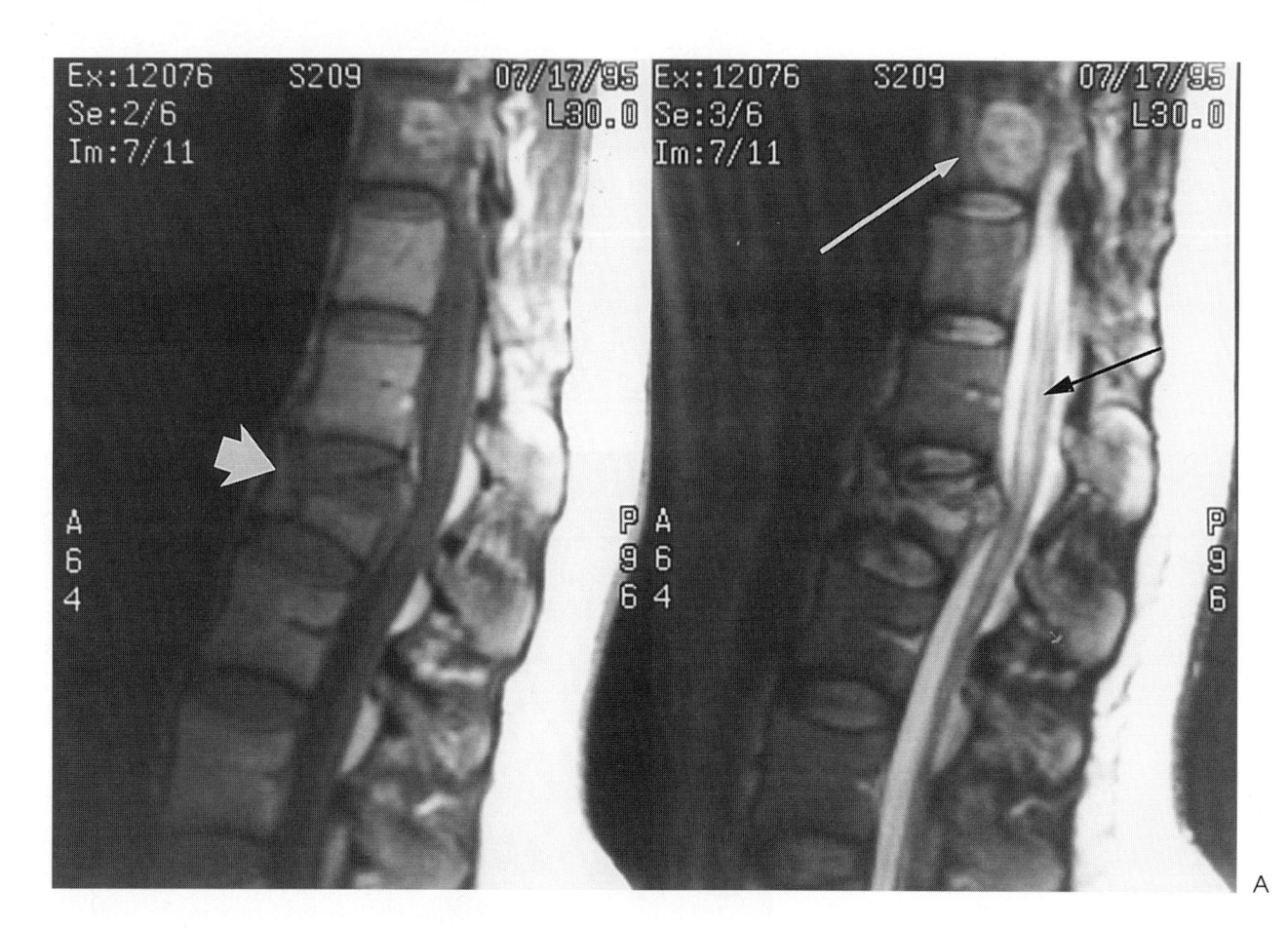

Radiologic Findings

Sagittal short (Fig. A, *left*) and long (Fig. A, *right*) TR images reveal a marked compression fracture of the L2 vertebral body (*left, arrow*). There is retropulsion of the posterior superior margin of the vertebral body into the vertebral canal. A linear area of increased signal intensity can be seen behind the vertebral body of L2. The long TR image reveals an area of increased signal intensity within the central portion of the distal spinal cord (*black arrow*). A rounded area of mottled but generally increased signal intensity is seen in the T11 vertebral body (*right, white arrow*).

TEACHING ATLAS OF SPINE IMAGING

B

C

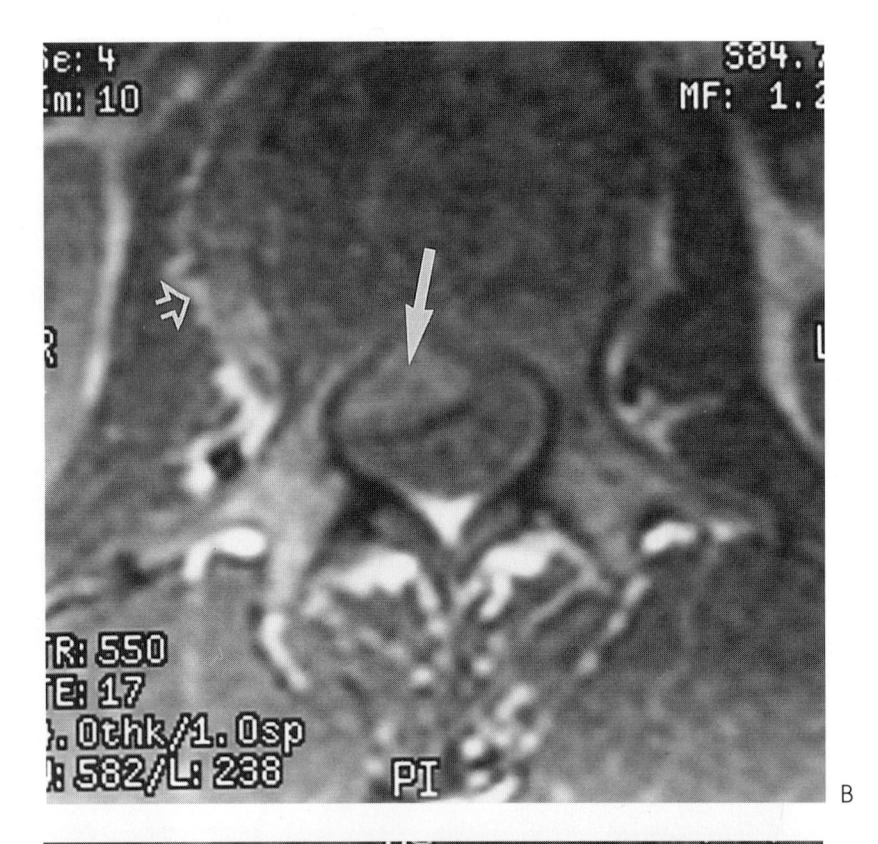

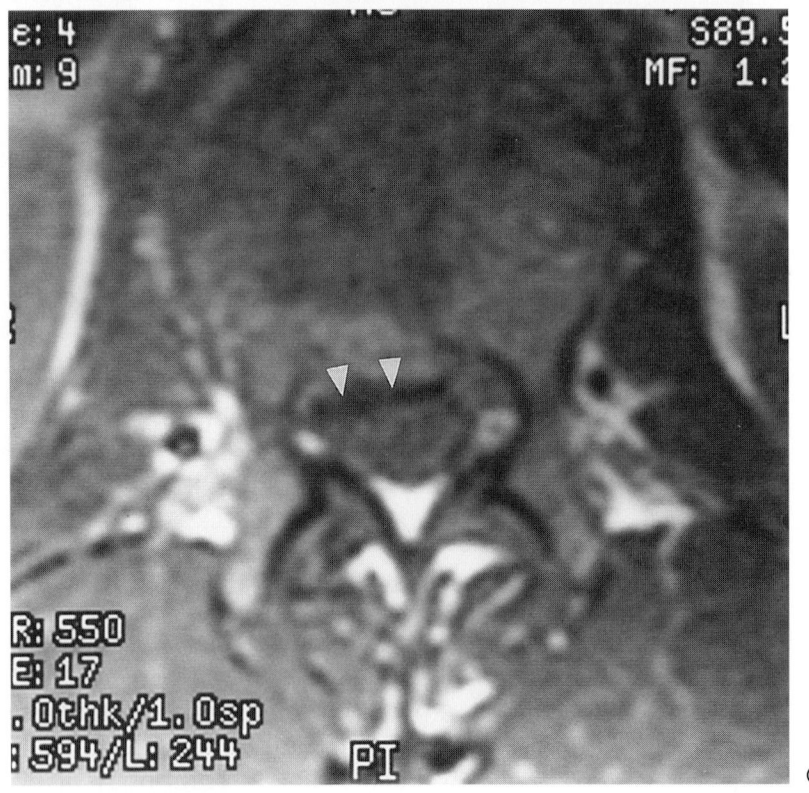

270

TRAUMA

Radiologic Findings (continued)

Axial short TR images at two different levels of L2 (Figs. B and C) reveal the posterior displacement of the posterior portion of the vertebral body into the vertebral canal (Fig. B, *solid arrow*). A similar appearance is present at a slightly lower level (Fig. C, *arrowheads*). There is a small paraspinal soft tissue mass on the right side (Fig. B, *open arrow*).

Diagnosis

Traumatic compression fracture with spinal cord edema.

Differential Diagnosis

- metastatic disease
- osteoporosis

Discussion

In a 45-year-old female, this type of compression fracture is unusual unless there is an underlying abnormality such as metastatic disease. This type of fracture may also occur in a patient with osteoporosis. Occasionally a traumatically herniated disc may occur; however, in this case, the encroachment upon the vertebral canal appears to be secondary to the bone of the vertebral body. The increased signal intensity within the thoracic spinal cord is secondary to a contusion and spinal cord edema. An incidental hemangioma is noted in the T11 vertebral body (Fig. A, right, *white arrow*).

There should be concern regarding the possibility of a pathologic fracture of the vertebral body. A radionuclide bone scan could be performed to evaluate the presence of other areas of bone involvement in addition to the fractured vertebral body. However, a fracture may occur even with a normal vertebral body if there is sufficient trauma.

PEARLS

- Computed tomographic scanning is useful to identify additional small fracture fragments that may affect the vertebral bodies.

- Magnetic resonance imaging is valuable because it provides a noninvasive method for evaluating the presence of injury to the spinal cord and also may be used to identify later changes, such as the presence of a syrinx cavity following trauma to the spinal cord.

PITFALL

- The spine should be evaluated for the presence of an underlying abnormality such as metastatic disease or osteoporosis.

TEACHING ATLAS OF SPINE IMAGING

Case 2

Clinical Presentation

The patient is a 42-year-old female seen in the emergency room following an automobile accident with roll-over. The patient was not wearing a seat belt. The patient sustained a liver fracture and hemorrhagic lung contusion with respiratory failure.

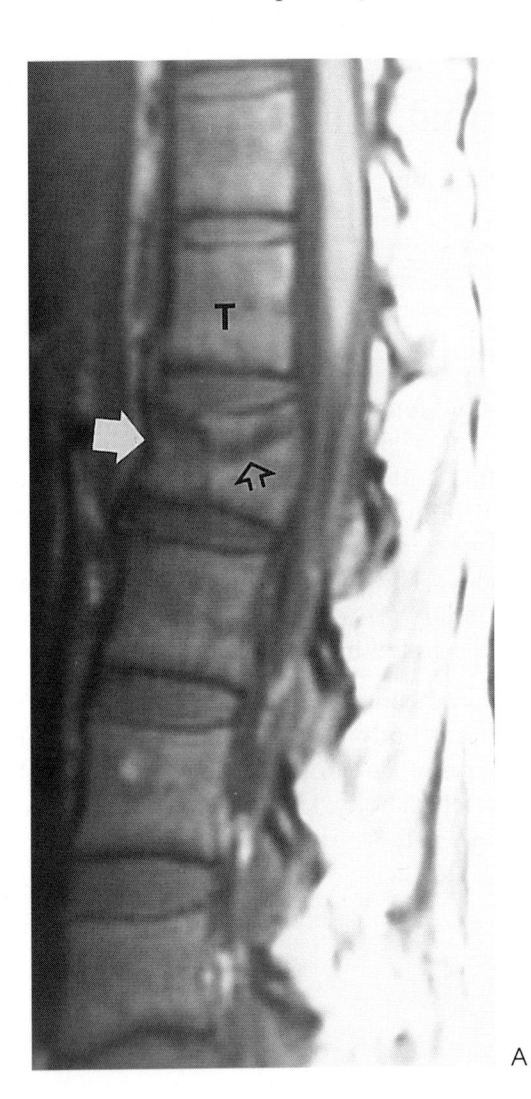

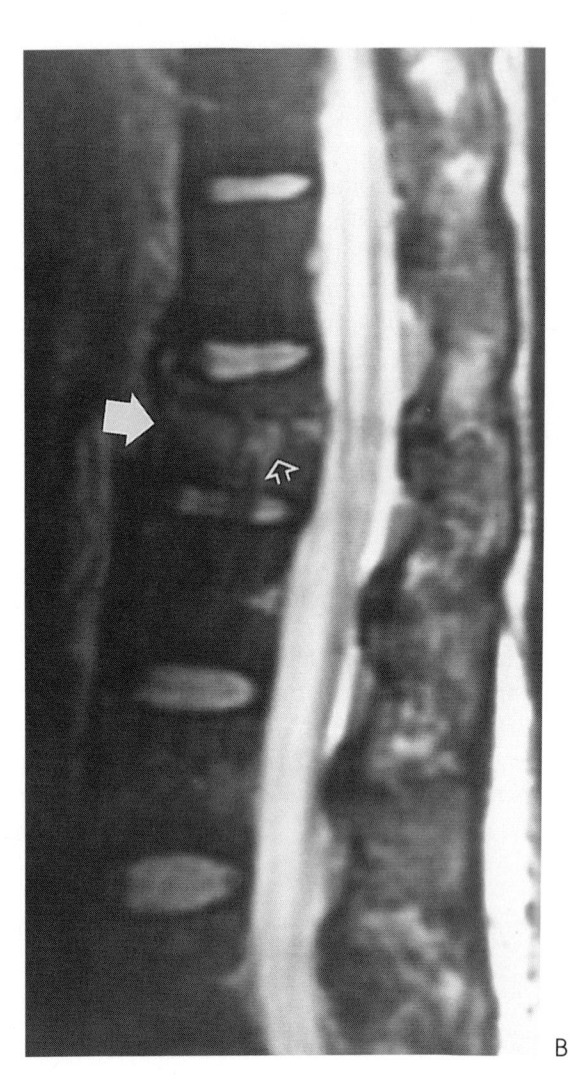

Radiologic Findings

Sagittal short TR image in the lumbar region (Fig. A) reveals loss of vertebral height at the L1 level (*white arrow*). There is a thin slightly irregular line in the upper one third of the vertebral body of L1 (*open arrow*). There is slight retropulsion of the posterior margin of the L1 vertebral body with slight compromise of the subarachnoid space at this level. The spinal cord is noted to end at the T12 level (*T*).

TRAUMA

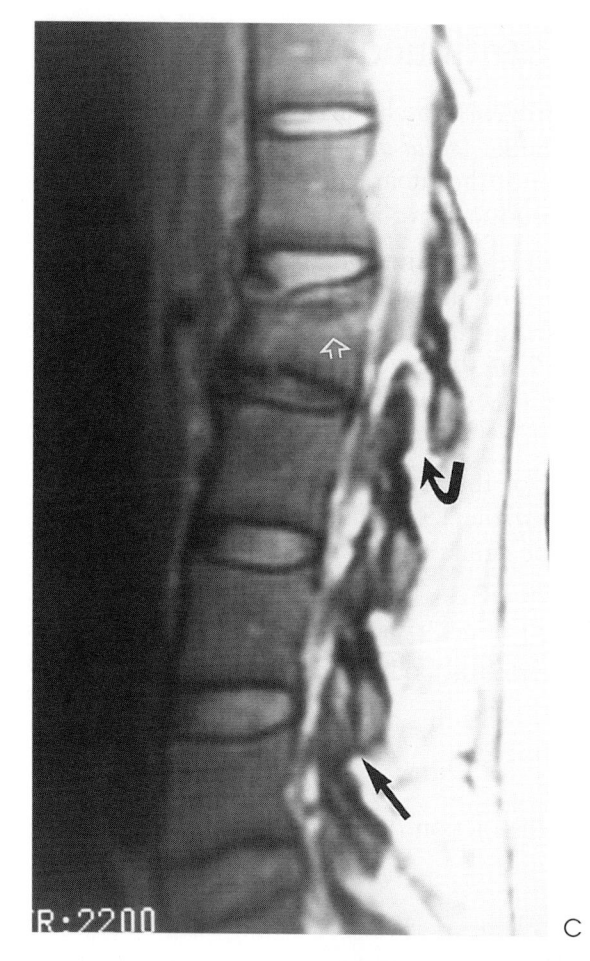

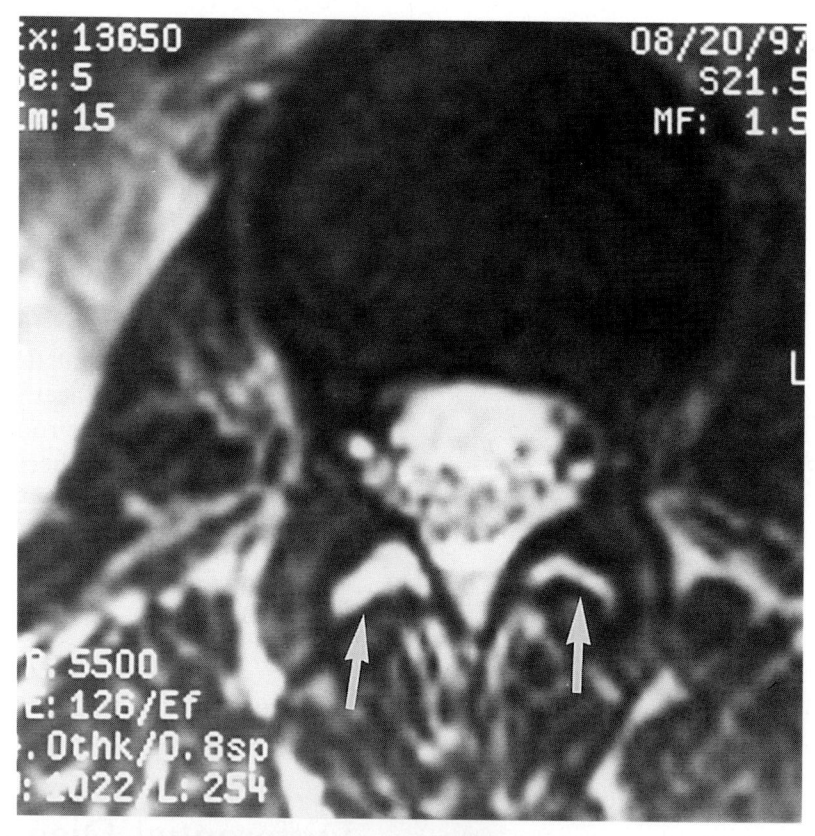

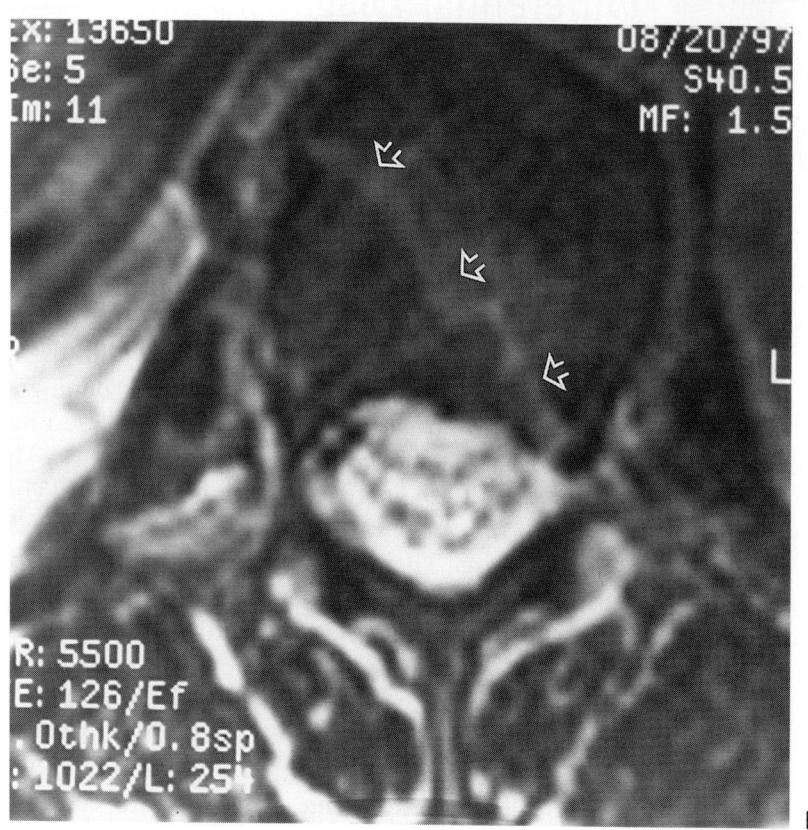

C

D

E

273

Radiologic Findings (continued)

Sagittal long TR image (Fig. B) reveals patchy areas of increased signal intensity in the upper portion of the L1 (*solid arrow*) vertebral body (*open arrow*). There is slight compromise of the subarachnoid space at this level. There is reversal of the normal lordotic curve at the L1 level.

Parasagittal long TR image (Fig. C) reveals the compression fracture of the L1 vertebral body (*open arrow*). The normal interfacet joint is seen at L3-4. The interfacet joint is widened at the L1-2 level (*curved solid arrow*). There is increased signal intensity at the level of the interfacet joint at L1-2. The normal interfacet joint is seen at the L3-4 level (*straight solid arrow*).

Axial long TR image at the level of the interfacet joint of L1-2 (Fig. D) reveals that the interfacet joints (*arrows*) are widened on the right more than the left. The nerve roots of the cauda equina are seen in the posterior portion of the lumbar thecal sac.

Axial long TR image at the level of L1 (Fig. E) reveals an oblique, increased signal intensity line through the vertebral body of L1 (*arrows*).

Diagnosis

Compression fracture of L1 and distraction of the interfacet joints at the L1-2 level.

Differential Diagnosis

- compression fracture
- Chance fracture

Discussion

This is a typical compression fracture of the lumbar spine. The decreased signal intensity line through the L1 vertebral body is secondary to edema or possibly compacted trabecular bone within the marrow of the vertebral body. The severe flexion has resulted in widening of the interfacet joint at the level of the fracture. There is also increased fluid within the interfacet joint and edema secondary to soft tissue injury. The combination of these changes results in increased signal intensity. Typically retropulsion of a portion of the vertebral body is seen when there is a compression fracture, as in this case. The retropulsion may result in spinal cord injury if it is sufficiently severe. This patient exhibits the fortunate anatomic variation of a high position of the conus medullaris such that the retropulsed portion of the bone does not damage the spinal cord. The normal termination of the distal end of the spinal cord is at the inferior end plate of L1 or the superior end plate of L2. Should the spinal cord be damaged, this results in edema or even the formation of a hematoma within the spinal cord. In addition, if there is edema or spinal cord contusion, this may ultimately result in the formation of a syrinx cavity within the damaged portion of the spinal cord.

PEARLS

- Computed tomographic (CT) scanning may also be helpful to evaluate the presence of comminuted fractures, which may be associated with this type of injury.

- CT scanning with sagittal reconstruction views greatly aids in identifying the separation of the interfacet joints. CT is also helpful for visualization of small bone fragments which may encroach upon the vertebral canal.

- Magnetic resonance imaging (MRI) is an ideal method for evaluating this type of fracture and is often used in conjunction with CT scanning.

PITFALLS

- Small bone fragments may not be demonstrated by MR scanning and are best evaluated by CT scanning.

- CT scanning does not demonstrate the spinal cord, therefore presence of spinal cord edema or hematoma cannot be evaluated by CT scanning.

A Chance fracture is a similar but slightly different fracture. A Chance fracture is also a flexion injury but occurs when the patient has a seat belt in place, and there is severe flexion over the seat belt. This results in a fracture through the midportion of the L1 vertebral body with extension through the vertebral body pedicle and lamina of the vertebral body. The end result is a separation between the upper and lower portions of the vertebrae. There is also soft tissue injury with a Chance fracture; this results in edema which appears increased signal intensity on long TR images.

TEACHING ATLAS OF SPINE IMAGING

Case 3

Clinical Presentation

The patient is a 27-year-old male who was involved in a motorcycle accident and was admitted with mild lower extremity weakness.

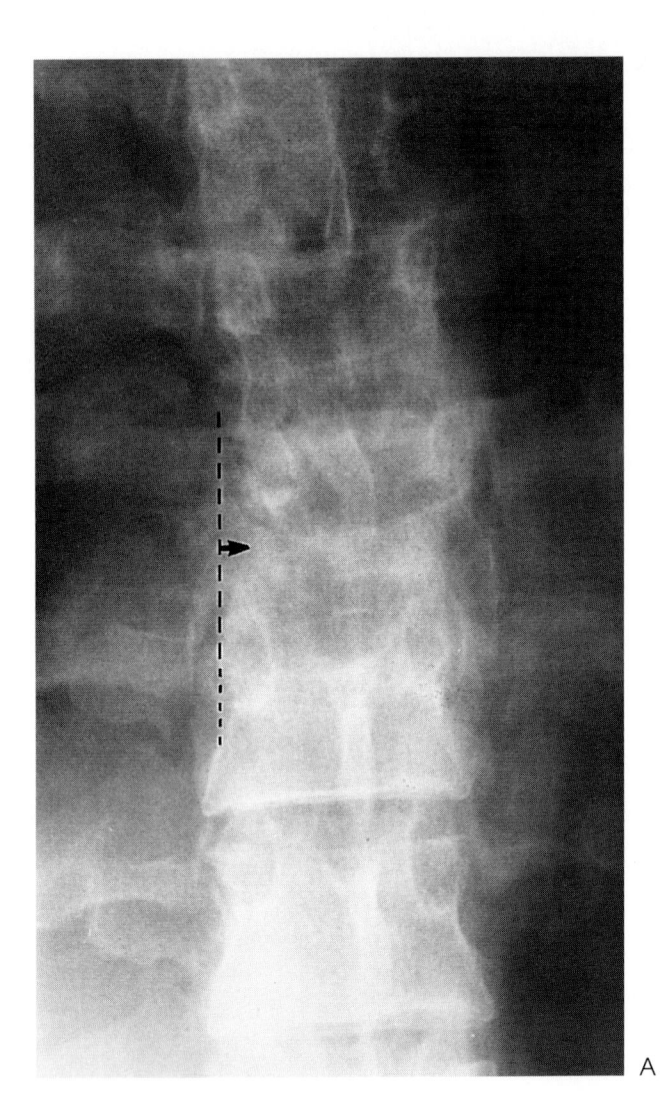

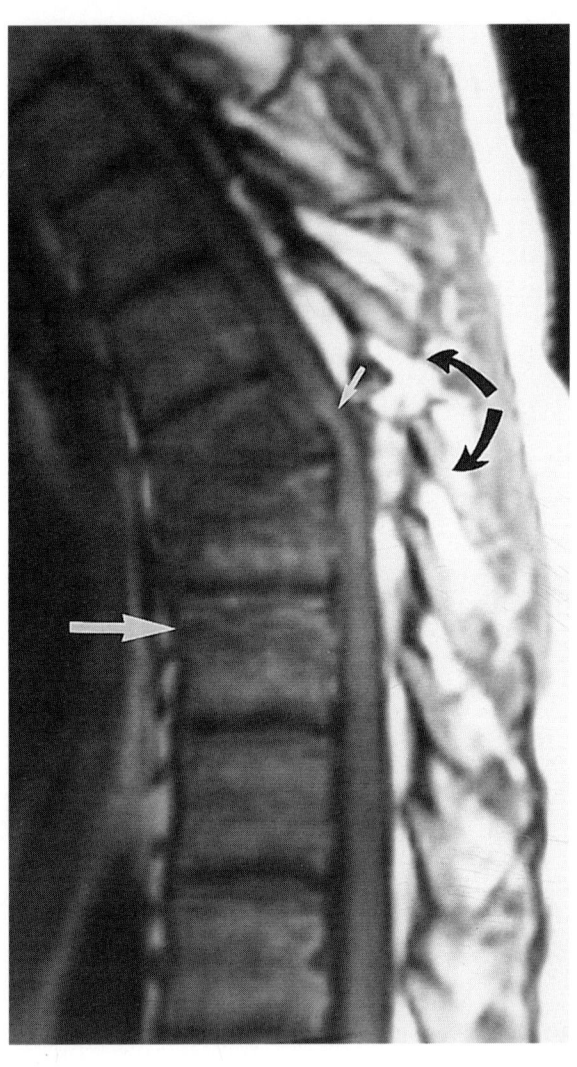

TRAUMA

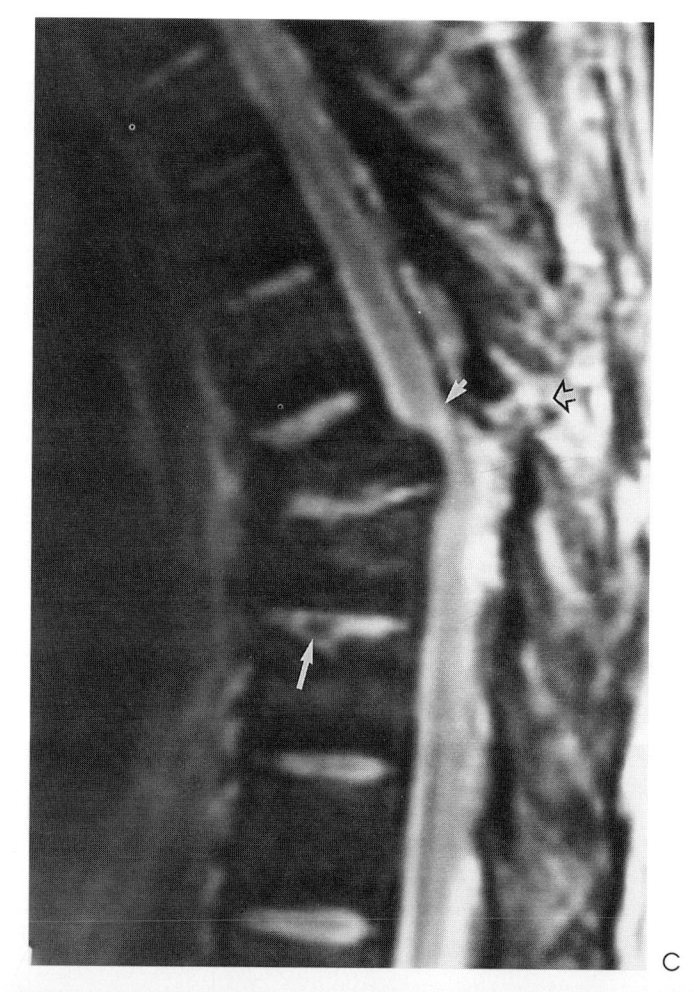

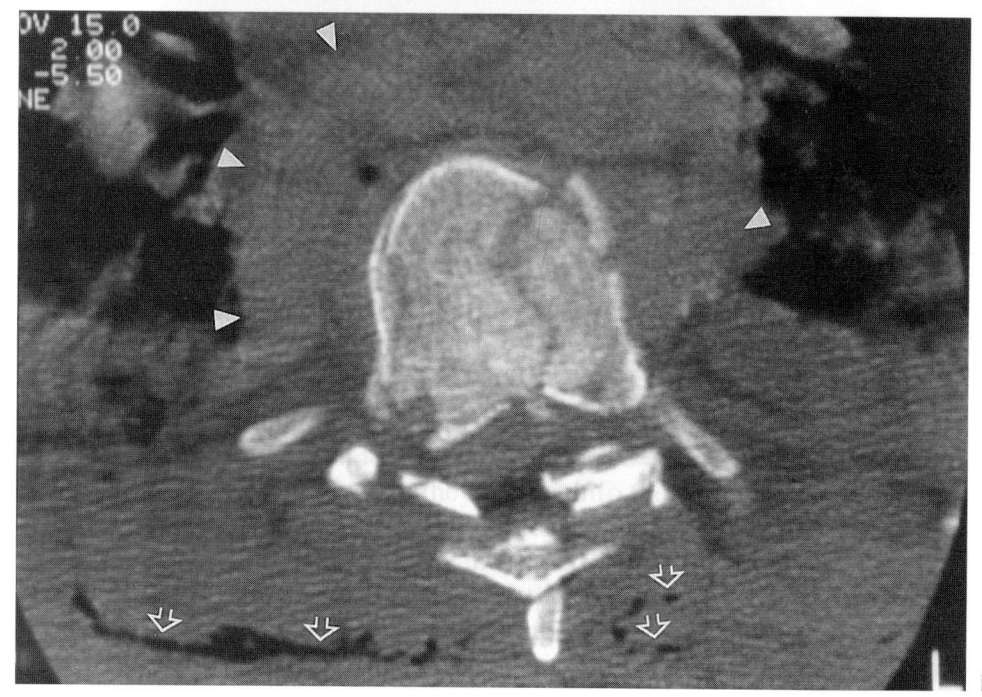

TEACHING ATLAS OF SPINE IMAGING

Case 6

Clinical Presentation

The patient is a 5-year-old female who presents with C5 radiculopathy following a motor vehicle accident.

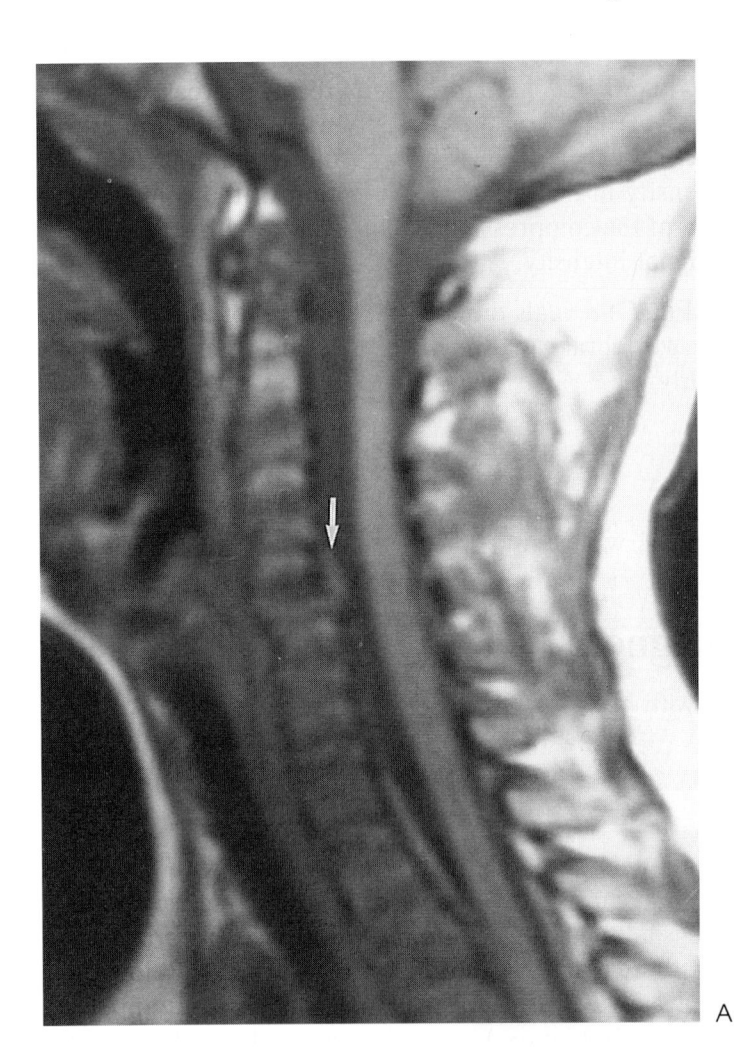

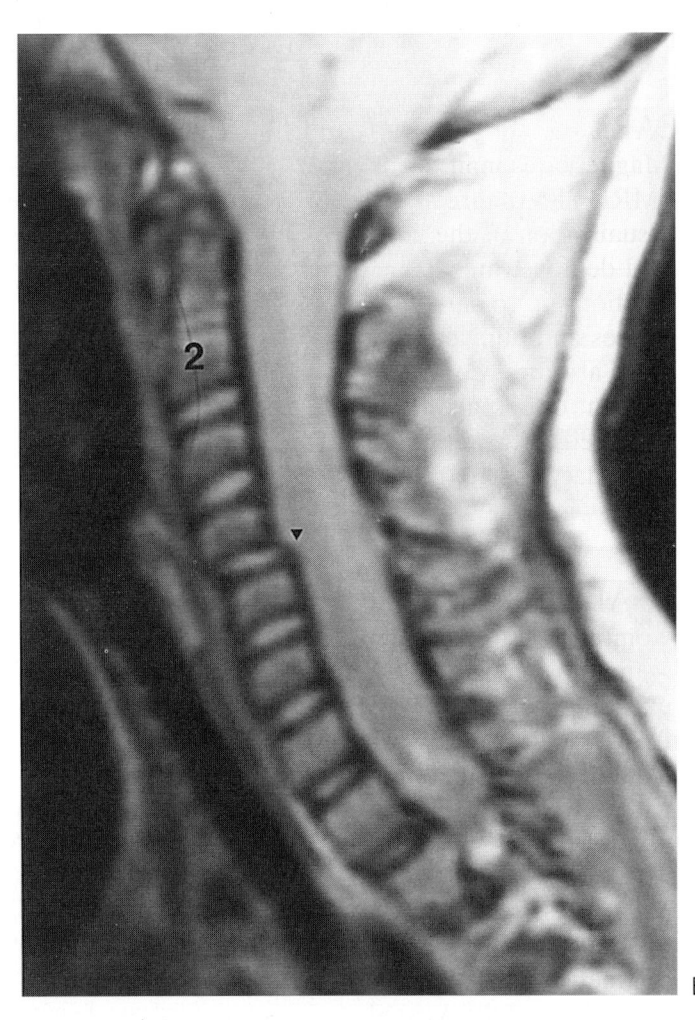

Radiologic Findings

Sagittal short TR image of the cervical spine (Fig. A) reveals forward subluxation of C4 on C5. The intervertebral disc at C4-5 protrudes posteriorly into the vertebral canal (*arrow*). There is straightening of the spine with loss of the normal cervical lordosis.

Sagittal long TR image (Fig. B) better demonstrates the forward displacement of C4 on C5. The arrowhead marks the posterior superior corner of the C5 vertebral body. The C2 vertebral body is identified with 2.

TRAUMA

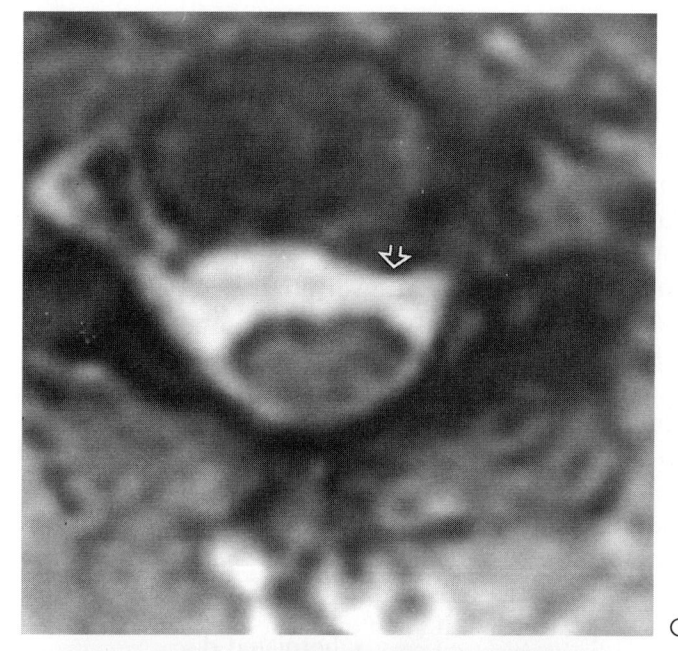

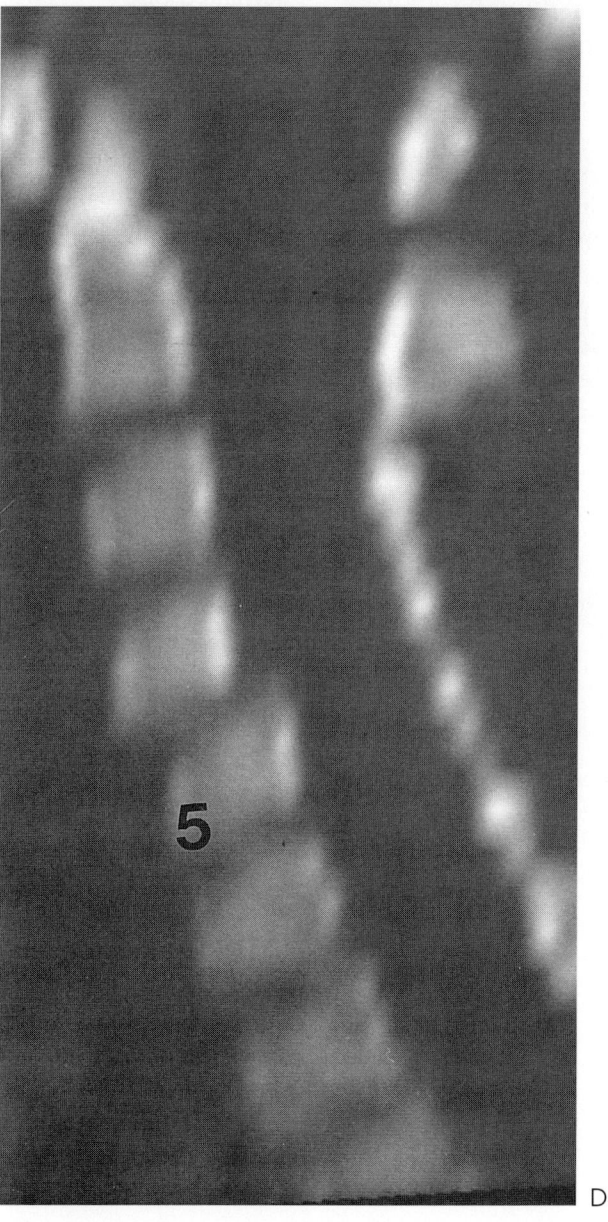

C

D

287

PEARLS

- MRI is the ideal method of evaluating this type of injury because it allows direct visualization of the spinal cord and its relationship with the surrounding bony structures. The presence of a hematoma can also be readily evaluated by the use of MRI.

- Long TR images may also demonstrate increased signal intensity surrounding the interfacet joints where there is soft tissue damage.

- Surgery can be performed, if necessary, based totally upon the findings in the MR images.

PITFALLS

- This study should be performed in conjunction with computed tomographic (CT) scanning to rule out the presence of fractures. Although demonstrable by MRI, facet dislocation, not seen in this patient, is also best demonstrated by CT scanning.

Radiologic Findings (continued)

Axial long TR image at the C4-5 level (Fig. C) reveals a decreased signal intensity soft tissue mass that encroaches upon the left anterior portion of the subarachnoid space (*open arrow*).

Sagittal midline reconstruction view of the cervical spine (Fig. D) reveals the forward displacement of C4 on C5. No fractures are seen. The C5 vertebral body is identified with 5.

Diagnosis

Traumatic anterolisthesis of C4 on C5 with a traumatically herniated disc on the left side at the C4-5 level.

Differential Diagnosis

- herniated disc

Discussion

Magnetic resonance (MR) imaging provides the ideal method for evaluating the presence of a herniated disc. The nucleus pulposus can be seen migrating from its normal location into the vertebral canal and superiorly behind the vertebral body of C4. The spinal cord is otherwise normal in size and configuration throughout. There is no abnormal signal intensity within the spinal cord to suggest that there is either hematoma or contusion within the cord. The herniated disc is also localized on the axial view where there is encroachment upon the intervertebral foramen. This encroachment would compress the nerve roots in the intervertebral foramen and cause this patient's symptoms.

TRAUMA

Case 7

Clinical Presentation

The patient is a 3-year-old who was brought to the emergency room by her parents who stated that she had fallen from the couch.

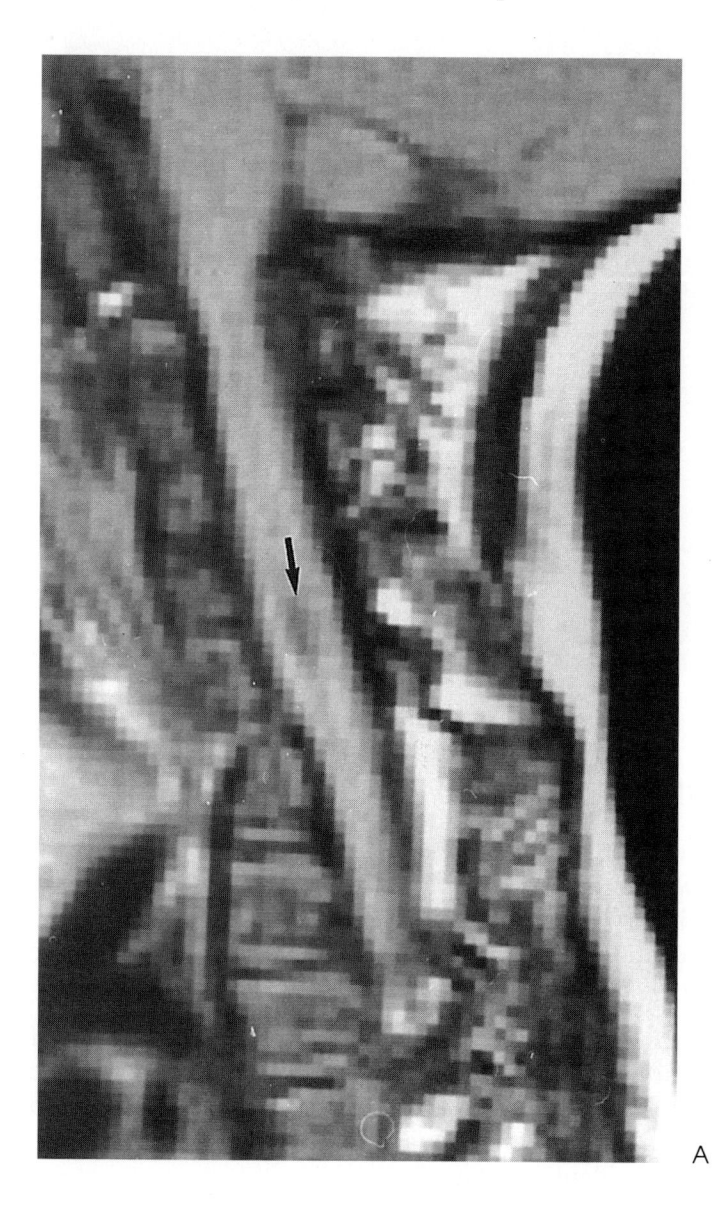

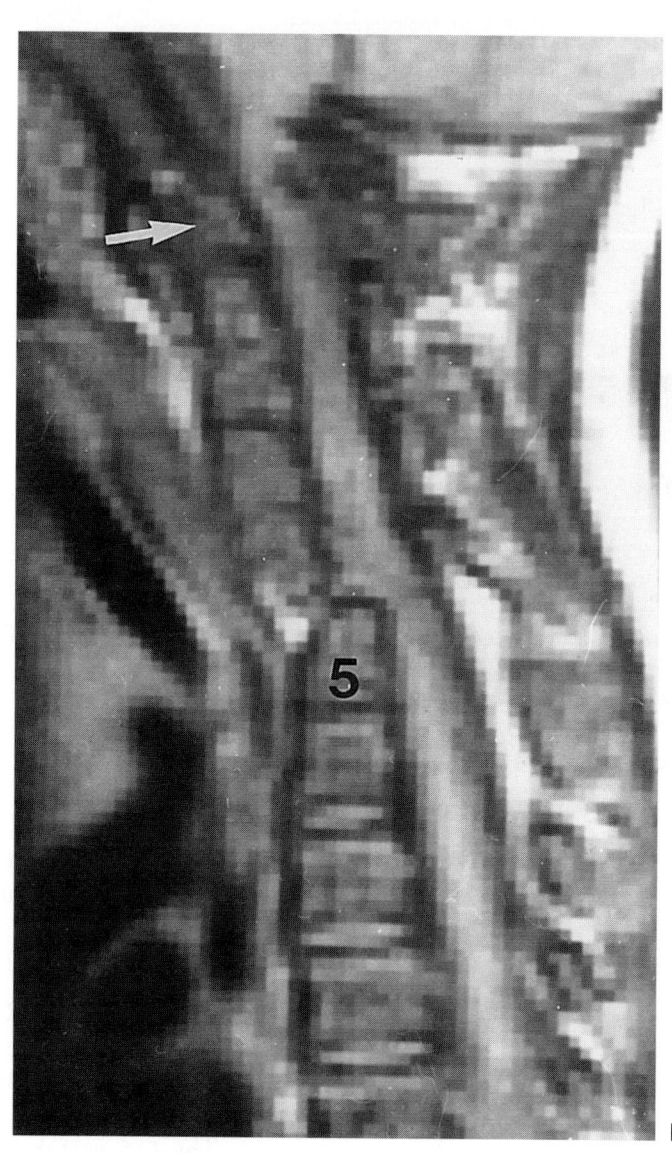

A

B

TEACHING ATLAS OF SPINE IMAGING

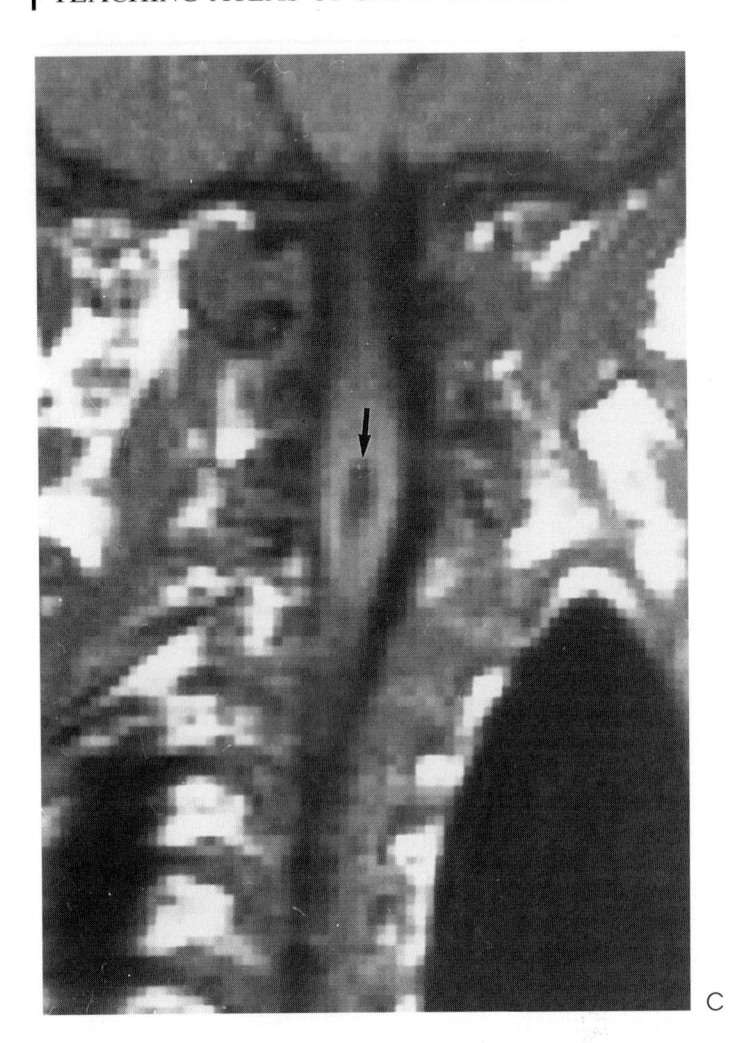

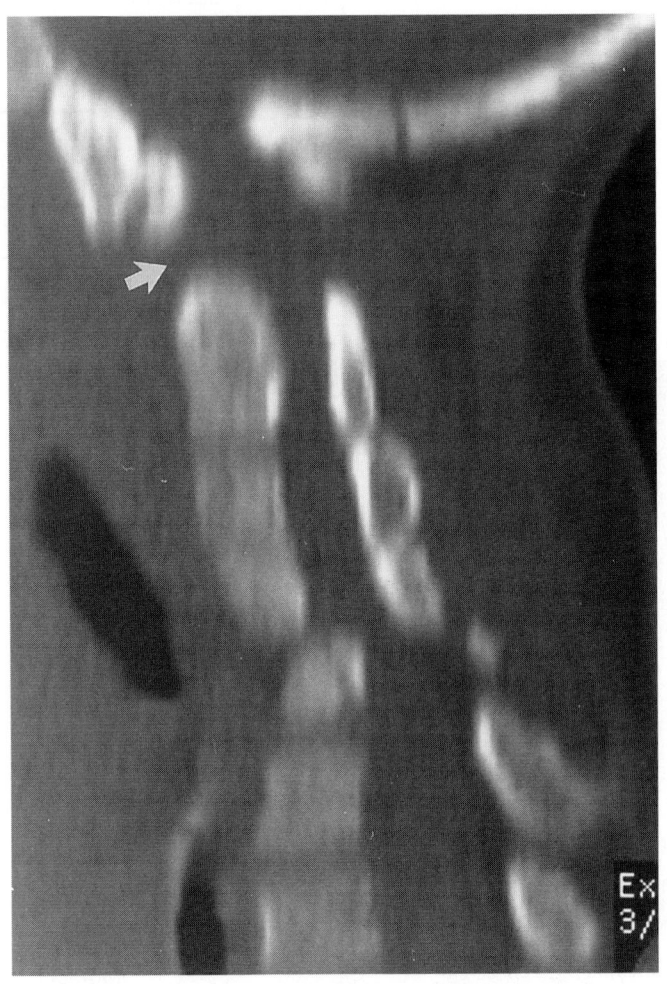

Radiologic Findings

Sagittal short TR image in the cervical region (Fig. A) reveals a small, low signal intensity area within the cervical spinal cord at approximately the C4 level (*arrow*). There is forward subluxation of the vertebral body of C4 on C5 and forward subluxation of the spinous processes of C4 on C5. There is a scoliosis of the cervical and thoracic spine.

Sagittal short TR image again (Fig. B) reveals the forward subluxation of C4 on C5. There is curvilinear distortion of the cervical spinal cord. The subarachnoid space is obliterated at the C5 level. There is a small rounded area with signal intensity similar to the remaining vertebral bodies (*arrow*). The C 5 vertebral body is identified with 5.

Coronal short TR image in the cervical region (Fig. C) reveals the decreased signal intensity area within the cervical spinal cord (*arrow*). The spinal cord is slightly expanded at this level.

Sagittal midline reconstruction images from a computed tomographic (CT) scan (Fig. D) reveal the forward subluxation of C4 on C5. There appears to be an oblique fracture of the posterior superior corner of the vertebral body of C5. The rounded edges suggest that this is old rather than acute. The posterior elements of vertebral bodies 1–4 are also displaced forward.

TRAUMA

Radiologic Findings (continued)

The odontoid process is separated from the body of C2 (*arrow*) and is in close proximity to the skull base. The posterior arch of C1 is adjacent to the occipital bone.

Diagnosis

Probably old fracture dislocation of C4 on C5 associated with a scoliosis and formation of a posttraumatic syrinx cavity at C4; presumed child abuse.

Differential Diagnosis

- old fracture

Discussion

The appearance of the fracture suggests that these changes are old. The formation of a syrinx cavity within the spinal cord also suggests that the change is old rather than acute. The anterolisthesis, involving the vertebral bodies as well as the posterior elements of C4 on C5, results in a severe spinal stenosis at the C5 level. Magnetic resonance imaging (MRI) nicely demonstrates the spinal cord and the surrounding bony structures as well as the syrinx cavity, which is probably a result of the trauma that caused the subluxation of C4 on C5.

There is also atlanto-occipital fusion with the anterior arch of C1 adherent to the bottom of the clivus and the posterior arch of C1 fused to the skull base. This is a congenital deformity and is possibly an incidental finding in this patient. However, the clinical history suggests that the child suffers from abuse; therefore, additional evaluation is advised.

There is a remote possibility that this represents a diagnostic consideration; however, this possibility seems unlikely. If tumor is a consideration, a postinfusion study should be performed as most spinal cord tumors will exhibit enhancement.

PEARLS
- The CT scan better demonstrates the fracture of the vertebral body of C5, which is not seen on the MR scan. MRI is the procedure of choice as it demonstrates the spinal cord relative to the surrounding structures.

- A posttraumatic lesion could cause subluxation at the C4-5 level; however, trauma would not cause the other anomalies.

PITFALL
- The syrinx cavity would not be demonstrated by CT scanning but is readily demonstrated by MRI.

TEACHING ATLAS OF SPINE IMAGING

Case 8

Clinical Presentation

The patient is a 27-year-old male who is a victim of battery who presented to the emergency room with a history of being hit on the back of the head with a board. The patient was quadriparetic.

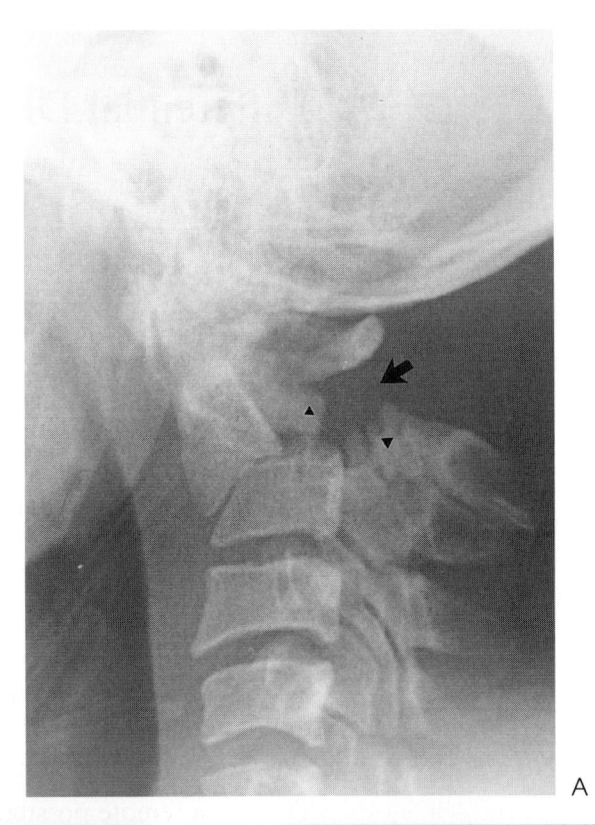

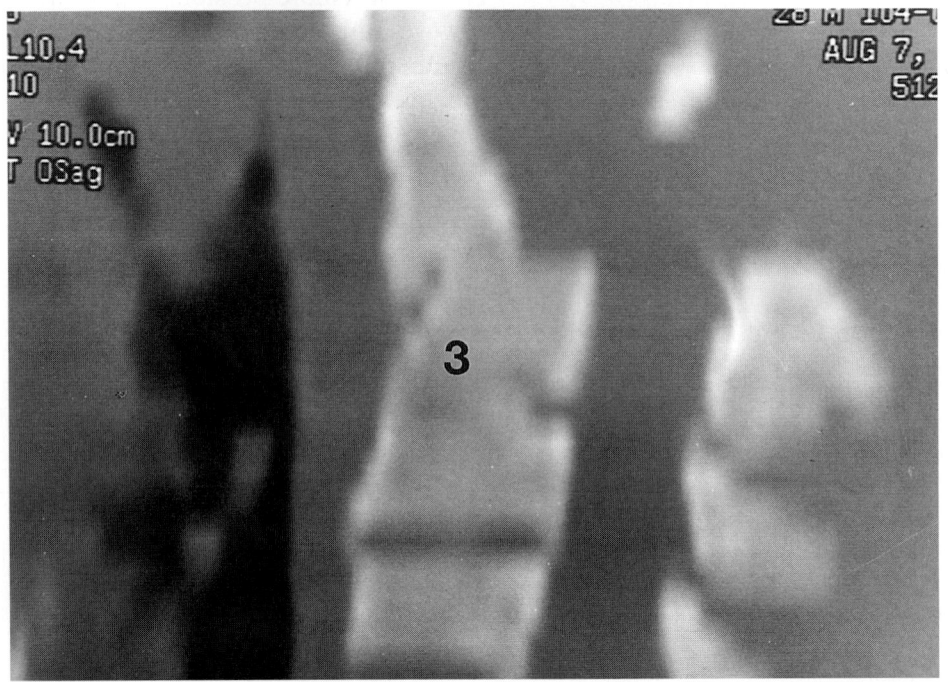

A

B

TRAUMA

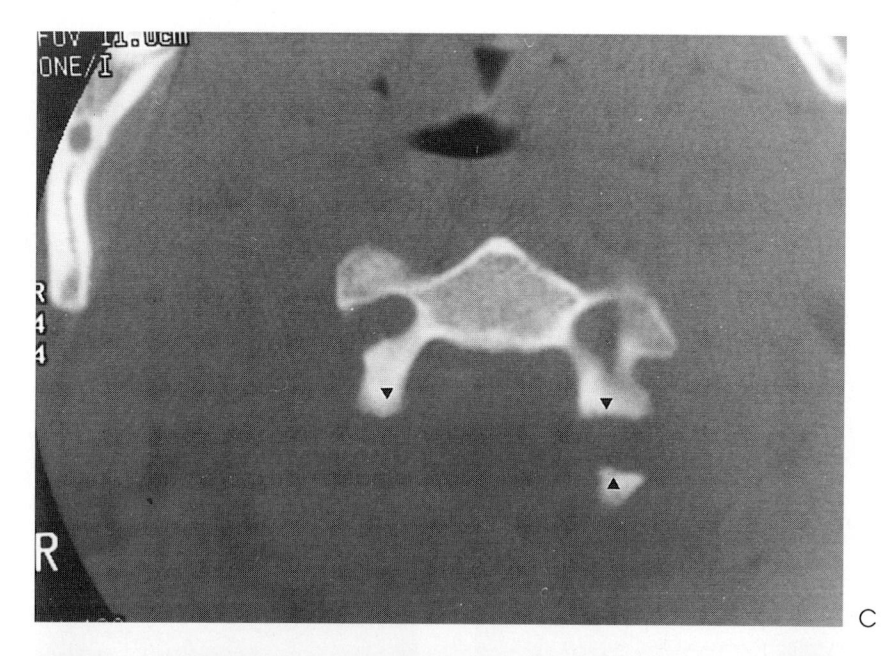

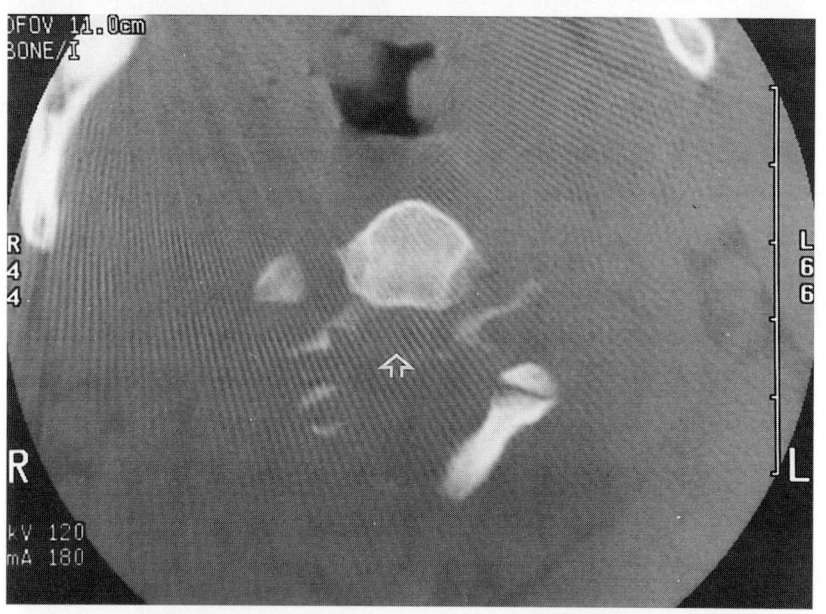

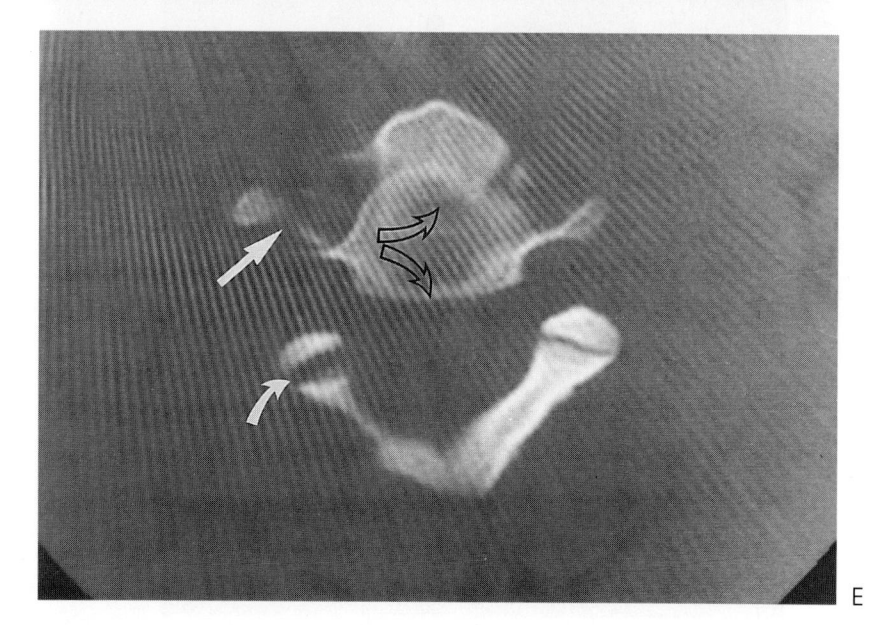

C

D

E

293

TEACHING ATLAS OF SPINE IMAGING

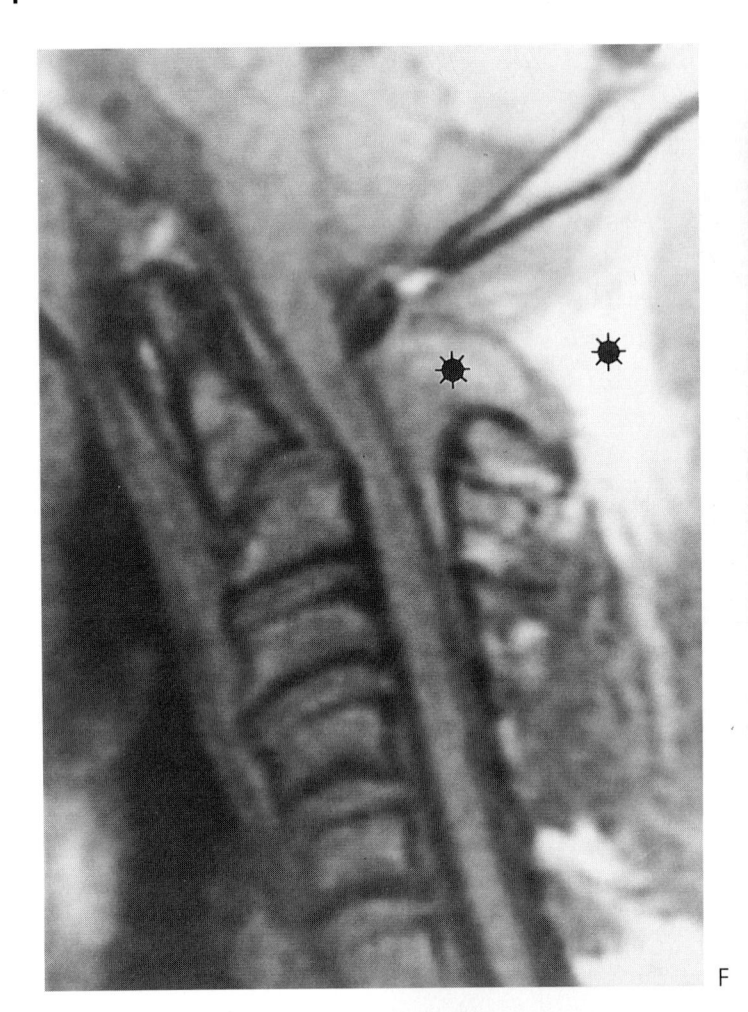

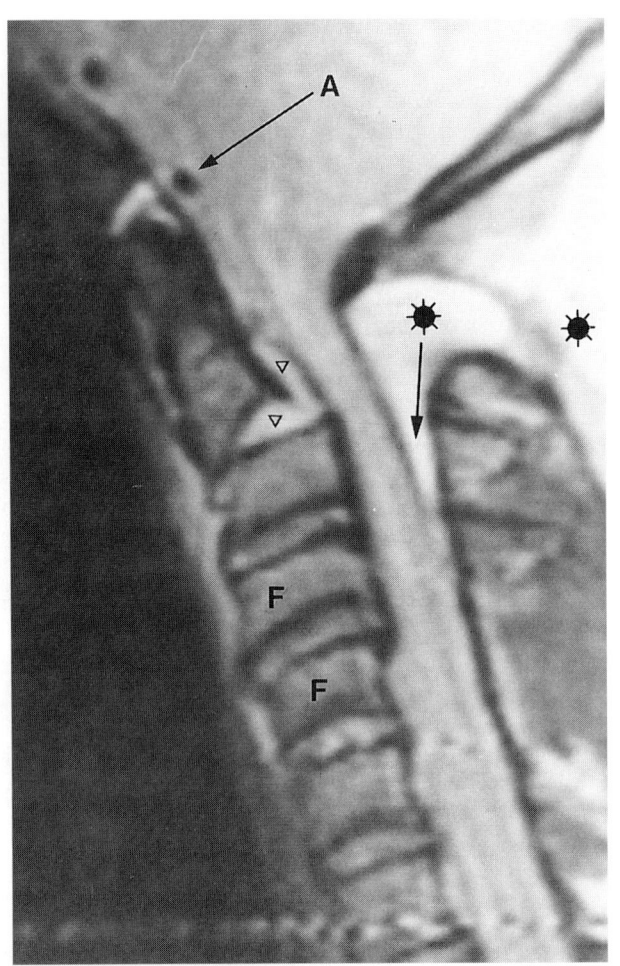

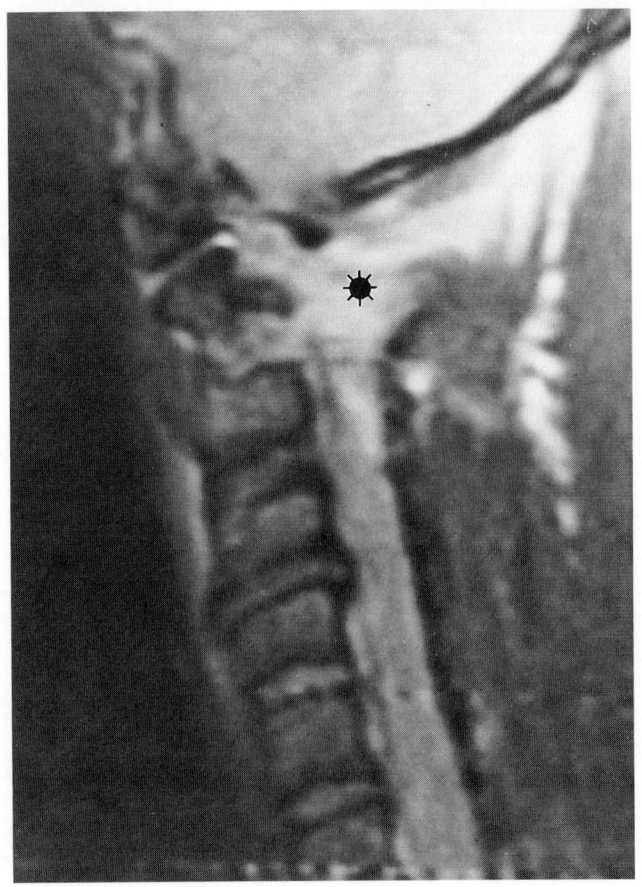

TRAUMA

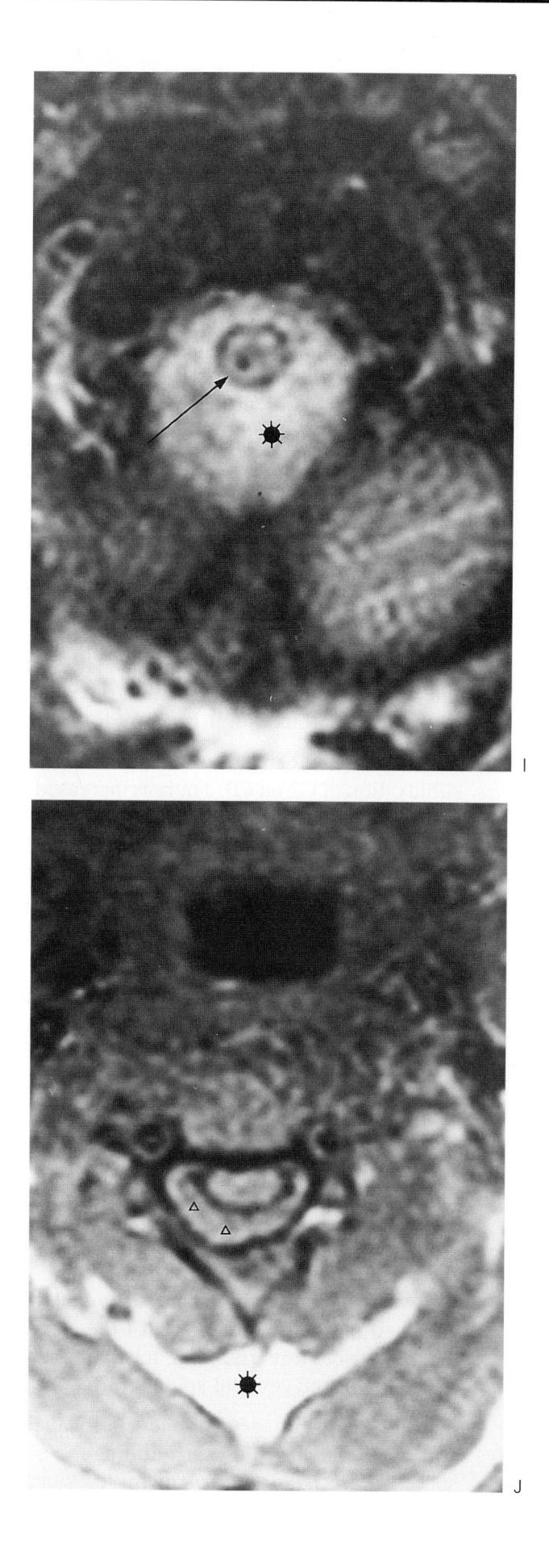

295

Radiologic Findings

Lateral view of the cervical spine (Fig. A) reveals a fracture dislocation at the C2-3 level. The body of C2 is markedly displaced forward over the vertebral body of C3. The posterior elements of C2 have been separated (*arrowheads*) by approximately 1 cm (*arrow*). There is posterior displacement of the spinous process of C2. The spinous processes of C2 and C3 are in close proximity to one another.

Sagittal midline reconstruction image from a computed tomographic (CT) scan (Fig. B) reveals findings similar to those seen on the plain film, but the posterior elements are not visualized on this midsagittal image. The C3 vertebral body is identified with 3.

Axial CT scan at the level of C2 (Fig. C) reveals the separation of the bony fragments of the C2 vertebral body (*arrowheads*).

Axial CT at the level of the body of C3 (Fig. D) reveals the comminuted fracture fragment of the posterior elements of the vertebral body on the right side. The posterior margin of the C2 vertebral body is faintly visualized posterior to the posterior margin of the C3 vertebral body (*arrow*).

Axial CT scan at the C2-3 level (Fig. E) reveals the forward displacement of C2 on C3 (*open black arrows*). The comminuted fracture fragments of the lateral mass of C2 are seen on the right side (*straight white arrow*). The distracted interfacet joint is seen on the right side (*curved white arrow*).

Sagittal short TR image in the cervical region (Fig. F) reveals the anterior subluxation of C2 on C3. There is increased signal in the soft tissues between the posterior arch of C1 and the spinous process of C2 extending back to the level of the nucal ligament (*). The intervertebral disc at the C2-3 level protrudes posteriorly into the vertebral canal and superiorly behind the vertebral body of C2. The spinal cord is compressed at the level of C3 and exhibits acute, focal reversal of the normal cervical lordotic curve.

Sagittal long TR image (Fig. G) reveals that the nucleus pulposus of the intervertebral disc protrudes posteriorly and superiorly (*arrowheads*). The areas of increased signal intensity dorsal to the dural extends in the epidural space behind C3 (*, *long arrow*) and appears increased signal intensity in the dorsal soft tissues (*). The vertebral artery appears as a rounded area of flow void (*A, long arrow*). The fourth and fifth vertebral bodies are identified with F.

Parasagittal long TR image (Fig. H) reveals increased signal intensity soft tissue surrounding the posterior arch of C2 (*). There are patchy areas of increased signal intensity in the soft tissues of the suboccipital region.

Axial short TR image at the level of the body of the second vertebrae (Fig. I) reveals increased signal intensity soft tissue (*) surrounding the spinal cord and marked compression of the cervical subarachnoid space (*arrow*). There is also a tiny, rounded, focal area of decreased signal intensity in the right side of the cervical spinal cord.

Axial short TR image at the level of C3 (Fig. J) reveals increased signal in soft tissue (*arrowheads*) surrounding the compressed cervical subarachnoid space. There is an area of increased signal intensity between the muscle layers of the cervical spine dorsally (*).

TRAUMA

> **PEARL**
> - Because there is a generous amount of subarachnoid space surrounding the spinal cord in the upper cervical region, a significant amount of distortion of the vertebral column and spinal cord may occur before the patient becomes symptomatic. However, MRI provides an ideal method of evaluation of changes related to trauma with or without hematoma formation.

> **PITFALL**
> - Life-threatening injuries may preclude the use of MRI in the acutely injured setting. However, if proper life support is available, MRI may be used for diagnosis and to direct surgery.

Diagnosis

Fracture dislocation of C2 on C3 in a "hangman's" type of fracture with a traumatically herniated disc at the C2-3 level.

Differential Diagnosis

- fracture dislocation
- herniated disc

Discussion

Magnetic resonance imaging (MRI) readily demonstrates the compression of the cervical spinal cord at the level of the fracture dislocation. Hematoma formation appears dorsally at the C2-3 level. The epidural hematoma extends behind the dural and beneath the spinous process of C2. There is also increased signal intensity hematoma in the soft tissues of the dorsal spine.

There is a high signal intensity traumatically herniated nucleus pulposus of the intervertebral disc at the C2-3 level. The small area of decreased signal intensity within the spinal cord seen in Figure I is a small area of magnetic susceptibility artifact secondary to hemorrhage and associated deposition of hemosiderin.

A hangman's fracture is defined as a fracture dislocation of C2 on C3 with involvement of the vertebral pedicles. A hangman's fracture is frequently a forced extension injury, as when the hangman's knot is placed under the victim's chin which is snapped back with the fall of the hanging and forces the vertebral body of C2 forward on C3. In this patient, the mechanism was somewhat different.

TEACHING ATLAS OF SPINE IMAGING

Case 9

Clinical Presentation

The patient is a 48-year-old alcoholic male who is status post fall and presents to the emergency room with neck pain.

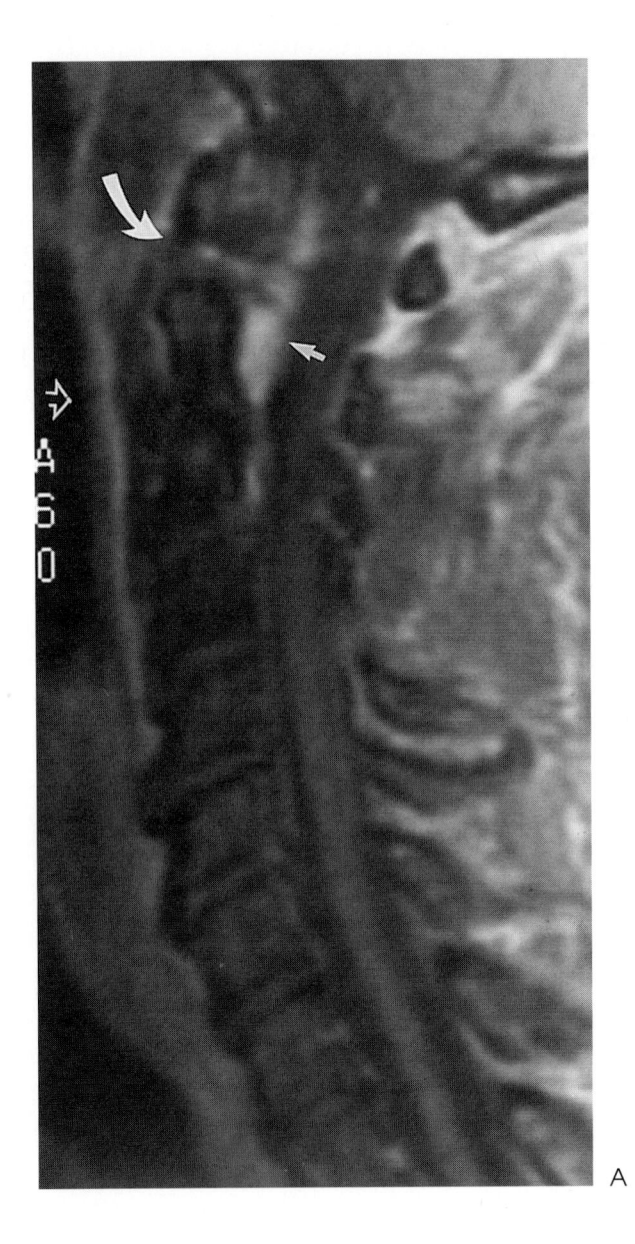

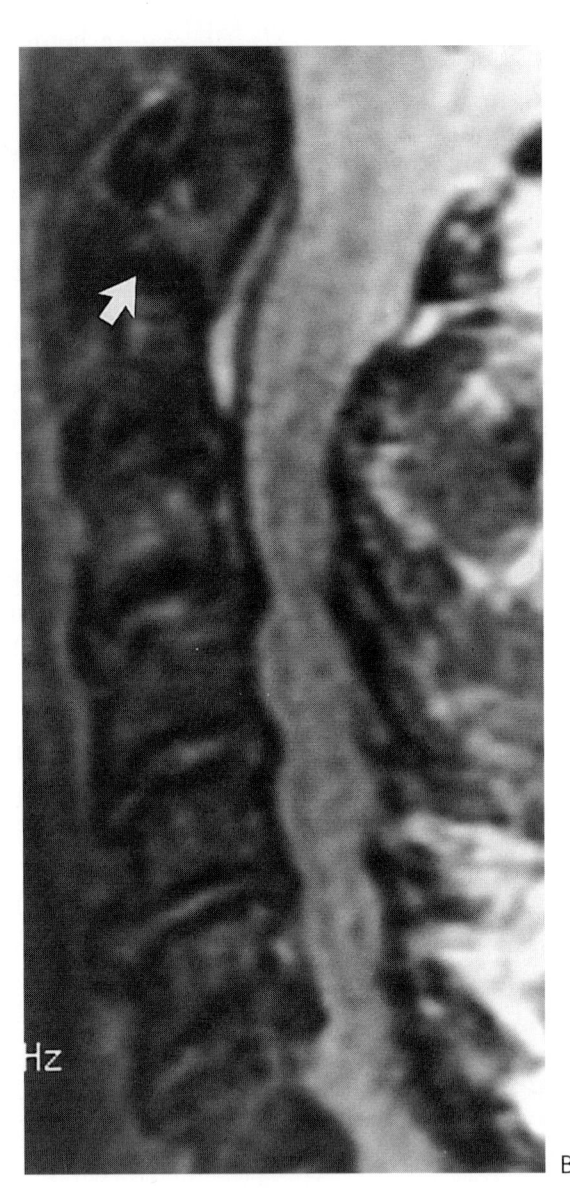

A

B

PEARLS

- Type I odontoid fractures involve the upper tip of the odontoid process. Type II odontoid fractures are broad based and extend into the upper portion of the C2 vertebral body.

- Because odontoid fractures frequently occur in the plane of the CT image slices, their presence may not be appreciated. Reconstruction images of the axial slices into the sagittal plane may provide better evaluation of the odontoid region.

PITFALLS

- Odontoid fractures are occasionally not visible acutely, so the index of suspicion must be high for this type of abnormality. The presence of soft tissue swelling is typically seen when there is an acute fracture.

- Because of the difficulty evaluating them, odontoid fractures are frequently the source of medical legal problems. Therefore, careful attention should be taken to rule out an odontoid fracture.

Radiologic Findings

Sagittal short TR image in the upper cervical region (Fig. A) reveals an area of increased signal intensity between the base of the odontoid process and the body of the C2 vertebrae (*curved arrow*). There is slight posterior displacement of the odontoid process relative to the body of C2. An area of increased signal intensity soft tissue appears behind the odontoid process and extends through the level of the body of C2 (*small arrow*). There is a slight scoliosis, and the cervical spinal cord is not seen on this image. Degenerative changes are noted throughout the remainder of the cervical spine with both anterior and posterior osteophytes. There is no widening of the prevertebral space (*open arrow*).

Sagittal long TR image (Fig. B) reveals multiple posterior osteophytes at all levels. There is indentation upon the subarachnoid space at multiple levels. The soft tissue at the base of the odontoid process remains decreased signal intensity (*arrow*).

Diagnosis

Old odontoid fracture; type II odontoid fracture.

Differential Diagnosis

- old fracture

Discussion

This fracture appears old because there are no areas of acute angulation at the ends of the fracture fragments. There is no prevertebral soft tissue swelling. There may be evidence of increased signal intensity hematoma formation behind the C2 vertebral body and odontoid process; however, fibrous scarring seems more likely. Computed tomographic (CT) scanning is helpful for evaluation of these fractures. They are occasionally difficult to demonstrate on plain film evaluation. The type III fractures extend into the vertebral body and, when impacted, are difficult to demonstrate on CT because the fracture is in the plane of imaging. The sagittal reconstruction views and the presence of prevertebral soft tissue swelling are helpful for the identification of these fractures. Fractures are usually associated with soft tissue prominence secondary to hematoma formation because of bleeding. Follow-up imaging is helpful and the patient should be immobilized in a collar if a fracture is suspected.

Case 10

Clinical Presentation

The patient is a 16-year-old male with neck pain following a football injury in which he sustained acute neck flexion.

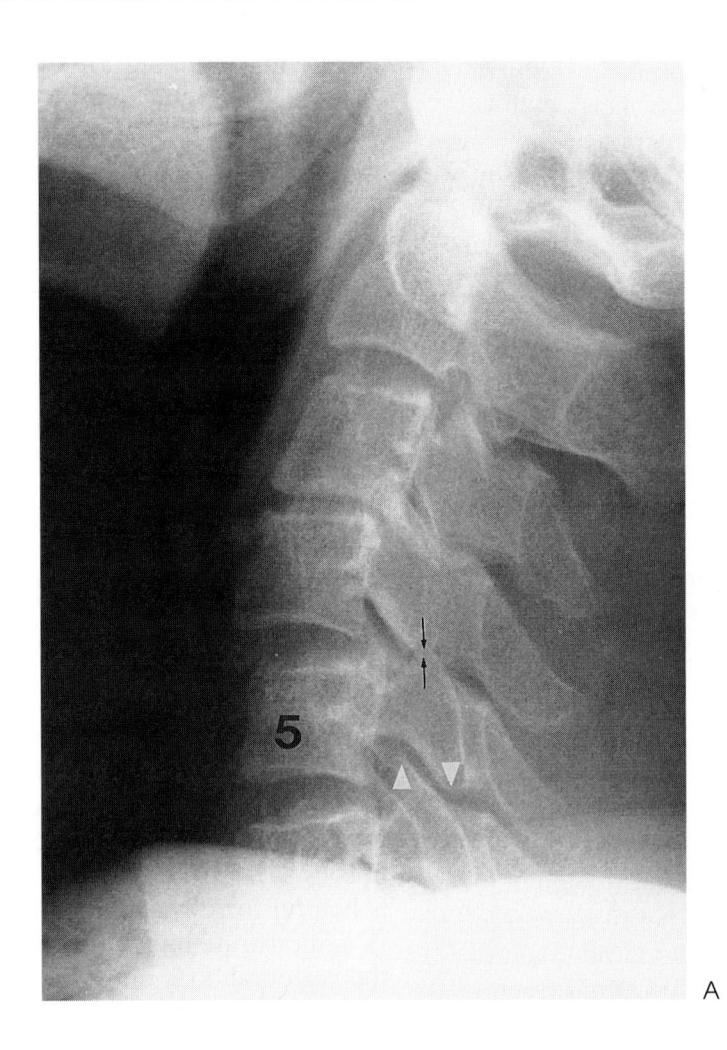

A

Radiologic Findings

Lateral plain film radiograph (Fig. A) reveals slight forward subluxation of C4 on C5. The normal relationship of the interfacet joint is present at C5-6 (*arrowheads*) where the facets rest adjacent to one another. At the C4-5 level, the inferior portion of the facet of C4 rests in direct apposition to the superior portion of the facet of C5 (*arrows*). The C5 vertebral body is identified with 5.

PEARLS

- Computed tomographic (CT) scanning may reveal additional small fractures which are not seen on the plain film radiography.

- MRI will demonstrate the exact relationship of the spinal cord to the surrounding bony structures and the presence or absence of abnormal signal within the spinal cord.

- Treatment can include follow-up imaging to determine if, after traction upon the cervical spine, there has been reduction in the facet dislocation. Therefore, follow-up imaging provides an ideal method of evaluation.

PITFALLS

- Small fractures may be missed without performing a CT scan.

- Because a syrinx cavity may occur after trauma even when there is no obvious damage to the spinal cord, follow-up with MRI is useful for additional evaluation.

Diagnosis

Bilateral perched facets.

Differential Diagnosis

- perched facets

Discussion

Radiculopathy may also occur if the nerve rootlets are compressed by the displaced bony structures. If viewed after 90 degree rotation of the radiograph, this results in a "bow tie" appearance, which is typical of perched facets. If unilateral, there is a scoliosis of the spine, and in this case, the anteroposterior view will reveal that the spinous processes are not aligned. Treatment is usually muscle relaxation and traction. If conservative treatment fails to return the facets to normal alignment, the facets are directly visualized and manipulated back into place with surgical tools. Magnetic resonance imaging (MRI) is an excellent method of evaluation and will reveal areas of increased signal intensity in the soft tissues where there has been sufficient damage to cause edema.

The patient should be evaluated to determine if there are bilateral or unilateral abnormalities involving the facets because the surgical approach will be different between the two.

TEACHING ATLAS OF SPINE IMAGING

Case 11

Clinical Presentation

The patient is a 17-year-old male victim of assault.

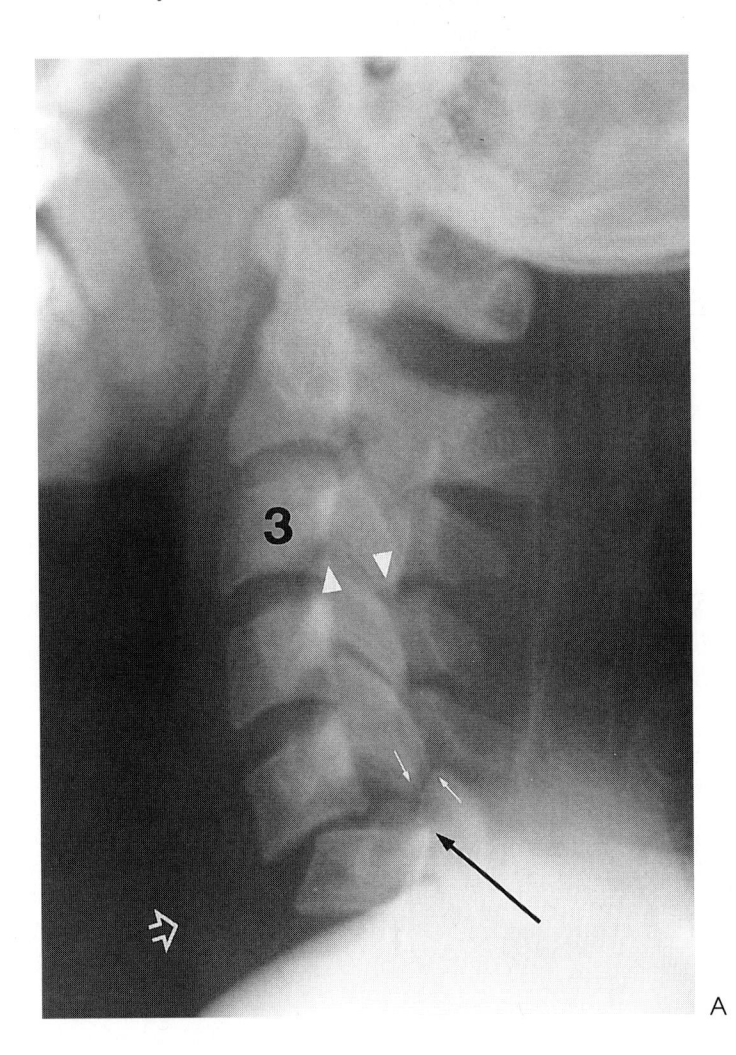

Radiologic Findings

Lateral plain film radiograph of the cervical spine (Fig. A) reveals marked forward subluxation of C5 on C6. The posterior superior corner of the C6 vertebral body is marked with the black arrow. The inferior portion of the facet at the C5 level is markedly displaced forward and is anterior to the superior portion of the articulating facet of C6 (*white arrows*). There is blunting of the ends of the facets. The identical anatomic areas are identified with small arrows at the C3 level white (*arrowheads*). There is prevertebral soft tissue swelling and the trachea is displaced far forward (*open arrow*). The C3 vertebral body is identified with 3.

TRAUMA

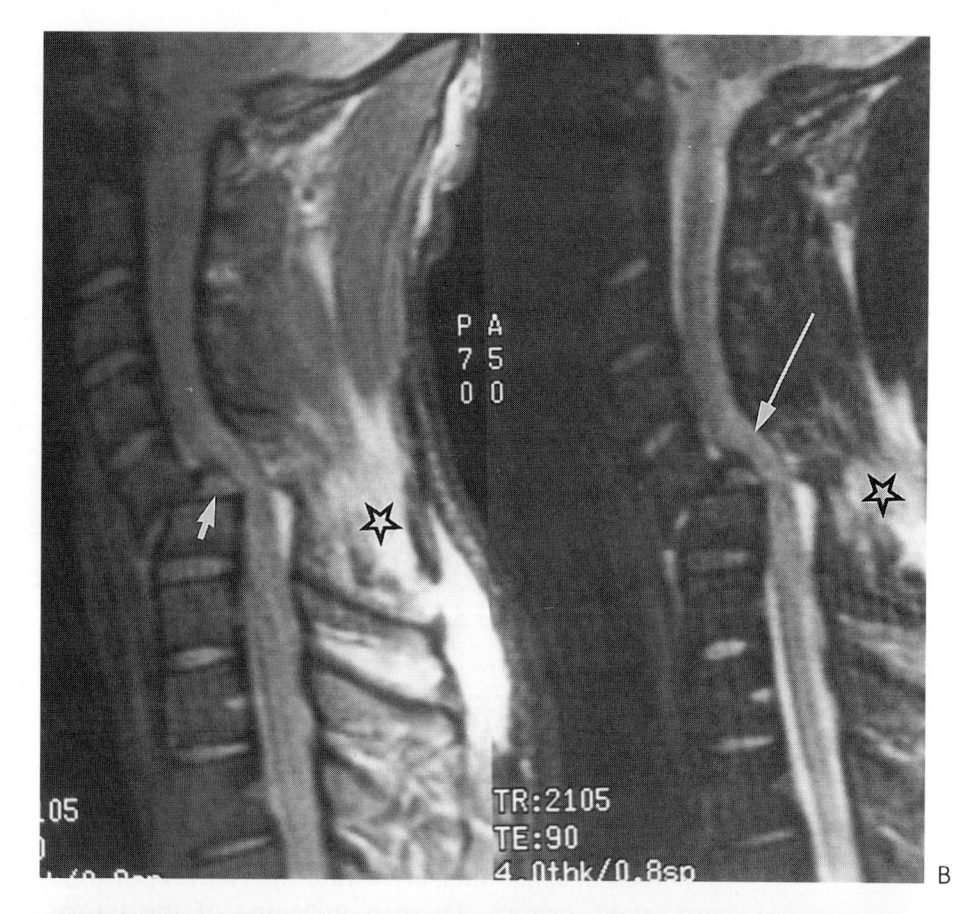

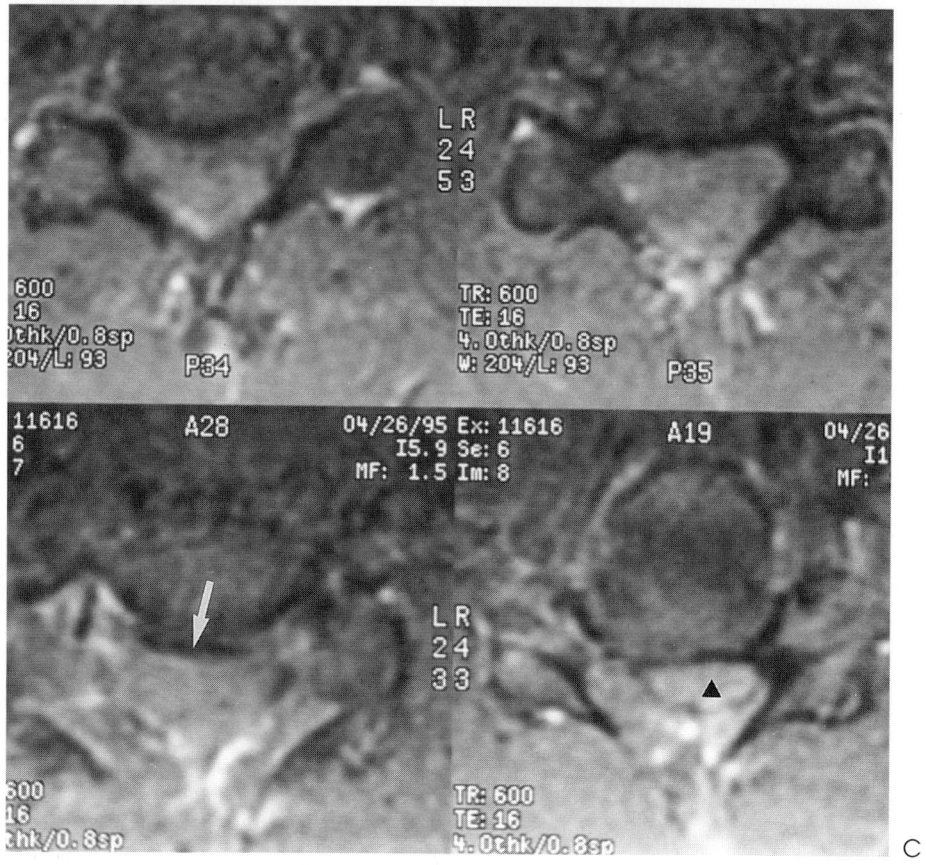

TEACHING ATLAS OF SPINE IMAGING

D

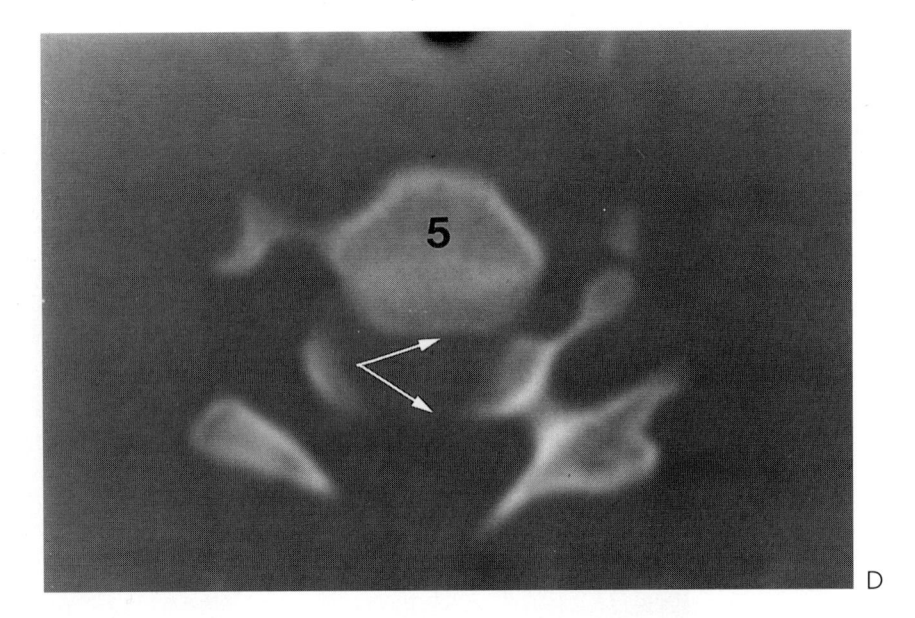

Radiologic Findings (continued)

Sagittal intermediate (Fig. B, *left*) and long (Fig. B, *right*) TR images reveal the forward subluxation of C5 on C6. There is prominence of the intervertebral disc at this level (*left, arrow*). On the long TR image, there is an area of increased signal intensity within the central portion of the cervical spinal cord (*right, arrow*). There is widening of the interspinous distance and increased signal intensity soft tissue between the spinous processes (*).

Axial short TR images (Fig. C) reveal complete obliteration of the normal high signal intensity fat that surrounds the thecal sac. There is a linear area of decreased signal intensity that projects behind the vertebral body of C5 (*bottom left, arrow*). The intervertebral disc seen in Figure B projects in the midline and toward the left side (*bottom right, arrowhead*) and markedly compresses the spinal cord. The thecal sac is surrounded by intermediate signal intensity soft tissue.

Axial computed tomographic (CT) scan (Fig. D) reveals the forward subluxation of C5 on C6; the posterior marking of the vertebrae are highlighted by the white arrows. The C5 vertebral body is identified with 5.

Diagnosis

Anterior dislocation of C5 on C6 with disruption of the nucal ligament and traumatic herniation of the intervertebral disc at the C5-6 level.

Differential Diagnosis

- herniated disc

- fracture dislocation

TRAUMA

PEARLS

- CT scanning reveals small fracture fragments better than MRI. Sagittal reconstruction views will also allow for evaluation of the amount of compromise of the vertebral canal.

- MRI demonstrates the presence of soft tissue swelling and/or hematoma formation. MRI readily demonstrates any change in the size of the spinal cord and whether it is related to edema or hematoma formation.

PITFALL

- While MRI is the method of choice for evaluation of the spinal cord, other life-threatening injuries may preclude the use of MRI in the acute setting.

Discussion

Magnetic resonance imaging (MRI) allows ready evaluation of the spinal cord and its relationship to the surrounding body structures. The area of increased signal intensity within the cervical spinal cord is an area of edema or contusion. The herniated disc also compresses the cervical spinal cord, and the combination of changes results in marked spinal stenosis at the C5-6 level. There is widening of the interspinous distance and a hematoma in the soft tissues between the spinous processes of C5 and C6, which appears as increased signal intensity. There is also soft tissue edema.

Both CT and MRI are excellent methods for evaluating the lower portions of the cervical spine when this area cannot be visualized by plane film evaluation. MRI is frequently more useful than CT scanning in many cases because, when the patient has very large shoulders, the lower cervical spine cannot be seen on CT images.

TEACHING ATLAS OF SPINE IMAGING

Case 12

Clinical Presentation

The patient is a 35-year-old female with continued back pain following epidural block for vaginal delivery. The patient developed a spinal headache, and blood patches were attempted to decrease the headache. The patient also has lower extremity weakness, which is greater in the right leg than the left.

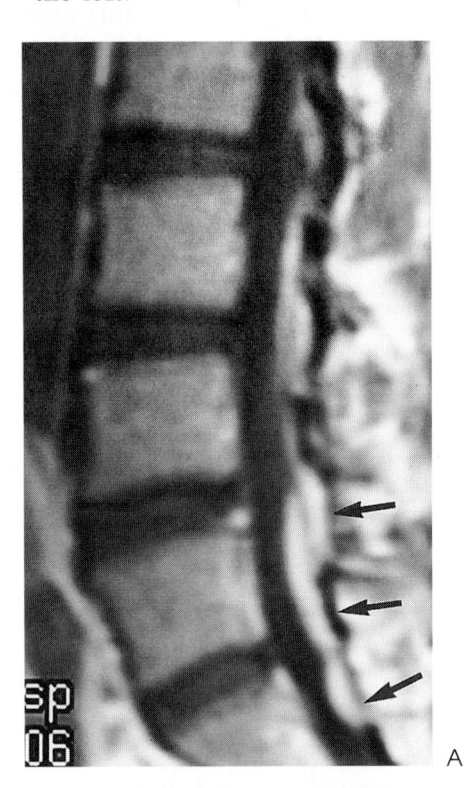

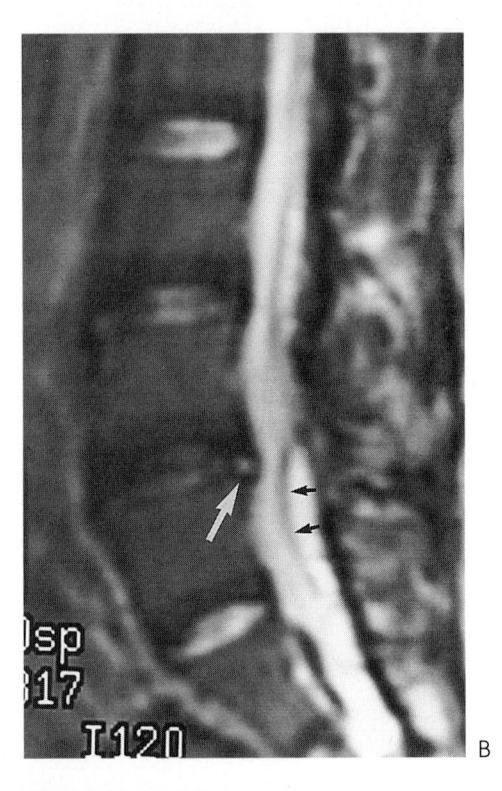

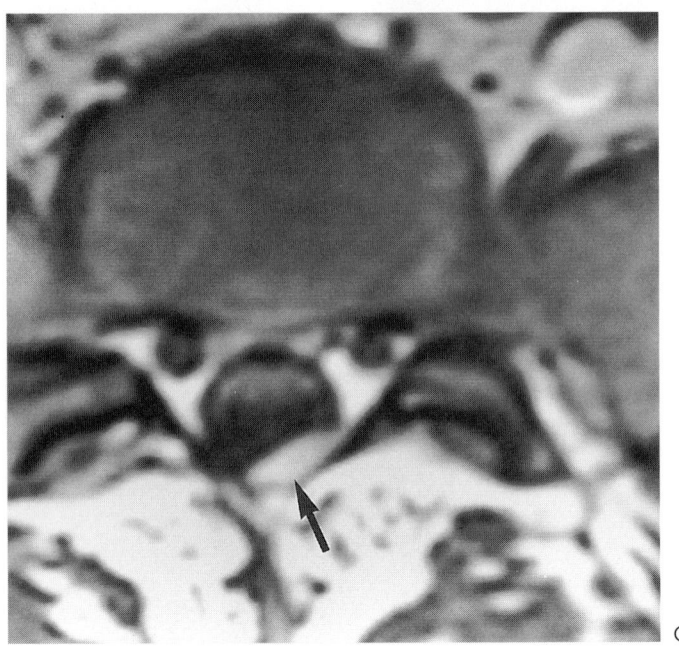

TRAUMA

Radiologic Findings

Sagittal short TR image in the lumbar region (Fig. A) reveals a lobulated area of increased signal intensity at the level of L5 and S1 (*arrows*).

Sagittal long TR image (Fig. B) reveals a thin curvilinear line of decreased signal intensity (*black arrows*) deep to the area of increased signal intensity seen in Figure A. There is also posterior extension of the intervertebral disc into the vertebral canal at the L4-5 level (*white arrow*).

Axial short TR image (Fig. C) reveals a lentiform area of increased signal intensity that encroaches upon the dorsal and left lateral aspect of the thecal sac (*arrow*).

PEARL
- Magnetic resonance imaging is the ideal method of evaluating this type of abnormality.

PITFALL
- Computed tomographic scanning will not demonstrate the presence of a hematoma.

Diagnosis

Small epidural hematoma.

Differential Diagnosis

- epidural hematoma
- epidural lipoma (unlikely)

Discussion

The epidural hematoma is methemoglobin, therefore, it appears increased signal intensity on short TR images. The decreased signal intensity line seen in Figure B is secondary to the dura, which is displaced anteriorly. It is unknown whether the epidural hematoma is secondary to the blood patch or the epidural anesthesia. There is also a herniated disc at the L4-5 level. In this patient, it is uncertain what the significance of the herniated disc is relative to the patient's back pain.

TEACHING ATLAS OF SPINE IMAGING

Case 13

Clinical Presentation

The patient is a 78-year-old male who developed severe back pain and inability to move his lower extremities following placement of an epidural catheter for spinal anesthesia for popliteal-femoral artery bypass.

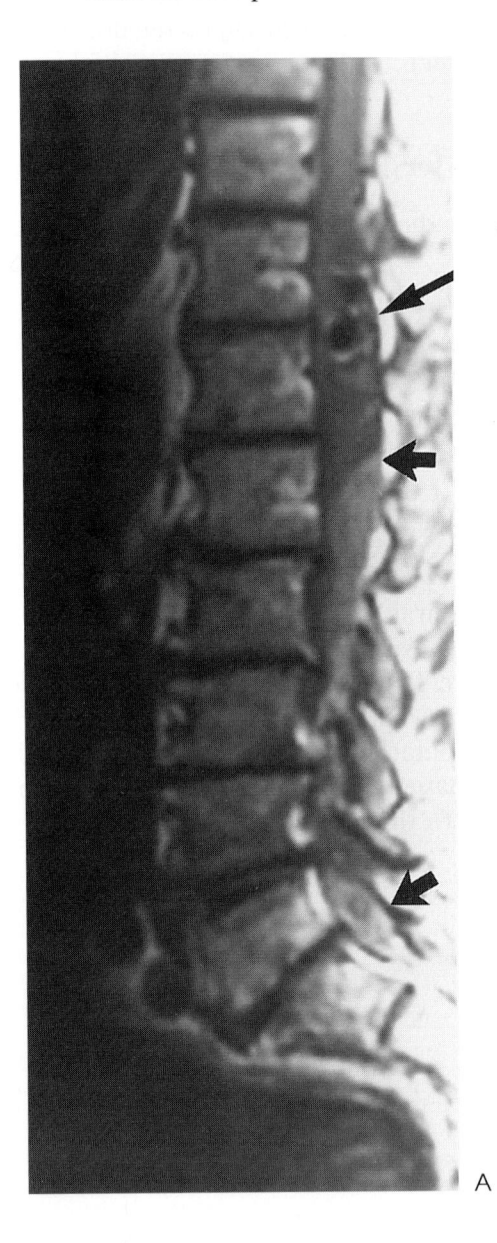

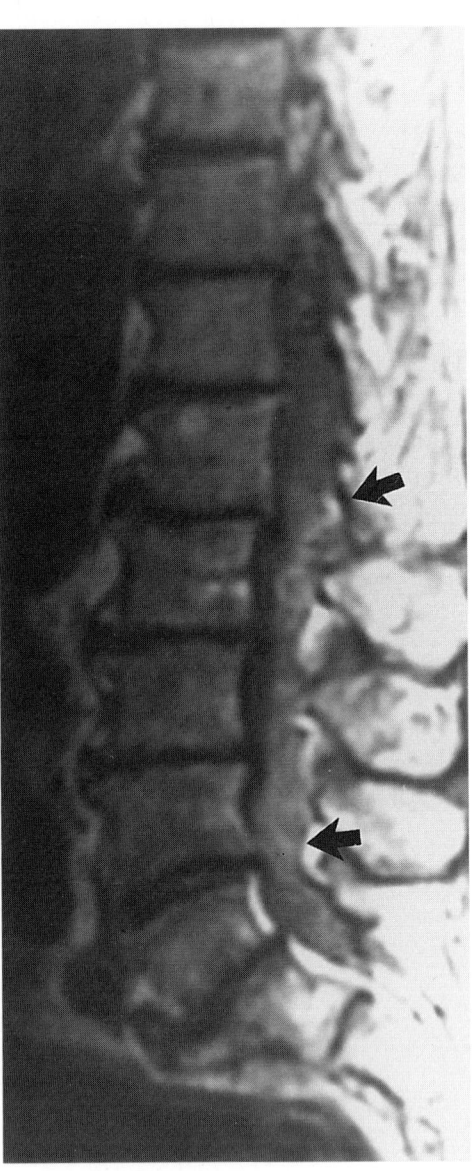

TRAUMA

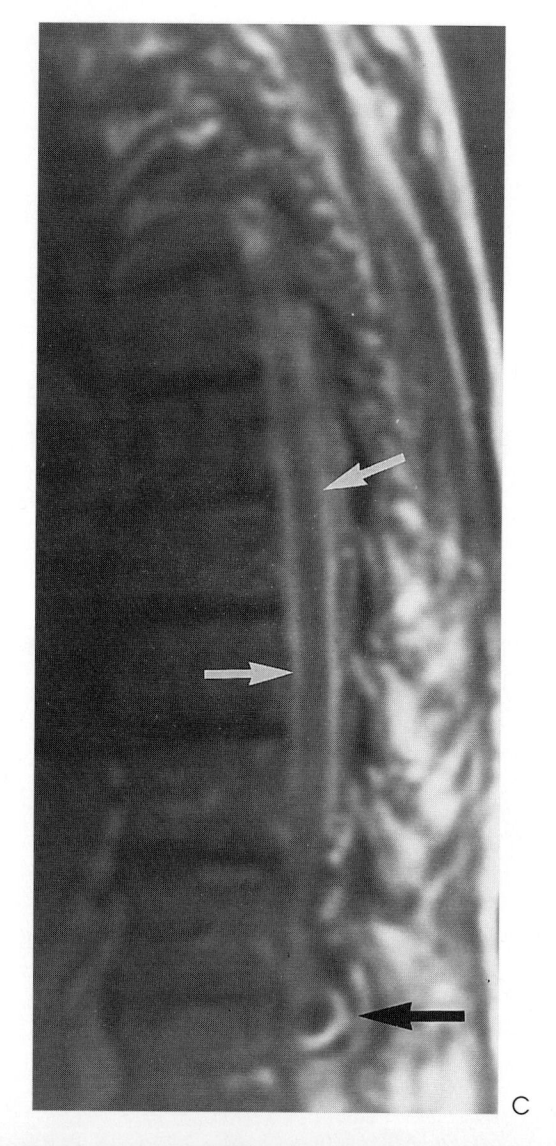

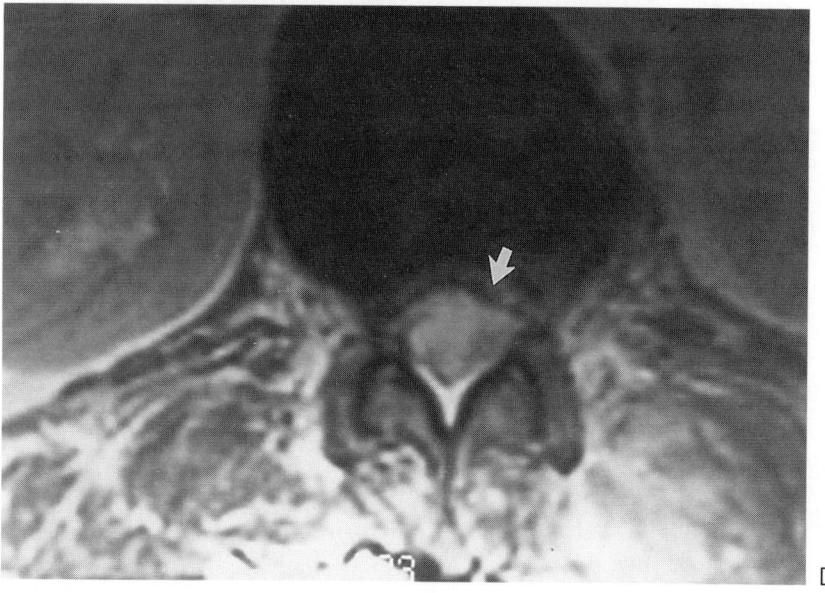

TEACHING ATLAS OF SPINE IMAGING

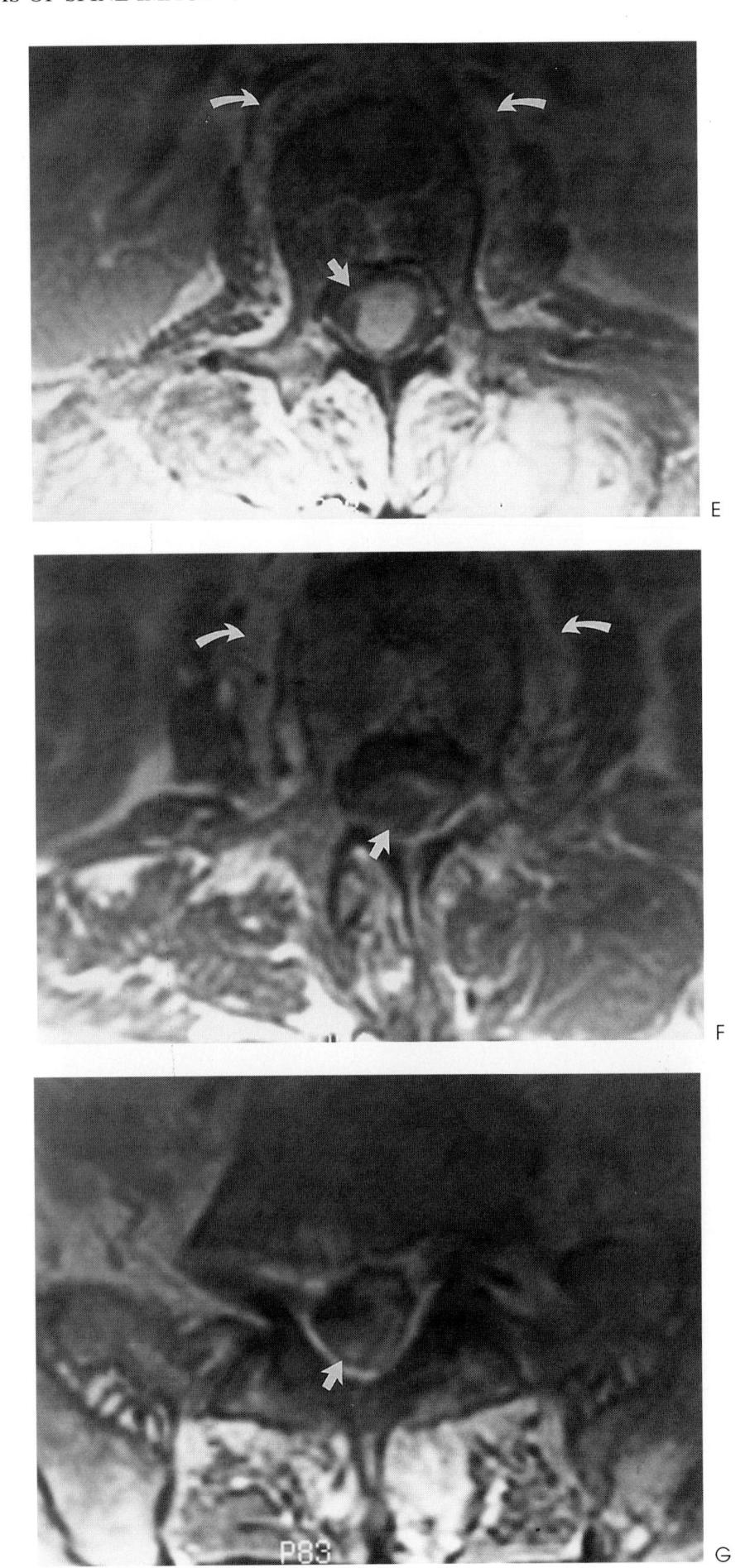

E

F

G

310

TRAUMA

Radiologic Findings

Sagittal short TR image in the lower thoracic and lumbar region (Fig. A) reveals two rounded areas of very decreased signal intensity at the level of T11-12 (*long black arrow*). A curvilinear area of increased signal intensity begins at the level of L1 (*upper short black arrow*) and extends to the lower end of the vertebral canal (*lower short black arrow*). There are degenerative changes with osteophytes at all levels of the lumbar spine.

Sagittal short TR image in a slightly different plane from Figure A (Fig. B) reveals that the area of increased signal intensity extends from L1 through S1 (*arrows*).

Sagittal short TR image in the thoracic region (Fig. C) reveals linear areas of increased signal intensity surrounding the thoracic spinal cord (*white arrows*). There are rounded and curvilinear areas of decreased signal intensity with partial halos of increased signal intensity in the lower thoracic region (*black arrow*).

Axial short TR image at the level of the kidneys (Fig. D) reveals that the thecal sac is not visualized and there is increased signal intensity soft tissue filling the vertebral canal (*arrow*).

Axial short TR image (Fig. E) reveals the thecal sac filled with increased signal intensity material (*straight arrow*). There are bilateral paraspinal curvilinear areas of increased signal intensity (*curved arrows*).

Bilateral curvilinear areas (Fig. F) of increased signal intensity (*curved arrows*) are visible at approximately the L3 level. The thecal sac is higher than normal signal intensity, and there is a surrounding halo of increased signal intensity (*straight arrow*).

At the L5 level, there is increased signal intensity soft tissue (Fig. G) which fills the thecal sac (*arrow*).

Diagnosis

Epidural hematoma; blood in the thecal sac; air in the vertebral canal in the lower thoracic region.

Differential Diagnosis

- epidural hematoma
- epidural inflammatory process

Discussion

When an epidural catheter is placed, it is threaded from the lumbar region superiorly into the lower thoracic region. Air can be injected into the catheter, and in this case appears as areas of markedly decreased signal intensity in the lower thoracic region. There is a halo of increased signal intensity

PEARLS

- Magnetic resonance imaging (MRI) is the procedure of choice for evaluation of blood or bleeding into the epidural space or into the thecal sac. Blood may exhibit a variety of signal intensities because of the phase of metabolism. Acute bleeding in the deoxyhemoglobin phase appears as decreased signal intensity, while subacute blood in the methemoglobin phase appears as increased signal intensity. Chronic blood in the hemosiderin phase (not seen in this patient) is decreased signal intensity.

- If surgery is performed for removal of a localized hematoma, MRI provides an ideal diagnostic method for follow-up.

PITFALL

- It is not always possible to determine the exact location of areas of hemorrhage or the exact anatomic compartment because the blood may compress and distort the thecal sac.

surrounding these areas because of magnetic susceptibility artifact. There is increased signal intensity blood surrounding the spinal cord in the thoracic region, probably in the subarachnoid space. In the lumbar region, the blood is both epidural and intrathecal. There are bilateral paraspinal hematomas in the midlumbar region as seen in Figures E and F.

An epidural inflammatory process is a remote consideration but appears unlikely in this clinical setting.

TRAUMA

Case 14

Clinical Presentation

The patient is an 87-year-old female who is taking coumadin and developed severe low back pain and lower extremity weakness.

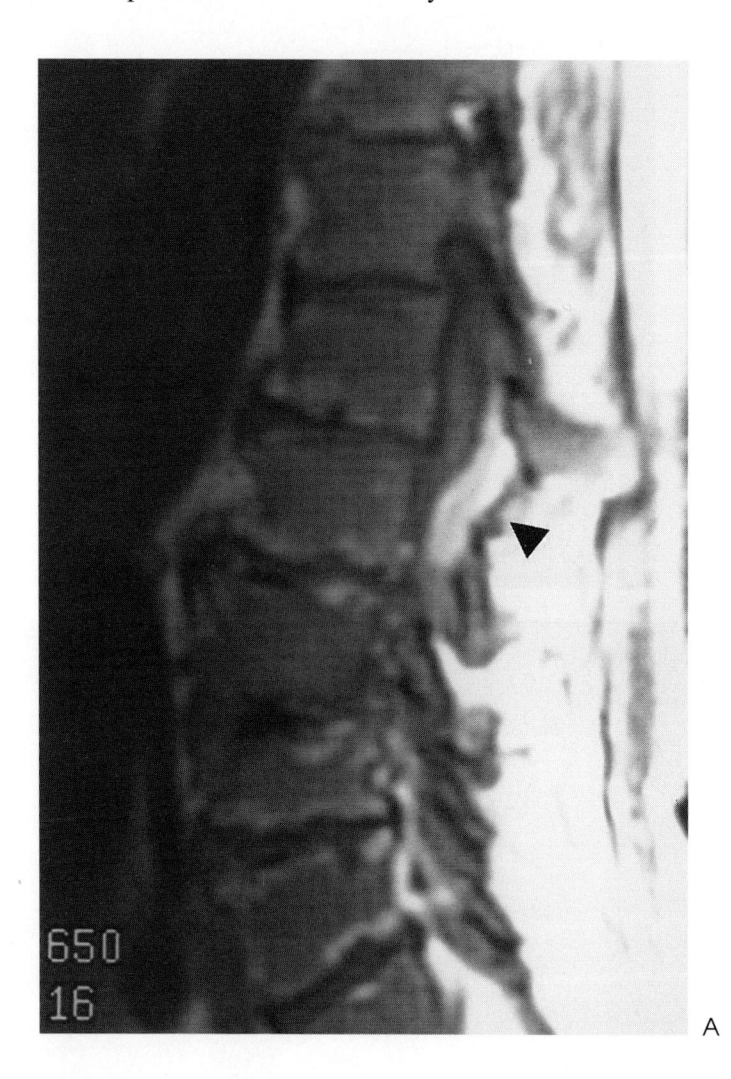

Radiologic Findings

Sagittal short TR image in the upper lumbar region (Fig. A) reveals an irregularly shaped area of increased signal intensity in the dorsal epidural space (*arrowhead*). There are severe degenerative changes in the spine.

TEACHING ATLAS OF SPINE IMAGING

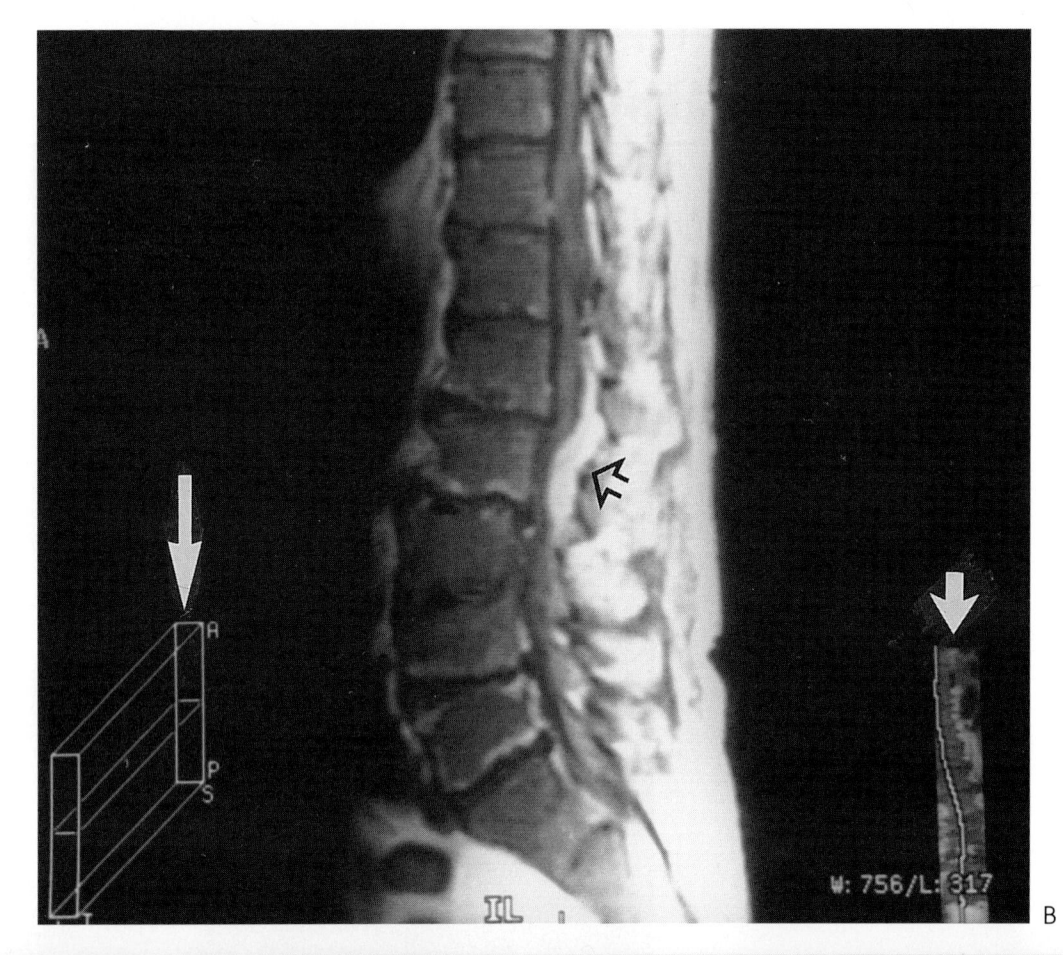

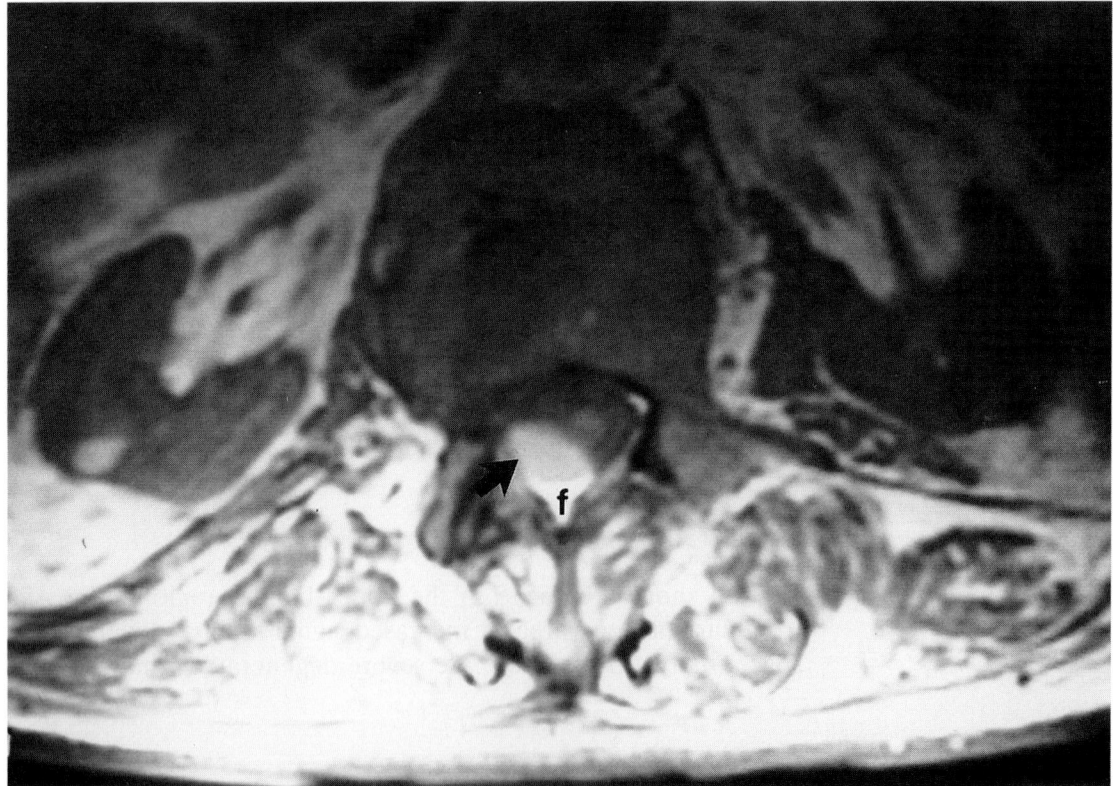

TRAUMA

D

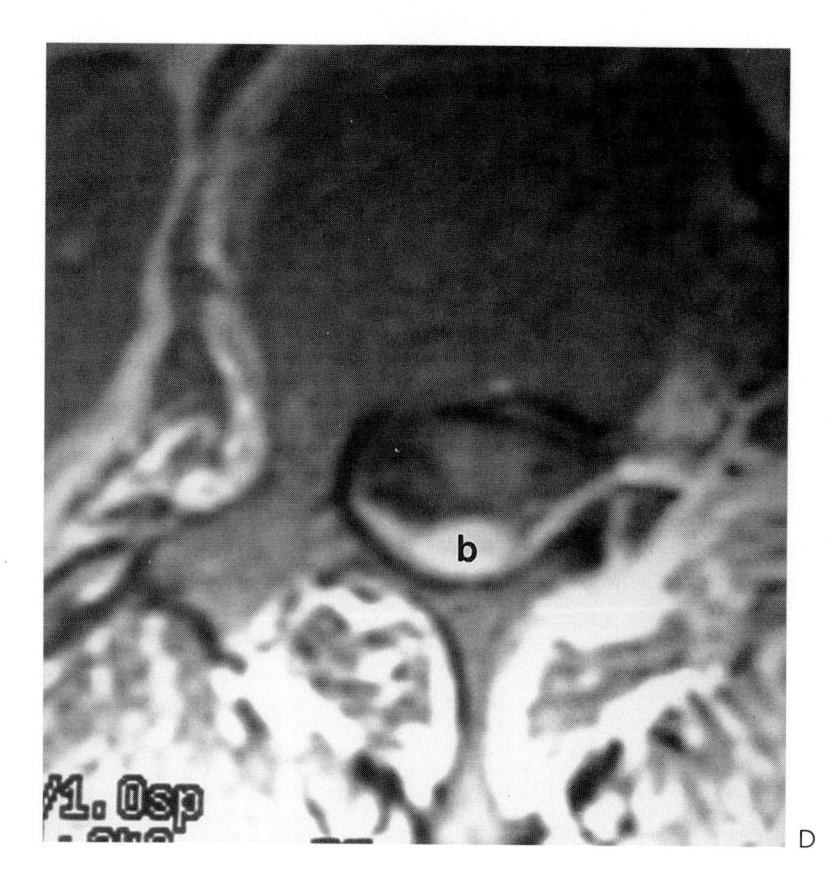

Radiologic Findings (continued)

Sagittal short TR image utilizing a "straightening" algorithm better (Fig. B) reveals the area of increased signal intensity in the dorsal epidural space at the L1-2 level (*open arrow*). The method of manual identification of the line of reconstruction is seen on the right side (*short arrow*), and the volume of tissue evaluated is seen on the left side (*long arrow*).

Axial short TR image at the level of L2 (Fig. C) reveals the lentiform area of increased signal intensity on the right side (*arrow*). The thecal sac is compressed and displaced to the left. The normal increased signal intensity fat is seen in the epidural space (*f*).

Axial short TR image at the level of L1 (Fig. D) reveals the lentiform area of increased signal intensity in the dorsal epidural space (*b*).

Diagnosis

Spontaneous epidural hematoma.

Differential Diagnosis

- epidural hematoma

TEACHING ATLAS OF SPINE IMAGING

PEARL
- Magnetic resonance imaging is the ideal method for evaluating areas of hemorrhage involving the spinal cord or the surrounding structures.

PITFALL
- Epidural fat, which also appears as increased signal intensity on short TR images, would have a similar appearance and would be a diagnostic consideration in another clinical setting.

Discussion

Patients who are treated with coumadin or other "blood thinners" may experience hemorrhages. In this case, the hemorrhage is into the epidural space resulting in spinal canal compromise. The straightening algorithm is very helpful for evaluation of this type of abnormality where the scoliosis may compromise the evaluation of the position of the lesion and its relationship to the surrounding structures. The clinical history of coumadin is very helpful for evaluation of the cause of this patient's epidural hematoma and resulting back pain.

TRAUMA

Case 15

Clinical Presentation

The patient is a 68-year-old male who presented with lower extremity weakness. The patient is taking coumadin and suffered a recent fall.

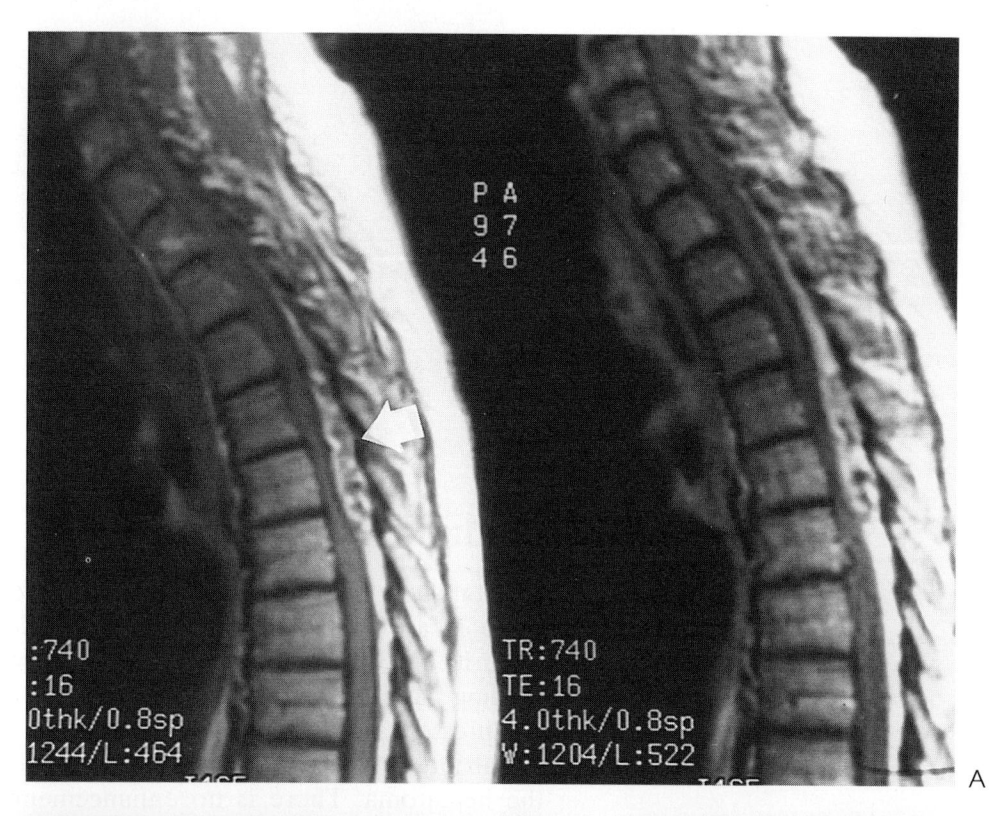

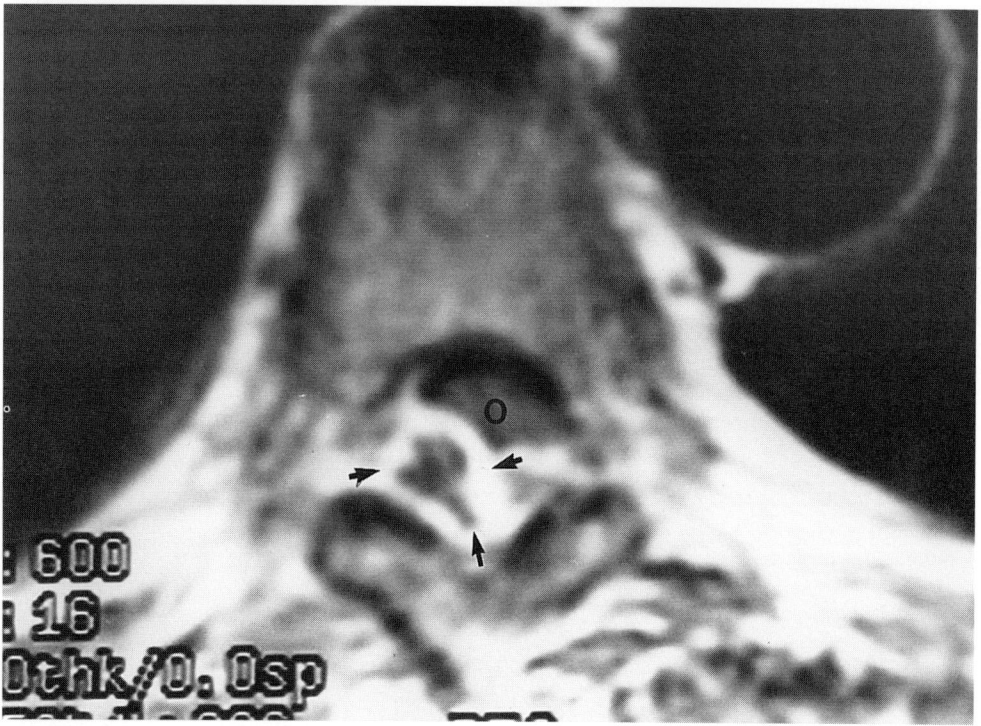

A

B

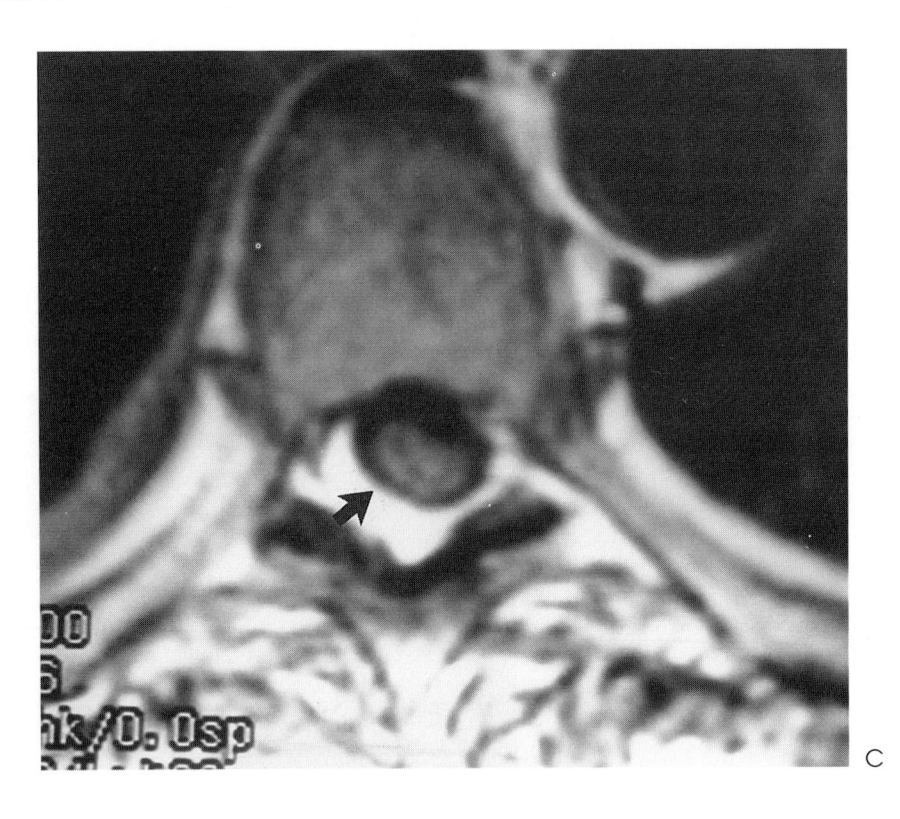

Radiologic Findings

Sagittal short TR images in the midthoracic region pre- (Fig. A, *left*) and postcontrast (Fig. A, *right*) injection reveal a mottled area of variable signal intensity in the epidural region (*left, arrow*) in the midthoracic spine extending from T3 through T7. The spinal cord is displaced anteriorly and compressed against the posterior margin of the spine. The normal high signal intensity of the thoracic epidural fat is obliterated at the level of the hematoma. There is no enhancement after the injection of contrast material (*right*).

Axial short TR image at the level of T5 (Fig. B) reveals the triangular-shaped area of increased signal intensity in the right dorsal aspect of the vertebral canal (*arrows*). There is a central area of decreased signal intensity. The spinal cord (*o*) is displaced anteriorly and to the left side.

Below the level of the area of increased signal intensity (Fig. C), the epidural fat is widened (*arrow*). The subarachnoid space is compressed.

Diagnosis

Spontaneous epidural hematoma in the midthoracic region secondary to coumadin treatment.

TRAUMA

PEARL
- CT scanning would not be helpful in the diagnosis or evaluation of the abnormality in this patient. Follow-up of resolution or response to surgery can be easily performed with MR evaluation.

PITFALL
- Epidural fat also appears as increased signal intensity on short TR images; however, this location is unlikely, and the clinical history is consistent with an area of hemorrhage.

Differential Diagnosis
- hemorrhage
- hemophilia

Discussion

Magnetic resonance imaging is the ideal method of evaluating the presence of an area of hemorrhage whether within the spinal cord or in the epidural space. The relationship of the area of blood collection is easily seen relative to the position of the spinal cord. The variable signal intensity in Figure A is secondary to the accumulation of both methemoglobin and deoxyhemoglobin. In Figure B, the central area of decreased signal intensity is deoxyhemoglobin, which is surrounded by increased signal intensity methemoglobin. Patients with hemophilia may also experience areas of hemorrhage. Knowledge of the clinical setting is important for accurate evaluation of the abnormality.

Case 16

Clinical Presentation

The patient is a 32-year-old female who is status post kidney transplant with severe and worsening back pain.

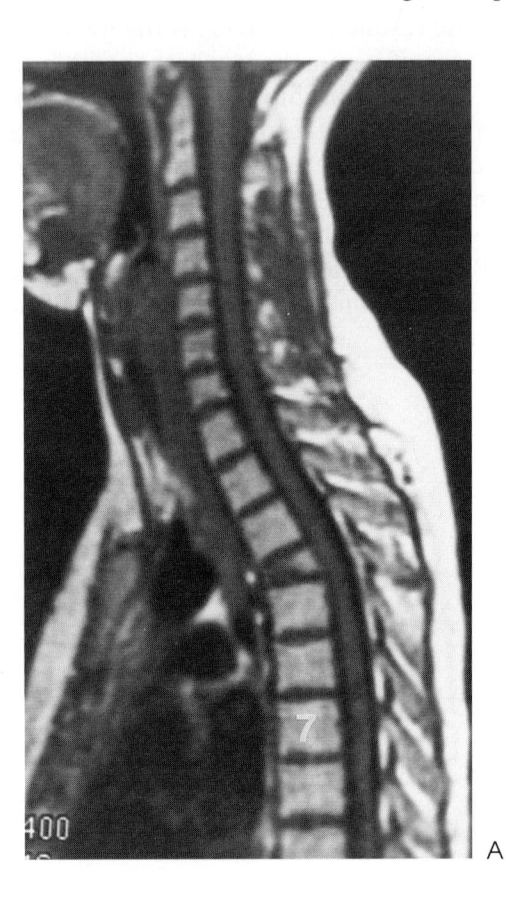

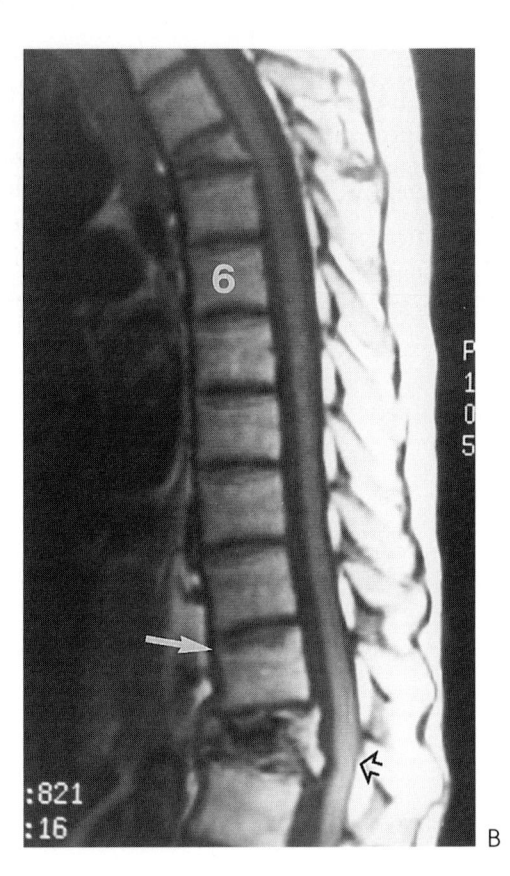

Radiologic Findings

Sagittal short TR image of the cervical and thoracic spine (Fig. A) reveals a compression fracture of the T4 vertebral body. The remainder of the vertebral bodies are normal. There is accentuation of the thoracic kyphosis at the T4 level. The T7 vertebral body is identified with 7.

Sagittal short TR image in the lower thoracic and lumbar region (Fig. B) reveals a marked compression fracture of the T12 vertebral body. The posterior margin of the T12 vertebral body is retropulsed into the vertebral canal, and curvilinear posterior displacement of the spinal cord is visible (*open arrow*). Compression deformity can be seen at the superior end plate of the T11 vertebral body (*solid arrow*). There is reversal of the normal lumbar lordosis because of the fracture. The T6 vertebral body is identified with 6.

TRAUMA

> **PEARL**
> - Magnetic resonance imaging is the ideal method of evaluation, and the entire vertebral column can be easily evaluated with the use of phased array coils.

> **PITFALL**
> - Evaluation should be made for possible metastatic disease. A radionuclide bone scan would be helpful to evaluate for the presence of other areas of increased signal intensity.

Diagnosis

Benign compression fractures of T4 and T12 secondary to osteoporosis.

Differential Diagnosis

- osteoporosis
- compression fracture
- metastatic disease

Discussion

There is diffuse increased signal intensity of the marrow of all the visualized vertebral bodies secondary to osteoporosis. The patient has been on steroids related to her kidney transplant. Otherwise there is no abnormal signal intensity within the vertebral marrow to suggest other underlying disease such as metastases. There is also widening of the interspinous distance at the T4-5 level because of the fracture.

Case 17

Clinical Presentation

The patient is a 73-year-old female with back pain.

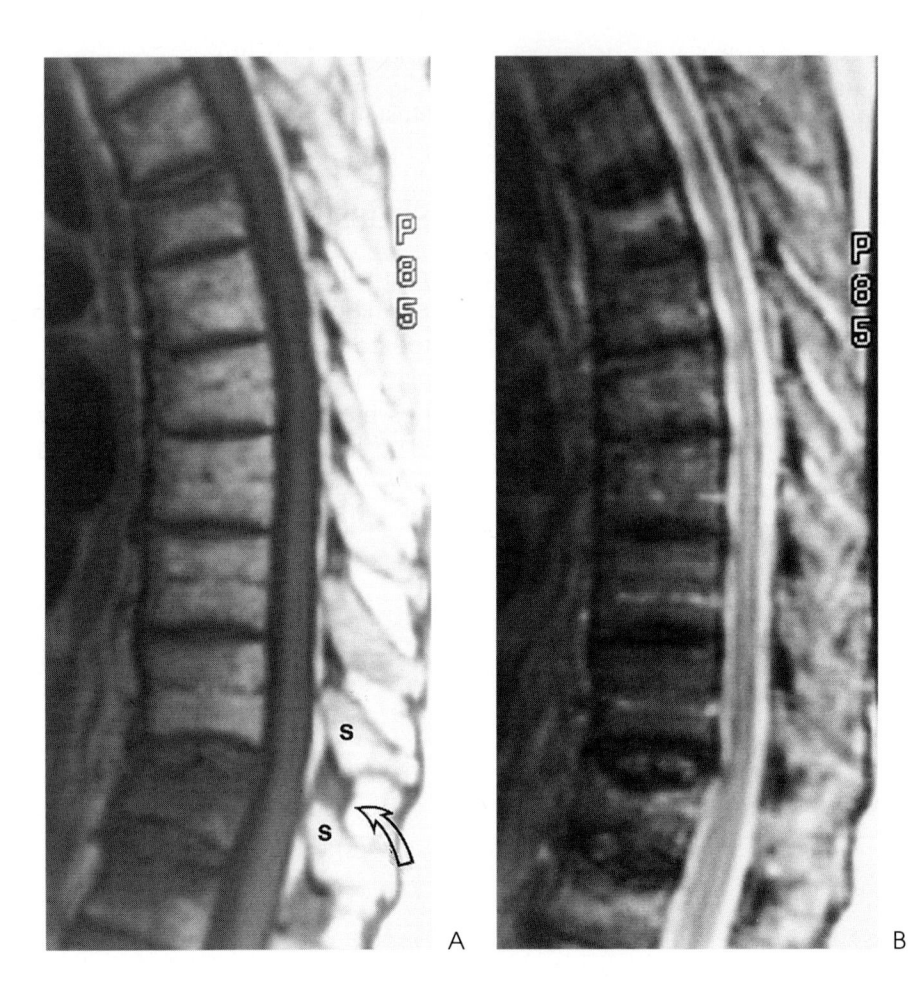

A

B

Radiologic Findings

Sagittal short TR image in the mid and lower thoracic region (Fig. A) reveals compression fractures of T4 (*open arrow*), T10, and T11. There are areas of decreased signal intensity involving the superior portions of the vertebral bodies at the levels of the fractures. There is slight irregularity of the superior end plates of the vertebral bodies of T10 and T11. There is an area of decreased signal intensity between the spinous processes (*s*), which is well seen at the T9-10 level.

Sagittal long TR image (Fig. B) reveals increased signal intensity of the areas of decreased signal intensity seen on the short TR images. There is slight compromise of the subarachnoid space at the T9-10 level but no abnormal signal intensity within the spinal cord.

TRAUMA

PEARL
- Magnetic resonance imaging is the ideal method of evaluation. In general, in the presence of a benign compression fracture, the vertebral body pedicle is normal; while in a pathologic fracture, the vertebral body pedicle is replaced by decreased signal intensity tumor. This is not always the case, and follow-up may be necessary for complete evaluation.

PITFALL
- The changes seen here could also be related to multiple myeloma, so correlation should be made with the analysis of the patient's serum chemical analysis.

Diagnosis

Multiple compression fractures.

Differential Diagnosis

- compression fractures
- metastatic disease
- osteoporosis

Discussion

These multiple compression fractures are secondary to osteoporosis. There is diffuse mottled increased signal intensity within the marrow of the visualized vertebral bodies. The soft tissue structure in Figure A is the ligamentum flavum and this is seen at multiple levels. The portions of the vertebral bodies that appear as decreased signal intensity on the short TR images become increased signal intensity on the long TR images. This change is secondary to edema related to these relatively acute fractures. The remote possibility of metastases is a consideration; however, the lack of focal areas of decreased signal intensity make this unlikely.

Case 18

Clinical Presentation

The patient is an 87-year-old female who presents with marked accentuation of the dorsal kyphosis.

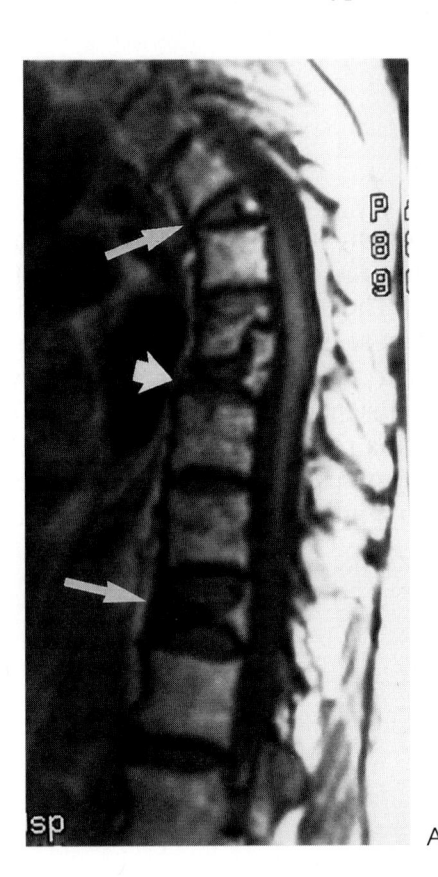

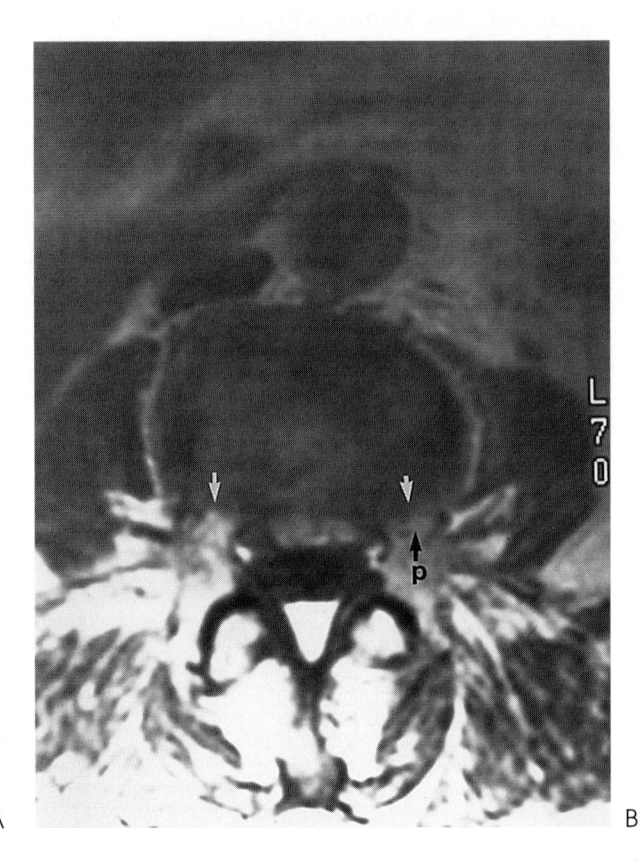

Radiologic Findings

Sagittal short TR image of the thoracic spine (Fig. A) reveals compression fractures of multiple thoracic vertebral bodies. There is complete loss of height of the vertebral body of T4 (*upper long arrow*). There is only a very small triangular area of increased signal intensity posteriorly, which represents the posterior portion of the vertebral body. The remainder is sufficiently compressed that it is no longer seen. The T7 vertebral body is likewise markedly compressed. The end plates are in apposition and appear as an area of linear decreased signal intensity (*short arrow*). A compression fracture of T6 is greater posteriorly than anteriorly. There is a marked compression fracture of T10 (*lower long arrow*).

Axial short TR image in the lumbar spine in the same patient (Fig. B) reveals that the vertebral body pedicle appears increased signal intensity (*p*).

TRAUMA

Diagnosis

Multiple benign compression fractures secondary to osteoporosis.

Differential Diagnosis

- osteoporosis
- metastatic disease

Discussion

The edema within the vertebral body is decreased signal intensity and extends to the base of the pedicle bilaterally (*arrows*, Fig. B). If the decreased signal intensity was secondary to metastatic disease, the pedicle would then also be decreased signal intensity secondary to this involvement with tumor. If the pedicle is not involved, this suggests a normal vertebral body.

The combination of all of these changes results in the accentuation of the dorsal kyphosis and the clinical appearance of the "dowager's hump."

PEARLS

- Magnetic resonance imaging (MRI) is the ideal method of evaluation of these abnormalities. The entire vertebral column can be easily evaluated.

- MRI allows ready evaluation of the vertebral body pedicles, which are important in the differentiation of benign versus malignant involvement of the vertebral body. MR also allows a noninvasive method of evaluation of encroachment upon the vertebral canal by retropulsed vertebral body fragments.

- Hematomas may occasionally occur and are also readily visualized by MRI.

PITFALLS

- In those cases where there is marked compression fracture of the vertebral body and complete loss of vertebral body height, the absence of the vertebral body may be difficult to appreciate. The accentuation of the kyphosis provides a clue to the diagnosis.

- Although involvement of the vertebral body pedicle with decreased signal intensity tumor is helpful for diagnosis, follow-up may be the only method by which an absolute diagnosis between benign and malignant compression fracture can be made.

Suggested Readings

Anderson LD, D'Alonzo RT. Fractures of the odontoid process of the axis. *J Bone Joint Surg Am.* 1974;56:1663–1674.

Becerra JL, Puckett WR, Hiester ED, et al. MR-pathologic comparisons of Wallerian degeneration in spinal cord injury. *AJNR.* 1995;16:125–133.

Brandser EA, El-Khoury GY. Thoracic and lumbar spine trauma. *Radiol Clin North Am.* 1997;35:533.

Caldemeyer KS, Mocharia R, Moran CC, et al. Gadolinium enhancement in the center of a spinal epidural hematoma in a hemophiliac. *JCAT* 1993;17:321

Castillo M, Mukherju SH. Vertical fracture of the dens. *AJNR.* 1996;17:1627–1630.

Coffin CM, Weill A, Miaux Y, et al. Posttraumatic spinal subarachnoid cyst. *Eur Radiol.* 1996;6:523–525.

Davis SJ, Khangure MS. Review of magnetic resonance imaging in spinal trauma. *Australas Radiol.* 1994;38:241.

Ehara S, El-Khoury GY, Clark CR. Radiologic evaluation of dens fracture: role of plain radiography and tomography. *Spine.* 1992;14:475–479.

El-Khoury GY, Kathol MH, Daniel WW. Imaging of acute injuries of the cervical spine: value of plain radiography, CT, and MR imaging. *AJR.* 1995;163:43–50.

Felsberg GJ, Tien RD, Osumi AK, et al. Utility of MR imaging in pediatric spinal cord injury. *Pediatr Radiol.* 1995;25:131–135.

Flanders AE, Schaefer DM, Doan HT, Mishkin MM, Gonzalez CF, Northrup BE. Acute cervical spine trauma: correlation of MR imaging findings with degree of neurologic deficit. *Radiology.* 1990;177:25–33.

Forster BB, Koopmans RA. Magnetic resonance imaging of acute trauma of the cervical spine: spectrum of findings. *Canad Assoc Radiol J.* 1995;46:168–173.

Gebarski SS, Maynard FW, Gabrielsen TO, Knake JE, Latack JT. Posttraumatic progressive myelopathy. *Radiology.* 1985;157:379–385.

Gundry DR, Heithoff KB. Epidural hematoma of the lumbar spine: 18 surgically confirmed cases. *Radiology.* 1993;187:427.

Hackney DB, Asato R, Joseph PM, et al. Hemorrhage and edema in acute spinal cord compression: demonstration by MR imaging. *Radiology.* 1986;161:387–390.

Hackney DB, Ford JC, Markowitz RS, et al. Experimental spinal cord injury: imaging the acute lesion. *AJNR.* 1994;15:960.

Harris JH Jr, Burke JT, Ray RD, et al. Low (type III) odontoid fracture: a new radiographic sign. *Radiology.* 1984;153:353–356.

Ito M, Ohki M, Hayashi K, Yamada M, Uetani M, Nakamura T. Trabecular texture analysis of CT images in the relationship with spinal fracture. *Radiology.* 1995;194:55.

Kang JD, Figgie MP, Bohlman HH. Sagittal measurements of the cervical spine in subaxial fractures and dislocations: analysis of two hundred and eighty-eight patients with and without neurological deficits (ab). *Radiololgy.* 1995;195:885.

Kerslake RW, Jaspan T, Worthington BS. Magnetic resonance imaging of spinal trauma. *Br J Radiol.* 1991;64:386–402.

Lee RR. MR imaging and cervical spine injury. *Radiology.* 1996;201:617.

Lövblad K-O, Baumgartner RW, Zambaz B-D, et al. Nontraumatic spinal epidural hernatomas: MR features. *Acta Radiol.* 1997;38:8–13.

McConnell CT Jr, Wippold FJ II, West OC, et al. "Open" exit foramen: new sign of unilateral interfacetal dislocation or subluxation in the lower cervical spine. *Emergency Radiol.* 1995;2:296.

McGrory BJ, Klassen RA, Chao EYS, et al. Acute fractures and dislocations of the cervical spine in children and adolescents (ab). *Radiology.* 1994;191:296.

Mirvis SE, Geisler FH, Jelinek JJ, Joslyn JN, Gellad F. Acute cervical spine trauma: evaluation with 1.5T MR imaging. *Radiology.* 1988;166:807–816.

Murphy MD, Batnitzky S, Bramble JM. Diagnostic imaging of spinal trauma. *Radiol Clin North Am.* 1989;27:855–872.

Noguchi K, Ogawa T, Inugami A, et al. Acute subarachnoid hemorrhage: MR imaging with fluid-attenuated inversion recovery pulse sequences. *Radiology.* 1995;196:773–777.

Nuñez DB Jr, Zuluaga A, Fuentes-Bernardo DA, Rivas LA, Becerra JL. Cervical spine trauma: how much more do we learn by routinely using helical CT? *RadioGraphics.* 1996;16:1307–1321.

Nussbaum ES, Sebring LA, Wolf AL, et al. Myelographic and enhanced computed tomographic appearance of acute traumatic spinal cord avulsion. *Neurosurg.* 1992;30:43–48.

Orrison WW Jr, Benzel EC, Willis BK, et al. Magnetic resonance imaging evaluation of acute spine trauma. *Emergency Radiol.* 1995;2:120.

Penning L. Prevertebral hematoma in cervical spine injury: incidence and etiologic significance. *AJNR.* 1980;1:557–565.

Petersilge CA, Lewin JS, Duerk JL, et al. Optimizing imaging parameters for MR evaluation of the spine with titanium pedicle screws. *AJR.* 1996;166:1213–1218.

Petersilge CA, Pathria MN, Emery SE, Masaryk TJ. Thoracolumbar burst fractures: evaluation with MR imaging. *Radiology.* 1995;194:49–54.

Post MJD, Becerra JL, Madsen PA, et al. Acute spinal subdural hematoma: MR and CT findings with pathologic correlates. *AJNR.* 1994;15:1895.

Quencer RM, Bunge Egnor M, Green BA, Puckett WR, Post MJD. Acute traumatic central cord syndrome: MRI-pathological correlation. *Neuroradiol.* 1992;34:85–94.

Reany SM, Parker MS, Mirvis SE, et al. Abdominal aortic injury associated with transverse lumbar spine fracture–imaging findings. *Clin Radiol.* 1995;50:834–838.

Reid AB, Letts RM, Black GB. Pediatric Chance fractures: association with intraabdominal injuries and seat belt use. *Trauma.* 1990;30:384–391.

Shanmuganathan K, Mirvis SE, Levine AM. Traumatic isolation of the cervical pillar: imaginary observations in 21 patients. *AJR.* 1996;166:897–902.

Stevens, Olney JF, Kendall BE. Post-traumatic cystic and non-cystic myelopathy. *Neuroradiol.* 1985;27:48–56.

Terae S, Takahashi C, Abe S, et al. Gd-DPTA-enhanced MR imaging of injured spinal cord. *Clin Imag.* 1997;21:82–89.

Terk MR, Hume-Neal M, Fraipont M, et al. Injury of the posterior ligament complex in patients with acute spinal trauma: evaluation by MR imaging. *AJR.* 1997;168:1481–1486.

Wallace SK, Cohen WA, Stern EJ, Reav DT. Judicial hanging: postmortem radiographic, CT, and MR imaging features with autopsy confirmation. *Radiology.* 1994;193:263.

Wasenko JJ, Hochhauser L, Holsapple JW, et al. MR of posttraumatic spinal cord lesions: unexpected improvement of hemorrhagic lesions. *Clin Imag.* 1997;21:246–251.

Weingardt JP, Rogers LF. Bilateral locked facets of the cervical spine: correlation between associated fractures and neurologic outcome. *Emergency Radiol.* 1994;1:172.

Section V

Spine Metastases

SPINE METASTASES

Case 1

Clinical Presentation

The patient is a 40-year-old female with a history of breast cancer diagnosed in 1989 and treated with modified radical mastectomy, chemotherapy and tamoxifen. The patient has subsequently been disease free. She presents with a recent history of low back pain.

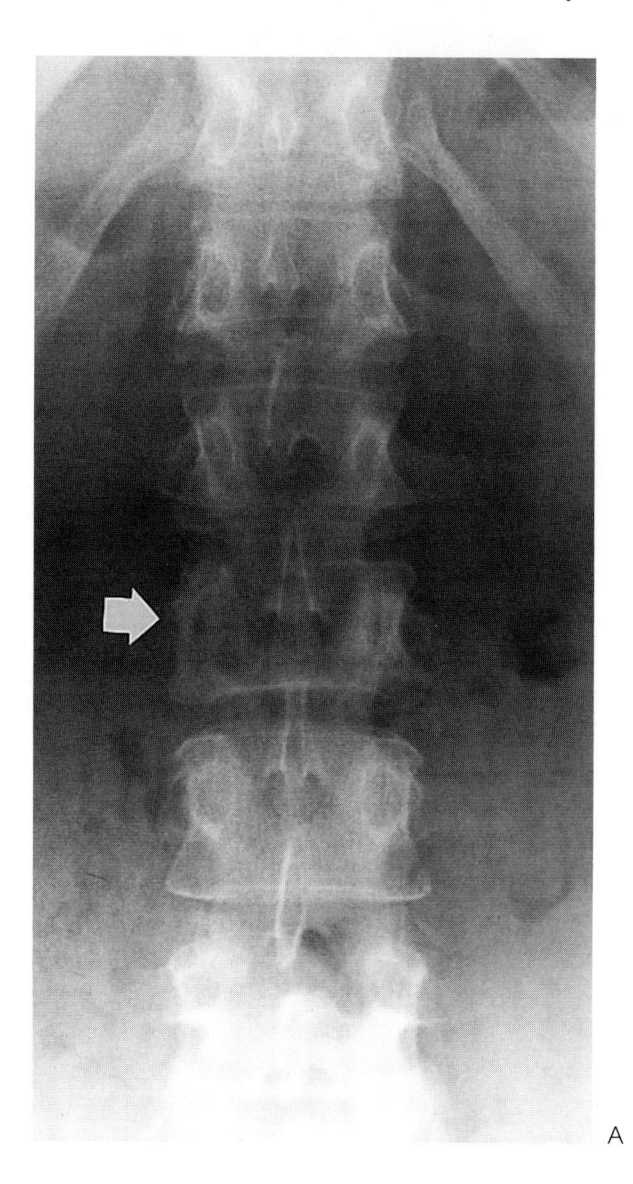

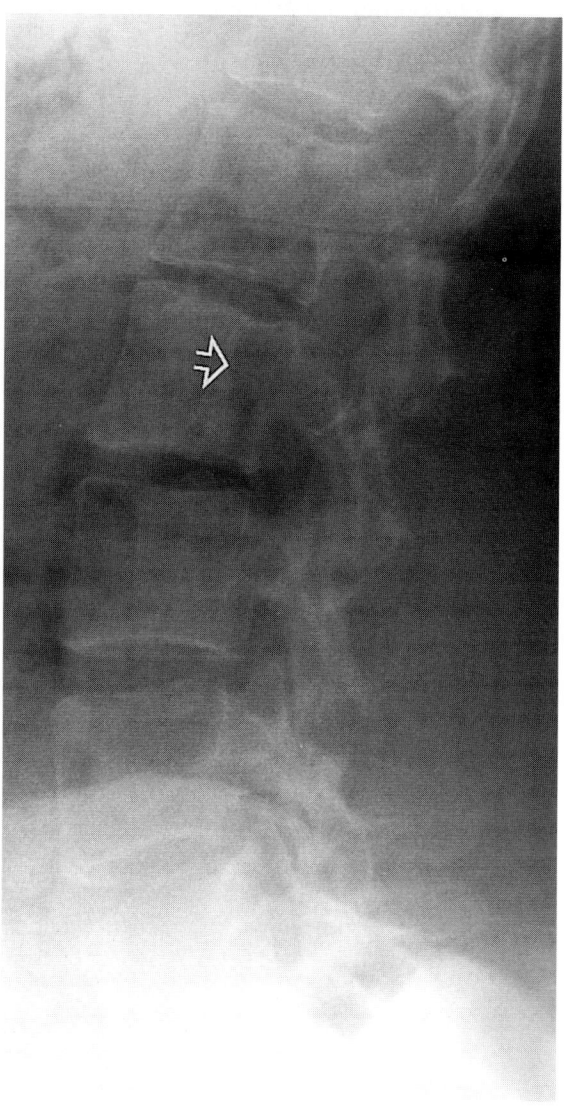

TEACHING ATLAS OF SPINE IMAGING

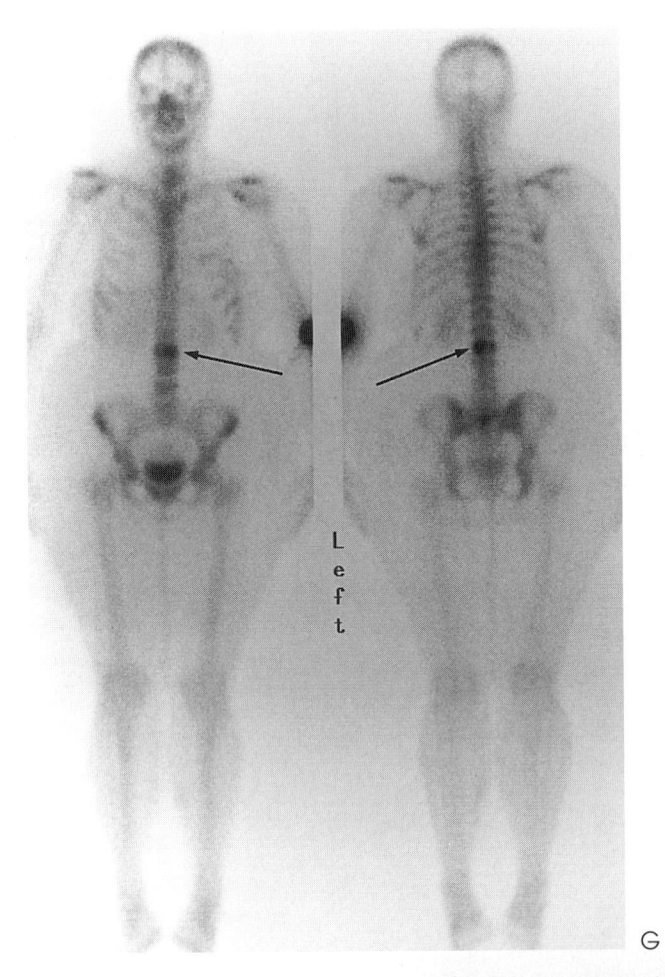

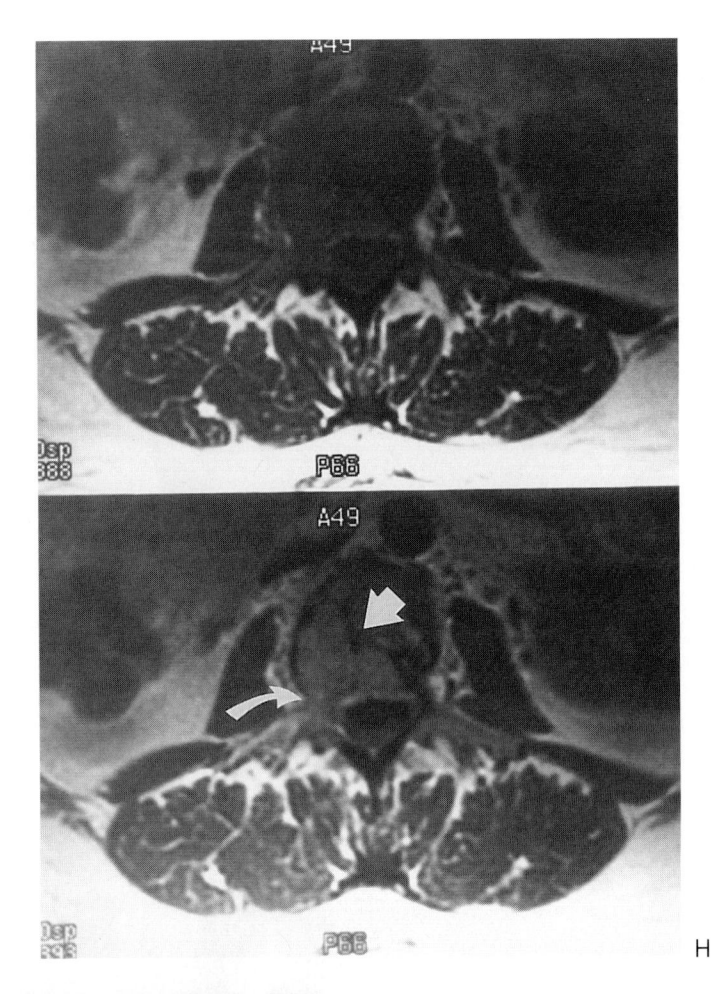

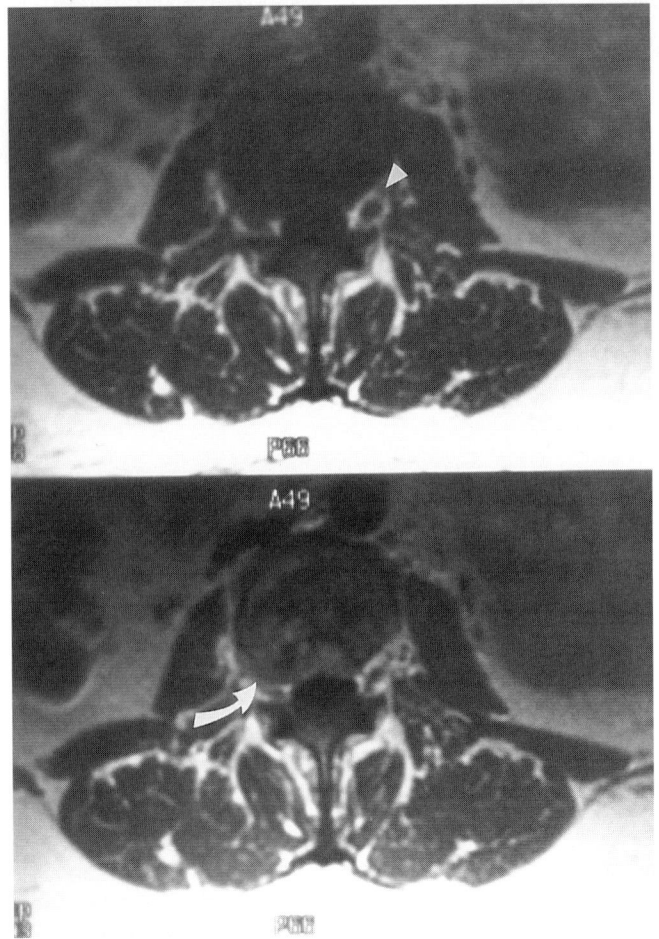

G

H

I

334

SPINE METASTASES

Radiologic Findings

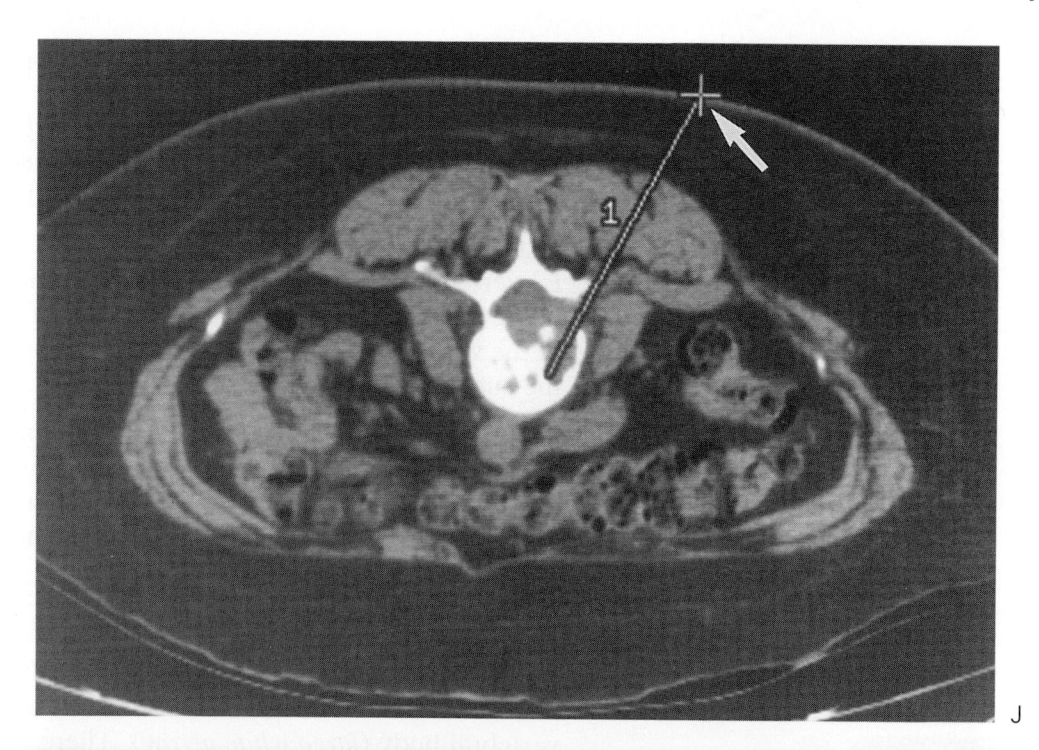

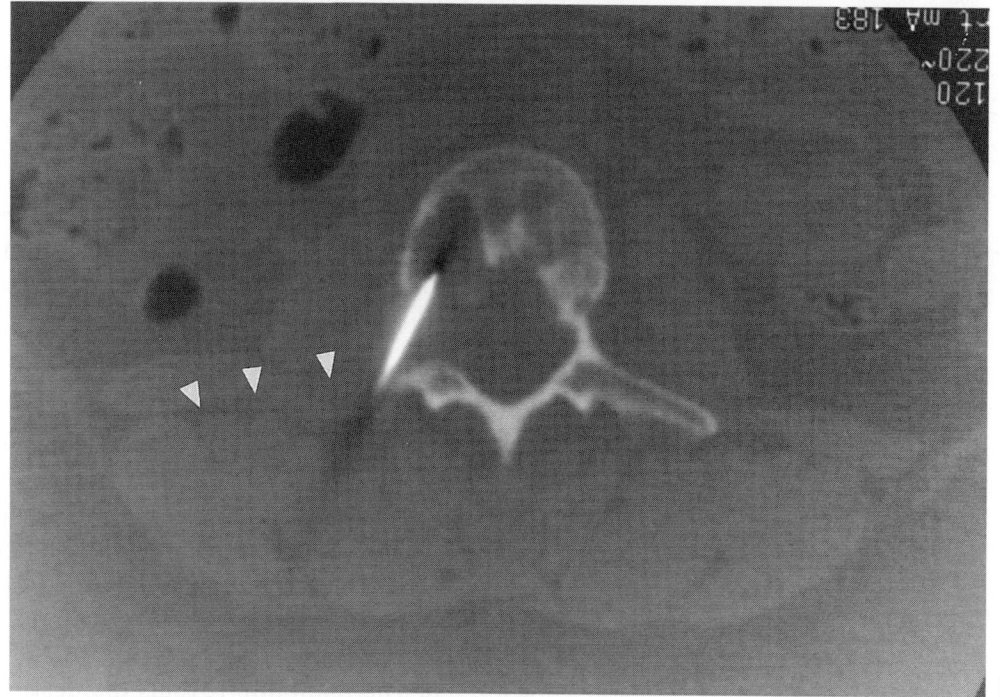

Lateral view of the lumbar spine (Fig. A) reveals that the pedicle on the right side is not seen at the L3 level (*white arrow*). The superior end plate of the L3 vertebral body is indistinct. The remainder of the vertebral bodies are normal.

Sagittal plain film view (Fig. B) reveals that there is a smoothly marginated area of decreased density in the posterior margin of the L3 vertebral body (*open arrow*). This low density extends posteriorly to involve the pedicle at the L3 level.

Radiologic Findings (continued)

Sagittal short TR image of the lumbar spine (Fig. C) reveals that the vertebral body of L3 exhibits diffusely decreased signal intensity. The remaining vertebral bodies appear normal in configuration and signal intensity.

Sagittal postcontrast short TR image (Fig. D) reveals enhancement of the L3 vertebral body. A mild compression fracture appears in the midportion of the L3 vertebral body. There is slight retropulsion of the posterior margin of the vertebral body into the vertebral canal and slight encroachment upon the subarachnoid space.

Sagittal intermediate TR and long TR images (Figs. E and F) reveal an area of higher than normal signal intensity in the posterior portion of the vertebral body of L3 (*white arrows*). There is expansion of the vertebral body and slight encroachment upon the subarachnoid space.

Anterior (Fig. G, *left*) and posterior (Fig. G, *right*) views of a technetium bone scan reveal an area of increased activity in the L3 vertebral body (*arrows*).

Pre- (Fig. H, *top*) and postcontrast (Fig. H, *bottom*) short TR axial images of the L3 vertebral body reveal enhancement of the right side of the L3 vertebral body (*large white arrow*). There is a small soft tissue component that extends beyond the margins of the vertebral body of L3 posteriorly (*curved arrow*) with slight encroachment upon the subarachnoid space anteriorly.

Pre- (Fig. I, *top*) and postcontrast (Fig. I, *bottom*) short TR axial images of the L3 vertebral body reveal enhancement in the posterior and right portion of the L3 vertebral body. There is also enhancement of the pedicle on the right side (*bottom, curved arrow*). The right transverse process also enhances. The dorsal root ganglion is well seen on the left side (*top, arrowhead*).

Clinical Course

Because the patient had no other evidence of disease, we elected to biopsy the L3 vertebral body using computed tomographic (CT) guidance. The distance from the patient's skin (+) to the vertebral body biopsy site is measured (Fig. J). The trajectory of the needle is determined and the bone biopsy needle is advanced into the area of bone destruction (Fig. K). Note that the bone of the transverse process has been destroyed (*white arrowheads*). The pedicle is not visible on the right side because it has been destroyed. The plain film reveals the destroyed pedicle on the right side as seen in Figure A. The biopsy should include the margin of the destroyed bone as well as an aspiration of any material within the central portion of the affected vertebral body.

Diagnosis

Isolated metastatic breast carcinoma to the L3 vertebral body, proved at biopsy.

PEARLS

- Cancer tends to affect the vertebral pedicle early in the course of metastatic spread. Particular attention should be paid to the vertebral pedicle because this may be the only sign of metastases.

- It has been reported that 50% destruction of the vertebral body is required before the destructive changes are apparent on the plain film evaluation.

PITFALLS

- Not all metastatic deposits enhance after contrast injection.

- Not all metastatic deposits appear increased signal intensity on the long TR images.

Differential Diagnosis

- metastatic disease

- multiple myeloma

Discussion

This patient presented with metastatic disease after an 8 year disease-free interval. This is not unusual; patients with metastatic breast cancer may present after a disease-free period of up to 20 years. Therefore, in a patient with new complaints, evaluation MUST be made for possible metastases. Magnetic resonance (MR) imaging is the most accurate method for evaluation of metastases. In general, a postinfusion scan is not necessary in the patient with only bony metastases. However, in the patient with a soft tissue component, the postinfusion MR scan better demonstrates the full extent of the soft tissue component. Metastatic deposits have a random distribution, and their location is not predictable.

The pedicles are a very vascular part of the vertebral body, so hematogenous spread of metastatic disease frequently affects this part of the vertebral body. In addition, this anatomic region is nicely evaluated by plain film evaluation as seen in Figure A, which shows the destruction of the superior end plate of the vertebral body. The changes of metastases, however, are apparent earlier on the MR scan; therefore, MR is the procedure of choice for the evaluation of the presence of metastases. Metastatic deposits replace the normal increased signal intensity fatty bone marrow with decreased signal intensity tumor. The extent and amount of these changes are readily apparent by MR imaging in the majority of cases.

Metastases have a variable response to the long TR sequences. In particular, osteoblastic metastases may appear very low in signal intensity on the various imaging sequences, with a decreased signal intensity appearance similar to cortical bone, while osteolytic metastases may appear as increased signal intensity on the long TR images and are more likely to reveal enhancement on the postcontrast images.

An additional method of evaluation is the use of fat-suppression short TR images after the infusion of contrast material. Using this technique, the fatty bone marrow is suppressed and appears as decreased signal intensity while the tumor enhances.

Metastatic disease is the most likely diagnosis in this patient; however, a primary bone tumor, such as osteogenic carcinoma, could have a similar appearance.

TEACHING ATLAS OF SPINE IMAGING

Case 2

Clinical Presentation

The patient is a 52-year-old female with a history of cervical cancer who now presents with low back pain.

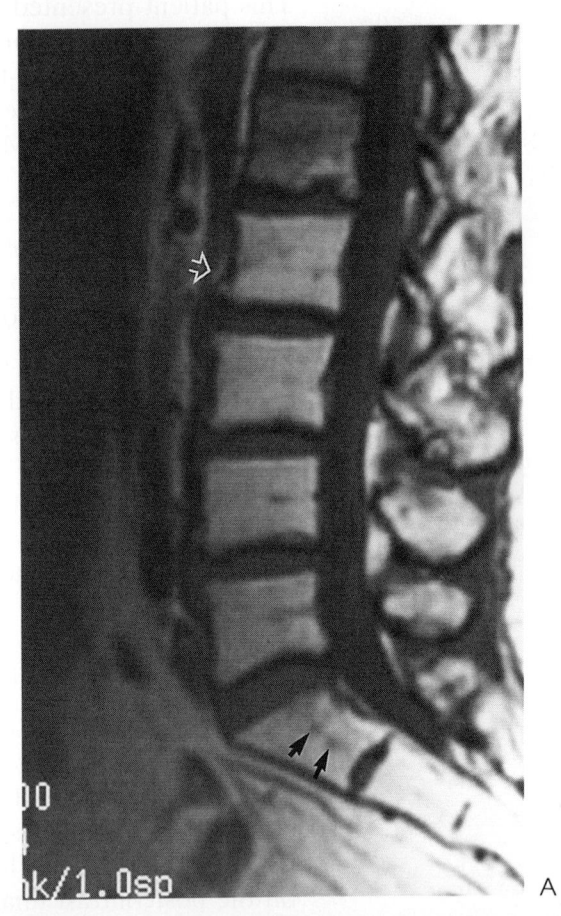

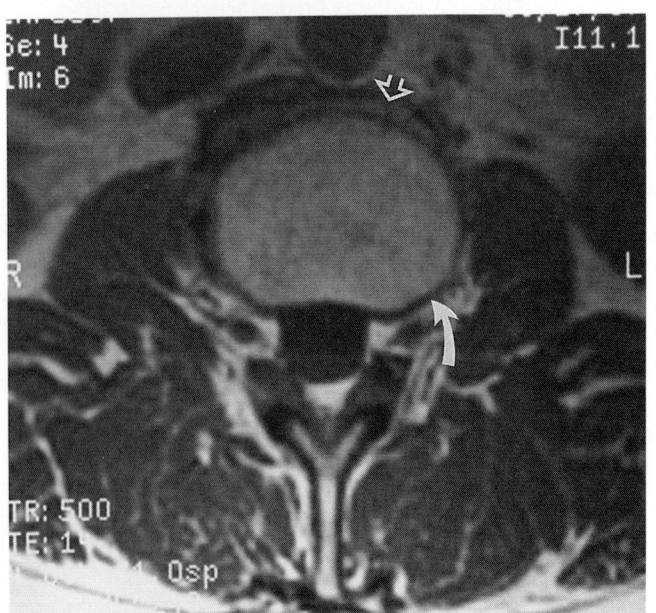

SPINE METASTASES

Radiologic Findings

Sagittal short TR image of the lumbar spine (Fig. A) reveals increased signal intensity within the vertebral bodies beginning at the level of the superior end plate of the L2 and extending through the sacrum. There are anterior osteophytes incidentally noted at the L2-3 level (*open arrow*). There is a Schmorl's node deformity in the inferior end plate of the L1 vertebral body. There are two small, ill-defined areas of decreased signal intensity within the vertebral body of S1 (*solid arrows*).

Axial short TR image at the level of L12 (Fig. B) reveals the anterior osteophyte at the L2 level (*open arrow*). The marrow appears as diffusely increased signal intensity, and this highlights the decreased signal intensity of the peripheral cortical margin of the vertebral body (*curved arrow*).

Diagnosis

Postradiation changes.

Differential Diagnosis

- postradiation changes
- paraspinal mass

Discussion

Clinical history is vital for absolute diagnosis in a case where postradiation changes are suspected. These postradiation changes of increased signal intensity become apparent approximately 4 weeks following radiation and persist indefinitely. Following radiation, there is an increase in the amount of fat within the bone marrow, which results in increased signal intensity on the short TR images. The areas of decreased signal intensity within the vertebral body of S1 are consistent with a "bone bruise" (Fig. A, *solid arrows*). These bone bruises are thought to be caused by internal areas of focal edema within the vertebral body. Compacted trabecular bone may also have a similar appearance.

Evaluation of the paraspinal area should also be performed to rule out a paraspinal mass. The radiated bone is weaker than the normal bone, so compression fractures may occur.

Schmorl's nodes are focal areas of herniation of the intervertebral disc into the vertebral body end plate.

The appearance is typical for postradiation change.

PEARL

- A clinical history of previous radiation is not always given; however, the straight margin of the area of increased signal is consistent with postradiation change and corresponds with the radiation port.

PITFALLS

- Postradiation changes may be more subtle than in this case.
- The postradiation changes may also be seen in association with marrow replacement by decreased signal intensity tumor.

Case 3

Clinical Presentation

The patient is a 65-year-old male with a history of prostate cancer with sudden onset of pain at the T4 level.

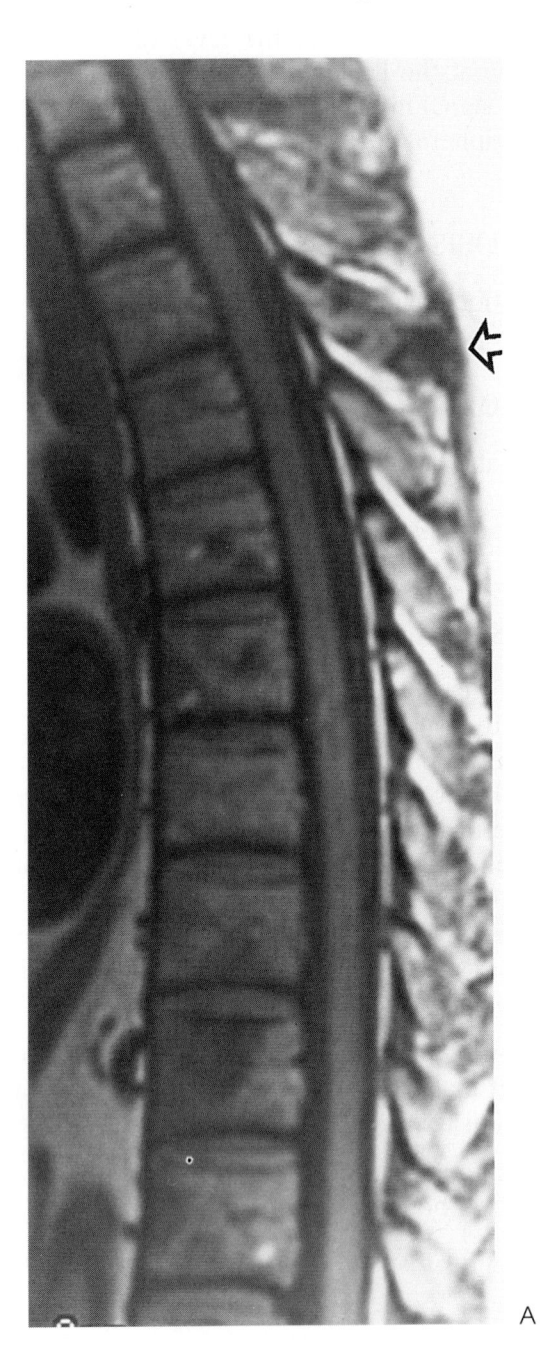

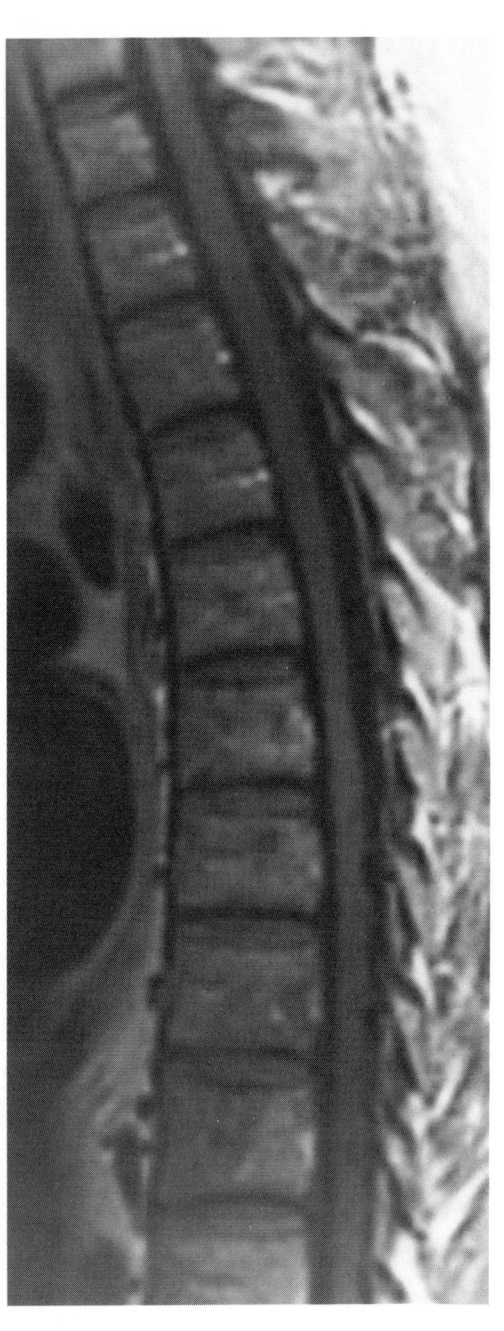

A

B

SPINE METASTASES

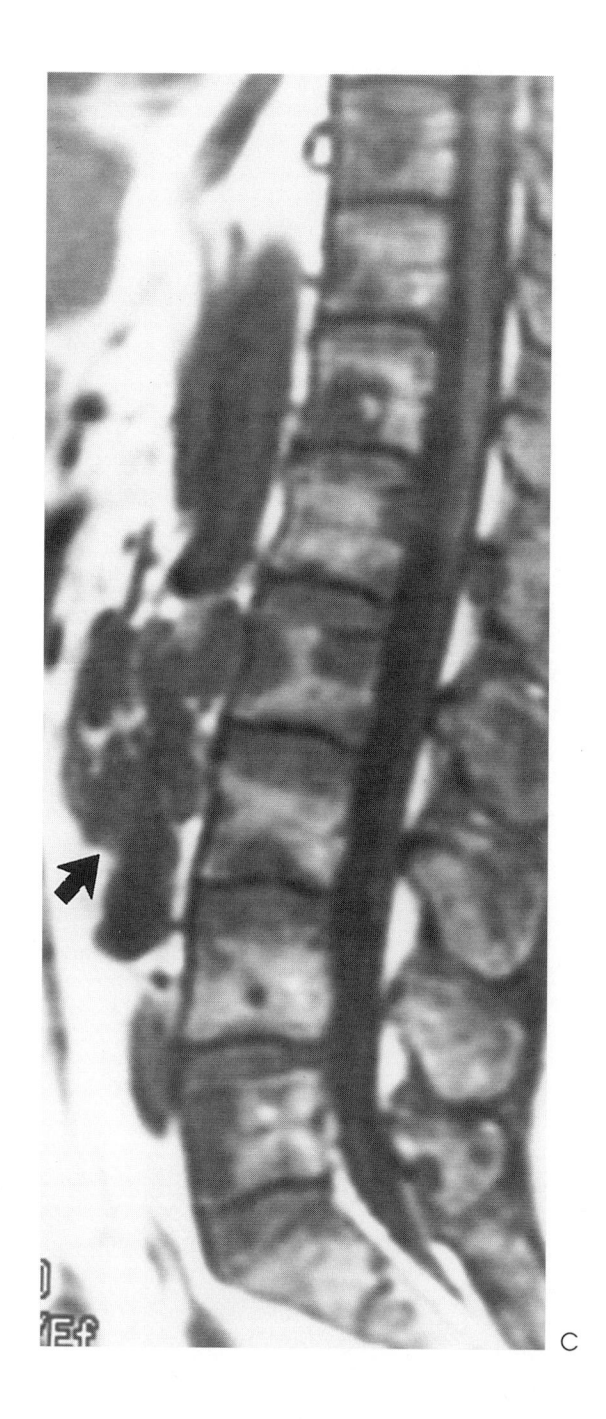

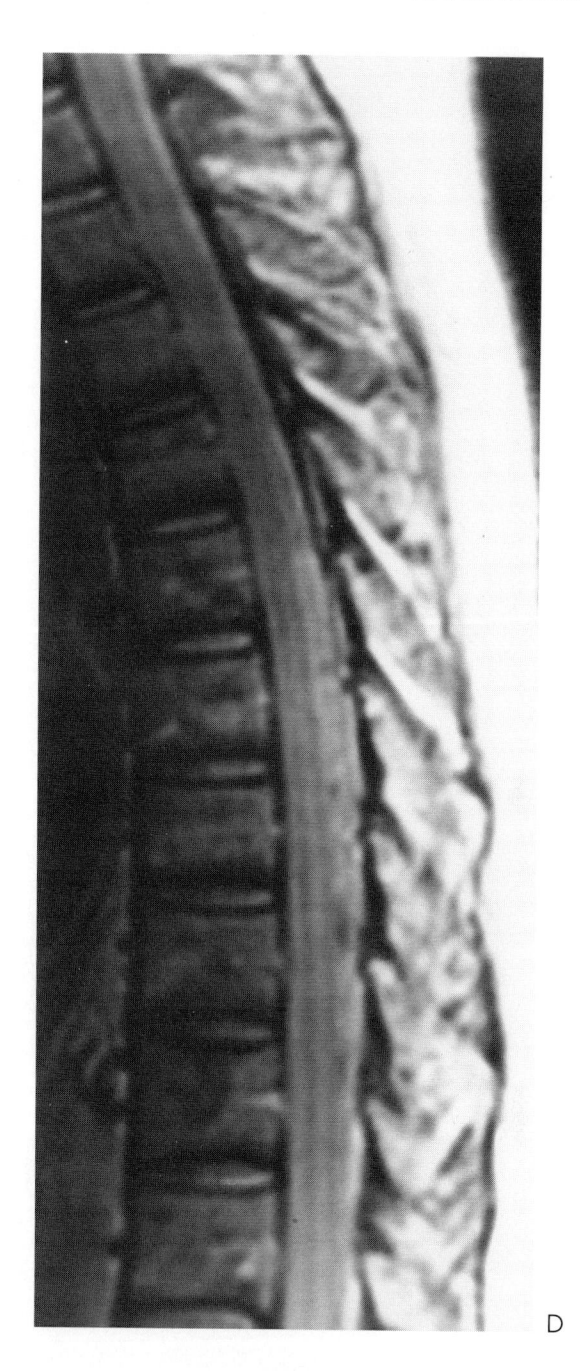

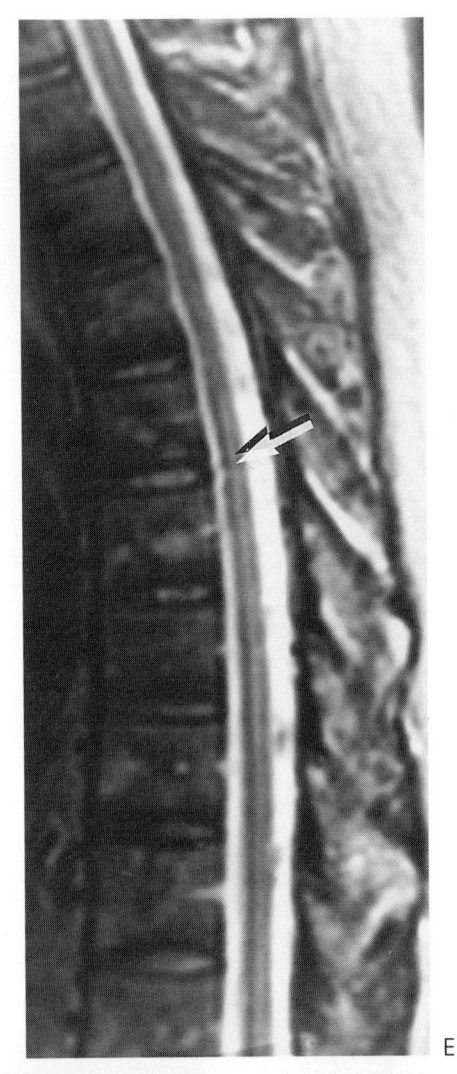

TEACHING ATLAS OF SPINE IMAGING

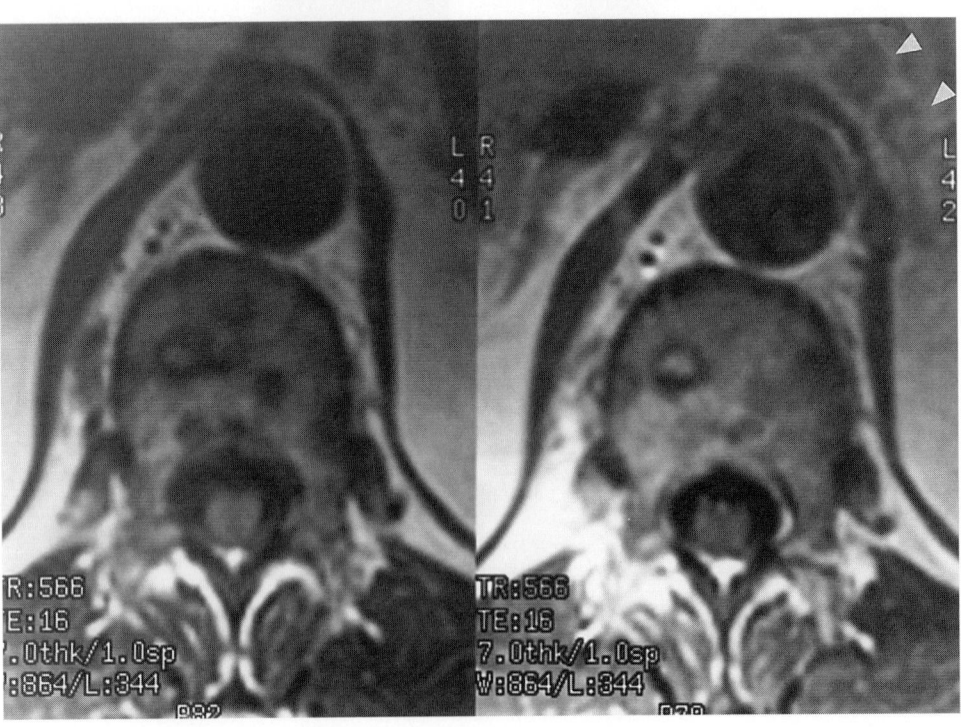

E

F

SPINE METASTASES

Radiologic Findings

Sagittal short TR image of the thoracic spine (Fig. A) reveals multiple rounded and irregularly marginated areas of decreased signal intensity within the vertebral body marrow at multiple levels. There is also decreased signal intensity within the spinous process of one of the upper thoracic vertebral bodies (*open arrow*). The spinal cord is demonstrated throughout its length and appears normal in size and configuration.

Short TR image postcontrast (Fig. B) reveals that there is enhancement and resulting partial obscuration of the multiple lesions demonstrated on the preinfusion scan.

Sagittal short TR image in the lumbar region (Fig. C) reveals multiple areas of decreased signal intensity that involve all of the visualized vertebral bodies. In addition, there are multiple soft tissue masses surrounding the abdominal aorta (*black arrow*).

Sagittal intermediate signal intensity image of the thoracic spine (Fig. D) reveals very faint scattered areas of increased signal intensity but is otherwise unremarkable.

Sagittal long TR image (Fig. E) reveals that the cerebrospinal fluid appears as increased signal intensity, mimicking the appearance of a myelogram. In the central portion of the thoracic spinal cord, there is a very faint line of increased signal intensity (*black and white arrows*). There are a few scattered areas of increased signal intensity within the marrow of several vertebral bodies.

Axial short TR image pre- (Fig. F, *left*) and postinfusion (Fig. F, *right*) reveals multiple areas of decreased signal intensity within the vertebral marrow of one of the upper lumbar vertebral bodies. The postcontrast (*right*) reveals enhancement and resulting obscuration of multiple lesions. Multiple soft tissue masses surround the abdominal aorta (*arrowheads*).

Diagnosis

Metastatic osteoblastic prostate cancer within the bone marrow; multiple para-aortic lymph nodes also show signs of metastatic disease.

Differential Diagnosis

- metastatic prostate cancer

Discussion

Metastatic prostate cancer is osteoblastic in greater than 85% of cases. Metastatic prostate carcinoma frequently exhibits diffuse bony involvement. Lymph node involvement may also be seen. Prostate cancer may be stable for long periods of time and multiyear survival is not uncommon. Many types of tumors may reveal this pattern of metastatic involvement.

PEARL

- The thin increased signal intensity line within the central portion of the thoracic spinal cord seen in Figure E is truncation artifact. The long TR image in the sagittal projection readily demonstrates the thoracic spinal cord and evaluates the presence or absence of spinal cord compression.

PITFALLS

- Postcontrast studies may reveal that the tumor is totally obscured by the enhancement. Therefore, it is important to obtain both pre- and postcontrast studies, and these images should be carefully compared side by side.

- The truncation artifact within the spinal cord may be mistaken for a true abnormality.

TEACHING ATLAS OF SPINE IMAGING

Case 4

Clinical Presentation

The patient is a 47-year-old female with known breast cancer who had previous surgery for spine stabilization.

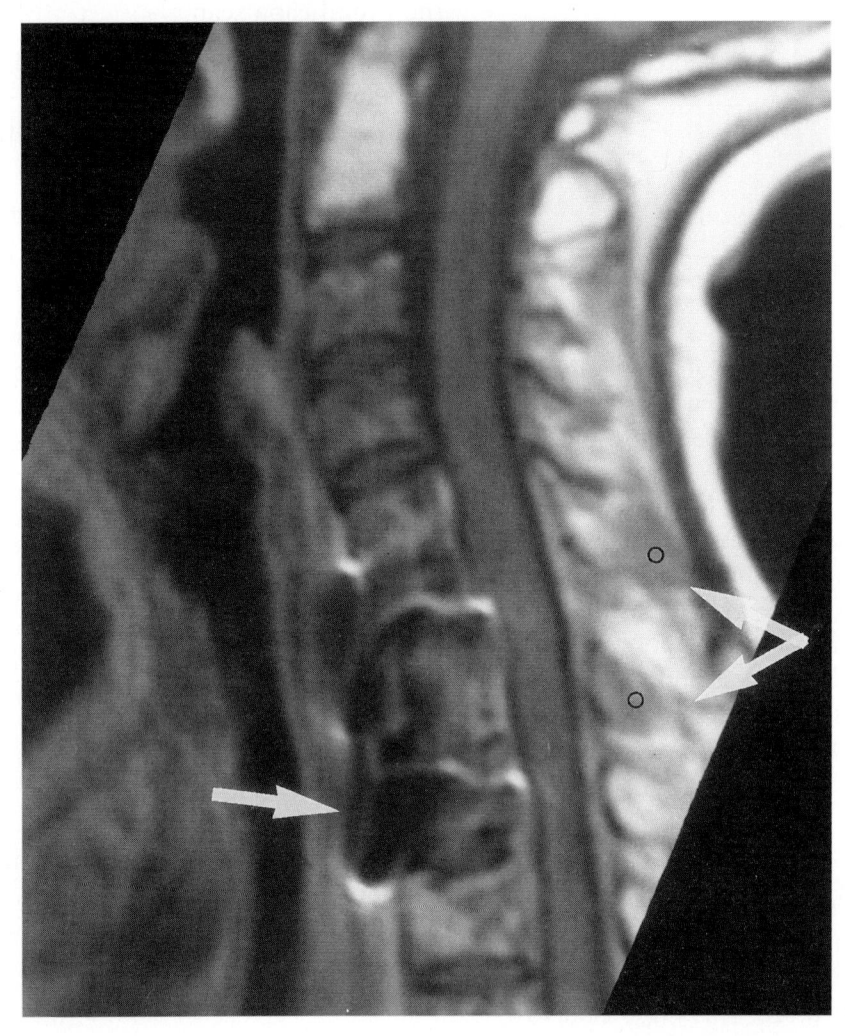

A

Radiologic Findings

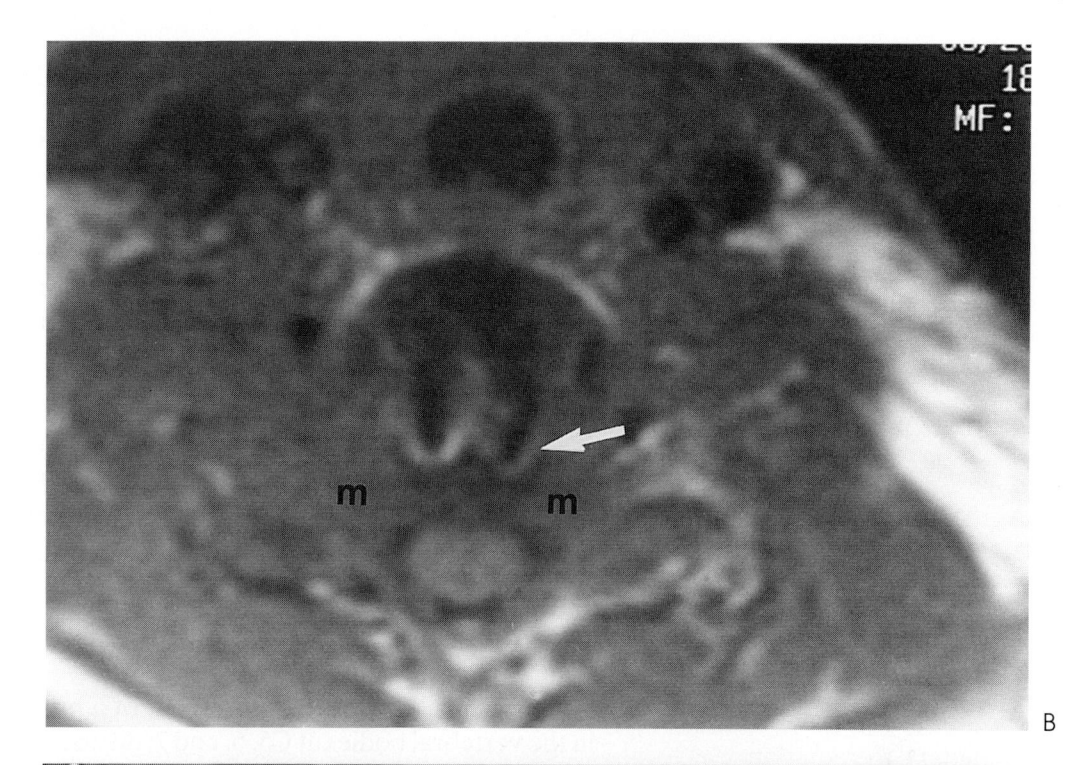

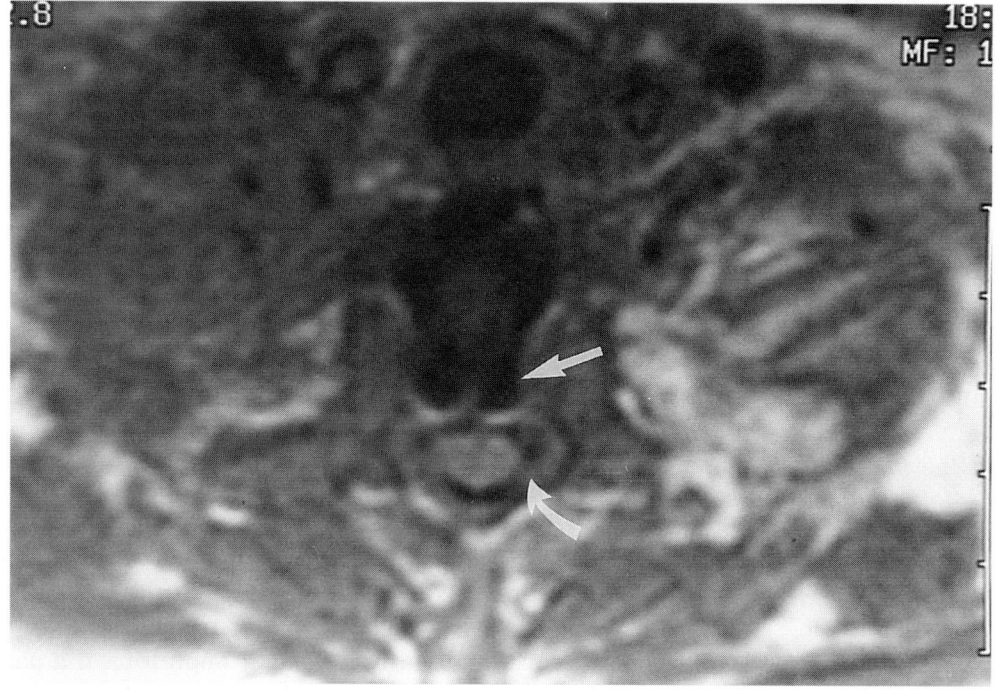

Sagittal short TR image (Fig. A) reveals distortion of the image at the site of the previous surgery at the C5-7 level. There are areas of decreased signal intensity with peripheral areas of curvilinear areas of increased signal intensity (*white arrow*). Although the images are somewhat distorted, forward subluxation of C5 on C6 is visible. The C2 vertebral body and odontoid reveal increased signal intensity, while the remainder of the vertebral bodies appear as diffuse, slightly irregular, decreased signal intensity throughout.

TEACHING ATLAS OF SPINE IMAGING

Radiologic Findings (continued)

The spinous processes of C5 and C6 (*open circles*) exhibit decreased signal intensity, and there is widening of the interspinous distance at the C5-6 level (*double arrow*).

Axial short TR image at the C5 level (Fig. B) reveals oval areas of decreased signal intensity surrounded by curvilinear areas of increased signal intensity in the anticipated area of the vertebral body (*white arrow*). Intermediate signal intensity soft tissue masses are visible in the region of the intervertebral foramen bilaterally (*m*).

Axial short TR images at the level of C7 (Fig. C) reveal intermediate signal intensity soft tissue material surrounding the cervical spinal cord (*curved arrow*). There is a bilobed area of decreased signal intensity in the vertebral body, with a curvilinear halo of increased signal intensity (*white arrow*).

PEARL

- The increased signal intensity within the marrow of C2 is secondary to radiation treatment. In addition, this vertebral body is not involved with decreased signal intensity metastatic disease.

Diagnosis

Postsurgical changes with placement of a metallic plate and multiple screws in the vertebral bodies at C5, 6, and 7; diffuse metastases to multiple vertebral bodies and spinous processes.

Differential Diagnosis

- metastatic disease
- multiple myeloma

PITFALLS

- A wide variety of metallic implants may be scanned without danger. When metallic implants are studied by MR imaging, there is some warming of the implant because of the radiofrequency waves. However, this heat is minor, dissipates rapidly, and does not cause harm to the tissues.

- If adequate demonstration the spinal cord and subarachnoid space are not possible with MR imaging, it may be necessary to perform a myelogram and a postmyelogram computed tomographic (CT) scan for complete evaluation. However, metallic implants also markedly degrade CT images.

Discussion

The widened interspinous distance seen in Figure A is secondary to forward subluxation of C5 on C6 and slight kyphosis at this level.

The metallic plate causes magnetic susceptibility artifact and results in distortion of the images. In spite of this the cervical spinal cord is fairly well demonstrated. The intermediate signal soft tissue masses seen in Figure B represent metastatic disease (*m*). The multiplanar imaging capability of magnetic resonance (MR) frequently allows demonstration of the spinal cord in at least one plane. Therefore, if a patient has metallic wires, plates, or screws, it is generally possible to evaluate the relationship of the spinal cord to the surrounding structures in at least one plane. The short TR images are the least susceptible to magnetic susceptibility artifact, long TR images next most susceptible and gradient echo images the most susceptible to magnetic susceptibility artifact. Because these metallic devices are firmly in place, they will not migrate in the magnetic field.

Metastatic disease is the most likely diagnosis. Multiple myeloma is a diagnostic consideration but is less likely. The MR appearance is typical of the distortion caused by magnetic susceptibility artifact. When in doubt, plain film evaluation will readily evaluate the postsurgical changes.

SPINE METASTASES

Case 5

Clinical Presentation

The patient is a 44-year-old female with a history of an abdominal mass who is status-post–bone marrow transplant with hip pain and leg pain of recent onset.

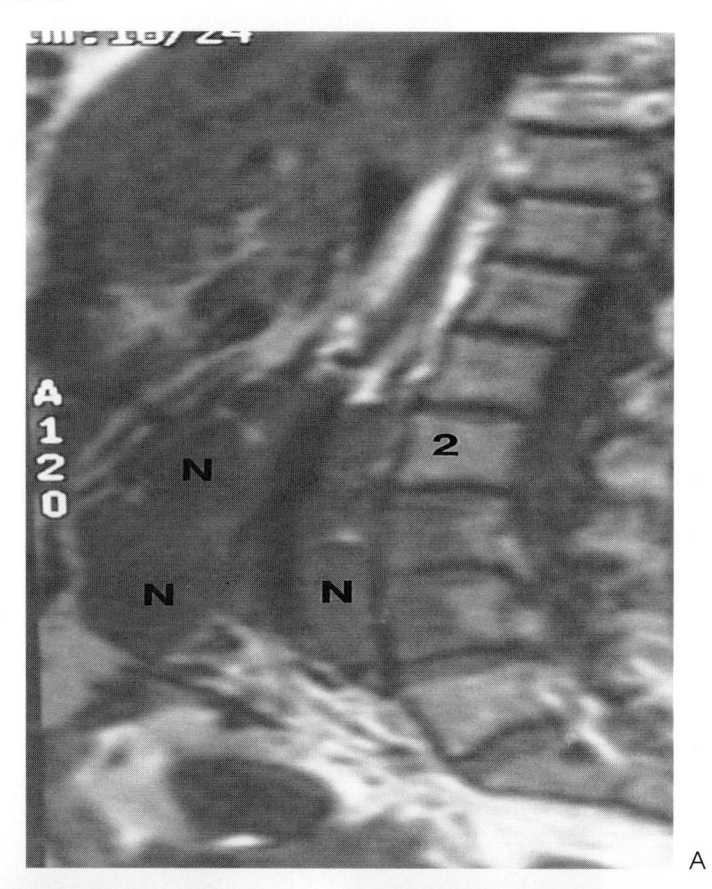

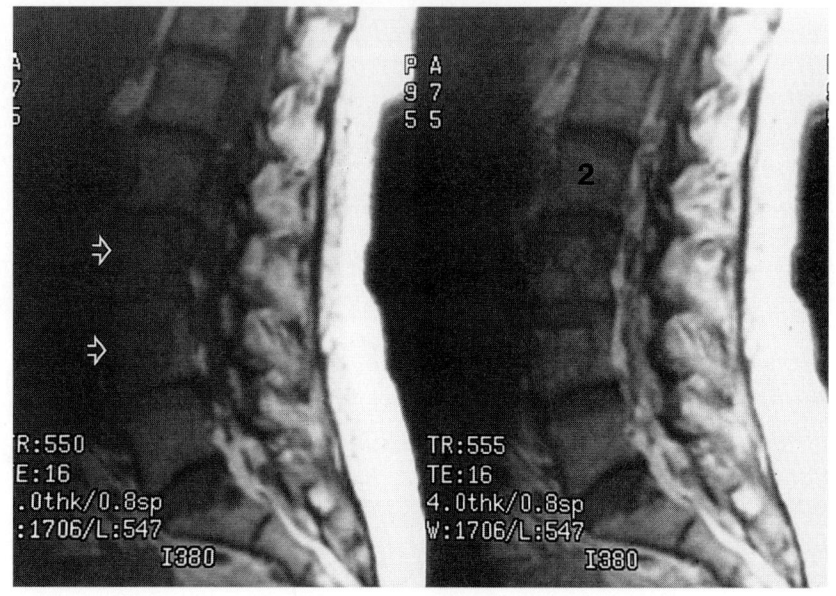

347

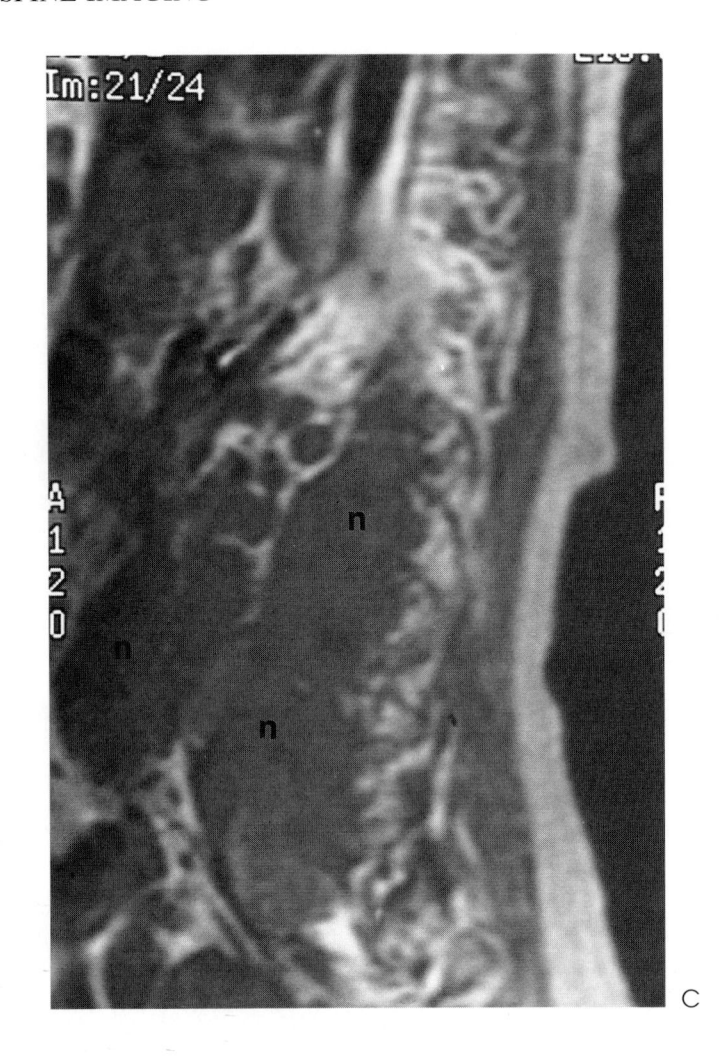

TEACHING ATLAS OF SPINE IMAGING

C

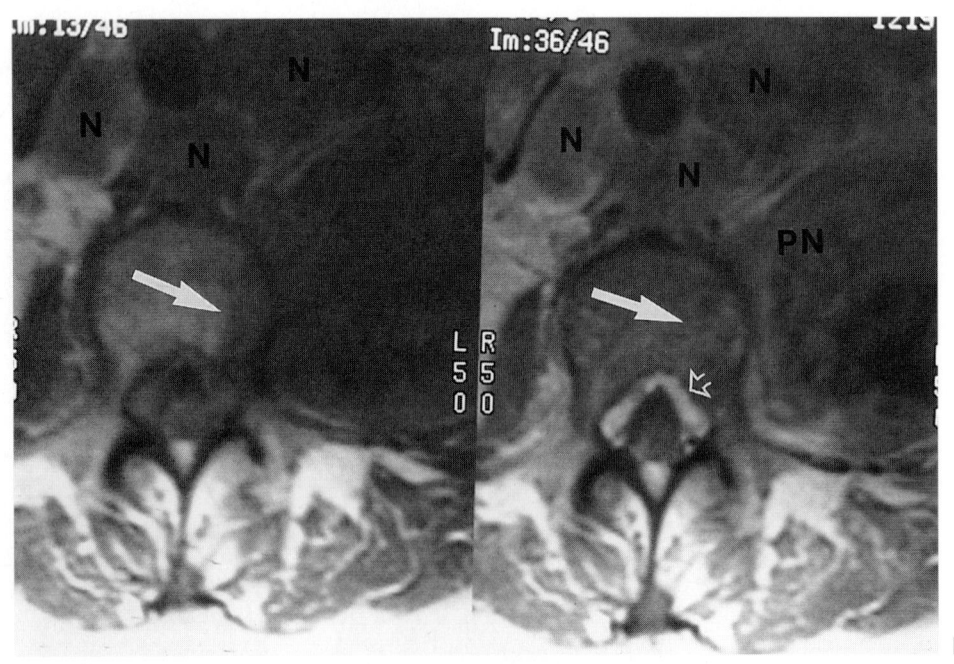

D

SPINE METASTASES

Radiologic Findings

Sagittal short TR image (Fig. A) reveals decreased signal intensity in the anterior half of the L3 and L4 vertebral bodies. In addition, there are multiple oval-shaped areas of soft tissue signal intensity surrounding the flow void of the abdominal aorta (*N*). The abdominal aorta appears as an area of flow void decreased signal intensity that is displaced anteriorly in the lower lumbar region. The L2 vertebral body is identified with 2.

Pre- (Fig. B, *left*) and postcontrast (Fig. B, *right*) sagittal short TR images reveal decreased signal intensity replacing the normal increased signal intensity of the marrow in the anterior three quarters of the vertebral bodies of L3 and L4 (*open arrows*). After the infusion of contrast material (*right*), there is almost complete obscuration of the appearance of the areas of decreased signal intensity. The L2 vertebral body is identified with 2.

Parasagittal short TR image (Fig. C) reveals multiple intermediate signal intensity soft tissue masses lateral to and anterior to the vertebral column (*n*).

Pre- (Fig. D, *left*) and postcontrast (Fig. D, *right*) axial short TR images reveal decreased signal intensity in the far lateral aspect of the vertebral body (*white arrows*). There is a large paraspinal intermediate signal intensity mass in the left paraspinal region as well as multiple rounded soft tissue masses anterior to the spine (*N*). All of these areas enhance after the infusion of contrast material (*right*). Bilateral epidural areas of enhancement anterior to the thecal sac are also visible on the postinfusion scan (*open arrow*).

PEARLS

- The postcontrast image results in an almost normal appearance of the vertebral bodies. For this reason, it is important to perform both pre- and postinfusion studies for complete evaluation.

- Additional history revealed that this patient had a diagnosis of non-Hodgkin's lymphoma.

PITFALL

- At the time of image evaluation, special attention should be paid to the paraspinal and prevertebral areas for the presence of masses or adenopathy.

Diagnosis

Vertebral metastases and multiple pathologically enlarged lymph nodes (*N, n*) secondary to non-Hodgkin's lymphoma.

Differential Diagnosis

- lymphoma
- metastases

Discussion

The appearance of the paraspinal adenopathy is typical of lymphoma. The para-aortic lymph nodes surround the flow void of the abdominal aorta and inferior vena cava. In a patient with neurofibromatosis type 1, this type of adenopathy could be interpreted as plexiform neurofibroma. Therefore, to ensure correct interpretation and diagnosis, it is important to be aware of the clinical history. The para-aortic area should be included in the final images so that the paraspinal region can be evaluated. In general, neurofibromas have a smoother margin and extend into the intervertebral foramen in a "dumbbell" type fashion rather than in a less well defined fashion as we see in this patient.

A variety of metastases, such as from breast, lung, or other soft tissue primary tumors, could cause a similar appearance. Lymphoma may also involve the vertebral bodies in a similar fashion to that illustrated in this case.

TEACHING ATLAS OF SPINE IMAGING

Case 6

Clinical Presentation

The patient is 78-year-old male with known prostate cancer who now presents with severe back pain.

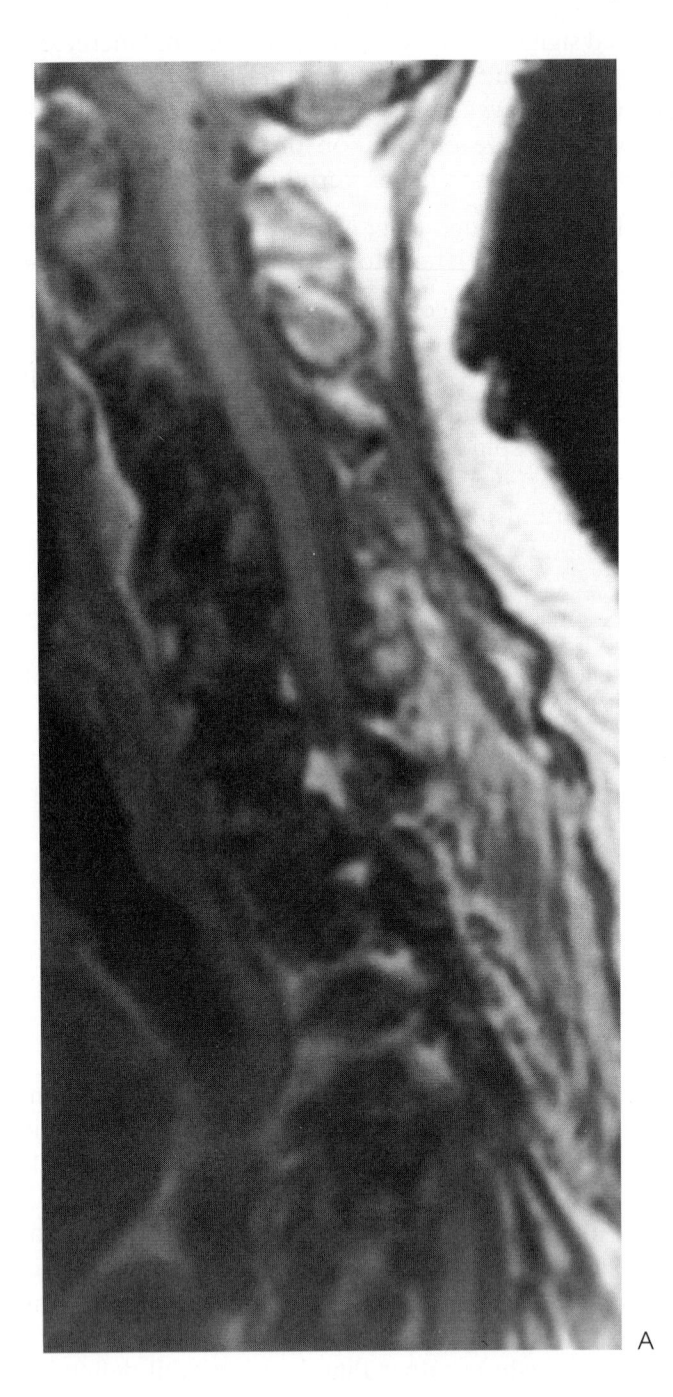

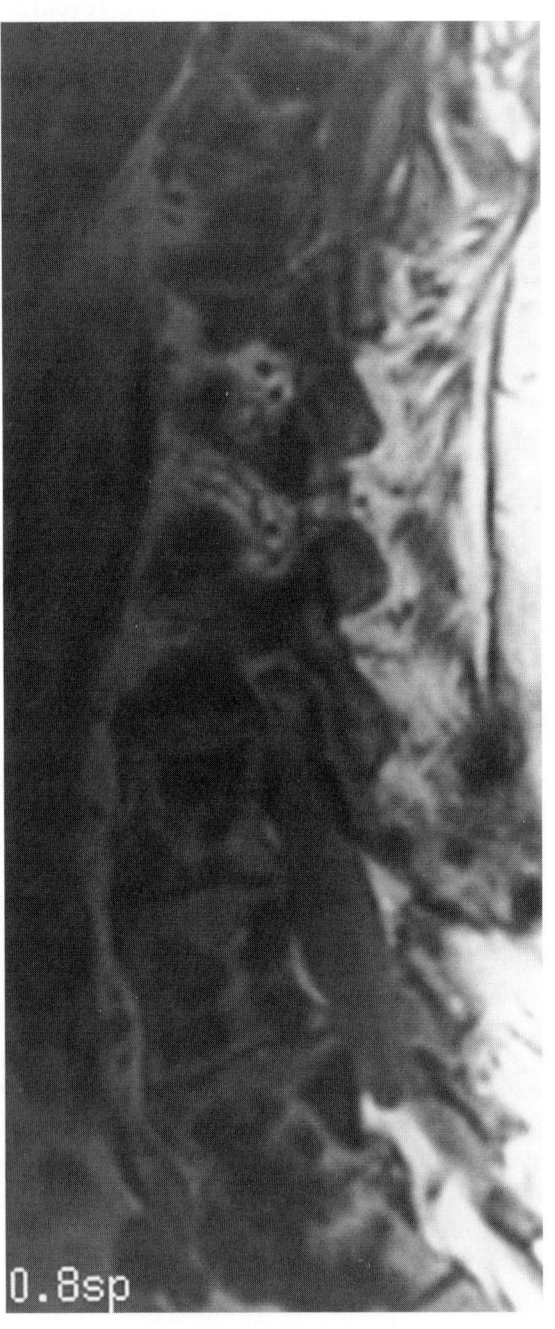

SPINE METASTASES

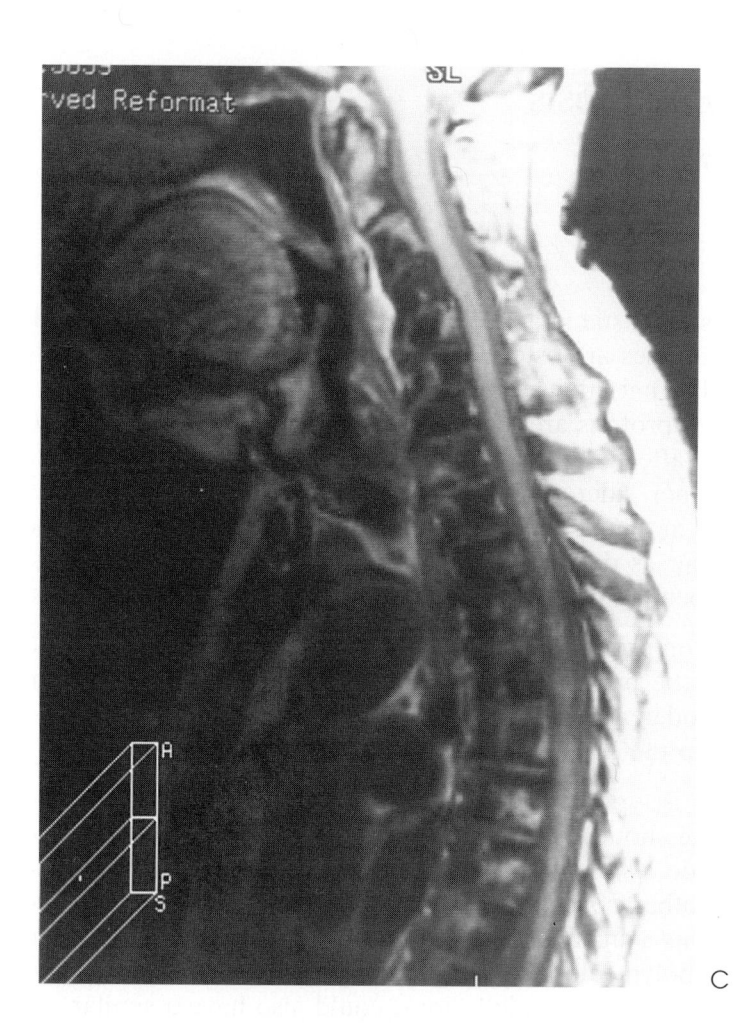

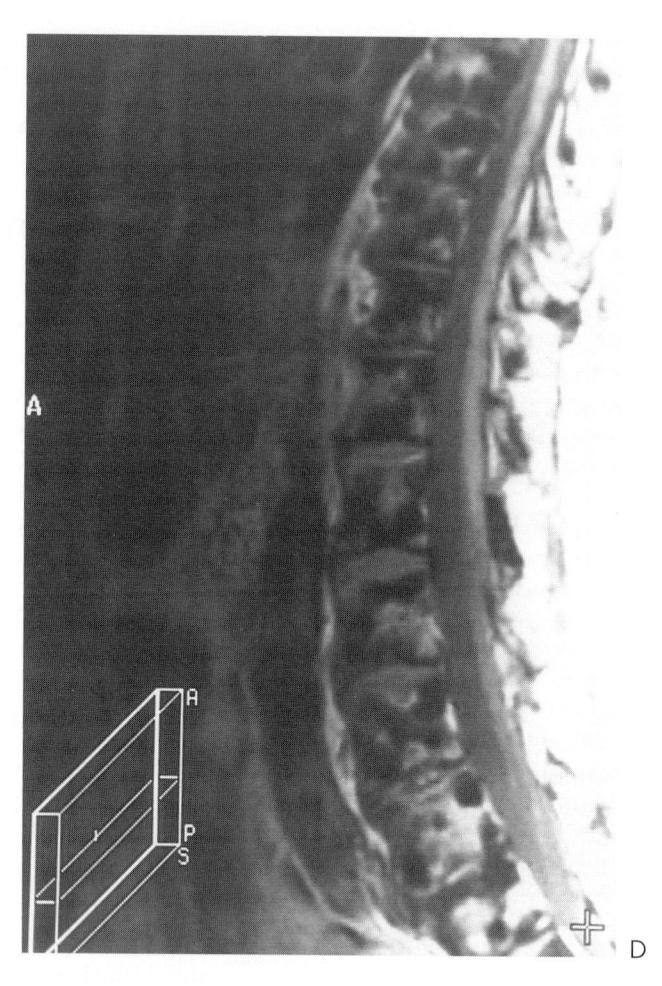

Radiologic Findings

Sagittal short TR image in the cervical and upper thoracic region (Fig. A) reveals that there is a marked scoliosis, and the spinal cord can be visualized in only a portion of its length. All the visualized vertebral bodies are involved with multiple, variable sized lesions that exhibit marked decreased signal intensity. There is reversal of the normal lordotic curve in the cervical region.

Sagittal short TR image in the lumbar region (Fig. B) reveals that the vertebral bodies are involved with variable sized rounded and irregularly shaped areas of markedly decreased signal intensity. The lumbar thecal sac is only seen in the lower lumbar region because of a scoliosis of the spine.

Sagittal short TR images following the use of a computer generated program that allows the images to be corrected for the presence of a scoliosis (Figs. C and D) reveals that the spinal cord is now demonstrable in its entirety.

Diagnosis

Diffuse metastases secondary to innumerable osteoblastic lesions related to the prostate cancer.

Differential Diagnosis

- osteoblastic metastases

Discussion

Prostate cancer is osteoblastic in approximately 85–90% of cases, although the remainder of the cases are osteolytic. Osteoblastic metastatic deposits remain as decreased signal intensity on all imaging sequences. This occurs because the hydrogen protons are locked in the crystal lattice of the bone matrix and cannot be affected by the radiofrequency waves of the magnetic resonance (MR) scanner. Therefore, they do not return a signal and appear markedly decreased in signal intensity. In general, osteolytic metastatic deposits, which appear as decreased signal intensity on short TR images, are more likely to appear as increased signal intensity on the long TR images.

The scoliosis correction program or curve reformat program is very helpful in the evaluation of the presence or absence of spinal cord compression. The use of this method generally allows the visualization of the spinal cord and its relationship to the surrounding bony structures.

The MR appearance is typical for osteoblastic metastases. Therefore, the greatest consideration should be for those primary tumors that will cause metastatic osteoblastic lesions, the most common of which is metastatic prostate cancer. Another consideration would be osteoblastic metastatic breast cancer, even in a male patient. Multiple myeloma in the clinical setting of POEMS (polymyelopathy, organomegaly, endocrinopathy, and myeloma), which causes osteoblastic lesions, could also have a similar appearance.

PEARL
- The use of a reformatting technique should be used for complete evaluation of the vertebral canal and to evaluate for cord compression.

PITFALL
- If a reformatting program is not available, it may be necessary to perform multiplanar imaging, including the coronal plane, for complete evaluation of the presence or absence of cord compression or compromise of the vertebral canal. In some cases, it may be necessary to perform a myelogram for complete evaluation.

SPINE METASTASES

Case 7

Clinical Presentation

The patient is a 43-year-old female with stage 1b uterine adenocarcinoma. The patient is status-post chemotherapy and radiation therapy to the pelvis and now presents with severe upper thoracic pain and paraplegia.

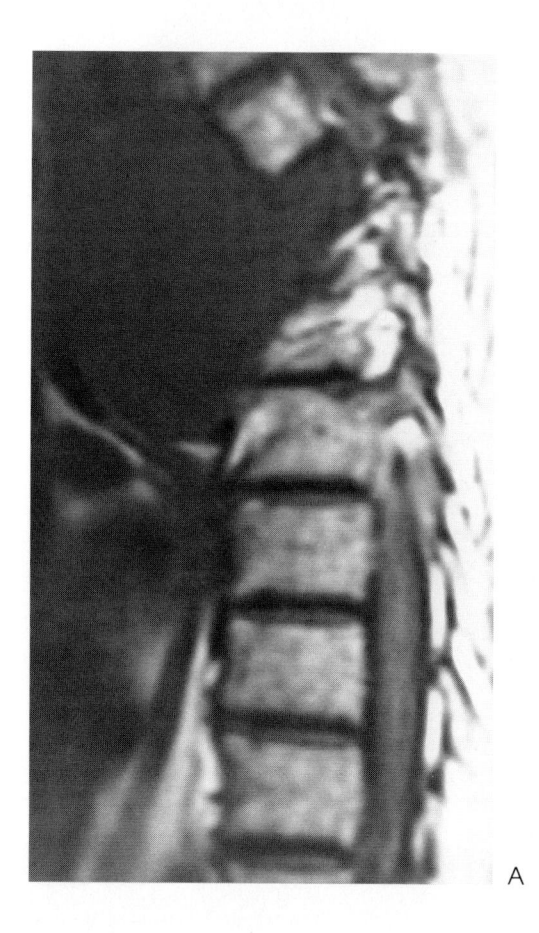

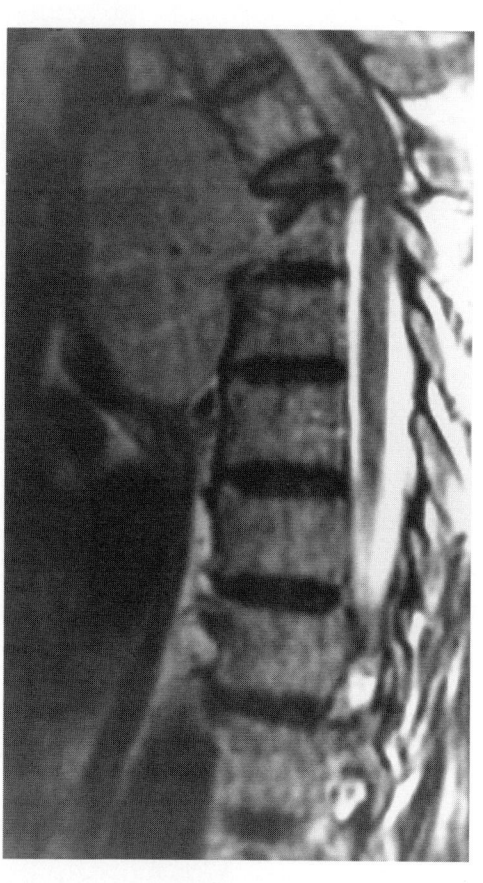

TEACHING ATLAS OF SPINE IMAGING

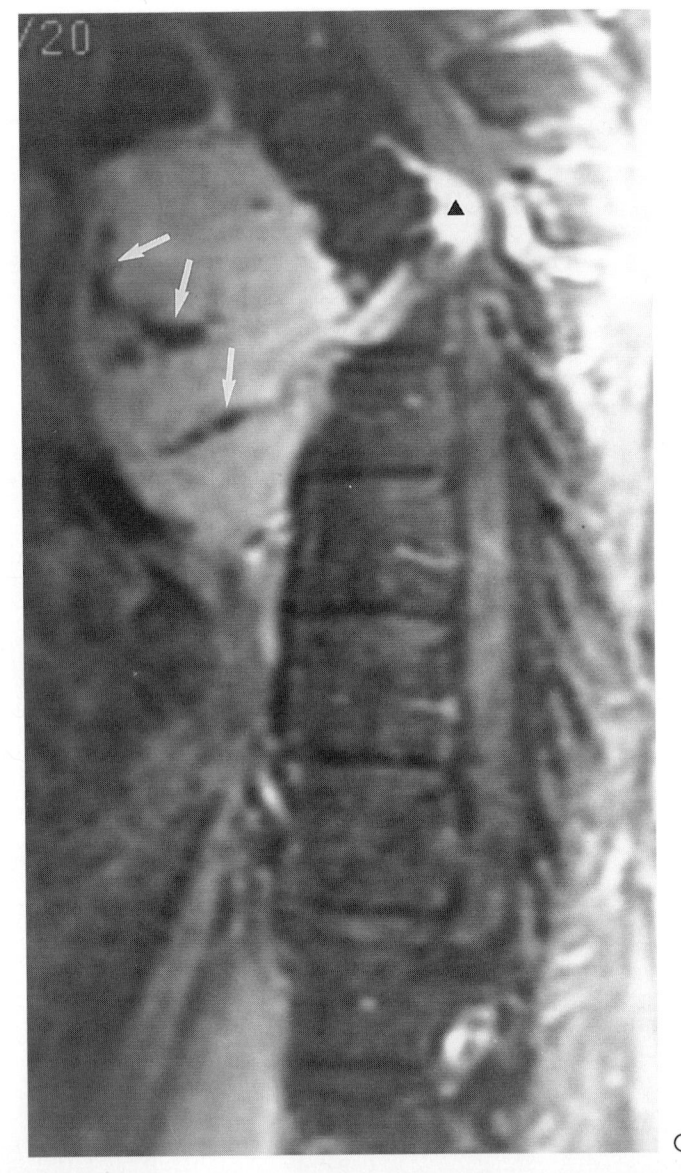

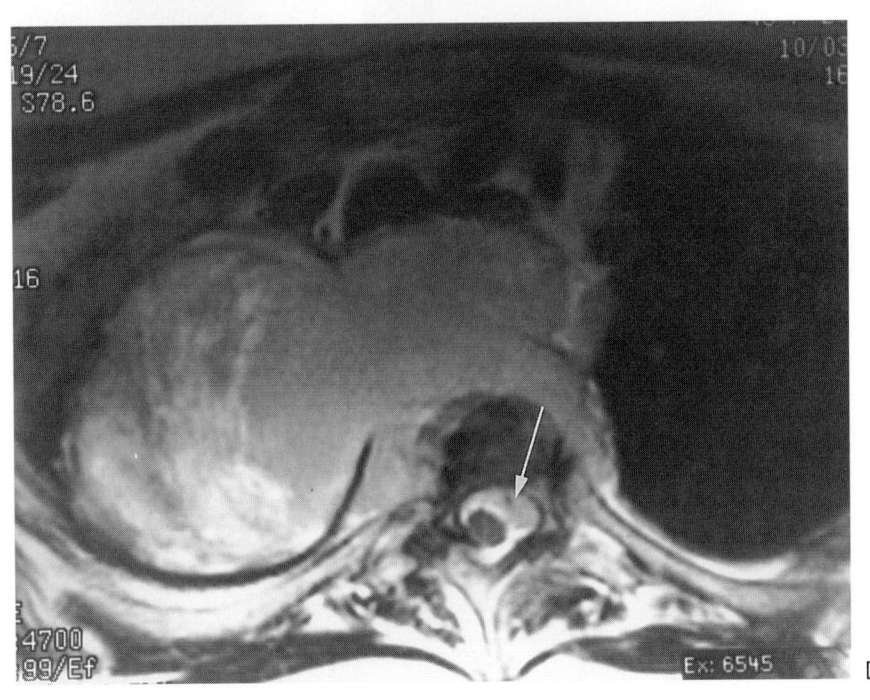

C

D

354

Radiologic Findings

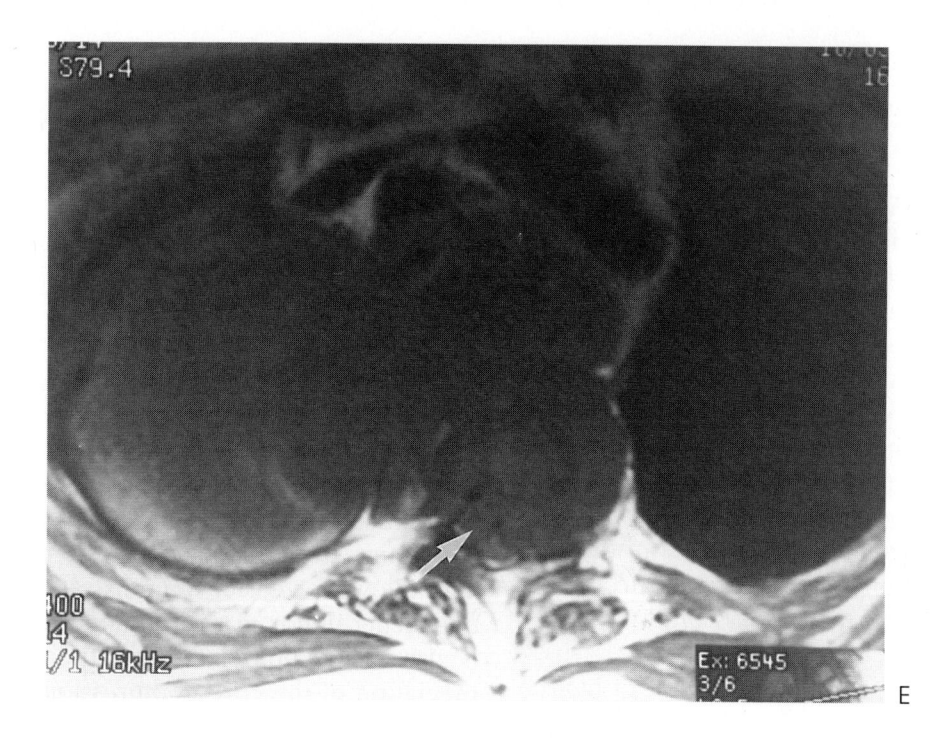

Sagittal short TR image (Fig. A) reveals a large tissue mass in the prevertebral area at the T3 level. There is marked accentuation of the thoracic kyphosis at this level, as well as anterior compression fracture of the T4 vertebral body and erosion of the anterior superior corner of the T5 vertebral body.

Sagittal long TR image (Fig. B) reveals that the mass appears slightly increased in signal intensity with some faint internal areas of decreased signal intensity. The spinal cord is displaced posteriorly. The T3 vertebral body is completely absent; this is at the level of the marked kyphosis.

Sagittal fat-suppressed image postcontrast (Fig. C) reveals that the mass enhances densely. There are curvilinear areas of internal decreased signal intensity (*arrows*). There is a streak-like area of increased signal intensity that extends into the vertebral column at the level of T3 and into the vertebral canal. The area of enhancement is in the vertebral canal and displaces the spinal cord posteriorly (*arrowhead*).

Axial short TR image precontrast (Fig. D) reveals a very large right paraspinal mass. The mass extends anterior to the vertebral column and surrounds the vertebral body at the T3 level. The mass extends into the vertebral canal from the left side (see Fig. E) where it obliterates the normal increased signal intensity fat in the intervertebral foramen and displaces the spinal cord (*arrow*) to the right.

Axial short TR image postcontrast (Fig. E) reveals inhomogeneous enhancement of the paraspinal and prevertebral component of the mass. The soft tissue component extending into the vertebral canal enhances and can be seen on the left side (*arrow*). The normal epidural fat is obliterated by the mass.

TEACHING ATLAS OF SPINE IMAGING

PEARL
- Note that in this patient the cerebrospinal fluid below the level of the cord compression in Figure C appears markedly increased in signal intensity. The cerebrospinal fluid above the level of the block appears relatively decreased in signal intensity. There are two reasons for this. The first is the fact that the cerebrospinal fluid below the level of the block contains an increased protein content. It contains an increase in the number of hydrogen protons and therefore is brighter. The second is that there is transmitted pulsation of heart beat and respiration, which results in motion of the cerebrospinal fluid above the level of the block. This motion causes the cerebrospinal fluid to appear decreased signal intensity.

PITFALLS
- In any patient with metastatic disease, the entire length of the vertebral column should be evaluated.

- When there is a marked compression fracture or extensive bony destructive change that completely destroys a vertebral body, the absence of this vertebral body may be difficult to appreciate. The only abnormality may be accentuation of the dorsal kyphosis.

Diagnosis

Metastatic adenocarcinoma with bone destruction and spinal cord compression.

Differential Diagnosis

- metastatic disease

Discussion

This type of metastatic deposit is unusual in a patient with uterine cancer. The fat-suppressed technique results in a low signal intensity of the fat containing structures, such as the normally high fat content bone marrow. This allows for easier demonstration of areas of enhancement such as the enhancing tumor in this patient. The presence of spinal cord compression is also easily appreciated. Multiplanar imaging allows for much easier appreciation of the cord compression.

Fat is an excellent intrinsic contrast material in magnetic resonance imaging; therefore, evaluation of the interruption or obliteration of this fat signal intensity is very helpful in evaluation of the changes that can be seen with metastatic disease.

Lung cancer would be a more likely tumor to result in this appearance. Other tumors, such as osteogenic sarcoma or even Ewing's sarcoma in a younger patient, could also have this appearance. Remotely, multiple myeloma might also have a similar appearance although the large soft tissue component would be unlikely.

SPINE METASTASES

Case 8

Clinical Presentation

The patient is a 51-year-old female with known breast cancer who now presents with neck pain and left upper extremity weakness.

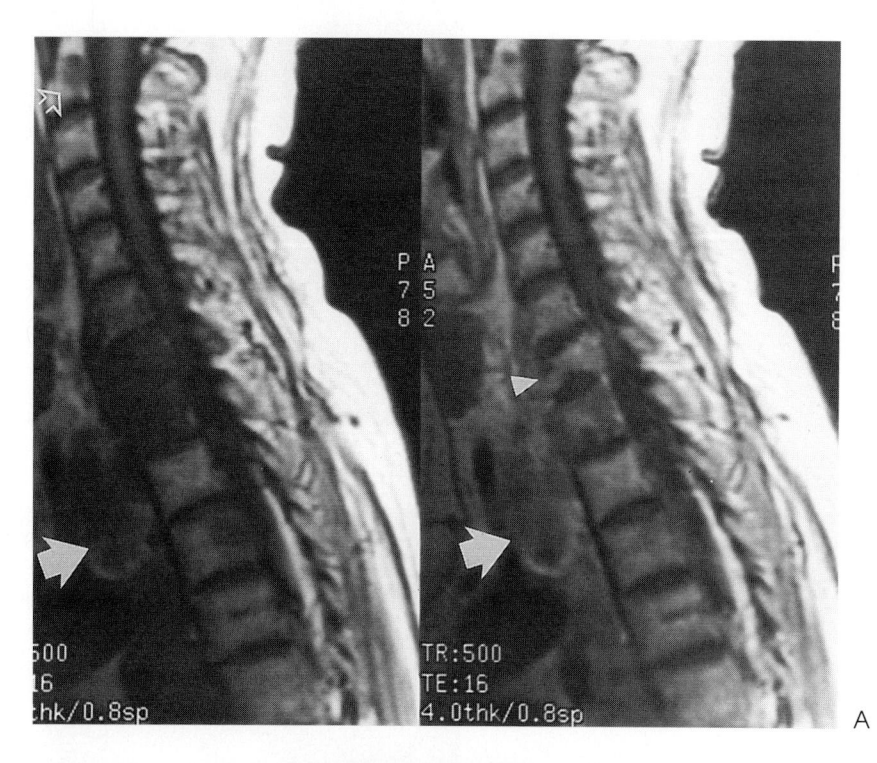

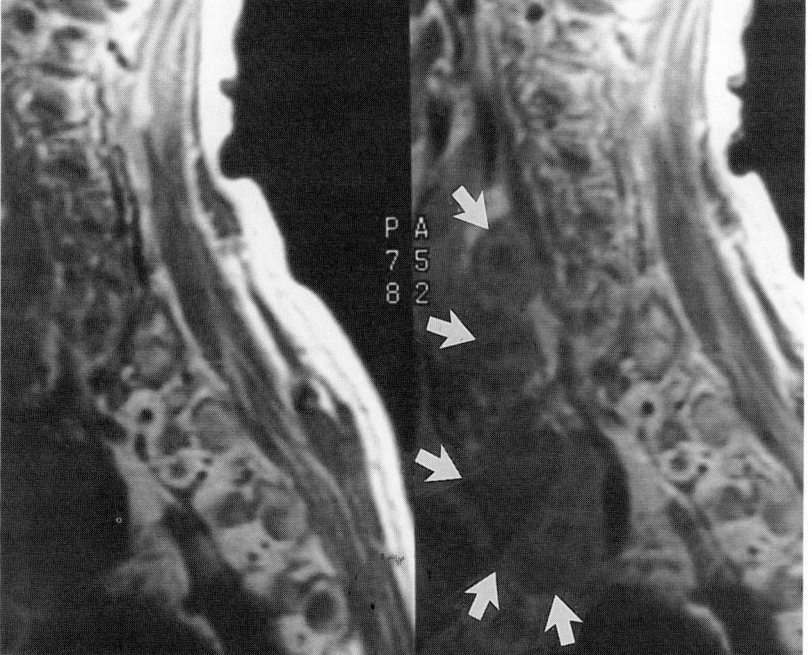

A

B

TEACHING ATLAS OF SPINE IMAGING

C

D

Radiologic Findings

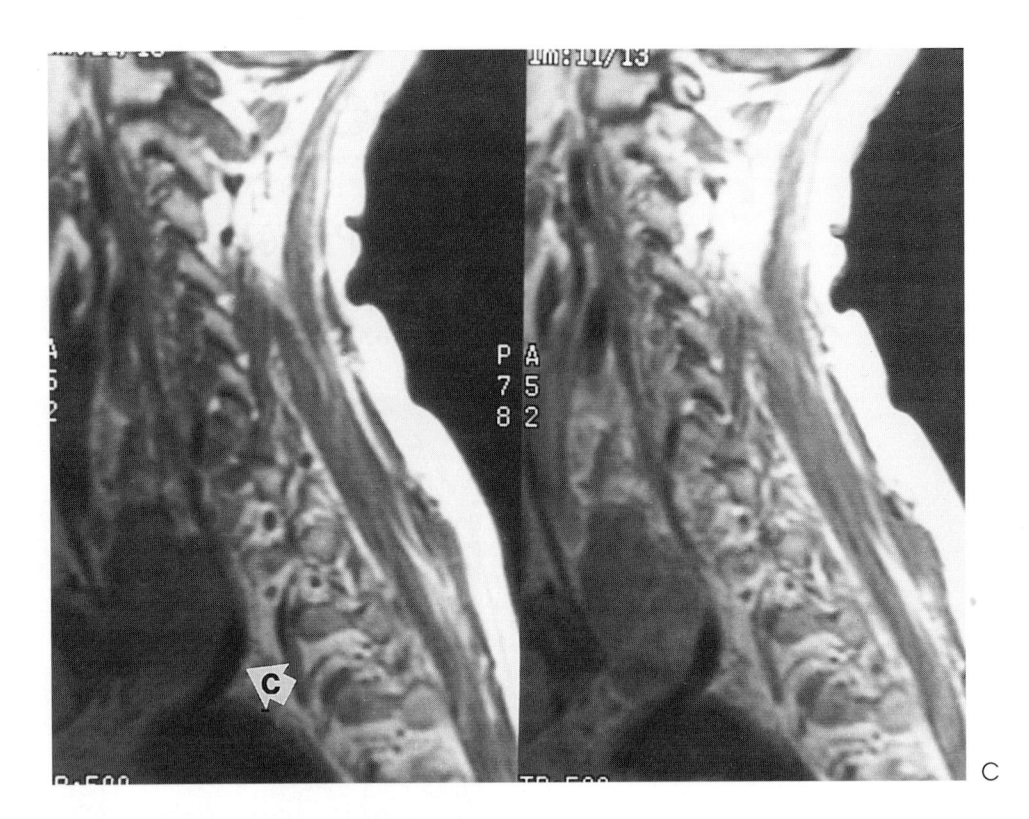

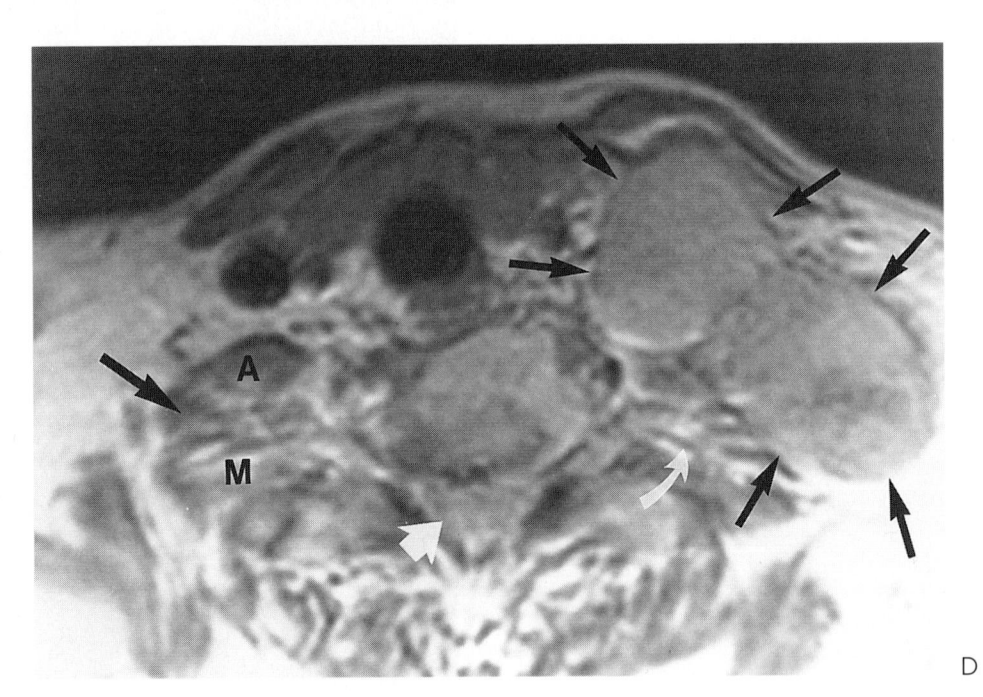

Pre- (Fig. A, *left*) and postcontrast (Fig. A, *right*) sagittal short TR images reveal a small area of decreased signal intensity in the vertebral bodies of C2 (*left, open arrow*). There is also decreased signal intensity replacing the vertebral bodies of C6 and C7 and the posterior portion of T1. An intermediate signal intensity mass anterior to the spine is visible at the T1-2 level

SPINE METASTASES

Radiologic Findings (continued)

(*left and right, white arrow*). The postcontrast study reveals enhancement of all of these areas. There is essentially complete disappearance of the T1 lesion (*white arrowhead*). There is a compression fracture of the T1 vertebral body with retropulsion of the posterior margin of the vertebral body into the vertebral canal.

Pre- (Fig. B, *left*) and postcontrast (Fig. B, *right*) parasagittal short TR images reveal multiple, rounded, intermediate signal intensity soft tissue masses projecting anterior and lateral to the spine (*arrows*).

Pre- (Fig. C, *left*) and postcontrast (Fig. C, *right*) parasagittal short TR images reveal a soft tissue mass anterior to the flow void of the carotid artery, which displaces the carotid artery posteriorly (*left, arrow-c*). The mass enhances on the postcontrast study.

Axial short TR image postcontrast at the level of C7 (Fig. D) reveals two large confluent masses on the left side (*long black arrows on right*) that exhibit enhancement. The nerve roots of the brachial plexus are displaced posteriorly by this mass (*curved arrow*). There is dense enhancement of the C7 vertebral body and compromise of the subarachnoid space with posterior compression of the cervical spinal cord (*white arrow*). The anterior scalenus muscle (*A*) and middle scalenus muscle (*M*) are seen on either side of the nerve roots of the brachial plexus on the right side (*black arrow on left*). The low signal intensity air filled trachea is displaced to the right.

PEARLS
- Remember that the brachial plexus extends from the level of the spinal cord to the level of the axilla.

- Vascular displacement as well as encroachment can be readily demonstrated by MR imaging.

PITFALL
- Evaluation should be made of the paraspinal area as well as the vertebral bodies.

Diagnosis

Metastatic breast cancer with vertebral body involvement and pathologic adenopathy.

Differential Diagnosis

- metastatic disease
- inflammatory process

Discussion

A clinical history of a primary tumor would be very helpful for accurate and complete evaluation. In this patient, there are multiple greatly enlarged metastatic lymph nodes in the neck in the supraclavicular region. There is compromise of the subarachnoid space and cord compression at the C7 level. The brachial plexus is also compressed by these pathologically enlarged supraclavicular lymph nodes. Although the remote possibility of an inflammatory process is a consideration, the adenopathy and lack of intervertebral disc involvement favor metastatic disease. Analysis of the cerebrospinal fluid may be helpful in differentiating between metastatic versus inflammatory disease.

Magnetic resonance (MR) imaging is the best method for evaluation of the brachial plexus. The entire course of the brachial plexus should be visualized for complete evaluation.

TEACHING ATLAS OF SPINE IMAGING

Case 9

Clinical Presentation

The patient is a 63-year-old female with known breast cancer who presents with left upper extremity weakness.

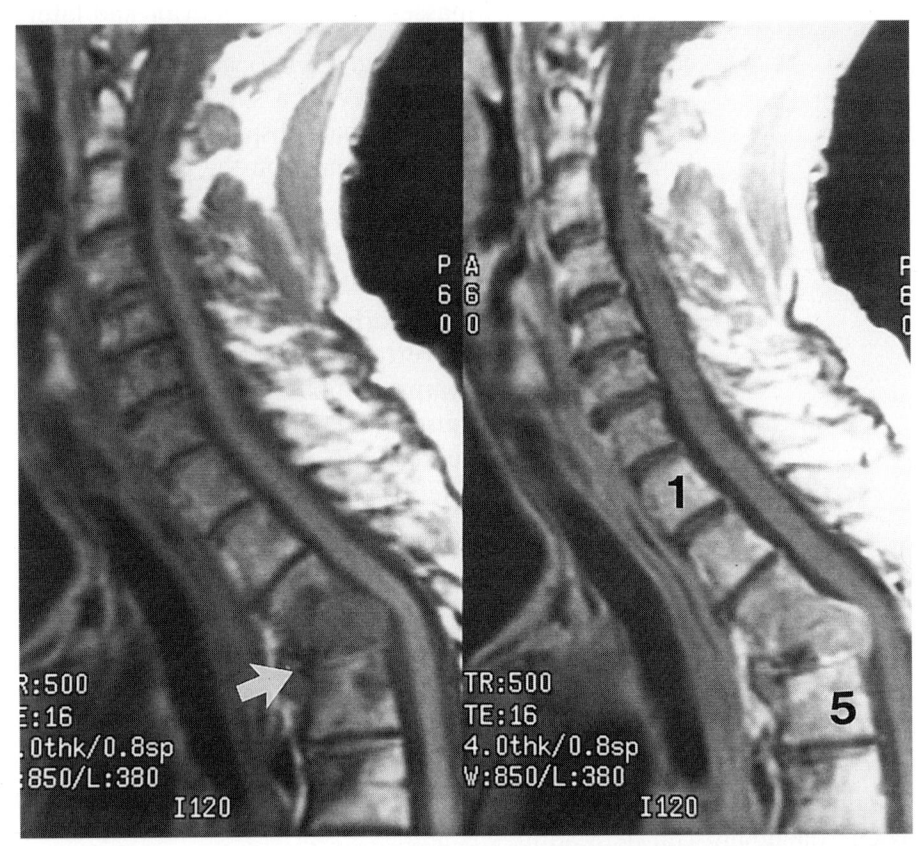

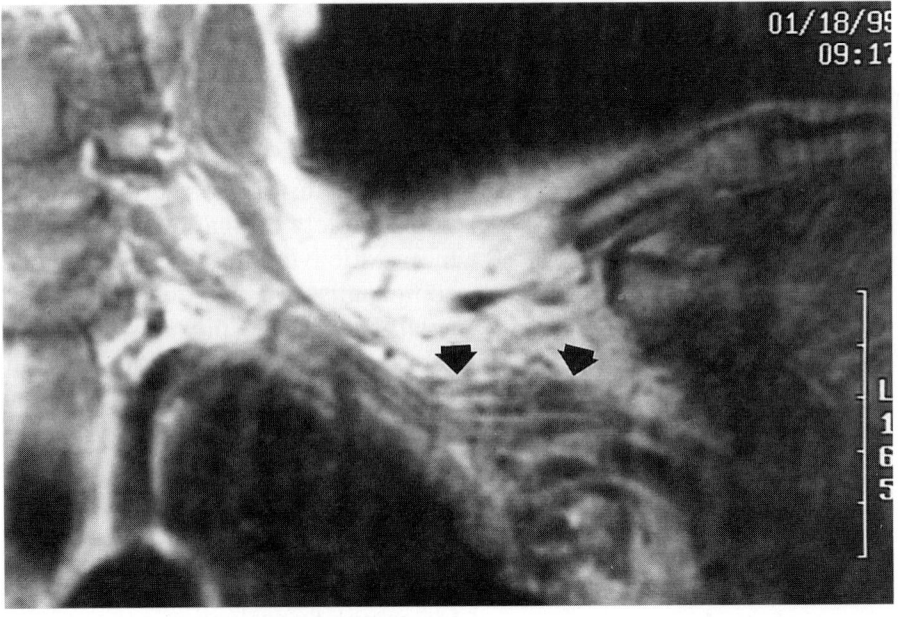

A

B

SPINE METASTASES

Radiologic Findings

Pre- (Fig. A, *left*) and postcontrast (Fig. A, *right*) sagittal short TR images reveal that multiple vertebral bodies are replaced by decreased signal intensity soft tissue. An acute kyphosis is visible at the T4 level, and there is marked destruction of the T4 vertebral body and retropulsion of the posterior margin of the vertebral body into the vertebral canal (*left, arrow*). The postcontrast study reveals extensive enhancement of the vertebrae at all levels. There is marked compromise of the subarachnoid space and curvilinear posterior displacement and indentation of the spinal cord at the level of maximal kyphosis. The L1 vertebral body is identified with 1, the L5 vertebral body with 5.

Coronal short TR image (Fig. B) reveals thickening of the nerve roots of the brachial plexus (*black arrows*) as they course just superior to the flow void of the subclavian artery.

Diagnosis

Metastatic breast cancer involving multiple vertebral bodies and the brachial plexus.

Differential Diagnosis

- metastatic disease

Discussion

The brachial plexus extends from the origin of the nerve roots from the spinal cord to the level of the axilla. Metastatic disease may affect the nerves at any location along the course of these nerves. Magnetic resonance imaging provides the best method of evaluating the brachial plexus. Studies may also be performed using the fat saturation technique. With this technique, the fat appears as decreased signal intensity, while enhancing lesions appear as increased signal intensity.

In this clinical setting, metastasis is the most probable diagnosis.

PEARL

- In cases where there is a severe pathologic fracture of the vertebral body with complete collapse, the resulting apparent absence of the vertebral body may not be appreciated. When there is marked collapse of a vertebral body, there is typically accentuation of the dorsal kyphosis.

PITFALLS

- The postcontrast study may give the appearance of totally normal vertebral bodies, so the studies should be performed both pre- and postcontrast.

- With such marked destruction, a missing vertebral body may not be appreciated on the images.

TEACHING ATLAS OF SPINE IMAGING

Case 10

Clinical Presentation

The patient is a 76-year-old previously healthy male with a history of 2 days of lower back pain and several months of anorexia. The patient also has a 50-year history of pipe smoking.

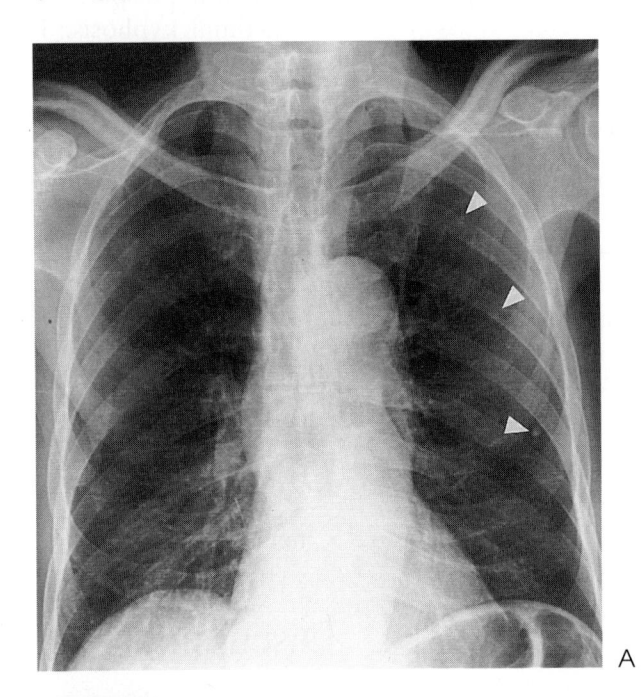

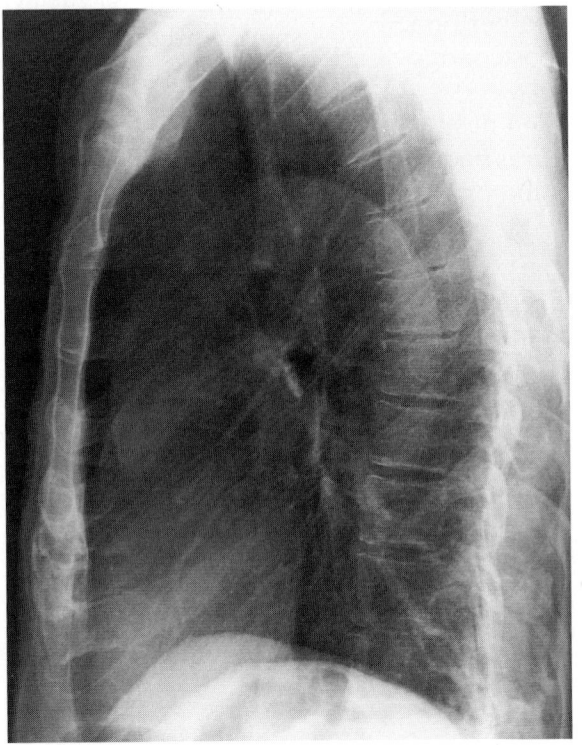

A

B

SPINE METASTASES

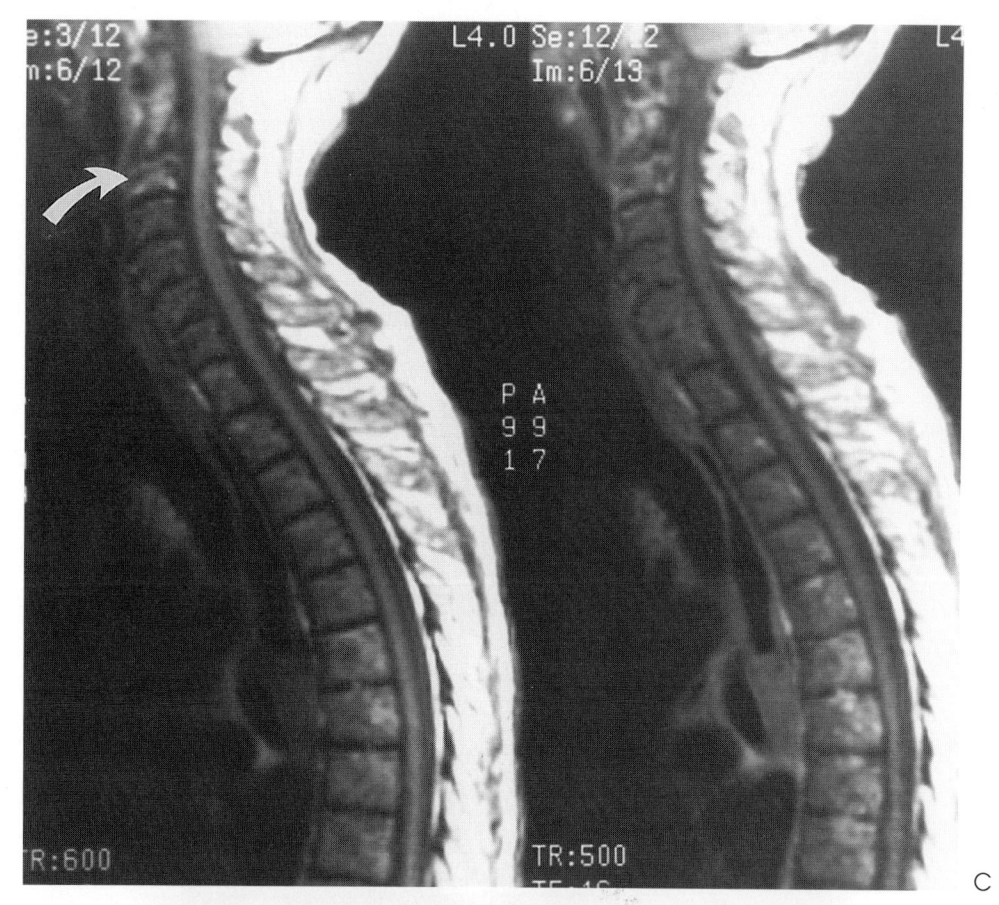

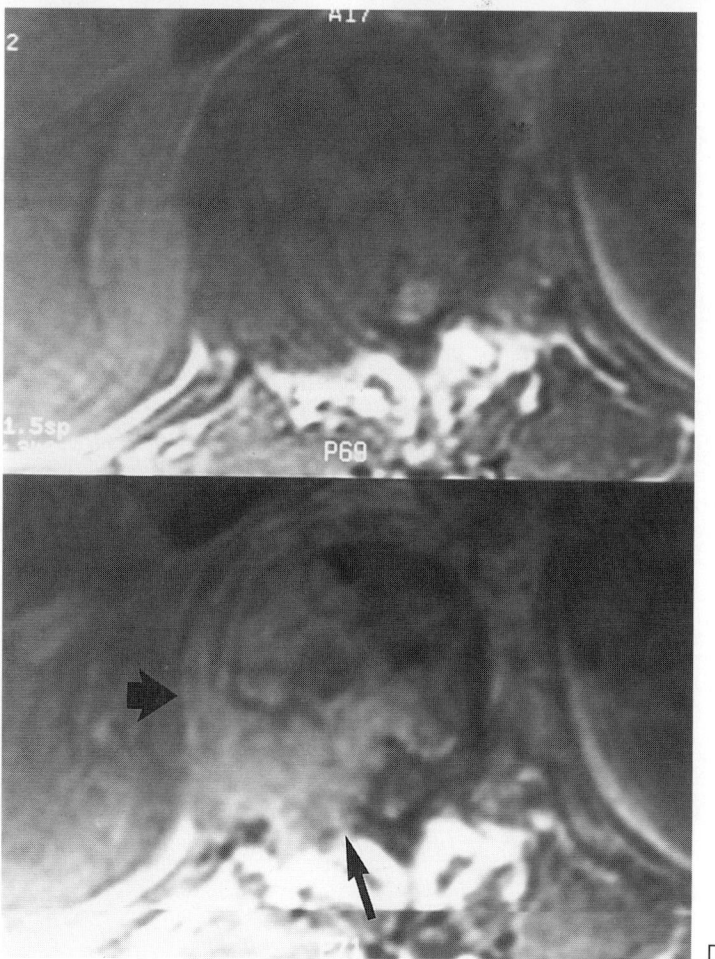

TEACHING ATLAS OF SPINE IMAGING

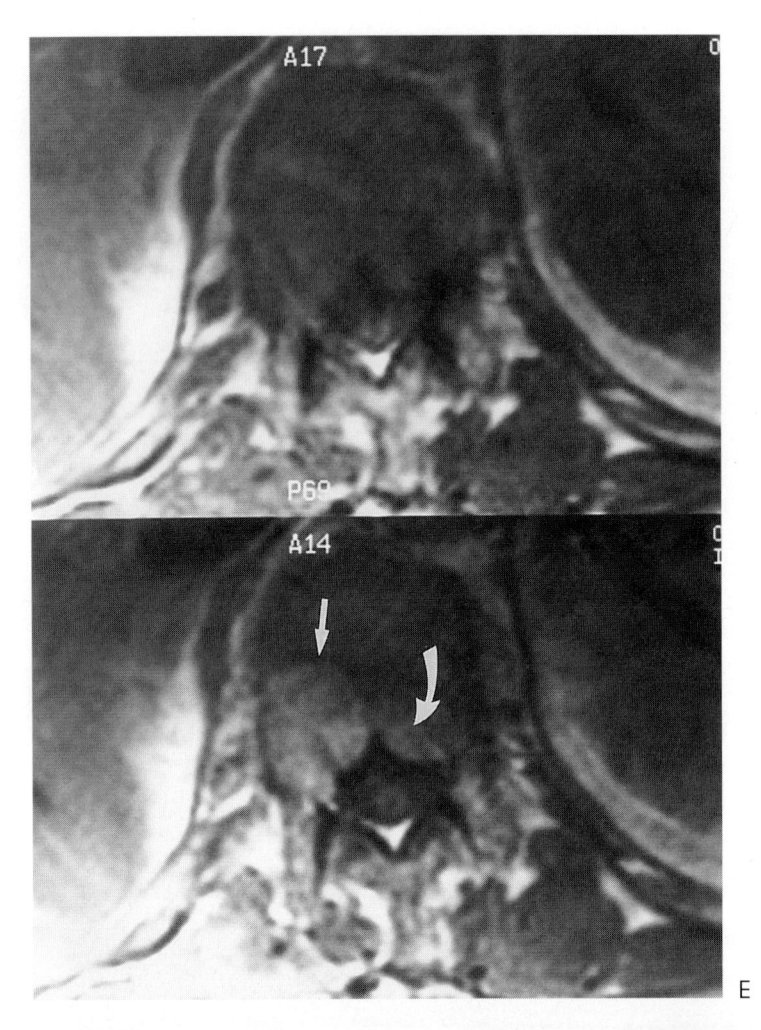

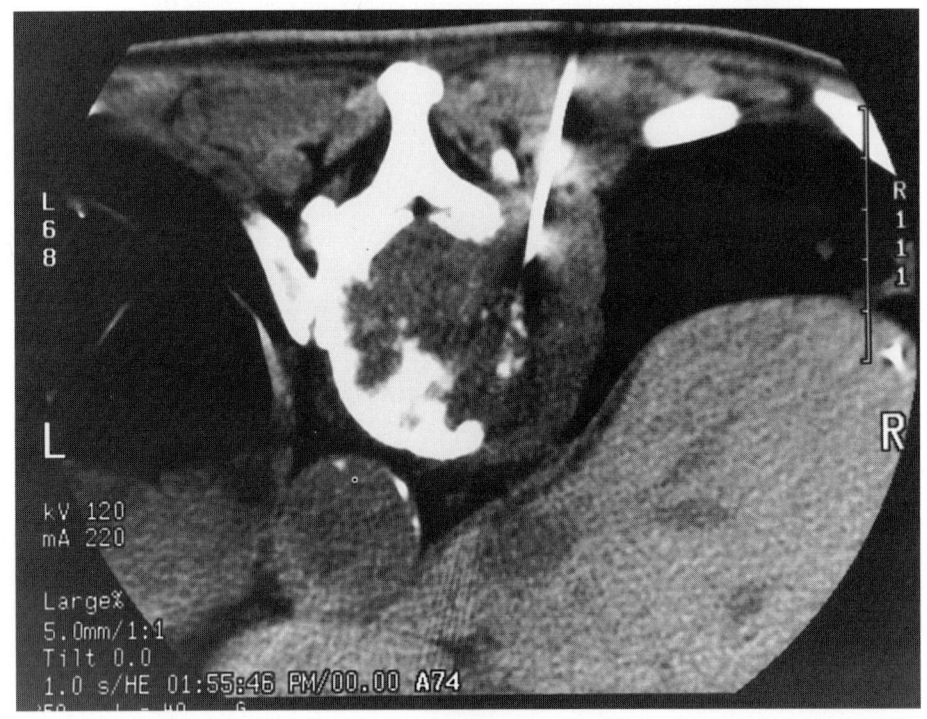

364

SPINE METASTASES

G

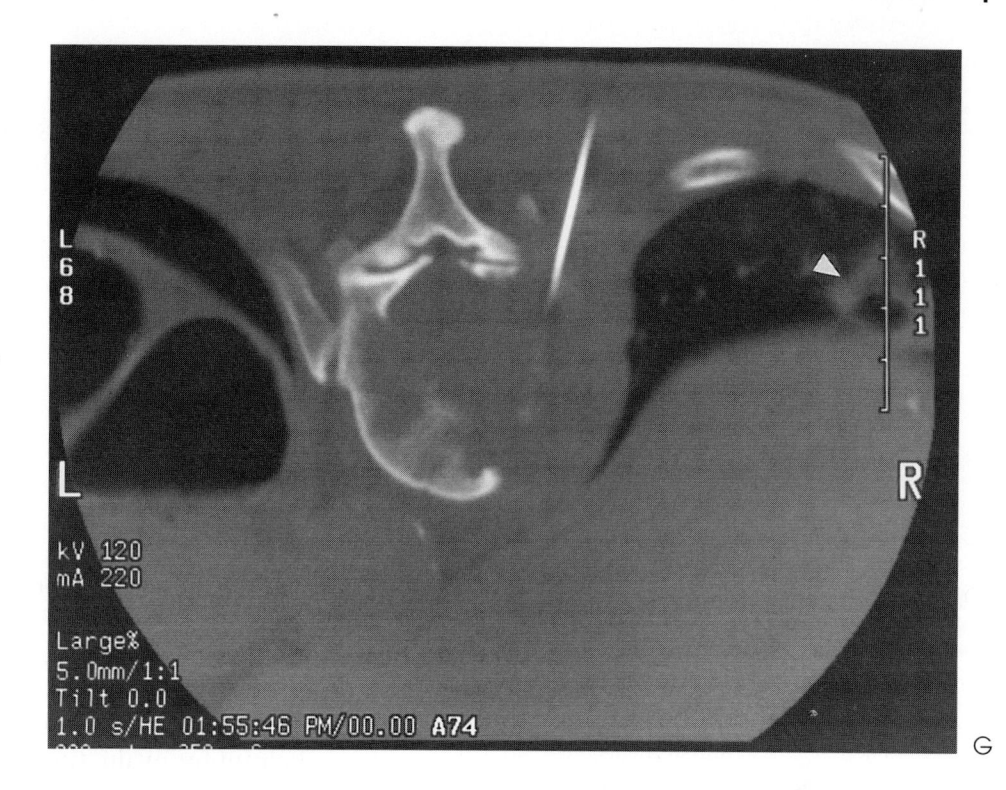

Radiologic Findings

Posteroanterior (Fig. A) and lateral (Fig. B) views of the chest reveal flattening of the hemidiaphragms bilaterally and three faint nodular densities in the left lung (Fig. A, *arrowheads*). The vertebrae appear normal on the lateral view.

Pre- (Fig. C, *left*) and postcontrast (Fig. C, *right*) sagittal short TR images reveal questionable loss of vertebral height at the C3 level. There is mottled signal intensity within the marrow of this vertebral body and questionable patchy enhancement (*left, curved arrow*). The vertebrae otherwise appear normal.

Pre- (Fig. D, *top*) and postcontrast (Fig. D, *bottom*) axial short TR images reveal extensive replacement of the vertebral body of T11 with decreased signal intensity soft tissue. This exhibits marked enhancement on the postcontrast study. There is expansion of the pedicle (*bottom, long black arrow*) and encroachment upon the right side of the thecal sac. The spinal cord is displaced to the left. There is also an enhancing soft tissue mass on the right side (*bottom, wide arrow*).

Pre- (Fig. E, *top*) and postcontrast (Fig. E, *bottom*) axial short TR images at a slightly different level reveals a bilobed, enhancing, soft tissue mass that encroaches upon the anterior aspect of the vertebral canal (*bottom, curved arrow*) and extends into the vertebral body (*bottom, straight arrow*).

Computed tomographic (CT) scan with CT-guided biopsy (Fig. F) reveals the soft tissue mass with the needle in place. The extensive destruction of the bone of the vertebral body can be appreciated. The soft tissue paraspinal component is readily visualized.

The wide window width image (Fig. G) better reveals the destructive process.

TEACHING ATLAS OF SPINE IMAGING

PEARL
- Occasionally, bony destructive changes are better appreciated on the CT scan than on the MR scan. This is because CT is more sensitive for destructive changes of the cortical bone, which may not be visible on the MR scan. In general, however, MR is the procedure of choice for the evaluation of the presence or absence of metastatic disease.

PITFALL
- The entire spine should be evaluated in a patient with possible metastatic disease.

Diagnosis

Metastatic lung cancer, biopsy proved. Multiple additional lung nodules were present on the chest CT scan. One is visible in the lung on the right side in Figure G (*arrowhead*).

Differential Diagnosis

- metastatic disease
- multiple myeloma

Discussion

Greater than 50% destruction of the vertebral body is necessary before these destructive changes can be identified. Magnetic resonance (MR) imaging is very sensitive to the presence of bony metastases and is positive in a high percentage of cases that have bony metastases. MR is more accurate than bone scanning because it is generally more specific. However, radionuclide bone scanning is helpful for evaluating other bony areas of involvement. In the patient who has back pain, MR is the imaging procedure of choice for evaluation of the presence of metastases.

Chest CT is more accurate than plain film in the evaluation of the presence of lung cancer or lung nodules secondary to metastatic disease.

Multiple myeloma could have a similar appearance. Metastases from any primary tumor could appear similar.

SPINE METASTASES

Case 11

Clinical Presentation

The patient is a 57-year-old with back pain and lower extremity weakness.

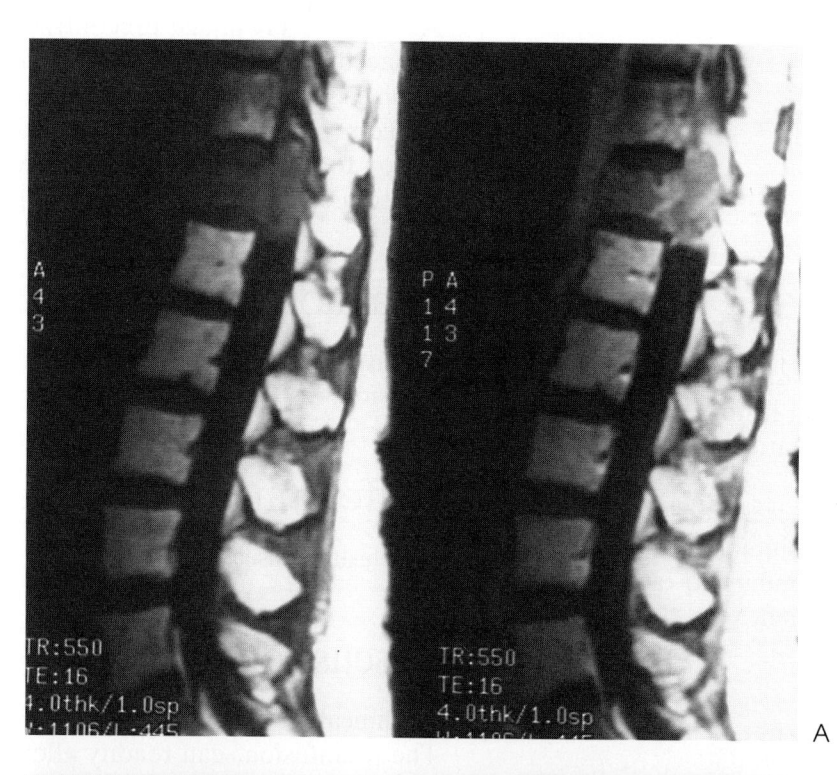

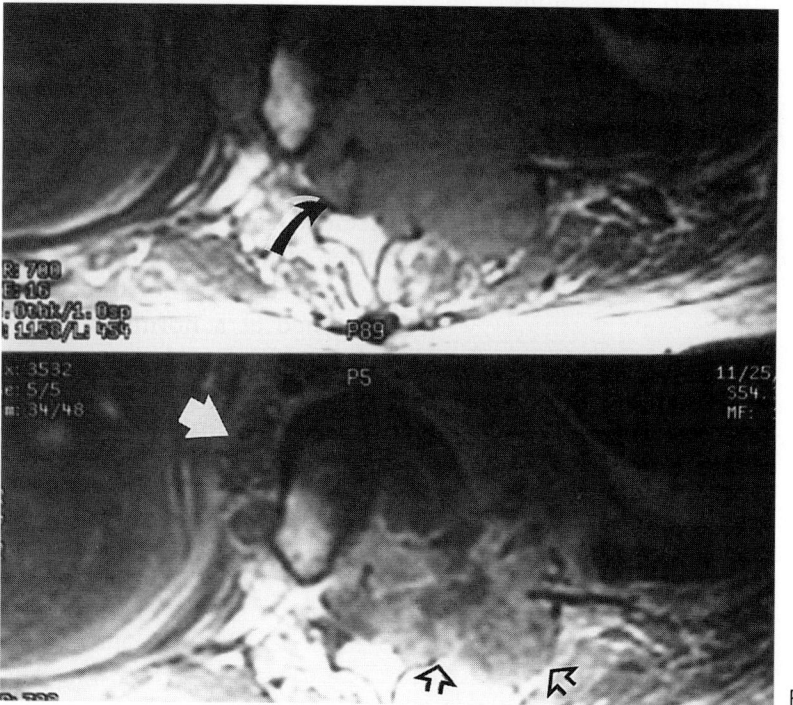

TEACHING ATLAS OF SPINE IMAGING

Radiologic Findings

Pre- (Fig. A, *left*) and postcontrast (Fig. A, *right*) sagittal short TR images reveal complete replacement of the T12 vertebral body with decreased signal intensity tumor. The remainder of the vertebral bodies are diffusely increased in signal intensity. The postcontrast image (*right*) reveals diffuse irregular enhancement of the T12 metastatic deposit. There is an enhancing soft tissue component that extends into and obliterates the vertebral canal.

Axial short TR image precontrast (Fig. B, *top*) reveals that the tumor has replaced the vertebral body of T12. The spinal cord is compressed and displaced to the far right (*curved double arrow*). Postcontrast (Fig. B, *bottom*) image reveals a tumor that extends laterally on the left into the paraspinal region to involve the ribs and the transverse process (*open arrows*). There is also a soft tissue mass in the right paraspinal area (*solid arrow*).

PEARLS
- Additional clinical history revealed that the patient had a known history of colon cancer metastatic to the liver.

- The increased signal intensity of the lumbar vertebral bodies is secondary to radiation treatment.

PITFALL
- The entire vertebral column should be evaluated to rule out the presence of other areas of involvement.

Diagnosis

Metastatic colon carcinoma to T12 with bone expansion and cord compression.

Differential Diagnosis

- metastatic disease

Discussion

A clinical history of a known primary tumor is important in this patient. The preinfusion scan readily allows one to make the correct diagnosis of a metastic deposit in the T12 vertebral body. While many primary tumors may metastasize and have a similar appearance, the known primary tumor makes this the most likely diagnosis. The postcontrast study is probably not necessary to make the diagnosis, but increases the conspicuity of the abnormality. The axial images are very distorted from normal, and the exact position of the spinal cord is difficult to determine based on one axial slice. Therefore, if a surgical approach is palnned, it is vital to determine the position of the spinal cord. Evaluation should be made of the images above and below the level of the abnormality, so the spinal cord position can be determined at a normal level and then followed down to the abnormal level. In this way, the exact location of the spinal cord can be accurately determined. A CT-guided biopsy may also be used to identify the nature of the abnormality and the source of the primary tumor.

Metastatic thyroid cancer, breast cancer, or lung cancer could have a similar appearance, as could a plasmacytoma or primary bone tumor.

SPINE METASTASES

Case 12

Clinical Presentation

The patient is a 24-year-old female with known Ewing's sarcoma with lower extremity weakness and a sensory level at T8.

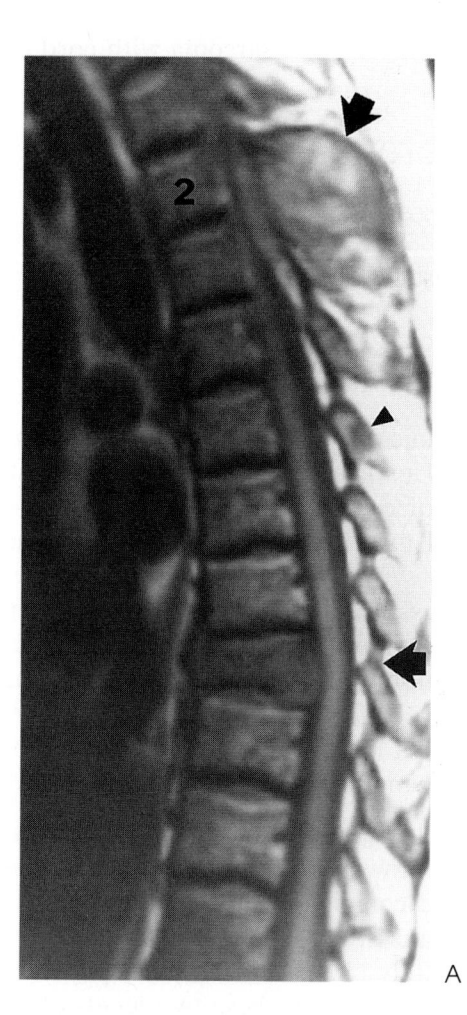

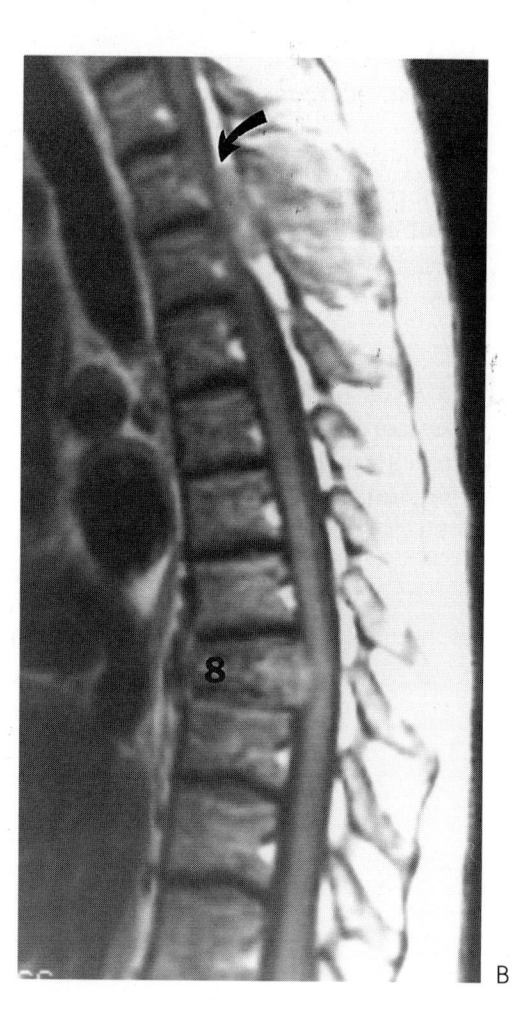

Radiologic Findings

Sagittal short TR image without contrast (Fig. A) reveals expansion of the spinous process at the T2 level (*upper arrow*). The normal epidural fat at the T2 (*2*) level is replaced by intermediate soft tissue signal intensity material. The T5 vertebral body spinous process reveals a rounded area of decreased signal intensity (*arrowhead*). There is a compression fracture at T8 with retropulsion of the posterior margin of the vertebral body into the vertebral canal (*lower arrow*).

Sagittal short TR image with contrast material (Fig. B) reveals enhancement of the soft tissue epidural mass at the T2 level (*arrow*). The normal epidural fat has been replaced by the soft tissue mass. The subarachnoid space dorsal to the spinal cord is compressed, and the spinal cord is compressed forward

Radiologic Findings (continued)

against the posterior margin of the vertebral body. There is diffuse enhancement of the T8 vertebral body (8). The spinal cord is compressed slightly along its anterior margin and displaced slightly posteriorly. There is obliteration of the subarachnoid space anterior to the spinal cord at this level.

Diagnosis

Metastatic Ewing's sarcoma with cord compression at the T2 level.

Differential Diagnosis

- Ewing's sarcoma
- metastatic disease

Discussion

The clinical examination does not always accurately reflect the anatomic level of involvement with tumor or metastases. This patient has two potential levels of cord compression. The T2 level appears to be the more severe area of involvement by magnetic resonance evaluation, while the T8 has greater symptoms in the clinical setting. In the patient with potential cord compression, the entire length of the vertebral column should be evaluated. This is best performed with short TR images with multiplanar imaging. The evaluation of the entire vertebral column determines if there is more than one level of cord compression or if the involvement is localized. Thus, treatment may be directed to the multiple areas involved. This patient is a good example of multiple abnormal levels with symptoms at only one level.

It should be noted that myelography may be performed in a patient such as this. However, if the study is performed via a lumbar tap, flow of contrast may be completely blocked at T8, the lower level of metastatic disease. When the study is performed via a cervical tap, flow of contrast may be completely blocked at T2, the upper level of spread of tumor. Therefore, the areas between these two levels of block to the flow of contrast would not be evaluated. Ewing's sarcoma typically may have an area of bone involvement with a much larger soft tissue component.

In this clinical setting of known Ewing's sarcoma, multiple metastases from the primary tumor are the most likely diagnosis.

PEARLS

- Ewing's sarcoma is a very malignant tumor, and metastatic disease is common.

- The postcontrast examination better evaluates the soft tissue component associated with the metastatic deposits.

PITFALL

- The cord compression is present at the T2 level, while the clinical level is at T8.

SPINE METASTASES

Case 13

Clinical Presentation

The patient is a 49-year-old female with renal cell cancer and new onset of upper back pain.

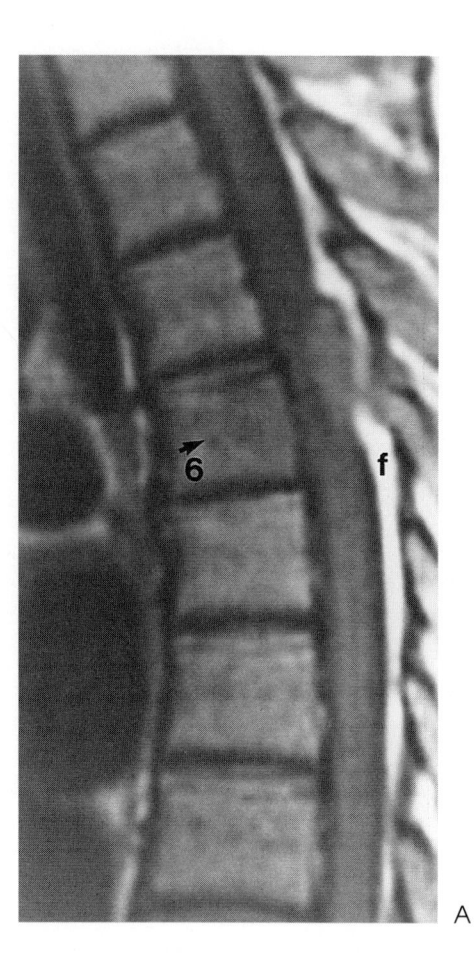

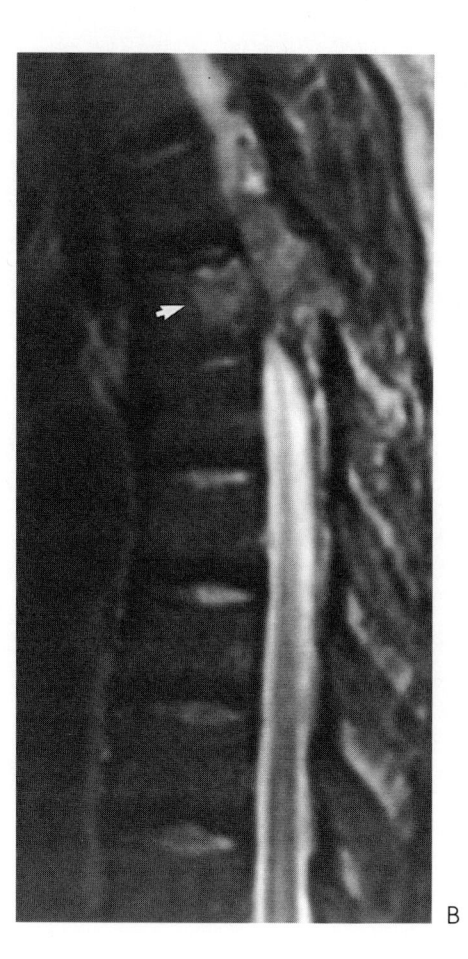

Radiologic Findings

Sagittal short TR image (Fig. A) reveals an intermediate signal intensity mass in the dorsal epidural space at the T6 level (*6*). The normal dorsal epidural fat (*f*) is obliterated. There is a very subtle area of decreased signal intensity in the posterior two thirds of the T6 vertebral body (*arrow*).

Sagittal long TR image (Fig. B) reveals that the soft tissue mass and the lesion in the posterior portion of T6 (*white arrow*) both become increased signal intensity.

TEACHING ATLAS OF SPINE IMAGING

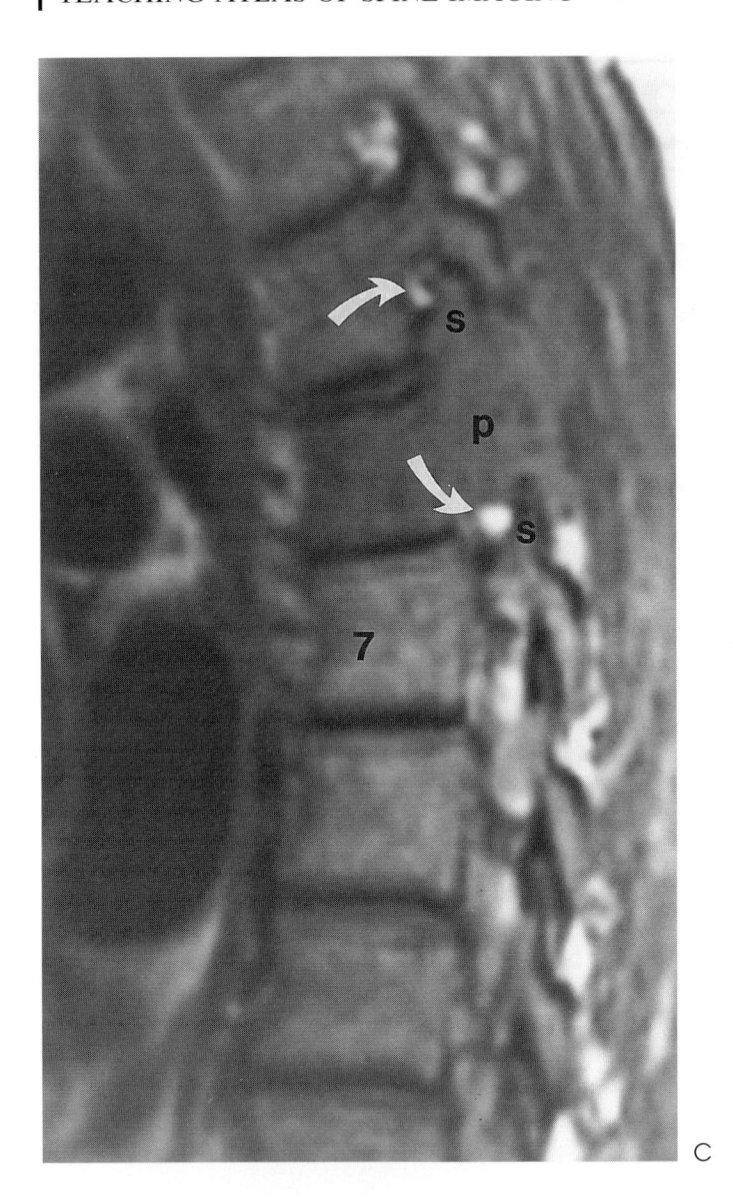

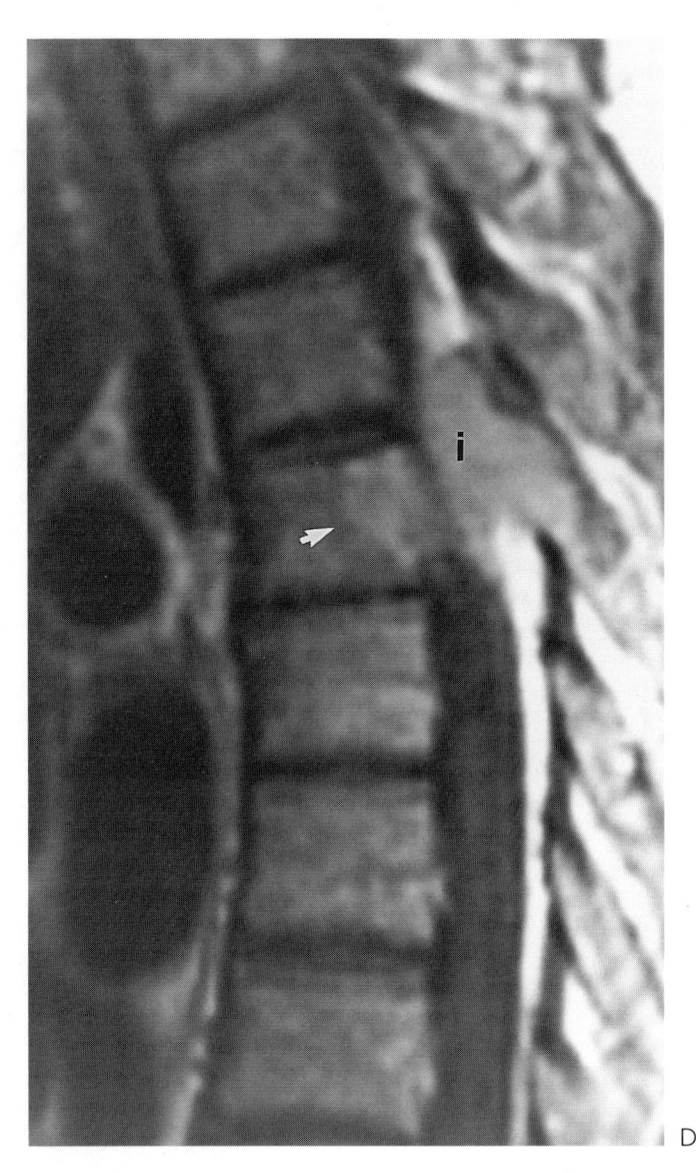

Radiologic Findings (continued)

Parasagittal short TR image (Fig. C) reveals expansion of the pedicle at the T6 level (*p*). This expansile process extends superiorly to involve the superior articulating facet and inferiorly to involve the inferior articulating facet. The upper *s* identifies the involved superior articulating facet, while the lower *s* identifies the normal superior articulating facet of the vertebral body below. The normal increased signal intensity fat in the intervertebral foramina at T5-6 and T6-7 is obliterated by the soft tissue mass (*curved arrows*). The T7 vertebral body is identified with 7.

Sagittal short TR image postcontrast (Fig. D) reveals enhancement of the soft tissue density material in the T6 vertebral body (*white arrow*) and the superior and inferior articulating facets (*i*).

SPINE METASTASES

Radiologic Findings (continued)

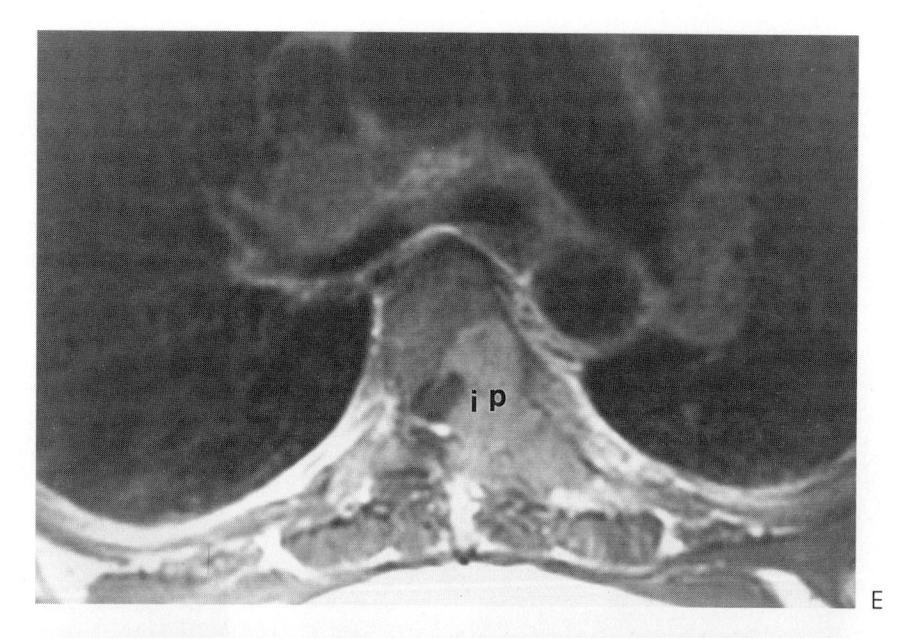

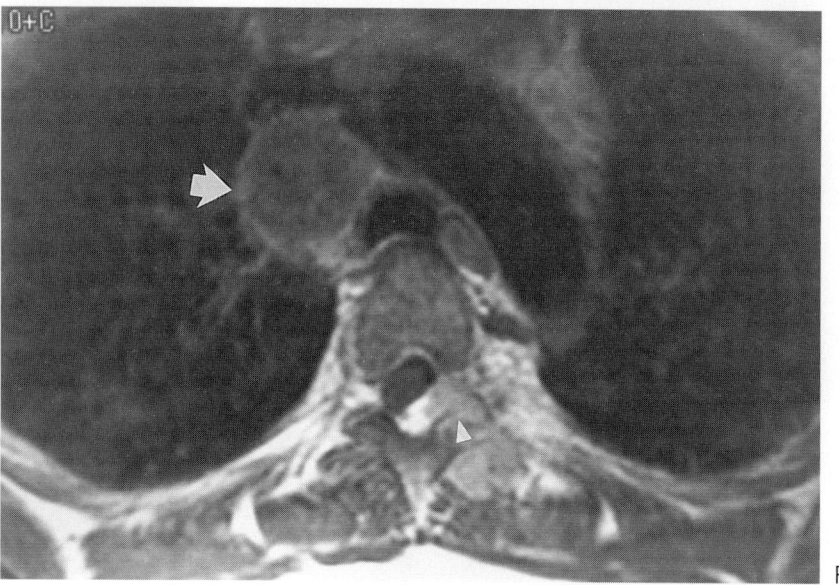

Axial short TR image postcontrast at the level of the vertebral body pedicle (Fig. E) reveals marked expansion of the pedicle (*p*) and superior articulating facet (*i*). Both reveal enhancement. The spinal cord is displaced toward to the right side and compressed. Multiple enlarged soft tissue masses surround the area of the tracheal bifurcation.

Axial short TR image (Fig. F) reveals a large soft tissue mass in the right lung (*white arrow*). The expanded inferior articulating facet is seen encroaching upon the left side of the vertebral canal (*white arrowhead*).

TEACHING ATLAS OF SPINE IMAGING

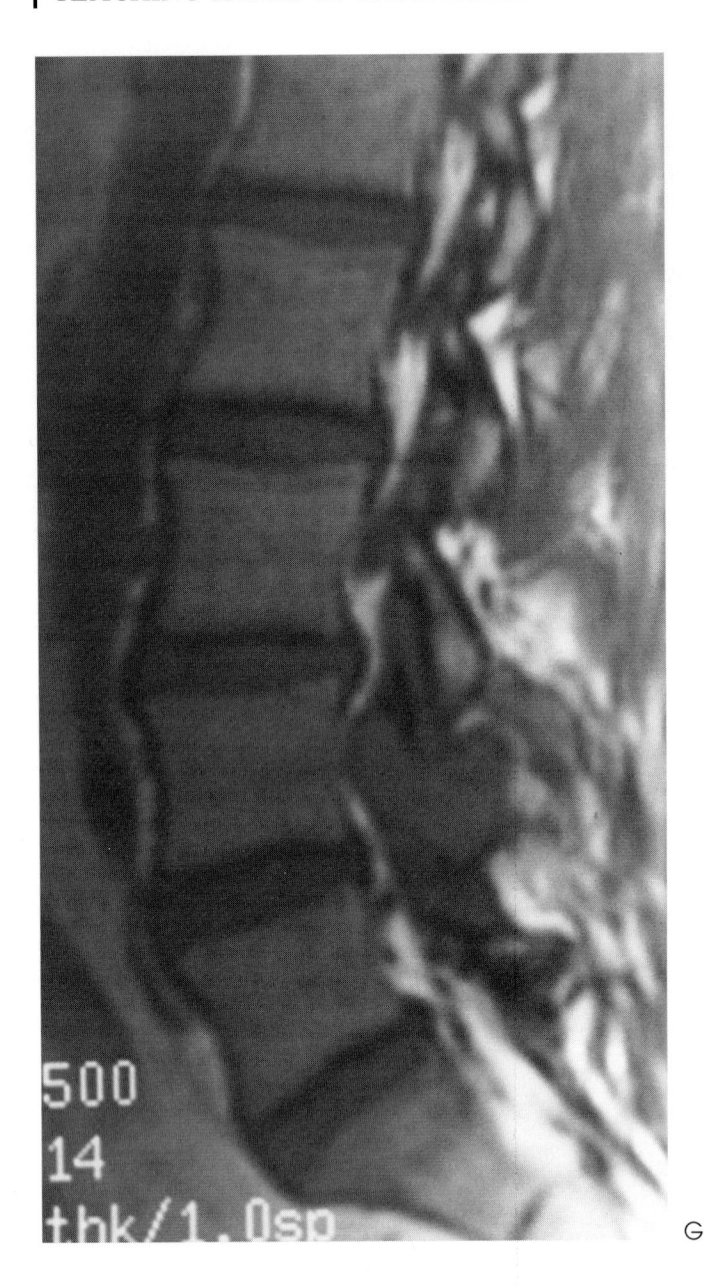

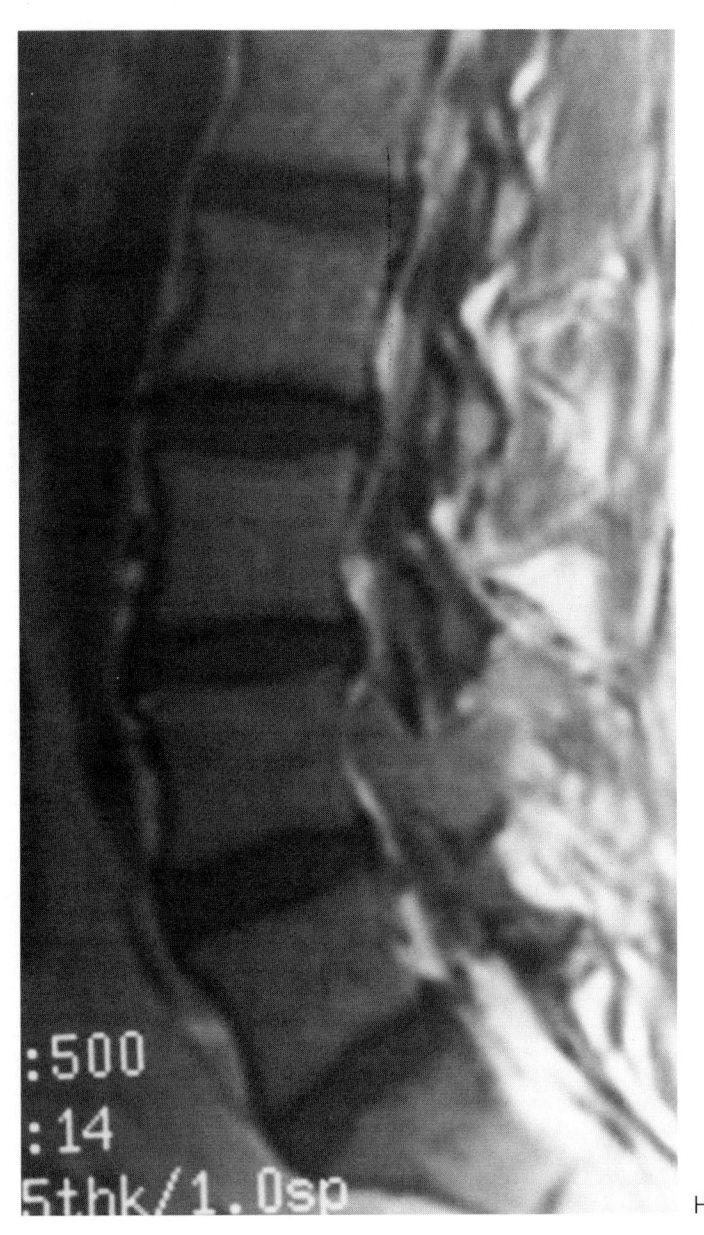

Radiologic Findings (continued)

Parasagittal pre- (Figs. G and I) and postcontrast (Figs. H and J) images reveal that the pedicle (Figs. I and J, *p*) and inferior articulating facet are replaced by soft tissue, which enhances postcontrast.

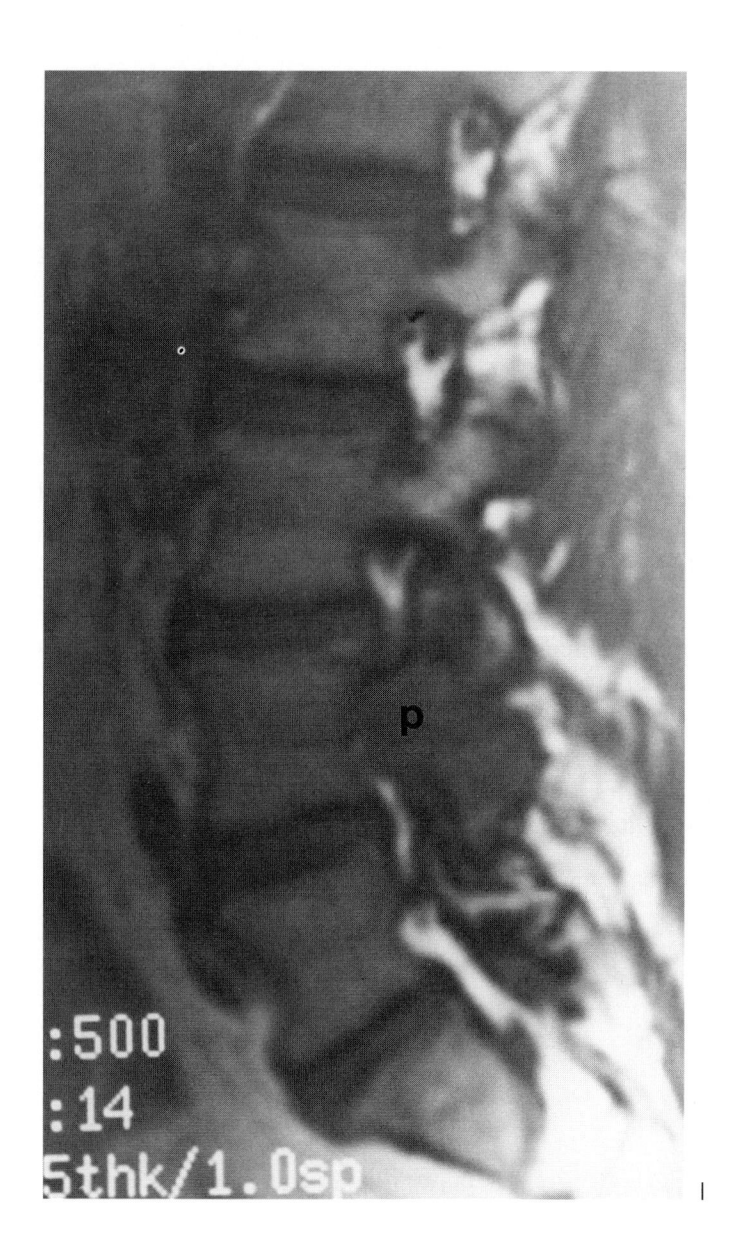

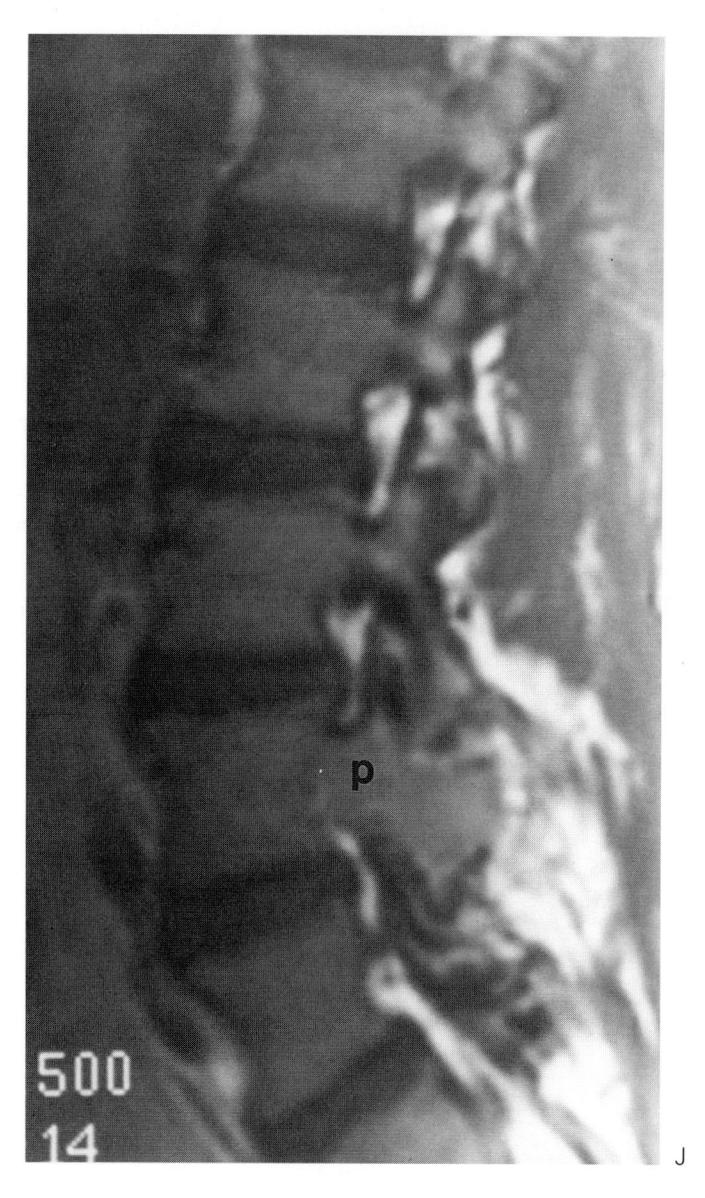

Diagnosis

Metastatic renal cell cancer to the right lung and the vertebrae in the thoracic and lumbar region and involving the paratracheal lymph nodes.

Differential Diagnosis

- metastatic disease from another primary
- multiple myeloma
- primary bone tumor

Discussion

Clinical history is helpful for diagnosis in this patient. The findings could also be related to metastatic lung cancer with the primary cancer in the

PEARL

- Evaluation of incidental findings on the image may be helpful and very rewarding for determining the patient's diagnosis and condition.

PITFALL

- The technique of filming may cause omission of the paraspinal areas, so sufficient attention should be paid to the paraspinal and prevertebral areas and should be included when indicated.

right lung field. The clinical history of back pain in any patient with known cancer warrants additional workup. Magnetic resonance (MR) is the best imaging method for evaluating these cases. The entire vertebral column should be evaluated, so treatment may proceed according to the abnormal findings. Surgery or radiation therapy may be planned based on the findings on the MR scan. MR imaging is also an excellent noninvasive method that may also be used for follow-up.

MR is superior to other diagnostic methods because the presence or absence of cord compression is also easily evaluated. In addition, treatment and follow-up can both be based upon the MR findings.

While myelography could be performed in a patient such as this and demonstrate a block to the flow of contrast material, the full extent of the spread of the disease can be best appreciated by MR imaging. Also MR is less invasive than myelography and postmyelography computed tomographic scanning.

Primary lung cancer, breast cancer, or any other soft tissue cancer, such as lymphoma, which may lead to metastatic disease may have a similar appearance.

SPINE METASTASES

Case 14

Clinical Presentation

The patient is a 25-year-old male with newly diagnosed acute myelogenous leukemia (AML), presenting with new neurologic deficit, with bilateral lower extremity weakness and right facial droop.

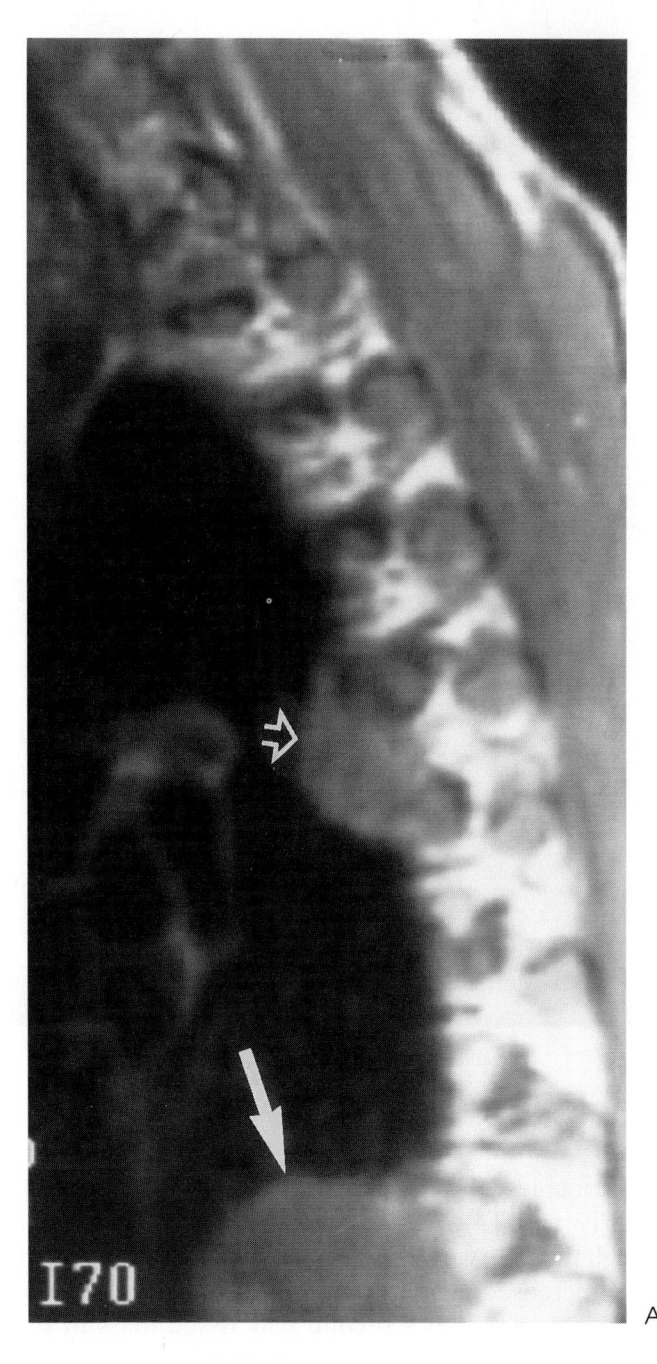

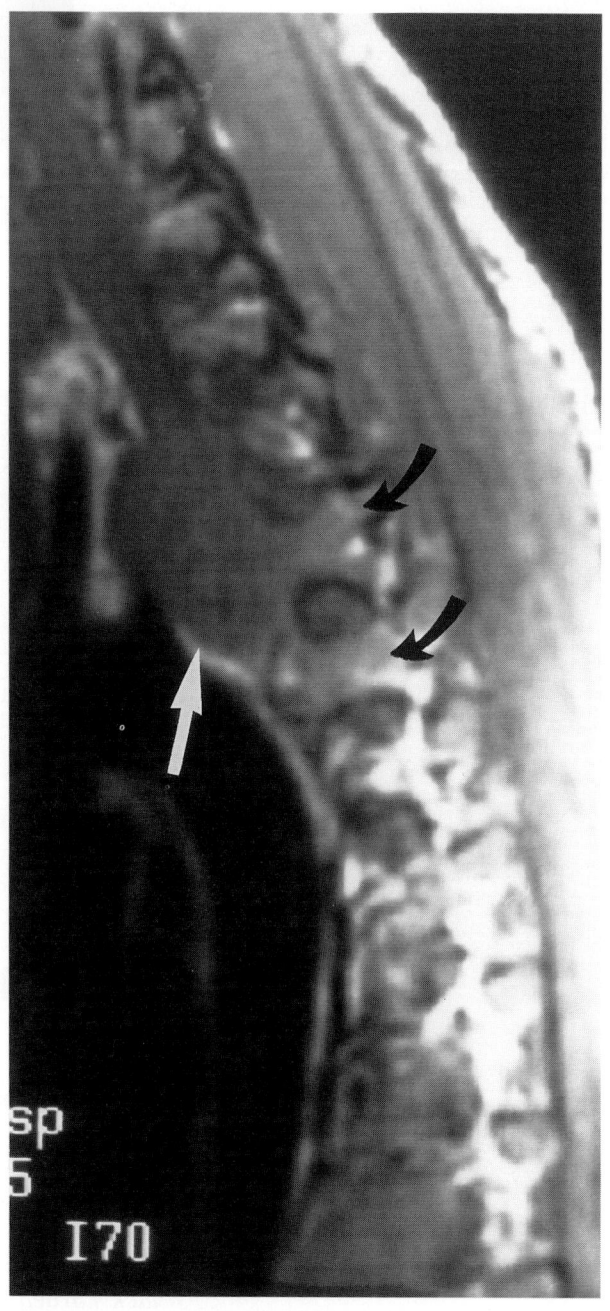

377

TEACHING ATLAS OF SPINE IMAGING

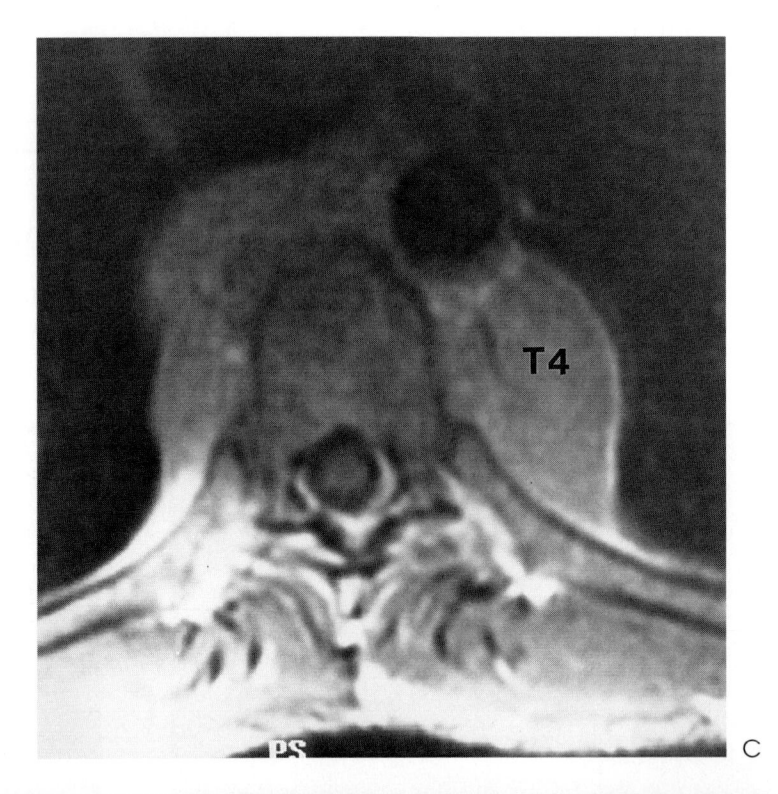

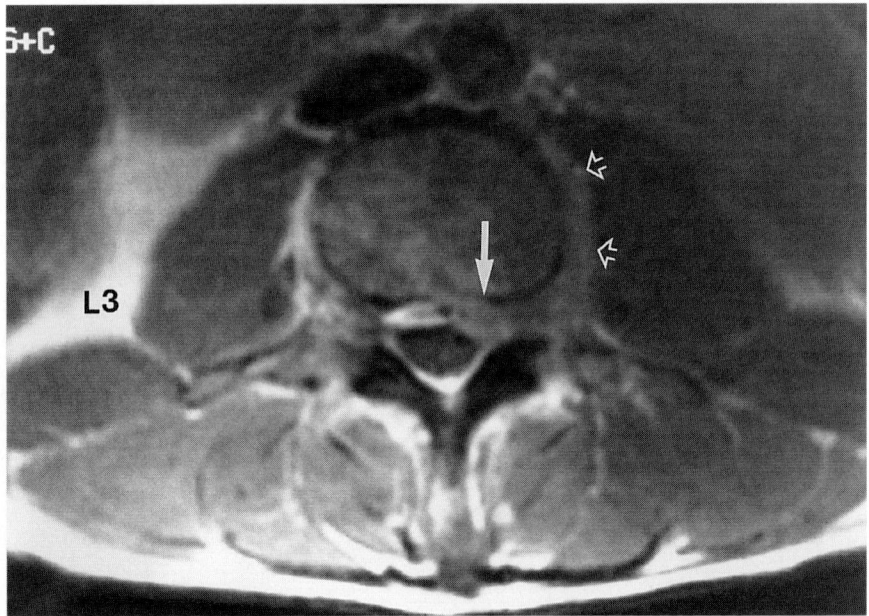

Radiologic Findings

Parasagittal short TR images (Figs. A and B) reveal a paraspinal soft tissue mass at the level of T3 and T4 (Fig. A, *open arrow*; Fig. B, *white arrow*), which extends through the intervertebral foramen and several levels, obliterating the perineural increased signal intensity fat at these levels (Fig. B, *black curved arrow*). There is also a second soft tissue mass in the lower thorax at approximately the T6-8 levels (Figs. A and B, *long white arrows*).

Axial short TR image at the T4 (T4) level (Fig. C) reveals bilateral paraspinal masses with anterior extension to surround the descending aorta (*arrows*). There is no involvement of the vertebral canal at this point.

SPINE METASTASES

Radiologic Findings (continued)

Axial short TR image at the L3 (L3) level (Fig. D) reveals a left paraspinal soft tissue mass that extends through the intervertebral foramen on the left side and into the vertebral canal (*solid arrow*) where there is obliteration of the normal epidural fat. There is slight effacement of the lumbar thecal sac anteriorly (*open arrows*).

> **PEARL**
> - Because of this patient's symptoms, the brain should also be evaluated for the presence of metastatic disease.

Diagnosis

Chloroma, secondary to AML.

Differential Diagnosis

- chloroma
- soft tissue tumor
- hematoma

> **PITFALL**
> - The entire spinal column should be evaluated.

Discussion

A chloroma is a mass of leukemic cells that may occur in any anatomic location; it has also been called granulocytic sarcoma. This mass has a greenish hue when visualized at the time of surgery and thus is called a chloroma.

Chloromas may occur in the central nervous system in the brain or spinal cord. In the spinal cord or spinal column area, chloromas may cause spinal cord compression. Diagnosis may be made at the time of surgery, or a needle biopsy may be performed.

Chloromas in the brain may present with the typical signs and symptoms of any other brain tumor. In these cases, the absolute diagnosis can be made only by biopsy. They may be seen in any age group. The development of a chloroma is a poor prognostic sign in patients with leukemia and is associated with a blast crisis. Chloromas may be single or multiple.

Any soft tissue tumor such as lung cancer or breast cancer could have a similar appearance, as could metastatic neuroblastoma, extramedullary hematopoesis, or even infarction. An inflammatory process is unlikely because of the lack of involvement of the intervertebral disc. A hematoma might also have a similar appearance and could potentially be included in the diagnosis; hematoma would not be anticipated to exhibit enhancement.

Case 15

Clinical Presentation

The patient is a 73-year-old female with a history of metastatic renal cell carcinoma to the liver who now presents with neck pain.

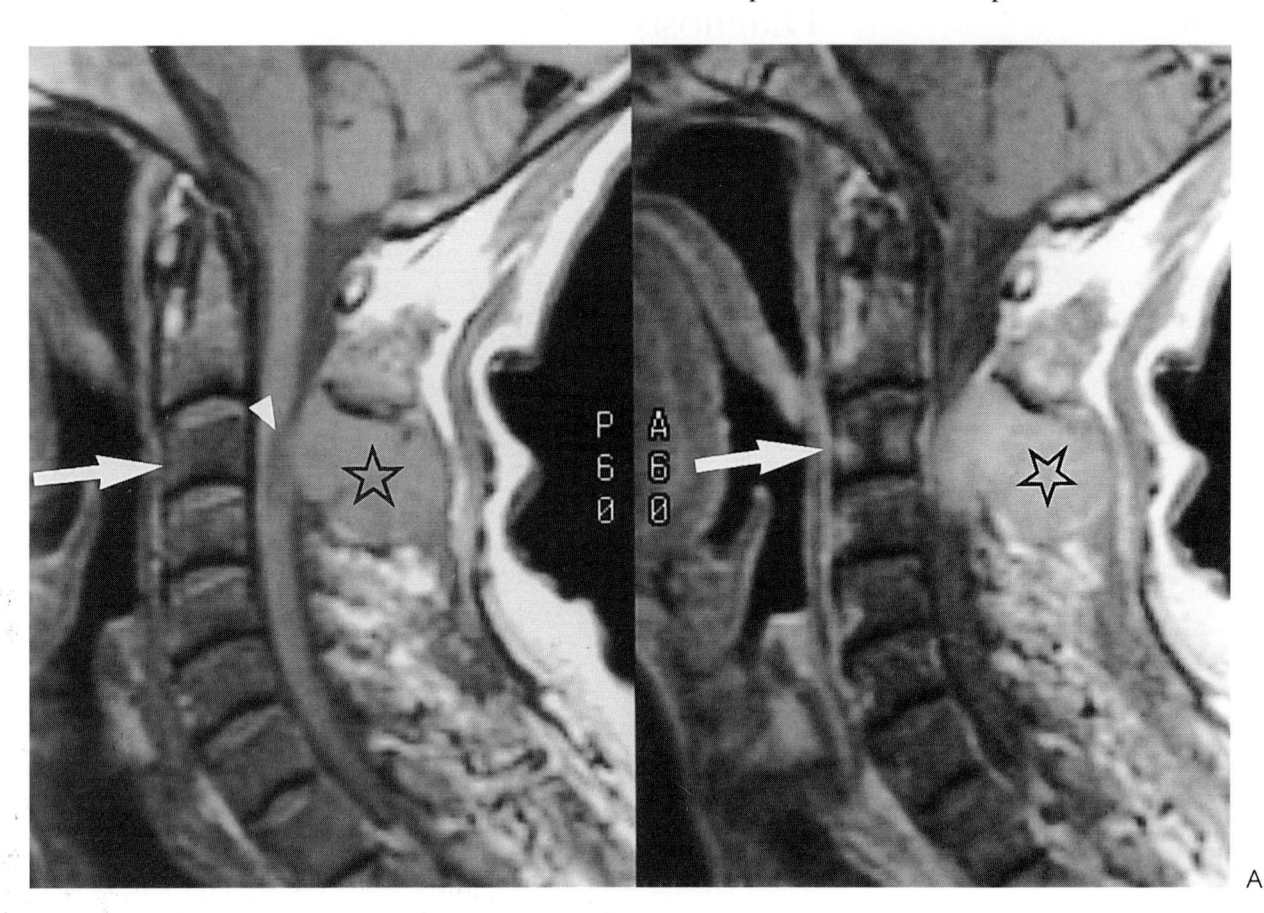

Radiologic Findings

Pre- (Fig. A, *left*) and postcontrast (Fig. A, *right*) sagittal short TR images reveal marked expansion of the spinous process of the C3 vertebral body (*right, **). The spinous process is also replaced by intermediate signal intensity material. Dorsal encroachment upon the subarachnoid space essentially completely obliterates the subarachnoid space. There is an area of decreased signal intensity within the cervical spinal cord at the C3 level (*left, arrowhead*), anterior to the expanded spinous process of the C3 vertebral body. The marrow within the cervical vertebral bodies is replaced by decreased signal intensity soft tissue. The postcontrast short TR image (*right*) reveals diffuse enhancement of the spinous process of C3. Patchy areas of enhancement in the vertebral bodies of C3 and C2 (*white arrow*) are also visible on pre- and postcontrast images.

SPINE METASTASES

B

Radiologic Findings (continued)

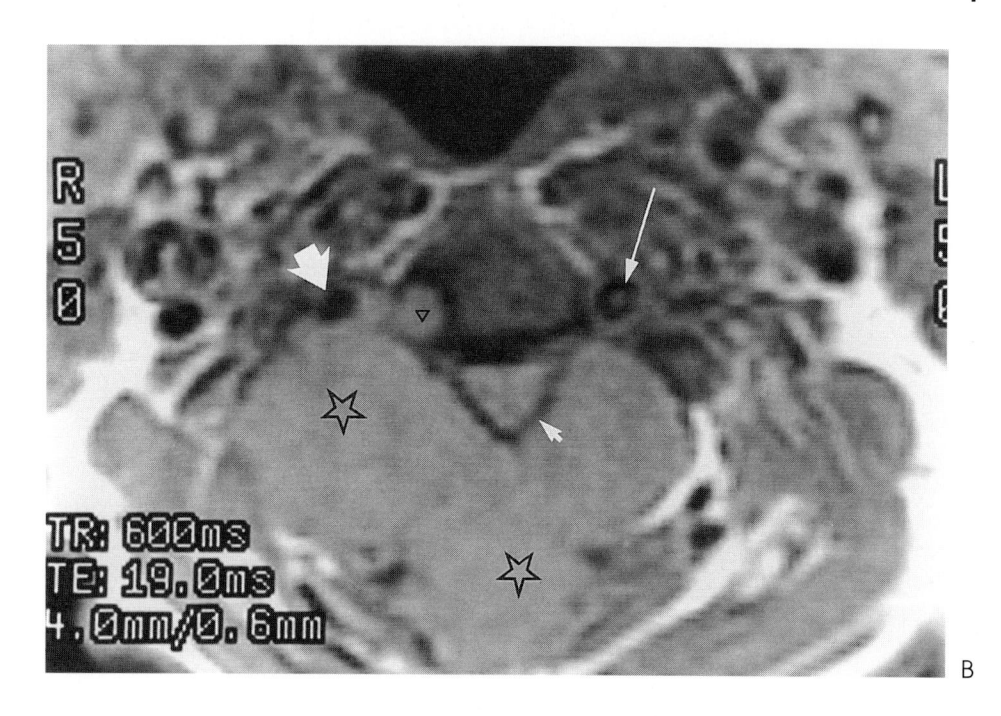

Axial short TR image precontrast (Fig. B) reveals that the spinous process, laminae, and lateral mass of C3 area are replaced by a decreased signal intensity process (*). There is obliteration of the subarachnoid space (*small arrow*). The area of enhancement in Figure A within the C3 vertebral body is identified in the right side of the vertebral body (*arrowhead*).

PEARL
• Treatment with radiation or surgery as well as follow-up can be based upon the magnetic resonance findings.

Diagnosis

Metastatic renal cell carcinoma involving the C3 vertebral body with cord compression.

Differential Diagnosis

• metastatic disease

PITFALL
• The marked compromise of the subarachnoid space is consistent with impending cord compression.

Discussion

The marrow of the vertebral bodies of C3 throughout the visualized cervical spine is probably replaced with decreased signal intensity tumor. There is only patchy enhancement of the areas of tumor involvement, except for the expanded tumor replaced spinous process of C3.

The vertebral artery appears as an area of flow void surrounded by tumor on the right side of the C3 vertebral body (Fig. B, *thick white arrow*). The left vertebral artery is seen with a central area of increased signal secondary to flow-related enhancement (Fig. B, *long thin arrow*).

The marrow of the vertebral bodies of C3 throughout the visualized cervical spine is probably replaced with decreased signal intensity tumor. This decreased signal intensity results in a "disc reversal" between the abnormal decreased signal marrow and the relatively increased signal intensity of the intervertebral disc. However, there is only patchy enhancement of the areas of tumor involvement, except for the expanded tumor replaced spinous process of C3. Note that the clivus is also replaced by decreased signal intensity tumor. The area of decreased signal intensity within the cervical spinal cord (seen in Fig. A) at the C3 level is secondary to edema.

Thyroid cancer metastatic to the bone could result in a similar appearance, as could a plasmacytoma. Metastatic lung or breast cancer are also considerations.

SPINE METASTASES

Case 16

Clinical Presentation

The patient is a 58-year-old female with lower extremity weakness.

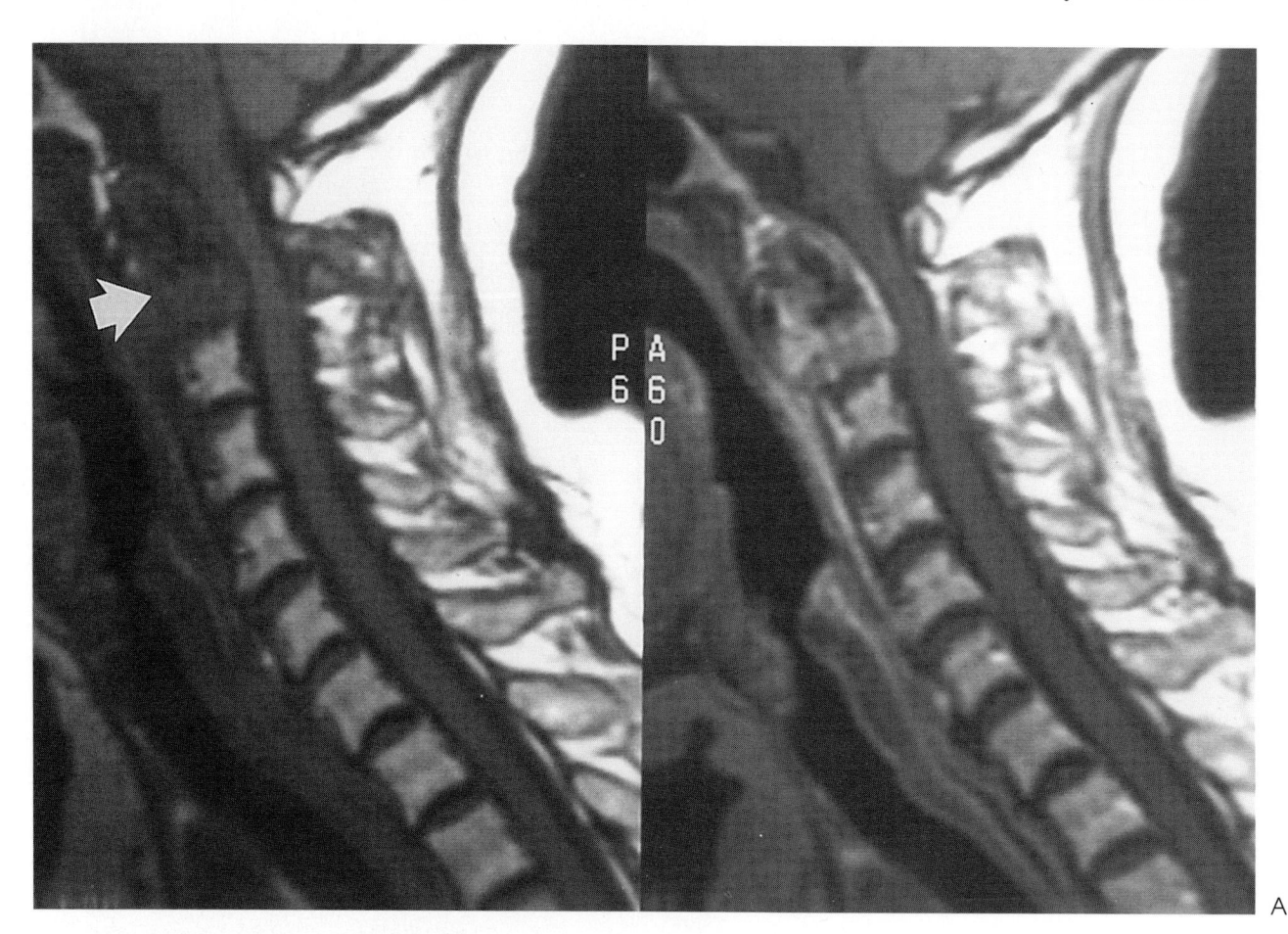

Radiologic Findings

Pre- (Fig. A, *left*) and postcontrast (Fig. A, *right*) sagittal short TR images reveal decreased signal intensity soft material replacing the odontoid process, the C2 vertebral body, and the posterior arch of C2 (*left, arrow*). The odontoid process is expanded and compromises the subarachnoid space, displacing the spinal cord posteriorly. The spinal cord is distorted in a curvilinear fashion at the C1-2 level. The postcontrast sagittal short TR image reveals dense enhancement of the peripheral margin of the odontoid process. The abnormality can be seen expanding the C2 vertebral body anteriorly and extending into the prevertebral space.

TEACHING ATLAS OF SPINE IMAGING

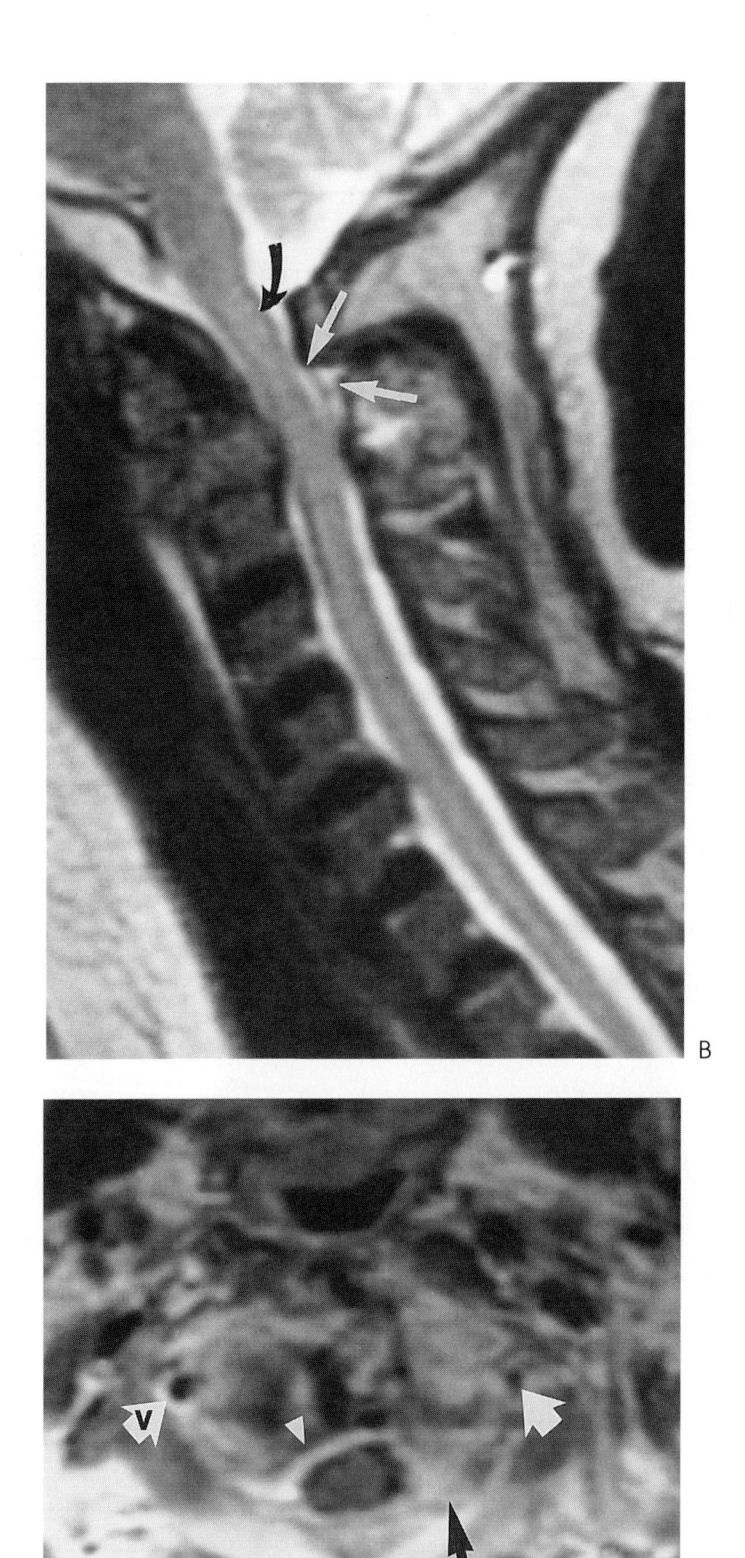

SPINE METASTASES

Case 22

Clinical Presentation

The patient, a 68-year-old male with known prostate cancer, presented 3 months ago with macroglobulinemia and new L1 level back pain without radicular component. He now presents with more marked low back pain.

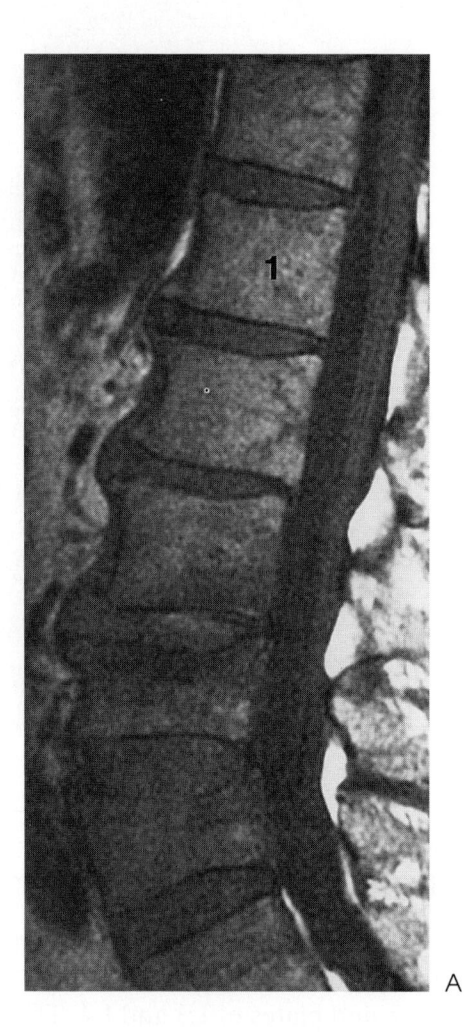

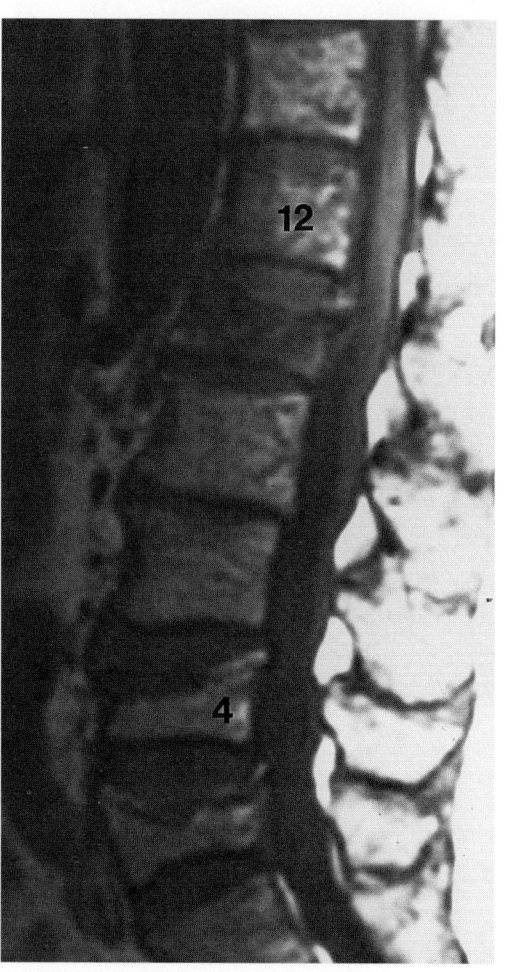

TEACHING ATLAS OF SPINE IMAGING

C

D

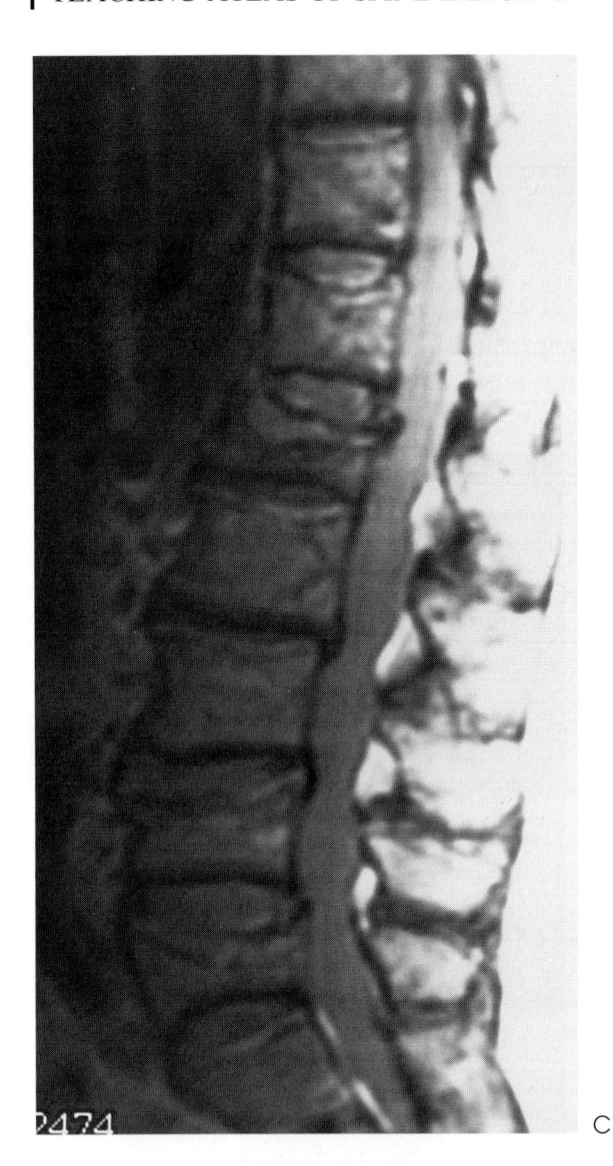

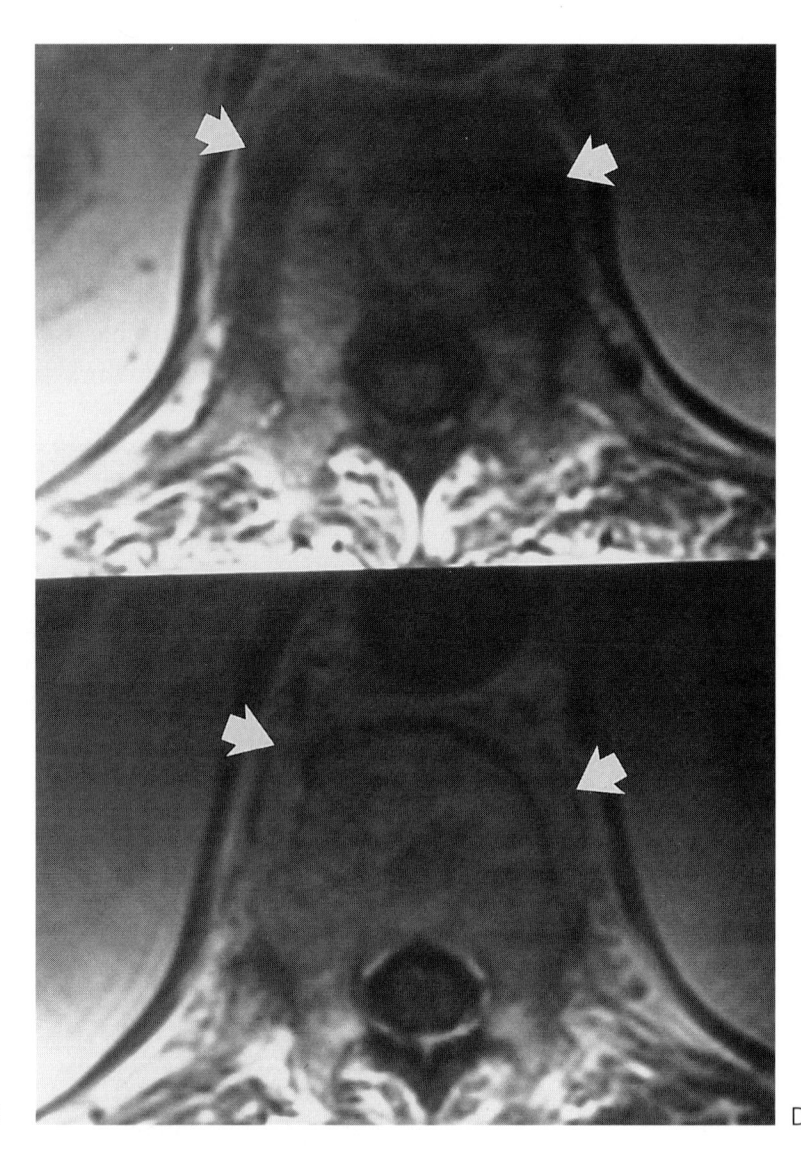

Radiologic Findings

Sagittal short TR image (Fig. A) reveals mild compression fractures of L4 and L5. There is decreased signal intensity of the vertebral body end plates adjacent to the end plates of L3 and L4. There is anterior herniation of the disc at the L3-4 level. The remainder of the vertebral bodies reveal a few minor scattered areas of decreased signal intensity. The L1 vertebral body is identified with 1.

Three months later the patient presents with even more marked low back pain. Sagittal short TR image at the time of follow-up (Fig. B) reveals a new compression fracture of L1. There is retropulsion of the posterior superior corner of the L1 vertebral body into the vertebral canal with obliteration of the subarachnoid space. There is encroachment upon the vertebral canal anteriorly at this level. The spinal cord is displaced posteriorly, and increased compression deformity of the L4 (*4*) and L5 vertebral bodies can be noted. The remainder of the vertebral bodies reveal mottled decreased signal intensity within the marrow spaces. The T12 vertebral body is identified with 12.

SPINE METASTASES

Radiologic Findings (continued)

Long TR image (Fig. C) reveals the mottled signal intensity of the marrow within the vertebral bodies and better demonstrates the encroachment upon the vertebral canal at L1. The vertebral pedicles are expanded bilaterally.

Pre- (Fig. D, *top*) and postcontrast (Fig. D, *bottom*) axial short TR images at the L4 level obtained reveal diffuse enhancement of the vertebral body on the postcontrast image. A small paraspinal mass that surrounds the vertebral body (*bottom, arrows*) is also visible. Importantly, there is destruction of the normally decreased signal intensity cortical margin of the vertebral body on the right side (*top, arrows*).

PEARL
- The diffuse involvement of all the visualized bony structures with very small decreased signal metastases is typical of myeloma.

PITFALL
- The patient could also have metastatic prostate cancer, as this cancer may metastasize with a similar appearing pattern. However, the cortical bone destruction is more in favor of multiple myeloma. Metastases from prostate cancer are more likely to be osteoblastic.

Diagnosis

Multiple myeloma with rapid progression.

Differential Diagnosis

- multiple myeloma
- metastatic disease

Discussion

The rapid progression may be seen in multiple myeloma. Clinical correlation should be performed with serum electrophoresis and identification of the typical Bence Jones proteins in urine. Metastatic prostate cancer would also be a consideration; however, no focal lesions are seen. The absence of focal lesions does not rule out metastatic prostate cancer, as occasionally the appearance could be similar to this case. Therefore, clinical correlation with the other laboratory tests, particularly protein electrophoresis, is necessary. The rapid progression could occur in either disease.

TEACHING ATLAS OF SPINE IMAGING

Case 23

Clinical Presentation

The patient is a 72-year-old male with a history of anemia and lower extremity weakness.

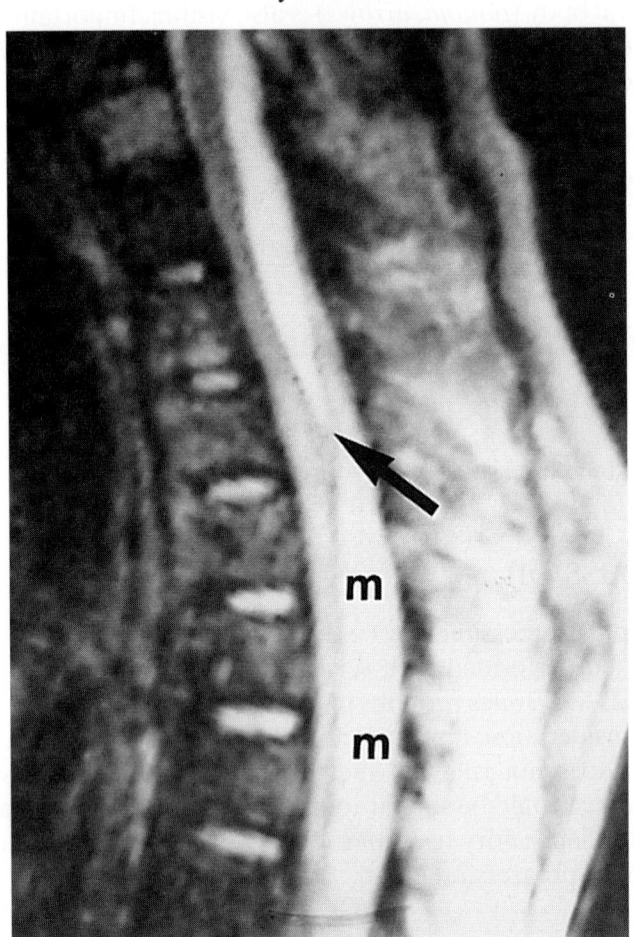

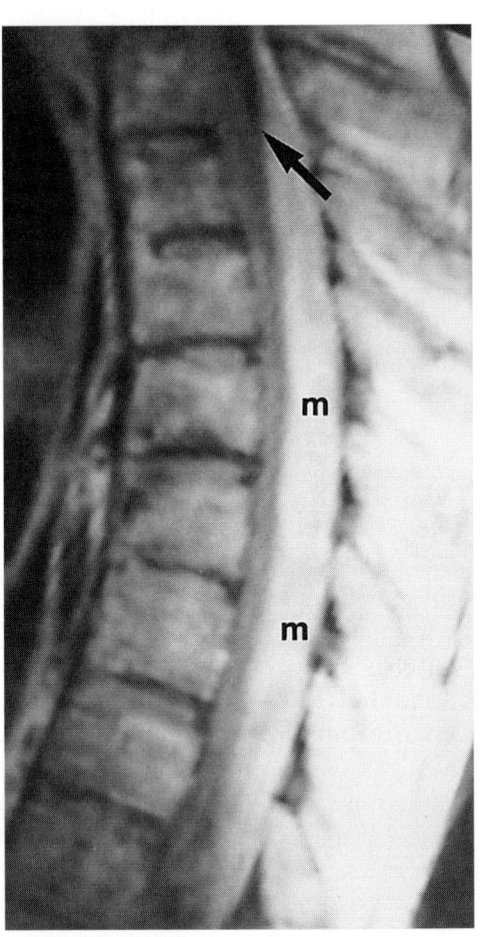

Radiologic Findings

Sagittal long TR image of the lower cervical and upper thoracic spine (Fig. A) reveals mottled signal intensity of multiple vertebral bodies. There is increased signal intensity in the C7 vertebral body. Incidentally noted are mild degenerative changes in the cervical spine. The spinous processes are also involved with decreased signal intensity metastatic disease. In the thoracic region, beginning dorsally at the T2-3 level, there is a soft tissue epidural mass (*m*) that extends inferiorly. The thoracic spinal cord is displaced anteriorly and compressed against the posterior margin of the thoracic vertebral bodies. The cerebrospinal fluid-containing space posterior to the spinal cord at the C7 through T2 level is enlarged. The spinal cord, soft tissue mass, and expanded cerebrospinal fluid space meet at the T3 level (*arrow*).

Sagittal short TR image after contrast enhancement (Fig. B) reveals dense homogeneous enhancement of the epidural mass (*m*). The thoracic spinal cord appears as an area of intermediate signal intensity compressed against

SPINE METASTASES

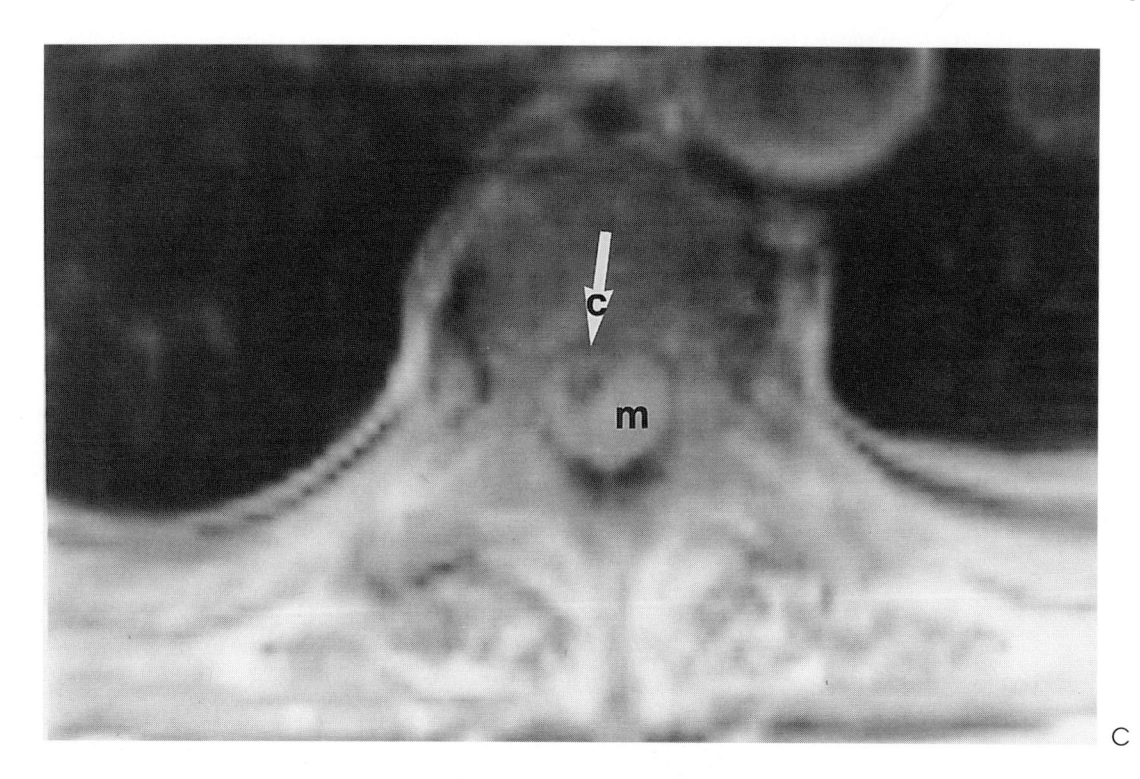

the posterior margin of the vertebral bodies. The narrowed subarachnoid space projects anterior to the mass and behind the spinal cord (*arrow*).

Axial short TR postcontrast image (Fig. C) reveals the soft tissue mass (*m*) almost totally surrounding the thoracic spinal cord (*arrow-c*). The spinal cord is compressed into a triangular shaped mass.

PEARLS
- Chloroma may also result in a similar appearance.
- Findings should be correlated with a history of any known primary cancer.

PITFALL
- Metastases of any type could cause a similar appearance.

Diagnosis

Multiple myeloma involving the bony structures and forming a soft tissue mass dorsal to the spinal cord resulting in cord compression.

Differential Diagnosis

- multiple myeloma
- chloroma
- metastatic disease

Discussion

Multiple myeloma is typically a disease of the marrow of the bones; however, it may occasionally present, as this patient did, with a soft tissue mass. Myeloma and plasmacytoma may also occur in the soft tissues remote from the bony structures. A chloroma or metastatic disease from a variety of primaries may also have a similar appearance. These include metastatic breast and lung cancer as well as more unusual primary tumors.

The diagnosis was confirmed at surgery, and CT-guided needle biopsy or open surgical biopsy may be necessary for final diagnosis.

Case 24

Clinical Presentation

The patient is a 68-year-old female with a severe low back pain and lower extremity weakness.

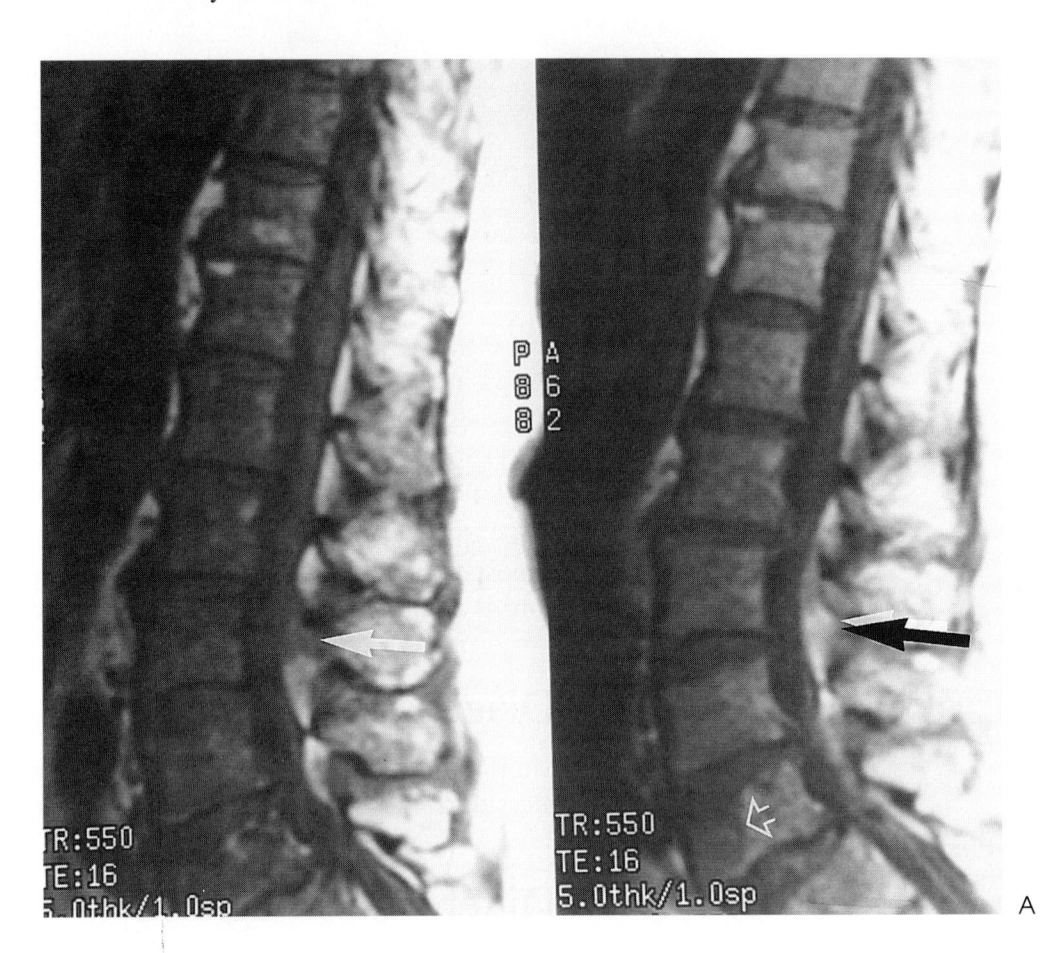

Radiologic Findings

Pre- (Fig. A, *left*) and postcontrast (Fig. A, *right*) sagittal short TR images reveal replacement of the normal high signal intensity epidural fat with decreased signal intensity tumor at the level of L3 (*left, white arrow*). This soft tissue mass enhances following the infusion of contrast material (*right, black and white arrow*). There is a compression fracture of the L5 vertebral body and a faint area of decreased signal intensity is seen in the anterior portion of the L5 vertebral body (*right, open white arrow*). Incidentally there are degenerative changes at multiple levels with anterior and posterior osteophytes. The marrow within the vertebral bodies reveals a faint pattern of mottled decreased signal intensity on the precontrast scan and diffuse enhancement post contrast.

SPINE METASTASES

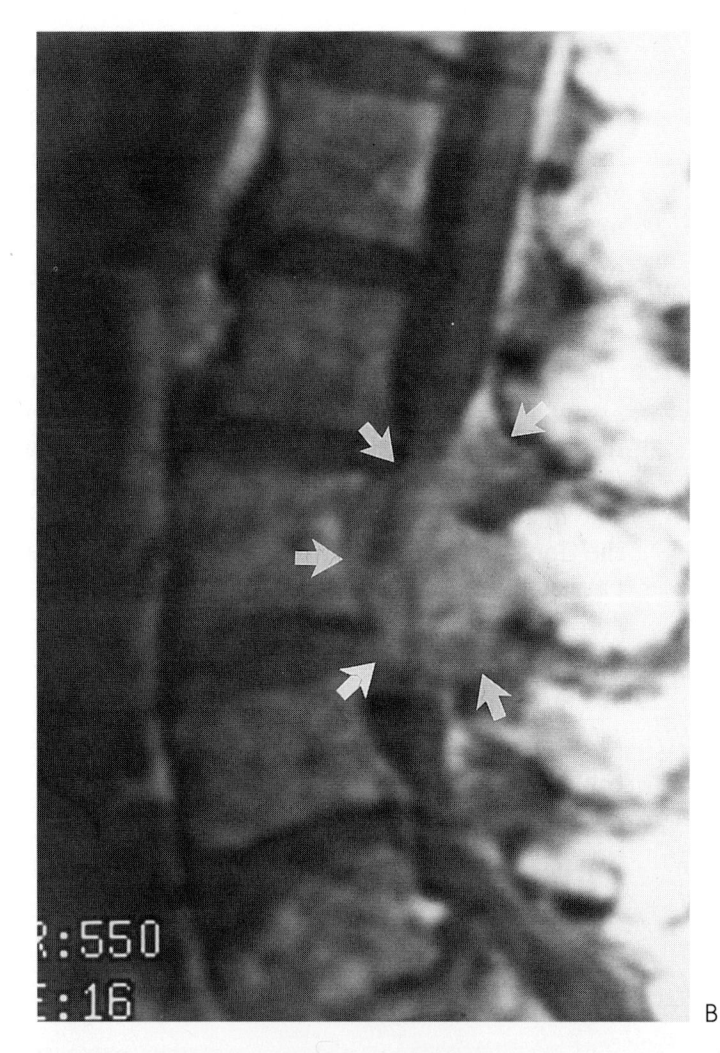

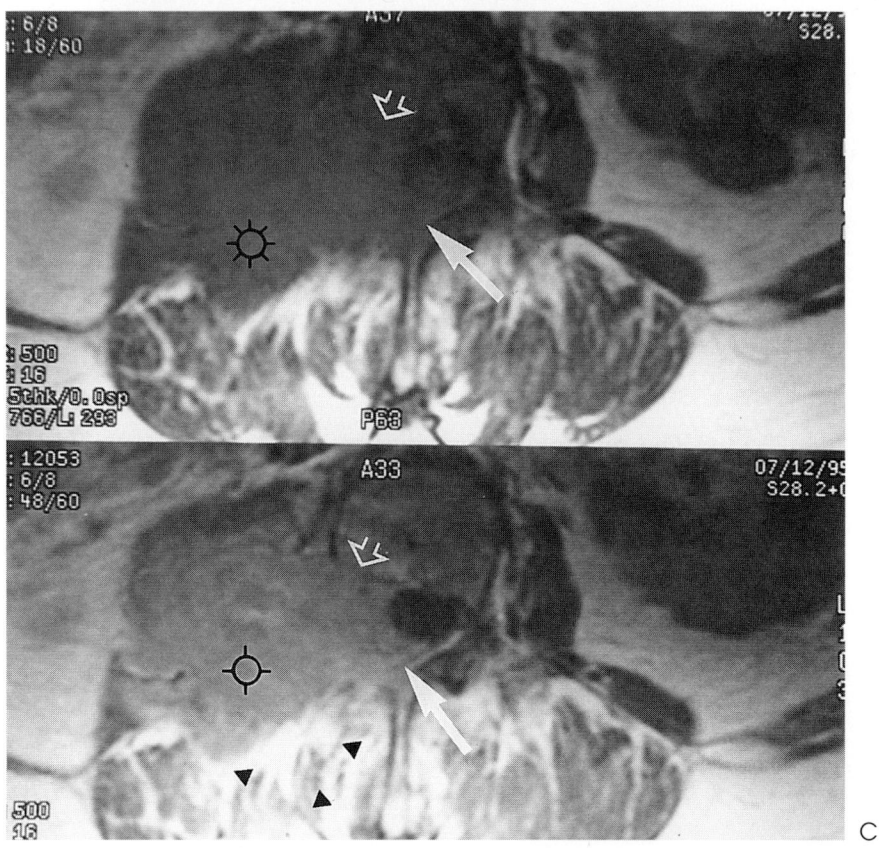

B

C

Radiologic Findings (continued)

Parasagittal postcontrast short TR image (Fig. B) reveals an enhancing soft tissue mass on the right side (*arrows*). The mass obliterates the normal epidural fat and compresses the thecal sac along the upper margin of the mass.

Axial short TR image obtained pre- (Fig. C, *top*) and postcontrast (Fig. C, *bottom*). There is a soft tissue mass in the right paraspinal region (*asterisk*) that extends medially into the vertebral canal via the intervertebral foramen. The mass erodes the posterior margin of the vertebral body (*open white arrow*) and extends into the vertebral canal. The mass extends dorsally within the vertebral canal to obliterate the dorsal epidural high signal intensity fat (*solid arrow*). This is at the level of L3, as identified on the sagittal view. The mass enhances post contrast (*bottom*). There is probably extension into the dorsal paraspinal muscles. There appears to be fatty infiltration of the paraspinal muscles (*top, arrowheads*).

PEARL
- The postcontrast appearance of the vertebral bodies is essentially normal. While this appearance may be seen with any metastatic tumor, multiple myeloma is the primary tumor that typically results in this diffuse homogeneous enhancement.

Diagnosis

Multiple myeloma with diffuse infiltration of the bone marrow of the vertebral bodies and with a soft tissue mass.

Differential Diagnosis

- metastatic disease
- multiple myeloma
- Ewing's sarcoma

PITFALLS
- Multiple myeloma may present with a wide variety of appearances. A number of metastatic tumors might have a similar appearance.

Discussion

In an elderly female patient, a disease such as metastatic breast or lung cancer are strong considerations. In a male patient, metastatic prostate carcinoma may have a similar appearance. A primary thyroid cancer with metastases could also have a similar appearance. In a much younger patient, Ewing's sarcoma might have a similar appearance. Ewing's sarcoma tends to have a small component extending into the vertebral canal, but a large soft tissue component.

The multiplanar imaging of magnetic resonance allows the evaluation of the paraspinal regions and the determination of the extent of the soft tissue component. The entire vertebral column should be evaluated.

Case 25

Clinical Presentation

The patient is a 69-year-old female with a rapidly progressive paraplegia and a history of chronic renal failure.

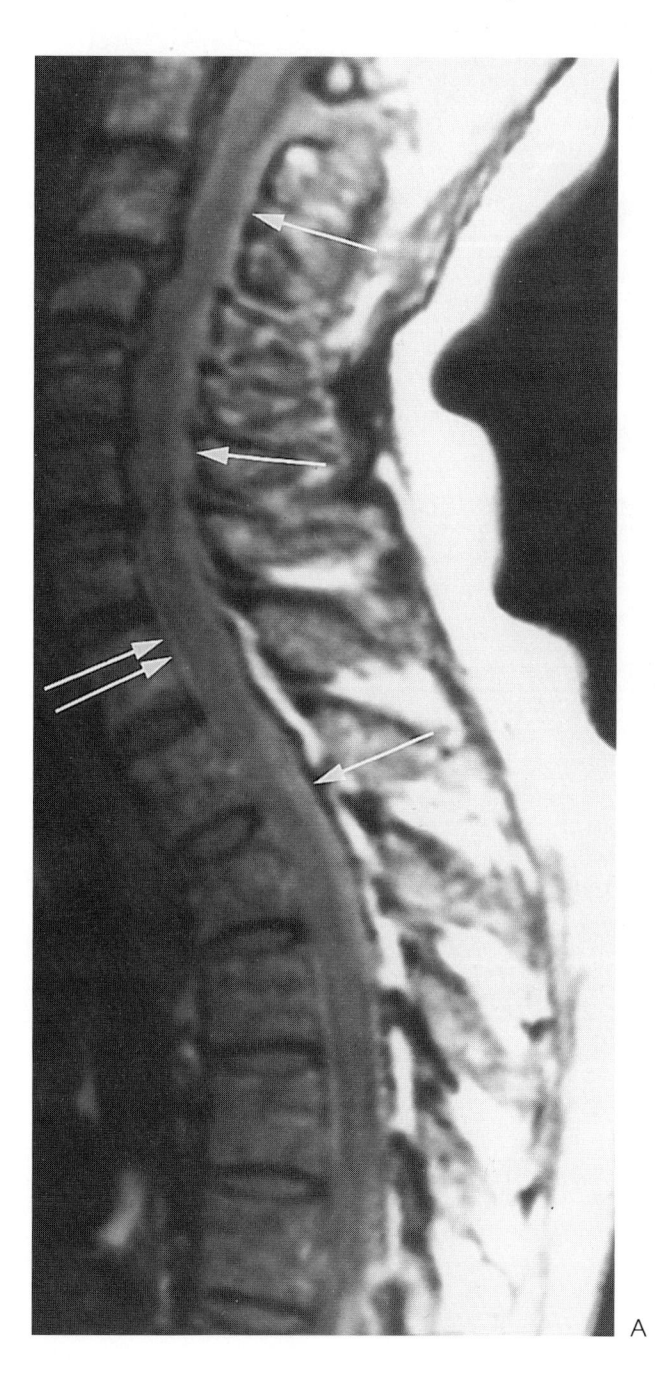

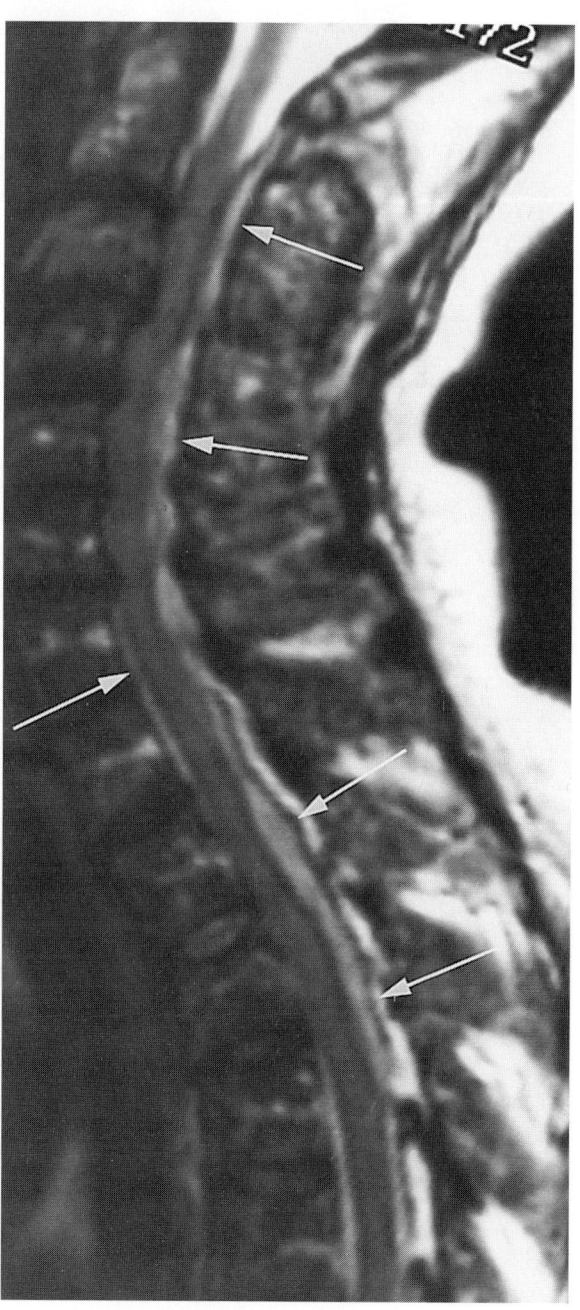

TEACHING ATLAS OF SPINE IMAGING

C

D

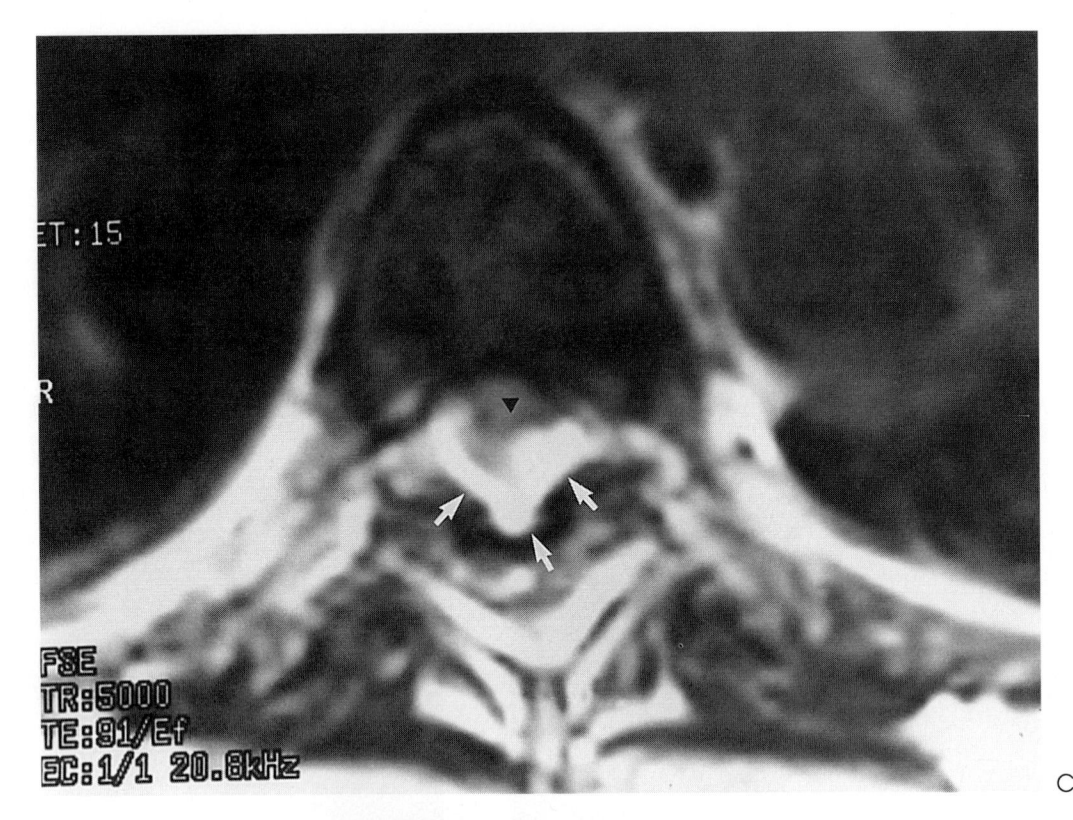

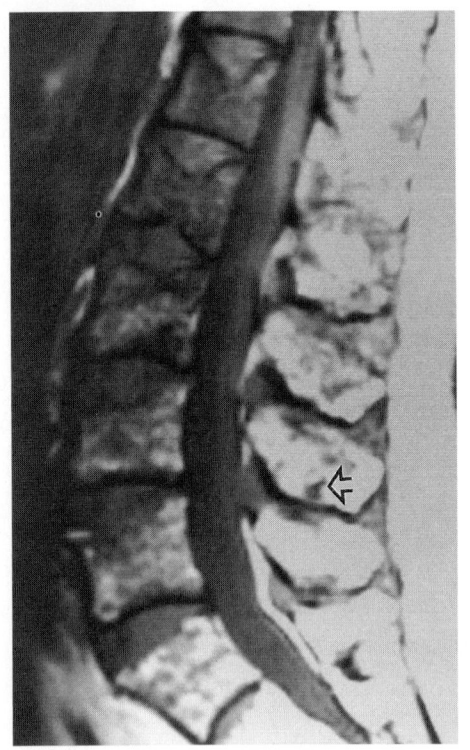

408

SPINE METASTASES

Radiologic Findings

Sagittal short TR image in the cervical and upper thoracic region (Fig. A) reveals a slightly irregularly marginated area of increased signal intensity dorsal to the spinal cord throughout the entire visualized length (*single arrows*). There is a smaller linear area of increased signal intensity anterior to the spinal cord at the C7-T1 level (*double arrows anteriorly*). The normal increased signal intensity epidural fat has been obliterated. The vertebral bodies reveal diffuse mottled decreased signal intensity.

Sagittal long TR image (Fig. B) reveals that the area of increased signal demonstrated in Figure A now appears even greater in increased signal intensity both anterior and posterior to the spinal cord (*arrows*). The vertebral marrow reveals patchy areas of increased signal intensity.

Axial short TR image (Fig. C) reveals bilateral areas of increased signal intensity masses (*white arrows*) that are displacing the cord (*black arrowhead anteriorly*) and compressing it. Increased signal intensity pleural effusions are visible bilaterally.

Sagittal short TR image in the lumber region (Fig. D) reveals that every visualized vertebral body contains small areas of decreased signal intensity. These areas are also present in the spinous processes. One is well demonstrated at the L4 level (*open arrow*). Compression fractures of multiple vertebral bodies can be noted.

Diagnosis

Multiple myeloma; multilevel epidural hematoma predominantly posteriorly, but also present anteriorly; bilateral bloody pleural effusions (Fig. C, *open arrows*).

Differential Diagnosis

- multiple myeloma

- metastatic disease

Discussion

Patients with multiple myeloma may have abnormalities of many organ systems. This patient exhibits the typical changes of multiple myeloma in the marrow of the vertebral bodies, but in addition, has an epidural hematoma secondary to low platelets that has resulted in spinal cord compression.

If a postinfusion-only magnetic resonance study is performed, one could mistake the increased signal intensity areas of blood for areas of enhancement. Therefore, a study should not be performed postinfusion only.

The subtle interruption of epidural fat may be difficult to appreciate but may be identified with careful evaluation.

Metastatic breast cancer in a female and metastatic prostate cancer in a male could also have a similar appearance as the bony changes in this patient. Epidural hematoma in a patient with multiple myeloma is a diagnostic consideration. Cases of multiple myeloma with masslike lesions may result in a similar appearance (see Case 23).

PEARLS

- Bleeding tendencies must be evaluated clinically.

- The possibility of two disease processes in a single patient, as seen in this case, must be considered.

PITFALL

- Osteoporosis, which may also lead to multiple compression fractures, results in increased signal intensity within the vertebral bodies secondary to increased fat deposition. Multiple myeloma results in decreased signal intensity tumor replacing the normal marrow.

TEACHING ATLAS OF SPINE IMAGING

Case 26

Clinical Presentation

The patient is a 68-year-old female with a clinical history of stiff neck and a 5-day history of increased neck pain with head rotation.

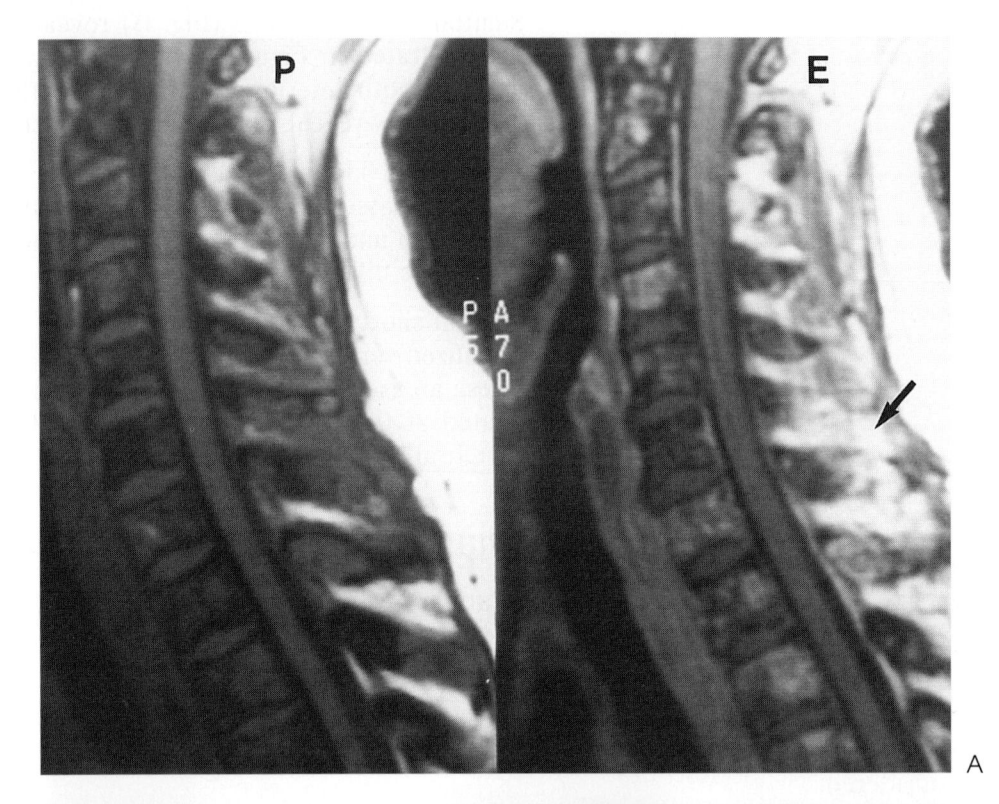

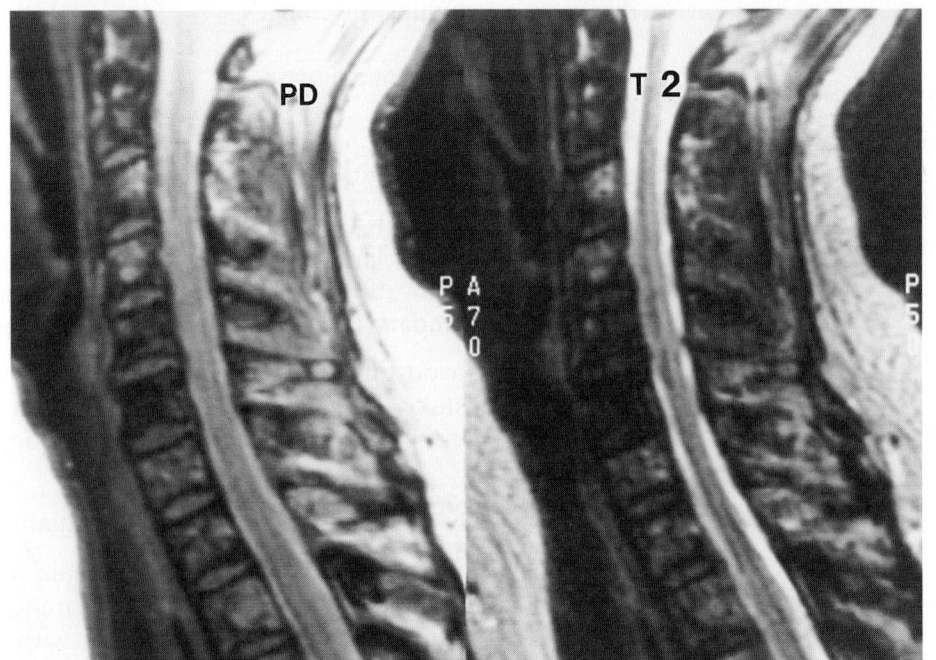

SPINE METASTASES

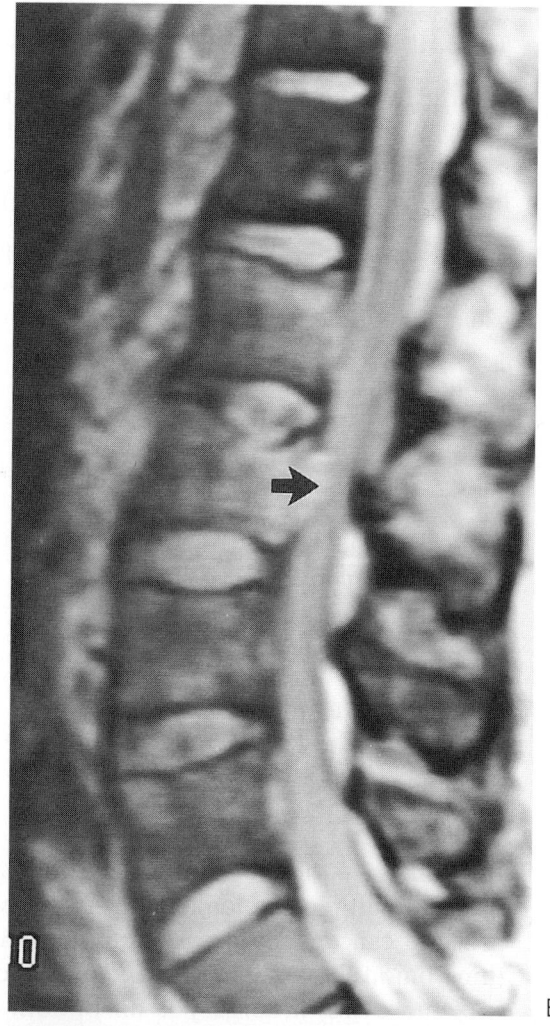

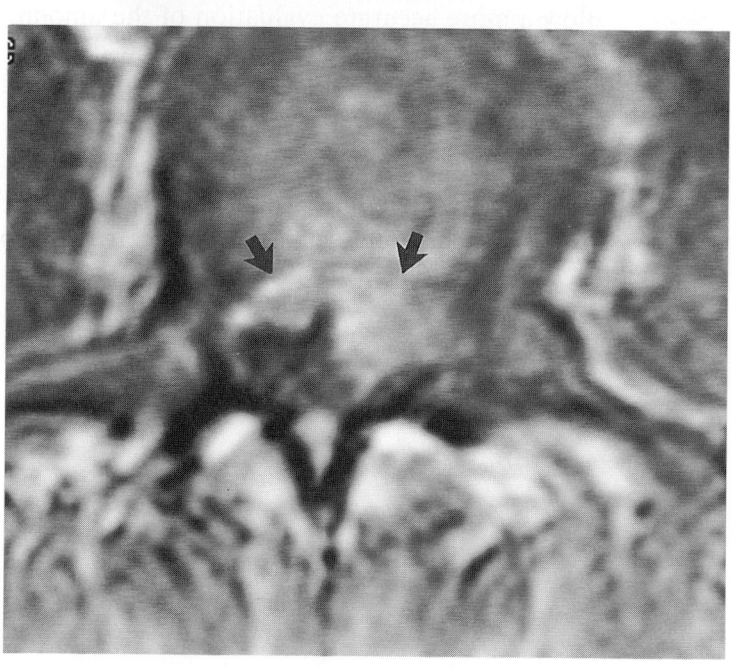

Radiologic Findings (continued)

Sagittal long TR image (Fig. B) reveals that there is variable increased signal intensity of the vertebral metastases. The para-aortic lymph nodes also become increased signal intensity. The retropulsed portion of the L3 vertebral body is seen in the vertebral canal (*arrow*).

Axial short TR postcontrast image (Fig. C) reveals lobulated tumor extending into the vertebral canal (*black arrows*) and compressing the thecal sac and cauda equina. There is involvement of the pedicle on the left side.

PEARL
- Fat saturation postcontrast study may better identify bony metastases.

PITFALL
- Magnetic resonance imaging may not allow differentiation between soft tissue metastatic disease versus bony metastases encroaching upon the vertebral canal. CT scanning may be necessary to differentiate between the two processes if surgery is contemplated for relief of symptoms of cord compression.

Diagnosis

Metastatic osteoblastic prostate carcinoma.

Differential Diagnosis

- metastatic disease
- multiple myeloma

Discussion

In addition to the most likely diagnosis of metastatic prostate cancer in this patient, multiple myeloma might also have a similar appearance. Metastatic prostate cancer may occasionally have very subtle presentation with very thin "onion skin paper"–like metastatic disease with expansion of the bone. In some cases, if surgery is an option, computed tomography (CT) may allow a more accurate evaluation of the amount of bone involvement with resulting compromise of the vertebral canal or spinal cord. In a female patient, metastatic breast cancer should also be considered in multiple myeloma.

A CT-guided bone biopsy or even open decompressive biopsy may be necessary for complete evaluation. Radionuclide scanning may also allow for a more accurate evaluation of the true extent of the disease.

SPINE METASTASES

Case 29

Clinical Presentation

The patient is a 43-year-old female with known diffuse osteoblastic bony metastases who now presents with severe low back pain and leg weakness.

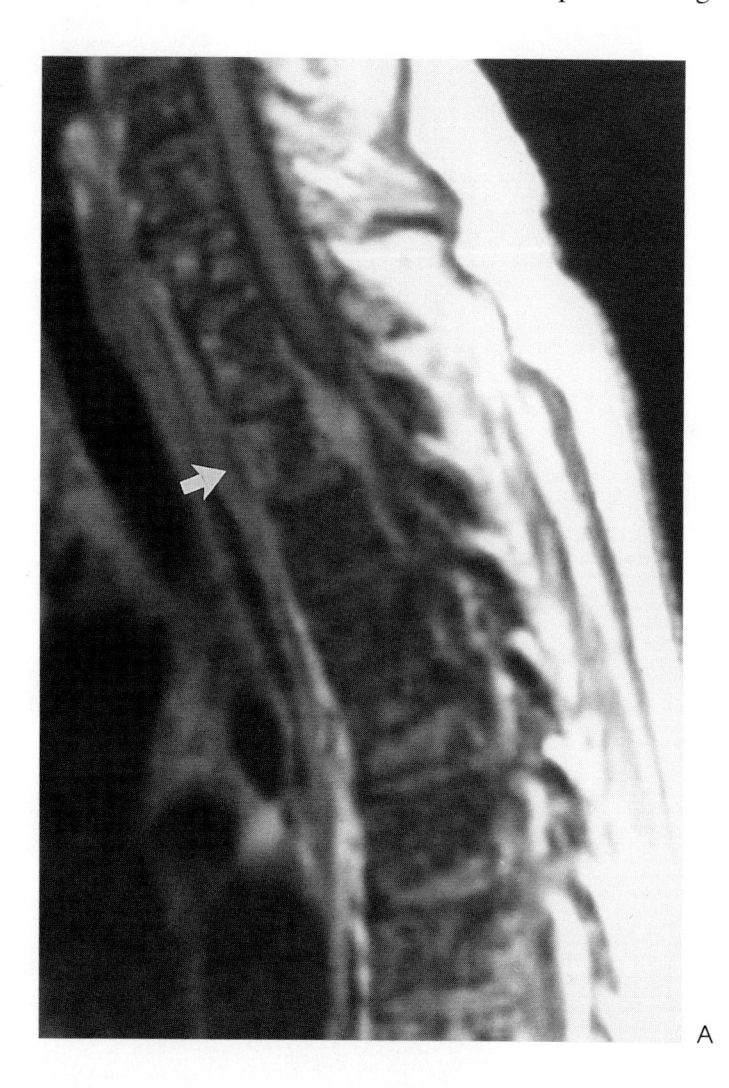

Radiologic Findings

Sagittal short TR image of the lower cervical and upper thoracic spine (Fig. A) reveals that all the vertebral bodies are diffusely replaced with decreased signal intensity soft tissue. In addition, there is a soft tissue component that encroaches upon the vertebral canal in the lower cervical region, obliterating the cervical spinal cord (*white arrow*). The spinous processes and the interfacet joints are also diffusely involved with low signal intensity soft tissue material.

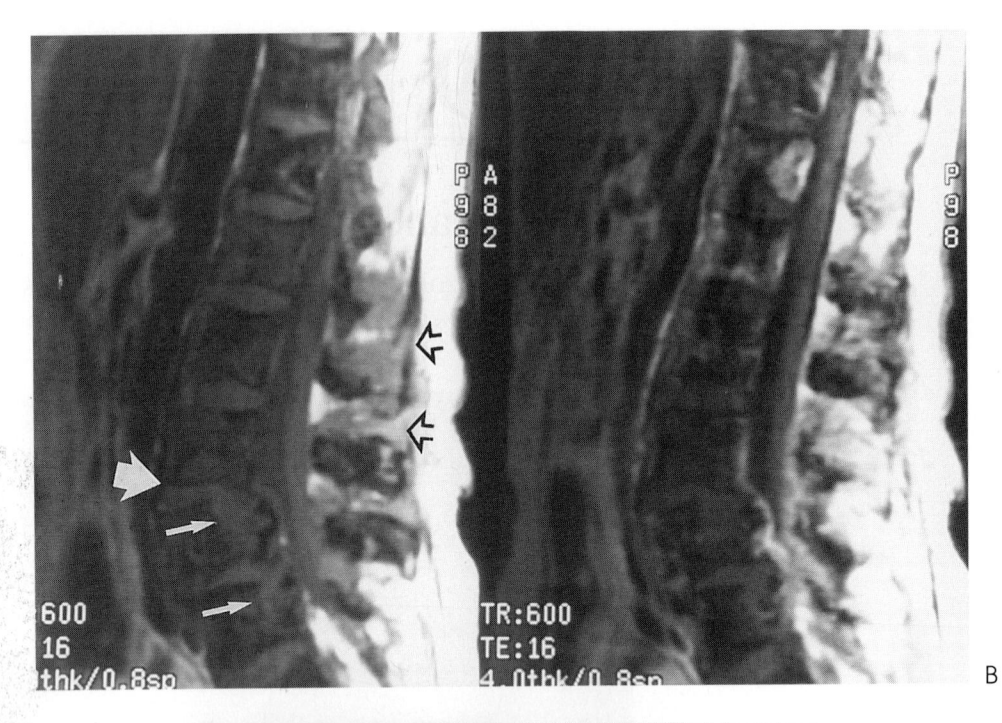

TEACHING ATLAS OF SPINE IMAGING

B

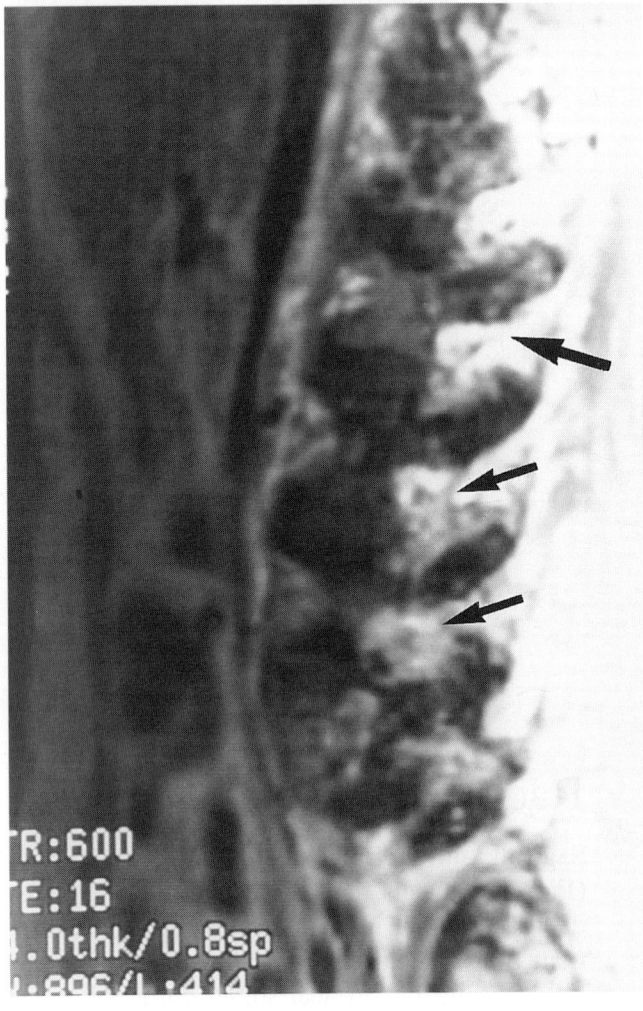

C

SPINE METASTASES

Radiologic Findings (continued)

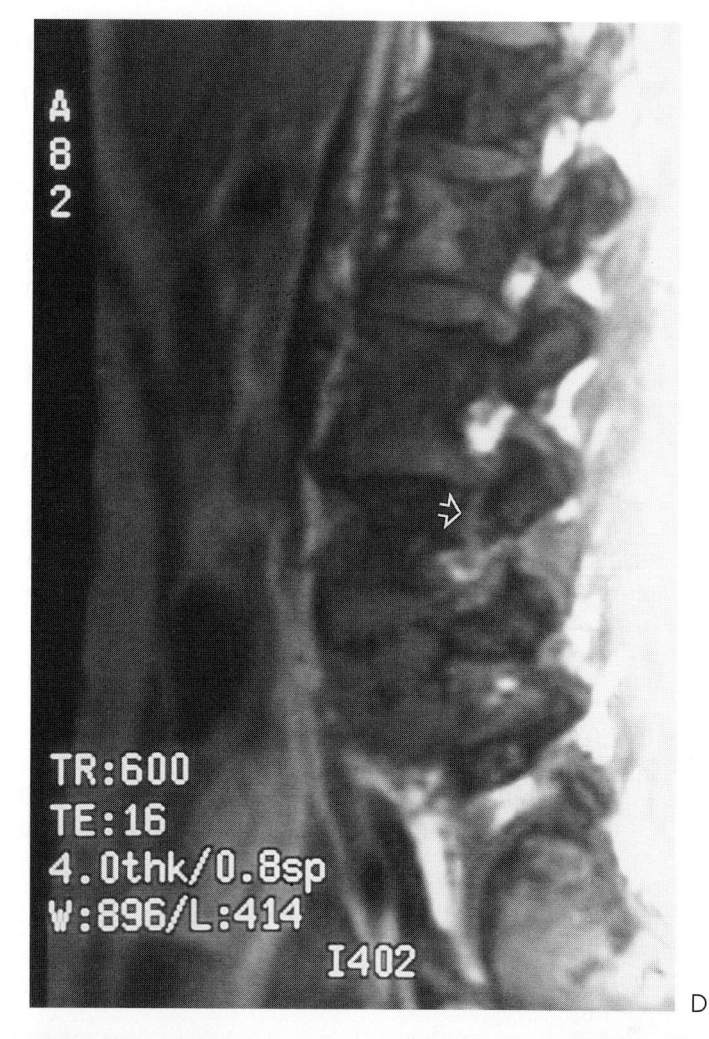

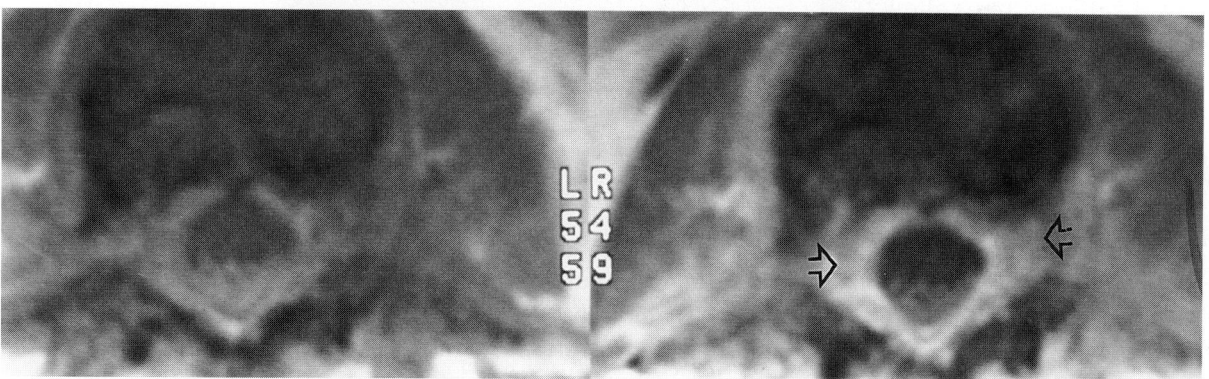

Sagittal short TR images in the lumbar region obtained pre- (Fig. B, *left*) and postcontrast (Fig. B, *right*) reveal diffuse replacement of all the visualized body structures, with decreased signal intensity soft tissue material metastases. There is intermediate signal intensity soft tissue density material surrounding the spinous processes at multiple levels (*left, open arrows*). There are vertical fractures through the L4 and L5 vertebral bodies (*left,*

TEACHING ATLAS OF SPINE IMAGING

Radiologic Findings (continued)

small solid arrows). There is forward displacement of L3 relative to L4 (*left, thick solid arrow*). The postcontrast images reveal variable enhancement.

Parasagittal short TR image postcontrast at the level of the lumbar intervertebral foramen (Fig. C) reveals a "halo" of soft tissue metastatic disease surrounding all the intervertebral foramen (*black arrows*). There is also encroachment upon the intervertebral foramen at all levels with enhancing soft tissue.

There is a fracture through the pedicle of the L3 vertebral body (Fig. D, *open arrow*).

Axial short TR images obtained pre- (Fig. E, *left*) and postcontrast (Fig. E, *right*) reveal diffuse involvement of the vertebral body with a soft tissue component. The postcontrast study reveals the paraspinal soft tissue component, which exhibits enhancement. The mass is larger on the left side than on the right side. There is extension into the intervertebral foramen bilaterally (*right, arrows*).

PEARLS
- The entire vertebral column should be evaluated in a patient with metastatic disease.
- Osteolytic metastases may become osteoblastic deposits after chemotherapy or radiation therapy when tumor growth has slowed sufficiently to allow bone growth.

PITFALL
- A surgical approach to a patient such as this would probably not be successful because there is no focal mass that could be removed.

Diagnosis

Diffuse osteoblastic metastatic disease with mild soft tissue component in the lower cervical region and multiple pathologic fractures.

Differential Diagnosis

- osteoblastic metastatic disease
- multiple myeloma
- metastatic disease

Discussion

Osteoblastic metastatic breast cancer may remain relatively stable in appearance for long periods of time. If sufficiently extensive, as in this patient, there may be a soft tissue component with extension into the vertebral canal and into the foramina, which results in severe constriction of the nerve structures. Such severe involvement, as in this case, is not amenable to surgical treatment. This patient's postinfusion scan highlights the soft tissue component of the soft tissues of the interspinous ligament. This latter finding is somewhat unusual. If involvement is sufficiently extensive, the scan may, in some patients with less advanced disease, appear almost normal. Therefore, the index of suspicion should be high and correlation performed with other tests, such as radionuclide scanning as well as CT-guided bone biopsy. In any patient with metastatic disease, the entire length of the vertebral column should be evaluated. In a male patient, metastatic prostate cancer would be the most likely diagnosis.

SPINE METASTASES

Case 30

Clinical Presentation

The patient is an 18-year-old with known osteogenic sarcoma of the lower extremity who now presents with lower extremity weakness.

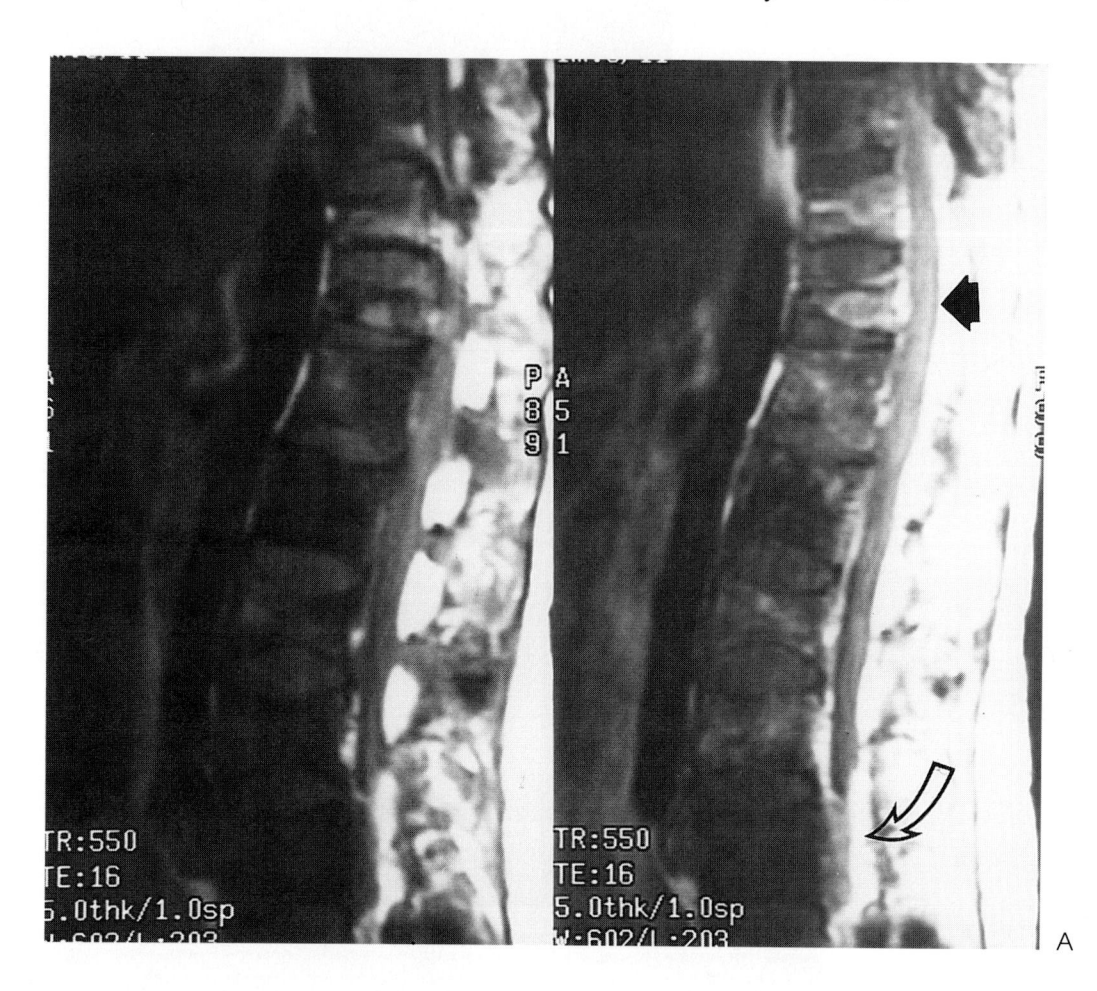

Radiologic Findings

Pre- (Fig. A, *left*) and postcontrast (Fig. A, *right*) sagittal short TR images of the lumbar spine reveal pathologic compression fractures of all of the lumbar vertebral bodies except L2 and L5. In addition, all the visualized vertebral bodies are replaced with markedly decreased signal intensity tissue. There is expansion of the L5 vertebral body with encroachment upon the lumbar subarachnoid space. The postcontrast study reveals enhancement of the T12 vertebral body (*right, broad arrow*) and enhancement of the tissue extending posterior to the vertebral body of L5 (*open curved arrow*).

421

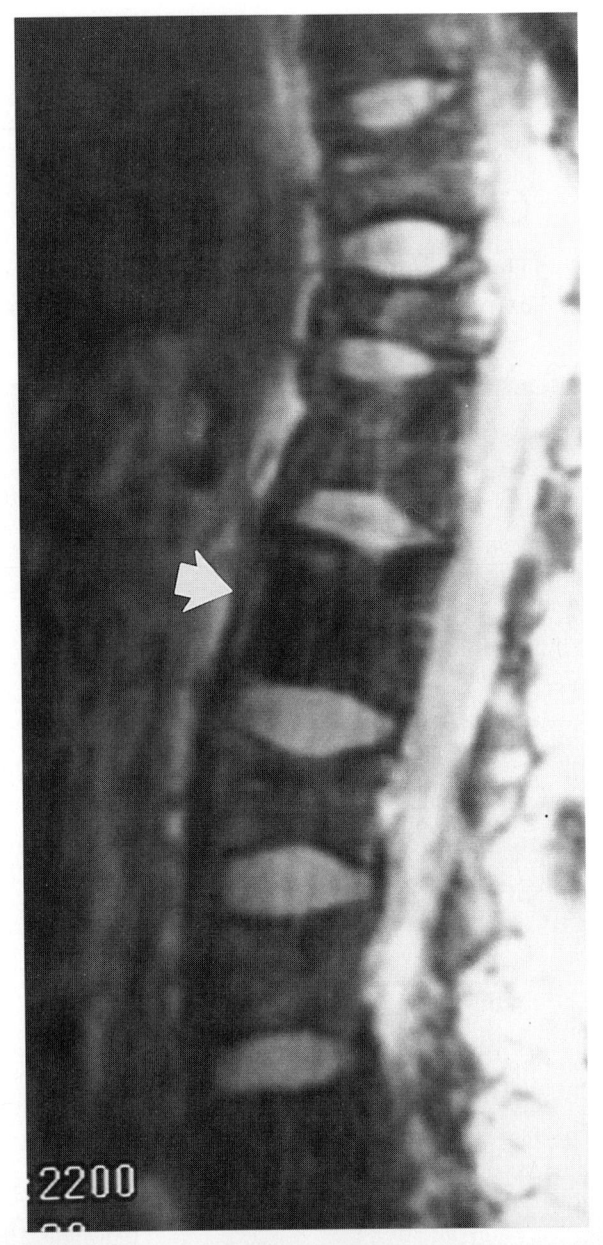

TEACHING ATLAS OF SPINE IMAGING

B

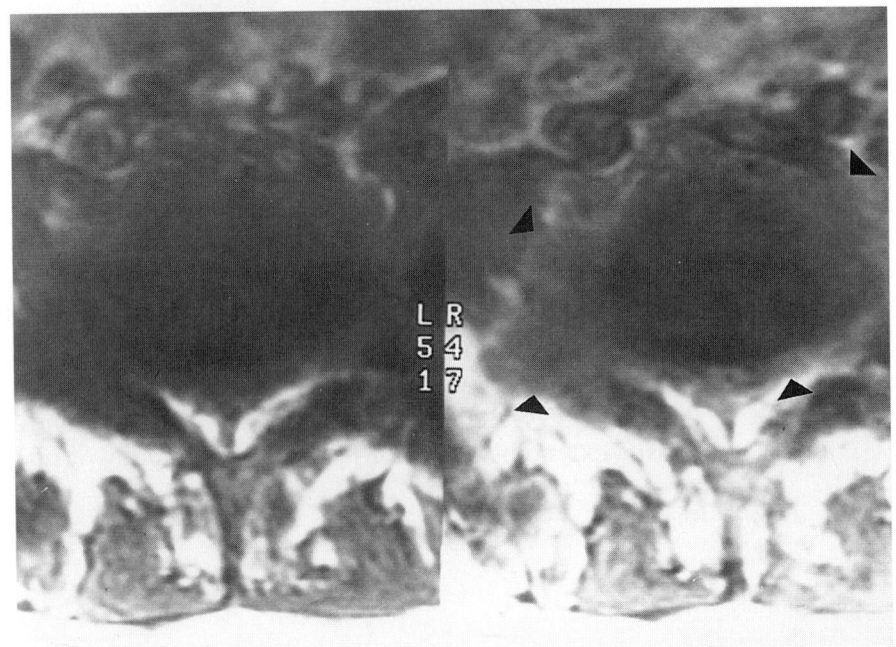

C

SPINE METASTASES

Radiologic Findings (continued)

Sagittal long TR image in the lumbar region (Fig. B) reveals that the intervertebral disc appear increased signal intensity. However the vertebral bodies continue to appear markedly decreased in signal intensity. There is retropulsion of the posterior margin of one of the upper vertebral bodies into the vertebral canal. The L2 vertebral body has *preservation* of the normal height but is markedly decreased in signal intensity (*arrow*).

Pre- (Fig. C, *left*) and postcontrast (Fig. C, *right*) axial short TR images reveal the ill-defined peripheral margin of the L5 vertebral body with the enhancing soft tissue surrounding the vertebral body (*right, arrowheads*).

> **PEARL**
> - Osteoblastic metastases reveal diffuse decreased signal intensity in response to all pulse sequences.

> **PITFALL**
> - If the involvement is diffuse and symmetric, the study could potentially appear normal.

Diagnosis

Diffuse osteoblastic metastases from the patient's known primary osteogenic sarcoma.

Differential Diagnosis

- osteoblastic metastatic disease

Discussion

In a young patient with less extensive disease, the decreased signal intensity marrow could be interpreted as normal. However, the presence of multiple compression fractures is definitely abnormal. Radionuclide bone scanning might be helpful for more complete evaluation.

In the presence of osteoblastic bony metastases, osteogenic sarcoma is a strong consideration. In the very young patient, medulloblastoma may also exhibit osteoblastic metastases and would be a consideration. Neuroblastoma may also exhibit diffuse involvement. The clinical history and evaluation of other organ systems would be helpful for more complete evaluation and would be necessary in any patient such as this.

In a female patient, metastatic osteoblastic breast cancer could have this appearance; while in a male, metastatic prostate cancer could have this appearance.

Suggested Readings

Abrahams JJ, Wood GW, Eames FA, Hicks RA. CT-guided needle aspiration biopsy of an intraspinal synovial cyst (ganglion): case report and review of the literature. *AJNR.* 1988;9:398–400.

Bender CE, Berquist TH, Wold LE. Imaging assisted percutaneous biopsy of the thoracic spine. *Mayo Clin Proc.* 1986;61:942–950.

Black P. Spinal metastasis: current status and recommended guidelines for management. *Neurosurgery.* 1979;5:726–746.

Boukobza M, Mazel C, Touboul E. Primary vertebral and spinal epidural non-Hodgkin's lymphoma with spinal cord compression. *Neuroradiol.* 1996;38:333–337.

Brugieres P, Gaston A, Heran F, Voisin MC, Marsault C. Percutaneous biopsies of the thoracic spine under CT guidance: transcostovertebral approach. *JCAT.* 1990;14:446–448.

Byrne TN, Waxman SG. Paraplegia and spinal cord syndromes. In: Bradley WG, Daroff RB, Fenichel GM, Marsden CE, eds. *Neurology in Clinical Practice: Principles of Diagnosis and Management.* 2nd ed. Boston, MA: Butterworth-Heinemann; 1996:345–358.

Chamberlain MC, Friedman HS. Leptomeningeal metastases: presentation, diagnosis, and management considerations. In: Levin VA, ed. *Cancer in the Nervous System.* New York, NY: Churchill Livingstone; 1996:281–290.

Constans JP, De Devitis E, Donzelli R, Spaziante R, Meder JF, Haye C. Spinal metastases with neurological manifestations: review of 600 cases. *J Neurosurg.* 1983;59:111–118.

Cotton A, Dewatre F, Cortet B, et al. Percutaneous vertebroplasty for osteolytic metastases and myeloma: effects of the percentage of lesion filling and the leakage of methyl methylacrylate at clinical follow-up. *Radiology.* 1996;200:525–530.

Crasto S, Duca S, Davini O, et al. MRI diagnosis of intramedullary metastases from extra-CNS tumors. *Eur Radiol.* 1997;7:732–736.

Cronquist S, Greitz D, Maeder P. Spread of blood in cerebrospinal fluid following craniotomy simulates spinal metastases. *Neuroradiol.* 1993;35:592–595.

Dunn RC, Kelly WA, Wohns RNW, Howe JF. Spinal epidural neoplasia: a 15-year review of the results of surgical therapy. *J. Neurosurg.* 1980;52:47–51.

Gangi A, Dietemann J-L, Schultz A, Mortazavi R, Jeung MY, Roy C. Interventional radiologic procedures with CT guidance in cancer pain management. *RadioGraphics.* 1996;16:1289–1306.

Gilbert RW, Kim JH, Posner JB. Epidural spinal cord compression from metastatic tumor: diagnosis and treatment. *Am Neurol.* 1978;3:40–51.

Haaga JR, Alfidi RJ. Precise biopsy localization by computed tomography. *Radiology.* 1976;118:603–607.

Jenkins CNJ, Colquhoun IR. Case report: symptomatic metastasis from a sacrococcygeal chordoma. *Clin Radiol.* 1995;50:416–417.

Jones KM, Schwartz RB, Mantello MT, et al. Fast spin-echo MR in the detection of vertebral metastases: comparison of three sequences. *AJNR.* 1994;15:401.

Laredo J-D, Lakhdari K, Bellaïche L, Hamze B, Janklewicz P, Tubiana J-M. Acute vertebral collapse: CT findings in benign and malignant nontraumatic cases. *Radiology.* 1996;199:541–549.

Lecouvet FE, Malghem J, Michaux L, et al. Vertebral compression fractures in multiple myeloma: part II. Assessment of fracture risk with MR imaging of spinal bone marrow. *Radiology.* 1997;204:201–205.

Lecouvet FE, Vande Berg BC, Maldague BE, et al. Development of vertebral fractures in patients with multiple myeloma: does MRI enable recognition of vertebrae that will collapse? *JCAT.* 1998;22:430–436.

Levitt LJ, Dawson DM, Rosenthal DS, Moloney WC. Central nervous system involvement in the non-Hodgkin's lymphomas. *Cancer.* 1980;45:545–552.

Livingston KE, Perrin RG. The neurosurgical management of spinal metastases causing cord and cauda equina compression. *J Neurosurg.* 1978;839–843.

Markus JB. Magnetic resonance imaging of intramedullary spinal cord metastases. *Clin Imag.* 1996;20:238.

Mascalchi M, Torselli P, Falaschi F, et al. MRI of spinal epidural lymphoma. *Neuroradiol.* 1995;37:303.

Case 1

Clinical Presentation

The patient is a 65-year-old female with a history of known breast carcinoma who now presents with increasing lower extremity weakness. Previous bone scan revealed abnormal uptake in L2 and L4.

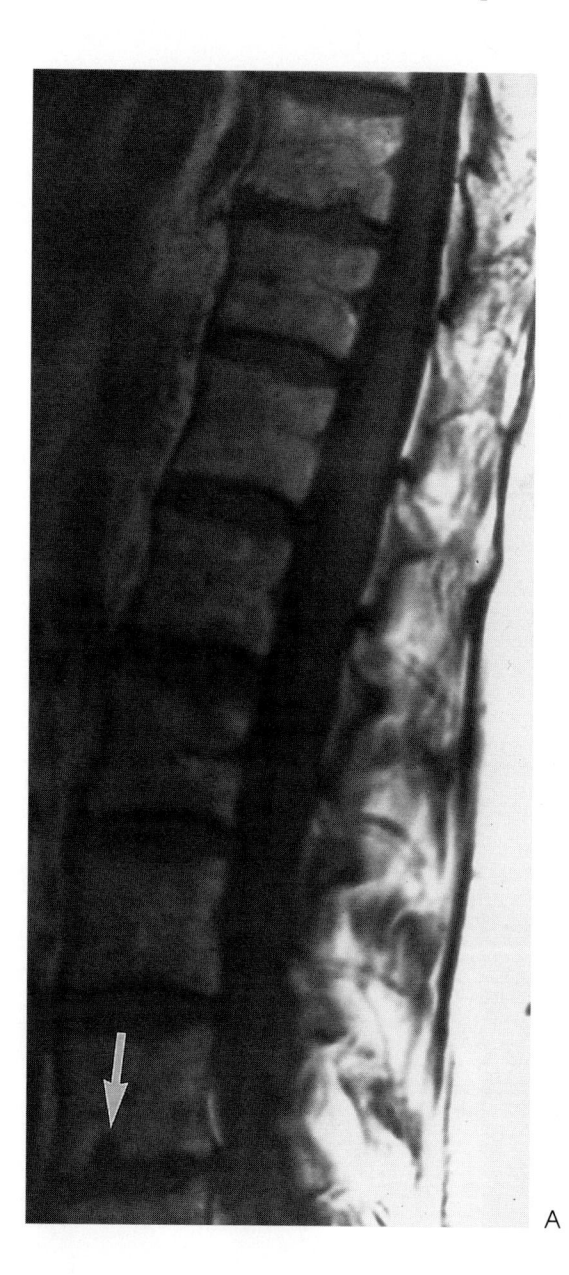

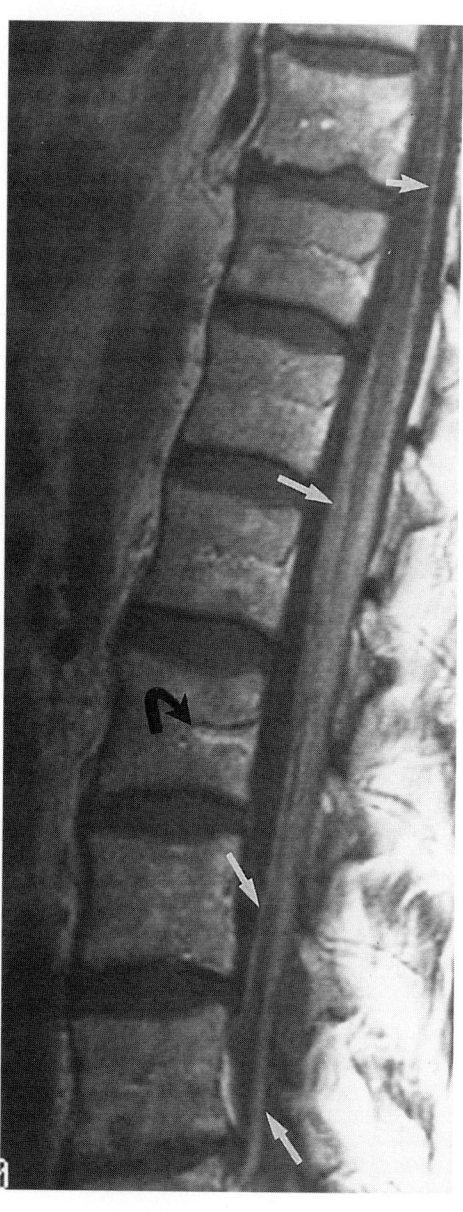

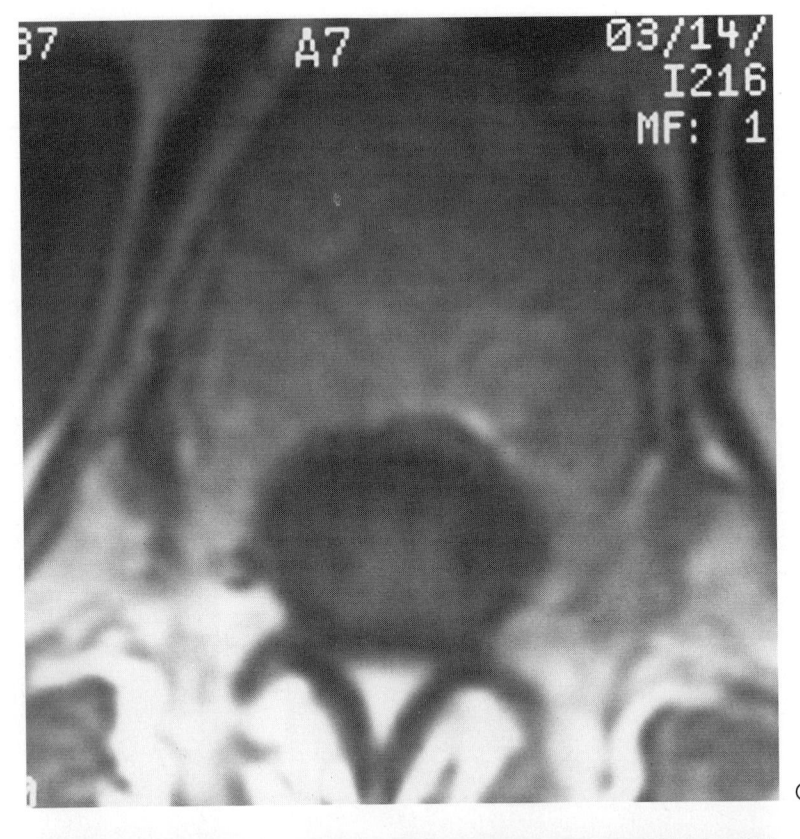

TEACHING ATLAS OF SPINE IMAGING

C

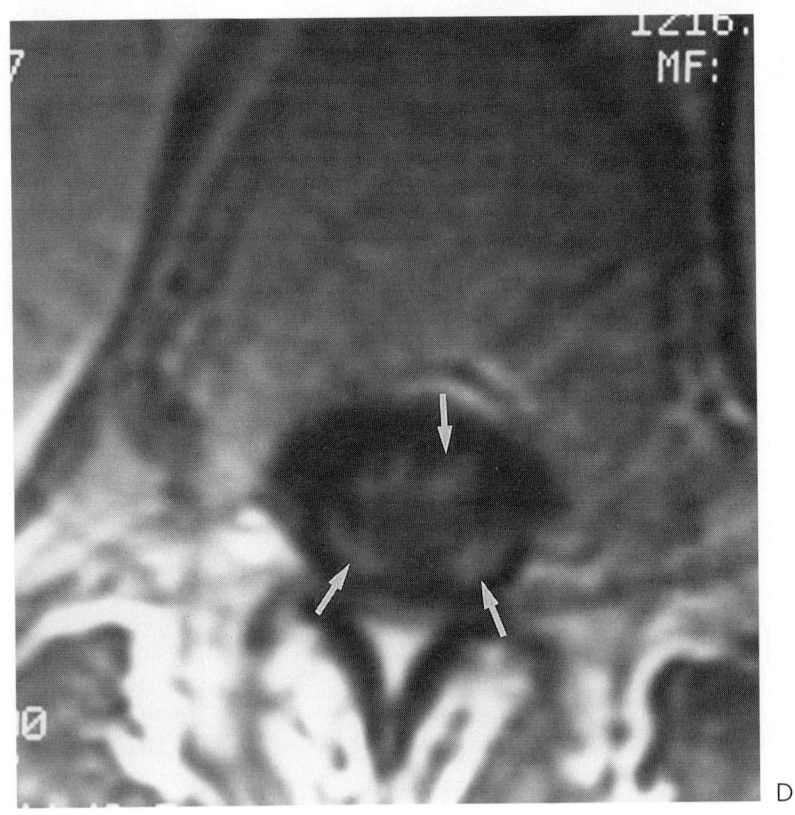

D

SPINAL MENINGEAL CARCINOMATOSIS

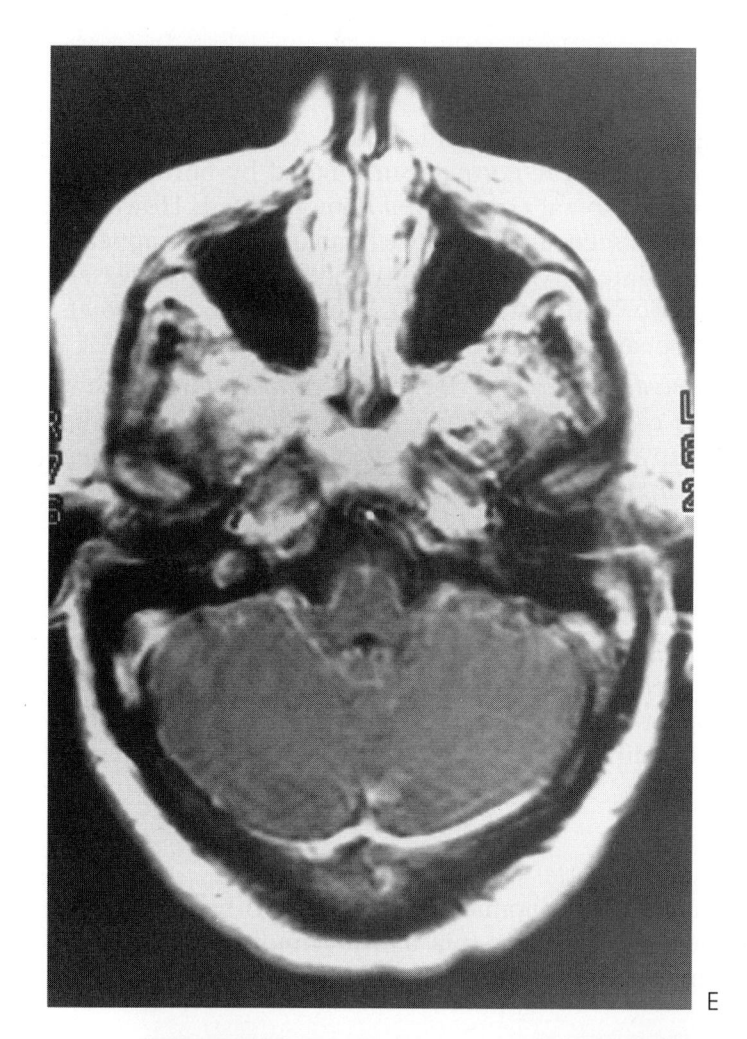

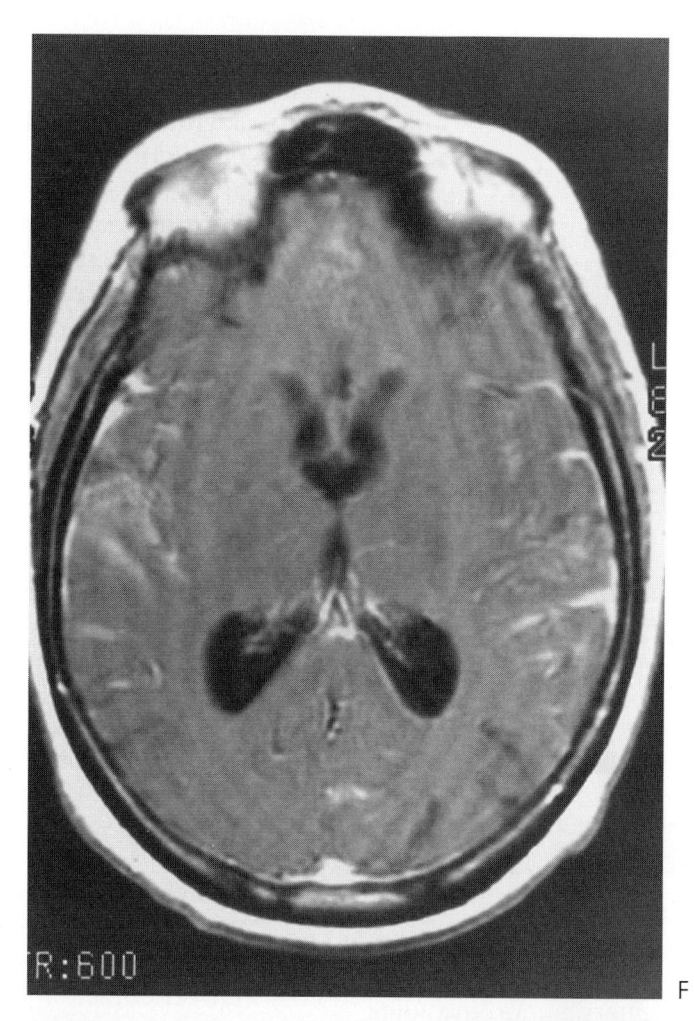

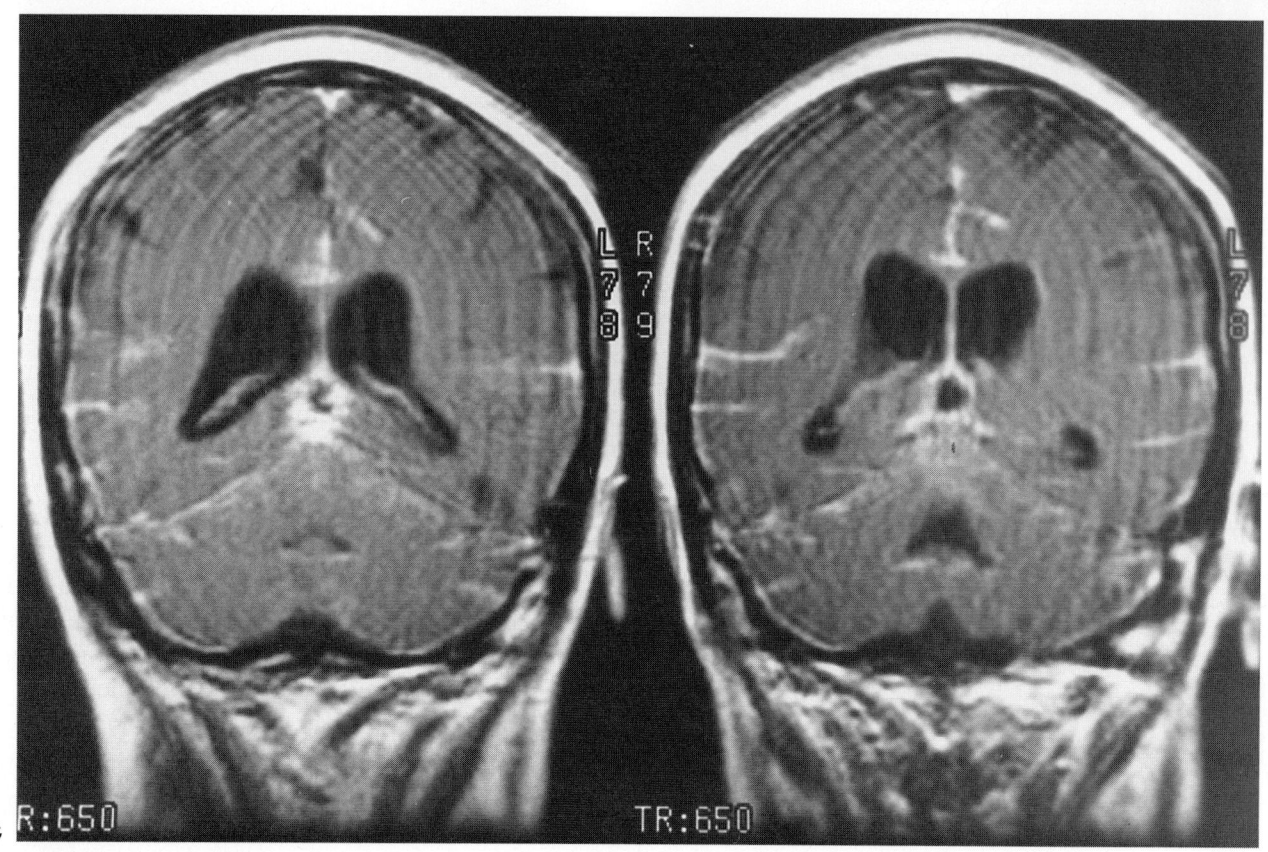

Radiologic Findings

Sagittal short TR image (Fig. A) reveals that the vertebral bodies and intervertebral disc spaces all appear normal. Surrounded by normal subarachnoid space, the thoracic spinal cord is well demonstrated. However, the cauda equina is never well seen, and the entire lumbar thecal sac appears diffusely increased in signal intensity. There is a rounded area of decreased signal intensity in the inferior end plate of the L4 vertebral body (*arrow*). The L2 vertebral body appears normal.

Sagittal short TR image postcontrast (Fig. B) reveals diffuse enhancement of the nerve roots of the cauda equina (*three bottom white arrows*). The distal spinal cord is also seen and is surrounded by a ring of densely enhancing soft tissue (*upper white arrow*). There is normal enhancement of the intervertebral basivertebral venous plexus (*curved black arrow at L2*).

Axial short TR image precontrast (Fig. C) reveals the distal end of the spinal cord and the nerve roots of the cauda equina.

Short TR image postcontrast (Fig. D) reveals dense enhancement of the nerve roots of the cauda equina (*arrows*).

Short TR images of the brain in the coronal (Figs. E and F) and axial (Fig. G) projections reveal diffuse enhancement of the cerebral meninges.

Diagnosis

Spinal and cerebral meningeal carcinomatosis secondary to breast cancer, with involvement of the leptomeninges (pia and arachnoid) of the spine and brain. Presumed metastatic deposit in the inferior end plate of the L4 vertebrae.

Differential Diagnosis

- meningeal carcinomatosis
- inflammatory meningitis
- lymphoma

Discussion

If meningeal carcinomatosis is a suspected clinical diagnosis, it is necessary to perform the examination with the infusion of contrast material. When the pattern of enhancement illustrated here is identified, a primary tumor must be sought. The primary tumor may be within the central nervous system, such as an ependymoma, medulloblastoma, pinealoma, or glioblastoma; or from a primary tumor outside of the nervous system, such as primary lung or breast cancer, or melanoma. The extension of the enhancement into the sulci of the brain confirm the involvement of the leptomeninges because it is the pial layer of the brain that extends deep into the sulci.

Meningeal carcinomatosis is the most likely diagnosis in this clinical setting. Inflammatory meningitis secondary to a bacterial organism, such as *Mycobacterium tuberculosis* or a similar organism, could have a similar appearance, as could lymphoma.

PEARL
- Inflammatory meningitis and lymphoma could also have a similar appearance, as could meningeal metastases from any primary tumor, including metastatic lung cancer or a tumor such as melanoma.

PITFALLS
- The only abnormalities present on the precontrast scan may be the inability to identify the individual nerve roots of the cauda equina and a relatively increased signal intensity of the spinal cerebrospinal fluid because of the presence of tumor replacing the cerebrospinal fluid.

- The index of suspicion needs to be high so that this diagnosis is not ignored and so that a postinfusion scan is obtained.

SPINAL MENINGEAL CARCINOMATOSIS

Case 2

Clinical Presentation

The patient is a 34-year-old male with glioblastoma multiforme of the left frontal lobe who is status post chemotherapy, radiotherapy, and surgery. The patient now presents with new onset of bladder and fecal incontinence as well as back pain.

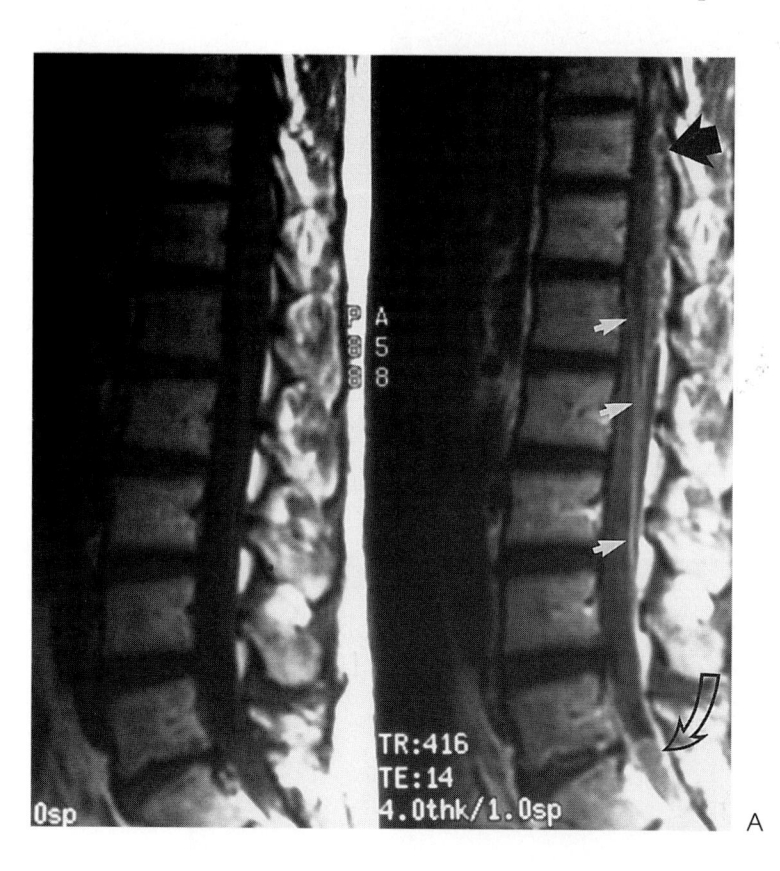

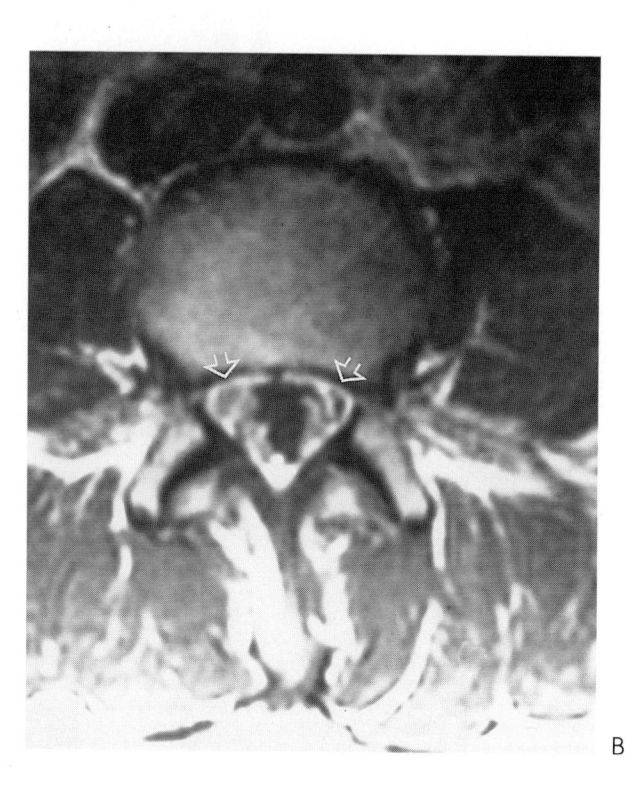

Radiologic Findings

Precontrast (Fig. A, *left*) sagittal short TR image in the lumbar region appears essentially normal. Postinfusion (Fig. A, *right*) sagittal short TR image reveals irregular enhancement of the meninges dorsal to the distal spinal cord (*black arrow*). There is enhancement along the surface of the distal spinal cord anteriorly and enhancement of the nerve roots of the cauda equina (*white arrows*). There is also tumor enhancing in the very distal end of the thecal sac (*curved open arrow*). Incidentally noted is narrowing of the L5-S1 intervertebral disc.

Axial short TR image in the lumbar region postcontrast (Fig. B) reveals dense enhancement of the nerve roots of the cauda equina (*open arrows*).

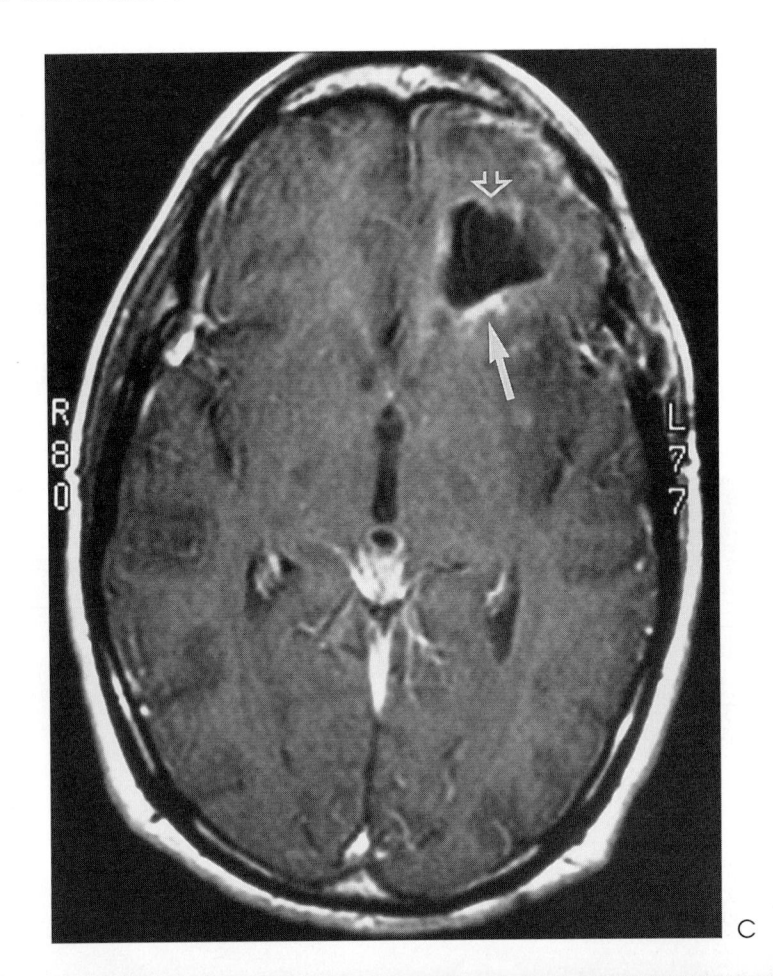

TEACHING ATLAS OF SPINE IMAGING

C

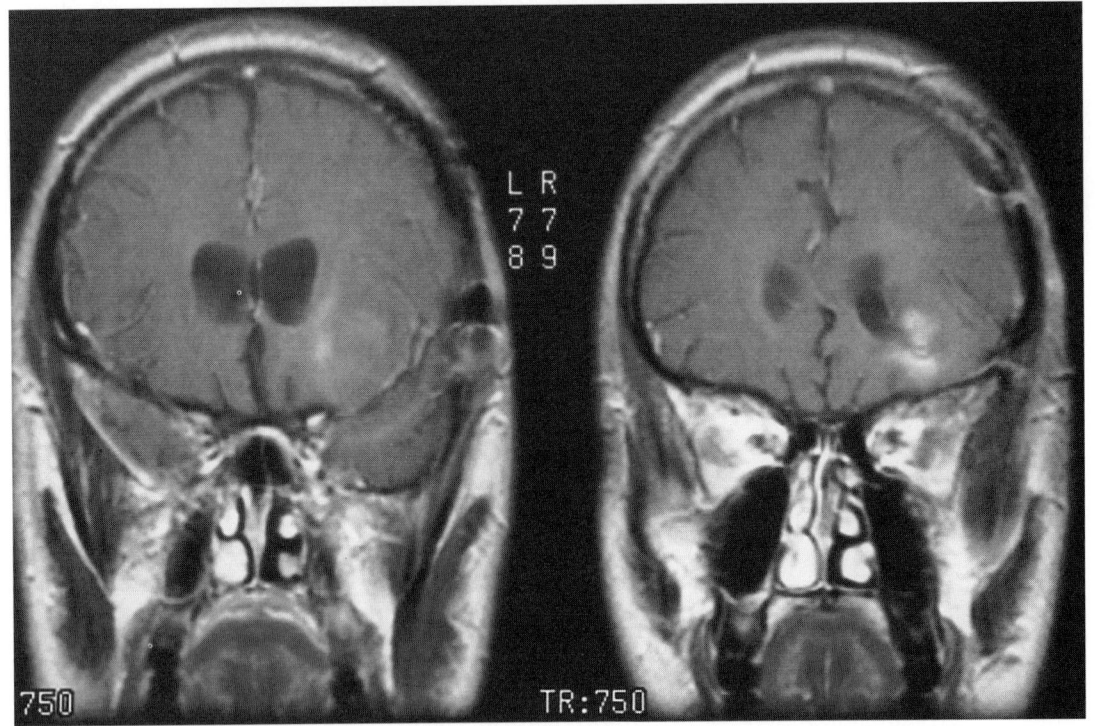

D

SPINAL MENINGEAL CARCINOMATOSIS

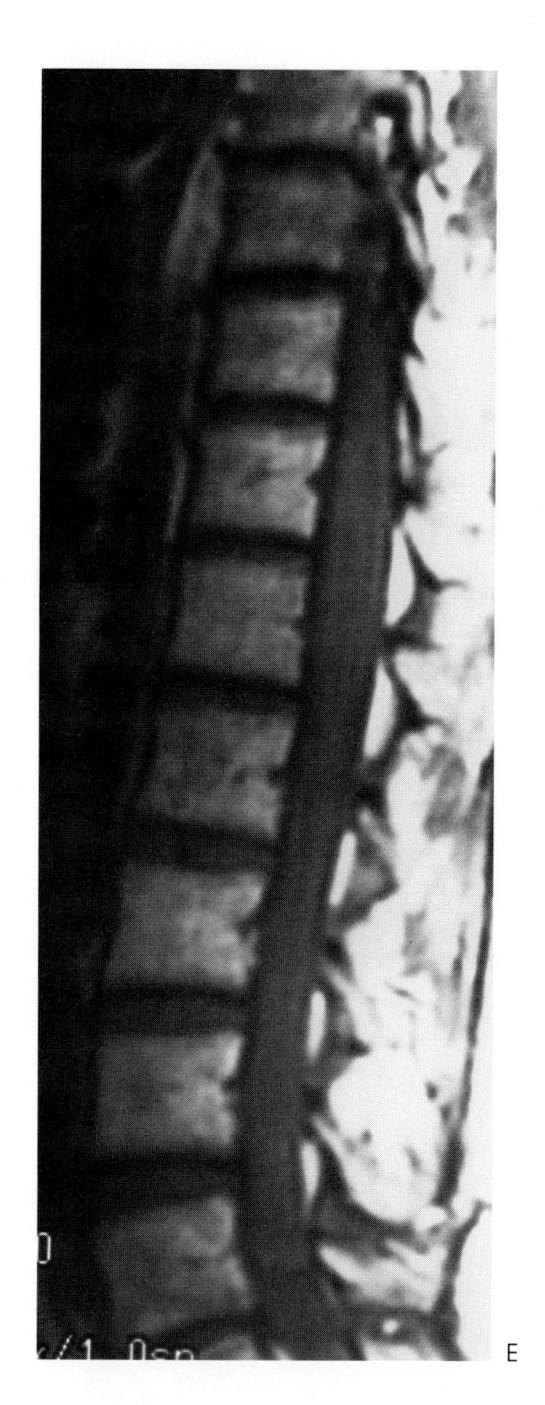

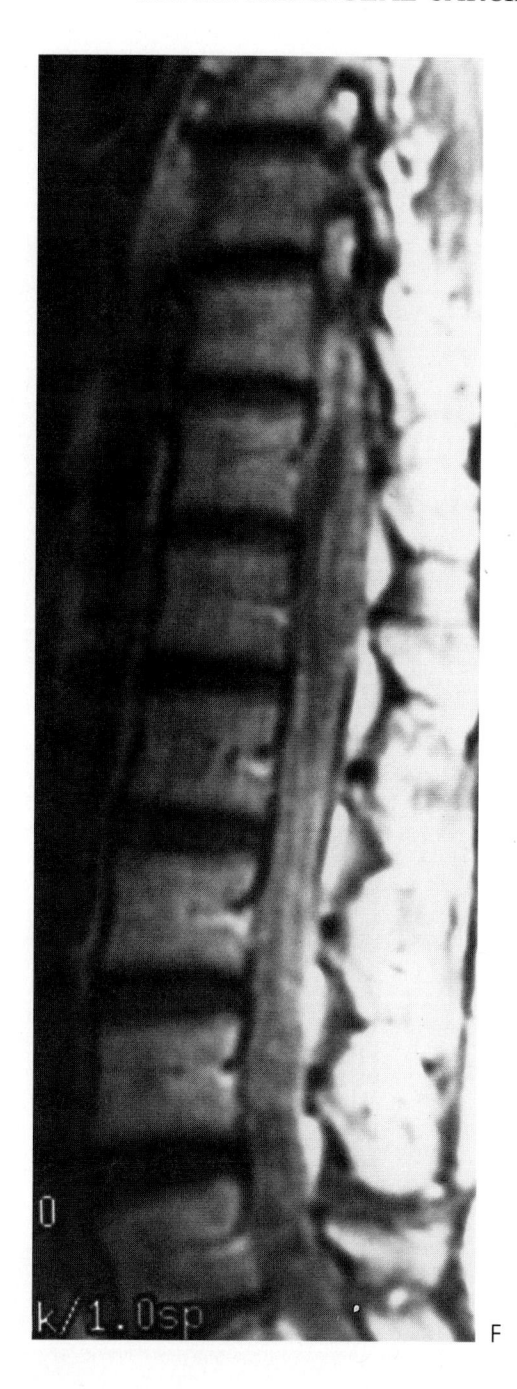

TEACHING ATLAS OF SPINE IMAGING

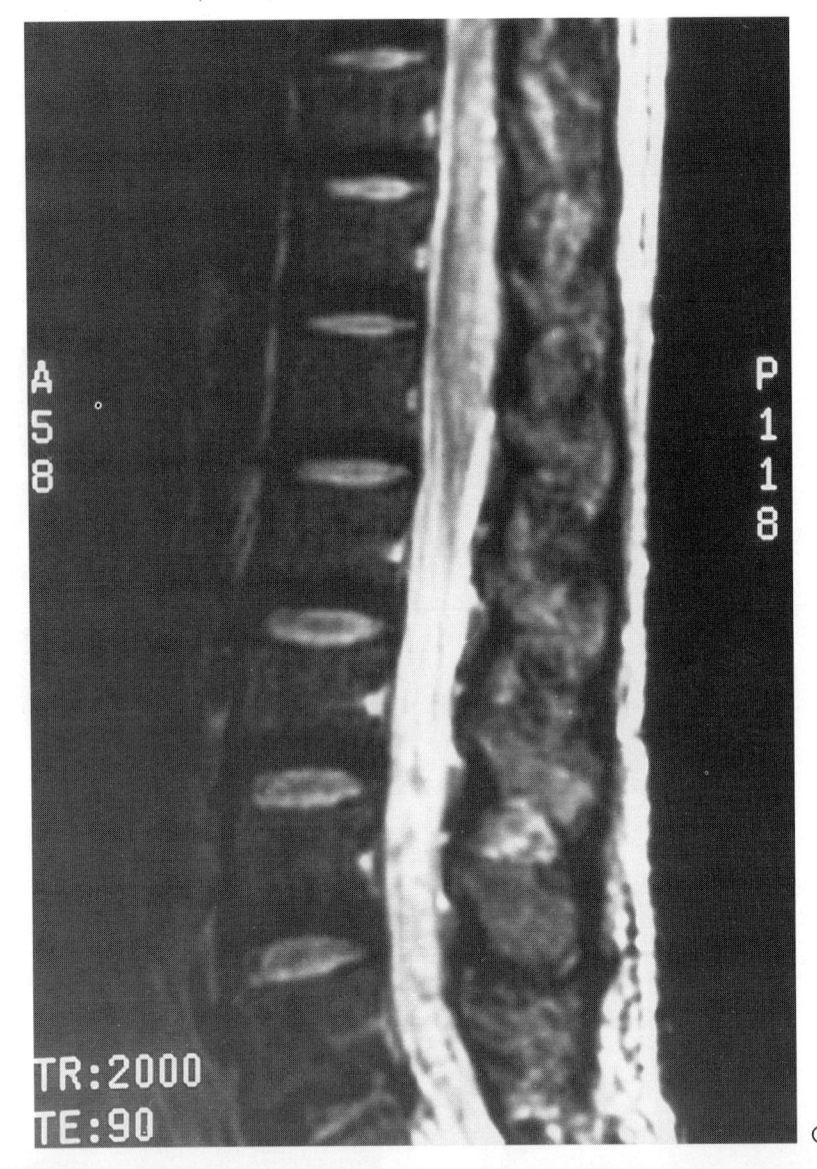

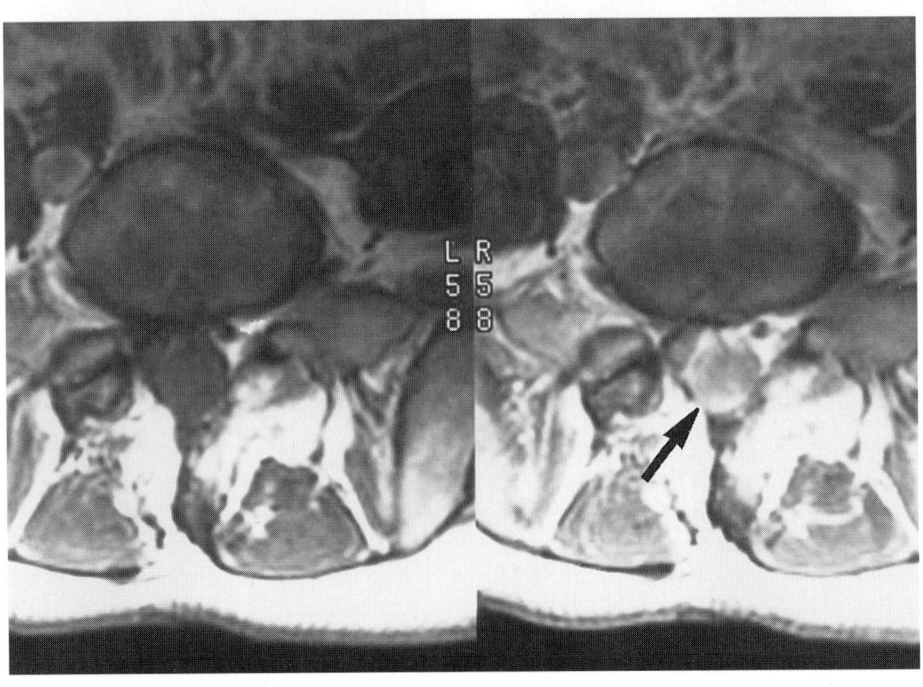

SPINAL MENINGEAL CARCINOMATOSIS

Radiologic Findings (continued)

Axial short TR image of the brain postcontrast (Fig. C) reveals postoperative changes in the left frontal region. There is a postoperative area of porencephaly that exhibits slightly irregular peripheral areas of enhancement with a thin rim anteriorly (*open arrow*) and a thicker rim posteriorly (*long arrow*). There is also mild edema posterior to the tumor and a few rounded areas of enhancement in the basal ganglia on the left. Although there is no mass (probably because of the decompression secondary to the surgery), the findings are highly suggestive of recurrent brain tumor.

Coronal short TR images postcontrast reveal (Fig. D) patchy, poorly marginated areas of enhancement in the left frontal lobe projecting just inferior and lateral to the frontal horn of the left lateral ventricle.

In spite of chemotherapy and radiation treatment, the patient's condition became worse and a follow-up scan was obtained 2 weeks later.

Sagittal short TR image in the lumbar region (Fig. E) reveals that the entire lumbar thecal sac is filled with intermediate signal intensity soft tissue. The nerve roots of the cauda equina cannot be visualized.

Sagittal short TR image postcontrast (Fig. F) reveals dense, linear, and patchy areas of enhancement throughout the lumbar thecal sac and surrounding the distal thoracic spinal cord.

Sagittal long TR image (Fig. G) reveals variable, scattered areas of decreased signal intensity in the distal thecal sac and patchy areas of increased signal intensity within the distal end of the spinal cord. Incidentally noted is a herniated disc at the L5-S1 level.

Pre- (Fig. H, *left*) and postenhancement (Fig. H, *right*) axial short TR images in at the S1 level reveal homogeneous signal intensity soft tissue material filling up the thecal sac on the preinfusion image and dense enhancement of this tissue postcontrast (*right, arrow*).

> **PEARL**
> - Although not common, glioblastoma multiforme may lead to drop metastases to the spinal meninges.

Diagnosis

Recurrent cerebral glioblastoma multiforme with drop metastases and resulting meningeal carcinomatosis.

Differential Diagnosis

- drop metastases with meningeal carcinomatosis
- infective meningitis

Discussion

Clinical information is vital for complete evaluation in this patient, especially in light of the rapid progression in the 2-week period between the initial scan and the follow-up scan 2 weeks later. Brain imaging may also be necessary in any patient in which meningeal carcinomatosis is a clinical

PITFALLS

- Meningeal carcinomatosis from a primary central nervous system tumor, such as a pinealoma, or metastases from tumor outside of the central nervous system, such as primary lung or breast cancer, lymphoma, or melanoma, could have a similar appearance.

- A postinfusion scan is absolutely necessary for complete evaluation of the patient with meningeal carcinomatosis. Without contrast enhancement, the presence of meningeal carcinomatosis of the spine or brain is usually not identified.

consideration. This rapid progression is unusual in a patient; however, with patients living longer because of better methods of treatment, we are seeing an increased incidence of meningeal carcinomatosis.

Drop metastases with meningeal carcinomatosis is the most likely diagnosis in this patient. In a pediatric patient, a PNET (primitive neuroectodermal tumor) could also result in a similar appearance. Infective meningitis could have a similar appearance but is unlikely in this clinical setting.

SPINAL MENINGEAL CARCINOMATOSIS

Case 3

Clinical Presentation

The patient is a 45-year-old female with breast cancer with widespread metastases, now presenting with headache and lower extremity weakness.

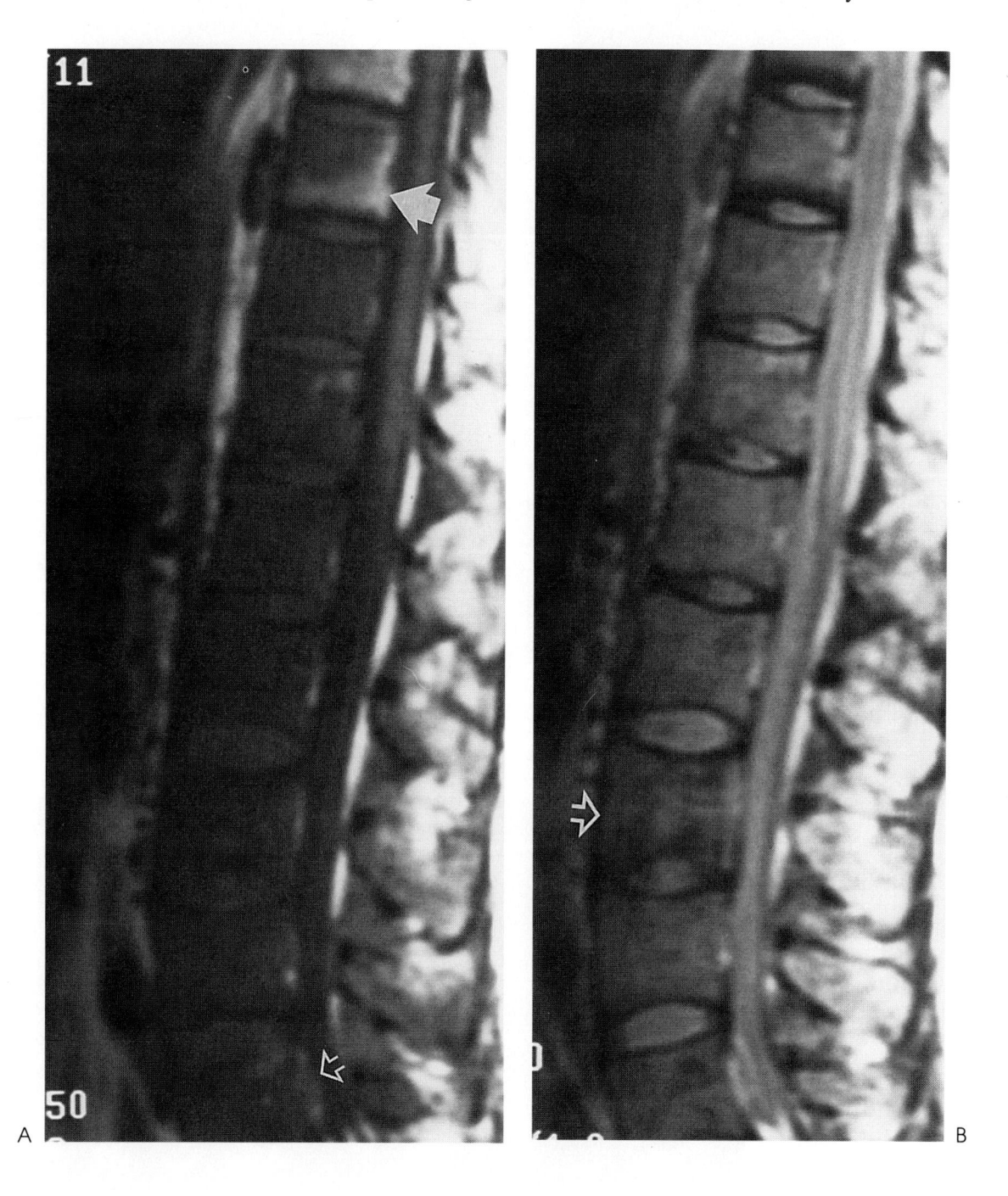

TEACHING ATLAS OF SPINE IMAGING

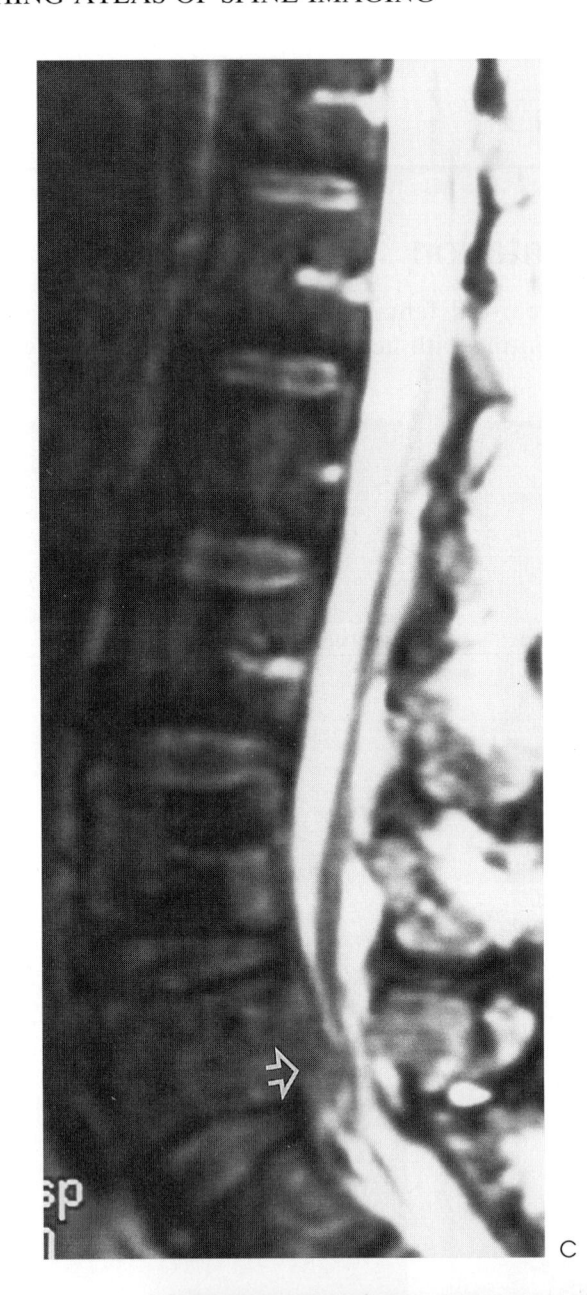

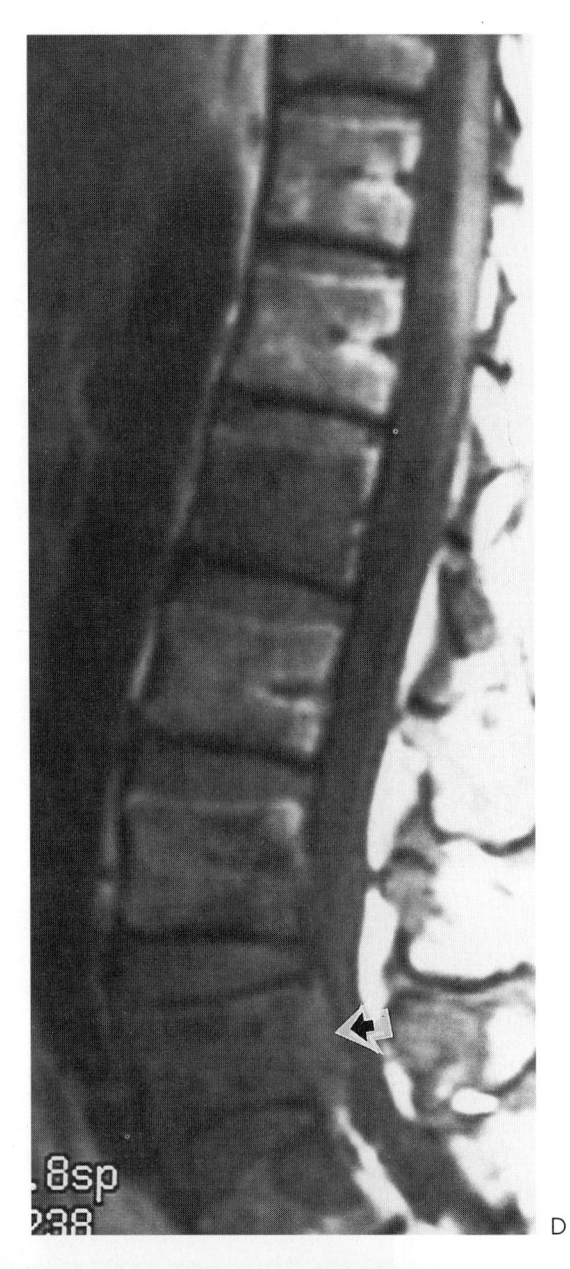

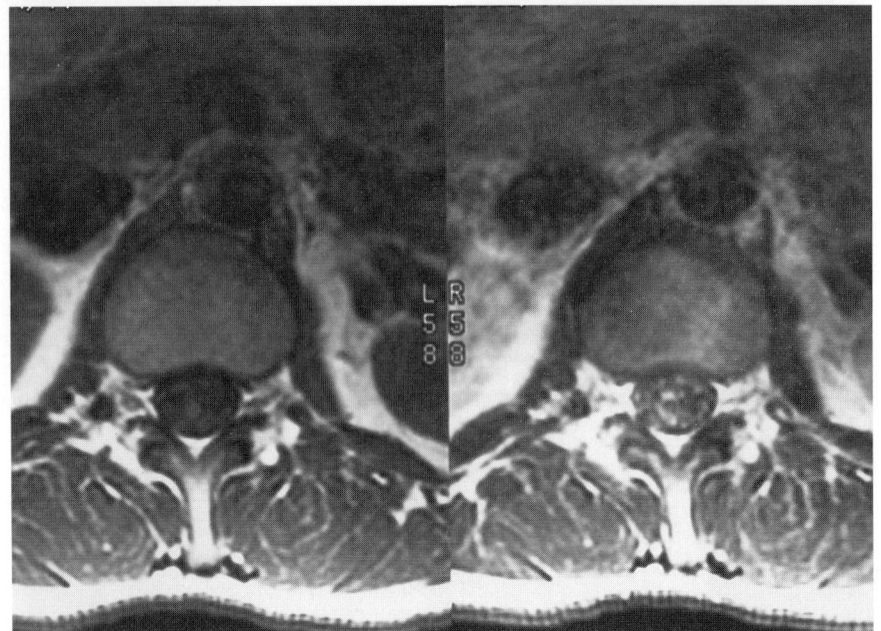

SPINAL MENINGEAL CARCINOMATOSIS

Radiologic Findings

Sagittal short TR image (Fig. A) reveals that the T11 through the S1 vertebral bodies are almost completely replaced by decreased signal intensity soft tissue. The upper anterior portion of T10 is also replaced by decreased signal intensity tumor (*white arrow*). The spinous processes exhibit mottled signal intensity. There is expansion of the L5 vertebral body with a soft tissue component (*open arrow*) that extends into the vertebral canal.

Sagittal intermediate TR image (Fig. B) reveals that the entire thecal sac appears homogeneous in signal intensity. The vertebral body marrow now reveal faint mottled decreased signal intensity within the L3 (*open arrow*) and T12 vertebral bodies.

Sagittal long TR image (Fig. C) reveals that the vertebral bodies now appear almost normal in signal intensity. Only L4 reveals faint mottled decreased signal intensity. The soft tissue expansion of the L5 vertebral body is seen extending into the vertebral canal (*open arrow*).

Sagittal short TR image postcontrast (Fig. D) reveals diffuse irregular enhancement of the marrow within the lumbar vertebral bodies. There is enhancement of the soft tissue mass behind the vertebral body of L5 (*arrow*).

Preinfusion (Fig. E, *left*) axial short TR image reveals that the nerve roots are well demonstrated as individual structures. Postcontrast (Fig. E, *right*) scan shows dense contrast enhancement of all of the nerve roots in the thecal sac. This change is secondary to meningeal carcinomatosis. This change is seen better on the axial than the sagittal images.

Diagnosis

Diffuse bone metastases and spinal meningeal carcinomatosis.

Differential Diagnosis

- meningeal carcinomatosis
- meningitis

Discussion

The brain was also involved with diffuse meningeal carcinomatosis. The only normal remaining marrow appears as areas of increased signal intensity as seen on Figure A (*white arrow*).

Meningitis could also have a similar appearance with the enhancement of the meninges; however, the combination of the involvement of the vertebral marrow as well as the enhancement of the meningitis is more consistent with meningeal carcinomatosis. These studies should also be correlated with cerebrospinal fluid analysis when appropriate.

PEARL
- Note that in the intermediate and long TR images, as well as in the postcontrast image, the diffuse bony metastases are partially obscured. This appearance is dramatic in this patient, but may be seen in many patients to a variable degree.

PITFALLS
- Because the vertebral marrow abnormality may be obscured, both pre- *and* postinfusion studies should be obtained. The presence of meningeal involvement with either tumor or inflammation may not be appreciated on the noninfused scan.
- When the cerebrospinal fluid appears homogeneous in signal intensity with the nerve roots of the cauda equina, the possibility of involvement with tumor or inflammation should be considered.

PEARLS

- Evaluate the paraspinal areas. The diffuse low signal intensity of the marrow of the vertebral bodies is secondary to replacement of the normal fatty marrow with leukemic cells.

- If meningeal carcinomatosis or drop metastases are suspected, a postinfusion study is required for complete evaluation.

PITFALL

- The slightly higher than normal tissue density soft tissue mass in the distal end of the thecal sac could be mistaken for a hematoma.

pathologic fracture of the L1 vertebral body. Metastases in the distal end of the thecal sac; meningeal carcinomatosis. Polycystic disease of the kidney (incidental finding).

Differential Diagnosis

- meningeal carcinomatosis
- infective meningitis

Discussion

Clinical history is vital in this patient to arrive at a correct diagnosis. The thickened roots of the cauda equina are consistent with meningeal carcinomatosis. In a patient with leukemia, evaluation should include the paraspinal area to rule out pathologic adenopathy. In this patient, there is no adenopathy; however, the kidneys have multiple cysts secondary to polycystic disease.

The decreased signal intensity seen in some AIDS patients within the marrow of the vertebral bodies could be mistaken for infiltration with tumor. Hemorrhage within the thecal sac could have a similar appearance; however, hemorrhage would not be expected to enhance.

SPINAL MENINGEAL CARCINOMATOSIS

Case 5

Clinical Presentation

The patient is a 65-year-old with colon cancer metastatic to the liver, lungs, and subcutaneous tissues now presenting with upper and lower extremity weakness.

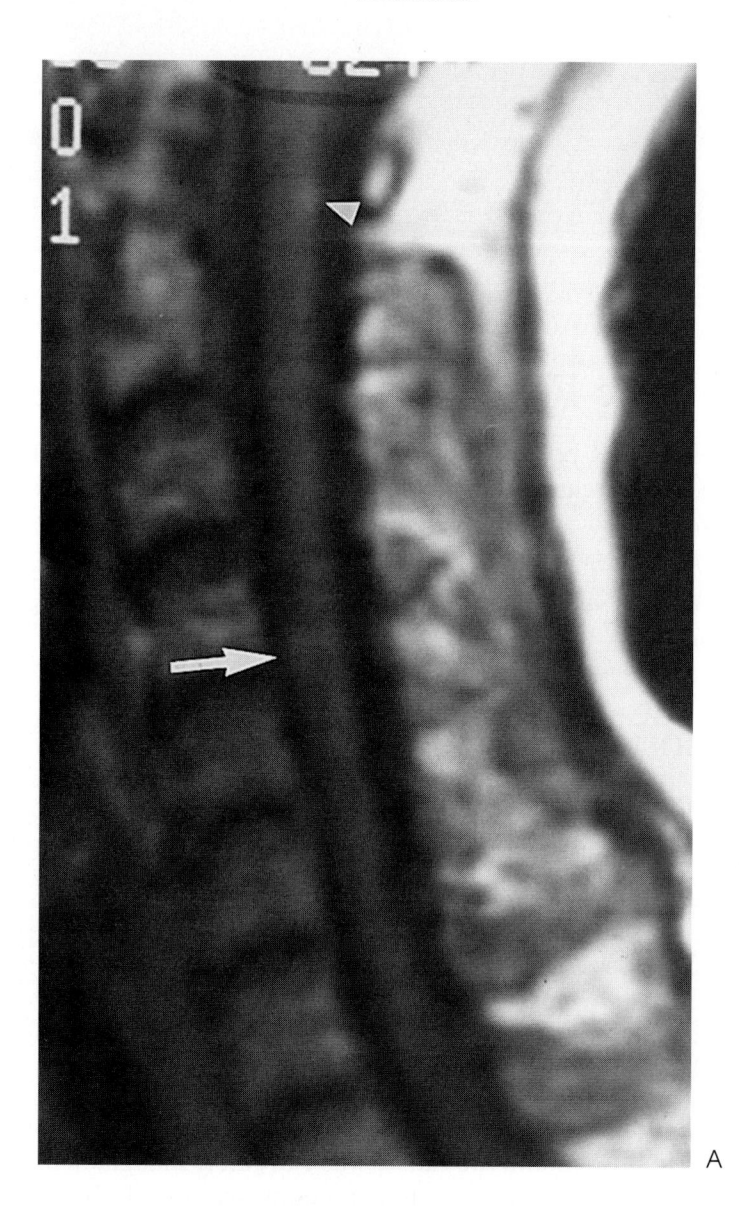

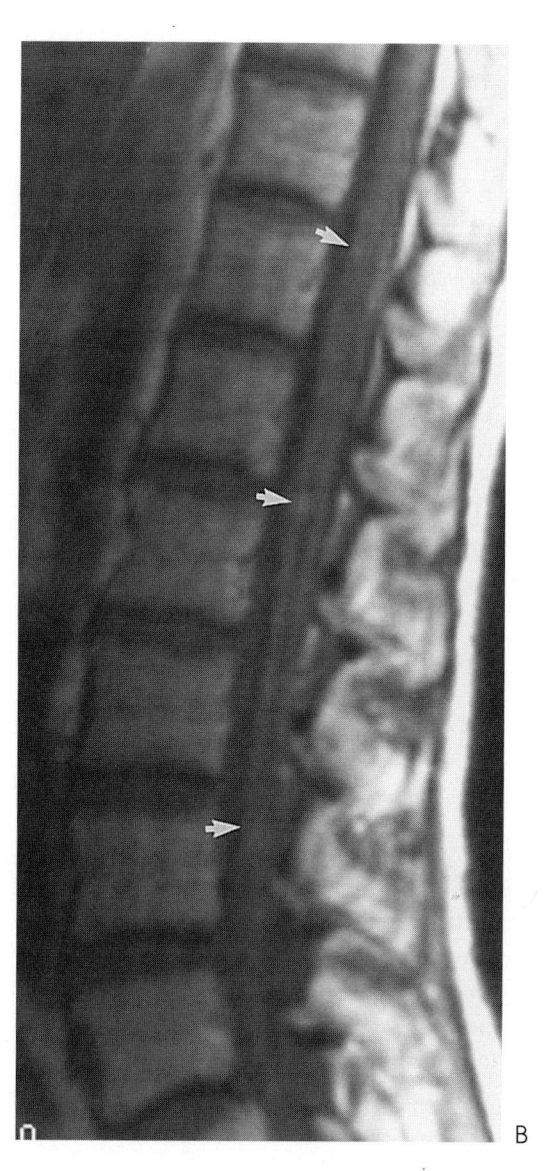

Radiologic Findings

Sagittal short TR postcontrast image at the level of the cervical spine (Fig. A) reveals multiple small rounded areas of enhancement in the subarachnoid space (*arrow at C4 ventrally and arrowhead at C2 dorsally*).

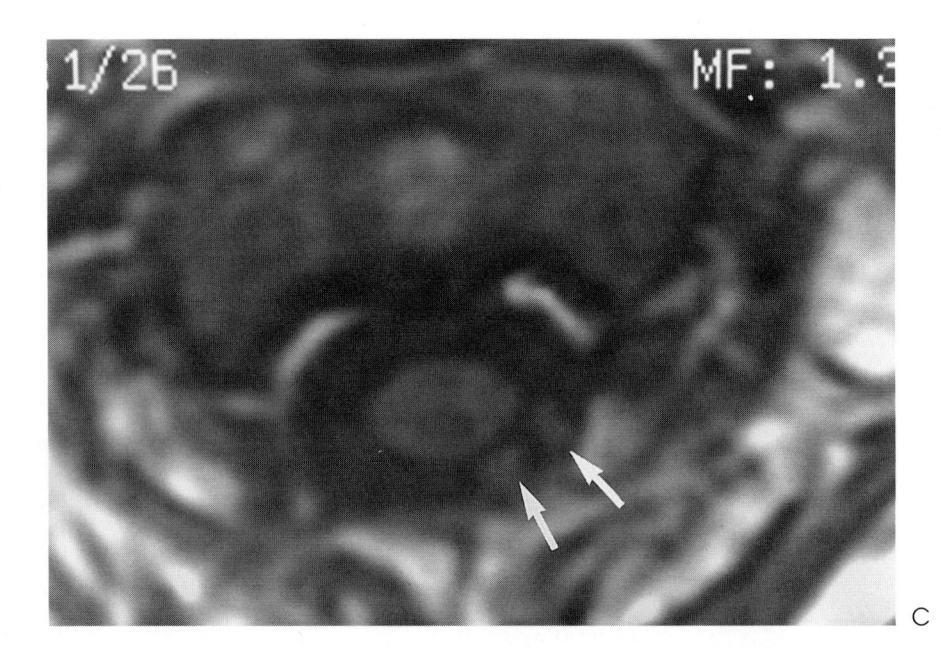

TEACHING ATLAS OF SPINE IMAGING

C

PEARLS
- Correlation should also be made with the evaluation of the cerebrospinal fluid.

- Close collaboration with the referring physicians is very helpful in these cases. If the clinical presentation is more ominous than the scan might suggest, a postinfusion scan is probably warranted to rule out the presence of an abnormality such as meningeal carcinomatosis.

PITFALLS
- The preinfusion scan in patients with meningeal carcinomatosis may be normal. Therefore, the index of suspicion must be high, and a postinfusion scan must be obtained for complete evaluation of these patients.

- As the distribution is not predictable and because the clinical symptoms may not correlate with the patient's symptoms, the entire vertebral canal should be evaluated. The brain and other intracranial contents should also be evaluated as appropriate.

Radiologic Findings (continued)

Sagittal short TR postcontrast image in the lumbar region (Fig. B) reveals multiple small areas of enhancement scattered in the lumbar subarachnoid space (*arrows*).

Axial short TR postcontrast image at the level of the C2 vertebral body (Fig. C) reveals two small enhancing metastases in the cervical subarachnoid space (*arrows*).

Diagnosis

Metastatic colon cancer in the subarachnoid space.

Differential Diagnosis

- metastatic disease

Discussion

This type of aggressive metastasis is very uncommon in colon carcinoma. However, in this patient, the tumor was extremely malignant and aggressive, including metastases to the subcutaneous tissues of the forearms. The changes of metastatic disease in the subarachnoid space may be very subtle. A postinfusion scan is absolutely necessary for complete diagnosis and for evaluation of the extent of disease. Other very aggressive types of primary tumors that may lead to this type of metastatic disease are lung cancer and breast cancer, as well as aggressive melanoma.

Other primary tumors, including primary lung or breast cancer or melanoma, may result in a similar appearance. Other primary CNS tumors, such as pinealoma or medulloblastoma, may also develop drop metastases.

SPINAL MENINGEAL CARCINOMATOSIS

Case 6

Clinical Presentation

The patient is a 6-year-old male presenting with headache and unsteady gait who had a primary medulloblastoma removed from the posterior fossa 1 year prior to this study.

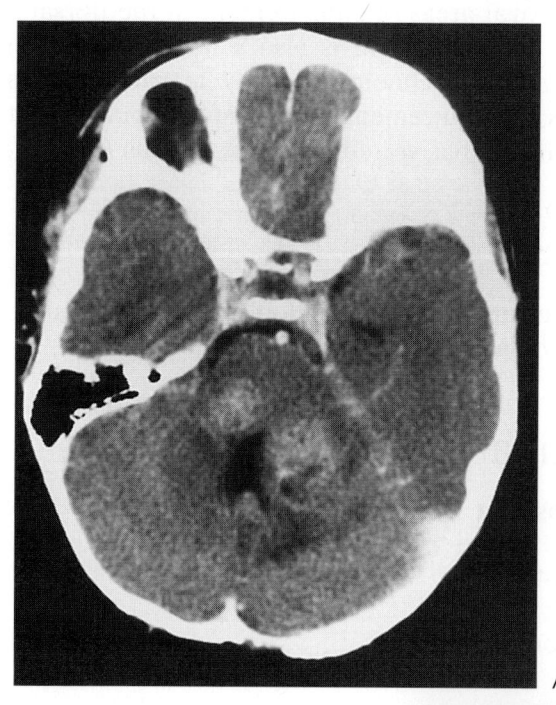

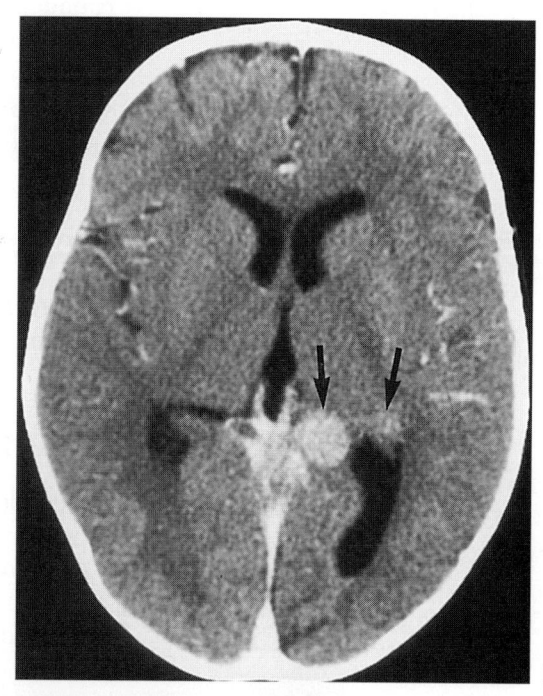

449

Radiologic Findings

Postinfusion computed tomographic scans (Figs. A and B) reveal postoperative changes in the occipital bone of the posterior fossa. There are rounded areas of enhancement in the posterior fossa, in the right side of the pons and in the left middle cerebellar peduncle. There are also modular lesions in the supratentorial region that reveal varying degrees of enhancement (*arrows* in Fig. B). There is mild ventricular enlargement.

Sagittal short TR image postcontrast (Fig. C) reveals multiple, varying sized, rounded and oval areas of enhancement in the dorsal spinal subarachnoid space (*open arrows*). There is also a larger area of enhancement in the upper thoracic subarachnoid space (*white arrow*). Rounded and triangular shaped areas of enhancement in the posterior portion of the vertebral bodies are the enhancing basivertebral venous plexus (*arrowhead*).

> **PEARL**
> - Hemorrhage may occur into these metastatic deposits and may lead to a patient's demise.

Diagnosis

Recurrent posterior fossa medulloblastoma with multiple drop metastases from medulloblastoma.

Differential Diagnosis

- medulloblastoma
- drop metastases
- inflammatory process

> **PITFALL**
> - Initial evaluation and staging as well as follow-up in these patients should also include evaluation of the spinal subarachnoid space.

Discussion

Metastases may occur into the supratentorial compartment as well as into the spine and subarachnoid space. Metastases from medulloblastoma may also spread superiorly into the supratentorial or infratentorial subarachnoid space, or into the cerebral parenchyma, as in this case. If metastases spread into the supratentorial compartment, it is not uncommon to find involvement of the suprasellar cistern. In these cases, the normal low density cerebrospinal fluid is replaced with increased density tumor. This tumor exhibits marked enhancement after the infusion of contrast material. In the absence of a known primary tumor, an inflammatory process, such as tuberculosis meningitis or some other inflammatory disease, would be a consideration.

Drop metastases from primary medulloblastoma are the most likely diagnosis in this patient.

SPINAL MENINGEAL CARCINOMATOSIS

Case 7

Clinical Presentation

The patient is a 5-year-old female with a history of headaches, lethargy, and lower extremity weakness.

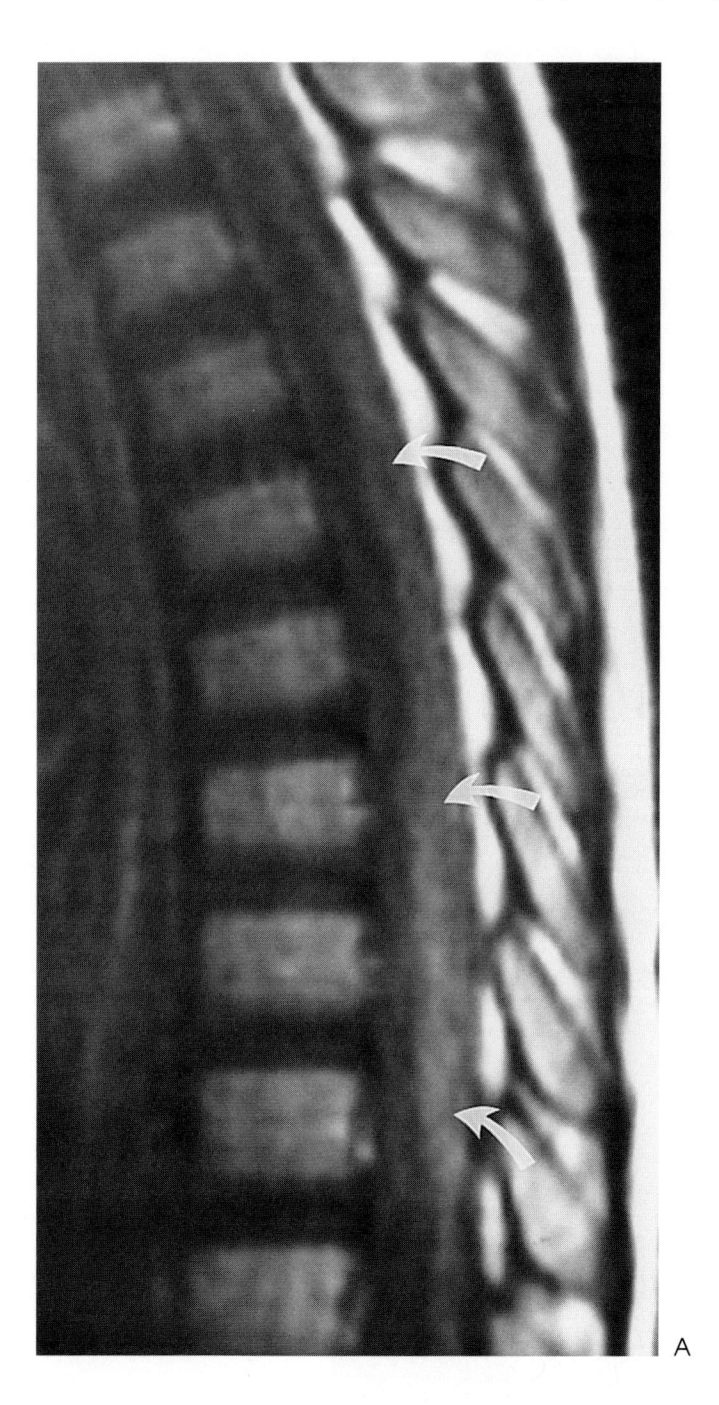

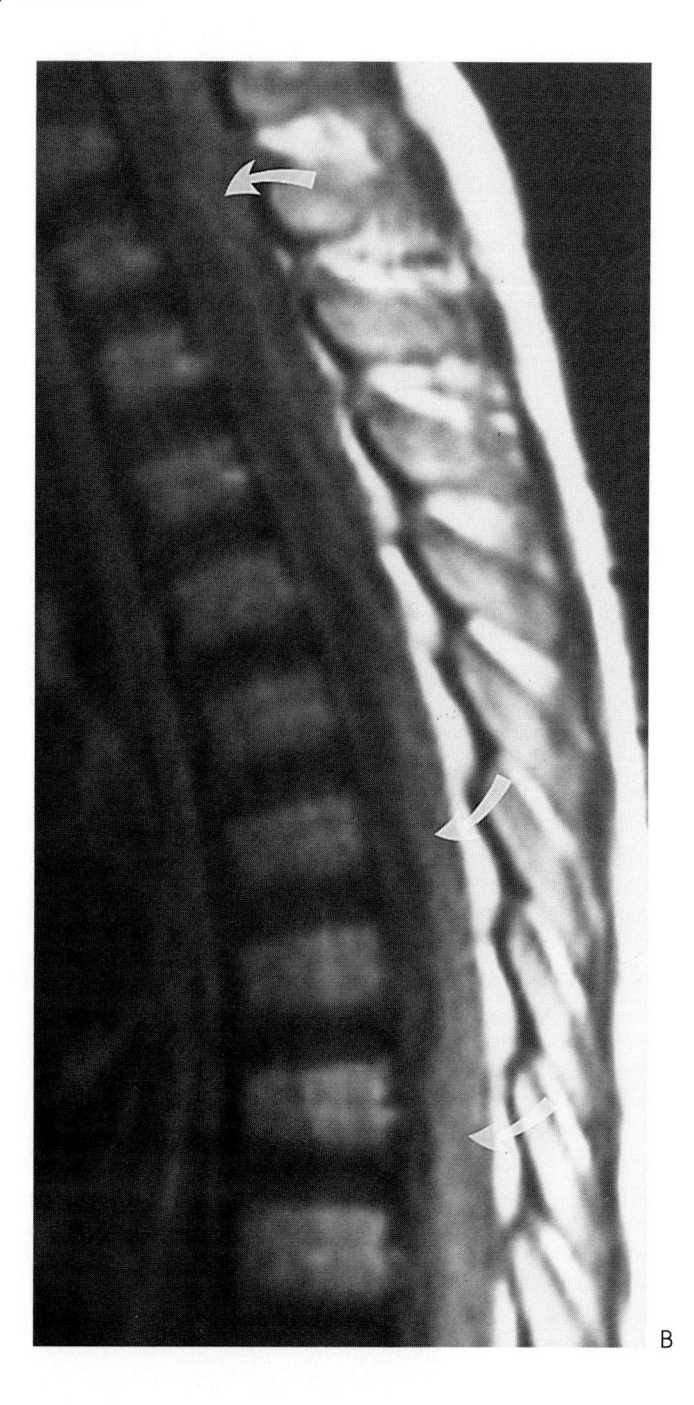

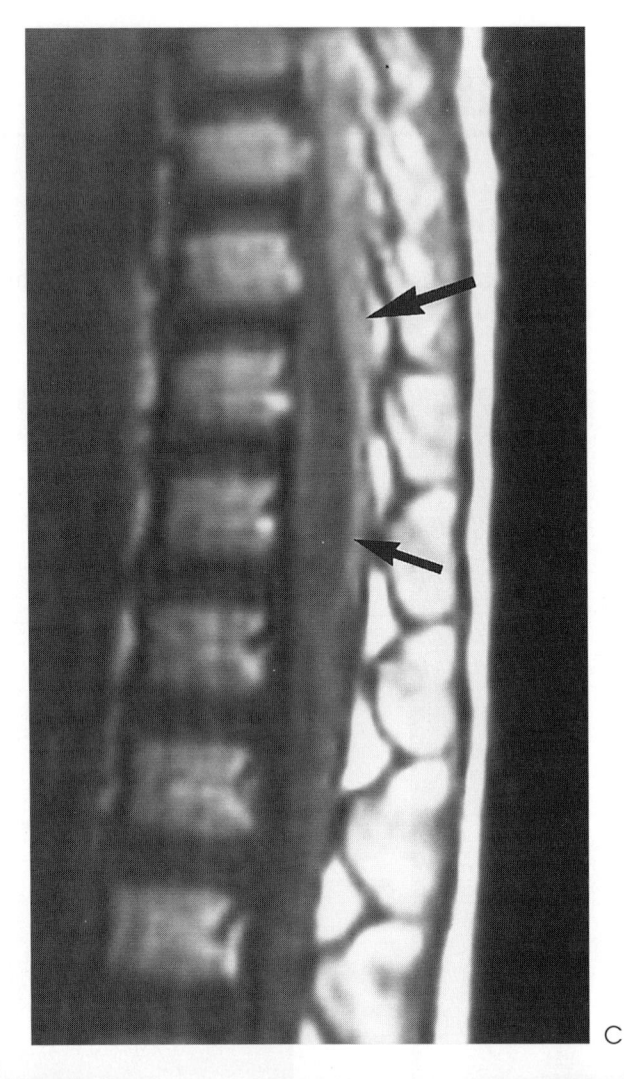

TEACHING ATLAS OF SPINE IMAGING

C

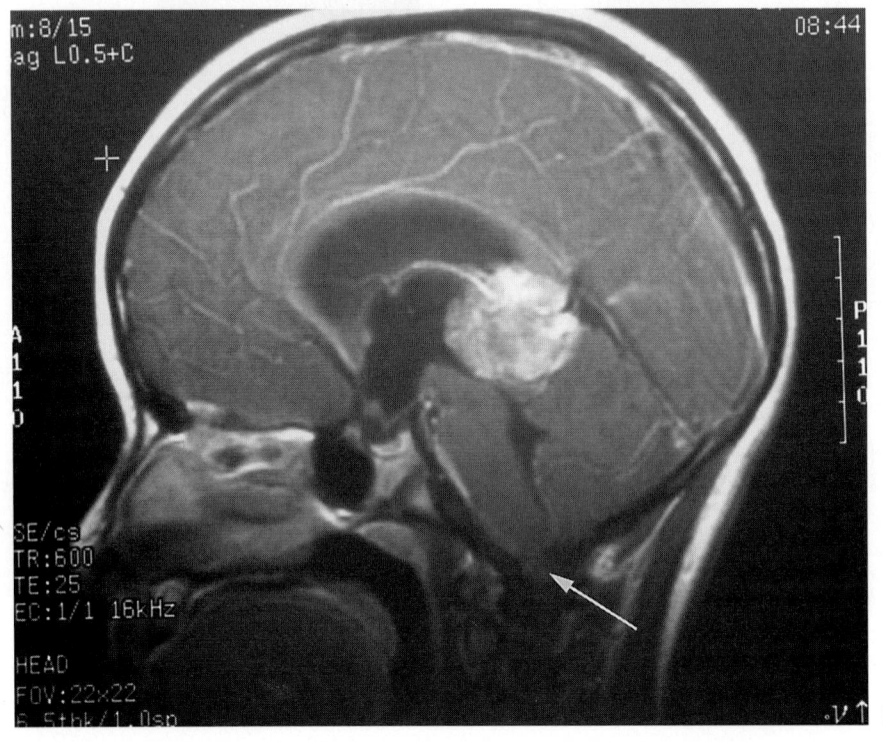

D

452

SPINAL MENINGEAL CARCINOMATOSIS

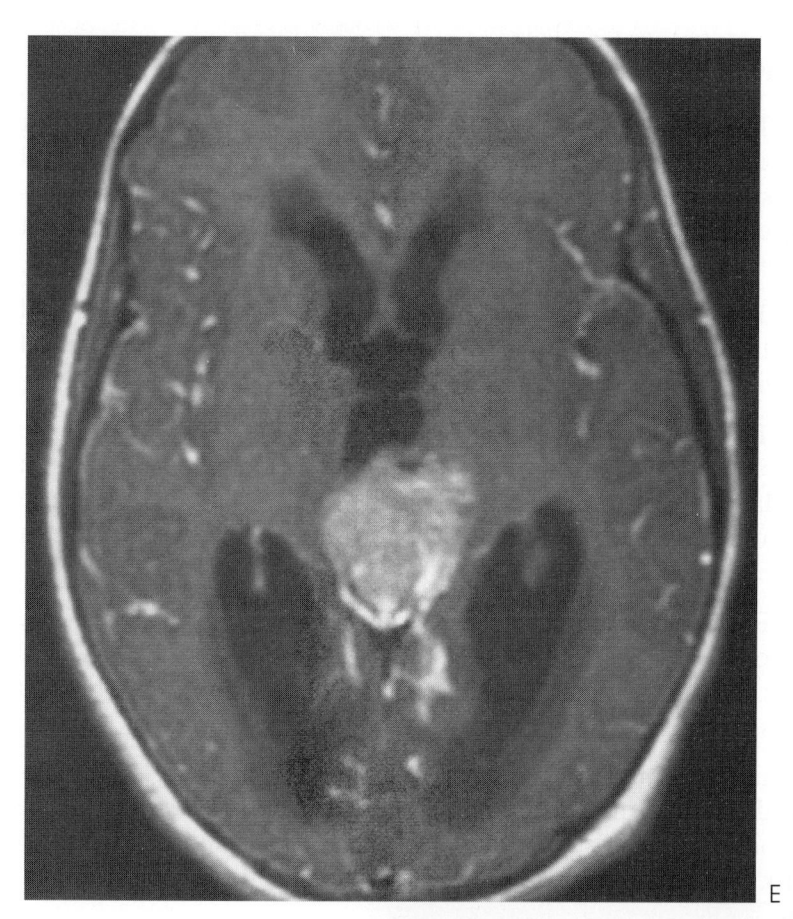

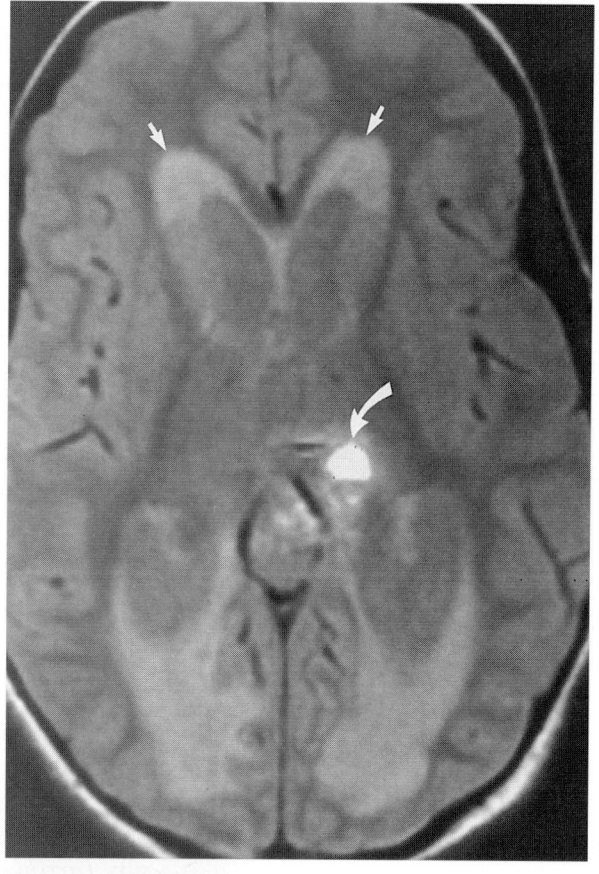

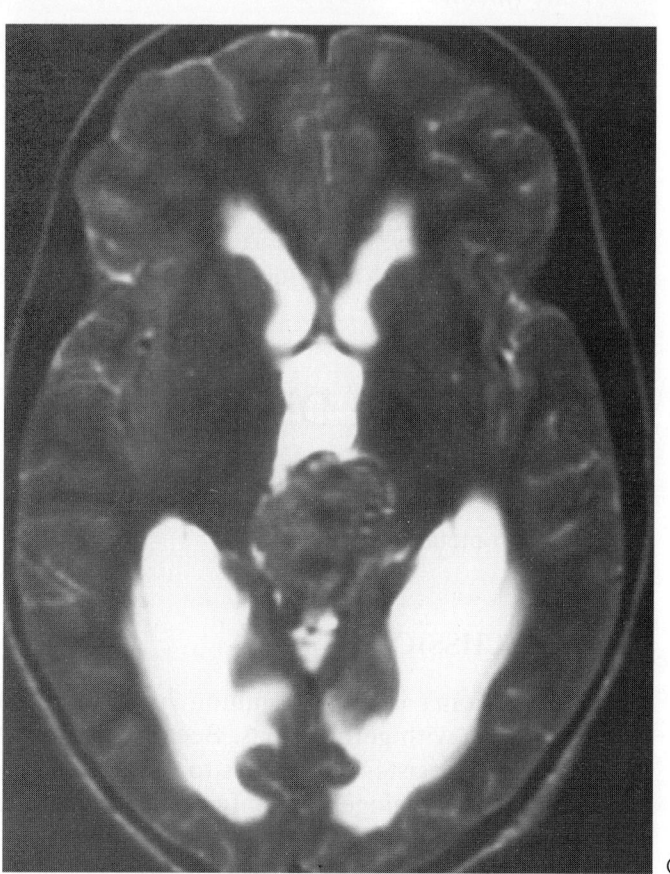

Radiologic Findings

Sagittal short TR images after the infusion of contrast material (Figs. A and B) reveal diffuse enhancement of long areas of scalloped marginated areas of soft tissue surrounding the spinal cord and obliterating the subarachnoid space. The normal spinal cord is never demonstrated with certainty at any level (*arrows*).

Sagittal short TR image at the level of the distal end of the spinal cord (Fig. C) reveals enhancement of a thick layer of tissue along the dorsal aspect of the distal spinal cord (*arrows*).

Sagittal short TR image of the brain postcontrast (Fig. D) reveals dense enhancement of a slightly irregularly marginated 3.5 cm mass in the region of the pineal gland. The lateral and third ventricles are enlarged. There are several small rounded areas of enhancement in the subarachnoid space at the level of the foramen magnum (*arrow*).

Axial short TR image of the brain postcontrast (Fig. E) reveals dense enhancement of a 3.5 cm oval-shaped mass in the region of the pineal gland. There is obstructive hydrocephalus with dilitation of the lateral and third ventricles.

Axial intermediate TR image at the level of the pineal gland (Fig. F) reveals an oval-shaped area of increased signal intensity (*curved arrow*) in the anterior portion of the mass identified in Figure E. A halo of increased signal intensity surrounds the frontal horns of the lateral ventricles bilaterally (*arrows*).

Axial long TR image at the level of the pineal gland (Fig. G) reveals that the mass remains as decreased signal intensity. The dilated lateral and third ventricles appear as increased signal intensity.

PEARLS
- Other tumors may occur in the region of the pineal gland, such as pineoblastomas and pinealocytomas; however, germinoma is the most likely tumor to develop drop metastases.

PITFALL
- Correlation with cerebrospinal fluid analysis should also be performed. However, in the case of a large intracranial mass lesion, a spinal tap should be performed only with great care and after consideration.

Diagnosis

Germinoma with drop metastases and resulting spinal meningeal carcinomatosis.

Differential Diagnosis

- germinoma
- drop metastases

Discussion

Germinoma is more common in males than in females. Metastases are common with germinomas. Because of the possibility of metastases to the suprasellar cistern as well as to other areas of the intracranial contents and the spinal meninges, postinfusion studies of the brain and spinal cord should be performed. This study should be performed at the time of initial diagnosis as well as at the time of follow-up.

SPINAL MENINGEAL CARCINOMATOSIS

Case 8

Clinical Presentation

The patient is a 32-year-old male with acute lymphocytic leukemia who is status post two episodes of bone marrow transplant. The patient now presents with a positive Babinski sign and lower extremity weakness.

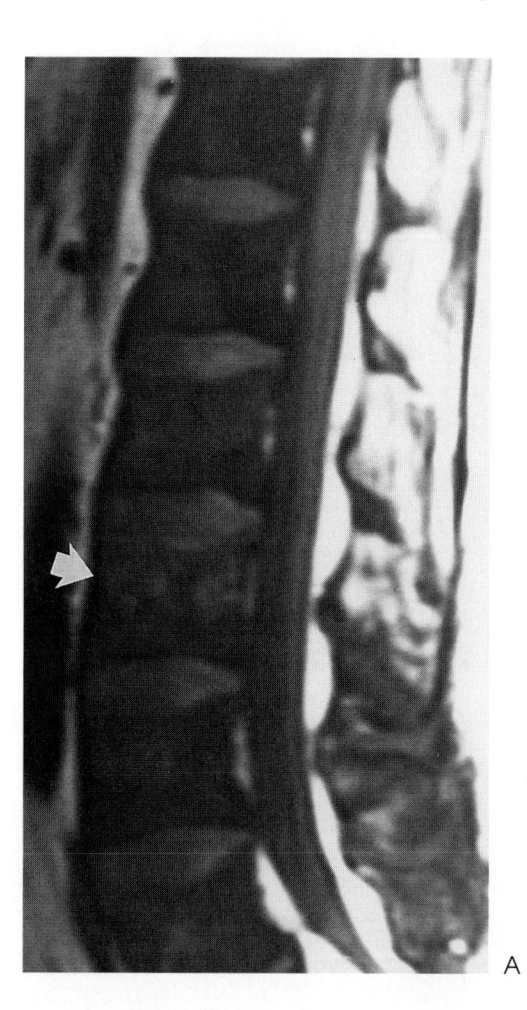

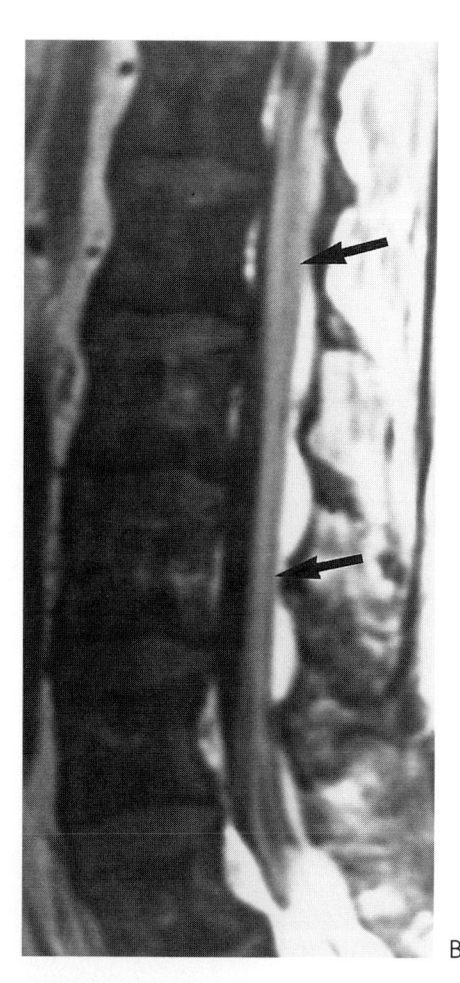

Radiologic Findings

Sagittal short TR image (Fig. A) reveals that the marrow within all of the vertebral bodies appears as decreased signal intensity. This replaces the normal increased signal intensity of the fatty bone marrow. There are small patchy areas of increased signal intensity within the L3 vertebral body (*arrow*).

Sagittal short TR image postinfusion (Fig. B) reveals that there is faint patchy enhancement within the marrow of the vertebral bodies, as well as dense, streaky enhancement of the nerve roots of the cauda equina and surrounding the terminal aspect of the spinal cord (*arrows*).

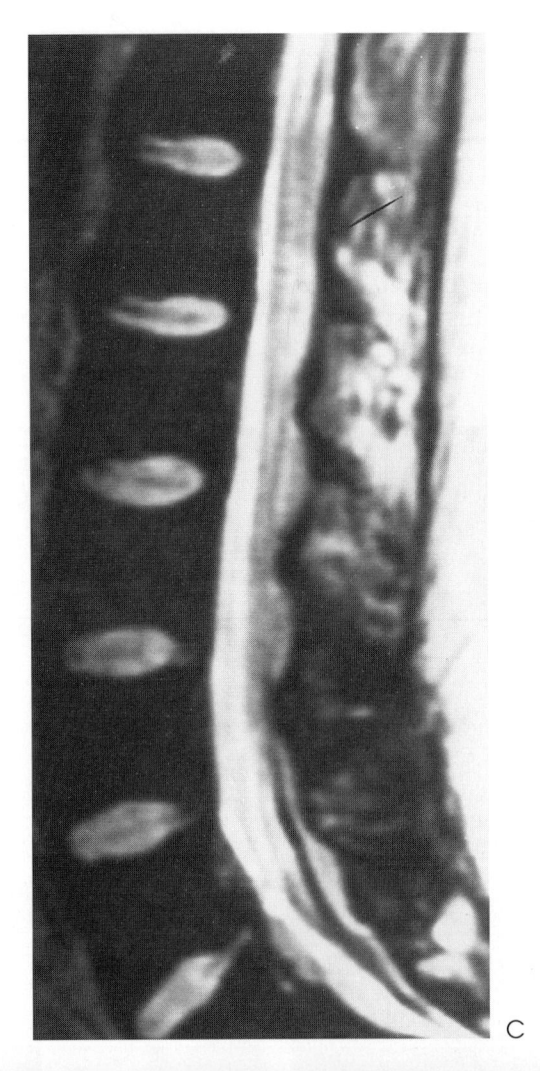

TEACHING ATLAS OF SPINE IMAGING

C

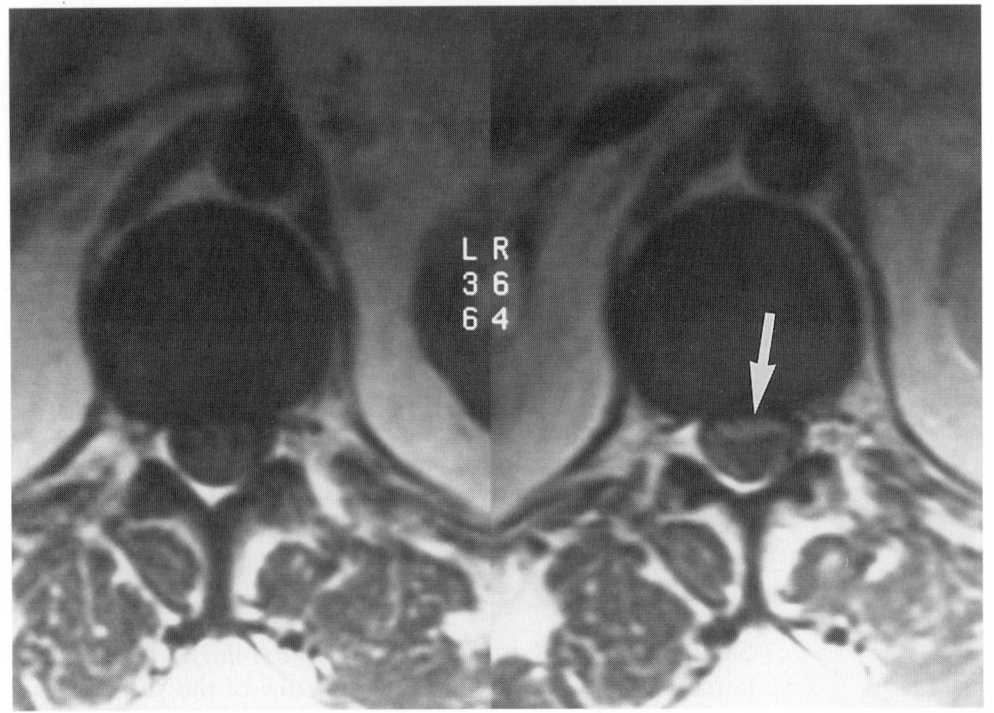

D

SPINAL MENINGEAL CARCINOMATOSIS

Radiologic Findings (continued)

Sagittal long TR image (Fig. C) reveals decreased signal intensity of the distal nerve roots of the cauda equina at the L5-S1 level (*arrows*).

Axial short TR preinfusion (Fig. D, *left*) image reveals decreased signal intensity of the marrow within the marrow of the vertebral body. Postinfusion (Fig. D, *right*) image shows diffuse enhancement of the nerve roots of the cauda equina (*arrow*).

Diagnosis

Leukemic infiltrate in the marrow of the vertebral bodies and meningeal carcinomatosis with enhancement of the nerve roots of the cauda equina.

Differential Diagnosis

- lymphoma or leukemia
- metastatic disease

Discussion

In the normal patient, the marrow should be higher in signal intensity than the intervertebral disc because it contains adipose tissue. The "disc reversal sign" occurs when the vertebral body bone marrow is lower in signal intensity than the intervertebral disc signal intensity. The disc reversal sign implies that there is a diffuse abnormality such as might be typically seen in a patient with a disease such as lymphoma or leukemia. The enhancement of the cauda equina is definitely abnormal and occurs because there is diffuse infiltration of the meninges by tumor. Metastatic prostate carcinoma might have a similar appearance; however, this does not usually exhibit meningeal carcinomatosis.

PEARL
- A postcontrast study is necessary for evaluation of the presence or absence of meningeal carcinomatosis.

PITFALL
- Because of the marrow's homogeneous nature, diffuse involvement of the marrow may be mistaken for normal. Correlation with other noninvolved areas of the body, such as the femur or femoral neck and head, may reveal a more normal appearing marrow and allow one to make a diagnosis of abnormal spinal marrow. Correlation with a radionuclide bone scan may also be helpful for more complete evaluation.

TEACHING ATLAS OF SPINE IMAGING

Case 9

Clinical Presentation

The patient is a 56-year-old female with known breast cancer who presents with back pain and lower extremity weakness.

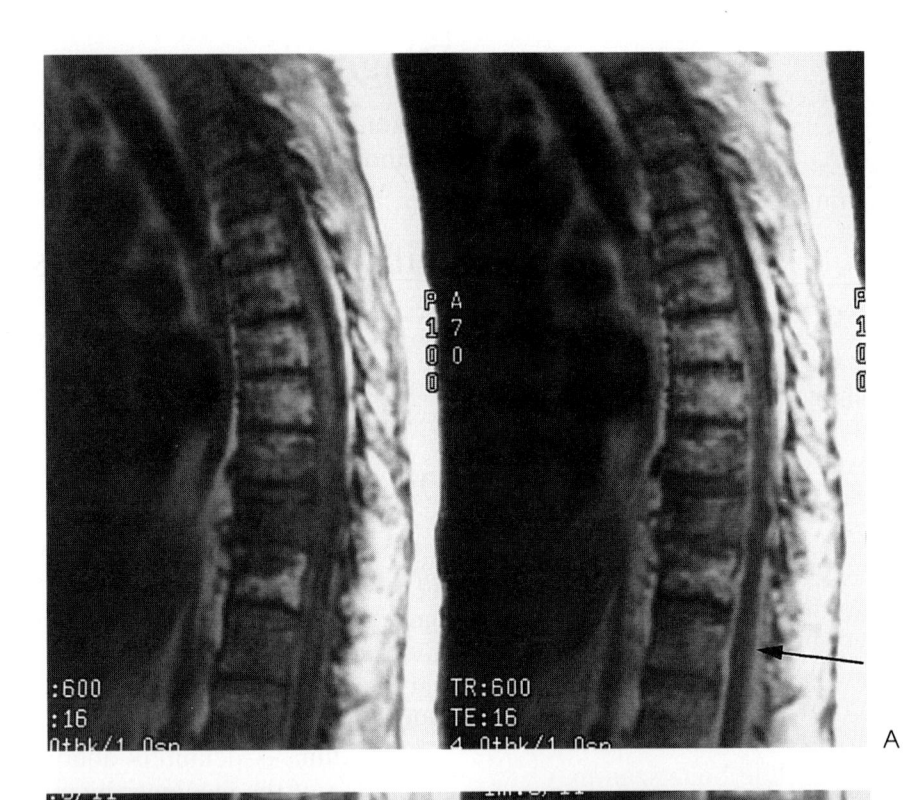

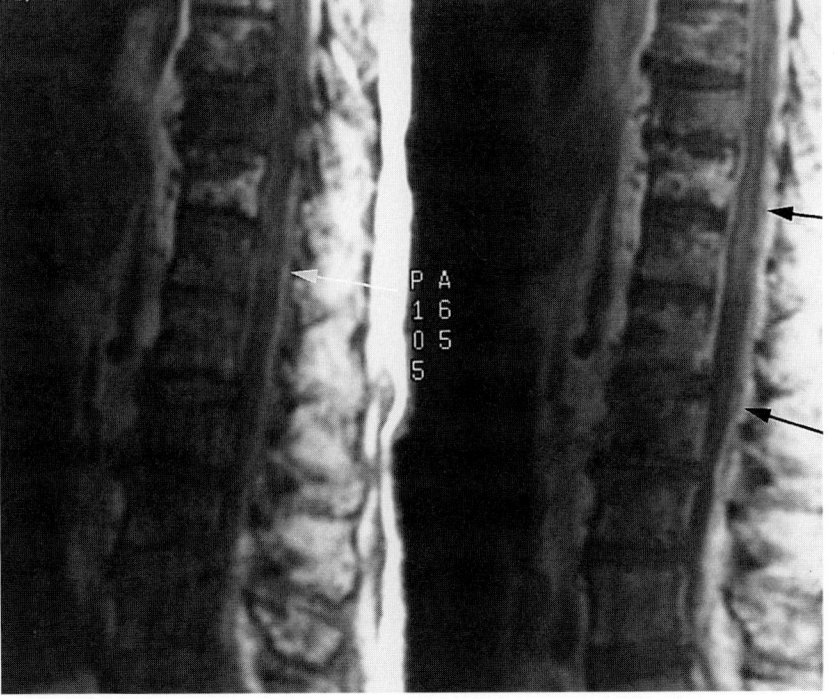

SPINAL MENINGEAL CARCINOMATOSIS

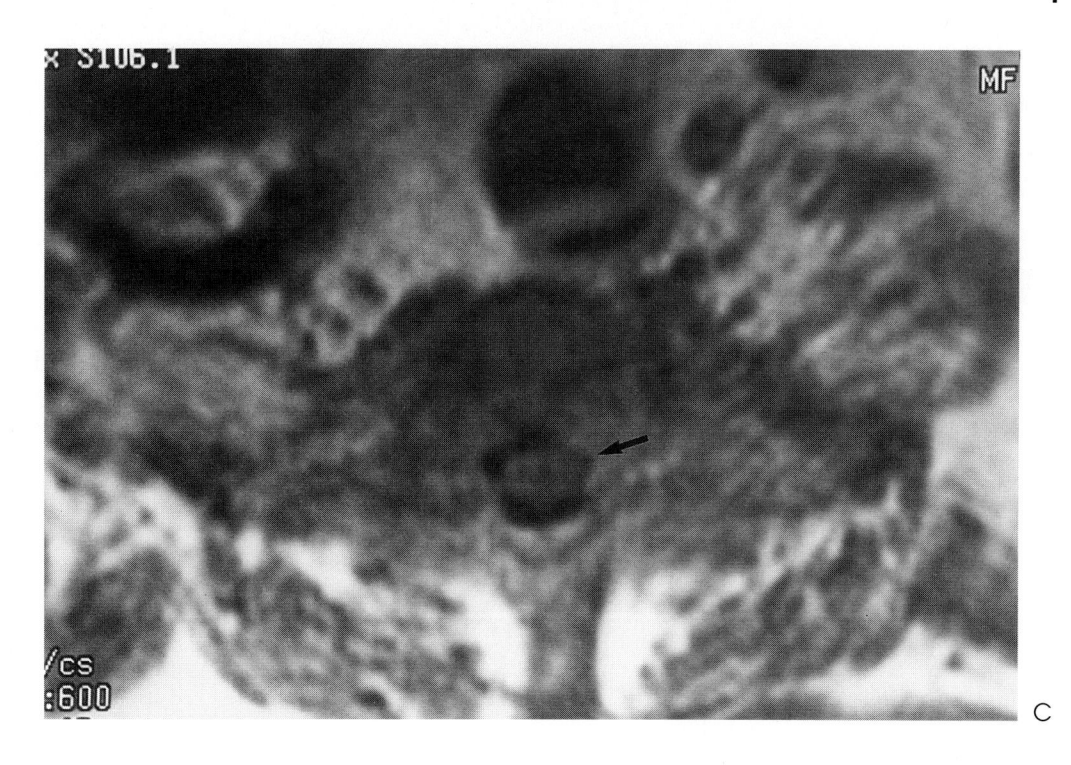

Radiologic Findings

Pre- (Fig. A, *left*) and postinfusion (Fig. A, *right*) sagittal short TR images in the upper thoracic region reveals diffuse patchy areas of decreased signal intensity in the marrow of all the visualized vertebral bodies and spinous processes. There are multiple patchy areas of interruption of the normal epidural fat. After the infusion of contrast (*right*), there is enhancement of a soft tissue mass dorsal to the spinal cord in the anticipated location of the normal epidural fat (*arrow*). Enhancement is also present anterior to the spinal cord.

Pre- (Fig. B, *left*) and postinfusion (Fig. B, *right*) sagittal short TR images in the lower thoracic region reveal patchy areas of decreased signal intensity in all the visualized bony structures. The normal high signal intensity of the epidural space is replaced by intermediate signal soft tissue (*left, white arrow*). The epidural areas of enhancement are again seen (*right, black arrows*).

Axial short TR image postinfusion at the level of the cervicothoracic junction (Fig. C) reveals expansion of the vertebral pedicle and circumferential encroachment upon the low signal intensity of the subarachnoid space. There is enhancement of the marrow in the vertebral body, the vertebral body pedicle with encroachment upon the lateral aspect of the subarachnoid space (*black arrow*), and the transverse processes, as well as in the visualized portions of the ribs.

Diagnosis

Metastatic breast cancer to the vertebral body marrow and the spinal epidural space.

PEARL
- The areas of high signal intensity within the vertebral marrow represent small areas of remaining normal vertebral marrow. Close evaluation for replacement of the normal high signal intensity fat will allow the more ready appreciation of replacement with metastatic tumor.

TEACHING ATLAS OF SPINE IMAGING

PITFALL
- There is variable enhancement after contrast enhancement. The pattern of enhancement from diffuse and homogeneous to the absence of enhancement are all possible in patients with metastatic disease.

Differential Diagnosis

- metastatic disease
- multiple myeloma

Discussion

Multiple myeloma could have a similar appearance, as could metastasis from any tumor that results in osteolytic or osteoblastic metastatic deposits. In the male patient, the most likely primary tumor would be prostate cancer.

SPINAL MENINGEAL CARCINOMATOSIS

Case 10

Clinical Presentation

The patient is a 53-year-old female with breast carcinoma now presenting with neck pain and a new right Horner's syndrome.

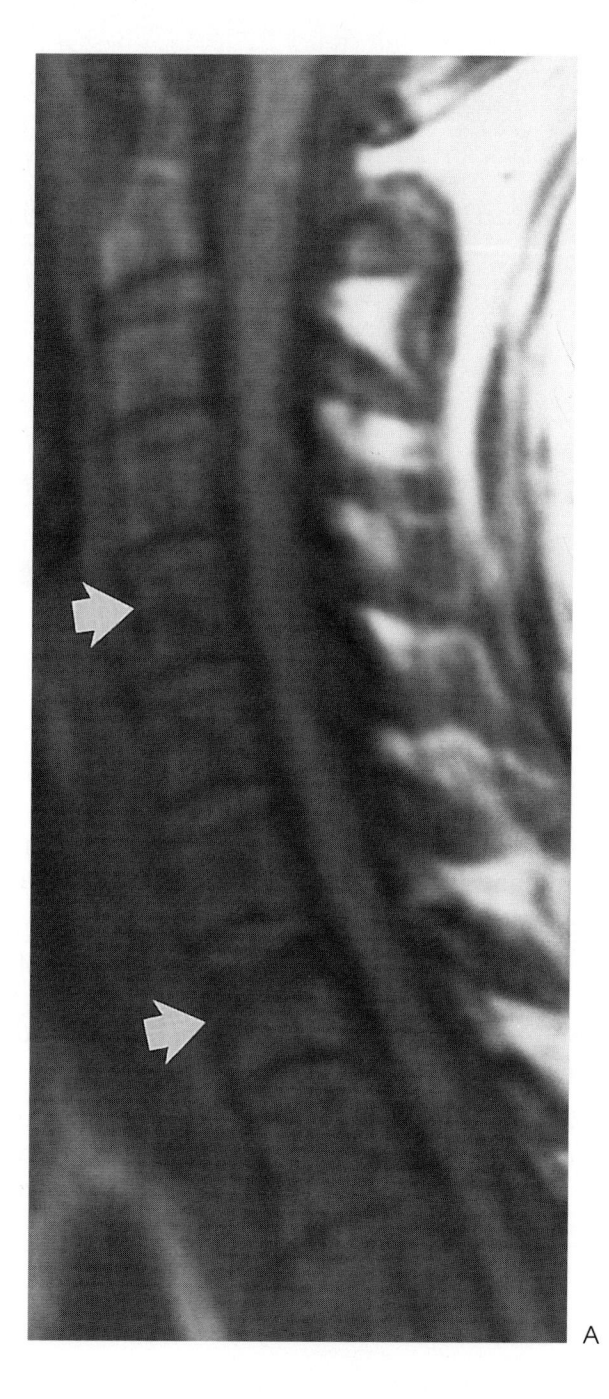

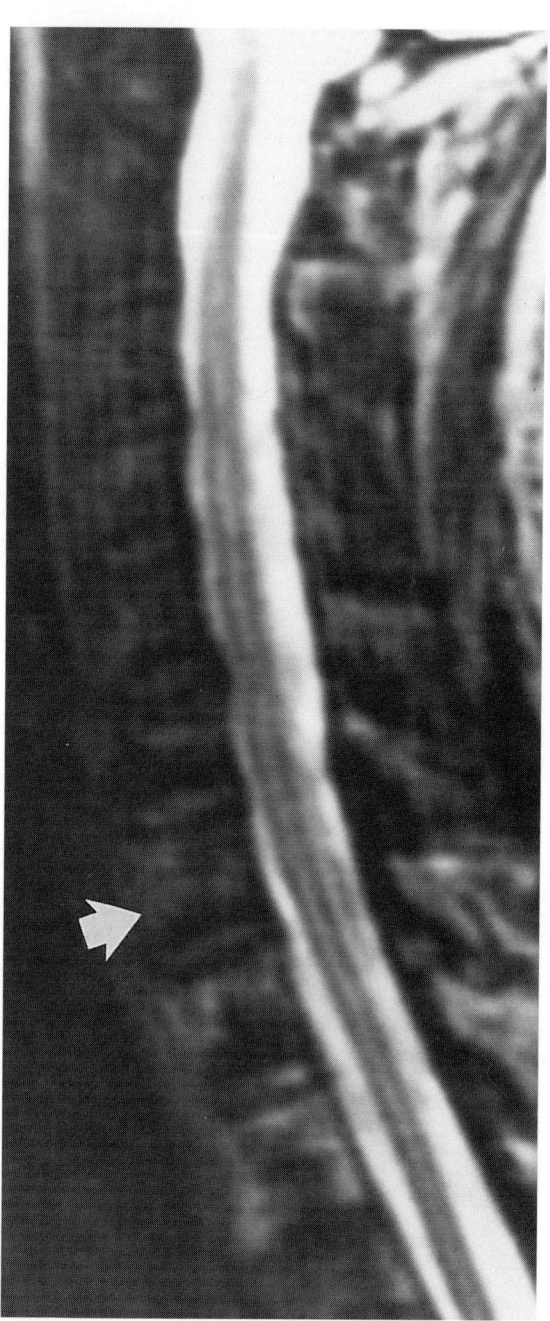

A

B

TEACHING ATLAS OF SPINE IMAGING

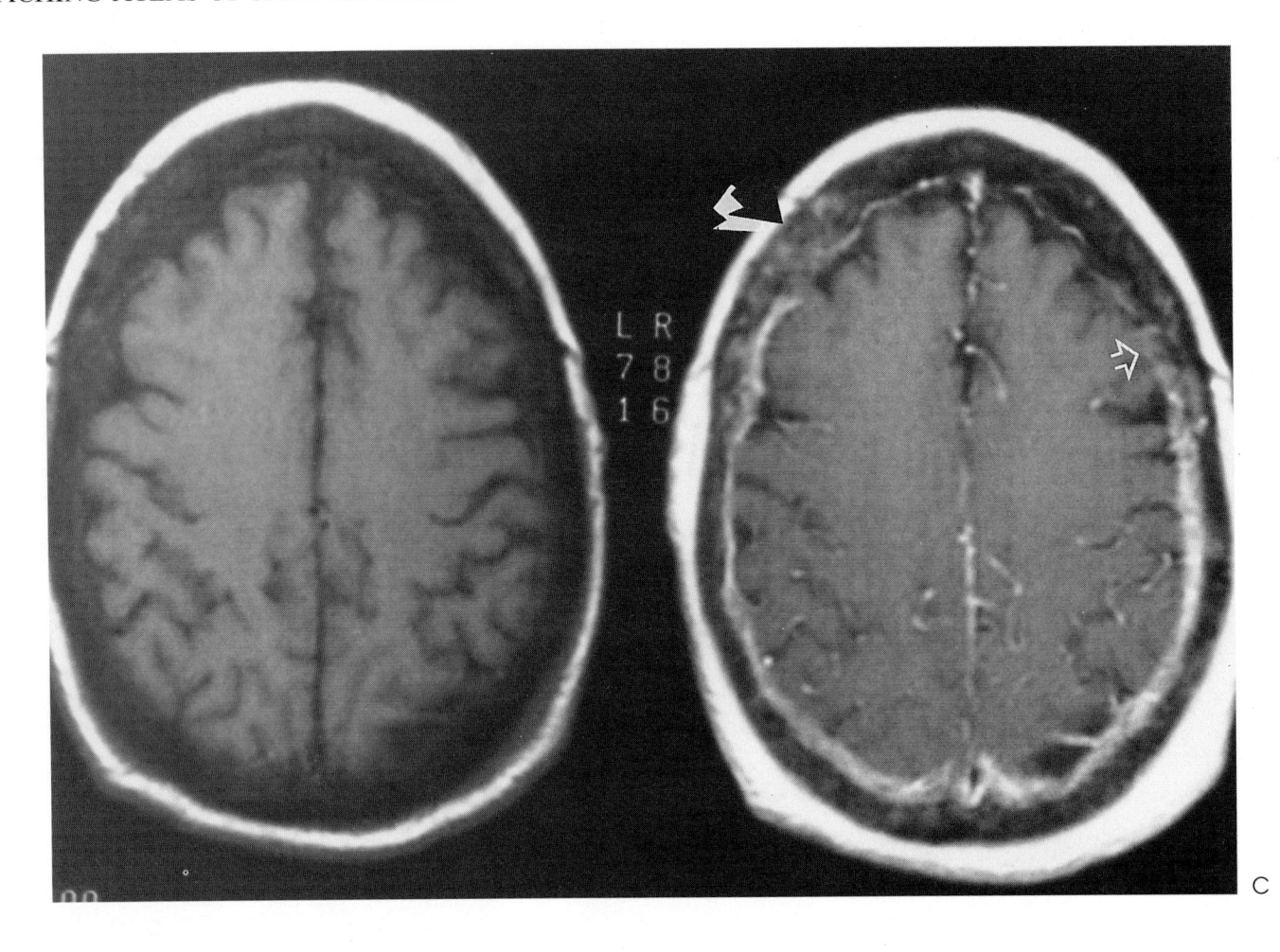

Radiologic Findings

Sagittal short TR image (Fig. A) reveals mottled areas of decreased signal intensity in the marrow of multiple vertebral bodies. This is seen in the midportion of C5 and in the upper half of the T1 vertebral body (*arrows*).

Sagittal long TR image (Fig. B) reveals persistent areas of decreased signal intensity throughout multiple vertebral bodies. The body of C7 reveals faint mottled areas of increased and decreased signal intensity (*arrow*). The T1 and T2 vertebral bodies reveal internal areas of increased signal intensity and decreased signal intensity.

Pre- (Fig. C, *left*) and postinfusion (Fig. C, *right*) axial short TR images of the brain reveal diffuse enhancement of the leptomeninges (*right, open arrow*). There are also patchy areas of expansion of the calvarium that reveal enhancement (*right, black and white arrow*).

Diagnosis

Diffuse osteoblastic and osteolytic metastatic deposits throughout the bony structures; cerebral meningeal carcinomatosis

PEARLS
- The mottled areas of variable decreased signal intensity area are secondary to mixed osteoblastic and osteolytic metastatic deposits.

- Osteolytic metastatic disease, such as breast cancer, may become osteoblastic after treatment. Treatment results in slowing of the destructive process and allows the bone to become osteoblastic.

SPINAL MENINGEAL CARCINOMATOSIS

PITFALL
- When the metastases are diffuse and relatively symmetric, the study may appear normal.

Differential Diagnosis

- metastatic disease
- multiple myeloma
- myelofibrosis

Discussion

Multiple myeloma would also be a possible diagnosis in this patient. Any primary tumor could result in a similar appearance. In the appropriate setting, the possibility of multiple marrow infarcts would also be a diagnostic consideration. Myelofibrosis that is idiopathic, secondary to a toxic chemical, or secondary to chemotherapy should also be considered.

Section VII

Inflammatory Diseases of the Spine

Section VII

Inflammatory Diseases of the Spine

INFLAMMATORY DISEASES OF THE SPINE

Case 1

Clinical Presentation

The patient is a middle-aged female with back pain.

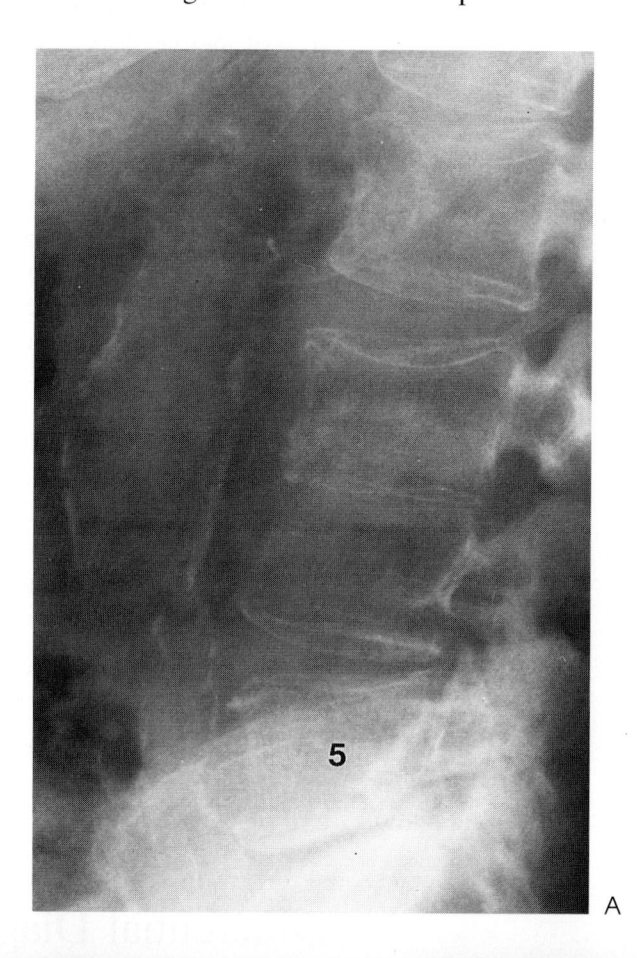

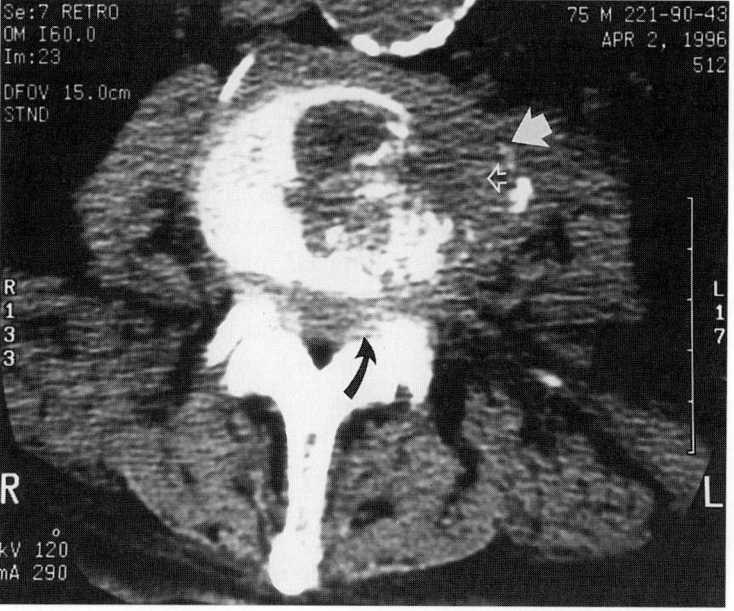

Radiologic Findings

Plain film evaluation (Fig. A) reveals narrowing of the intervertebral disc space between the L3 and L4 vertebral bodies. There is sclerosis of the lower half of the L3 vertebral body and indistinctness of the superior end plate of the L4 vertebral body. The anterior superior corner of L4 is not visualized. A slight loss of height of the L3 vertebral body can be noted. Degenerative changes with anterior osteophytes are noted at L5 (5). An area of increased bone density extends from the inferior end plate to the midportion of the vertebral body of L3. A calcified abdominal aortic aneurysm is displaced anteriorly by a soft tissue mass that extends from the inferior end plate of L2 through the inferior end plate of L4.

Computed tomography (CT) at the level of the L3-4 intervertebral disc (Fig. B) reveals irregularity of the visualized vertebral body endplate. There is anterior and left paraspinal expansion of the disc. The anterior and left lateral margins of the vertebral body are absent, as seen on the plain film evaluation. The anticipated margin of the vertebral body is identified by the open arrow and the bulging disc and soft tissue are identified by the large white arrow. The soft tissue component extends anteriorly to the vertebral body as well. The calcified wall of the abdominal aorta projects anteriorly. The soft tissue extends posteriorly into the vertebral canal and obliterates the thecal sac, resulting in a severe spinal stenosis at this level. The mass also obliterates the left intervertebral foramen (*curved arrow*). Incidentally there are degenerative changes involving the interfacet joints bilaterally.

Diagnosis

Discitis with soft tissue component and destruction of the vertebral body end plate.

Differential Diagnosis

- metastases

Discussion

The involved disc exhibits decreased signal intensity on short TR images and may appear widened or narrowed depending on the stage of involvement. On long TR images, the intervertebral disc appears as increased signal intensity because there are an increased number of protons in the form of increased edema and pus. Typically there is irregularity of the adjacent end plates. This aids in the differentiation of the discitis from a simple degenerative disc. With an infected disc, enhancement is usually visible on the postinfusion portion of the examination; the amount of enhancement is highly variable. There may be paraspinal abscess formation that also exhibits enhancement. In addition, there may be extension in to the psoas muscle when the lumbar spine is involved. Therefore, specific evaluation should be made for psoas muscle involvement.

PEARLS

- CT-guided needle aspiration is helpful for diagnosis.

- Incidental abdominal aortic aneurysm is displaced anteriorly away from the anterior margin of the spine by soft tissue mass associated with the infected intervertebral disc.

- It is also important to evaluate the paraspinal regions in any patient in whom an inflammatory process is suspected.

INFLAMMATORY DISEASES OF THE SPINE

> **PITFALLS**
>
> - Early or subtle changes related to discitis may be mistaken for degenerative disc disease. However, in degenerative disc disease, signal intensity is typically decreased on long TR images; when there is inflammation, signal intensity is generally increased on long TR images.
>
> - MR with contrast infusion is the procedure of choice for evaluation and reveals enhancement of the infected disc and the associated soft tissue component.

Diagnosis may be confirmed by blood cultures or, even more accurately, by direct needle aspiration of the involved disc level. Note that the organism may not be identified or cultured following needle aspiration because the patient has typically been partially or extensively treated with broad spectrum antibiotics by the time needle aspiration is performed. However, in occasional cases where there has been incomplete or no response to antibiotics, the needle aspiration may identify an organism not previously suspected and not responsive to the antibiotics that have been given to that point. CT-guided needle biopsy and/or disc space aspiration is strongly suggested in cases that do not respond to antibiotics.

Prior to magnetic resonance (MR) imaging, discitis was evaluated with plain film examination and CT scanning, and occasionally nuclear medicine studies, which revealed increased activity. The early changes with plain film examination were often subtle and difficult to identify. Plain film changes were frequently not obvious until the disease had progressed to a late stage. The bone sclerosis (Fig. A) involving the inferior half of the L3 vertebral body is secondary to reactive bone formation and may have preceded the inflammatory process.

Compacted trabecular bone and an entity called "bone bruising" may also exhibit a similar appearance. Bone bruising is probably secondary to edema within the bone marrow after bone trauma. Bone bruises may also be seen with athletic injuries.

TEACHING ATLAS OF SPINE IMAGING

Case 2

Clinical Presentation

The patient is a 16-year-old male who developed back pain following a football game in which he was tackled very hard. There was no history of drug abuse.

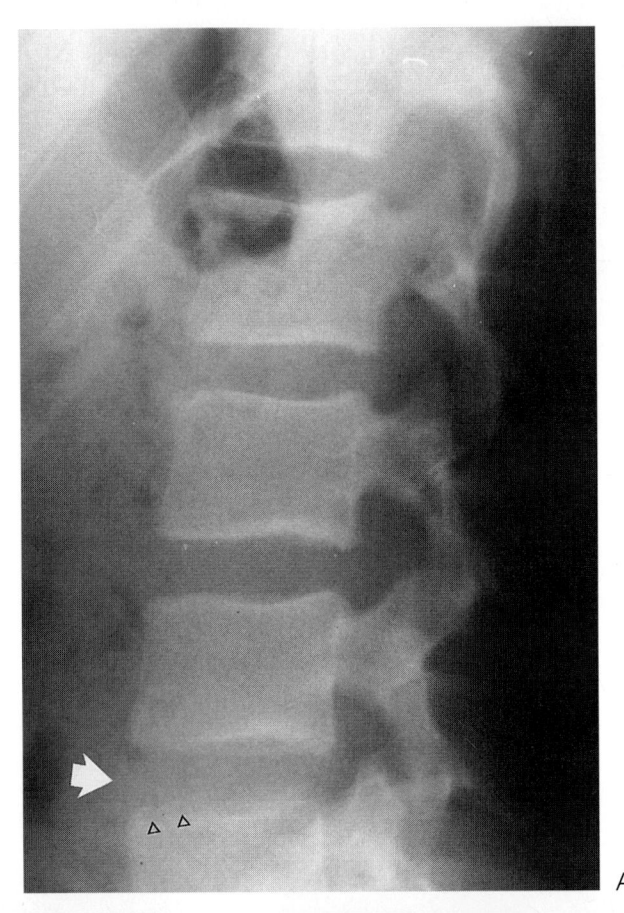

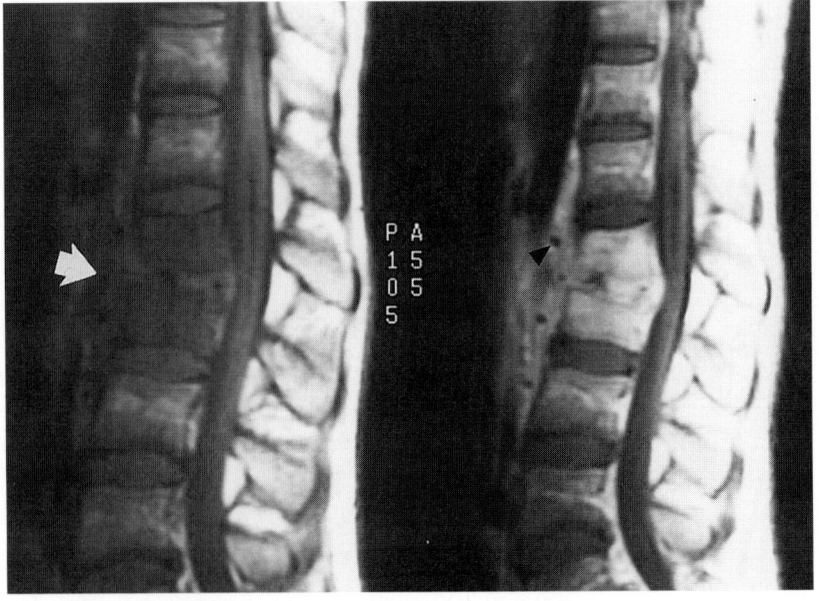

INFLAMMATORY DISEASES OF THE SPINE

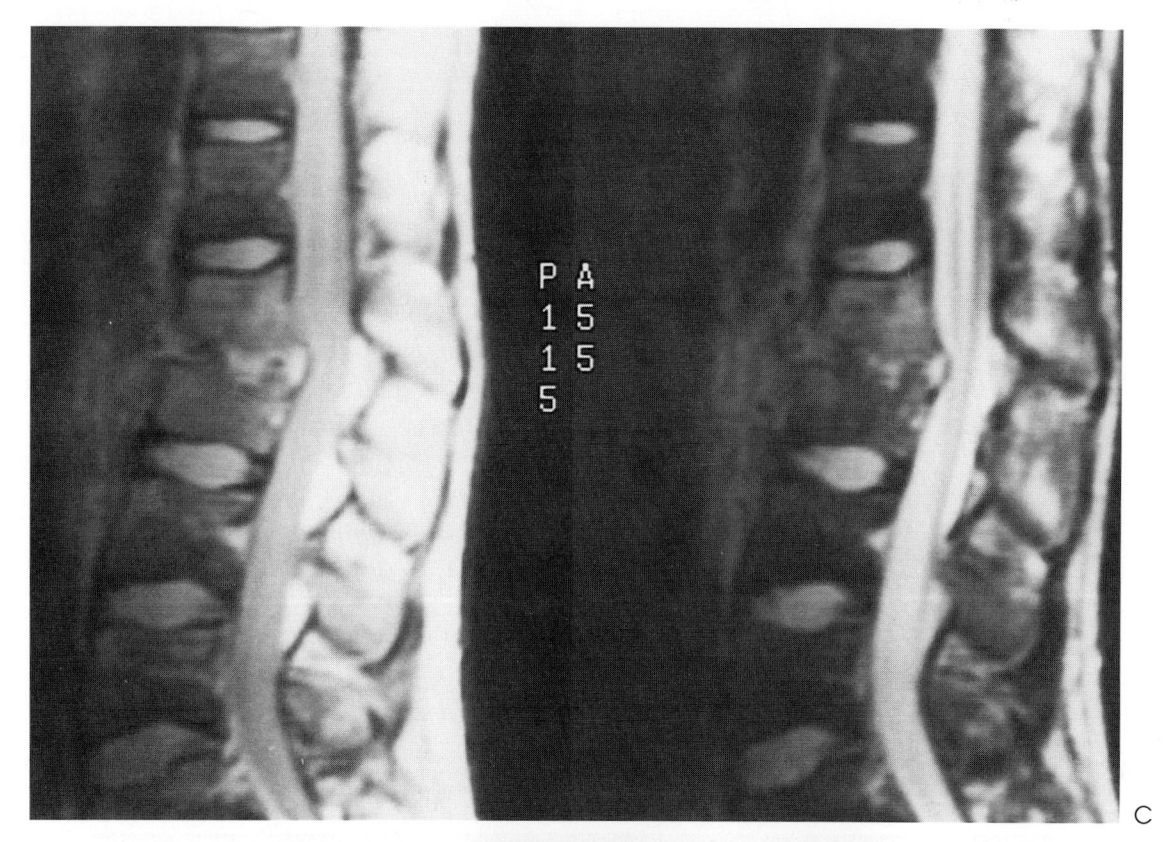

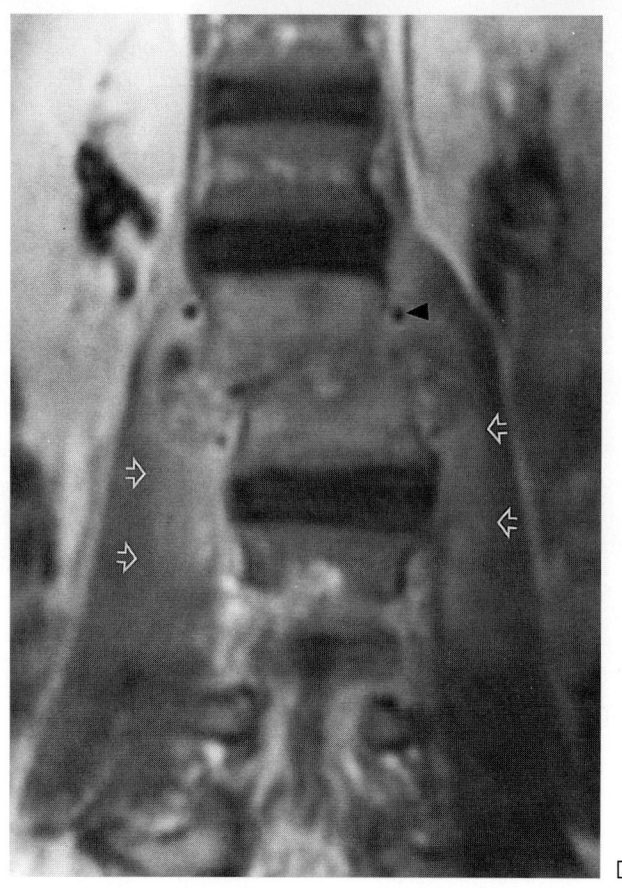

TEACHING ATLAS OF SPINE IMAGING

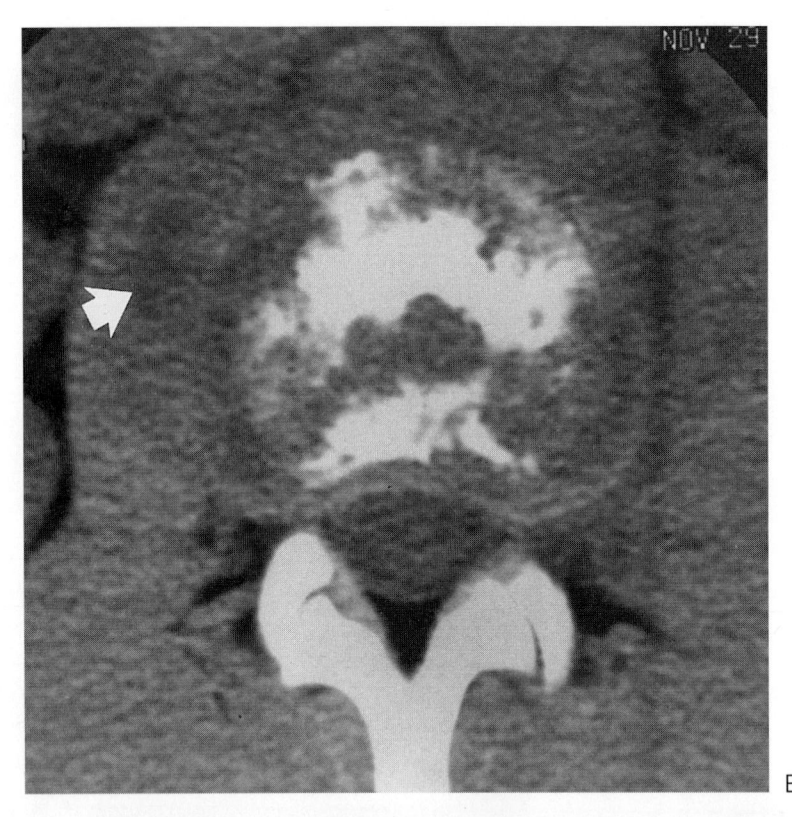

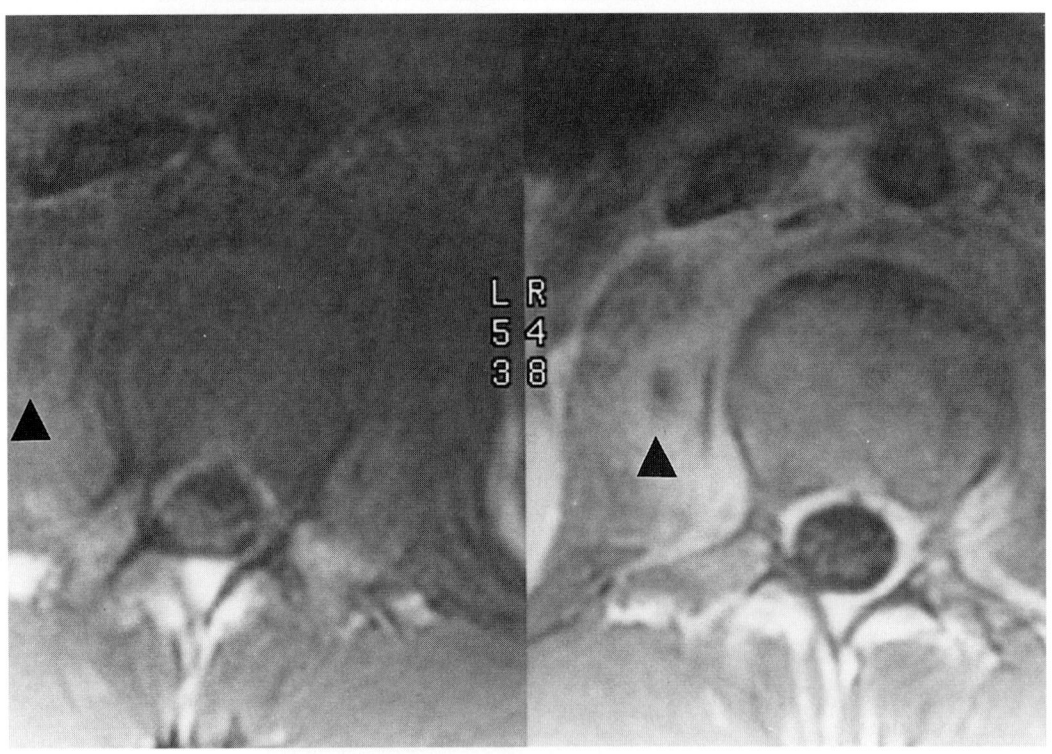

INFLAMMATORY DISEASES OF THE SPINE

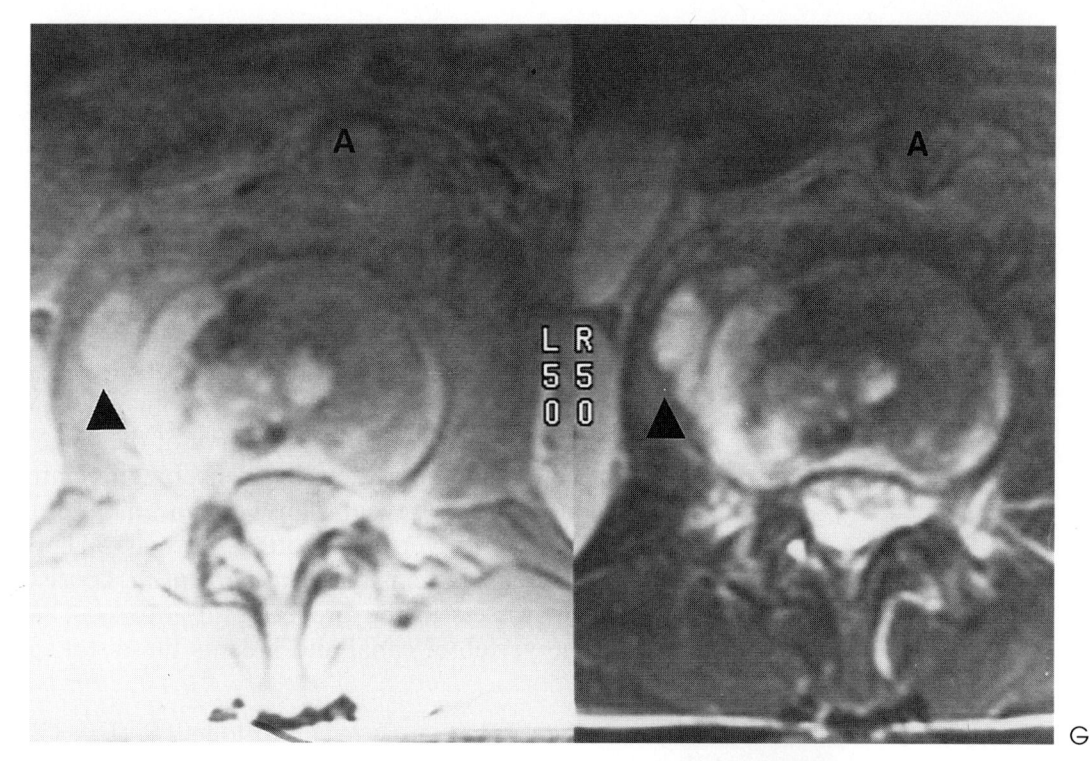

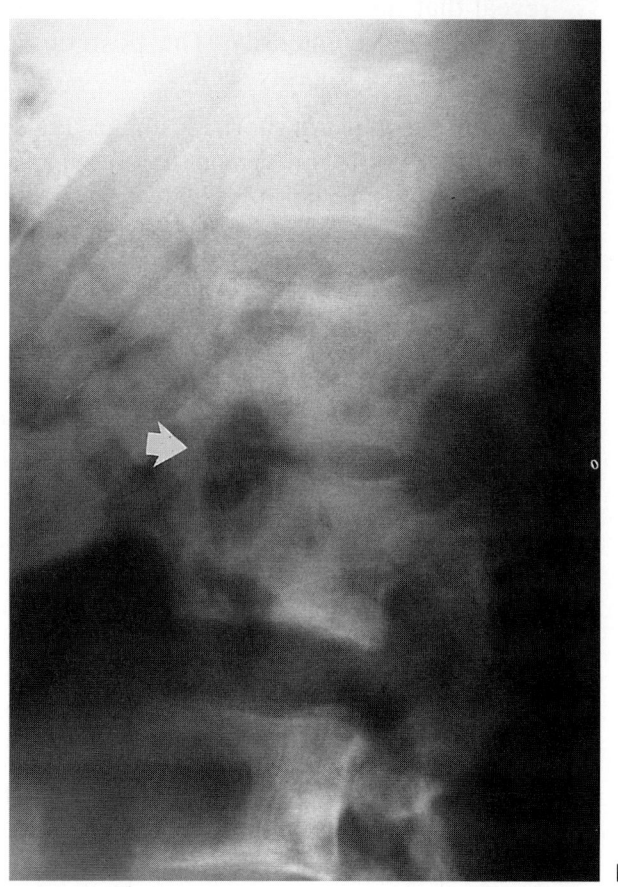

473

Radiologic Findings

Initial lateral plain film radiograph (Fig. A) of the spine was obtained approximately 2 weeks following the injury. At the level of the L3-4, the scan of the intervertebral disc (*white arrow*) reveals that the superior end plate of the L3 vertebral body (*open arrowheads*) is indistinct compared to the remaining normal vertebral body endplates.

Pre- (Fig. B, *left*) and postcontrast (Fig. B, *right*) sagittal short TR images approximately 1 month following the plain spine evaluation reveal narrowing of the intervertebral disc space with destruction of the adjacent vertebral body endplates (*left, white arrow*). A small anterior paraspinal soft tissue mass is visible, and there is reversal of the curve of the spine and posterior displacement of the vertebral body and intervertebral disc into the vertebral canal. The postcontrast study reveals dense enhancement of the intervertebral disc as well as the prevertebral soft tissue mass. There are internal areas of rounded low signal intensity (*right, arrowhead*) consistent with areas of flow void within vessels in the prevertebral abscess. The disc projects posteriorly into the vertebral canal and indents the distal spinal cord and cauda equina.

Sagittal intermediate TR (Fig. C, *left*) and long TR (Fig. C, *right*) images reveal that the intervertebral disc and the prevertebral abscess all exhibit increased signal intensity. The posterior projection of the disc into the vertebral canal is easily seen.

Coronal postcontrast short TR image (Fig. D) reveals the right lateral offset of L3 relative to L4. There are large mottled areas of increased signal intensity with internal areas of decreased signal intensity in the psoas muscles bilaterally at the level of the intervertebral disc and extending inferiorly (*open white arrows*). A small rounded area of flow void is (*black arrowhead*) is seen within the area of soft tissue prominence.

Computed tomographic (CT) scan (Fig. E) at the same time as the magnetic resonance (MR) scan reveals the irregular, "moth eaten" appearance of the vertebral body end plate adjacent to the abnormal intervertebral disc. There is an ill-defined area of low density faintly visible in the psoas muscle on the right side (*white arrow*).

Pre- (Fig. F, *left*) and postcontrast (Fig. F, *right*) axial short TR images reveal the diffusely bulging disc with some encroachment on the anterior aspect of the thecal sac. The decreased signal intensity cystic cavity is seen in the right psoas muscle (*arrowhead*) surrounded by an increased signal intensity thick walled rim that exhibits dense enhancement on the postinfusion scan. There is extension into the left psoas muscle as well as seen on the coronal images.

Axial intermediate (Fig. G, *left*) and long (Fig. G, *right*) TR images reveal that the intervertebral disc and the psoas muscle lesion all exhibit increased signal intensity. There is a rounded area of increased signal intensity in the right psoas muscles (*arrowhead*). The aorta (*A*) is displaced anteriorly and surrounded by intermediate signal intensity soft tissue.

The lateral radiograph (Fig. H) reveals that the intervertebral disc space is increasingly narrowed (*white arrow*).

INFLAMMATORY DISEASES OF THE SPINE

PEARLS

- In the patient who does not improve with treatment or in the patient in whom the diagnosis is in question, CT-guided biopsy is helpful, and strongly advised, for complete evaluation.

- Enhancement of the intervertebral disc is a typical finding of an inflammatory process. Metastatic disease would be very unlikely.

PITFALLS

- The index of suspicion must be high in cases of infection, so an MR scan can be obtained early in the course of the patient's illness.

- Evaluation by CT scanning may mimic the appearance of severe degenerative disc disease.

Diagnosis

Discitis, following trauma, with an unusual organism as the etiologic agent. There are bilateral psoas abscesses and an abscess surrounding the abdominal aorta.

Differential Diagnosis

- discitis
- metastases
- degenerative disc disease

Discussion

Plain spine imaging was essentially normal in this patient early in the course of the illness. Because MR imaging was not performed initially, it is uncertain if it would have been normal or abnormal. However, MR imaging in general is more sensitive than plain film evaluation and should be performed early in the course of an illness if an inflammatory process is suspected. The late follow-up in this patient revealed complete fusion between the two vertebral bodies, which is a known result of an inflammatory process involving the intervertebral disc.

The pre- and postcontrast MR images (Fig. F) reveal that the process in the psoas muscle is a thick walled psoas abscess. The pus filled abscess cavity is demonstrated as a central area of decreased signal intensity (Fig. F, *arrowhead*) and increased signal intensity in the intermediate and long TR images (Fig. G). On postcontrast enhancement, there is dense peripheral enhancement of a thick wall surrounding the psoas abscess (Fig. G, *right*). The nerve roots of the cauda equina also appear prominent, probably secondary to an element of meningitis involving the leptomeninges.

Following the abnormal MR scan the patient was initially placed on high doses of broad spectrum antibiotics, but did not improve. Therefore, after a follow-up MR scan did not reveal improvement, a CT-guided biopsy was obtained with aspiration of material from the psoas muscle abscess. Aspiration revealed that the etiologic agent was *Pseudomonas aeurginosa*. With this diagnosis, the antibiotic was changed to a more appropriate one, and the patient improved.

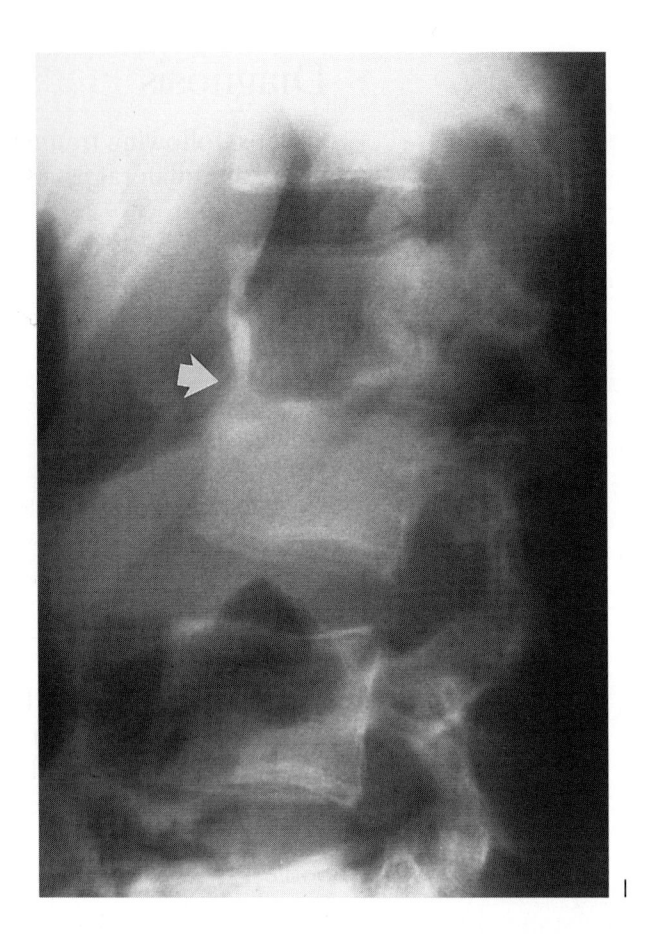

Figure I is the final follow-up spine film and reveals fusion between the L3 and L4 vertebral bodies (*arrow*).

INFLAMMATORY DISEASES OF THE SPINE

Case 3

Clinical Presentation

The patient is a 50-year-old male with a history of intravenous drug abuse, presenting with bilateral lower extremity weakness.

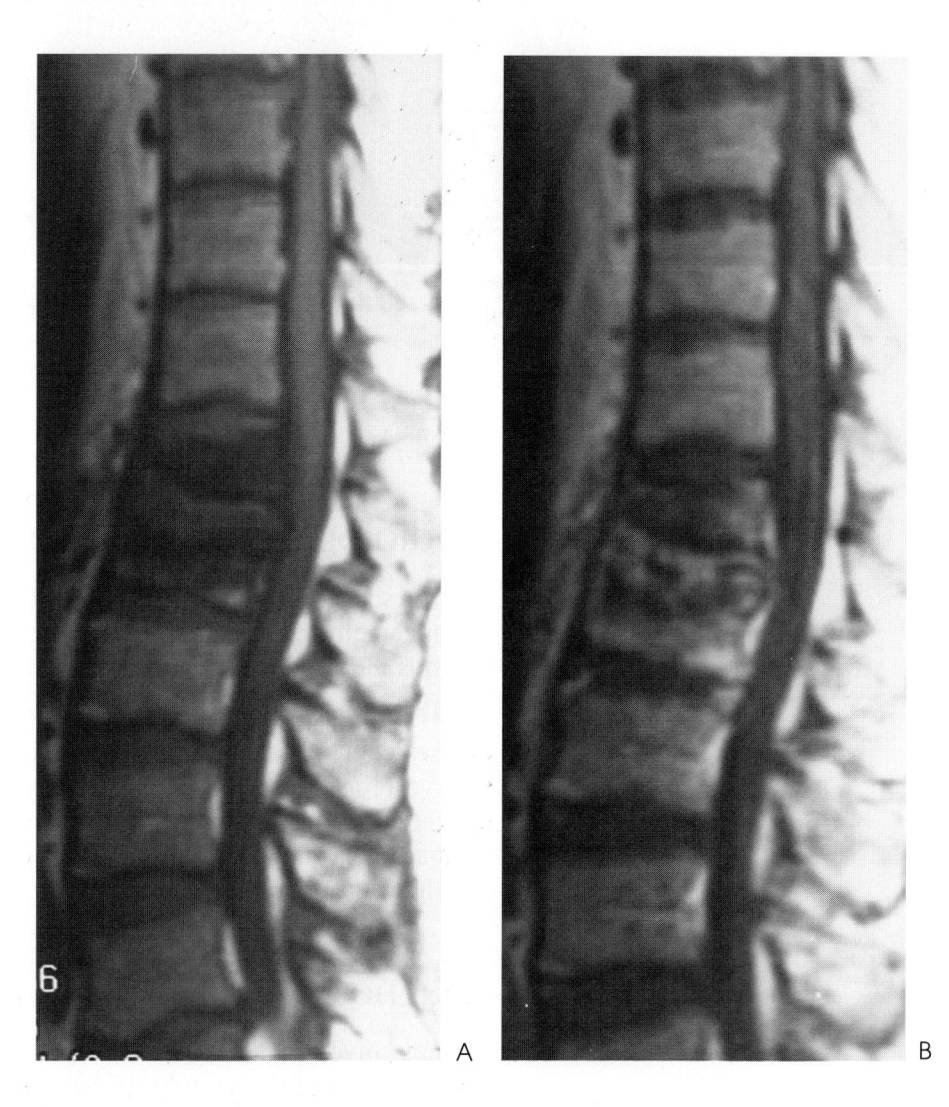

Radiologic Findings

Sagittal short TR image (Fig. A) reveals loss of height of the L1 and L2 vertebral bodies anteriorly and apparent disproportionate widening of the intervertebral disc. There is destruction of the inferior end plate of the L1 vertebral body and of the superior end plate of the L2 vertebral body. There is reversal of the normal lordotic curve at the L1-2 level. There is encroachment upon the anterior epidural space and curvilinear posterior displacement of the spinal cord.

TEACHING ATLAS OF SPINE IMAGING

C

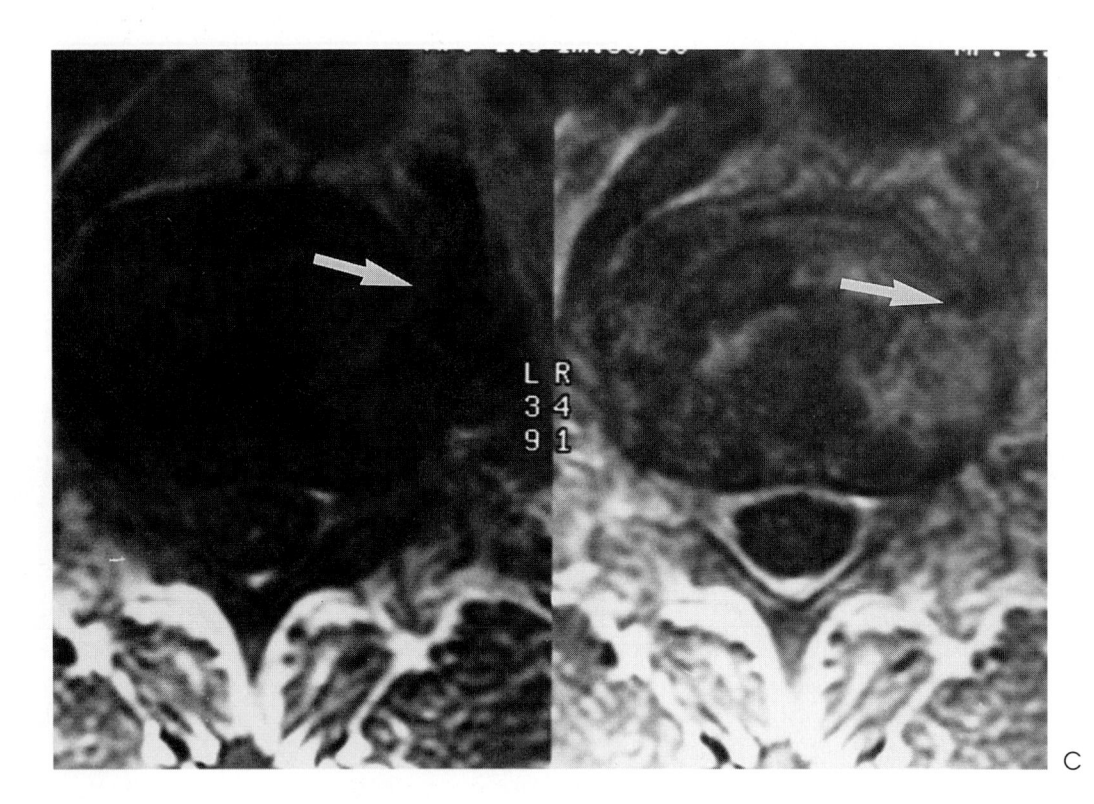

Radiologic Findings (continued)

Sagittal short TR image postcontrast (Fig. B) reveals dense slightly irregular enhancement of the intervertebral disc at the L1-2 level. The enhancement extends into and involves the superior end plate of the L2 vertebral body.

Pre- (Fig. C, *left*) and postcontrast (Fig. C, *right*) axial short TR images at the level of the intervertebral disc reveal dense enhancement of the intervertebral disc with extension into the dorsal paravertebral muscles on the left side (*white arrow*). There is diffuse enhancement surrounding the lumbar thecal sac. The normal high signal intensity epidural fat surrounding the thecal sac is obliterated.

Diagnosis

Discitis, involving the intervertebral disc with paraspinal extension. The enhancement of the vertebral body reflects the presence of vertebral osteomyelitis.

Differential Diagnosis

- discitis

- degenerative disc disease

INFLAMMATORY DISEASES OF THE SPINE

PEARLS
- Care should be taken that an infected disc is not mistaken for a degenerated disc. A degenerated disc generally does not enhance on the postcontrast study.

- CT-guided aspiration and culture of the disc space is helpful for more complete evaluation.

PITFALL
- Metastases to not typically affect the intervertebral body and adjacent disc spaces.

Discussion

If there is question regarding an individual case, and if there is a need to differentiate between infection and degenerative changes, it may be necessary to evaluate the patient with other tests such as radionuclide bone scanning or gallium scanning. In some cases, a final diagnosis may not be possible at the time of the initial study, and the patient may need to return for additional follow-up at a later date. The studies should be performed without and with the infusion of contrast material. Because these patients are frequently treated with high doses of broad spectrum antibiotics prior to attempted biopsy with aspiration, the cultures are frequently negative even in the presence of an inflammatory process. However, even if no organism is cultured, the aspirate may reveal inflammatory cells consistent with infection.

Typical organisms include *Staphalococcus aureus* or Streptococcus; however, in an immunocompromised patient, the organism may include various fungal organisms such as aspergillosis. In the AIDS, patient there is an increased incidence of involvement with *Mycobacterium avium intracellulare* and *Mycobacterium tuberculosis*.

CT-guided biopsy with aspiration of cells as well as fluid is very helpful for complete evaluation and frequently eliminates the need for open surgical biopsy. Care must be taken to send the samples for aerobic as well as anaerobic bacteriological analysis.

TEACHING ATLAS OF SPINE IMAGING

Case 4

Clinical Presentation

The patient is a 60-year-old female with a history of recent surgery for herniated disc and a new history of severe low back pain and a draining surgical incision.

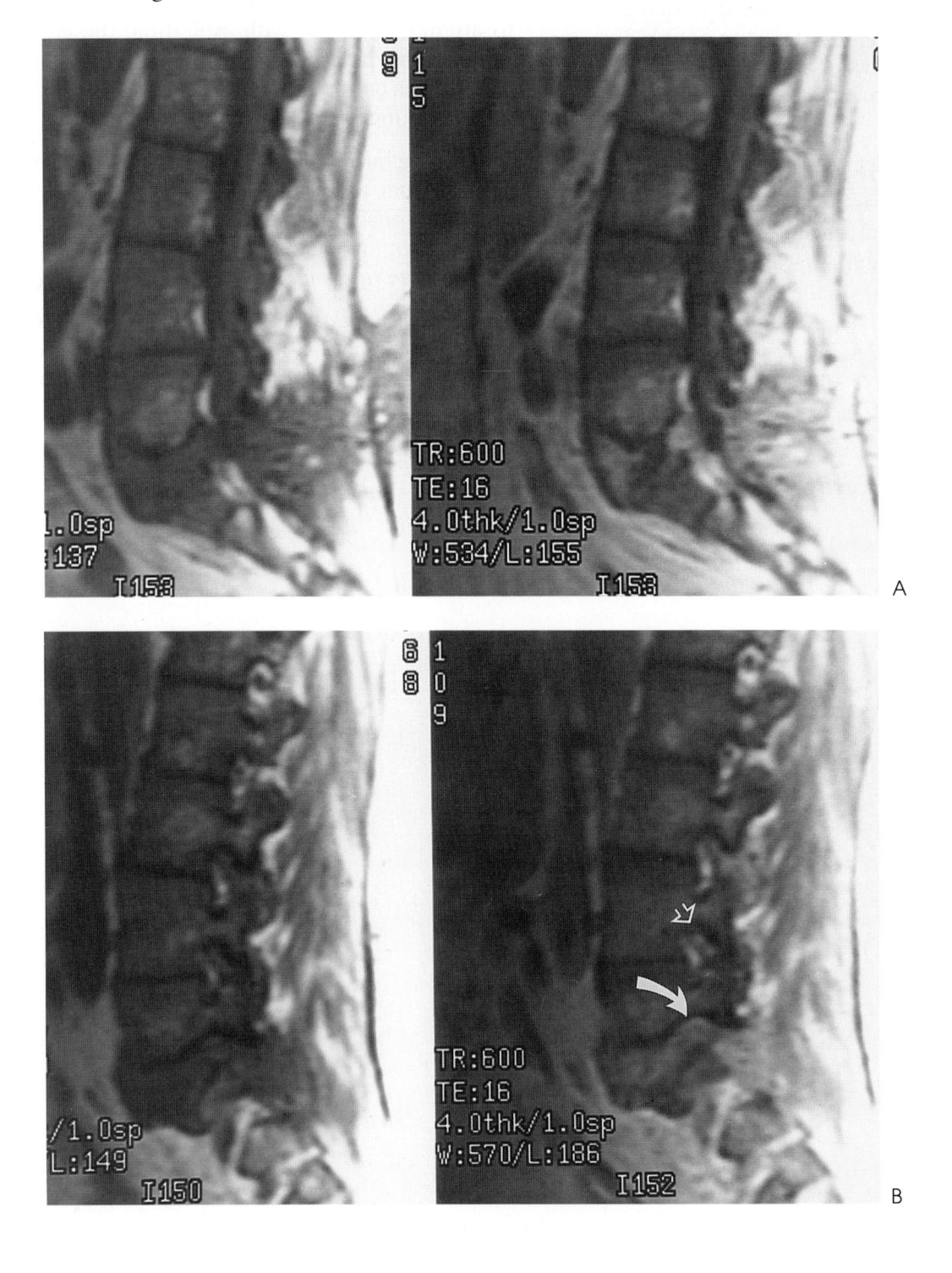

INFLAMMATORY DISEASES OF THE SPINE

C

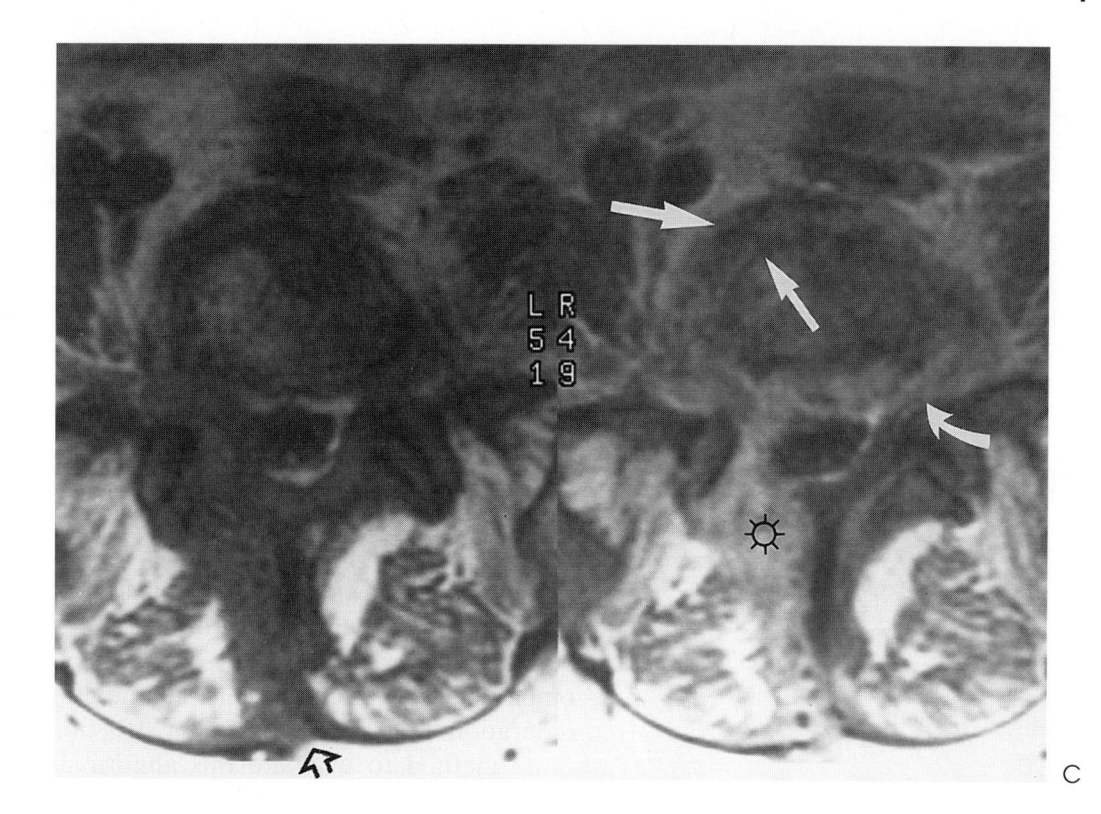

Radiologic Findings

Pre- (Fig. A, *left*) and postcontrast (Fig. A, *right*) sagittal short TR images. The precontrast study reveals expansion of the intervertebral disc at the L5-S1 level. There is irregularity of the superior end plate of the S1 vertebral body, and there is both anterior and posterior prominence of the intervertebral disc. There are postsurgical changes in the soft tissues of the back with disruption of the normal configuration of the dorsal paraspinal muscles of the back. The postcontrast study reveals dense enhancement of the intervertebral disc. The disc is distorted into a "butterfly" configuration, extending posteriorly into the vertebral canal where it compresses the thecal sac. The soft tissues in the lower spinal region dorsal to the thecal sac also enhance.

Pre- (Fig. B, *left*) and postcontrast (Fig. B, *right*) parasagittal short TR images reveal dense enhancement of the intervertebral disc. There is also extension of the enhancement into the intervertebral foramen (*right, curved arrow*). The intervertebral foramen is obliterated with enhancing soft tissue; the normal intervertebral foramen is seen as an area of increased signal fat surrounding the normal dorsal root ganglion (*right, open arrow*). This enhancement extends into the soft tissues of the back.

Pre- (Fig. C, *left*) and postcontrast (Fig. C, *right*) axial short TR images reveal enhancement and diffuse bulging of the disc. The enhancement is also present in the intervertebral foramen bilaterally (*right, curved arrow*). There is prevertebral soft tissue component which extends beyond the margin of the vertebral body (*right, white arrows*), and enhancement of the muscles in the dorsal paraspinal region on the right side (*right, asterisk*), which extends up to the level of the skin. The point of drainage on the skin is also identified (*left, open arrow*).

PEARL
- MR imaging is the most efficient method to evaluate discitis. The convenient multiplanar capability of MR to image the spine and discs allows accurate evaluation both for diagnosis as well as follow-up.

PITFALL
- The patient who does not respond to antibiotics should be considered for CT-guided biopsy so that treatment may be altered appropriately depending upon the organism that is identified.

Diagnosis

Postoperative wound infection with draining sinus tract and postoperative disc infection. The inflammatory process extends into the soft tissues of the back and into the intervertebral foramenae bilaterally.

Differential Diagnosis

- discitis
- epidural abscess

Discussion

Severe pain, as seen in this patient, is a very common clinical symptom in a patient with discitis or epidural abscess. However, the absence of pain makes the diagnosis less likely. In a patient with a draining wound, with a compatible clinical course, an inflammatory process is a strong clinical consideration. Magnetic resonance (MR) imaging is the most sensitive and accurate method to evaluate this abnormality. Because of the extension into the intervertebral foramenae, radicular pain would also be a common symptom in a patient presenting like this.

CT-guided biopsy with culture as well as histology is very helpful for complete diagnosis.

INFLAMMATORY DISEASES OF THE SPINE

Case 5

Clinical Presentation

The patient is a 48-year-old male presenting with a history of intravenous drug abuse and active pulmonary tuberculosis. The patient has a new history of a sensory level with decreased sensation at the level of T4 to T8. There is progressive weakness in the lower extremities.

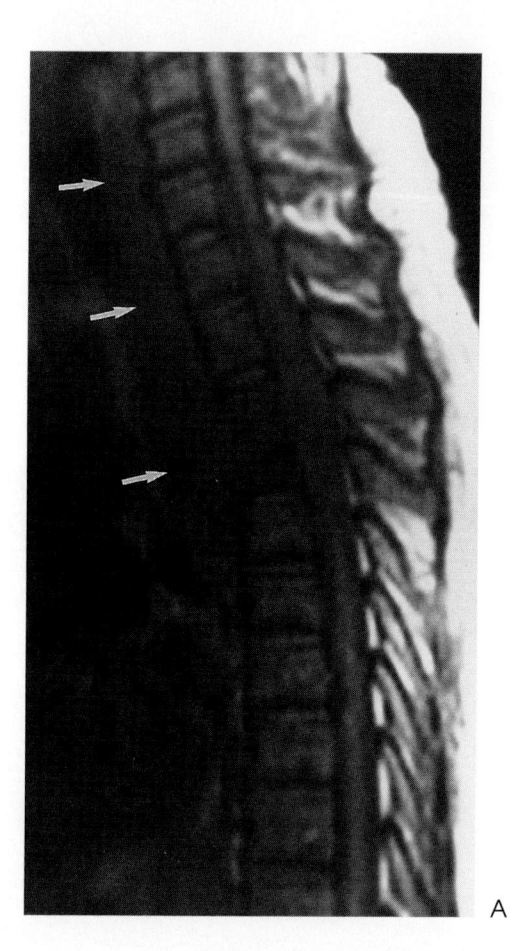

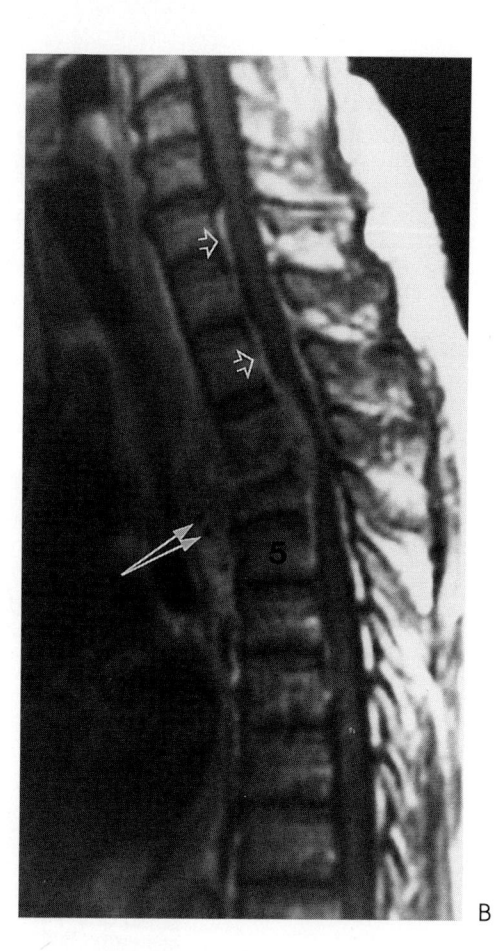

Radiologic Findings

Sagittal short TR image (Fig. A) reveals decreased signal intensity in the T3 and T4 vertebral bodies. There is anterior loss of vertebral body height and poor definition of the intervertebral disc space. An approximately 2-cm-wide anterior prevertebral mass, which extends from approximately C6 through T6 (*arrows*), is visible. The spinal cord is poorly seen from the level of T2 through T5. There is anterior kyphosis at the T3-4 level.

483

TEACHING ATLAS OF SPINE IMAGING

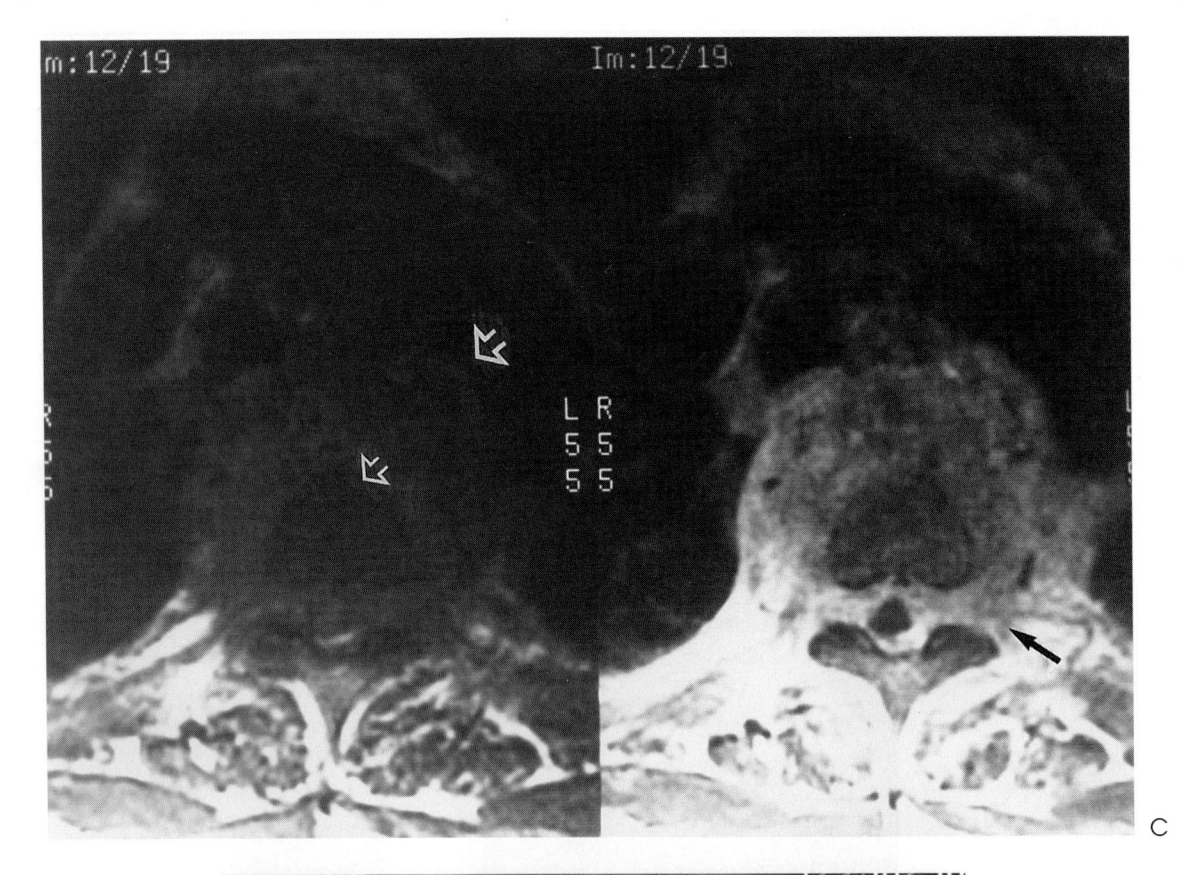

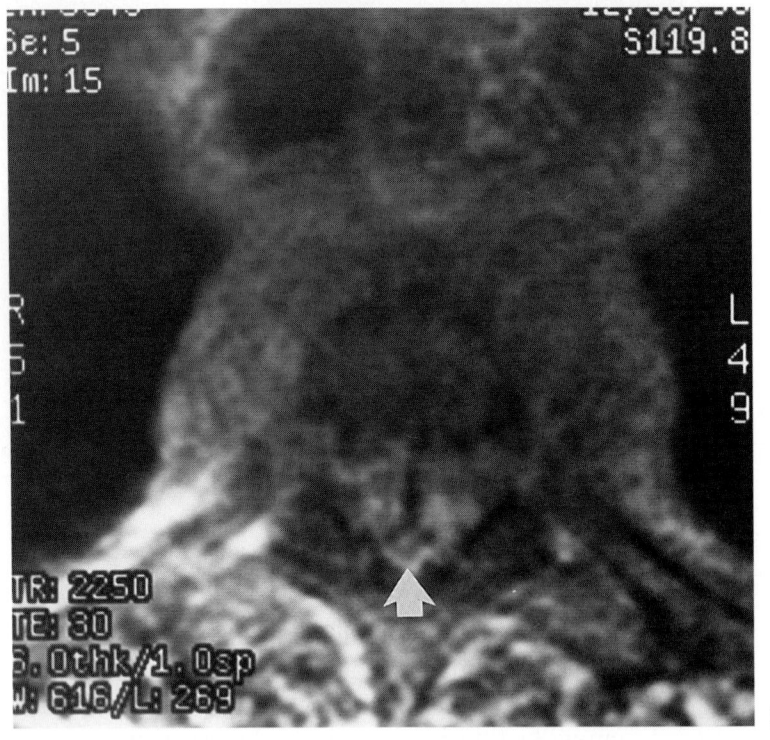

INFLAMMATORY DISEASES OF THE SPINE

Radiologic Findings (continued)

Sagittal short TR image (Fig. B) reveals enhancement of the intervertebral disc at the T3-4 level. The prevertebral soft tissue mass exhibits enhancement with streaks of decreased signal intensity. Small vessels within the anterior soft tissue mass appear as rounded areas of decreased signal intensity flow void (*solid white arrows*). There is also a crescent shaped area of enhancement that extends into the vertebral canal at the T3-4 intervertebral disc level and extends both above and below the disc level posterior to the vertebral bodies. There is a linear area of enhancement that extends superiorly in the epidural space up to the level of C7 (*open arrows*). The T5 level of the spine is identified by 5.

Pre- (Fig. C, *left*) and postcontrast (Fig. C, *right*) axial short TR images reveal a large paraspinal area of enhancement surrounding the T3 vertebral body. The open white arrows identify the edge of the vertebral body and the edge of the paraspinal mass. There is extension into the intervertebral foramen on the left side (*right, black arrow*). The transverse aorta is displaced anteriorly.

Axial short TR image at T4 (Fig. D) reveals marked compression of the thecal sac (*white arrow*) by the large anterior soft tissue mass.

Diagnosis

Discitis and epidural and paraspinal abscess secondary to *Mycobacterium tuberculosis*.

Differential Diagnosis

- discitis

Discussion

The imaging appearance is typical of discitis secondary to *Mycobacterium tuberculosis* (TBc). The illness progresses so slowly that patients may experience mild symptoms relative to the degree of abnormality demonstrated on the images. An inflammatory process is the most likely diagnosis in this patient. A CT-guided biopsy with aspiration is helpful to identify the organism that is causing the inflammatory process. In addition to the involvement of the intervertebral disc, there may also be a paraspinal abscess; therefore, evaluation and filming should be performed to include these areas in the final images.

PEARLS

- There may be multiple levels of involvement with *Mycobacterium tuberculosis* (TBc).

- The entire vertebral column should be evaluated at the time of initial evaluation.

PITFALL
- At surgery, the anterior vertebral body soft tissue component may represent only granulation tissue and not a true abscess.

A chest x-ray should be obtained in any patient with a suspect diagnosis of *Mycobacterium tuberculosis*. Chest x-ray in these patients will typically reveals evidence of an inflammatory process consistent with tuberculosis. In the acquired immunodeficiency syndrome patient, however, the x-ray may be negative even in the presence of an active infection.

In addition, follow-up after a suitable period of medical management is also helpful for patient management. Magnetic resonance imaging with contrast enhancement is the most sensitive method of evaluation.

INFLAMMATORY DISEASES OF THE SPINE

Case 6

Clinical Presentation

The patient is a 28-year-old male with a history of intravenous drug abuse who presented with fever, severe back pain, and paraplegia.

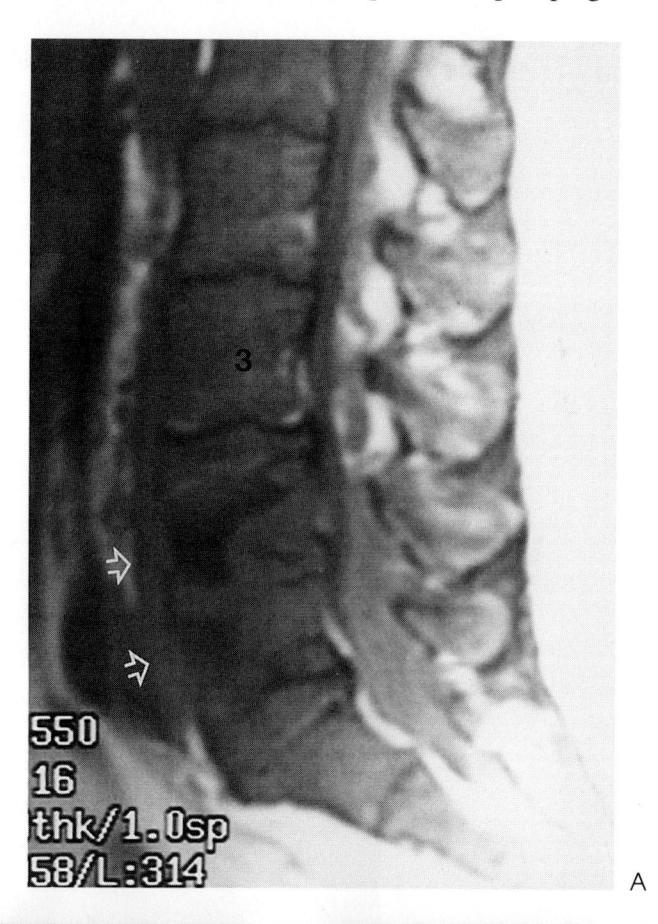

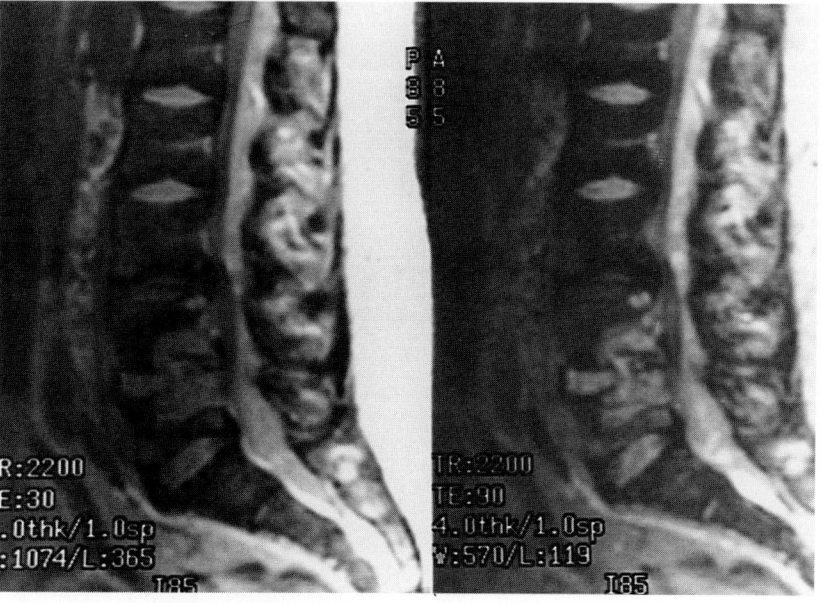

487

TEACHING ATLAS OF SPINE IMAGING

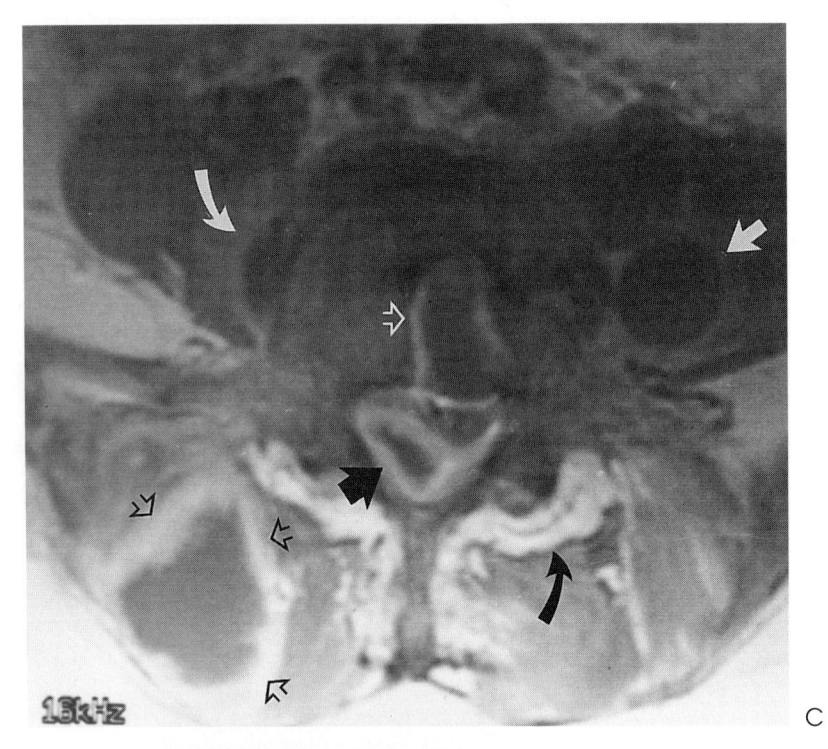

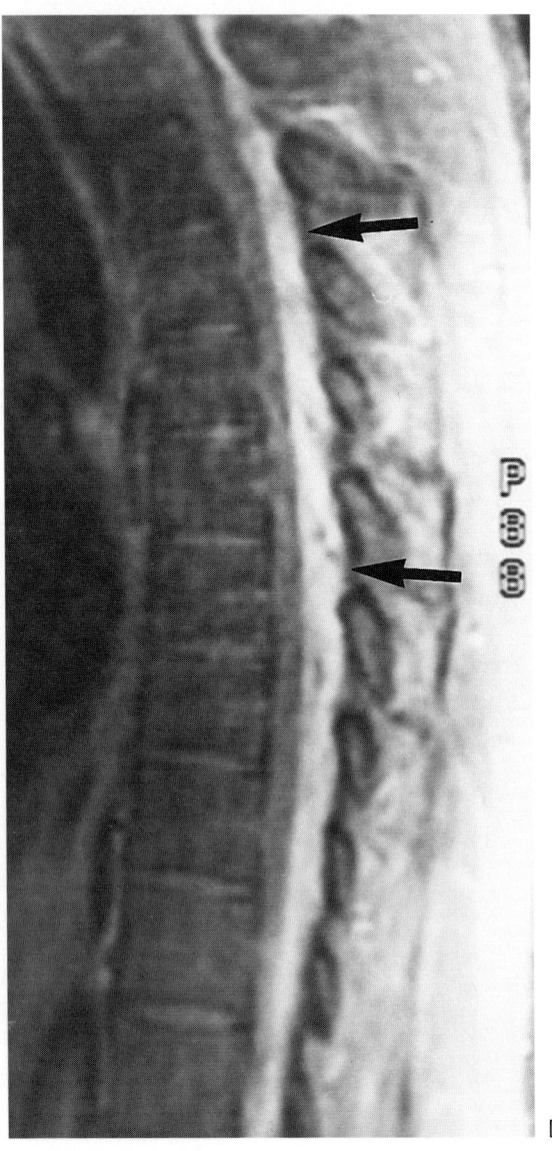

INFLAMMATORY DISEASES OF THE SPINE

Radiologic Findings

Sagittal short TR image (Fig. A) reveals disc space narrowing at the L4-5 level. An intermediate signal intensity soft tissue mass, anterior to the vertebral bodies in the lower lumber region (*open arrows*). There is a low signal intensity mass that exhibits a scalloped margin extending from L4 through L5. This process obliterates the normal dorsal epidural fat and compresses the lower end of the lumbar thecal sac. Areas of intermediate signal intensity involving the inferior end plate of L4 and superior end plate of L5 are adjacent to the intervertebral disc. The anterior margins of both L4 and L5 appear as decreased signal intensity, and this decreased signal intensity also involves the superior end plate of the L4 vertebral body. The L3 vertebral body is identified by 3.

Intermediate (Fig. B, *left*) and long (Fig. B, *right*) TR images reveal that the intermediate signal intensity areas demonstrated on the short TR images now appear as increased signal intensity, as does the intervertebral disc at L4-5. A soft tissue mass of intermediate signal intensity projects posteriorly to the L4 vertebral body and slightly compresses the thecal sac.

Axial short TR image postcontrast (Fig. C) reveals a "U" shaped area of enhancement in the region of the intervertebral disc (*open white arrow*). Areas of enhancement are seen in the region of the left psoas muscle (*solid straight white arrow*) and in the region of the right psoas muscle (*curved white arrow*). A triangular shaped area of enhancement is dorsal to the thecal sac on the right side (*thick black arrow*), and a broad curvilinear area of enhancement is dorsal to the intervertebral facets (*curved black arrow*). A densely enhancing, thick-walled, irregularly margined area of enhancement in the paraspinal muscles on the right (*open black arrows*) is also demonstrated. There is a central area of decreased signal intensity.

Fat-suppressed sagittal short TR image (Fig. D) reveals diffuse enhancement of tissue dorsal to the thecal sac throughout the entire thoracic region (*arrows*).

Diagnosis

Discitis, vertebral osteomyelitis, bilateral psoas abscesses, epidural abscess extending from the lumbar region through the thoracic spine, and thick-rimmed thoracic paraspinal muscle abscess.

Differential Diagnosis

- discitis

Discussion

The intravenous drug abuser is susceptible to a variety of infectious diseases in various organ systems. Spinal infections may also occur, and they may be caused by unusual organisms. In addition, there has been a recent increase in the occurrence of infection with such previously uncommon organisms as *Mycobacterium avium intracellularae*. Infection with *Mycobacterium tuber-*

PEARL
- Multiplanar imaging using short TR sequences without and with contrast enhancement is very helpful in the evaluation of any multilevel inflammatory process. Because contrast was injected prior to evaluation of the thoracic region in this patient, it was elected to perform fat-suppressed short TR images to determine the superior extent of the inflammatory process. The normally increased signal intensity fat is therefore suppressed while the areas of enhancement—in this case a multilevel area of enhancement—appear as areas of increased signal intensity.

TEACHING ATLAS OF SPINE IMAGING

PITFALL
- Abscesses in the paraspinal muscles may not be appreciated because they are remote from the normal anticipated areas of involvement. Images should be obtained that include sufficient paraspinal tissue for evaluation of these abnormalities.

culosis may also occur. In those cases, aspiration biopsy is strongly suggested, so the causative organism can be identified, and the correct treatment instituted. It should be noted that *Mycobacterium avium intracellularae* is a common organism in the environment and becomes a pathogen in only the immunocompromised host. Of some concern is that this organism is known to be drug resistant in both immunocompetent and immunocompromised hosts.

The areas of decreased signal intensity in Figure A are presumably related to reactive bony sclerosis. The area of decreased signal intensity behind the vertebral body of L4 in Figure B is the compressed, anteriorly compressed nerve roots of the cauda equina.

Follow-up scanning with magnetic resonance with contrast infusion is the ideal method of following the clinical response of these patients to treatment.

INFLAMMATORY DISEASES OF THE SPINE

Case 7

Clinical Presentation

The patient is a 57-year-old male with a history of diabetes mellitus who was admitted with complaints of right lower back pain, diabetic ketoacidosis, and methacillin resistant *Staphylococcus aureus* bacteremia with persistent fevers while on antibiotics. There is increased pain in the cervical and lumbar regions and weakness in the lower extremities.

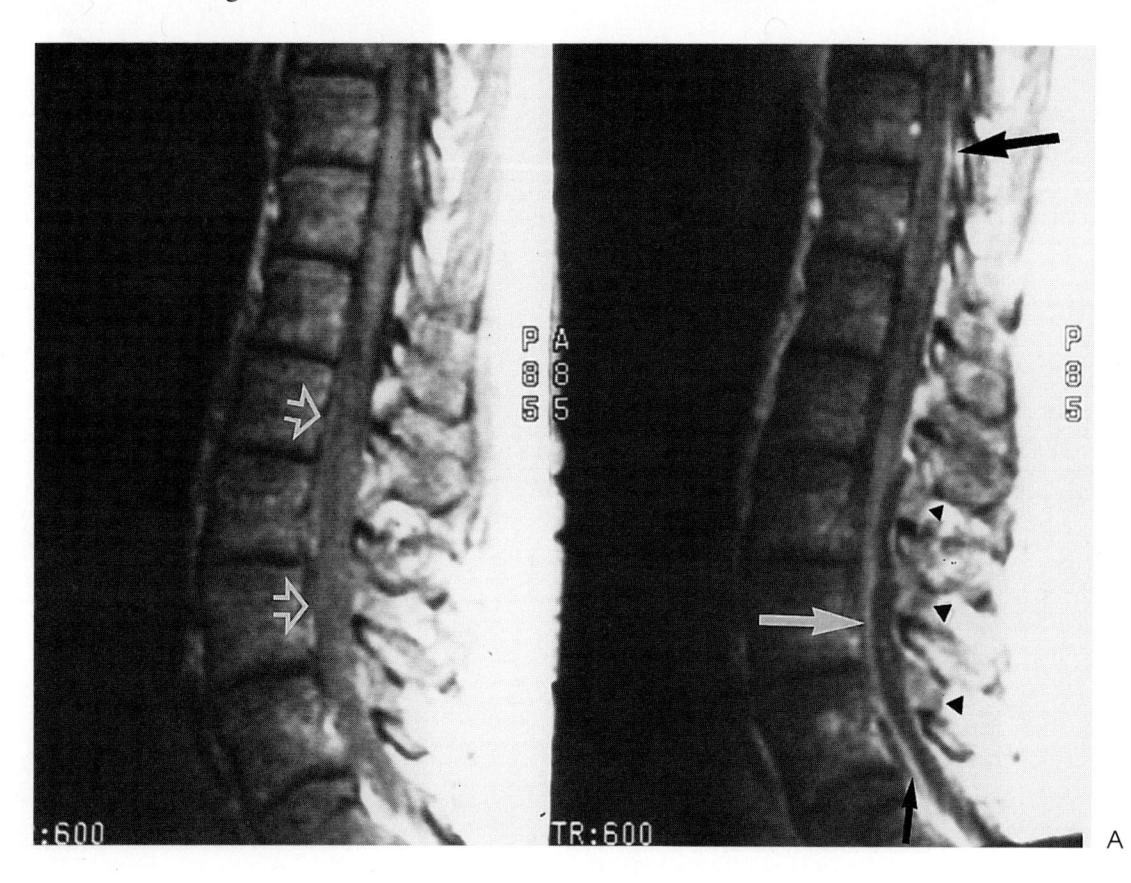

Radiologic Findings

Sagittal short TR image preinfusion (Fig. A, *left*) image reveals that the entire lumbar subarachnoid space is isointense with the signal intensity of the spinal cord (*open arrows*). The normal cerebrospinal fluid (CSF) is not visible surrounding the spinal cord. A postcontrast image (Fig. A, *right*) reveals linear enhancement of the meninges in the lumbar region (*white arrow*). This extends superiorly to the level of the thoracic spine, where a thin line of enhancement is seen along the ventral and dorsal aspects of the thoracic spinal cord. There is enhancement dorsal to the thecal sac in the lower thoracic region (*black arrow* at T11). The enhancement extends inferiorly in the epidural space down to the level of L5 (*black arrowheads* L3 to L5). A linear area of low signal intensity is posterior to the vertebral body of L5 (*black arrow on right*).

TEACHING ATLAS OF SPINE IMAGING

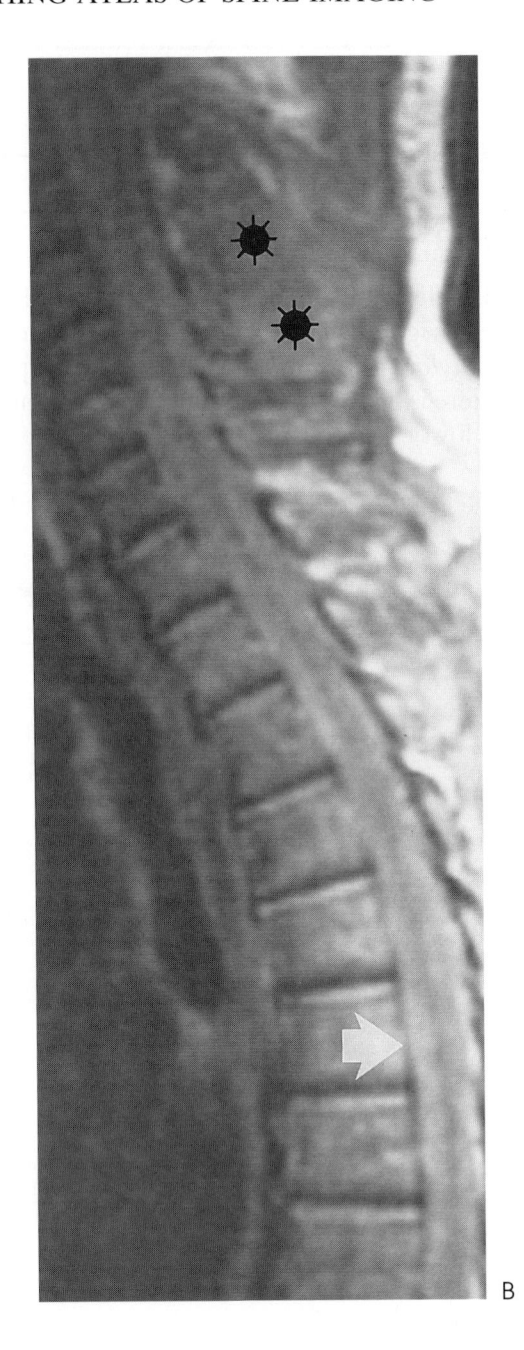

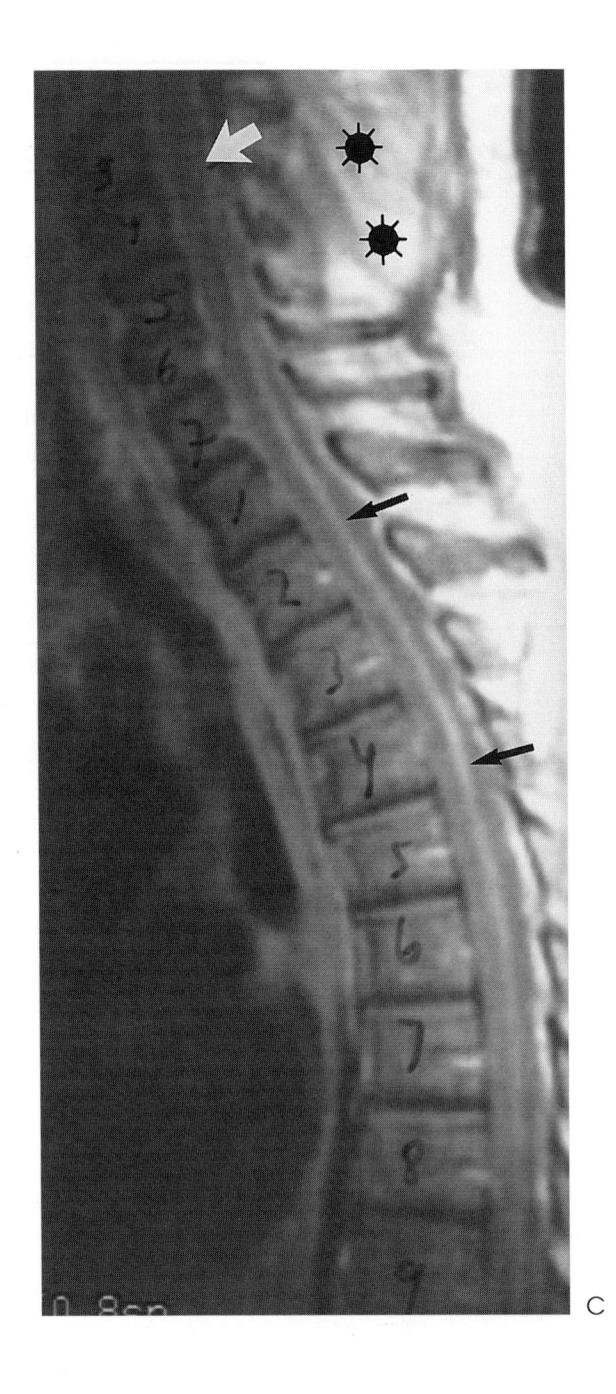

INFLAMMATORY DISEASES OF THE SPINE

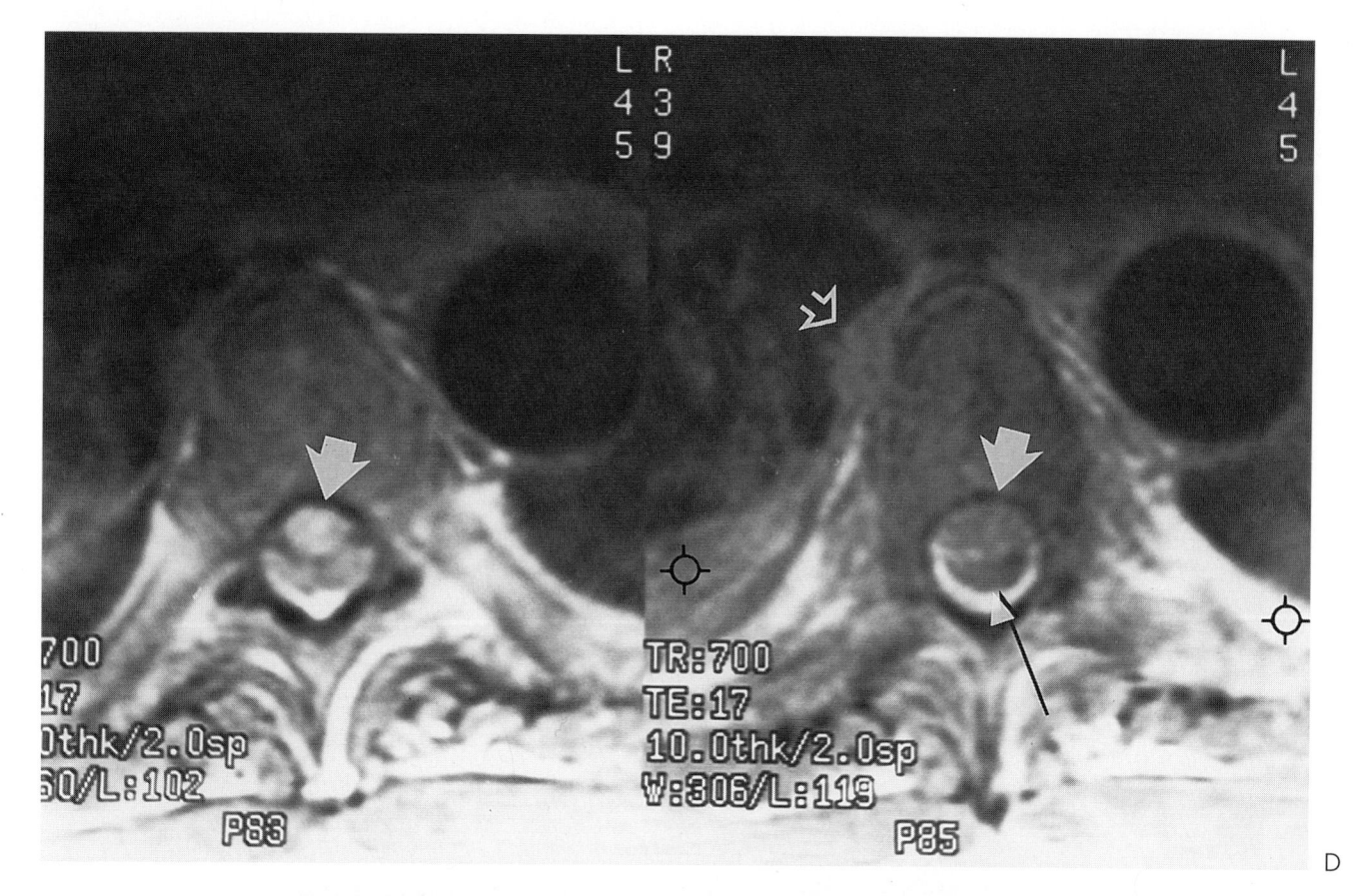

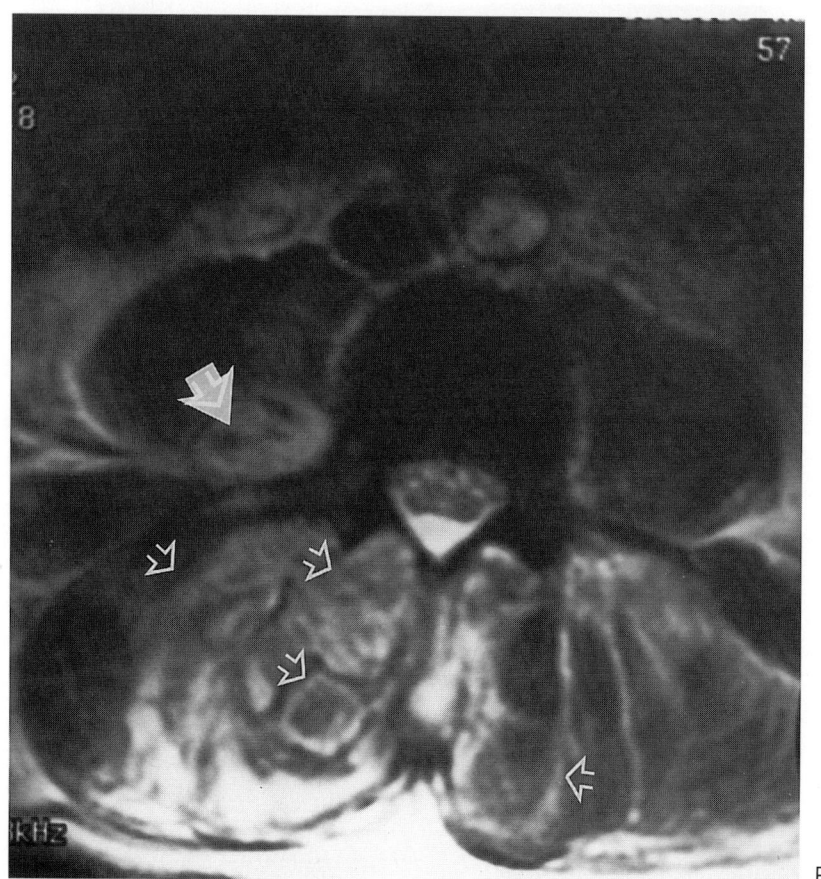

493

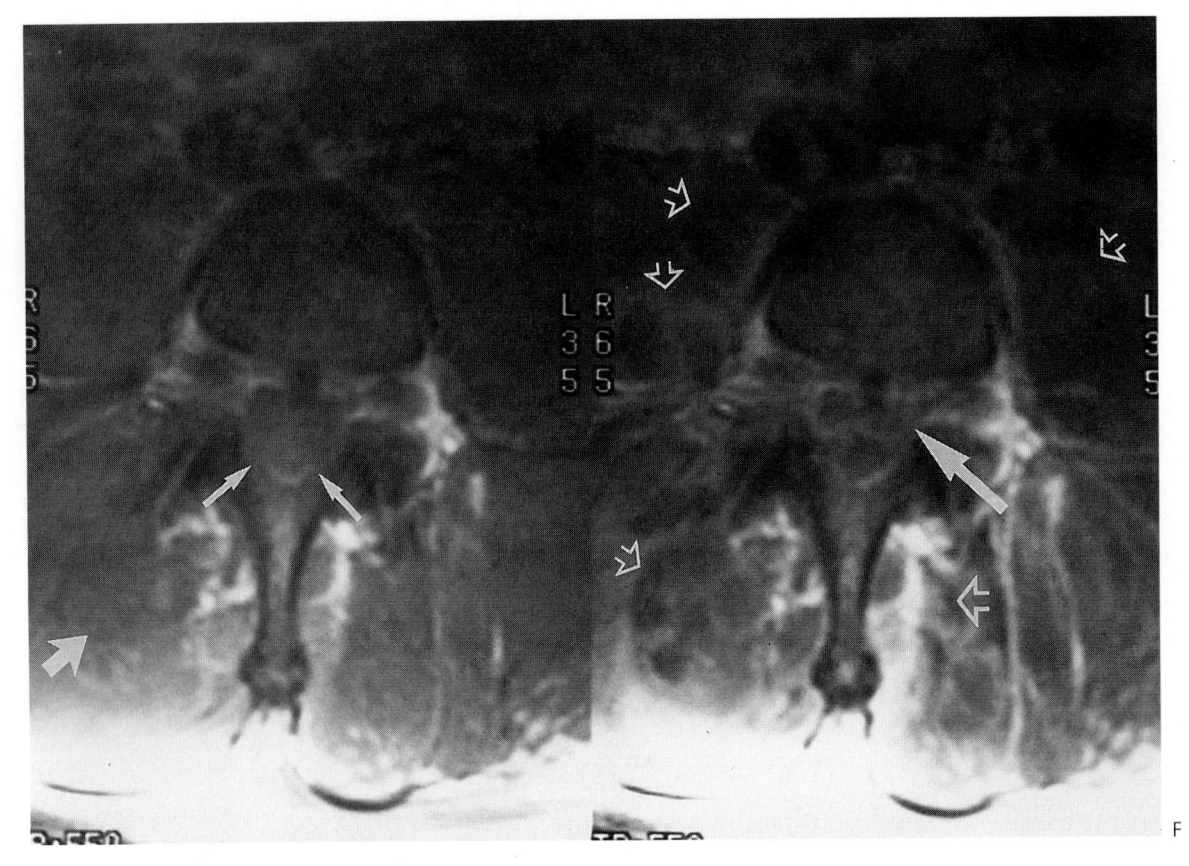

TEACHING ATLAS OF SPINE IMAGING

F

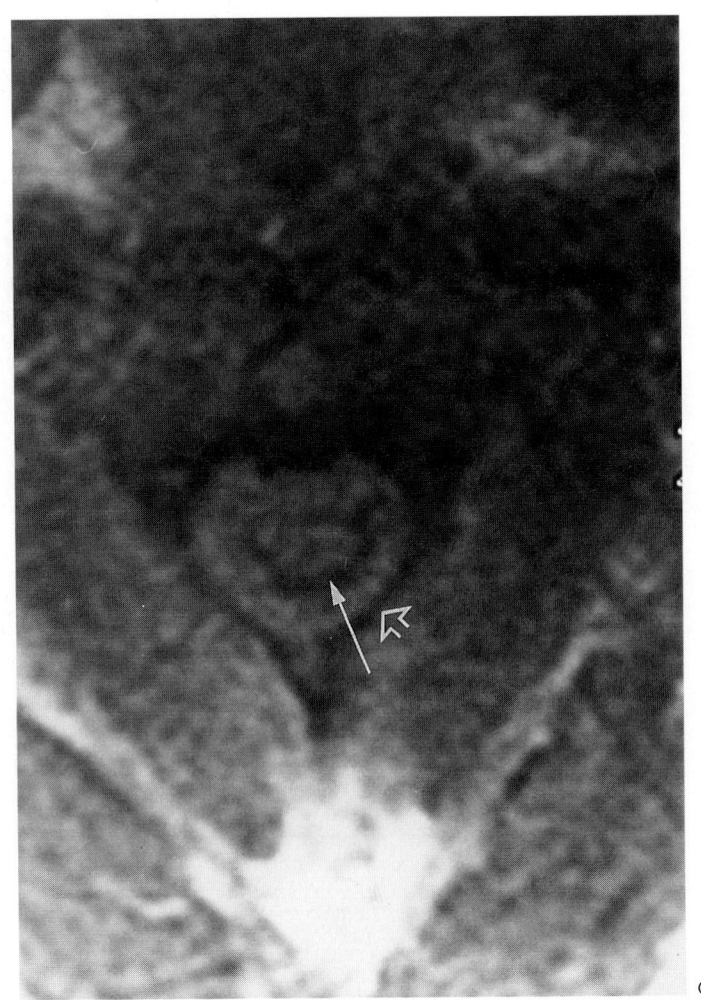

G

INFLAMMATORY DISEASES OF THE SPINE

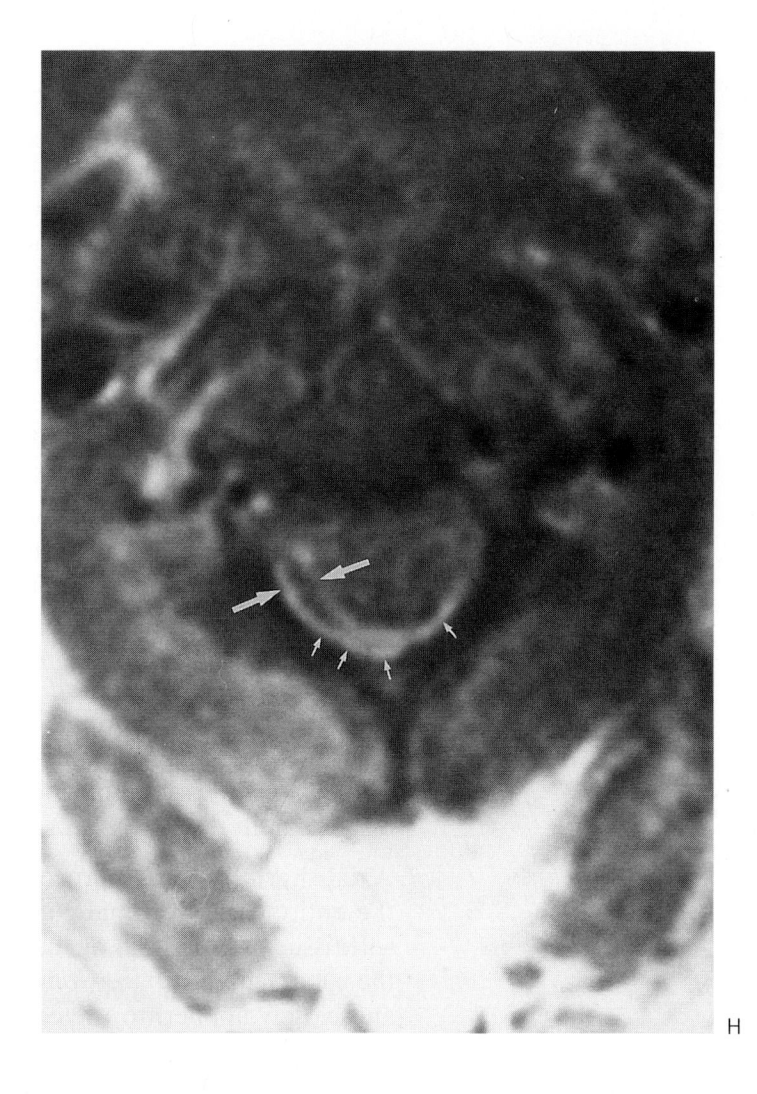

H

Radiologic Findings (continued)

Sagittal short TR image (Fig. B) in the thoracic region reveals that the normal spinal cord is never demonstrated. The entire subarachnoid space is obliterated. Diffuse increased signal intensity soft tissue material in the anticipated position of the subarachnoid space extends throughout the thoracic region and superiorly into the cervical region. (T6 is identified with a *white arrow*.) There is a soft tissue intermediate signal intensity mass in the cervical region at the level of C3-5 (*asterisks*). The normal epidural fat at all levels in the thoracic spine and cervical region is obliterated.

Sagittal short TR image postcontrast (Fig. C) reveals enhancement of the membrane associated with the vertebral canal extending throughout the entire length of the vertebral canal (*black arrows*). In the cervical region, the intermediate signal intensity spinal cord (*white arrow*) can be seen to be displaced anteriorly and compressed against the posterior margin of the cervical vertebral bodies. The dorsal epidural soft tissue mass at C3-6 is enhancing (*asterisks*).

495

TEACHING ATLAS OF SPINE IMAGING

Radiologic Findings (continued)

Axial short TR images postcontrast at the level of T6 (Fig. D) reveals the rounded area of enhancement of a soft tissue mass (*left, white arrow*). Just inferiorly, the area of enhancement is again seen (*right, white arrow*). The spinal cord is noted to be displaced posteriorly (*right, long black arrow, white arrowhead*). A right-sided paraspinal mass (*right, open arrow*) and bilateral pleural effusions (*right, asterisks*) are visible.

Axial long TR image in the lumbar region (Fig. E) reveals multiple, curvilinear, patchy areas of increased signal intensity in the paraspinal muscles of the back of the spine (*small open arrows*). There is also a rounded area of increased signal in the psoas muscle on the right side (*solid arrow*).

Pre- (Fig. F, *left*) and postcontrast (Fig. F, *right*) axial short TR images in the lumbar region. The precontrast (*left*) image reveals complete obliteration of the normal epidural fat (*thin white arrows*) within the vertebral canal by an intermediate intensity soft tissue mass. A rounded, intermediate signal intensity paraspinal mass is also seen disrupting the normal architecture of the paraspinal muscles (*left, large white arrow*). Postcontrast (*right*) there are irregularly marginated ring-shaped areas of enhancement surrounding bilateral psoas and paraspinal muscle cystic areas (*open arrows*). Enhancement of an anterior epidural abscess (*right, long white arrow*) with posterior displacement of the thecal sac is also visible.

Axial short TR image precontrast at the level of C2 (Fig. G) reveals that the entire cervical spinal cord is encircled by intermediate signal intensity soft tissue. The lamina of the vertebral body is marked by the open arrow; the subarachnoid space (*long white arrow*) is circumferentially compressed and closely applied to the cervical spinal cord.

Axial short TR image postcontrast (Fig. H) reveals curvilinear areas of enhancement dorsal to the spinal cord (*small white arrows*) and enclosing a low signal intensity area dorsal and to the right of the cervical spinal cord (*long white arrows*). Minimally enhancing soft tissue is anterior to the cervical spinal cord.

Diagnosis

Multilevel anterior and posterior epidural abscess, meningitis and multiple dorsal and paraspinal, and psoas muscle abscesses.

Differential Diagnosis

- inflammatory process
- meningitis
- metastases, meningeal carcinomatosis

INFLAMMATORY DISEASES OF THE SPINE

PEARL

- Evaluation of the entire length of the spine is vital to determine the extent of involvement. Multilevel laminectomy may be performed, as in this patient, if appropriate; the exact levels of involvement should be identified prior to surgery.

PITFALLS

- This case illustrates the need for multiplanar imaging at all levels of abnormality.

- It is best to obtain pre- and postcontrast images so a more accurate evaluation of the level of the abnormalities can be made.

Discussion

The clinical history is particularly helpful here as it leads one to suspect an inflammatory process. The sagittal short TR images (Figs. A, B, and C) revealed that the normal CSF surrounding the spinal cord is not seen because the entire subarachnoid space has been obliterated by the space-occupying epidural abscess. In addition, the lumbar subarachnoid space is diffusely increased in signal intensity because of the involvement of the nerve roots with an inflammatory process and because of the increased protein content. A meningitis could have a similar appearance to that seen in the lumbar subarachnoid space; however, the epidural component would be more consistent with an epidural abscess. Metastases would not be likely to give this appearance on imaging.

In this patient the clinical symptoms were confined to the lumbar region. For this reason, contrast material was injected prior to evaluation of the thoracic region. Therefore, the fat saturation images were obtained to demonstrate the possible areas of enhancement. This fat suppression technique results in suppression of the normally increased signal intensity of the epidural fat. Therefore, the area of increased signal intensity in the dorsal epidural space is secondary to enhancement and not epidural fat because normal epidural fat would have been suppressed by using the fat suppression technique.

A spinal tap with cerebrospinal fluid analysis would be helpful for more complete evaluation.

The extent of this process is unusual. Its treatment would require a wide, multilevel laminectomy to remove the purulent material and to relieve the cord compromise.

TEACHING ATLAS OF SPINE IMAGING

Case 8

Clinical Presentation

The patient is a 75-year-old male with a history of right sided weakness. Previous computed tomographic (CT) neck scan revealed a retropharyngeal abscess.

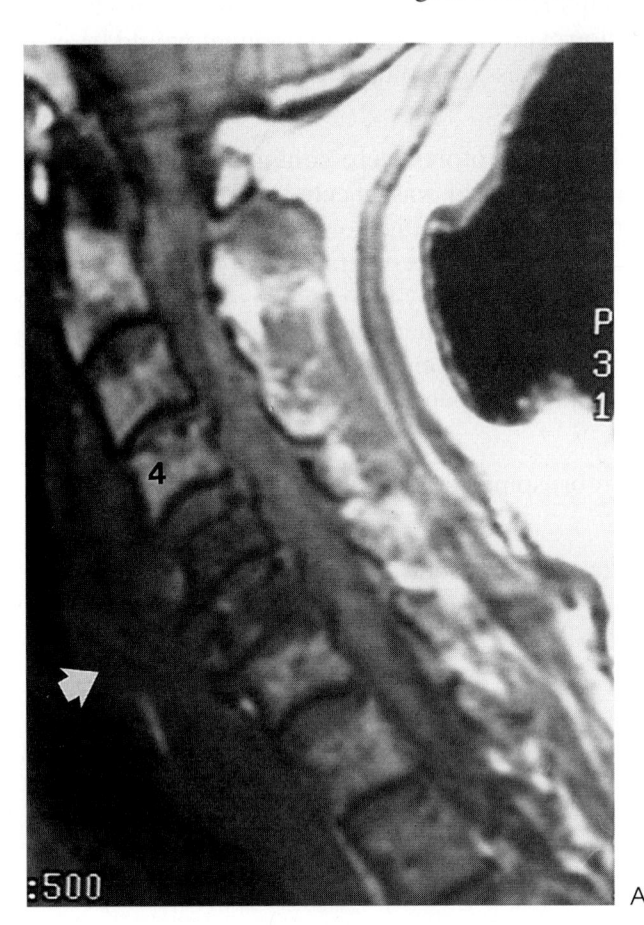

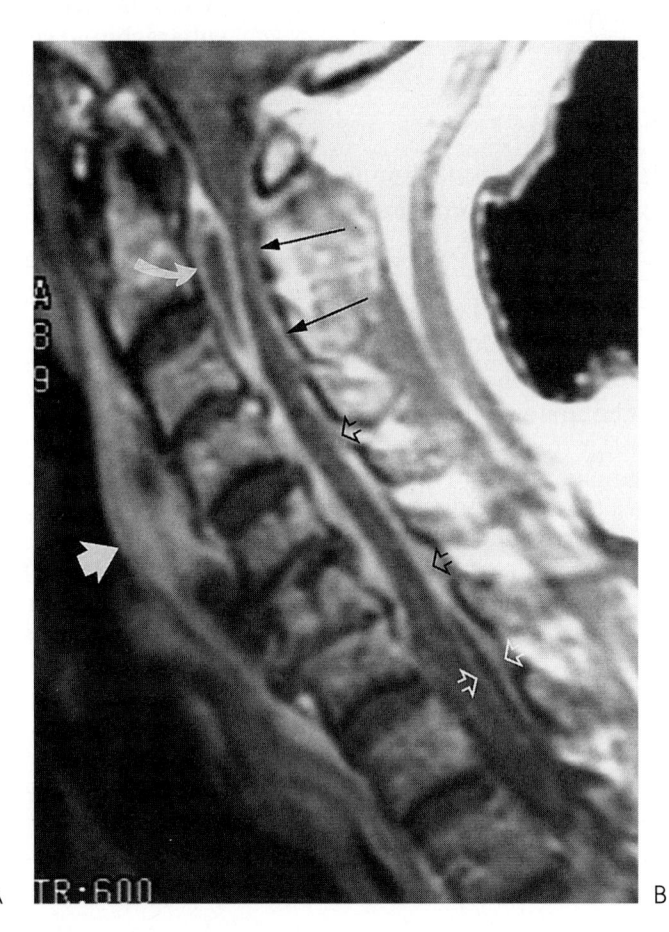

Radiologic Findings

Sagittal T1W image of the cervical spine (Fig. A) reveals that the normal cervical spinal cord is not visualized. The entire subarachnoid space is filled with material that is isointense to the cervical spinal cord. The C5 and C6 vertebral bodies are decreased in signal intensity, and there is narrowing of the C5-6 intervertebral disc space. Incidentally, note the degenerative changes in the cervical spine with both anterior and posterior osteophytes at multiple levels. A streaklike area of decreased signal intensity at the c2-3 level is parallel to the cervical spinal cord. There is a large prevertebral soft tissue mass (*white arrow*); the trachea is displaced anteriorly. The C4 vertebral body is identified with 4.

INFLAMMATORY DISEASES OF THE SPINE

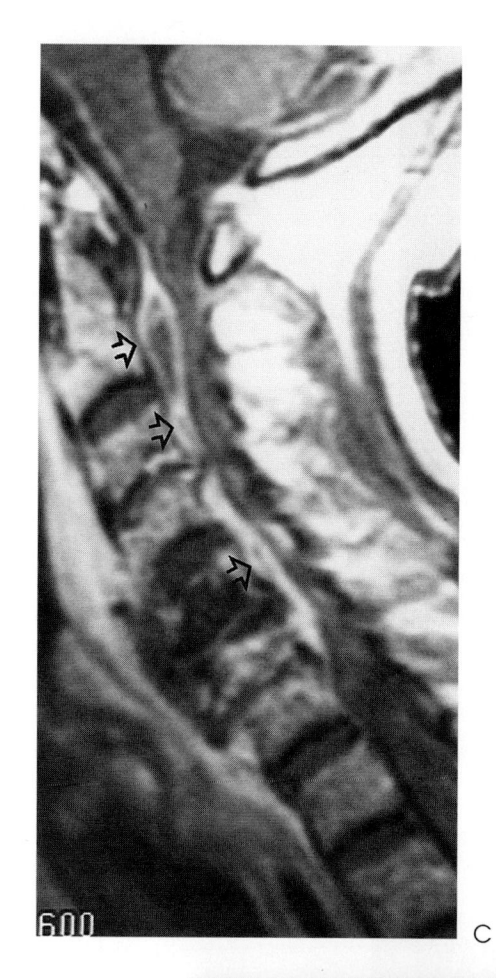

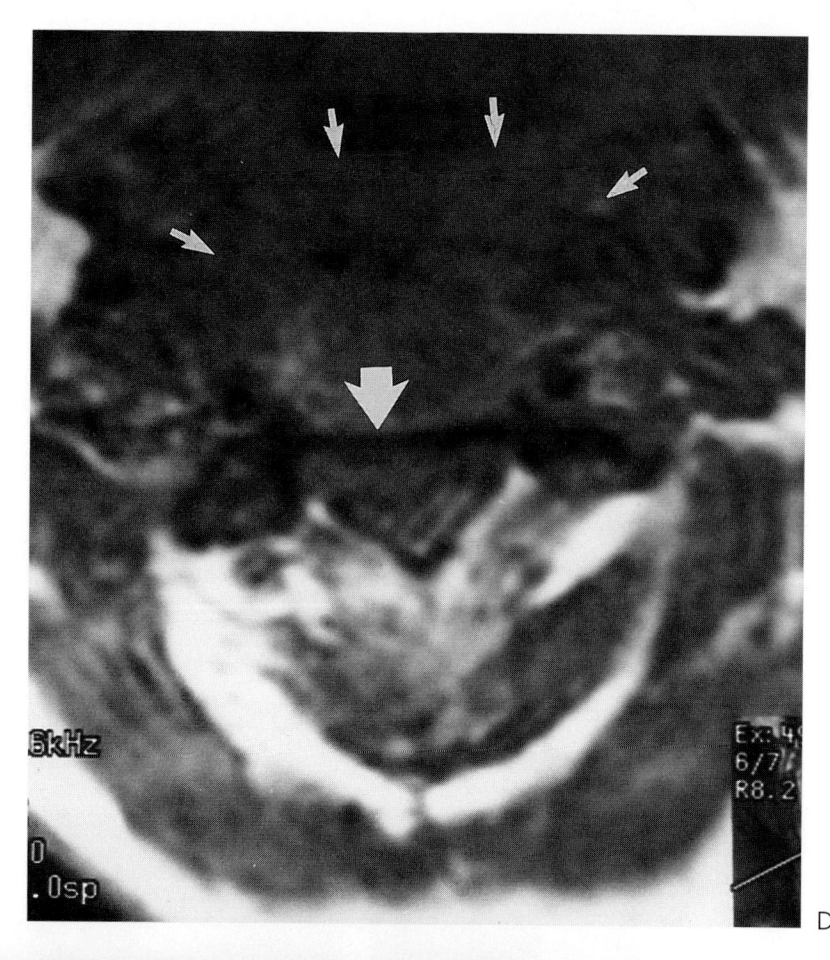

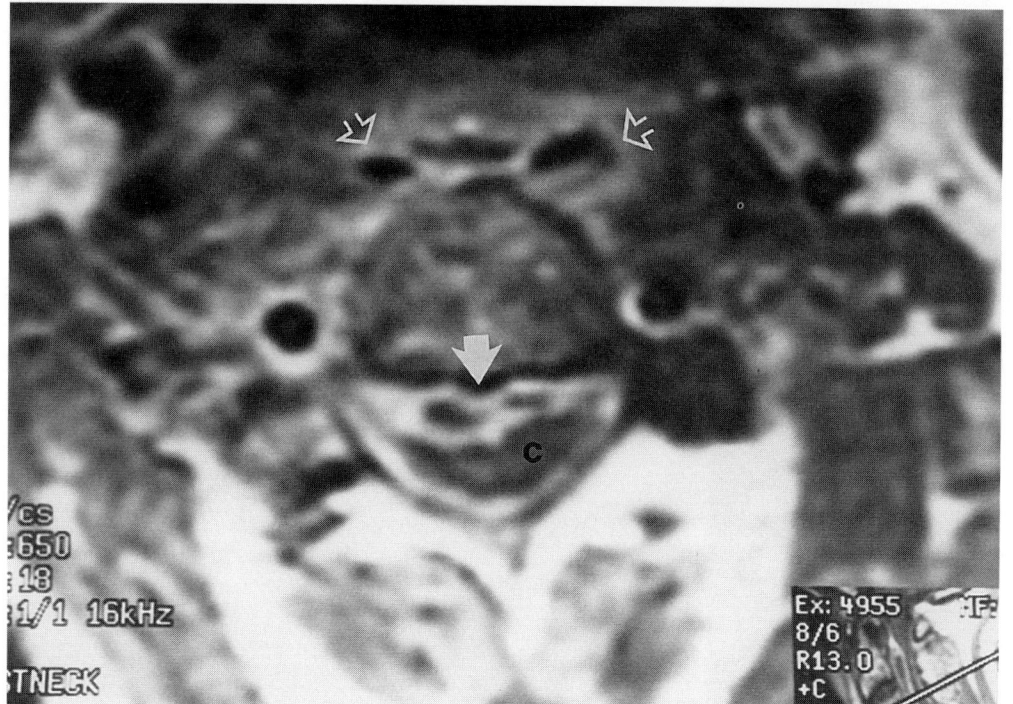

499

TEACHING ATLAS OF SPINE IMAGING

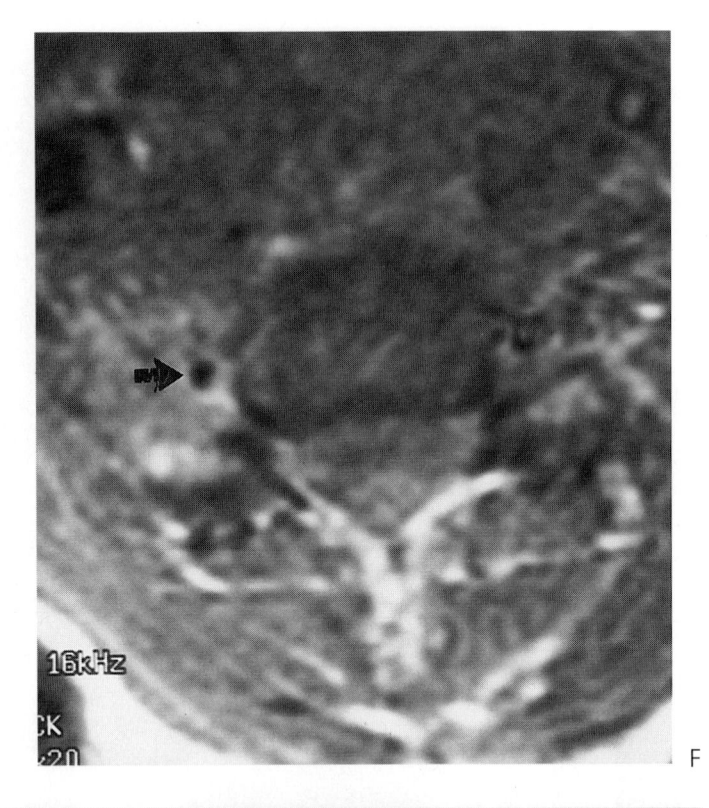

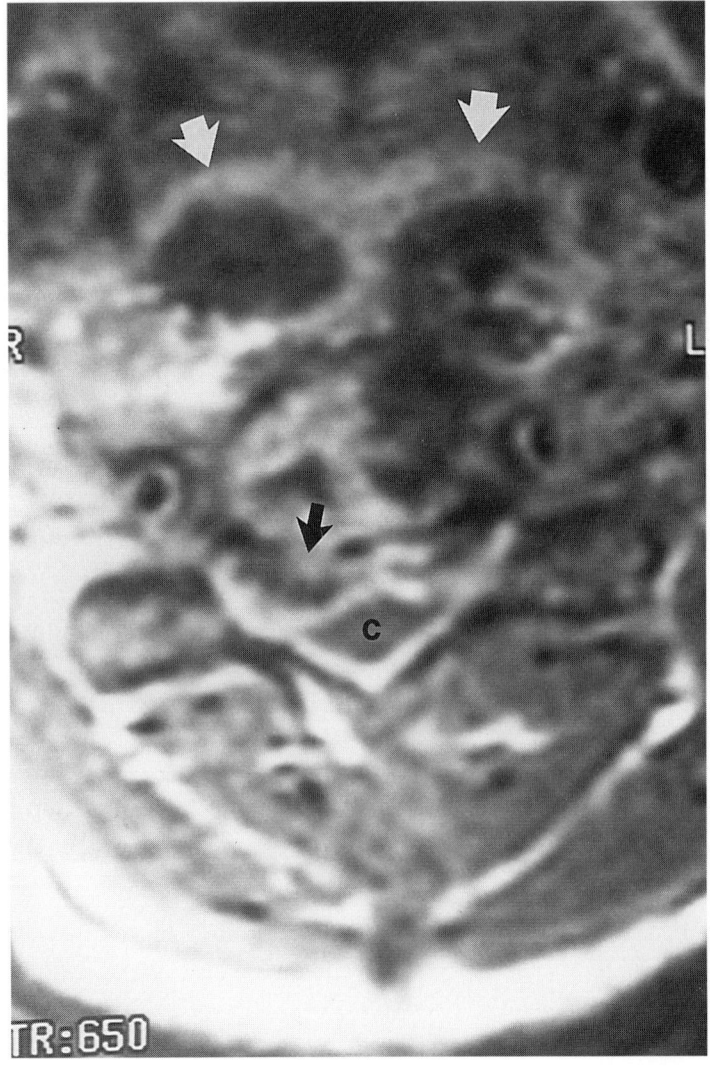

Radiologic Findings (continued)

Sagittal short TR image postcontrast (Fig. B) reveals an area of enhancement posterior to the vertebral bodies of C2-3 (*curved arrow*); this enhancement extends inferiorly to the level of C7. The cervical spinal cord is compressed and displaced posteriorly. There is dense enhancement of the C5 and C6 vertebral bodies. Anterior to the intervertebral disc at the C5-6 level, there is a low signal intensity oval-shaped area; this is surrounded by enhancement of the prevertebral soft tissue mass (*solid white arrow*). Dorsal to the spinal cord at the T1 level, there are two parallel lines of enhancement (*open white arrows*) that surround an area of decreased signal intensity. The enhancement extends superiorly in the dorsal epidural space to the level of C4 (*open black arrows*) and continues as a thin line of enhancement in the epidural space (*long black arrows*). There is dense enhancement of the intervertebral discs at C5-6 and C6-7. At T1, there is an elongated area of decreased signal intensity surrounded by two areas of enhancement (*open white arrows*).

Parasagittal postcontrast image (Fig. C) reveals the loculated area of enhancement in the anterior epidural space (*black arrows*). Multiple small internal areas of decreased signal intensity can be identified. The low signal intensity central portion of the prevertebral soft tissue mass can be seen in the retropharyngeal space anterior to C5 and C6. The prevertebral enhancing soft tissue mass extends superiorly to the level of C2 and inferiorly to the level of C7. There is persistent decreased signal intensity within the lateral portion of the C5 vertebral body. The trachea is displaced anteriorly.

Axial short TR image in the upper cervical region at the C3 level (Fig. D) reveals that the spinal cord is displaced markedly posteriorly by a soft tissue mass anterior to the spinal cord (*thick white arrow*) and compressed into a seminar configuration. There is also a prevertebral soft tissue mass in the prevertebral/retropharyngeal space (*small white arrows*).

Axial short TR image postcontrast in the midcervical region (Fig. E) reveals the peripherally enhancing loculated soft tissue mass in the anterior epidural space. The abscess is slightly larger on the right side (*solid arrow*). There is also a bilobed prevertebral/retropharyngeal soft tissue mass that exhibits peripherally enhancing margins and bilateral low signal intensity areas (*open arrows*) and linear dense dorsal enhancement in the epidural space. The spinal cord (*c*) is compressed more on the left side than the right and displaced dorsally and to the left. The trachea is displaced anteriorly.

Axial short TR image in the cervical region (Fig. F) reveals the vertebral artery surrounded by soft tissue (*arrow*).

Axial short TR image postcontrast (Fig. G) reveals dense enhancement of a curvilinear dense wall of enhancement with decreased signal intensity central areas (*white arrows*). There is a lobulated area of peripheral enhancement in the anterior epidural space (*black arrow*). The cervical spinal cord is compressed posteriorly into a diamond shape (*c*).

Diagnosis

Loculated, multilevel anterior and posterior epidural abscess secondary to retropharyngeal abscess. The etiologic organism was not cultured.

TEACHING ATLAS OF SPINE IMAGING

Retropharyngeal abscess with bilateral loculated accumulations, discitis at multiple levels, vertebral osteomyelitis at the C5 and C6 levels, loculated anterior and posterior epidural abscesses.

Differential Diagnosis

- discitis

- osteomyelitis

Discussion

In this diabetic patient, the most likely diagnosis is that of a retropharyngeal abscess that has progressed to discitis involving the C5-6 intervertebral disc. Progression then led to anterior and posterior epidural abscesses and vertebral osteomyelitis.

There is decreased signal intensity pus within the loculated abscesses (Figs. B, C, E, and G). The vertebral bodies of C5 and C6 enhance densely (Fig. B), a finding consistent with vertebral osteomyelitis. The midline post-contrast image reveals enhancement of the margins of a loculated anterior epidural abscess that projects behind the body of C2-3 and extends inferiorly to the level of T1. There is also a dorsal epidural loculated abscess cavity (Fig. B).

Dense enhancement of a prevertebral/retropharyngeal abscess extends from the level of C2 through the level of the thoracic inlet (*white arrows* in Figs. A and B). There is a persistent area of low signal intensity just anterior to C5 and C6, consistent with a pus-filled abscess cavity.

Incidentally, a small oval area of decreased signal intensity in the posterior aspect of the intervertebral disc at the C5-6 level is an area of vacuum degenerative change.

It is important to perform a postinfusion scan to completely evaluate a case such as this. The decreased signal intensity central areas surrounded by dense enhancement are consistent with pus-containing abscess cavities. The C5 vertebral body contains areas of decreased signal intensity most likely secondary to bony sclerosis.

Although metastatic disease could be a possible diagnosis, the combination of findings with the prevertebral abscesses make this diagnosis unlikely.

PEARLS
- The entire length of the spinal column should be evaluated to determine the extent of the abscess.

- CT-guided aspiration of the abscess in the retropharyngeal space may allow identification of the etiologic organism.

PITFALL
- If the spinal cord is not demonstrated or visible on the short TR images, this implies that the CSF containing subarachnoid space is replaced by intermediate signal intensity material. A postcontrast study is necessary for complete evaluation.

INFLAMMATORY DISEASES OF THE SPINE

Case 9

Clinical Presentation

The patient is a 5-year-old male with headache and emesis. The patient had a history of Chiari type 1 malformation and is status postcraniotomy.

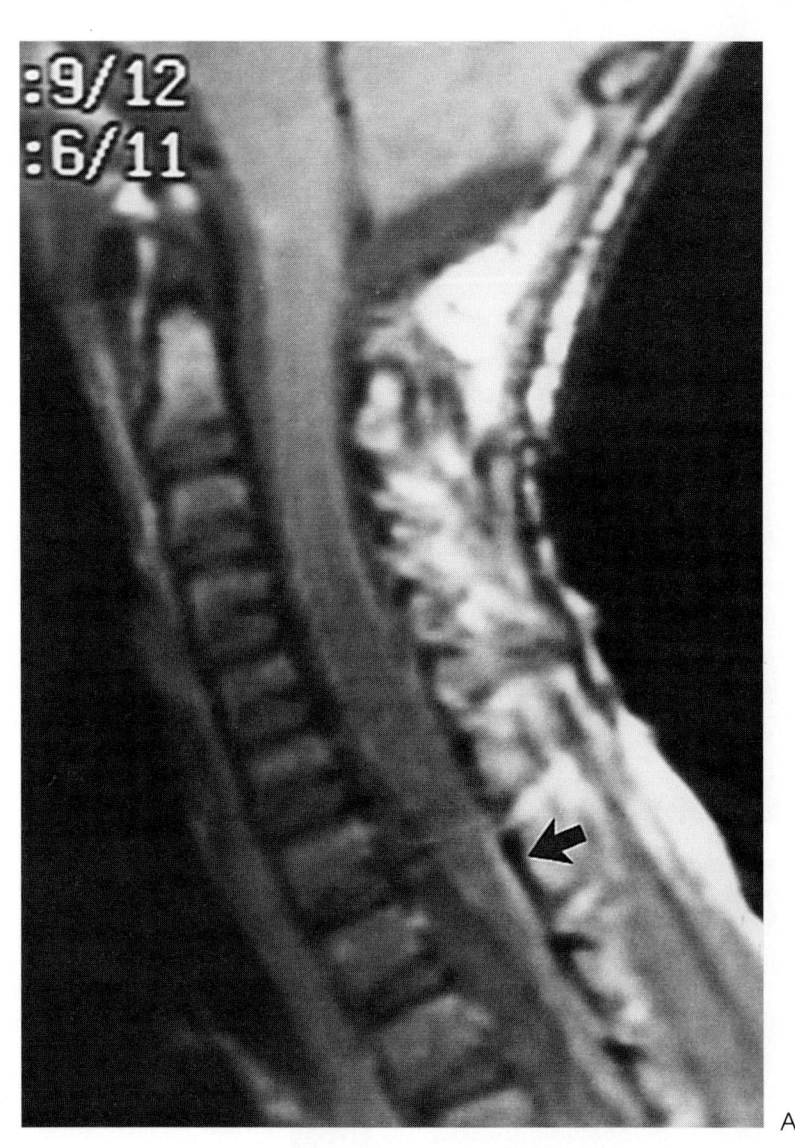

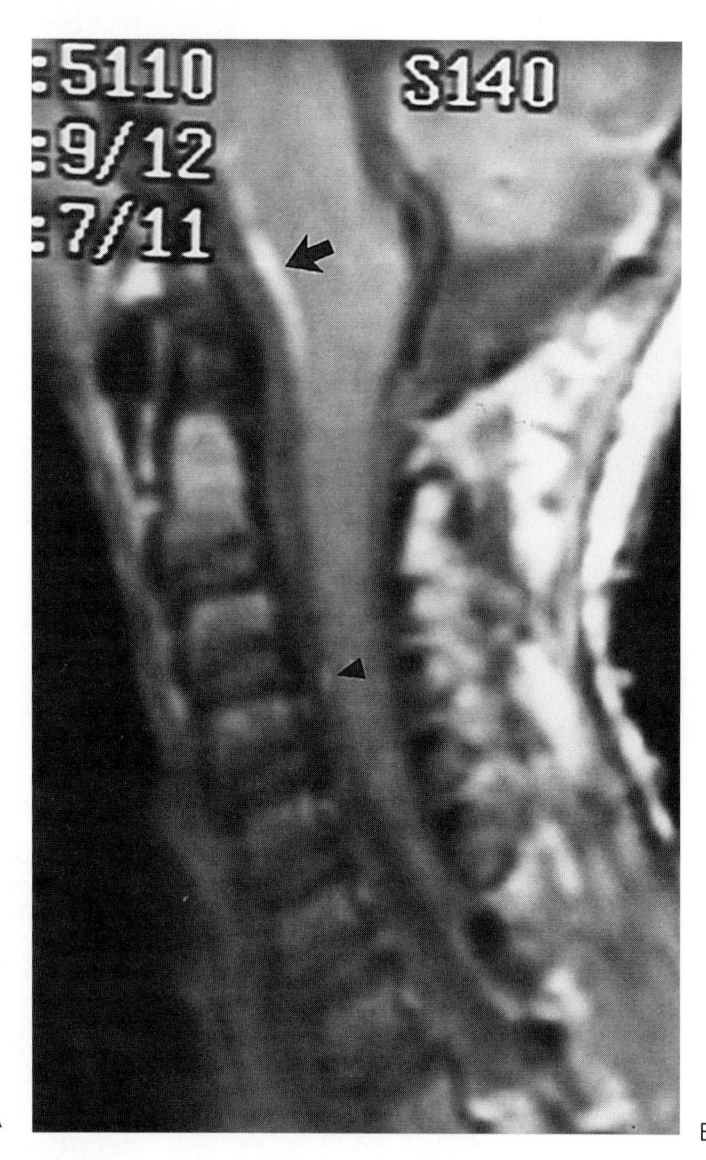

Radiologic Findings

Sagittal short TR images postcontrast enhancement (Figs. A and B) reveal diffuse enhancement of the meninges, which extends superiorly intracranially to involve the meninges of the anterior aspect of the pons (*arrows*). The inferior portion of the occipital bone and the posterior margin of the foramen magnum has been surgically removed.

TEACHING ATLAS OF SPINE IMAGING

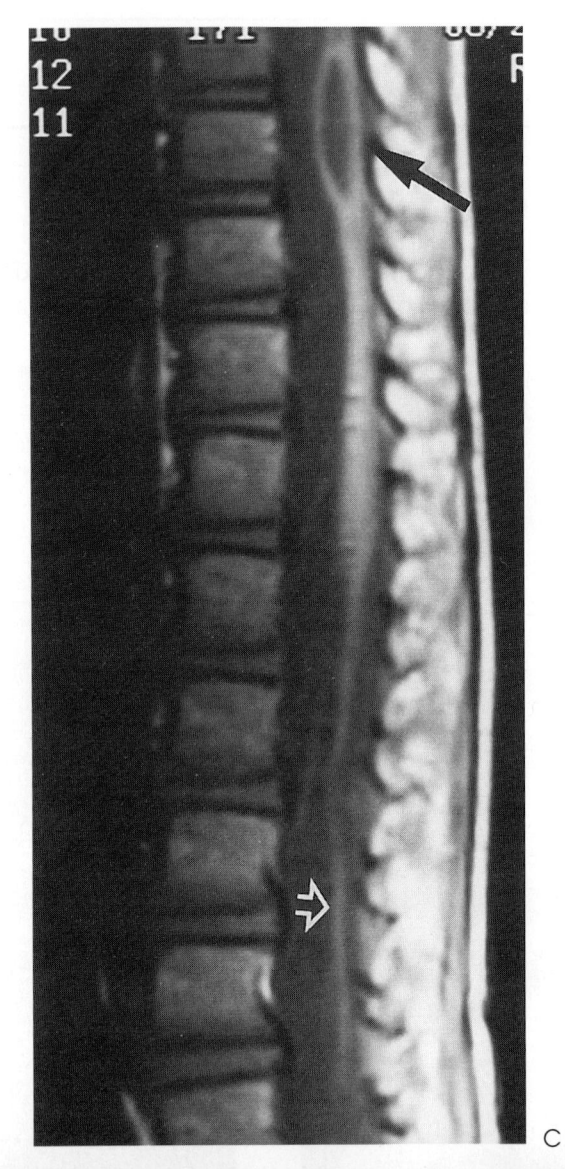

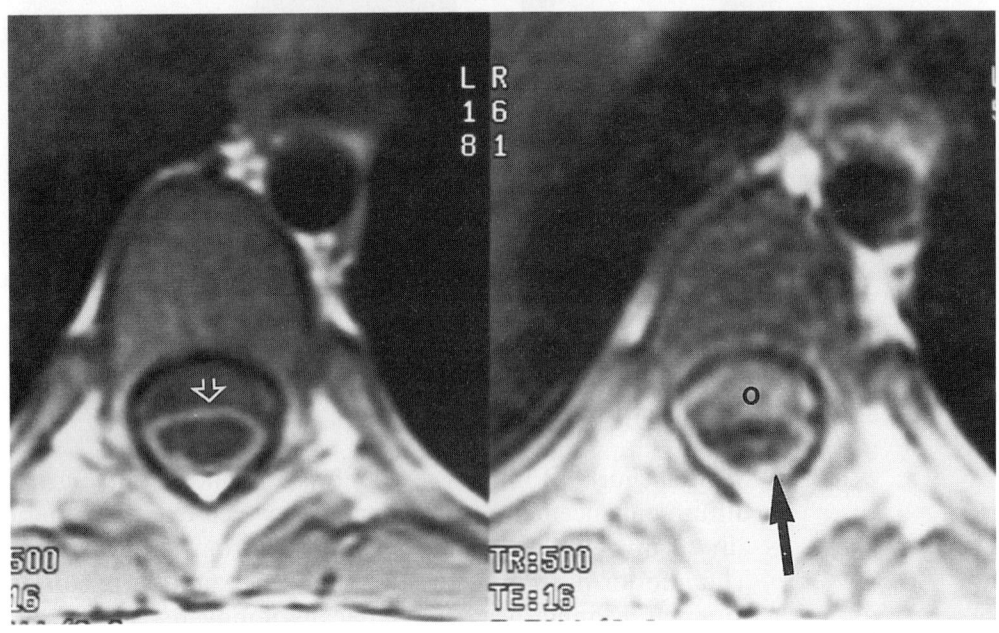

C

D

504

INFLAMMATORY DISEASES OF THE SPINE

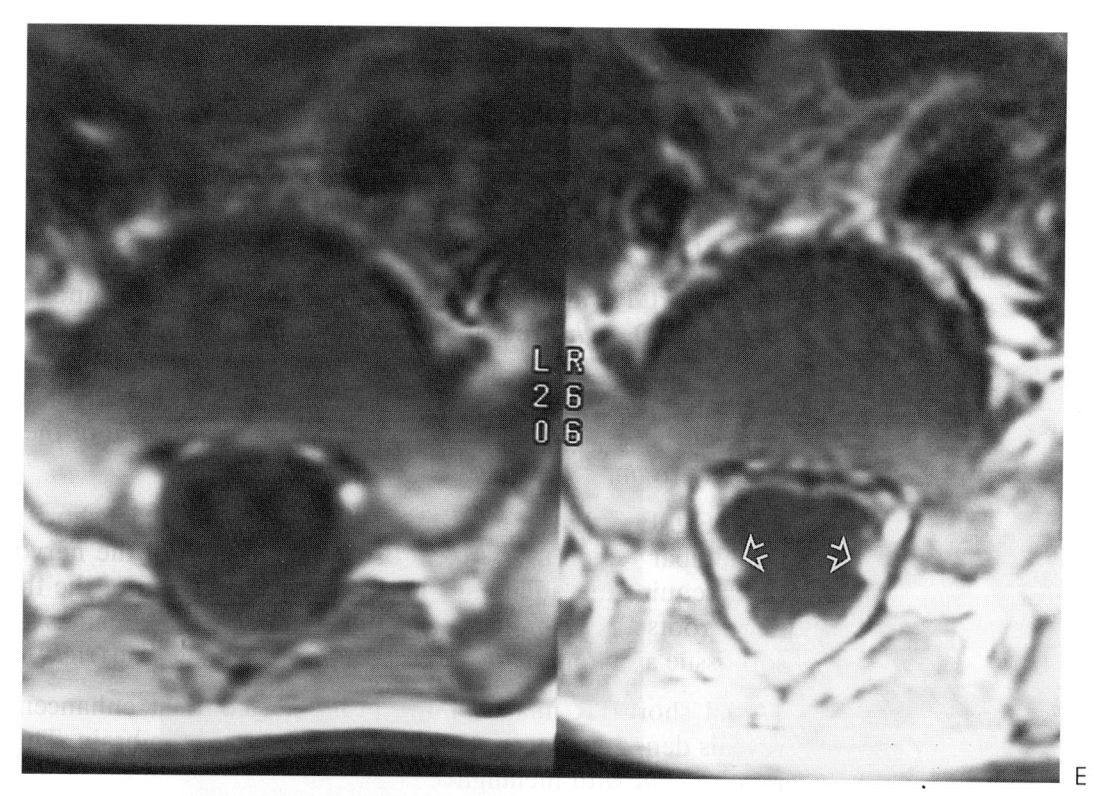

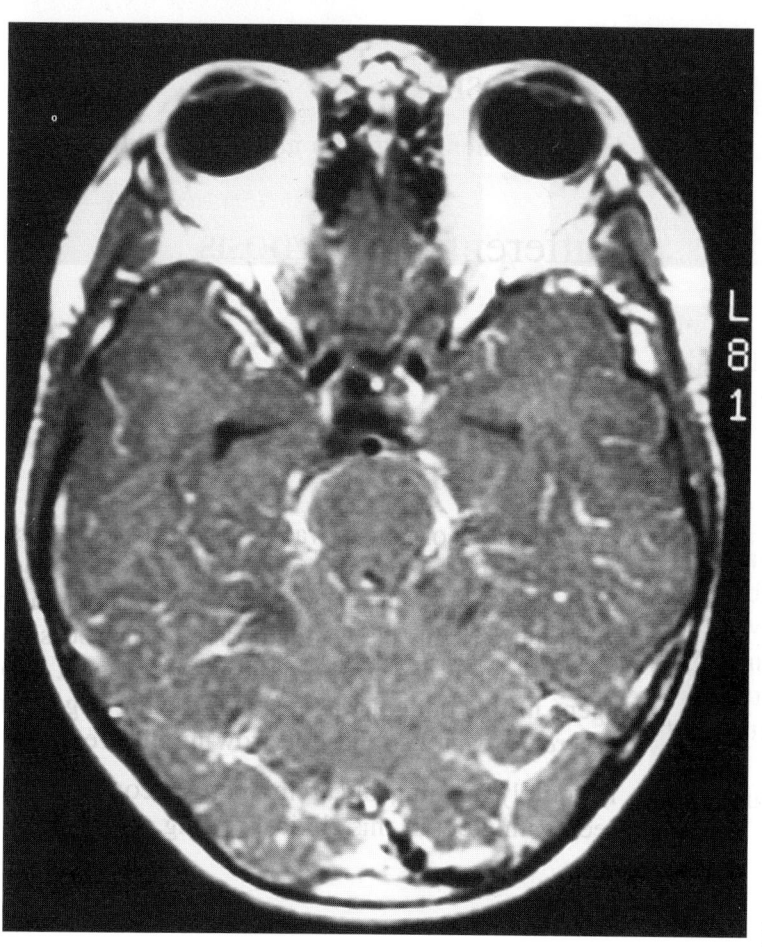

505

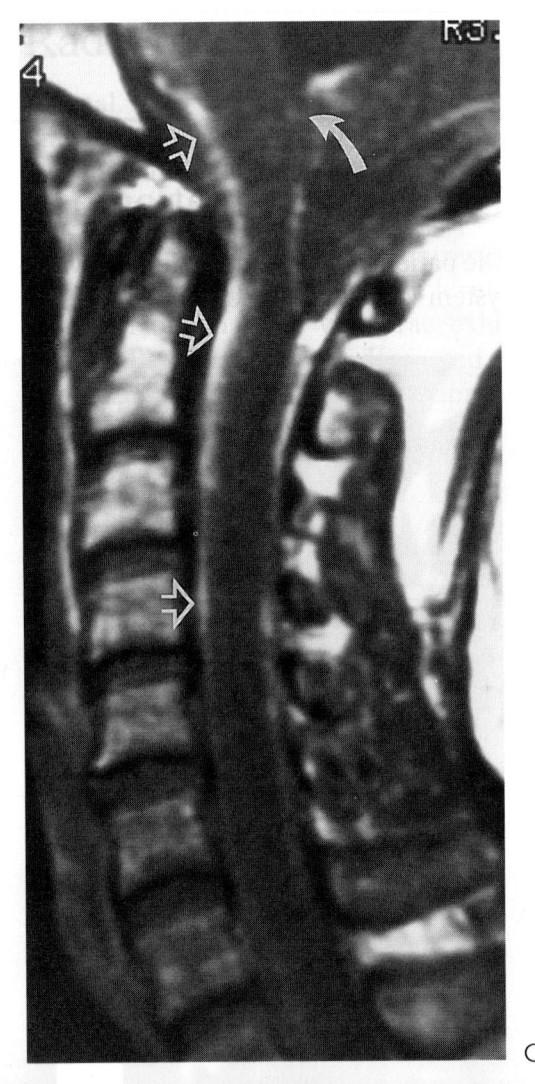

TEACHING ATLAS OF SPINE IMAGING

C

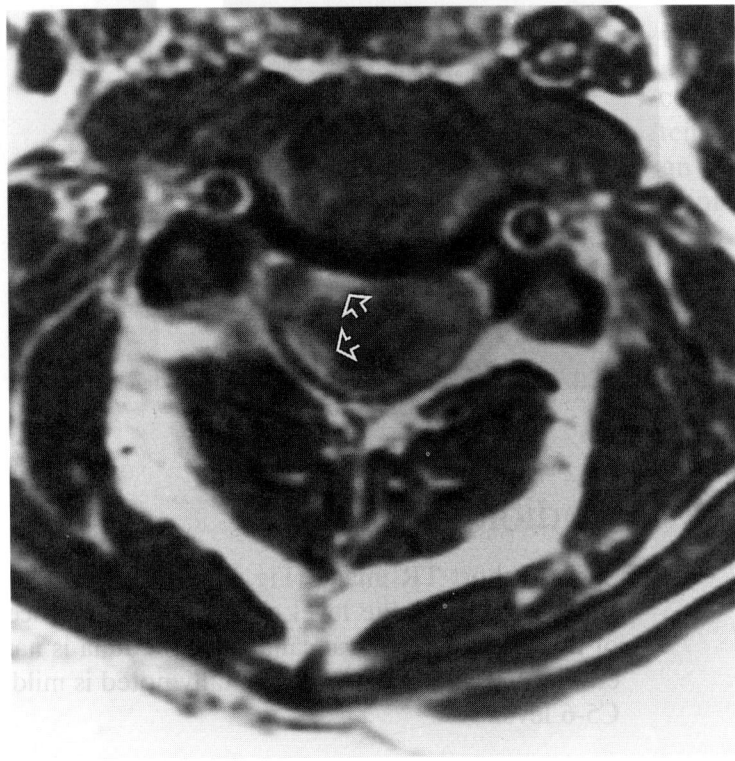

D

510

INFLAMMATORY DISEASES OF THE SPINE

Radiologic Findings (continued)

Sagittal short TR image postcontrast (Fig. B) reveals dense enhancement of the soft tissue at the T8 level (*8, solid arrow*). The pedicle enhances along its lower margin (*open arrow*).

Pre- (Fig. C, *above*) and postcontrast (Fig. C, *below*) axial short TR images at the level of the pedicle of the T8 vertebral body reveal soft tissue signal intensity material that extends into the vertebral canal and obliterates the normal epidural high signal intensity fat along the lateral margin of the epidural space (*long white arrow*). This soft tissue extends into the paraspinal area on the left side (*thick white arrow*). The postinfusion images reveal enhancement of the areas of abnormal soft tissue.

Parasagittal short TR image in the paraspinal area of the lumber spine (Fig. D) reveal that the interfacet faint at the T12-L1 level is indistinct (*black arrow*). There is a rounded area of decreased signal intensity in the posterior inferior portion of the T12 vertebral body (*open arrow*).

Parasagittal short TR image postcontrast enhancement (Fig. E) reveals enhancement of the interfacet joint at T12-L1 (*black arrow*). The area of decreased signal in the T12 vertebral body enhances (*open arrow*).

Pre- (Fig. F, *upper*) and postcontrast (Fig. F, *lower*) axial short TR images reveals the enhancement of the interfacet joint on the left side (*long white arrow*), and reveals that there is a small associated soft tissue component (*top, thick white arrow; bottom, black arrow*) that exhibits enhancement.

PEARLS
- The radionuclide bone scan was also abnormal at these two levels.
- Cerebrospinal fluid analysis may be helpful for complete evaluation, although infection may be present with an organism such as *Mycobacterium tuberculosis* and still be normal.

PITFALL
- Subtle abnormalities such as this could be easily overlooked during routine evaluation. Care should be taken to be aware of the other abnormalities in this type of patient, so a correlation may be made with the neuroradiologic imaging abnormalities.

Diagnosis

Mycobacterium tuberculosis in the interfacet joints in the thoracic and lumber regions.

Differential Diagnosis

- inflammatory process
- metastases

Discussion

This patient had no known risk factors and did not have AIDS. However, he was also found to have involvement of the right temporal bone with TBc. This temporal bone involvement ultimately led to an intracerebral brain abscess secondary to the TBc organism. Multiple levels of involvement with TBc are not uncommon in the spine. Careful evaluation should be made for additional areas of involvement.

Metastases would be very unlikely with a presentation such as this. An inflammatory process is the most likely diagnosis. The previous history of a cerebral abscess secondary to TBc was particularly helpful in this patient. The final diagnosis would be found at the time of surgery or CT-guided needle aspiration with culture.

TEACHING ATLAS OF SPINE IMAGING

Case 13

Clinical Presentation

The patient is a 35-year-old female with progressive mild upper extremity weakness.

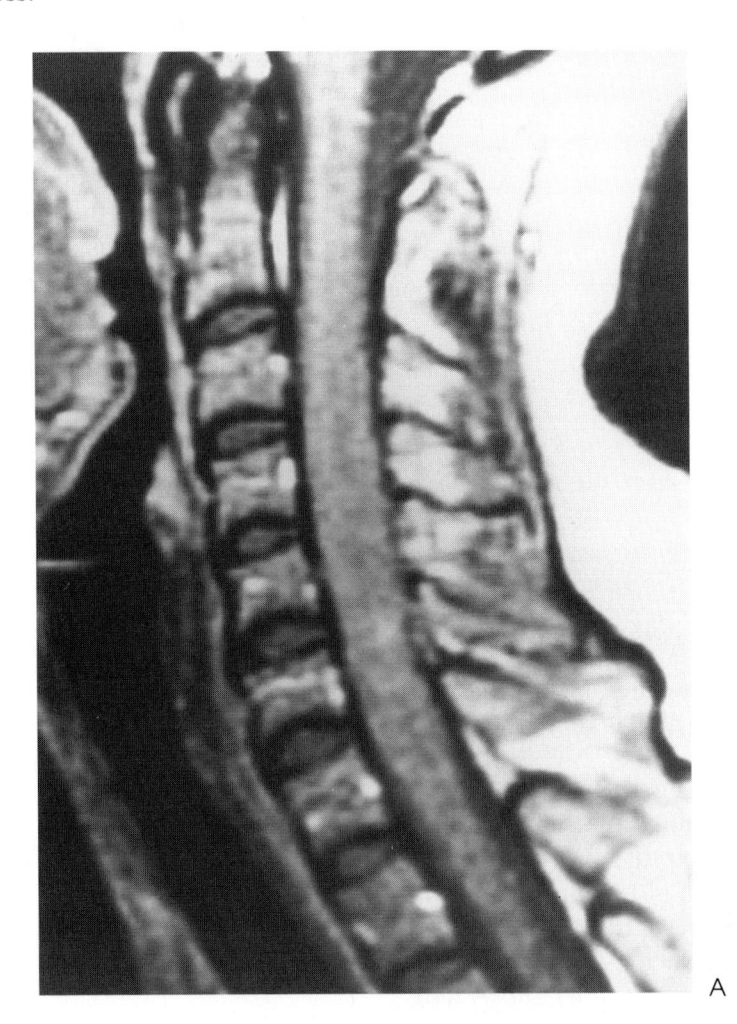

Radiologic Findings

Sagittal short TR image (Fig. A) reveals that the cervical spinal cord is diffusely enlarged in size. There is compromise of the subarachnoid space throughout the length of the cervical subarachnoid space.

Sagittal short TR image postcontrast (Fig. B) reveals dense slightly lobulated enhancement in the dorsal aspect of the cervical spinal cord that extends from the level of C4 through the level of C6. The area of enhancement is in the dorsal aspect of the spinal cord. Other areas of the cervical spinal cord that are edematous do not exhibit areas of enhancement.

Axial short TR image postcontrast (Fig. C) reveals dense enhancement of a rounded area in a white matter distribution (*arrows*).

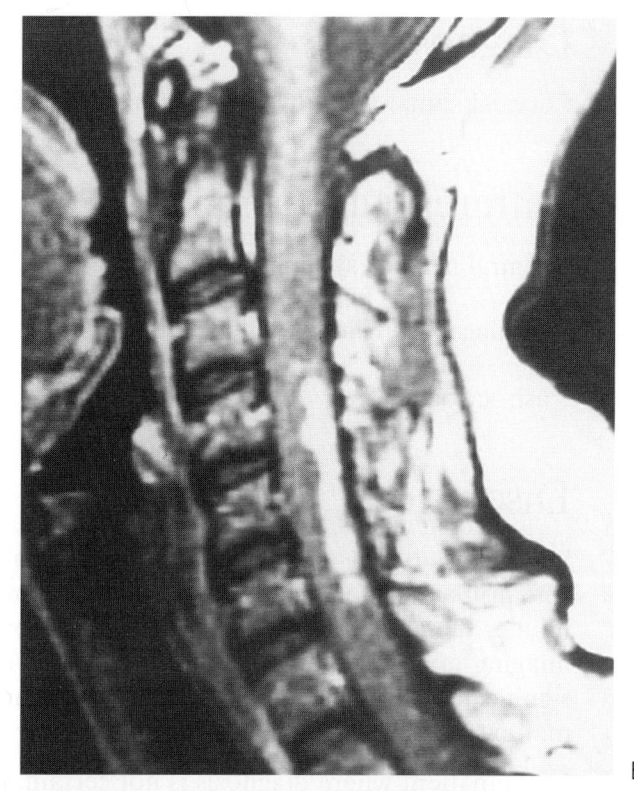

INFLAMMATORY DISEASES OF THE SPINE

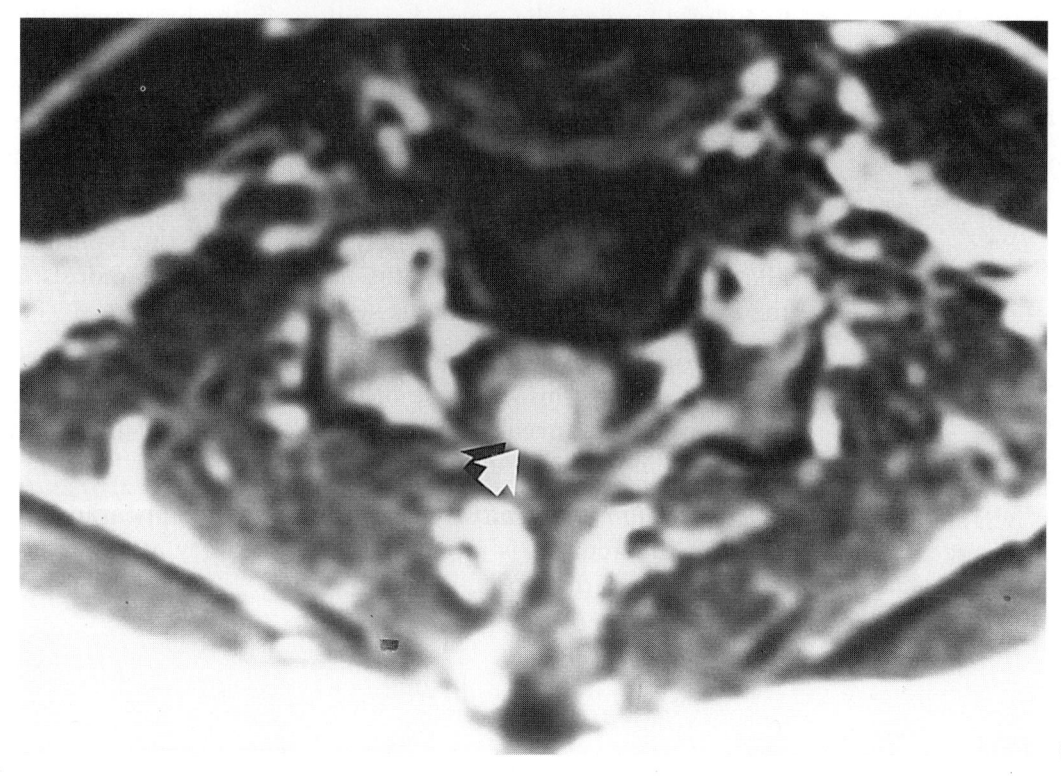

517

Diagnosis

Cervical spinal cord involvement with sarcoidosis.

Differential Diagnosis

- central nervous system (CNS) sarcoidosis
- meningeal carcinomatosis
- astrocytoma

Discussion

Sarcoidosis of the spinal meninges may exhibit a variety of appearances. The primary pattern may be that of diffuse meningeal enhancement, which mimics the appearance of meningeal carcinomatosis. In other patients, the imaging appearance is very similar to that illustrated in this example. A significant clue is that the clinical symptoms are minor relative to the abnormal extent of the imaging appearance.

In the patient where diagnosis is not certain, imaging of the brain may also be helpful for final diagnosis. Sarcoidosis in the brain typically involves the pituitary stalk, which appears thickened and to exhibits dense enhancement on the postcontrast study. In other cases, there may be mass-like areas within the parenchyma of the brain. In some patients, there is a diffuse nodular/meningeal pattern of enhancement. These imaging changes should be correlated with cerebrospinal fluid analysis.

Correlation with a chest x-ray may demonstrate the typical appearance of hilar and paratracheal adenopathy that is seen in sarcoidosis. This confirms the diagnosis of central nervous system sarcoidosis.

Spinal cord tumor such as astrocytoma would be a strong consideration in a patient such as this. Because of this possibility, the area of enhancement was biopsied and revealed sarcoidosis. Cerebrospinal fluid analysis is important for complete evaluation.

Mycobacterium tuberculosis may also mimic the appearance of sarcoidosis. Because tuberculosis is a treatable disease every attempt should be made to rule out this diagnosis.

PEARLS

- The enhancement is in a white matter distribution in the cervical spinal cord.
- At the time of spine imaging, the area of the sella turcica may be visualized, and this should be evaluated for possible enhancement of the pituitary stalk that would substantiate the diagnosis of sarcoidosis.

PITFALL

- A spinal cord tumor could have this appearance; however, the white matter distribution of enhancement and the very mild clinical symptoms relative to the size of the lesion make the diagnosis of an inflammatory process in this case more likely.

INFLAMMATORY DISEASES OF THE SPINE

Case 14

Clinical Presentation

The patient is a 3-year-old with a history of amyelogenous lymphatic leukemia who is status postchemotherapy with new onset of inability to walk.

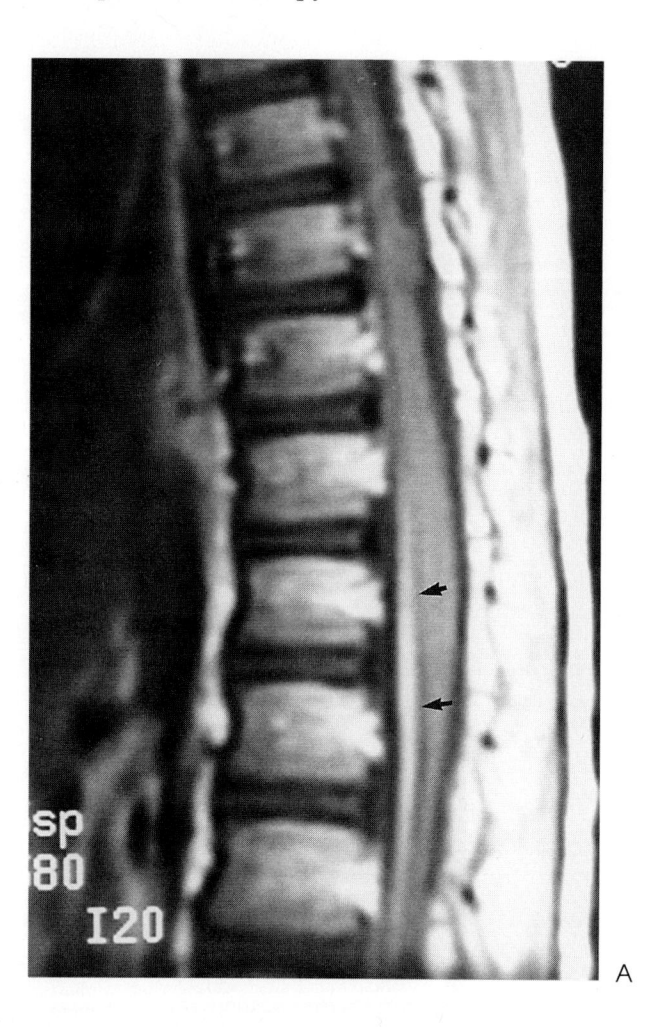

Radiologic Findings

Sagittal short TR image postcontrast (Fig. A) reveals enhancement anteriorly in the lower thoracic and upper lumbar region (*arrows*).

TEACHING ATLAS OF SPINE IMAGING

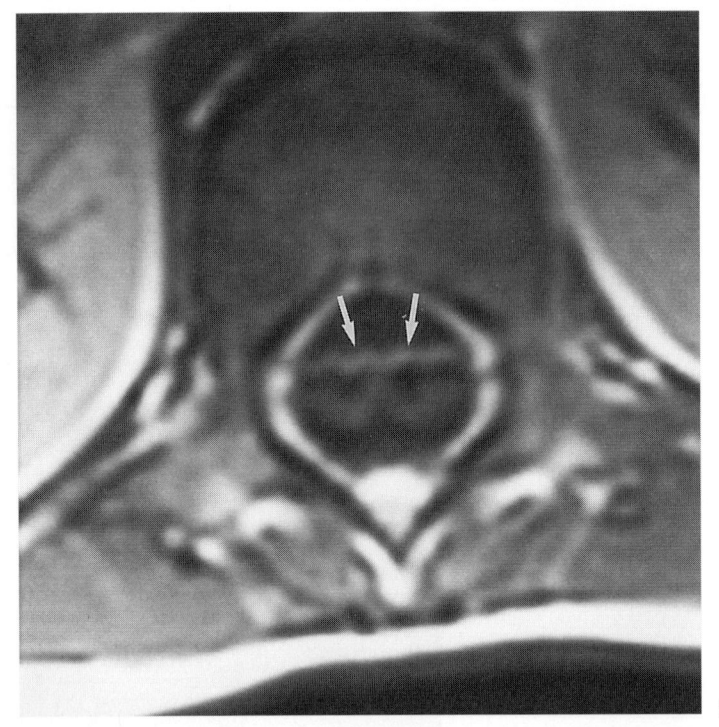

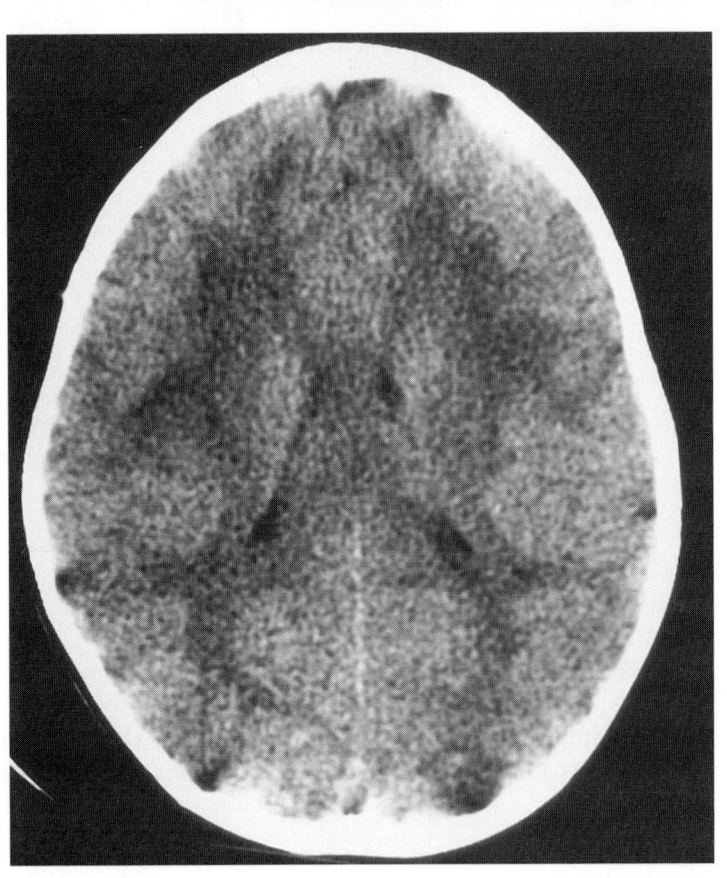

B

C

520

INFLAMMATORY DISEASES OF THE SPINE

Radiologic Findings (continued)

Axial short TR image postcontrast (Fig. B) reveals that the enhancement seen on the sagittal view is actually the nerve roots of the cauda equina (*arrows*).

Computed tomographic (CT) scan of the brain (Fig. C) reveals diffuse low density throughout the brain in a white matter distribution. This is thought to be secondary to involvement of the cerebral tissue with the cytomegalovirus (CMV) virus.

Diagnosis

CMV radiculitis.

Differential Diagnosis

- CMV radiculitis
- cerebral ventriculitis
- meningeal carcinomatosis

PEARL
- Meningeal carcinomatosis of the spinal cord could have a similar appearance; therefore, evaluation should be made for a primary tumor within or outside of the central nervous system.

PITFALL
- The CT appearance of the brain has been reported in Guillain-Barré syndrome; however, this is a very rare clinical syndrome.

Discussion

Clinical history would be vital in this patient to arrive at a correct diagnosis. Analysis of the cerebrospinal fluid would also allow more accurate evaluation. Such analysis should include aerobic and anaerobic cultures, cell count, and cytology for complete evaluation. CMV radiculitis has also been reported in AIDS patients. In these cases, there is typically enhancement involving the nerve roots of the cauda equina.

Cerebral ventriculitis is a typical inflammatory process that may affect the central nervous system. In these cases, the postinfusion scan reveals dense periventricular enhancement.

Meningeal carcinomatosis with limited involvement of the spinal meninges would also be a diagnostic consideration in this patient. A typical primary tumor would be medulloblastoma or pinealoma.

In addition, the CT appearance of the brain could suggest a disease process such as a metabolic or degenerative disease.

Suggested Readings

Angtuaco EJC, McConnell JR, Chadduck WM, Flanigan S. MR imaging of spinal epidural sepsis. *AJNR.* 1987;8:879–883.

Baker AS, Ojemann RG, Swartz MN, Richardson EP Jr. Spinal epidural abscess. *N Eng J Med.* 1975;293:463–468.

Barakos JA, Mark AS, Dillon WP, Norman D. MR imaging of acute transverse myelitis and AIDS myelopathy. *JCAT.* 1990;14:45–50.

Bertino RE, Porter BA, Stimac GK, Tepper SJ. Imaging spinal osteomyelitis and epidural abscess with short T1 inversion recovery (STIR). *AJNR.* 1988;9:563–564.

Bonaldi VM, Duong H, Starr MR, et al. Tophaceous gout of the lumbar spine mimicking an epidural abscess: MR features. *AJNR.* 1996;17:1949–1952.

Bushara KO, Petermann G, Waclawik AJ, et al. Sarcoidosis of the spinal cord with extensive vertebral involvement: case report. *Comput Med Imag Graph.* 1995;19:443–446.

Danner RL, Hartman BJ. Update of spinal epidural abscesses: 35 cases and review of the literature. *Rev Infect Dis.* 1987;9:265–274.

Davis WL, Harnsberger HR. CT and MRI of the normal and disease perivertebral space. *Neuroradiol.* 1995;37:388–394.

Demaerd P, Wilms G, Van Lierde, S. et al. Lyme disease in childhood presenting as primary leptomeningeal enhancement without parenchymal findings on MR. *AJNR* 1994;15:302–304.

Enzman DR, DelePaz RL, Rubin JB. Infection and inflammation. In: *Magnetic Resonance of the Spine.* St. Louis, MO: CV Mosby; 1990.

Feder HM, Zalneriatis EL, Reik L. Lyme disease: acute focal meningoencephalitis in a child. *Pediatrics.* 1988;82:931–934.

Feydy A, Carlier R, Mompoint D, et al. Brain and spinal cord MR imaging in a case of acute disseminated encephalomyelitis. *Eur Radiol.* 1997;7:415–417.

Friess HM, Wasenko JJ. MR of staphylococcal myelitis of the cervical spinal cord. *AJNR.* 1997;18:455–458.

Georgy BA, Chong BW, Chamberlain M, et al. MR of the spine in Guillain-Barré syndrome. *AJNR.* 1994;15:300–301.

Gero B, Sze G, Sharif H. MR imaging of intradural inflammatory disease of the spine. *AJNR.* 1991;12:1009–1019.

Graham E, James DG. Neurosarcoidosis. *Sarcoidosis.* 1988;5:125–131.

Heenan SD, Britton J. Septic arthritis in a lumbar facet joint: rare cause of an epidural abscess. *Neuroradiol.* 1995;37:462–464.

Hirai T, Korogi Y, Hamatake S, et al. Case report—varicella-zoster virus myelitis—serial MR findings. *Br J Radiol.* 1996;69:1187–1190.

Jinkins JR, Bazan C III, Xiong L. MR of disc protrusion engendered by infectious spondylitis. *JCAT.* 1996;20:715–718.

Kircun R, Shormaker EI, Chovanes GI, Stephens HW. Epidural abscesses of the cervical spine: MR findings in five cases. *AJR.* 1992;158:1145–1149.

Lang IM, Hughes DG, Jenkins JPR, et al. MR imaging appearances of cervical epidural abscess. *Clin Radiol.* 1995;50:466–471.

Lexa FJ, Grossman RI. MR sarcoidosis of the brain and spine: spectrum of manifestations and radiographic response to steroid therapy. *AJNR* 1994;15:973.

Loke TKL, Ma HTG, Chan CS. Magnetic resonance imaging of tuberculous spinal infection. *Australas Radiol.* 1997;41:7–12.

Modic MT, Feiglin DH, Piraino DW, et al. Vertebral osteomyelitis: assessment using MR. *Radiology.* 1985;157:157–166.

Muder RR, Lumish RM, Corsello GR. Myelopathy after herpes zoster. *Arch Neurol.* 1983;40:445–446.

Nesbit GM, Miller GM, Baker GL, Ebersold MJ, Scheithauer BW. Spinal cord sarcoidosis: a new finding at MR imaging with Gd-DTPA enhancement. *Radiology.* 1989;173:839–843.

Post MJD, Quencer RM, Montalvo BM, et al. Spinal infection: evaluation with MR imaging and intraoperative US. *Radiology.* 1988;169:765–771.

Post MJD, Sze G, Quencer RM, et al. Gadolinium-enhanced MR in spinal infection. *JCAT.* 1990;14:721–729.

Quencer RM, Post MJD. Spinal cord lesions in patients with AIDS. *Neuroimag Clin North AM.* 1997;7:359–373.

Rieger J, Hosten N. Spinal cord sarcoidosis. *Neuroradiol.* 1994;36:627.

Rozenblit A, Wasserman E, Marin ML, et al. Infected aortic aneurysm and vertebral osteomyelitis after intravesical bacillus Calmette-Guérin therapy. *AJR.* 1996;167:711–713.

Sadato N, Numaguchi Y, Rigamonti D, et al. Spinal epidural abscess with gadolinium-enhanced MRI: serial follow-up studies and clinical correlations. *Neuroradiol.* 1994;36:44–51.

Sandhu FS, Dillon WP. Spinal epidural abscess: evaluation with contrast-enhanced MR imaging. *AJNR.* 1982;12:1087–1093.

Schellinger D. Patterns of anterior spinal canal involvement by neoplasms and infections. *AJNR.* 1996;17:953–959.

Sharif H, Clark DC, Aabed MY, et al. Granulomatous spinal infections: MR imaging. *Radiology.* 1990;177:101–107.

Sze G, Sloetsky S, Bronen R, et al. MR imaging of the cranial meninges with emphasis on contrast enhancement and meningeal carcinomatosis. *AJNR.* 1989;10:965–975.

Talpos D, Tien RD, Hesselink JR. Magnetic resonance imaging of AIDS-related polyradiculopathy. *Neurology* 1991;41:1995–1997.

Thrush A, Enzman DR. MR imaging of infectious spondylitis. *AJNR.* 1990;11:1171–1180.

Thurnher MM, Jinkins JR, Post MJD. Diagnostic imaging of infections and neoplasms affecting the spine in patients with AIDS. *Neuroimag Clin North Am.* 1997;7:341–357.

Violon P, Patay Z, Braeckeveldt J, et al. Atypical infectious complication of anterior cervical surgery. *Neuroradiol.* 1997;39:278–281.

Yunten N, Alper H, Zileli M, et al. Tuberculosis radiculomyelitis as a complication of spondilodiscitis: MR demonstration. *J Neuroradiol.* 1996;23:241–244.

Section VIII

Cervical Disc Disease

Section VIII

Cervical Disc Disease

CERVICAL DISC DISEASE

Case 1

Clinical Presentation

The patient is a 39-year-old male with a clinical history of 7 days of right neck, shoulder, arm, and hand pain and numbness in the C6 distribution. No history of trauma.

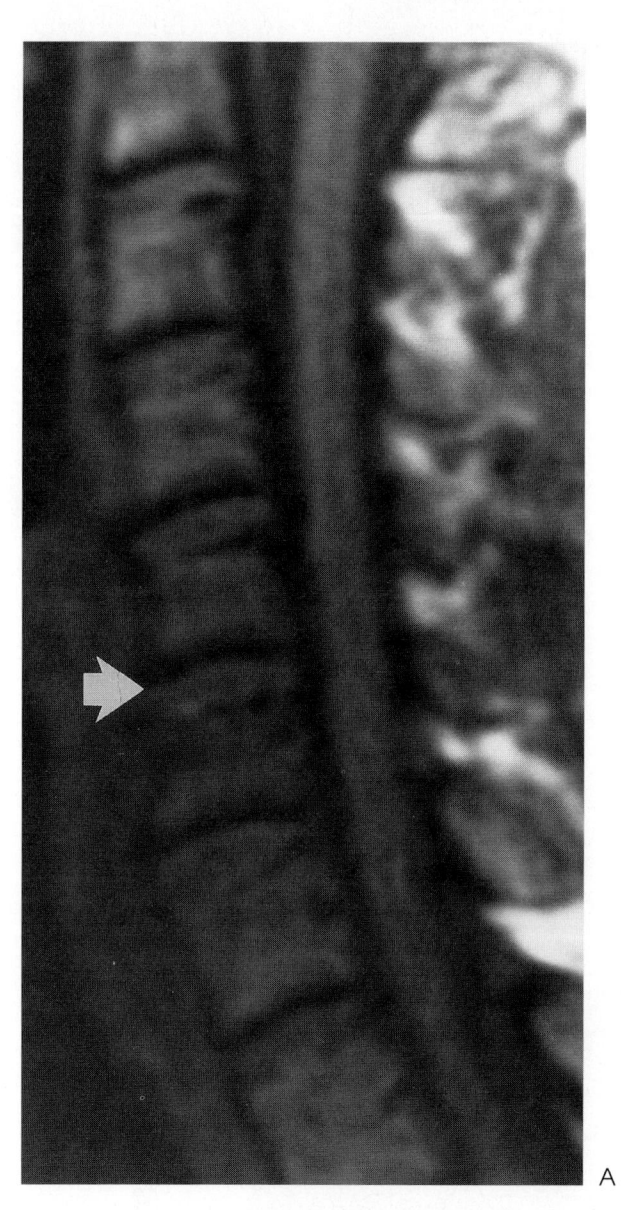

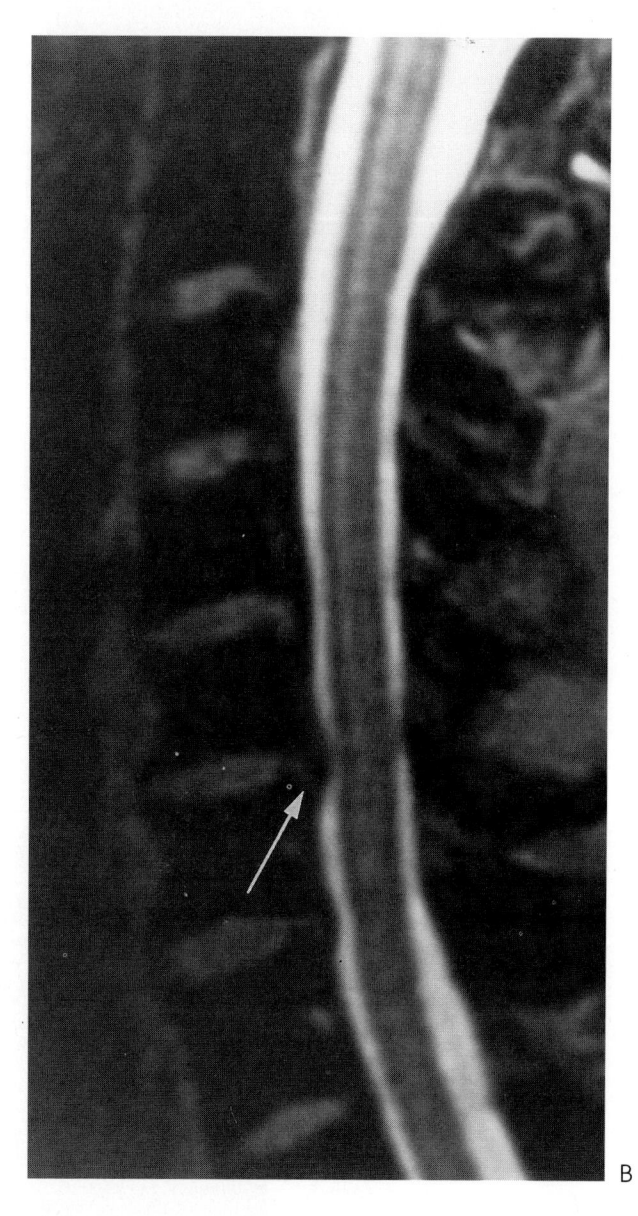

Radiologic Findings

Midsagittal short TR image in the cervical spine (Fig. A) reveals very slight narrowing of the intervertebral disc space at the C5-6 level (*arrow*).

Midsagittal long TR image (Fig. B) reveals slight disc space narrowing and a small bulging disc at the C5-6 level (*arrow*).

TEACHING ATLAS OF SPINE IMAGING

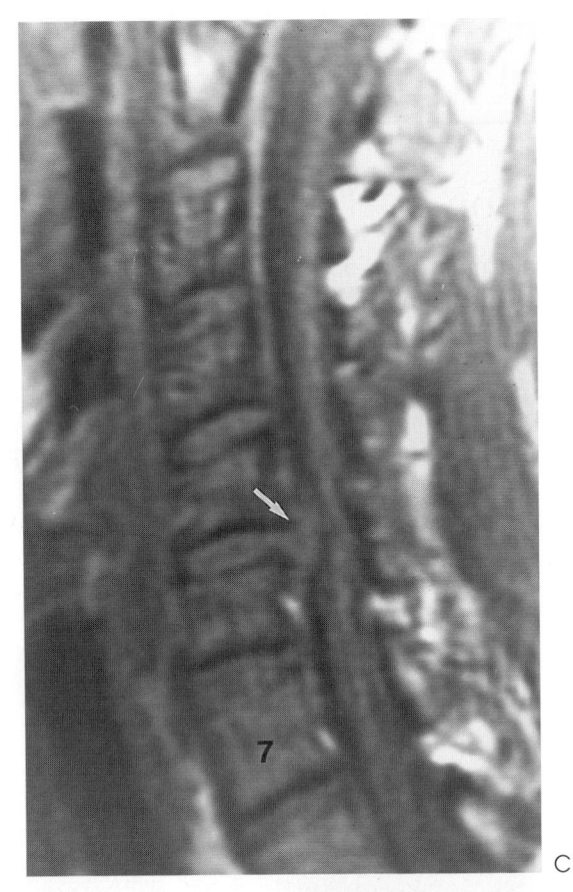

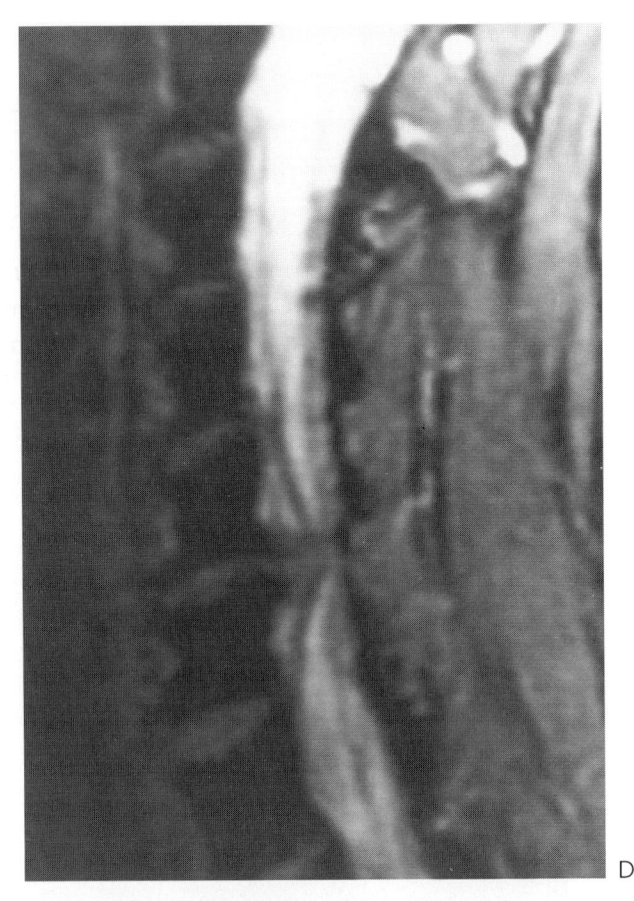

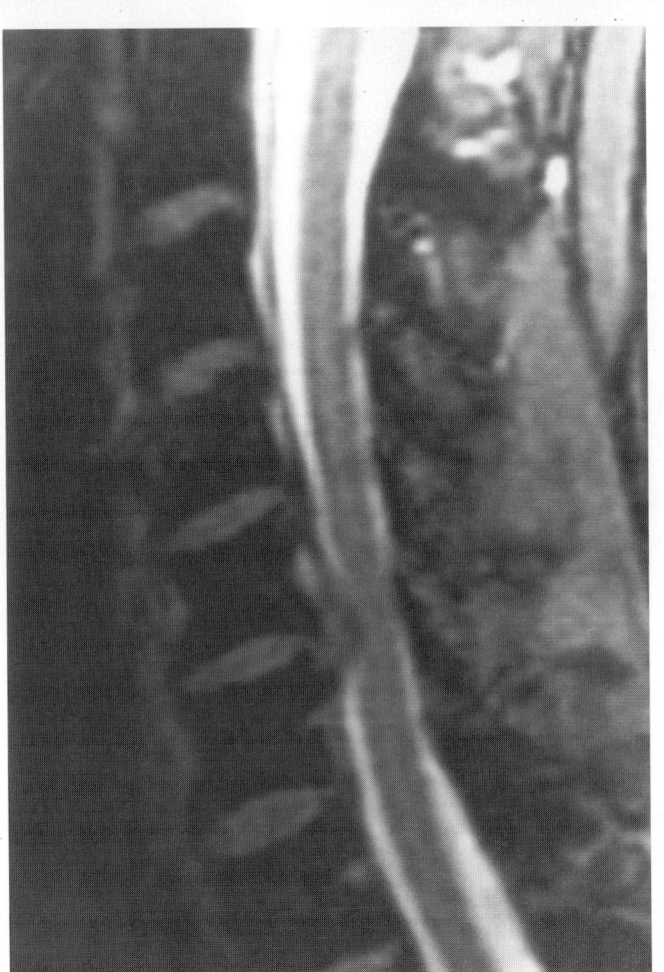

CERVICAL DISC DISEASE

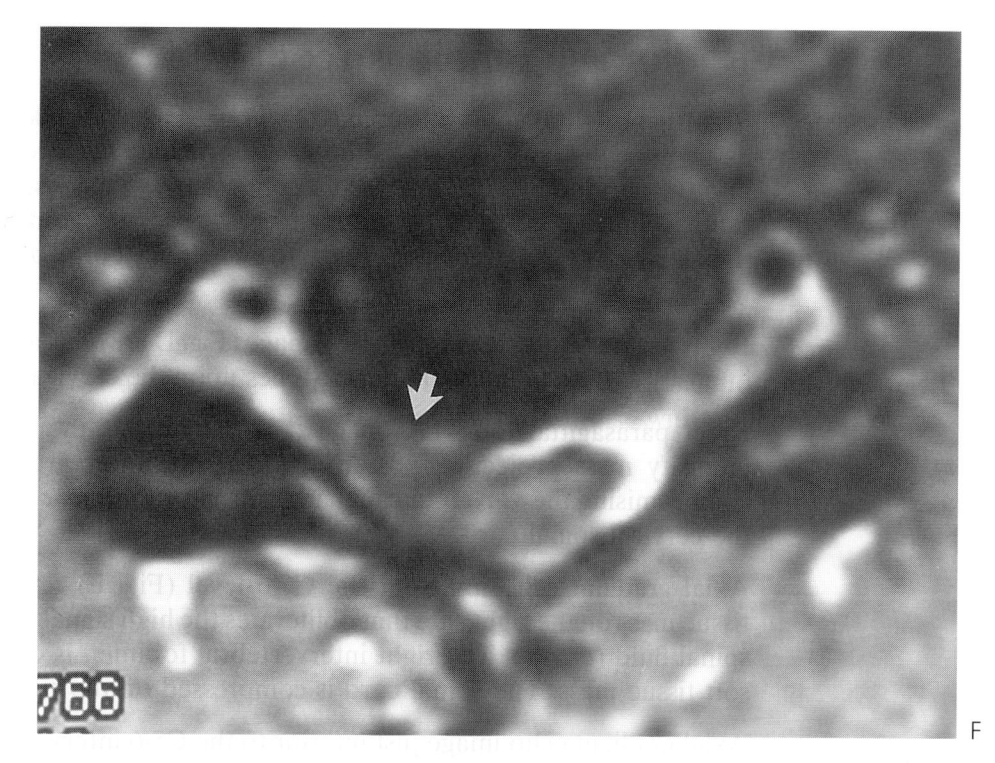

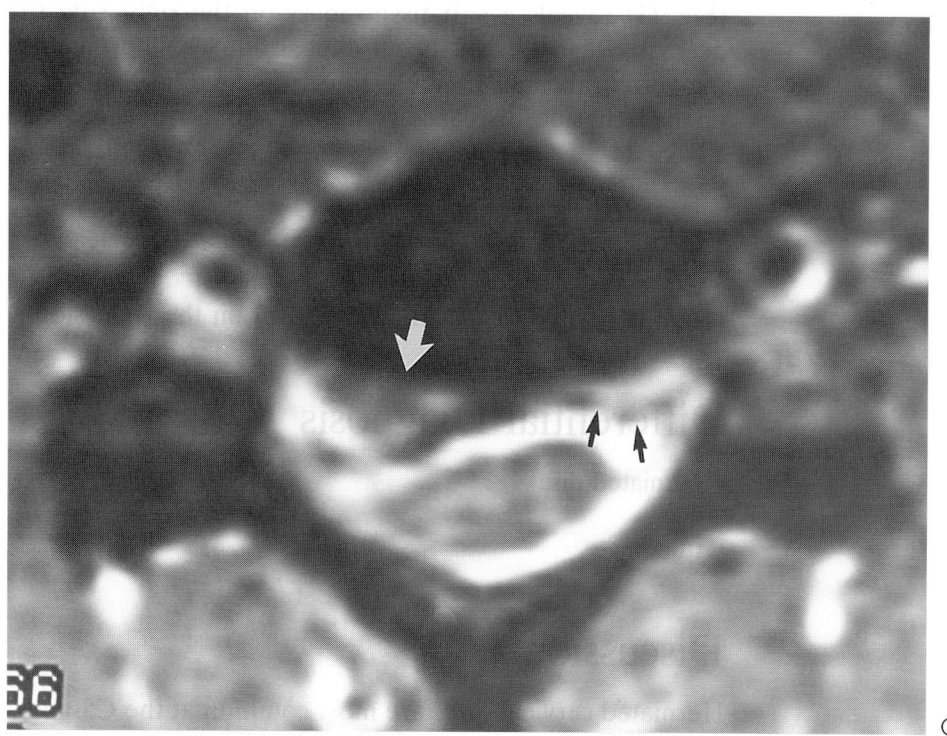

TEACHING ATLAS OF SPINE IMAGING

Case 2

Clinical Presentation

The patient is a 40-year-old female with a clinical history of right C6 radiculopathy, pain, and weakness.

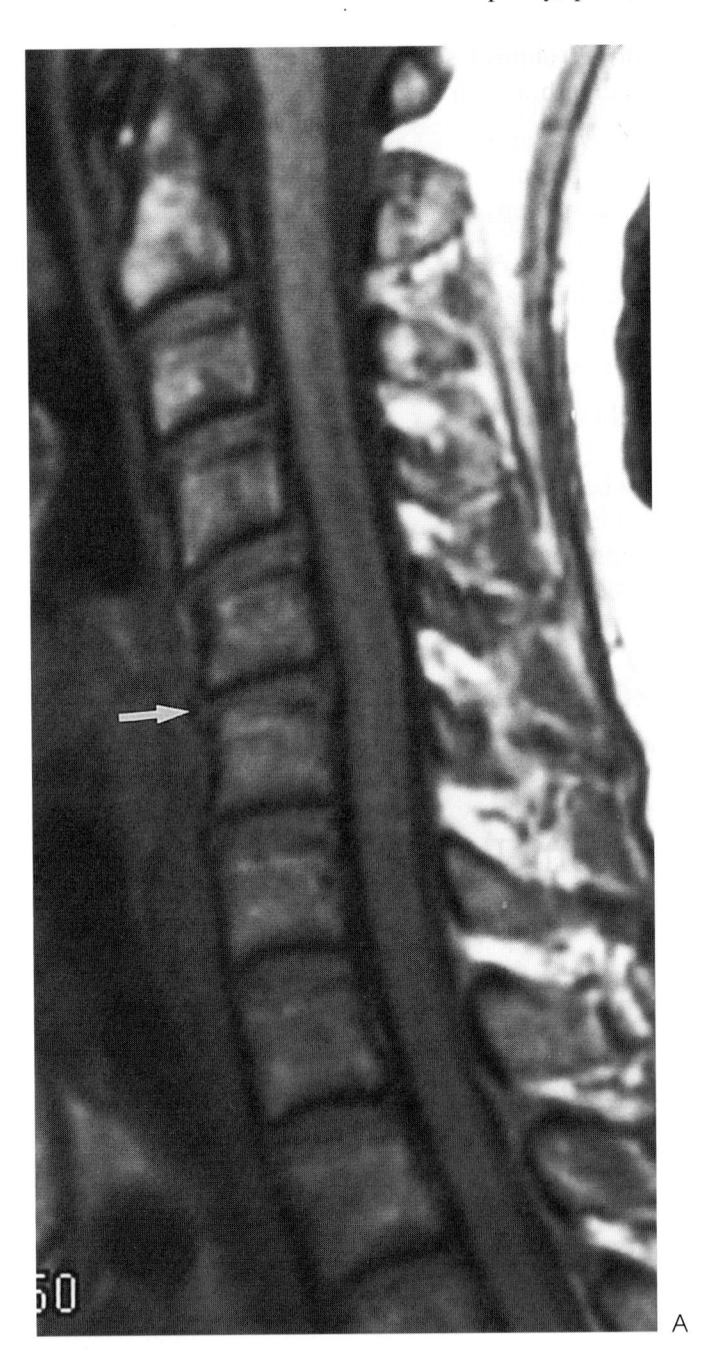

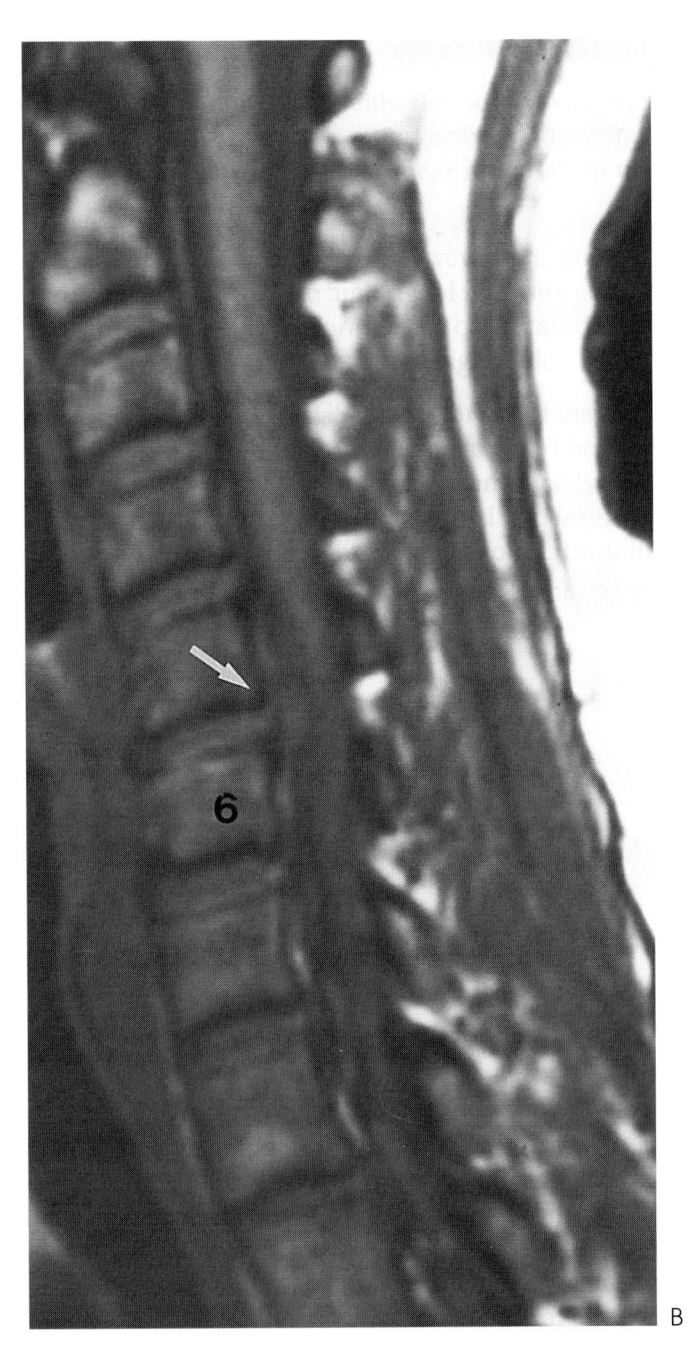

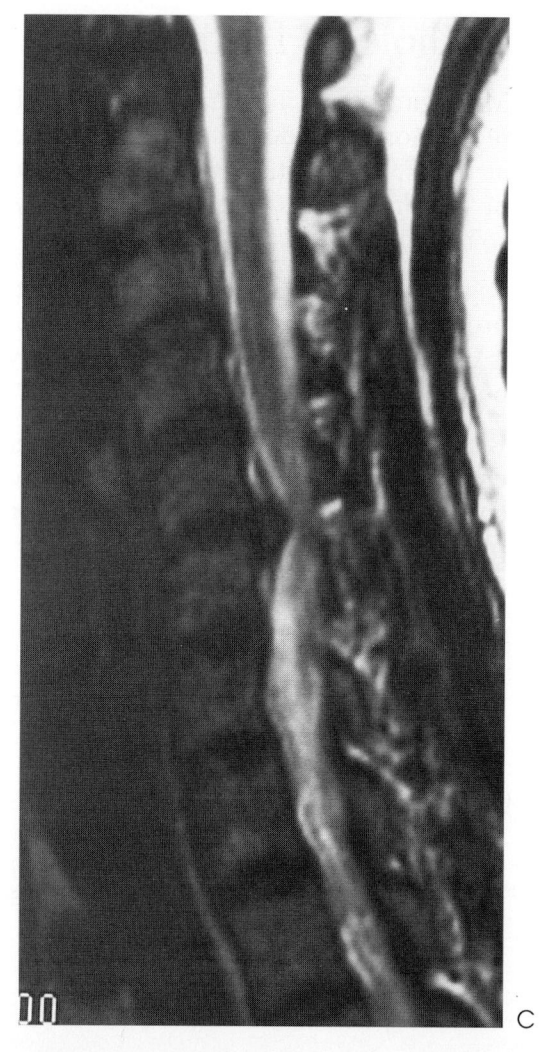

CERVICAL DISC DISEASE

C

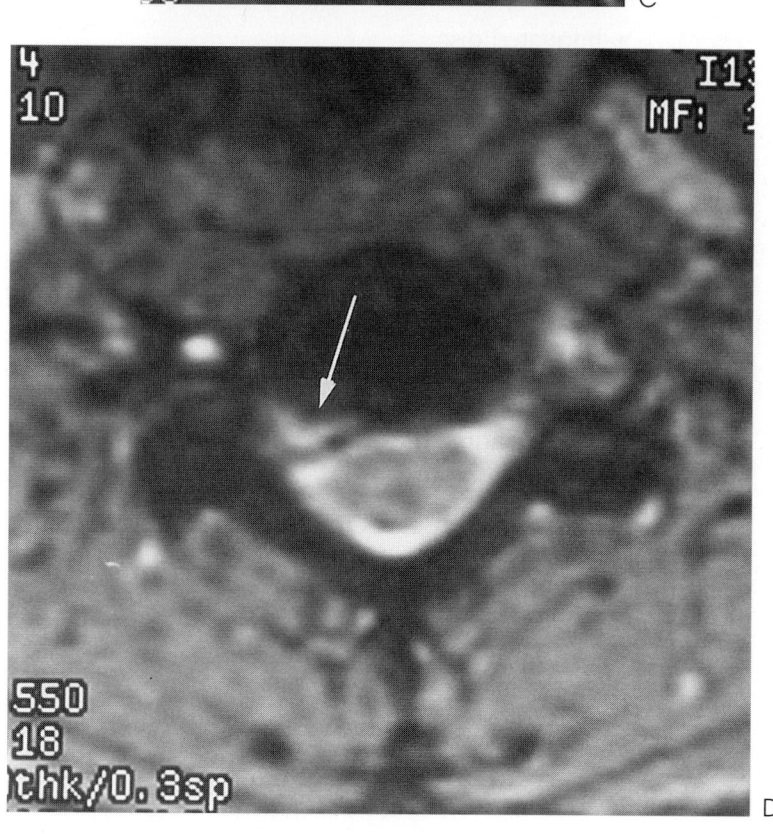

D

TEACHING ATLAS OF SPINE IMAGING

Radiologic Findings

Midsagittal short TR image in the cervical region (Fig. A) reveals reversal of the normal lordotic curve. There is narrowing of the intervertebral disc at the C5-6 level (*arrow*) with slight *anterior* as well as posterior bulging of the disc at this level. There is curvilinear indentation of the cervical spinal cord.

Right parasagittal short TR image (Fig. B) reveals a soft tissue mass that projects posteriorly into the vertebral canal at the C5-6 level (*arrow*). There is curvilinear indentation upon the cervical spinal cord. The C6 vertebral body is identified with 6.

Right parasagittal long TR image (Fig. C) reveals a soft tissue mass encroaching upon the cervical vertebral canal at the C5-6 level. The spinal cord is compressed and displaced laterally toward the left side out of the plane of imaging.

Axial gradient echo image at the C5-6 level (Fig. D) reveals a high signal intensity soft tissue mass on the right side (*arrow*). The normal high signal intensity cerebrospinal fluid is obliterated. There is effacement of the right, anterior margin of the cervical spinal cord and obliteration of the intervertebral foramen on the right side.

Diagnosis

Right-sided herniated intervertebral disc at the C5-6 level.

Differential Diagnosis

- herniated disc
- tumor

Discussion

The appearance is very typical of a herniated cervical disc. The C5-6 level in the most common level of a herniated cervical disc. The radicular pain is secondary to the mechanical compression of the nerve roots as they exit from the intervertebral foramen. The loss of lordotic curve and narrowing of the intervertebral disc are changes that can be appreciated on the plain film evaluation; these findings can be utilized to predict the possible presence of a herniated disc.

The appearance does not suggest a tumor. The soft tissue mass arises from the intervertebral disc and is herniated both anteriorly and posteriorly. In general, progressive weakness is a more typical clinical presentation for a herniated disc, while neck pain and radiculopathy are more typical presentations for a patient with a herniated disc.

PEARLS

- Surgery can be performed based on the magnetic resonance imaging (MRI) findings because MRI accurately reflects the anatomic deformities.

- The long TR images should be carefully evaluated for the presence of abnormal signal intensity in the spinal cord. These changes are thought to be secondary to vascular compromise or possibly direct trauma to the spinal cord.

PITFALLS

- Computed tomographic (CT) scanning in association with myelography can be used for diagnosis; however, MRI has proved to be an accurate method to evaluate cervical disc disease.

- CT is more sensitive than MRI for the identification of small bony osteophytes and so may be performed in conjunction with MRI for evaluation of bony encroachment. Myelography and postmyelography also may be used for more complete evaluation.

CERVICAL DISC DISEASE

Case 3

Clinical Presentation

The patient is a 45-year-old left-handed female with sudden onset of severe pain and weakness in the left arm after playing tennis.

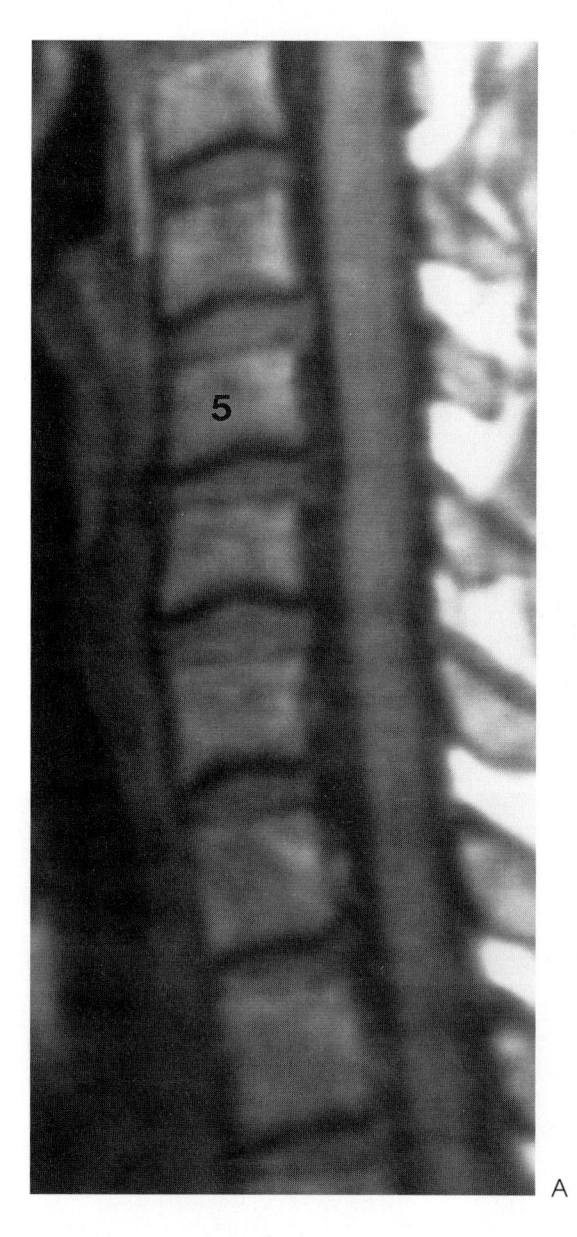

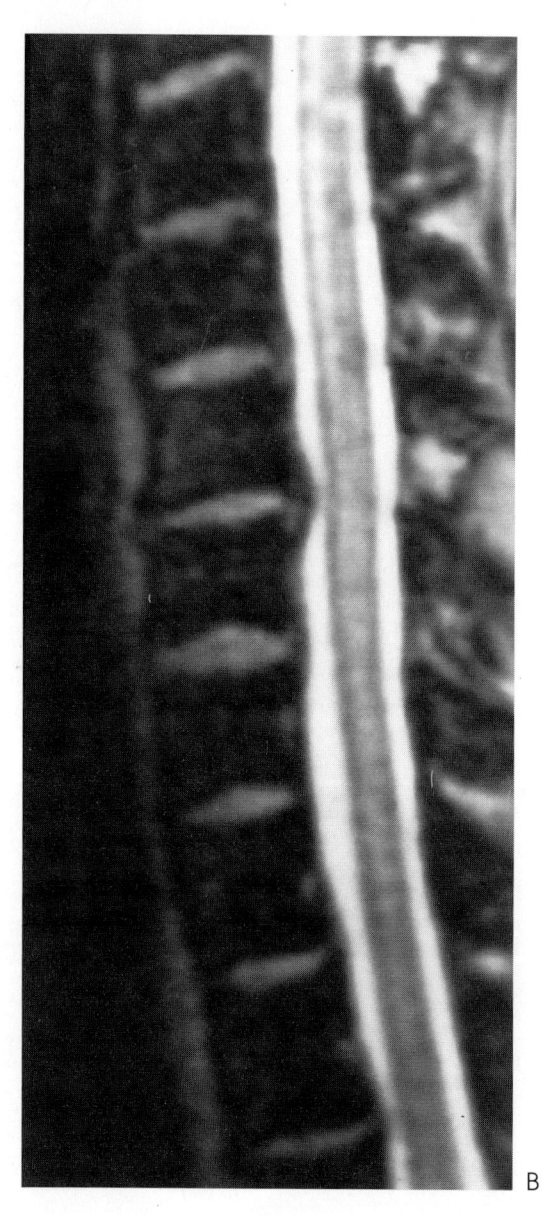

Radiologic Findings

Midsagittal short TR image (Fig. A) reveals straightening of the spine. There is a bulging disc at the C4-5 level with encroachment upon the cervical subarachnoid space. There is also disc prominence at the C5-6 level with slight encroachment upon the cervical subarachnoid space. The C5 vertebral body is identified with 5.

TEACHING ATLAS OF SPINE IMAGING

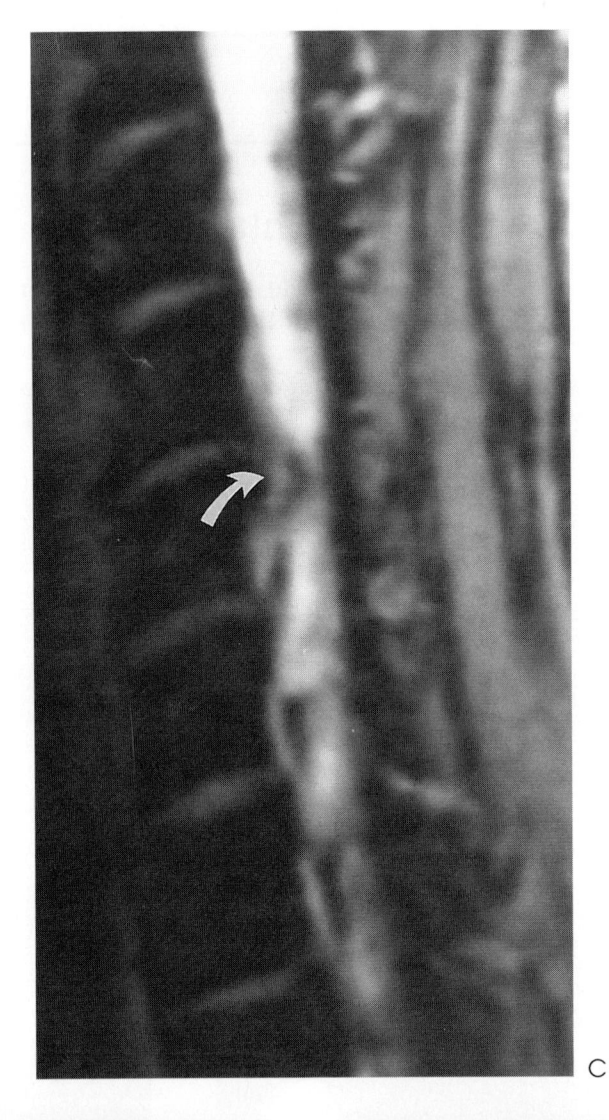

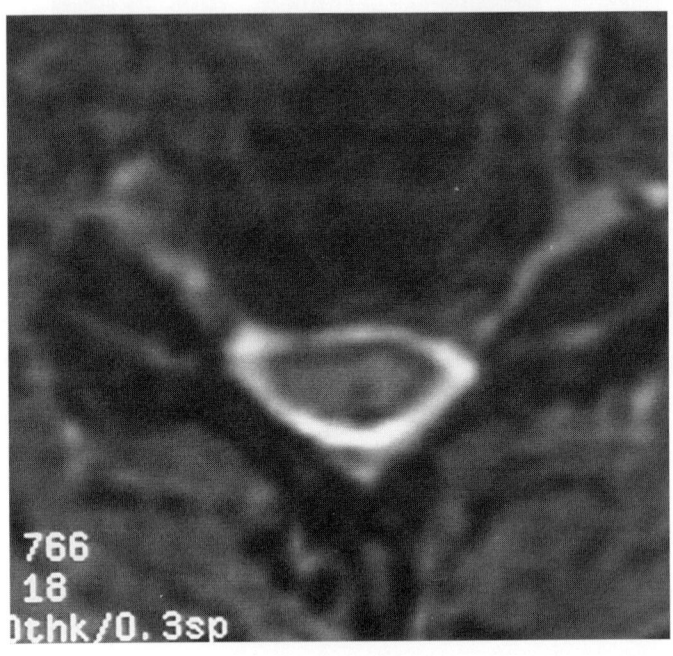

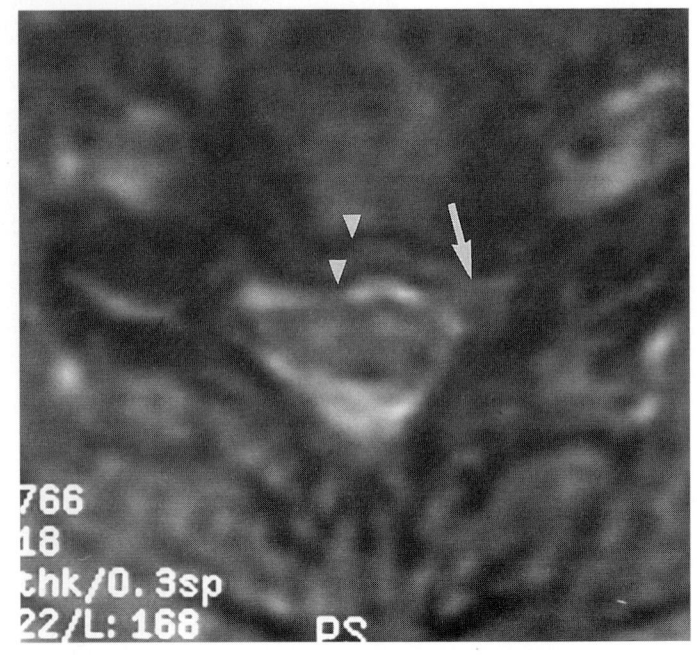

CERVICAL DISC DISEASE

Radiologic Findings (continued)

Midsagittal long TR image (Fig. B) reveals that the disc at C5-6 appears more prominent than the disc at the C4-5 level. Note the slight anterior disc herniation at the C5-6 level. There is slight loss of intervertebral disc height at the C3-4, C4-5, and C5-6 levels. There is no abnormal signal within the cervical spinal cord. Long streaks of increased signal intensity within the spinal cord are secondary to truncation artifact.

Parasagittal T2W image (Fig. C) reveals evidence of a far laterally placed soft tissue mass at the C5-6 level (*arrow*). There is encroachment upon the cervical subarachnoid space.

Axial gradient echo image (Fig. D) reveals bulging of the disc at the C4-5 level. There is slight encroachment upon the cervical subarachnoid space and slight compression of the cervical spinal cord.

Axial gradient echo image at the C5-6 level (Fig. E) reveals definite encroachment upon the cervical subarachnoid space. The normal high signal intensity epidural fat in the intervertebral foramen at the C5-6 level of the left side (*arrow*) is obliterated. There is a double signal intensity area where the disc extends beyond the posterior margin of the vertebral body (*arrowheads*). There is slight effacement of the left lateral margin of the cervical spinal cord.

Diagnosis

Left lateral herniated disc at the C4-5 level.

Differential Diagnosis

- herniated disc
- schwannoma

Discussion

The midsagittal images in this case appear almost normal, or suggest only a small abnormality of the disc at the C4-5 level. However, close evaluation of the parasagittal images reveals the presence of a soft tissue mass encroaching upon the subarachnoid space. The axial images are also subtle and reveal the soft tissue mass obliterating the epidural fat on the left side. The normal high signal intensity of the epidural fat provides the perfect contrast material when using magnetic resonance imaging (MRI). The herniated disc also obliterates the high signal intensity fat in the intervertebral foramen, as seen on Figure E. Because the nerves must exit via these foramina, a herniated disc will lead to severe radicular pain.

The possibility of a schwannoma at the C5-6 level is a consideration; however, the broad base arising from the intervertebral disc space favors a herniated cervical disc.

PEARL
- Careful evaluation of the parasagittal images are very helpful in the accurate diagnosis of a laterally herniated disc in the cervical region.

PITFALL
- Computed tomographic (CT) scanning with myelography will demonstrate failure of filling of the nerve root sleeve at the level of the herniation on the myelogram and an extradural defect by CT scanning; however, accurate interpretation of the noninvasive MRI scan will preclude the use of myelography for diagnosis in most cases.

Case 4

Clinical Presentation

The patient is a 43-year-old female with a history of neck pain.

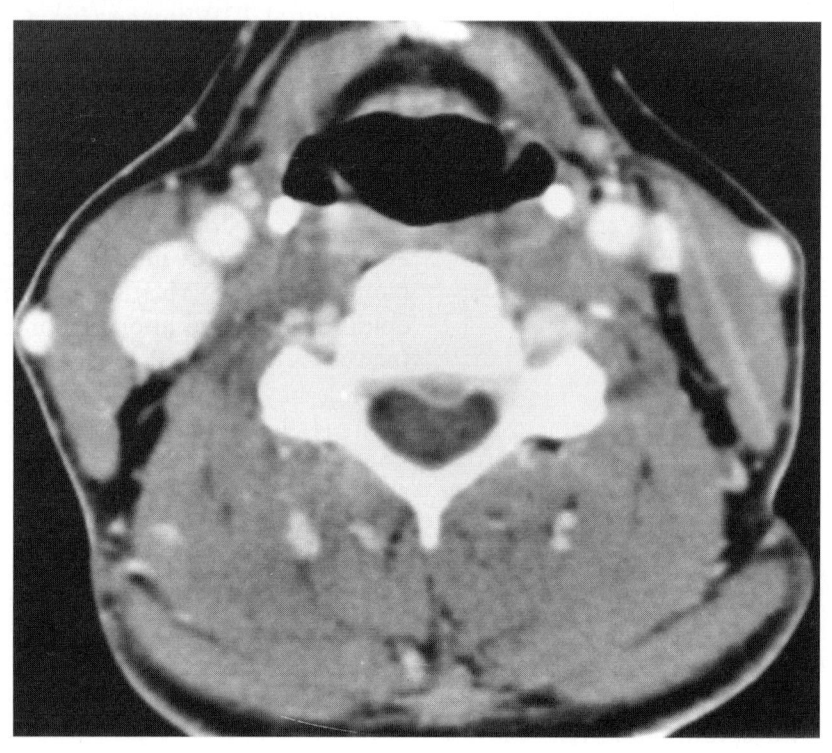

A

Radiologic Findings

Axial postenhancement with iodinated contrast material computed tomographic (CT) scan (Fig. A) reveals a low density curvilinear area projecting behind the intervertebral disc space at the C4-5 level. A peripheral high density margin surrounds this structure. The subarachnoid space is compromised, and the cervical spinal cord is slightly indented..

Incidentally, there is also enhancement of the carotid arteries and jugular veins as well as other branch vessels in the neck.

Diagnosis

Herniated midline and left paracentral cervical disc at the C4-5 level.

Differential Diagnosis

- herniated disc
- epidural abscess

CERVICAL DISC DISEASE

PEARLS

- Herniated discs may be seen even in asymptomatic patients. Therefore, care must be taken to interpret the presence of a herniated disc in the clinical setting of the patient's symptoms.

- While CT scanning can be used for the evaluation and diagnosis of herniated cervical discs, MRI is the more accurate and less invasive method.

PITFALLS

- A small epidural abscess could have a similar appearance, so correlation should be performed with the clinical setting of the patient's presentation.

- CT scanning may be used for diagnosis; however, it is best performed with the use of an infusion of contrast material. Therefore, MRI is recommended as the procedure of choice for evaluation because MRI in this clinical setting does not require the use of contrast material.

Discussion

Prior to the development of magnetic resonance imaging (MRI), various methods were attempted to identify herniated cervical discs. One of these methods was the use of CT scanning in association with contrast enhancement. The cervical venous plexus is very vascular and therefore enhances with contrast infusion. In this case, the venous plexus appears as a curvilinear area of increased density surrounding the relatively low density herniated disc. In those patients with a pure soft herniated disc that is not associated with osteophyte formation, this method is a useful tool, particularly if MRI is not available or the patient is not able to undergo MRI.

Herniated discs in the cervical region may be in the midline, off to one side (in which case they are termed paracentral), or far laterally placed. Herniated discs that are off the midline may cause encroachment upon the nerve roots as they exit in the intervertebral foramen.

The remote possibility of an epidural abscess is a consideration. However, the abnormality is centered at the level of the intervertebral disc, and the absence of a clinical history of fever or pertinent clinical setting such as drug abuse makes this diagnosis unlikely.

MRI is the procedure of choice for the evaluation of herniated cervical discs; however, in some patients a myelogram with postmyelogram CT scanning may be necessary to better define the anatomic location of a disc.

Case 5

Clinical Presentation

The patient is a 37-year-old female with a history of a motor vehicle accident with a whiplash injury.

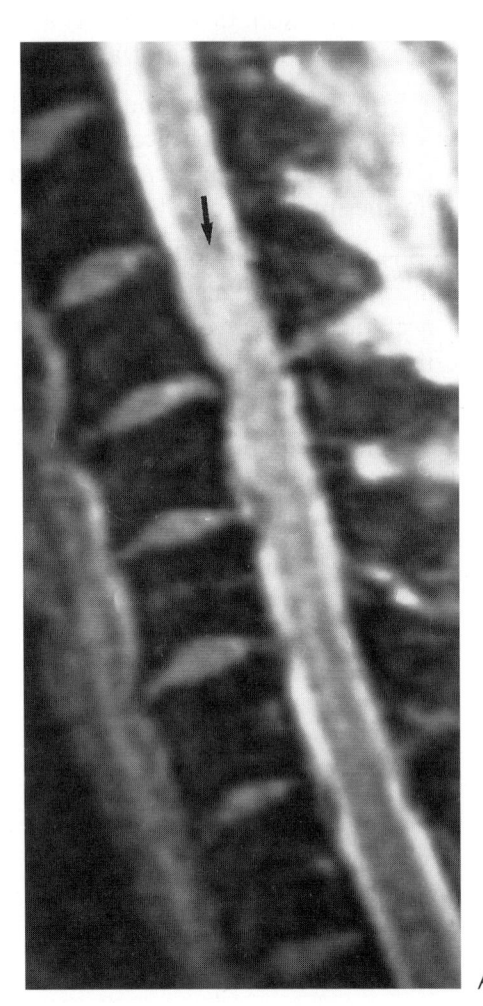

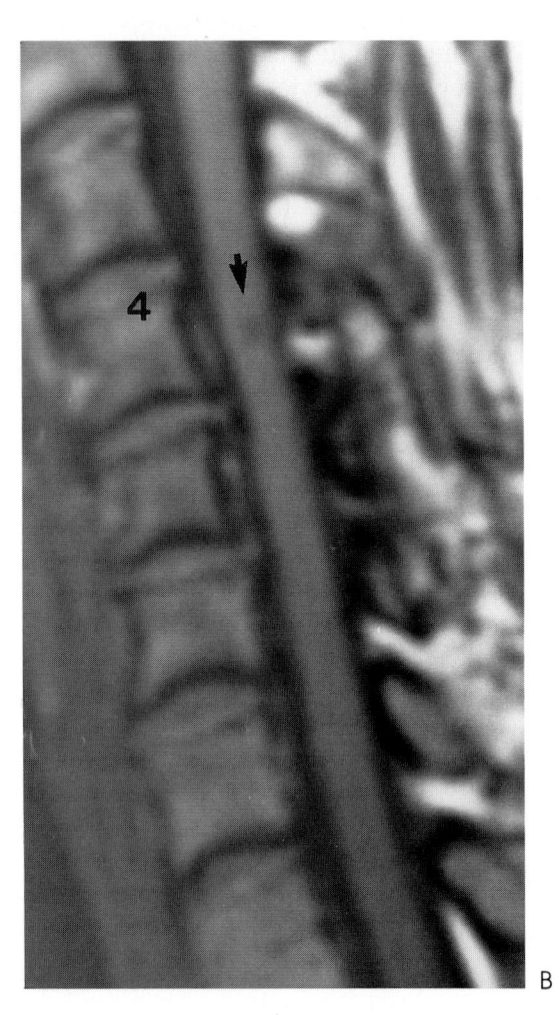

Radiologic Findings

Sagittal long TR image (Fig. A) reveals a small herniated disc at C4-5 and C5-6 and disc bulges at C6-7 and C7-T1. An oval area of increased signal intensity is just superior to the herniated disc at the C4-5 level (*arrow*). There is anterior prominence of the disc at the C4-5 level and reversal of the curve of the cervical spine.

Sagittal short TR image obtained approximately 4 months later (Fig. B) reveals an increase in the disc space narrowing at C4-5 and C5-6. There is a small oval area of decreased signal intensity that projects at the level of the midbody of the C4 vertebra (*arrow*). The C4 vertebral body is identified with 4.

CERVICAL DISC DISEASE

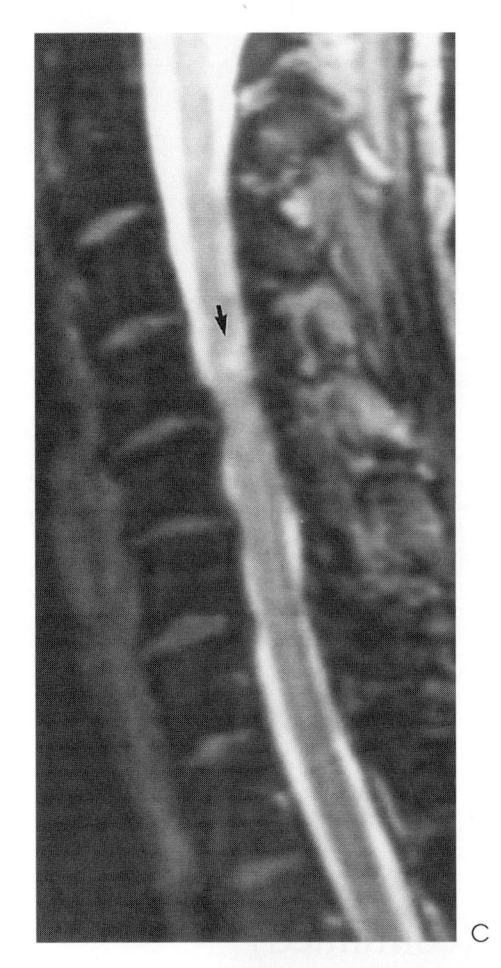

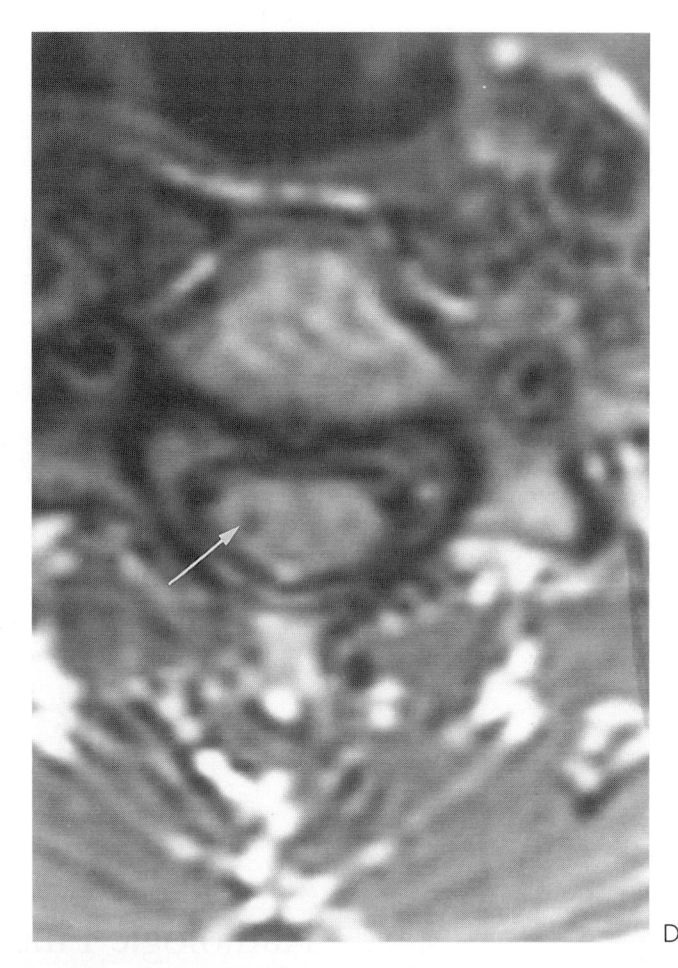

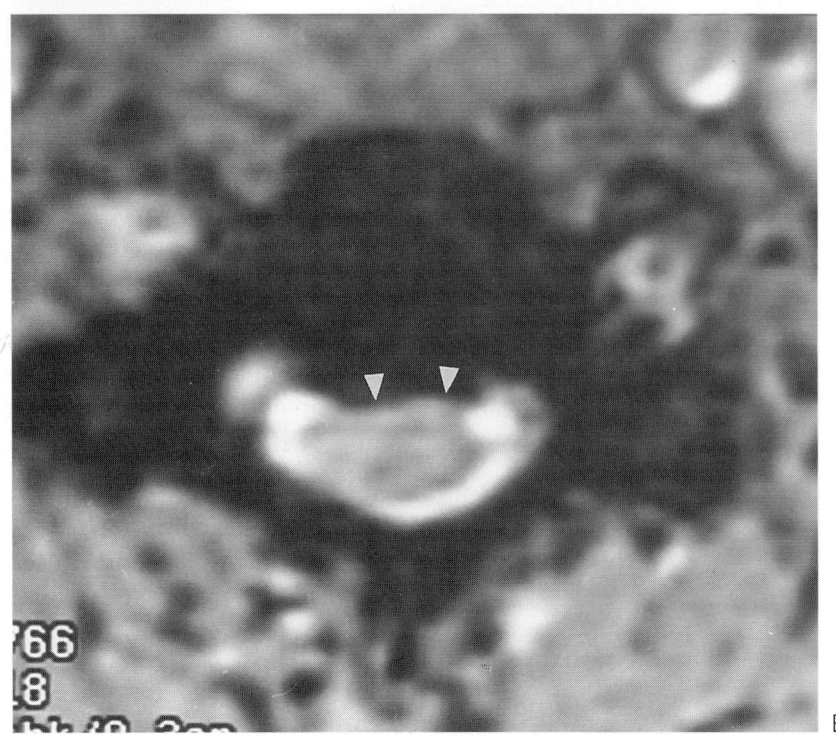

F

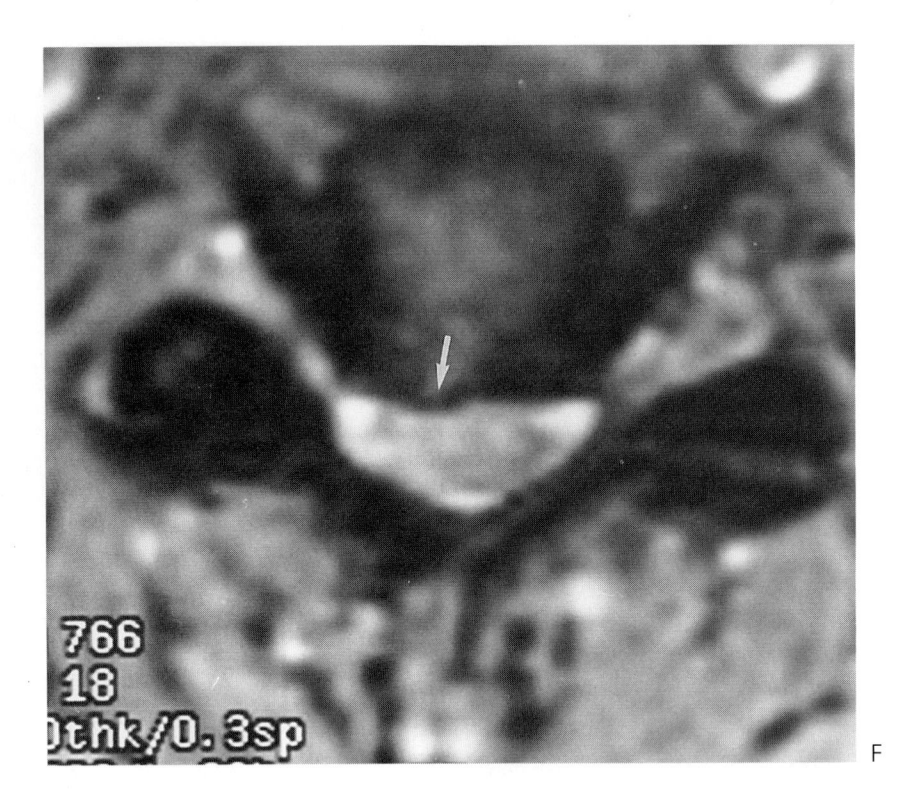

Radiologic Findings (continued)

Sagittal long TR image (Fig. C) reveals that the small area of decreased signal intensity now appears as a focal area of increased signal intensity (*arrow*). There is intervertebral disc space narrowing at multiple levels and encroachment upon the subarachnoid space at multiple levels.

Axial short TR image (Fig. D) reveals the area of decreased signal intensity in the right side of the cervical spinal cord (*arrow*). This presumably represents an area of myelomalacia. These areas are thought to be secondary to either repeated trauma or vascular compromise.

Axial gradient echo image obtained just above the level of the disc at the C4-5 level (Fig. E) reveals the decreased signal intensity of an osteophyte projecting from the posterior margin of the vertebral body (*arrowheads*). There is slight compromise of the cervical subarachnoid space at this level.

Axial short TR image at the C4-5 level (Fig. F) reveals a small right sided herniated disc (*arrow*). This results in compromise of the subarachnoid space at this level and flattening of the cervical spinal cord.

Diagnosis

Degenerative changes with osteophyte formation and trauma resulting in myelomalacia.

CERVICAL DISC DISEASE

PEARL
- Magnetic resonance imaging (MRI) is the ideal method for initial evaluation of these patients. MRI also aids in evaluating the presence of a hematoma following trauma. Initially these patients may do well clinically only to develop symptoms at a later date, so MRI is the ideal method for follow-up.

PITFALL
- Myelography and postmyelography CT scanning will not generally reveal these areas of myelomalacia. If a syrinx cavity forms, delayed CT scanning approximately 8 hours following a myelogram may reveal the concentration of contrast material within a syrinx cavity.

Differential Diagnosis
- myelomalacia

Discussion

At the time of initial trauma, this patient presumably sustained a contusion of the spinal cord at the C4 level secondary to the bony osteophyte. Over the succeeding 4 months, this area of contusion or edema progressed to an area of focal myelomalacia or a small syrinx cavity. Although the exact cause of these areas of myelomalacia is uncertain, one theory is that they are secondary to direct trauma to the spinal cord or secondary to vascular compromise. In some cases, these areas of initial increased signal intensity revert to normal, while in other patients, they progress to areas of myelomalacia. Small syrinx cavities may also form.

The tiny syrinx cavity seen here could have been a pre-existing lesion, but the proximity to the osteophyte and the herniated disc are more suggestive that the tiny cavity is related to the disc.

TEACHING ATLAS OF SPINE IMAGING

Case 6

Clinical Presentation

The patient is a 72-year-old female with a history of neck pain and numbness. The patient was in an automobile accident approximately 1 year prior to this study.

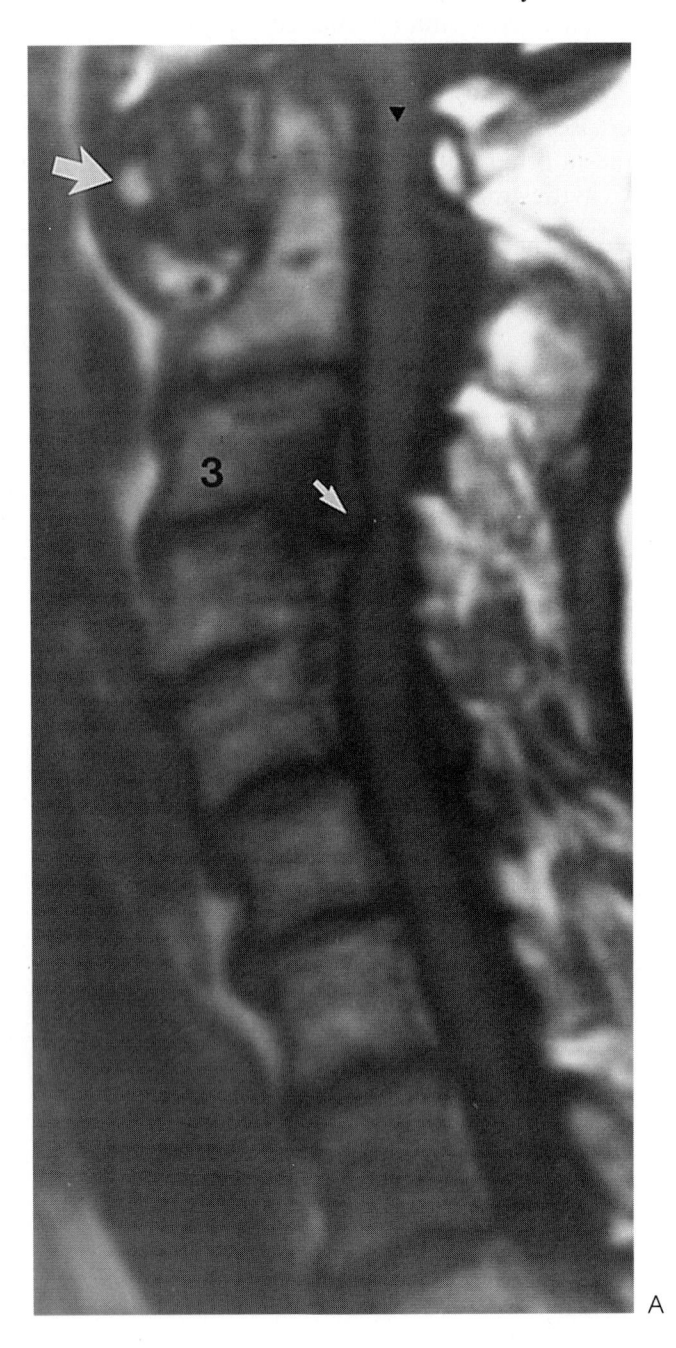

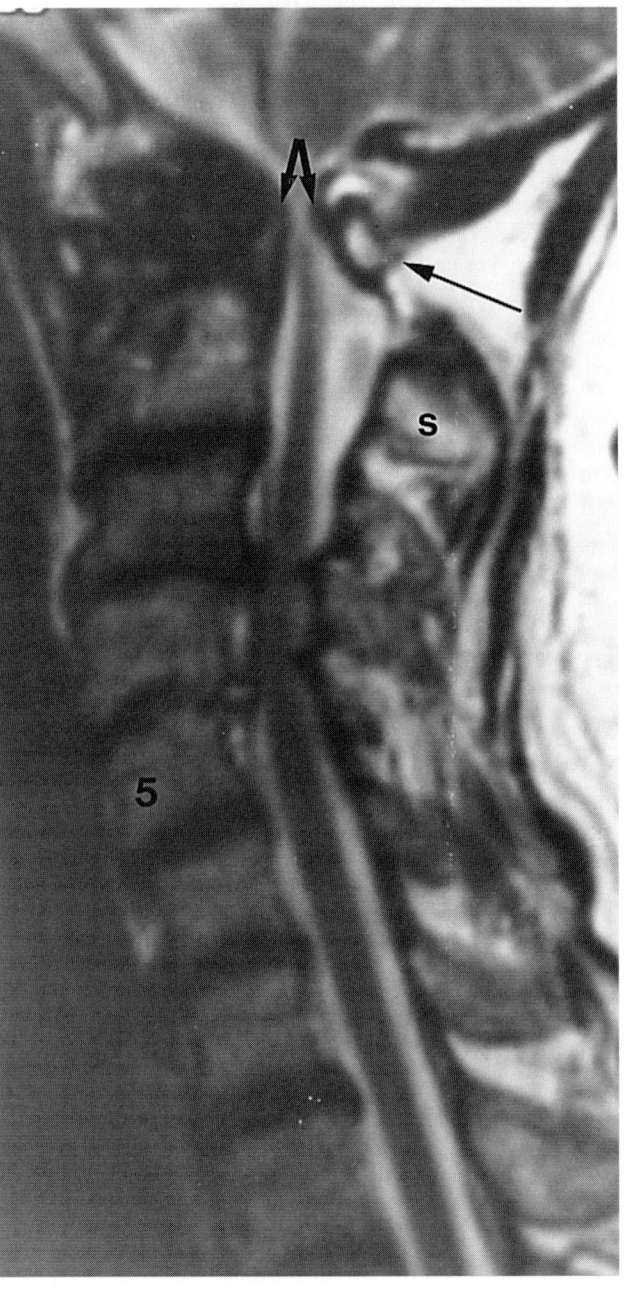

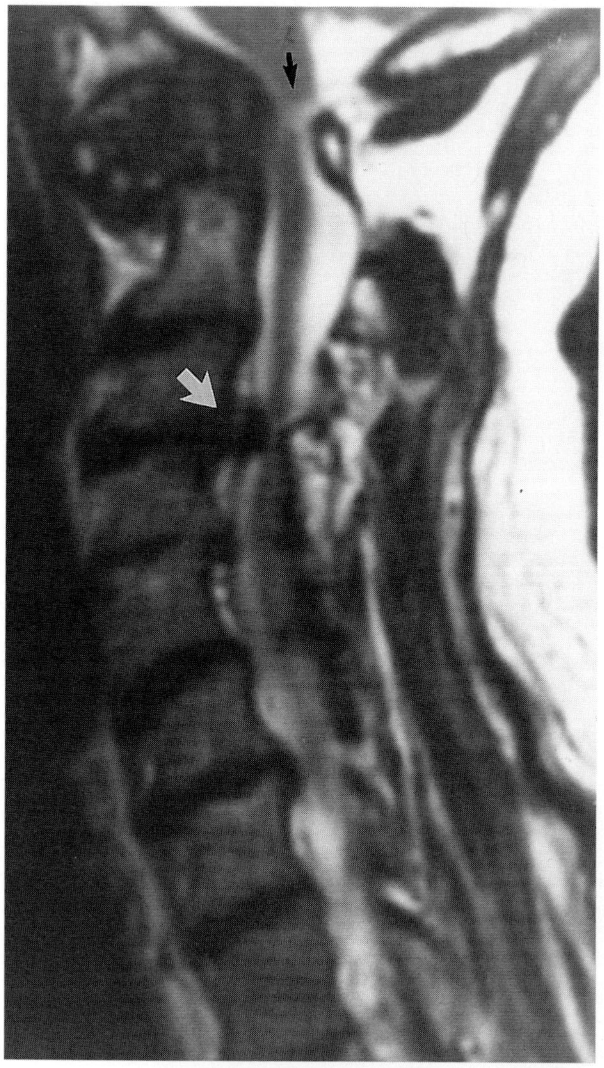

C

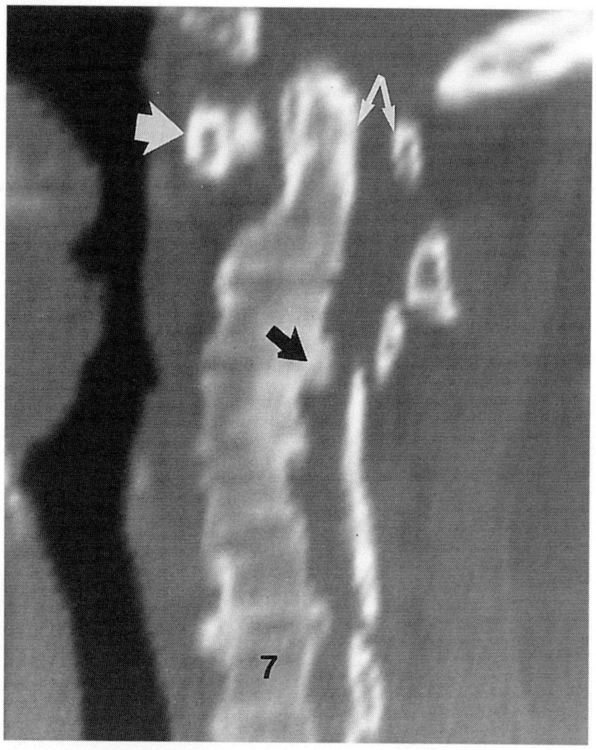

D

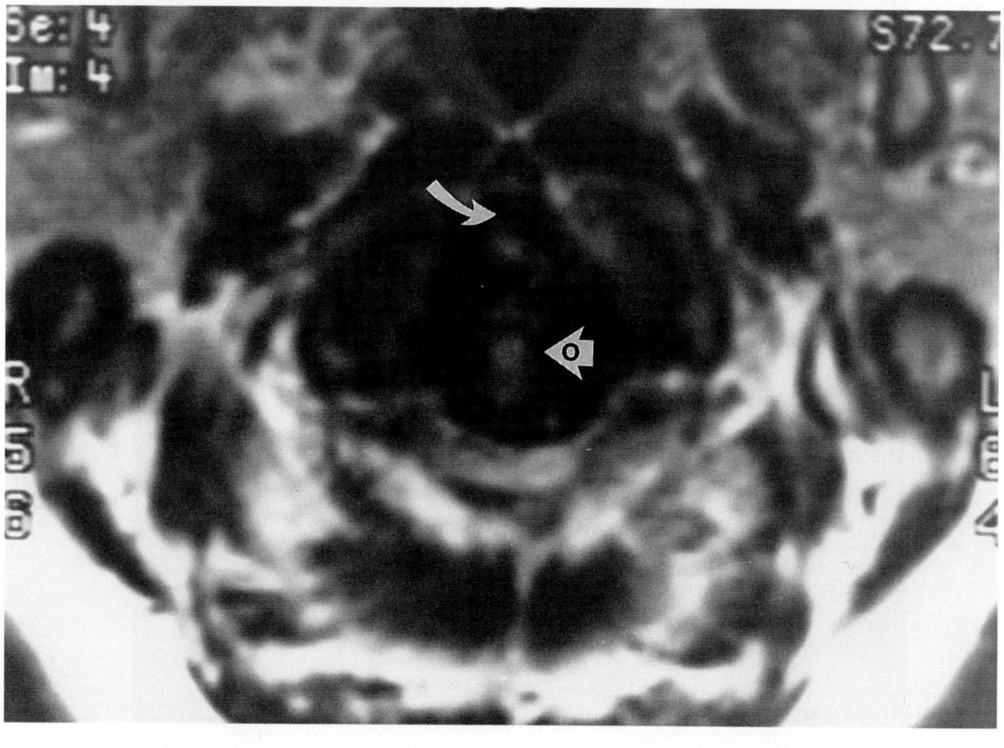

E

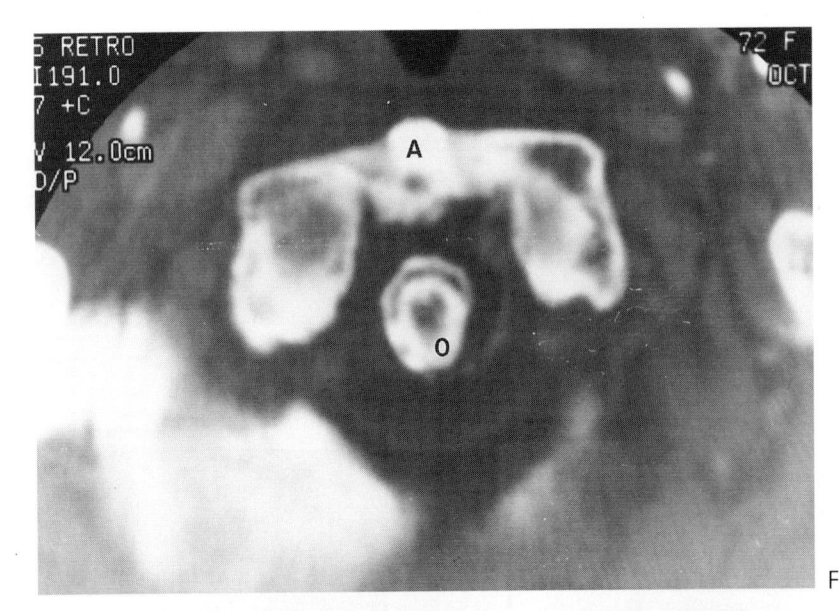

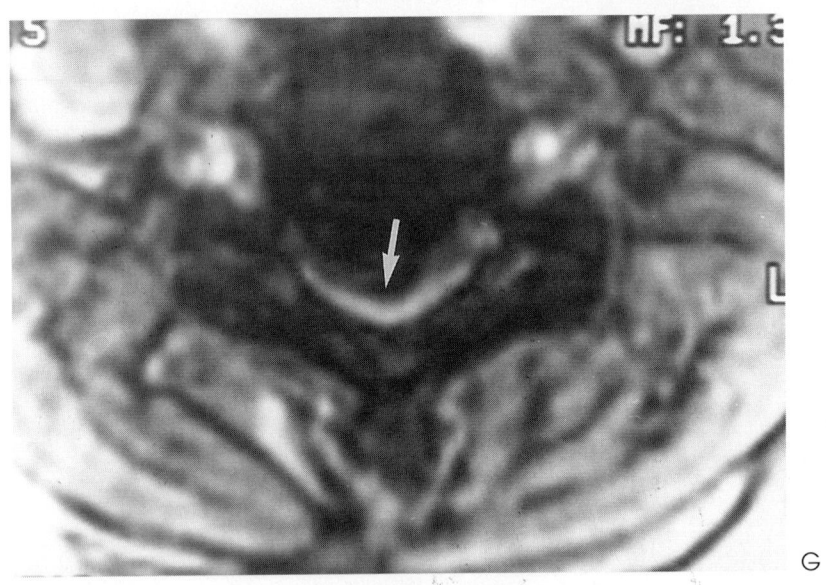

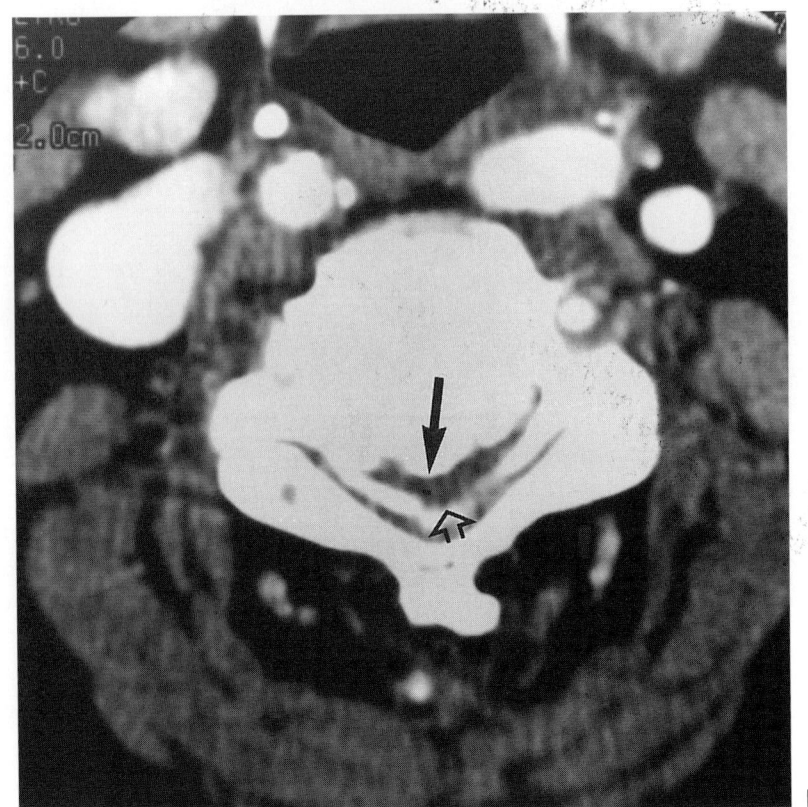

F

G

H

CERVICAL DISC DISEASE

Radiologic Findings

Sagittal short TR image (Fig. A) reveals that the odontoid processes are displaced posterior to the anterior arch of the C1 vertebral body. The anterior arch of C1 appears as an oval area of increased signal intensity (*large white arrow*). There is a mottled, lower than normal signal intensity mass posterior to the arch of C1 and anterior to the odontoid process. The spinal cord at the level of the cervicomedullary junction (*black arrowhead*) is markedly compressed. At the C3-4 level, a large herniated disc projects posteriorly into the vertebral canal and narrows the spinal cord at the C3-4 level (*small white arrow*). The C3 vertebral body is identified by 3.

Midsagittal long TR image (Fig. B) reveals anterior displacement of the posterior arch of C1 (*long black arrow*) relative to the spinous process of C2 (*s*). The posterior displacement of the odontoid process and the anterior displacement of the posterior arch of C2 result in a severe stenosis at this level (*double black arrows*). The spinal cord is markedly compressed at this level. There is also marked canal compromise at the C3-4 and C4-5 levels secondary to prominent intervertebral discs at both of these levels. The C5 vertebral body is identified with 5.

Parasagittal long TR image (Fig. C) reveals more marked prominence of the intervertebral disc at the C3-4 level off toward the right side (*white arrow*). The spinal cord at the level of the cervicomedullary junction is markedly compressed and exhibits a tiny focal area of increased signal intensity within the spinal cord (*black arrow*). The odontoid process is displaced posteriorly and superiorly.

Sagittal reconstruction image of the cervical spine (Fig. D) reveals the anterior arch of C1 (*large white arrow*). There is an oval shaped area of increased density posterior to the arch of C1. The distance between the posterior arch of C1 and the odontoid process is markedly narrowed (*double white arrows*). There is an osteophyte that arises from the posterior margin of the C3 vertebral body and extends into the vertebral canal (*black arrow*) at the C3-4 level. There is a small posterior osteophyte at the C4-5 level and anterior and posterior osteophytes at the C6-7 level. The C7 vertebral body is identified with 7.

Axial short TR image (Fig. E) reveals posterior displacement of the odontoid process (*o, with straight arrow*) relative to the anterior arch of the C1 vertebral body (*curved arrow*). The osteophyte projects behind the anterior arch of C1 and appears as a rounded area of increased signal intensity.

Axial computed tomographic (CT) scan at the level of C2 (Fig. F) reveals that the odontoid process is displaced posteriorly away from its normal anticipated position behind the anterior arch of C1 (*A*). The bony osteophyte seen in the sagittal reconstruction image projects behind the anterior arch of C1. The odontoid process is identified with O.

Axial long TR image at the level of the C3-4 intervertebral disc (Fig. G) reveals a large decreased signal intensity mass that projects posteriorly into the vertebral canal and markedly narrows the cervical vertebral canal. The spinal cord (*arrow*) is compressed into to a crescent shaped structure posteriorly in the vertebral canal.

Postmyelogram axial CT scan at the level of C3-4 (Fig. H) reveals a large osteophyte that markedly encroaches upon the vertebral canal (*solid arrow*). The spinal cord is compressed posteriorly into a crescent shape (*open arrow*).

Diagnosis

Rheumatoid arthritis with C1-2 dislocation; herniated disc at the C3-4 and C4-5 levels.

Differential Diagnosis

- rheumatoid arthritis

- pseudogout

Discussion

The patient had a known history of rheumatoid arthritis. The soft tissue mass posterior the anterior arch of C1 is pannus formation related to the rheumatoid arthritis. Laxity of the transverse and cruciate ligaments which normally hold the odontoid process in close proximity to the posterior arch of C1 is also associated with rheumatoid arthritis in this patient. The relative posterior displacement of the odontoid process and C2 vertebral body as compared to the relative anterior displacement of the C1 vertebral body and the skull base results in a severe stenosis of the vertebral canal. This narrowing is visible on the CT scan (Fig. D); however, the magnetic resonance imaging (MRI) scan better reveals that this stenosis is even more severe than appreciated by the CT scan because the additional soft tissues can be seen by MRI as compared to CT scanning (see Fig. C). In addition the patient also has a large herniated disc and accompanying osteophyte at the C3-4 level. The sagittal MRI scan also reveals a herniated disc at the C4-5 level (Fig. C). Note that the CT scan better demonstrates the bony abnormalities, while MRI is superior in identifying the soft tissue abnormalities and the relationship of the spinal cord to the surrounding bony and soft tissue abnormalities.

Calcium pyrophosphate deposition disease (pseudogout) could have a similar appearance; however, patients with rheumatoid arthritis generally have a more typical clinical presentation with involvement of the joints of the extremities.

The patient did not develop quadriplegia with the marked compression of the spinal cord because the changes occurred over a prolonged period of time. When the compression happens very slowly, the spinal cord is allowed to atrophy without catastrophic clinical symptoms. On the other hand, rapid development of spinal compression would result in quadriplegia.

PEARLS

- MRI is the procedure of choice for the evaluation of rheumatoid arthritis.

- In addition to static images, images can also be obtained using short TR images in flexion and extension views to reveal the amount of motion at the C1-2 level and to determine the effect upon the cervical spinal cord.

PITFALLS

- These patients are a difficult management problem because of the multilevel abnormalities and because of the longstanding nature of the subluxation with compression atrophy of the cervical spinal cord.

- Care must be taken clinically when attempting to manipulate these patients because the patients themselves assume a position that is comfortable for them. Manipulation of the head and neck in a stressful way that is uncomfortable may have dire neurological consequences, including quadriplegia.

CERVICAL DISC DISEASE

Case 7

Clinical Presentation

The patient is a 54-year-old male with longstanding neck stiffness and recent acute neck pain.

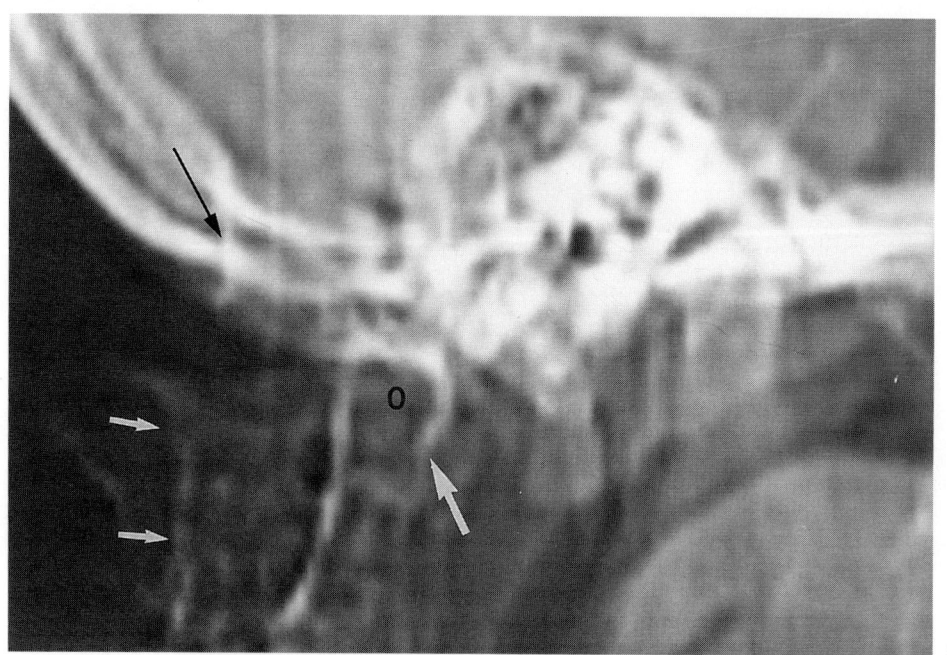

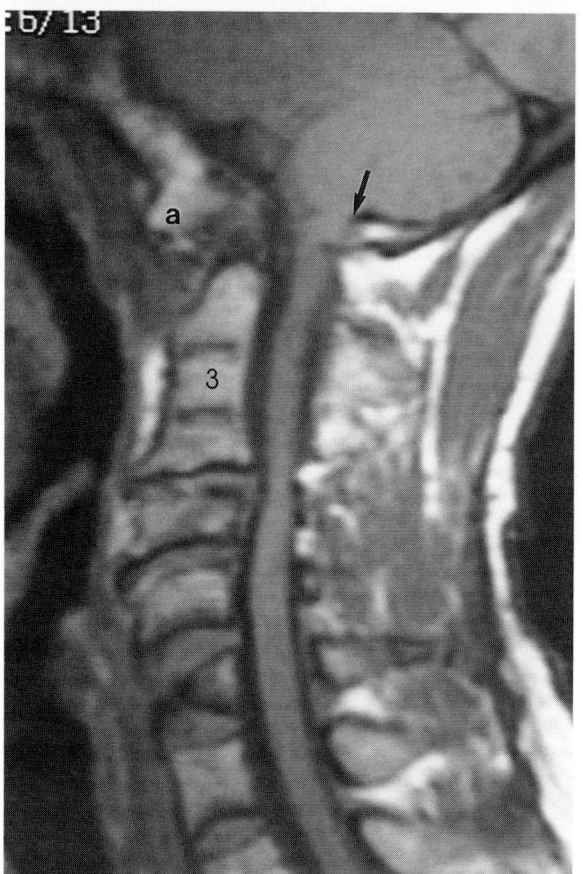

549

TEACHING ATLAS OF SPINE IMAGING

C

D

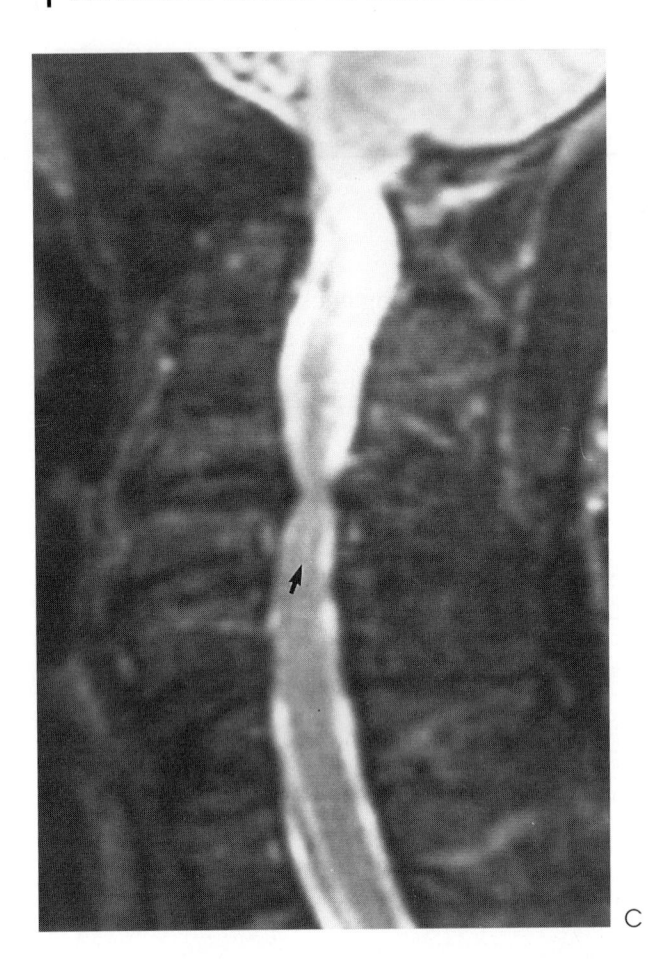

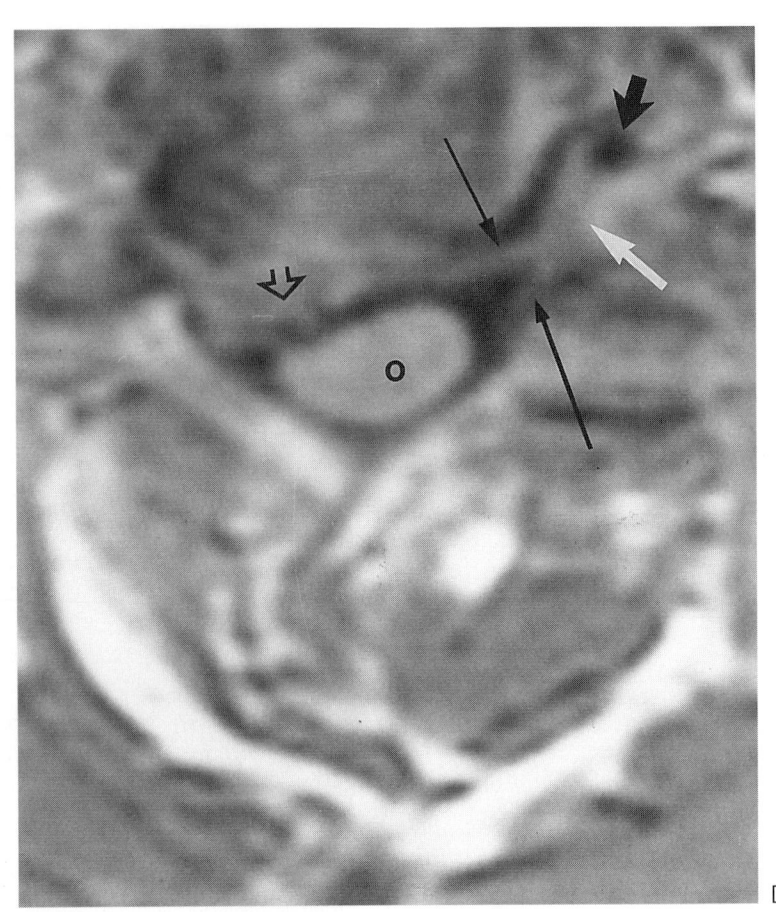

Radiologic Findings

Lateral view of the cervical spine from the digital image obtained at the time of computed tomographic (CT) scanning (Fig. A) reveals posterior and superior displacement of the odontoid process (*O*) relative to the anterior arch of C1. The large white arrow identifies the base of the odontoid process. Neither the anterior arch nor the posterior arch of C1 are well visualized. There is failure of segmentation (fusion) between the vertebral bodies and spinous processes of C2 through C4 (*small white arrows*). The black arrow identifies the posterior margin of the foramen magnum.

Sagittal short TR image of the cervical spine (Fig. B) reveals that the C1 vertebral body is not seen. The posterior arch of the C1 vertebral body is fused and incorporated into the occipital bone at the skull base. The anterior arch of the C1 vertebral body (*a*) is fused to the inferior aspect of the clivus. There is widening of the space between the odontoid process and the anterior arch of the C1 vertebral body. The odontoid process is displaced posterior and superior to its normal anticipated position. Anterior osteophytes are visible at the C4-5, C5-6, and C6-7 levels. There is loss of anterior vertebral body height at the C7 level. The C3 vertebral body is identified with 3.

Sagittal long TR image of the cervical spine (Fig. C) reveals a ventral indentation upon the subarachnoid space at the C4-5 level. The vertebral canal is narrowed to 5 mm at this level. There is a small "streak-like"

CERVICAL DISC DISEASE

Radiologic Findings (continued)

area of increased signal intensity within the cervical spinal cord at the C5 level (*arrow*).

Axial short TR image at the C4-5 level (Fig. D) reveals an intermediate area of soft tissue prominence at the C4-5 level which is largest the right side and extends to the midline (*open arrow*). There is compromise of the subarachnoid space and compression of the cervical spinal cord (*o*) on the right side. The afferent (*long thin black arrow*) and efferent (*short thin black arrow*) nerve roots of the cervical spinal cord are well demonstrated. The nerve root ganglion is also seen at the level of the intervertebral foramen lateral to the afferent and efferent nerve roots (*white arrow*). The flow void of the vertebral artery is seen in the foramen transversaria (*short solid black arrow*). The afferent nerve is carrying impulses toward the spinal cord while the efferent nerve is carrying nerve impulses away from the spinal cord.

PEARL
- The vertebral body and spinous process fusion is generally well demonstrated by plain film evaluation. In this case, the fusion between the vertebral bodies is well demonstrated on the MR images.

PITFALL
- These patients may be difficult to manage because of the multiple congenital anomalies.

Diagnosis

Atlantoaxial fusion; Klippel-Feil anomaly; right-sided herniated disc at the C4-5 level.

Differential Diagnosis

- atlantoaxial fusion
- Klippel-Feil anomaly

Discussion

The C1 vertebral body is completely fused to the skull base. This anomaly is called atlantoaxial fusion, and it is a congenital anomaly. In addition, there is laxity of the transverse and cruciate ligaments that fix the odontoid process to the anterior arch of C1. This allows the odontoid process to migrate superiorly and posteriorly. This migration results in marked compromise of the foramen magnum and compression of the cervical spinal cord at the level of the foramen magnum.

The Klippel-Feil anomaly is also a congenital deformity with fusion of multiple cervical vertebral bodies. This fusion of the vertebral bodies causes limitation of motion of the cervical spine in the upper cervical region. This limitation translates the stress to the adjacent intervertebral disc, in this case C4-5, which is just below (or above in some cases) the fused vertebral body segments, resulting in a herniated disc at the C4-5 level. This translation of stress can also be seen in patients who have had surgical fusion between the vertebral bodies; herniated discs may be seen above and/or below the level of the fusion.

Fusion of the vertebral bodies following a surgical procedure would result in the obliteration of the intervertebral disc spaces.

TEACHING ATLAS OF SPINE IMAGING

> **PITFALL**
> - The full extent of the abnormality may not be demonstrated by MRI.

decreases the ability of MRI to demonstrate this abnormality. However, the diagnosis may be suspected because of secondary changes, such as interruption of the subarachnoid space and spinal cord compression. The axial images are also helpful for demonstration of changes in the posterior longitudinal ligament.

The appearance is very typical of the diagnosis. The cause of the increased signal intensity within the spinal cord seen on the sagittal short TR image in Figure A is uncertain. It could be related to hemorrhage, or more, likely to increased protein content within the spinal cord.

CERVICAL DISC DISEASE

Case 9

Clinical Presentation

The patient is a 68-year-old female with neck pain and limitation of motion.

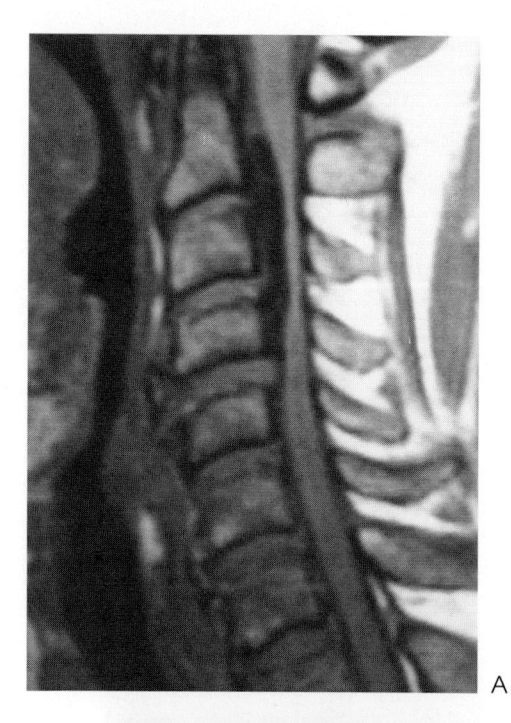

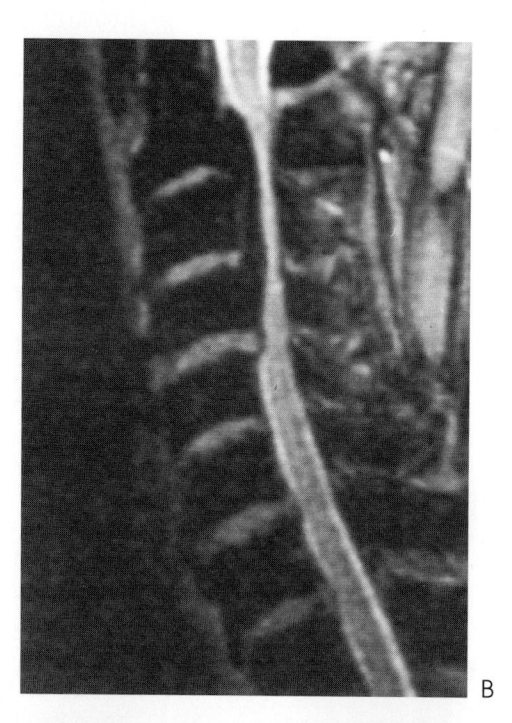

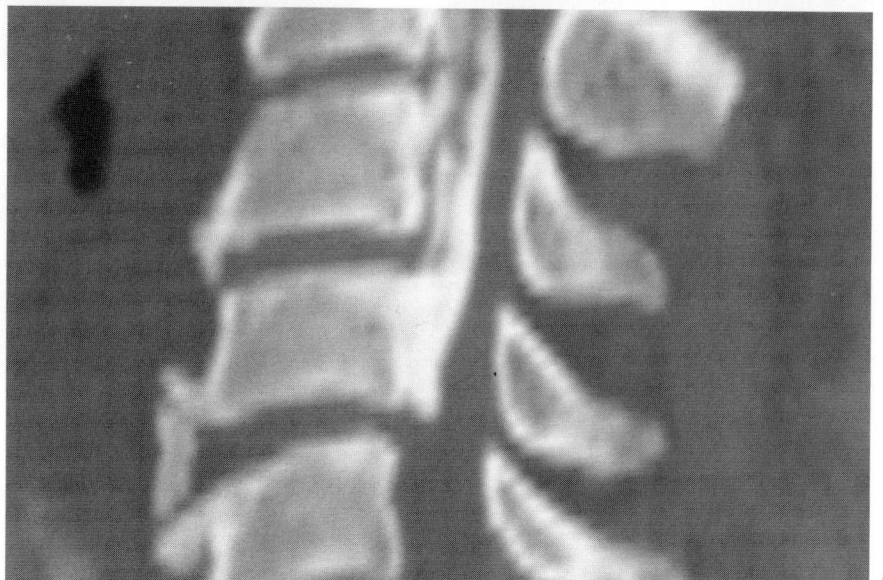

TEACHING ATLAS OF SPINE IMAGING

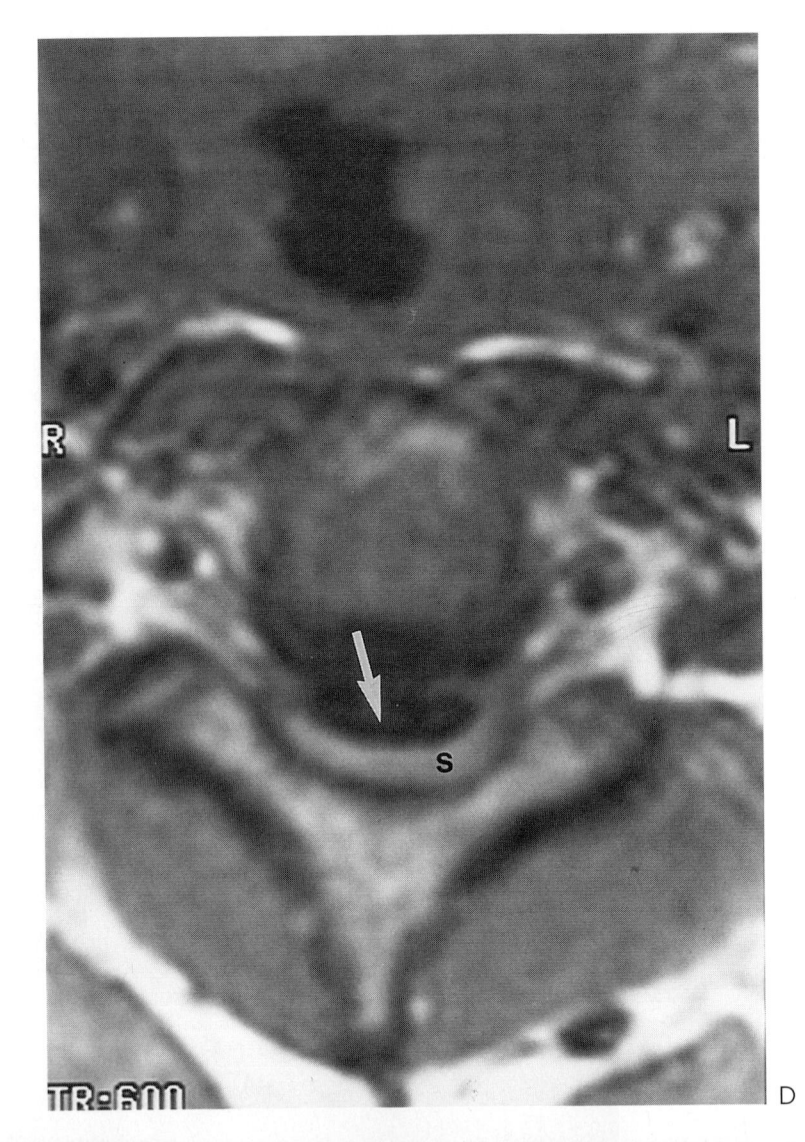

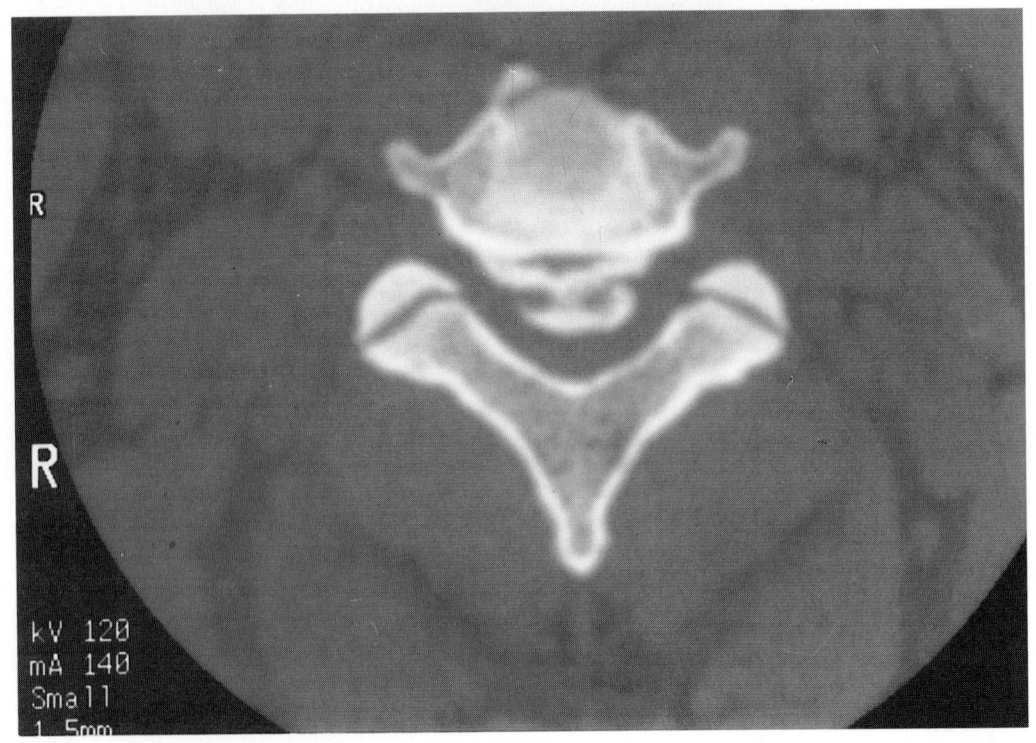

CERVICAL DISC DISEASE

Radiologic Findings

Sagittal short TR image of the cervical spine (Fig. A) reveals a dense ridgelike area of marked decreased signal intensity behind the cervical vertebral bodies of C2 through C4. The spinal cord is displaced markedly posteriorly and compressed at the C2 through C4 levels. There are anterior osteophytes at C4-5, C5-6, C6-7, and C7-T1. There is loss of the normal cervical lordotic curve.

Sagittal long TR image (Fig. B) reveals that the area of decreased signal intensity seen in Figure A remains decreased signal intensity on the long TR image. The spinal cord is compressed to a "ribbonlike" structure. There is mild bulging of the intervertebral disc at the C4-5 level.

Sagittal reconstruction image of a computed tomographic (CT) scan (Fig. C) reveals the dense linear, laminated appearing area of calcification/ossification posterior to the vertebral bodies of C2 through C4. There are large bridging osteophytes anteriorly at the C4-5 level. The cervical vertebral canal is narrowed to 4 mm in the anteroposterior dimension.

Axial gradient echo image at the C3 level (Fig. D) reveals a pancake-shaped area of decreased signal intensity projecting posterior to the vertebral body (*arrow*). The spinal cord (*S*) is markedly flattened into a curvilinear configuration posteriorly in the vertebral canal.

Axial CT scan at the same level as Figure D (Fig. E) reveals the laminated-appearing areas of calcification/ossification projecting posterior to the vertebral bodies. The vertebral canal is markedly compromised.

Diagnosis

Posterior longitudinal ligament calcification/ossification.

Differential Diagnosis

- posterior longitudinal ligament ossification

Discussion

Posterior longitudinal ligament ossification is nicely demonstrated by the CT scan in this patient. The laminated nature of this type of calcification is well demonstrated by the CT scan. The overhanging edges of the ossified areas are also well demonstrated in this case. These appear as areas of intermediate signal intensity by short TR magnetic resonance imaging (MRI) or linear areas of increased signal intensity by long TR MR images. CT scanning is unable to directly demonstrate the appearance of the cervical spinal cord. MRI has the advantage of being able to directly visualize the spinal cord and its relationship to the surrounding vertebral canal. MRI thus allows for direct noninvasive visualization of the anatomic position of the spinal cord.

PEARL
- The marked compression of the spinal cord is sufficiently severe that any areas of increased signal intensity present in the spinal cord may not be visualized.

PITFALL
- Both CT and MRI may be necessary for complete evaluation. In this patient, there is excellent correlation between the CT scan and the MR scan; however, posterior longitudinal ligament calcification is often not well demonstrated by MRI and is generally better demonstrated by CT scanning. MRI, on the other hand, demonstrates the exact relationship between the spinal cord and the surrounding bony structures; this relationship is not demonstrated by CT scanning.

Radiologic Findings

Sagittal short TR images (Fig. A) in the cervical region reveal that bony fusion plugs have been placed at the level of the intervertebral discs at the C4-5 and C5-6 levels (*arrows*). At the C5-6 level, there is a cleft of decreased signal intensity that probably represents an area of gas accumulation. The bony plugs extend slightly posterior to the posterior margins of the vertebral bodies. There is slight straightening of the cervical spine and loss of the normal cervical lordosis. The C3 vertebral body is identified with 3.

Sagittal postcontrast infusion short TR image (Fig. B) reveals enhancement of the bony fusion plugs at both the C4-5 and the C5-6 levels (*arrows*). The C5 vertebral body is identified with 5.

Diagnosis

Recent surgery for disc removal at the C4-5 and C5-6 levels with bony fusion plugs in place.

Differential Diagnosis

- bony fusion plugs

Discussion

The magnetic resonance imaging (MRI) study reveals that there is no migration of the bony fusion plugs, which enhance on the postinfusion study. Ideally, the plugs should not extend posterior to the posterior margin of the vertebral body. MRI provides the ideal method for follow-up of these patients. Surgical complications include anterior slippage or migration of the bony fragments out of the intervertebral disc space. Posterior migration into the vertebral canal may also occur but is less common. Posterior migration of the bony plug would jeopardize the cervical spinal cord. Note the mild prevertebral soft tissue swelling because of the recent surgery.

PEARL
- MRI is the ideal method of evaluation of the postoperative patient.

PITFALL
- If injury to the spinal cord occurred at the time of surgery, the area of increased signal intensity may be seen in the cervical spinal cord on long TR images. Therefore, long TR images should be obtained in these patients for complete evaluation.

CERVICAL DISC DISEASE

Case 11

Case Presentation

The patient is a 56-year-old male with increasing weakness in the upper extremities bilaterally, and numbness in the upper and lower extremities bilaterally. Weakness on the left is greater than on the right.

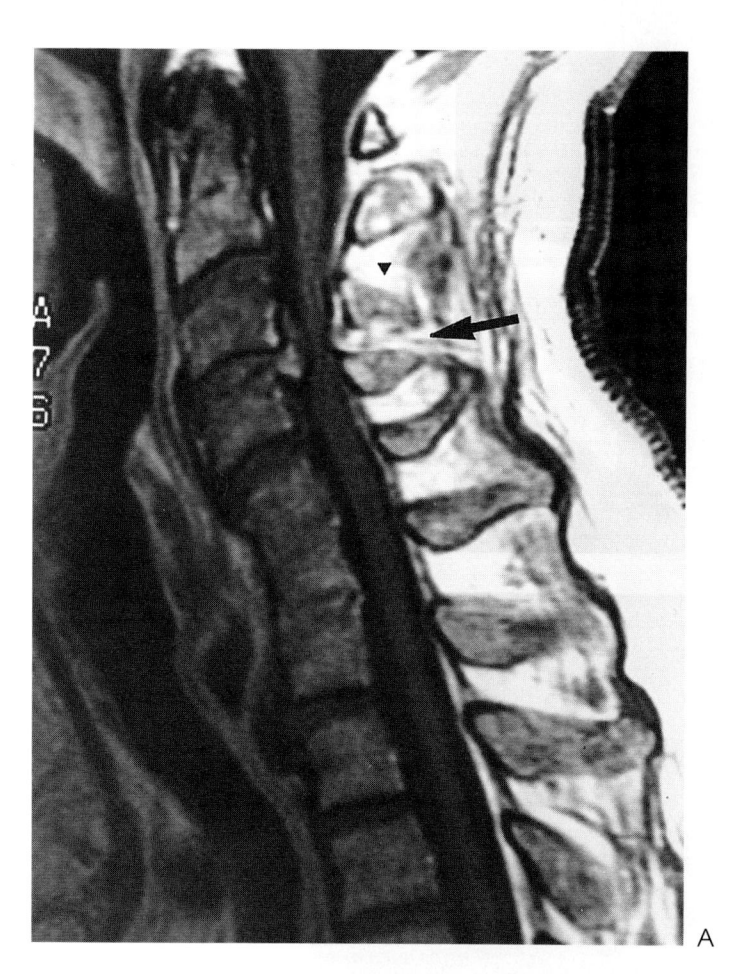

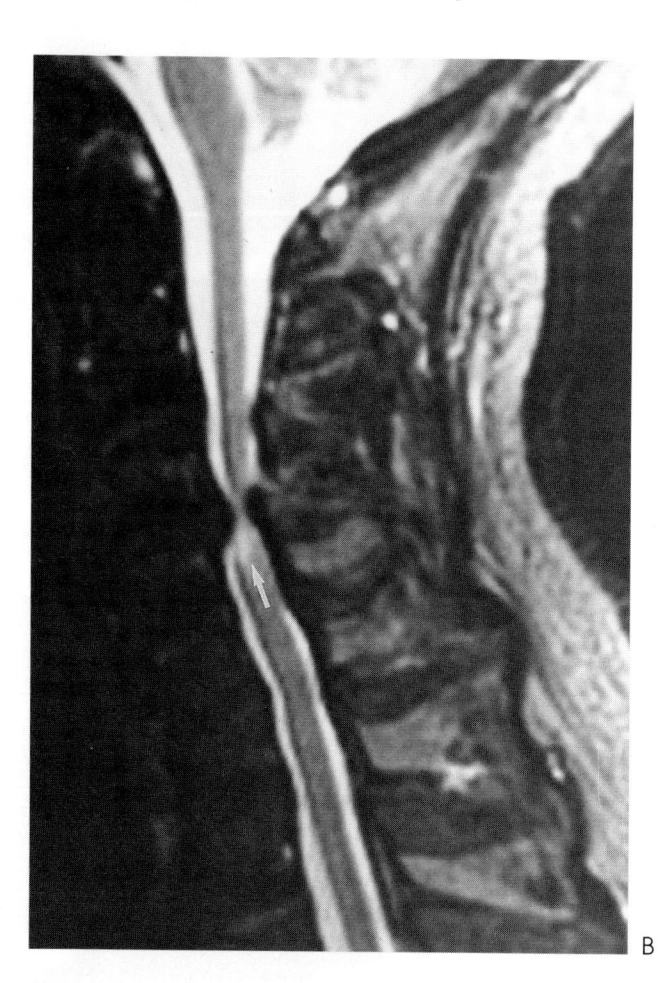

Radiologic Findings

Sagittal short TR image (Fig. A) reveals a large herniated disc at the C3-4 level. There is marked extension into the cervical vertebral canal, obliteration of the subarachnoid space anterior to the spinal cord, and compression of the cervical spinal cord. There is straightening of the cervical spine. Incidentally noted are postoperative changes with fusion between the C5, C6, and C7 vertebral bodies. There is focal reversal of the curve of the cervical spine at this level and narrowing of the interspinous distance at the C3-4 level (*black arrow*) and widening of the interspinous distance at the C2-3 level (*arrowhead*).

TEACHING ATLAS OF SPINE IMAGING

Diagnosis

Large, midline herniated disc at the C3-4 level; postoperative changes with fusion at the C5-6 and C6-7 levels.

Differential Diagnosis

- herniated disc

Discussion

Following fusion of the cervical spinal vertebral bodies, herniation of a cervical disc just above or just below the level of the fusion frequently occurs. This appears to be because the stress is translated to the levels above or below the fusion. In this patient, there is a very old fusion between the C5-6 and C6-7 vertebral bodies. Marked cord compression is visible at the C3-4 level secondary to the herniated soft disc. There is also prominence of the posterior elements, which cause dorsal encroachment upon the cervical subarachnoid space as seen in Figure B. The resulting myelomalacia appears as an area of increased signal intensity. The cause of the increased signal intensity could be secondary to direct trauma and resulting edema, myelomalacia, or even a small syrinx cavity. The decreased signal intensity areas identified in Figure E suggest that these are small syrinx cavities.

The changes seen in this patient are those that may typically occur in a patient with a previous spinal surgery. Herniated discs occur above and below the fusion levels because stress is translated to these levels when there is fusion between the vertebral bodies.

PEARLS

- Note the widening of the interspinous distance between C6 and C7 spinous processes. This is because of the reversal of the curve of the normal cervical lordosis.

- MRI is the procedure of choice for the evaluation of the presence of myelomalacia and syrinx cavity formation.

PITFALL

- It is not possible to differentiate with absolute certainty between myelomalacia and a syrinx cavity.

CERVICAL DISC DISEASE

Case 12

Clinical Presentation

The patient is a 42-year-old male with a clinical history of previous spine surgery with anterior cervical discectomy and fusion, now with recurrent pain in the left shoulder and arm.

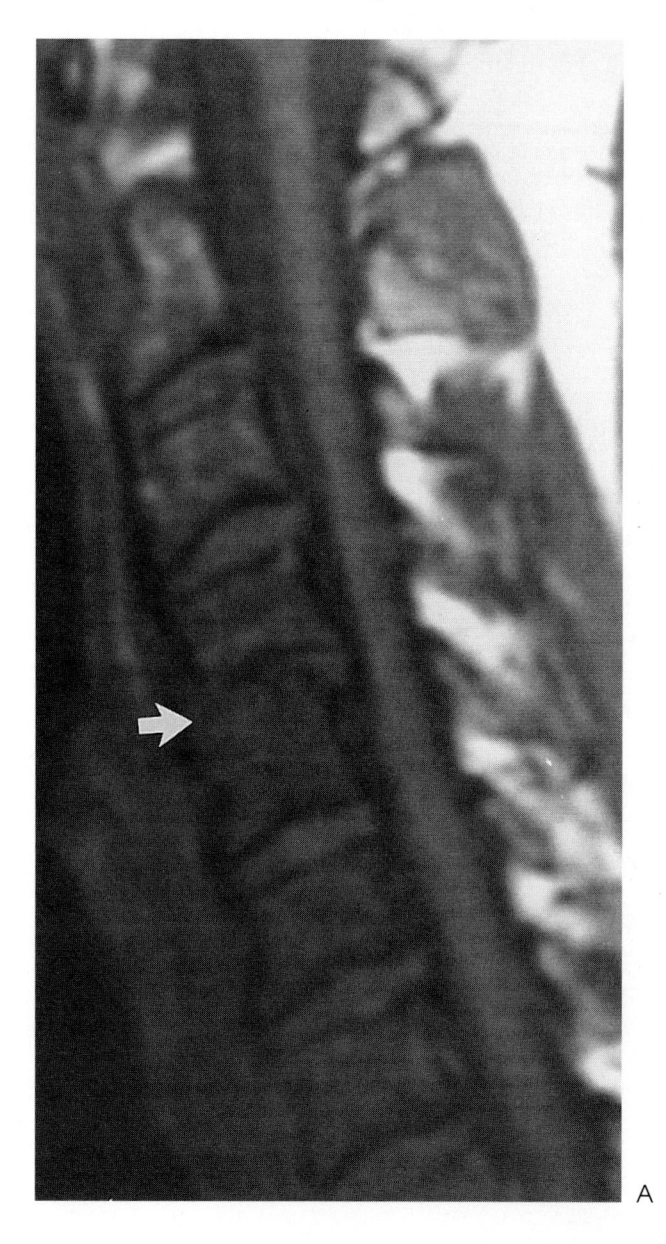

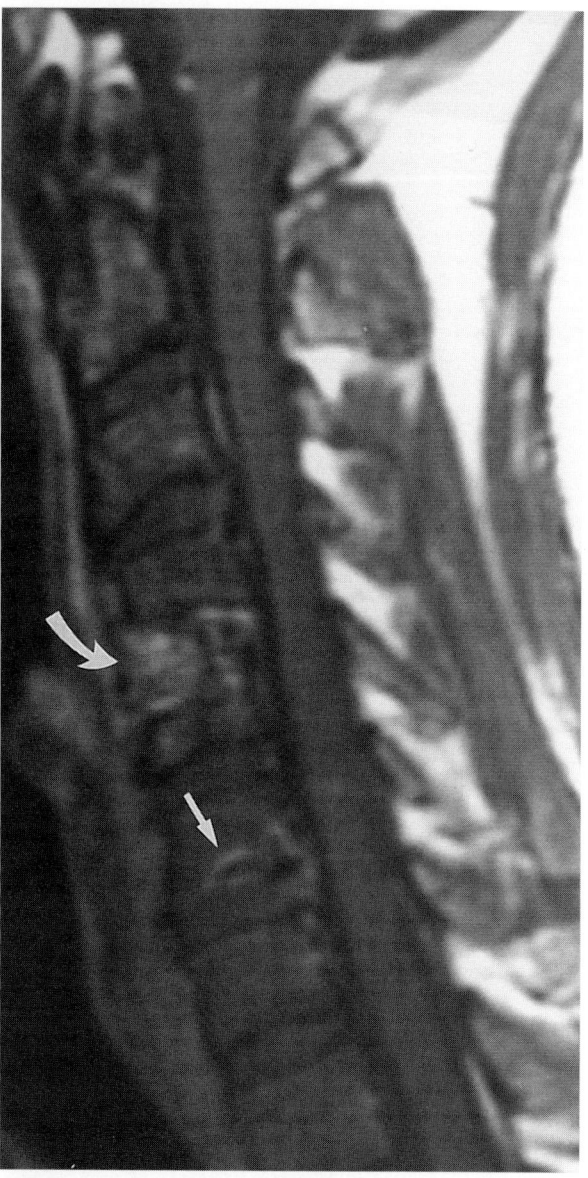

TEACHING ATLAS OF SPINE IMAGING

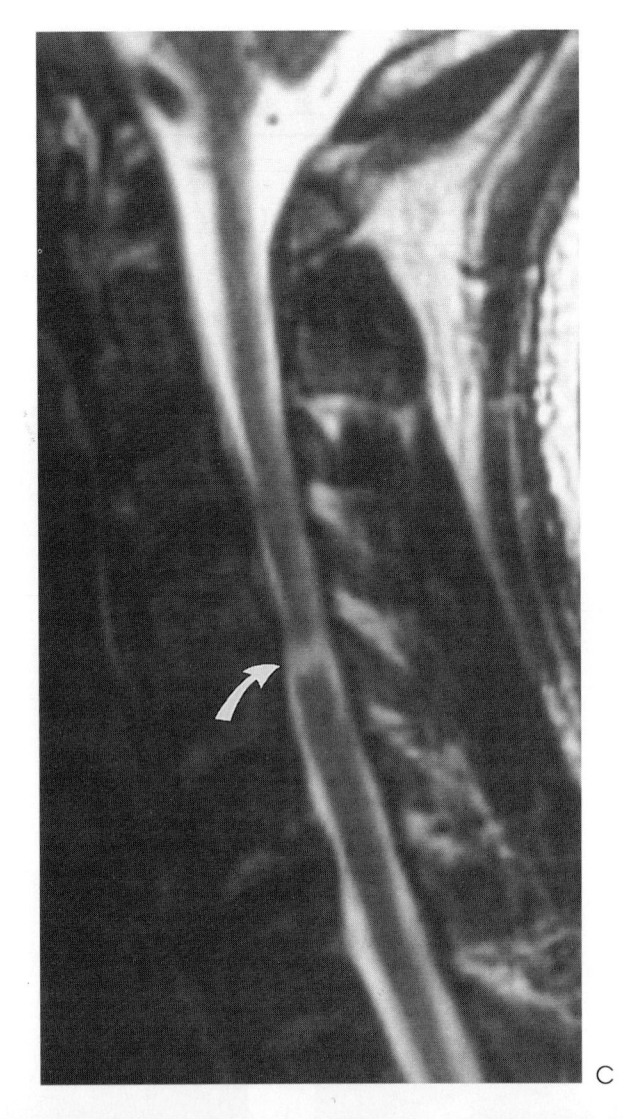

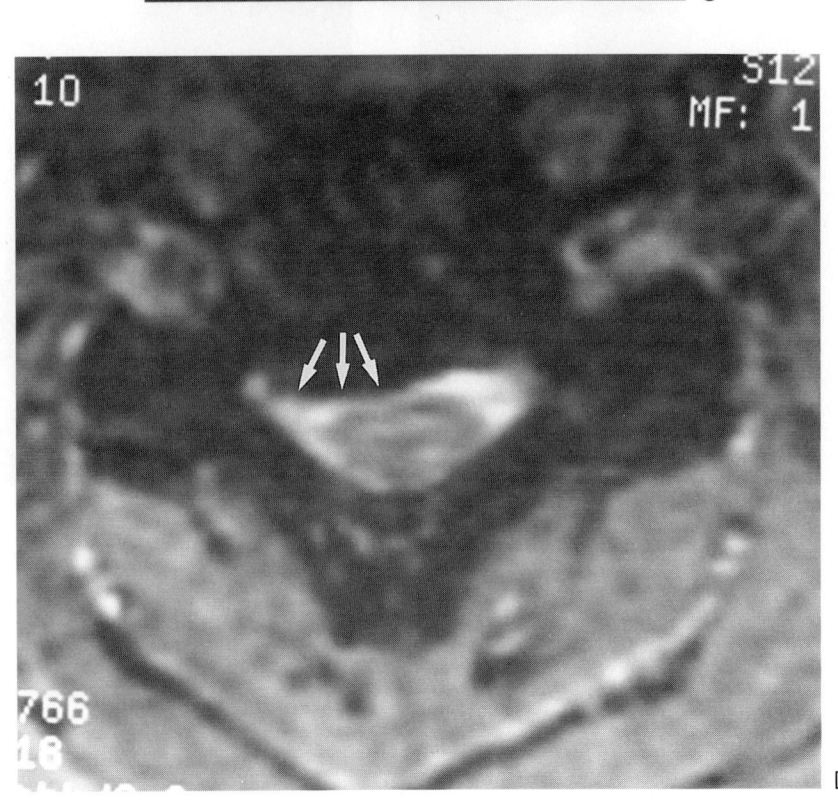

CERVICAL DISC DISEASE

Radiologic Findings

Sagittal short TR image of the cervical spine (Fig. A) reveals straightening of the spine. Postsurgical change with obliteration of the intervertebral discs space is visible at the C4-5 level (*arrow*). There is slight retrolisthesis of C4 on C5 and prominence of the intervertebral disc at the C4-5 level.

Sagittal short TR image postcontrast (Fig. B) reveals enhancement of the inferior end plate of the C 6 vertebral body (*straight arrow*). The bony fusion plug between the C4 and C5 vertebral bodies is enhanced (*curved arrow*). There is also compromise of the subarachnoid space behind the vertebral bodies of C4 and C5, and curvilinear compression of the spinal cord from C3 through C5.

Sagittal long TR image (Fig. C) reveals a rounded area of increased signal intensity within the cervical spinal cord at the C4-5 level (*arrow*).

Axial gradient echo image (Fig. D) reveals a barlike area of decreased signal intensity at the C4-5 level in the midline and extending to the right side (*arrows*). There is compromise of the increased signal intensity cerebrospinal fluid at this level.

Diagnosis

Postoperative changes with fusion at C4-5; bony osteophyte at the C4-5 level with compromise of the subarachnoid space; area of myelomalacia at the C4-5 level.

Differential Diagnosis

- postoperative changes secondary to fusion
- bony osteophyte
- myelomalacia

Discussion

The postoperative changes are secondary to a fusion between the C4 and C5 vertebral bodies. A bony osteophyte remains at the C4-5 level, and there is an area of myelomalacia (cord softening) at the C4-5 level secondary to repeated trauma of the herniated disc. Degenerative changes are visible at the C6-7 level. The area of myelomalacia occurred either because of direct trauma from the herniated disc, which was present before surgery, or because of direct injury to the spinal cord at the time of surgery. The anterior spinal artery is located along the midline in the anterior aspect of the spinal cord and is therefore at risk from a herniated disc or surgery. Note that at the C4-5 level the cervical spinal cord is compressed slightly on the right side and displaced slightly toward the left side of the vertebral canal. There is also a mildly bulging disc at the C6-7 level in this patient.

PEARLS

- It is not uncommon for degenerative changes to occur at a level above or below the level of a previous cervical spine fusion. This occurs because the fusion at one level causes the stress to be translated to a different level.

- These bony fusion plugs often reveal enhancement postinfusion, although the exact reason for this is unclear. An inflammatory process is a consideration; however, there is no associated soft tissue swelling, and the patient did not have a febrile clinical course.

PITFALL

- Multilevel spinal fusion causes marked limitation in a patient, and the patient is at a markedly increased risk in the event of an automobile accident or any other cause of a "whiplash" type of injury.

TEACHING ATLAS OF SPINE IMAGING

Case 13

Clinical Presentation

The patient is a 44-year-old male who originally presented with a history of neck pain and a herniated disc, and was treated with discectomy and anterior cervical fusion. The patient presents for follow-up.

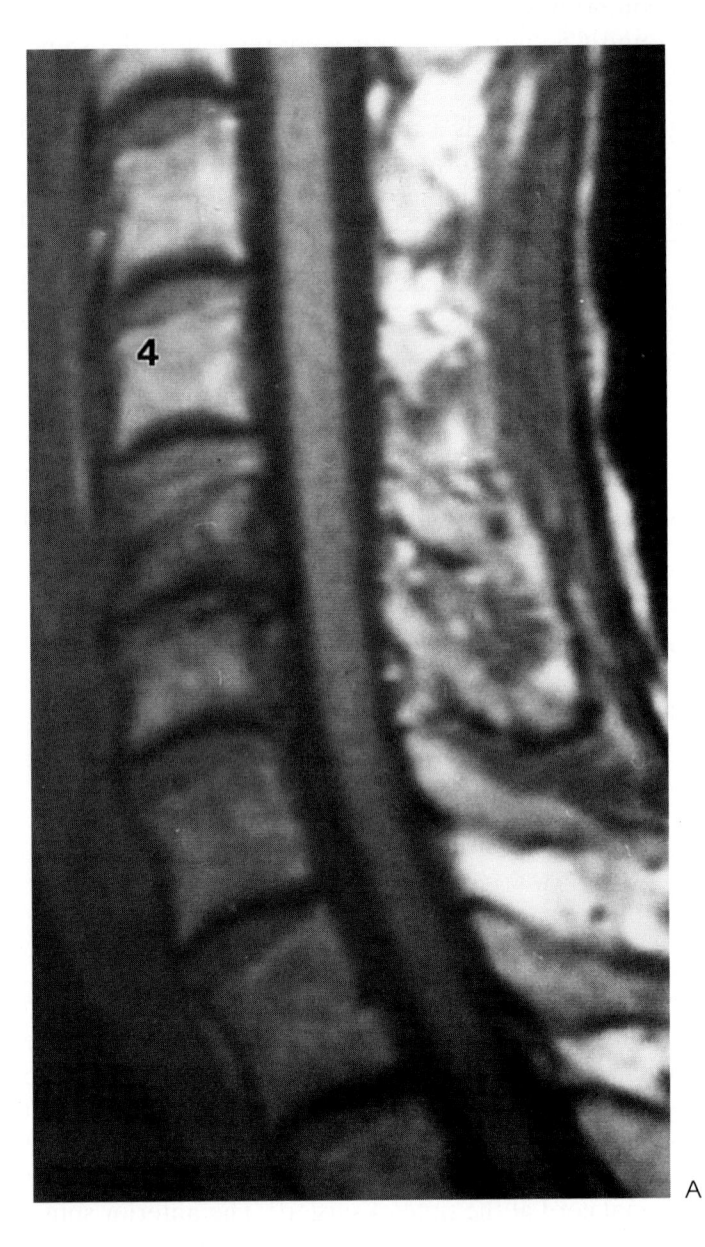

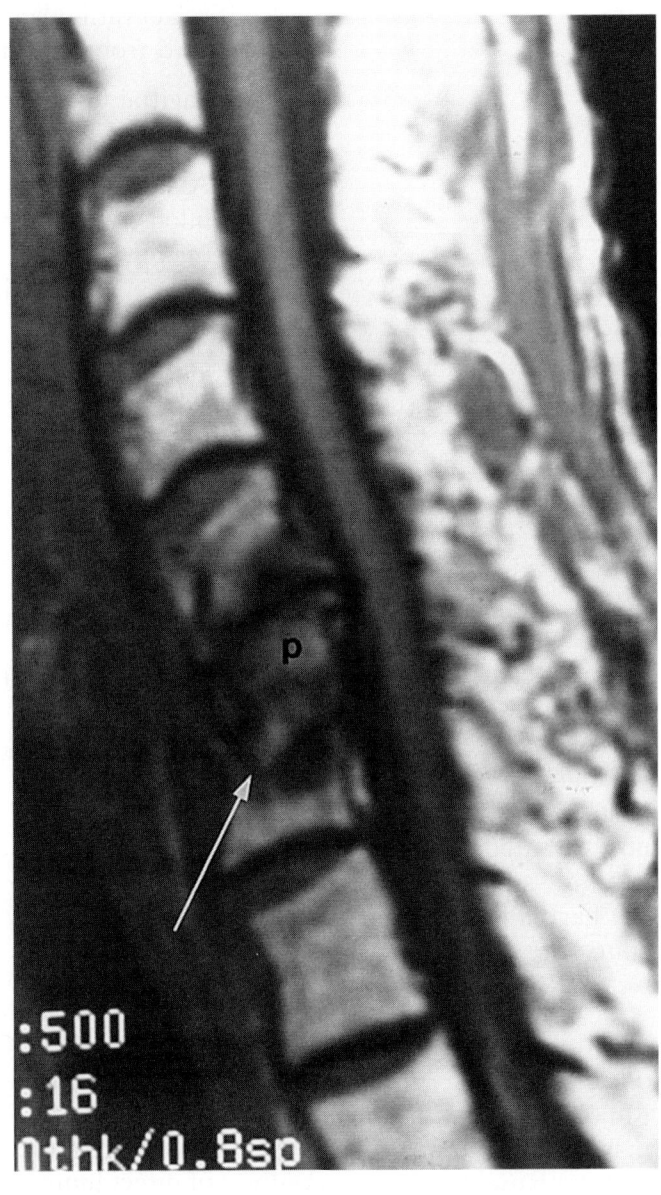

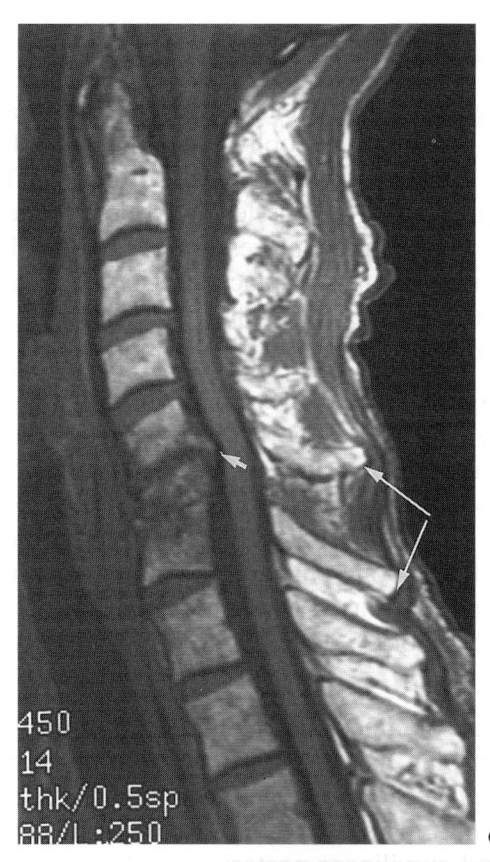

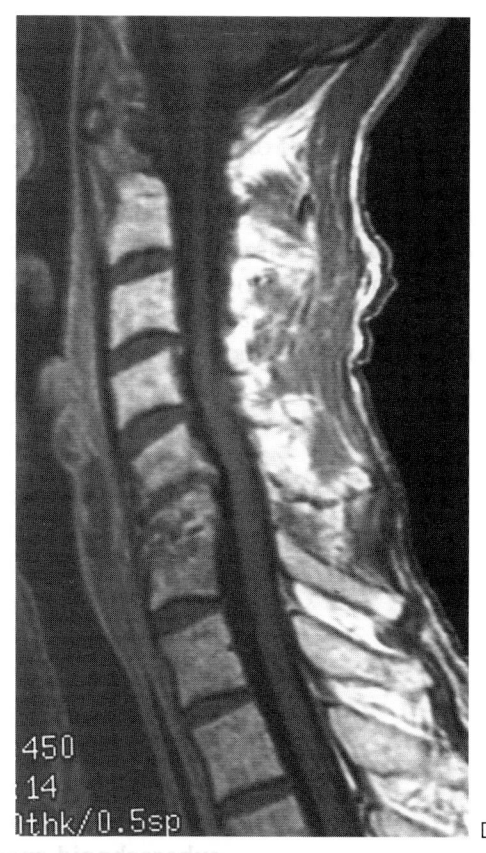

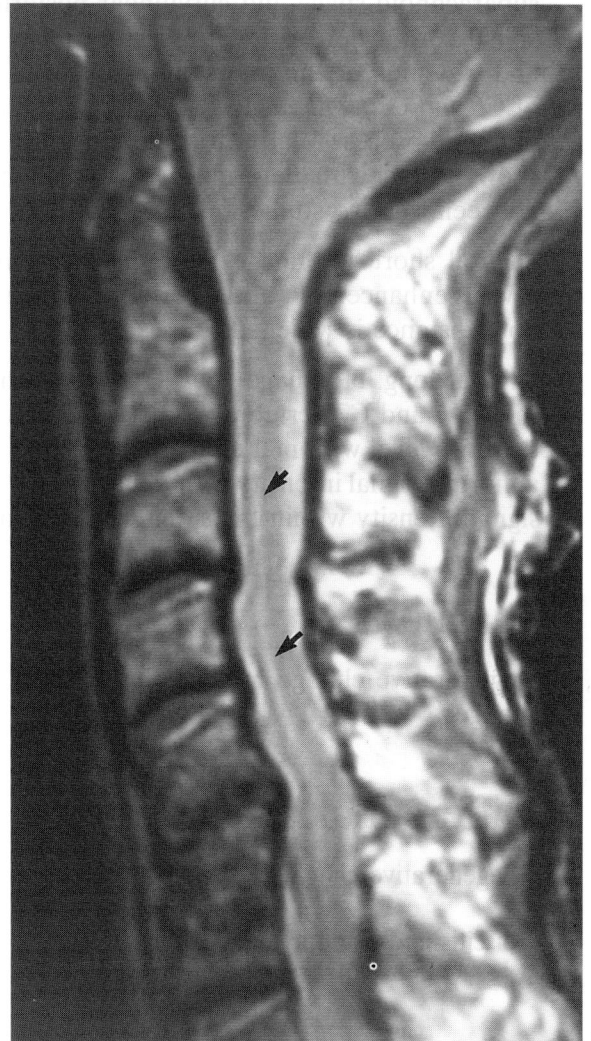

CERVICAL DISC DISEASE

TEACHING ATLAS OF SPINE IMAGING

Case 14

Clinical Presentation

The patient is a 55-year-old female with a history of tingling in the arms when she moves her head from side to side.

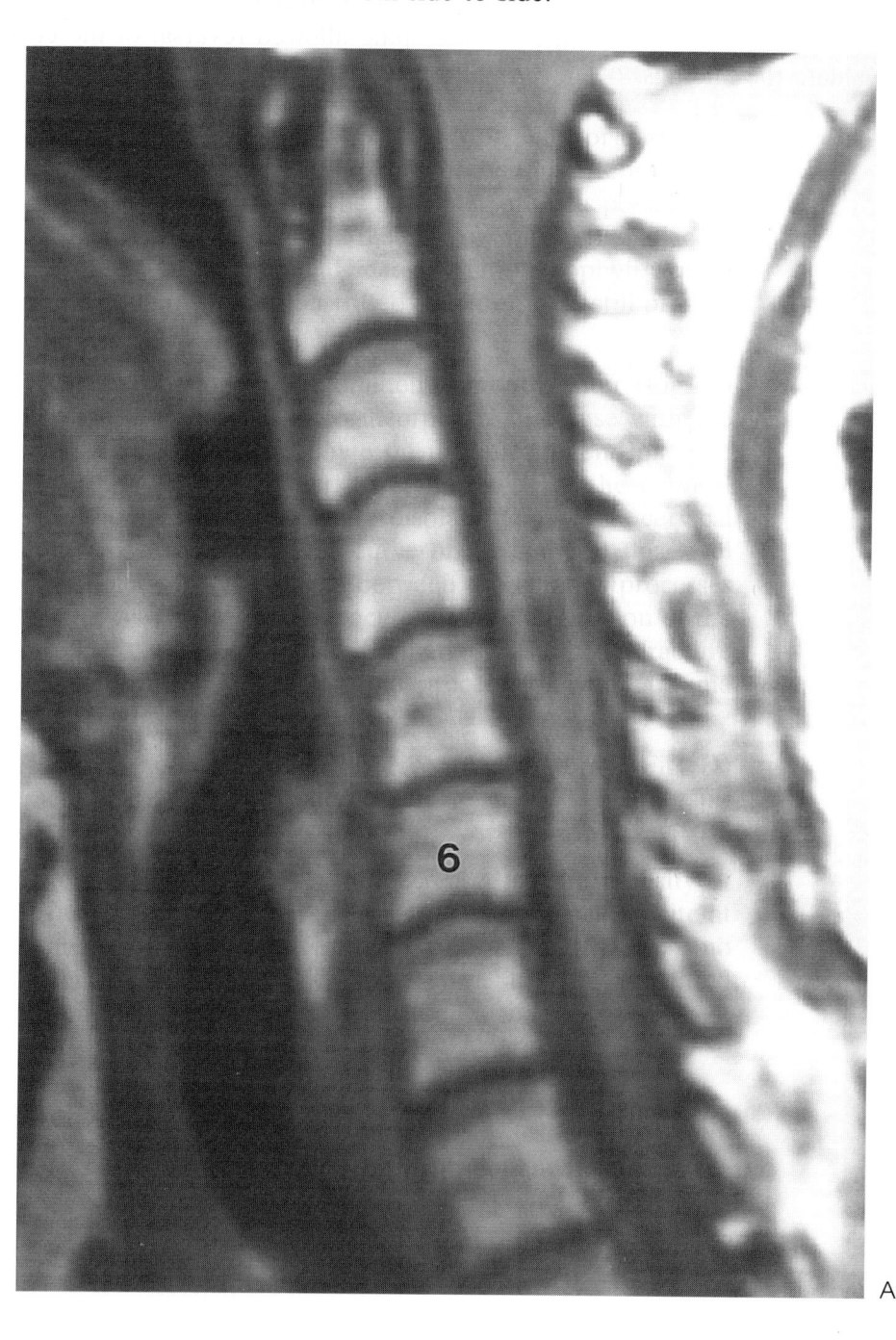

A

CERVICAL DISC DISEASE

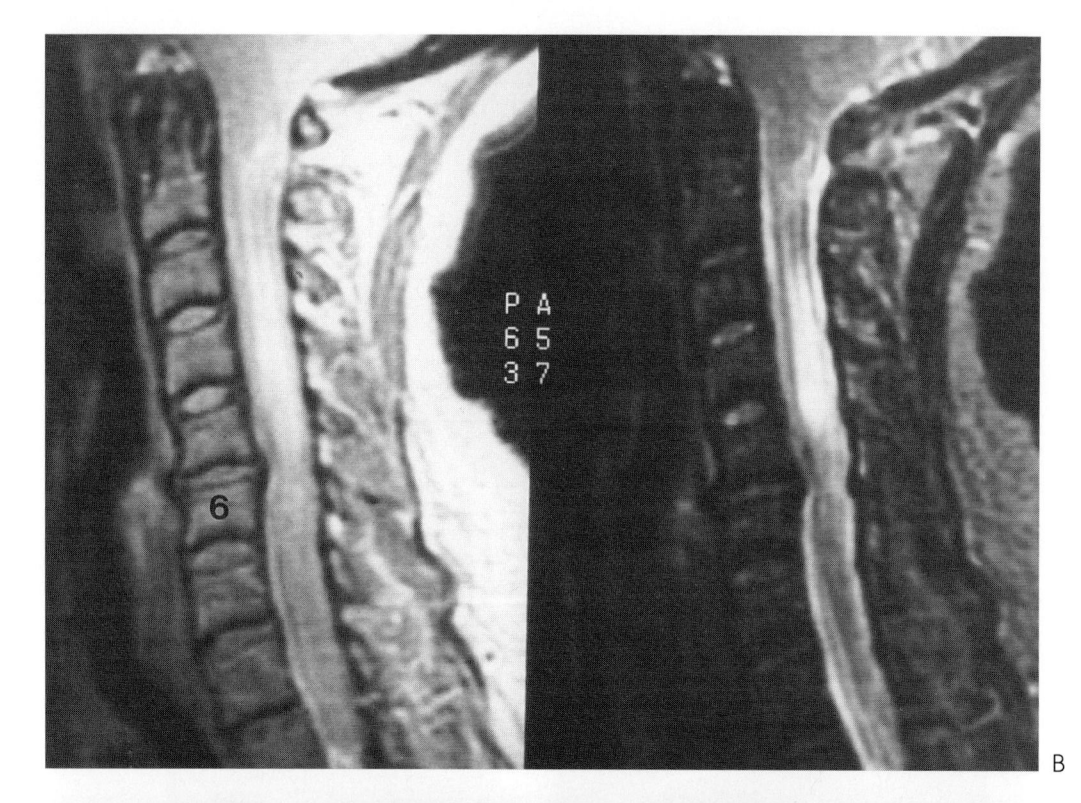

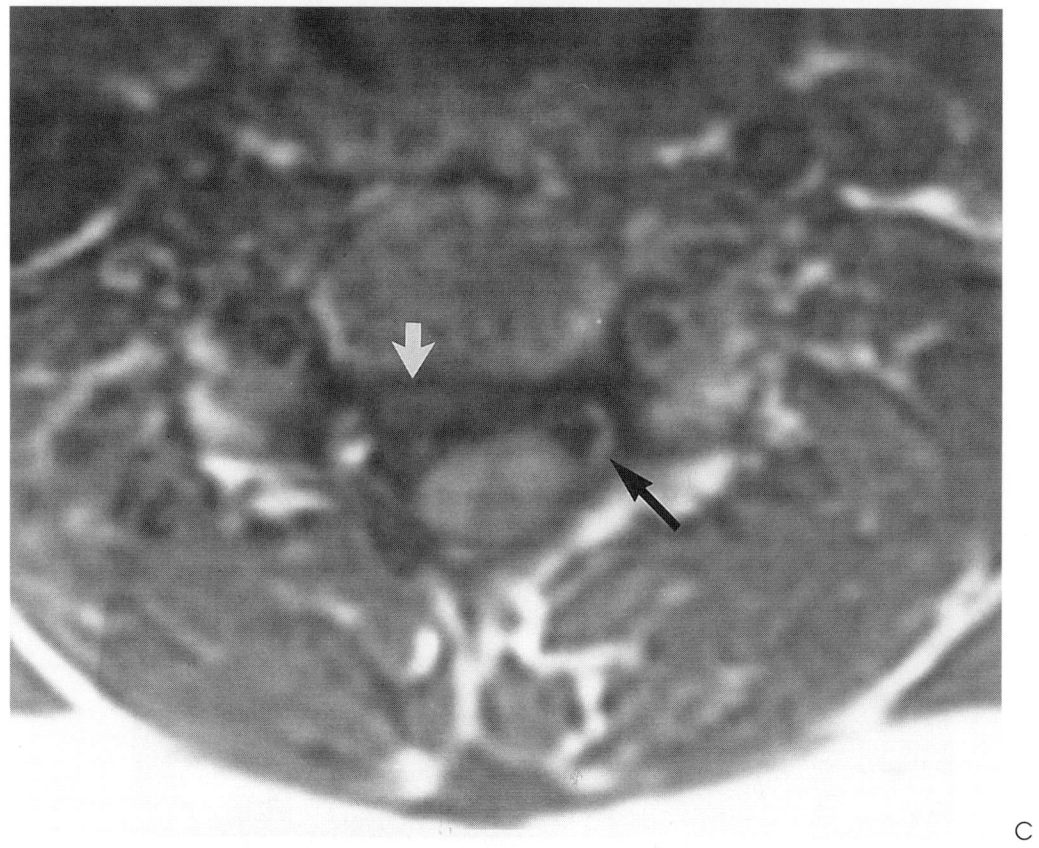

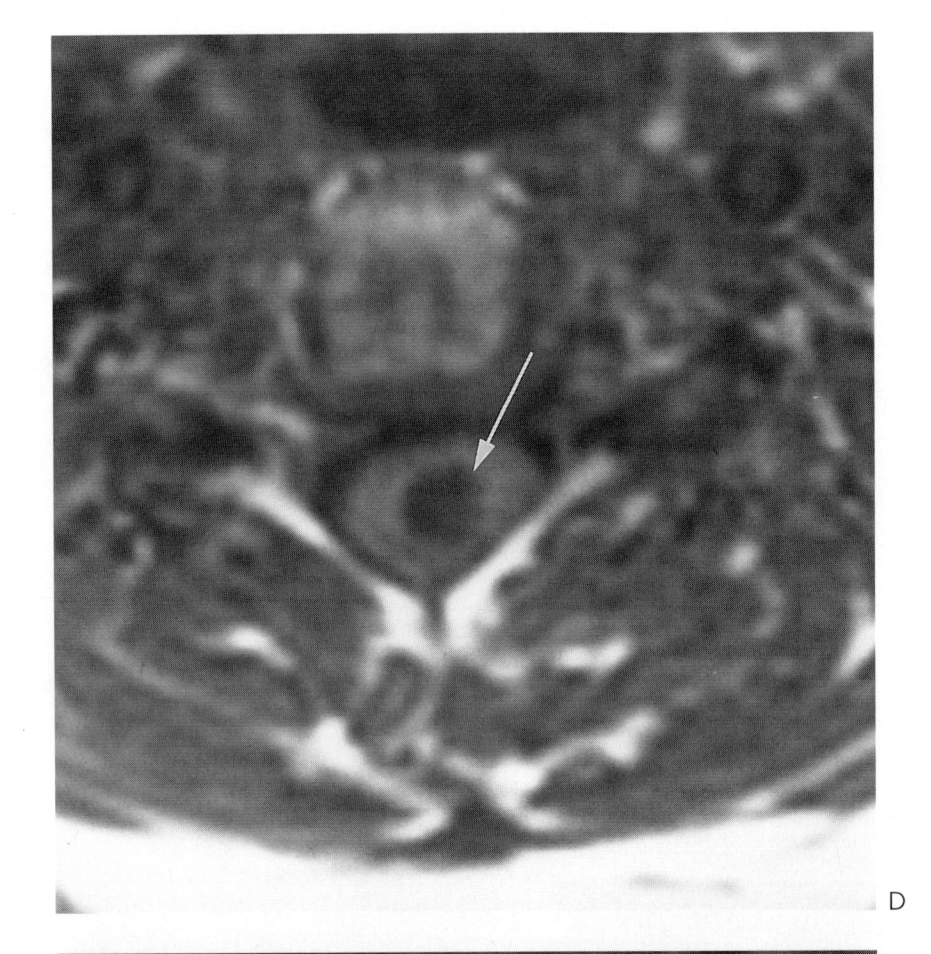

TEACHING ATLAS OF SPINE IMAGING

D

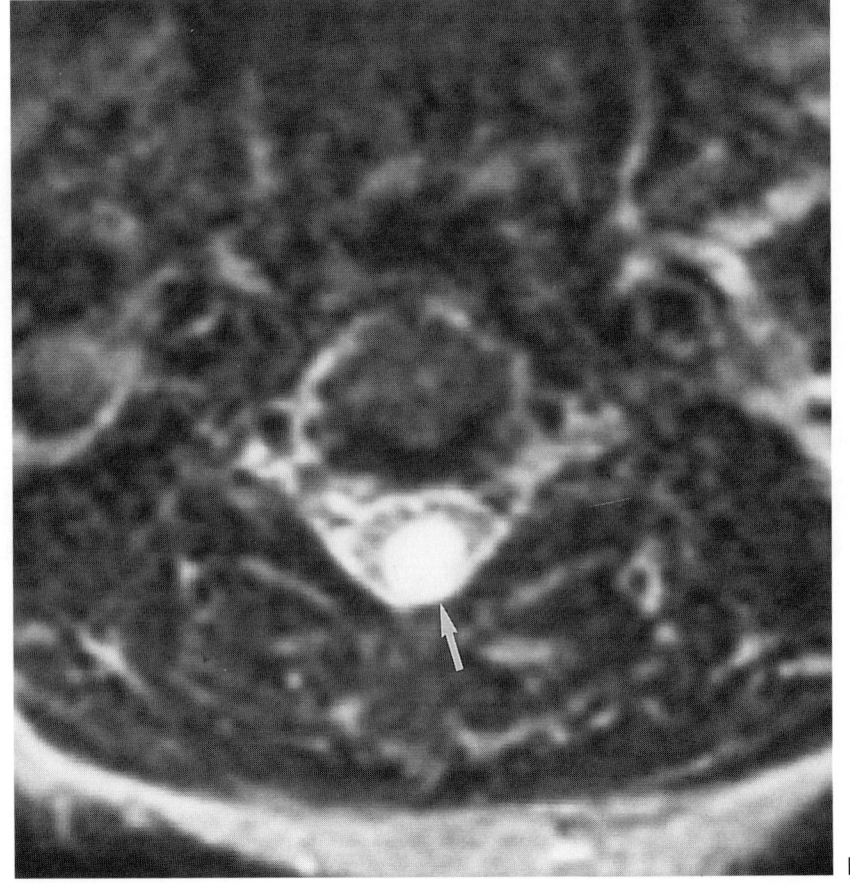

E

576

CERVICAL DISC DISEASE

Radiologic Findings

Sagittal short TR image (Fig. A) reveals a small oval area of decreased signal intensity in the central portion of the cervical spinal cord at the C4-5 level. There is reversal of the curve of the cervical spinal cord at the C5-6 level and slight compression of the cervical spinal cord at the C5-6 level secondary to a bulging herniated disc. The C6 vertebral body is identified with 6.

Sagittal intermediate (Fig. B, *left*) and long TR (Fig. B, *right*) images reveal a larger area of increased signal intensity in the cervical spinal cord, which extends from C3 through C5-6. The herniated cervical disc is now seen to better advantage. Anterior herniation of the disc can also be seen at the C5-6 level. The C6 vertebral body is identified with 6.

Axial short TR image (Fig. C) reveals a right-sided intermediate signal intensity soft tissue mass (*white arrow*). The spinal cord is rotated away from the herniated disc. The afferent nerve root is seen in the subarachnoid space (*black arrow*).

Axial short TR image (Fig. D) reveals the central location of the area of decreased signal intensity (*arrow*).

Axial gradient echo image (Fig. E) reveals an area of increased signal intensity in the central portion of the spinal cord (*arrow*).

Diagnosis

Right-sided herniated nucleus pulposus at C5-6 and resulting myelomalacia.

Differential Diagnosis

- herniated disc
- myelomalacia

Discussion

The midsagittal image in Figure A also reveals anterior prominence of the intervertebral disc at the C5-6 level. The axial image (Fig. C) better demonstrates the presence of the herniated disc on the right side with compression of the spinal cord. This probably is not as well demonstrated on the sagittal images because of the partial volume effect and the finite limitation of the thinness of the sagittal images, which obscures demonstration of the focal lateral herniated disc. The area of decreased signal intensity within the spinal cord seen on the short TR images is thought to represent an area of myelomalacia secondary to the herniated disc. The exact cause of this is uncertain but is thought to be secondary to direct trauma or vascular compromise. This could also represent a small syrinx cavity and differentiation between the two is not always possible. An area of myelomalacia not related to the herniated disc is also a consideration but appears less likely.

PEARL
- Follow-up examination may be helpful for more complete evaluation in this patient.

PITFALL
- An area of myelopathy (previously called myelitis) might have a similar appearance. MRI of the brain to evaluate for the presence of areas of increased signal intensity secondary to demyelination might also be helpful for more complete evaluation.

If a syrinx cavity associated with a spinal cord tumor is a consideration, a postinfusion study should be performed. Spinal cord tumors exhibit enhancement in the majority of cases; therefore, if enhancement is demonstrated, the possibility of a tumor would be a strong consideration.

In the correct clinical setting, an area of demyelination in association with acute disseminated encephalomyelitis might be a consideration, but seems unlikely in this patient.

CERVICAL DISC DISEASE

Case 15

Clinical Presentation

The patient is a 62-year-old male with a history of discectomy and fusion. The patient now presents with upper extremity weakness.

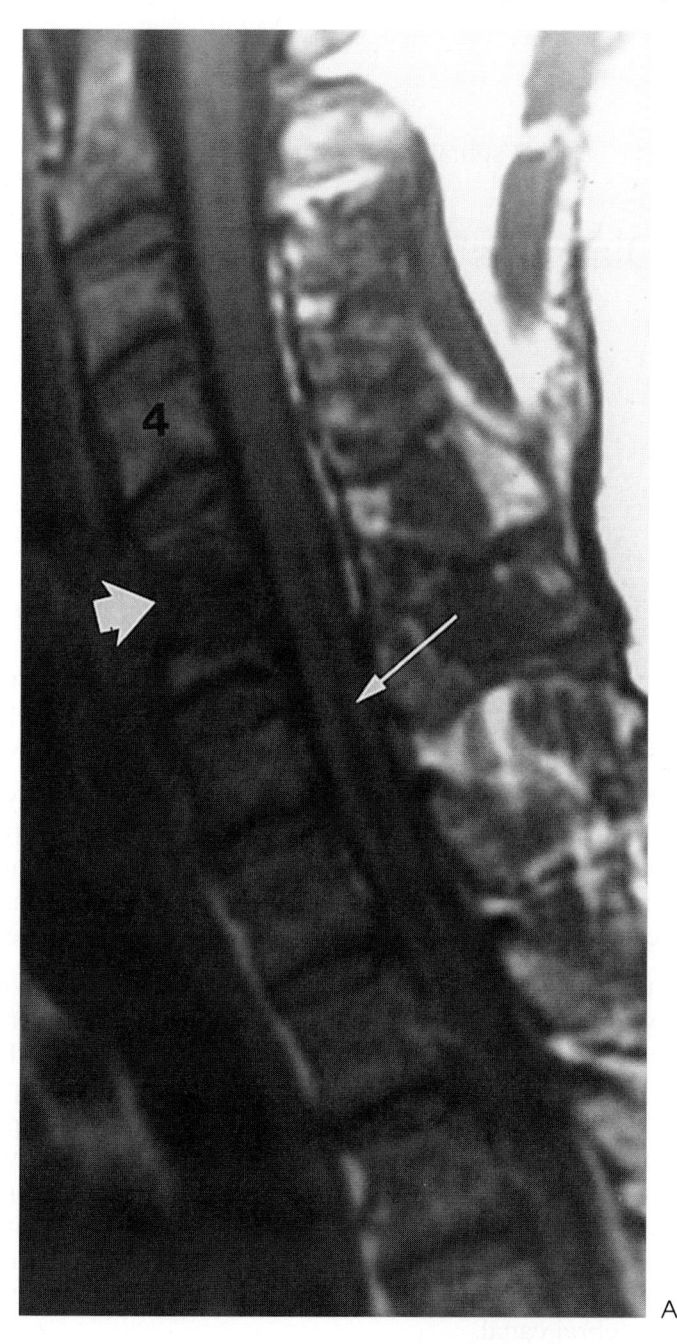

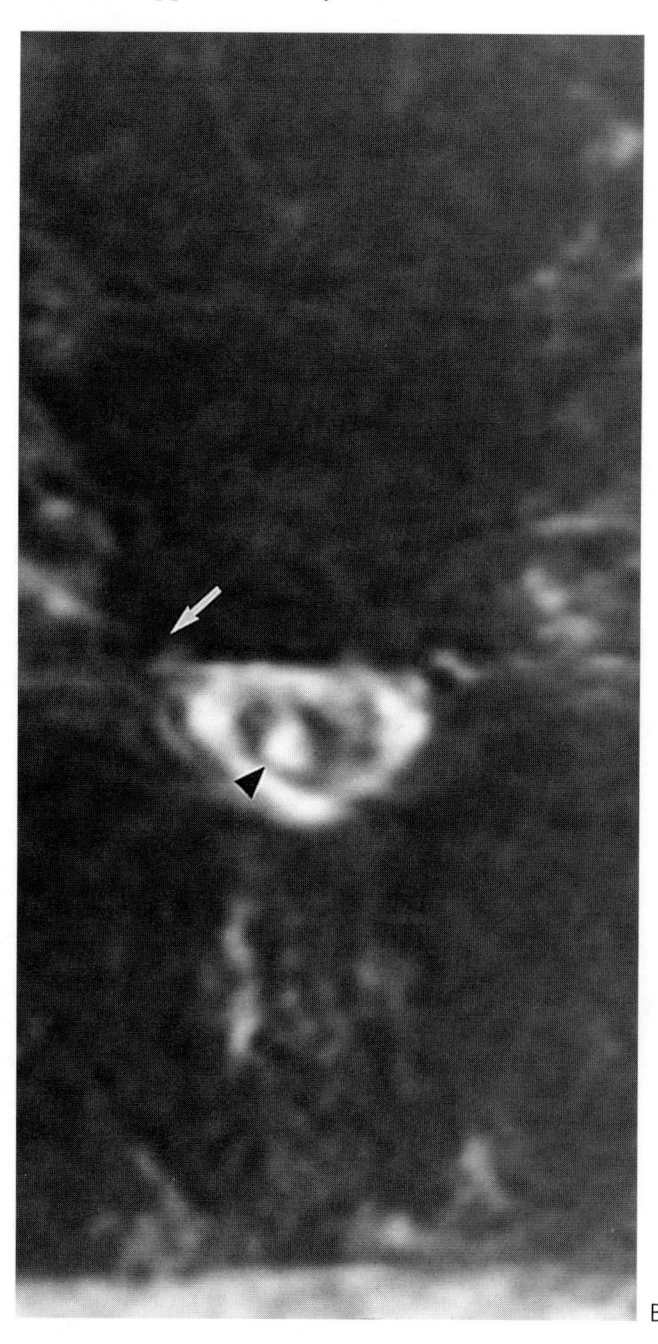

Radiologic Findings

Sagittal short TR image (Fig. A) reveals postoperative changes with a fusion between the D5 and C6 vertebral bodies (*wide arrow*). A long area of decreased signal intensity within the cervical spinal cord extends from the

TEACHING ATLAS OF SPINE IMAGING

Radiologic Findings (continued)

C5-6 level through the T1-2 level (*thin arrow at C7*). The C4 vertebral body is indicated by 4.

Axial gradient echo image at the C6 level (Fig. B) reveals a rounded area of increased signal intensity within the right side of the cervical spinal cord (*arrowhead*). There is also an increase in the amount of bone formation surrounding the vertebral body, resulting in encroachment on the intervertebral foramen on the right side (*arrow*).

Diagnosis

Postoperative changes; cervical spinal cord syrinx.

Differential Diagnosis

- syrinx cavity
- spondylosis
- spinal cord tumor

Discussion

The cause of the syrinx cavity is unclear. The syrinx cavity was not present preoperatively. One hypothesis is that trauma to the spinal cord by the herniated disc was present prior to the surgery for spinal fusion. A second is that direct trauma to the cervical spinal cord during surgery with resulting vascular compromise progressed to myelomalacia and then to a syrinx cavity.

The hypertrophic changes seen in Figure B are secondary to osteophytes surrounding the uncinate processes of the vertebral body. The hypertrophic changes result in encroachment upon the vertebral foramen and may cause radicular pain. The normal foramen is filled with increased signal intensity fat; in most cases, the individual afferent and efferent nerve roots can be seen.

A commonly used term for degenerative changes of the spine is cervical spondylosis. Spondylosis is an inclusive term that includes a number of changes that may be associated with degenerative changes in the spine. This term often includes a combination of disc space narrowing, hypertrophic bony osteophytes surrounding the uncinate processes, and hypertrophic osteophytes arising from the vertebral body end plates either anteriorly or posteriorly. The term tends to imply bony changes rather than herniation of the intervertebral discs. It should also be noted that individual degenerative changes or a combination of these changes will be more significant in a patient with a congenitally small vertebral canal than in a patient with a congenitally large vertebral canal.

Because computed tomography (CT) is more sensitive than magnetic resonance imaging (MRI) for evaluation of bone, CT is recommended for determination of the amount of bone encroachment by osteophyte formation prior to surgery. This best performed in conjunction with myelography so that contrast material outlines the subarachnoid space.

PEARLS
- Correlation should be performed with any preoperative MR scans if they are available as the syrinx cavity could have been present preoperatively.
- The remote possibility of a spinal cord tumor with a cystic component is a consideration, and a postcontrast study would reveal an area of enhancement in this clinical setting.

PITFALL
- If the patient did not have a preoperative MR scan, the syrinx cavity could have been present preoperatively and not appreciated.

CERVICAL DISC DISEASE

Case 16

Clinical Presentation

The patient is a 72-year-old male with limitation of motion of the cervical spine.

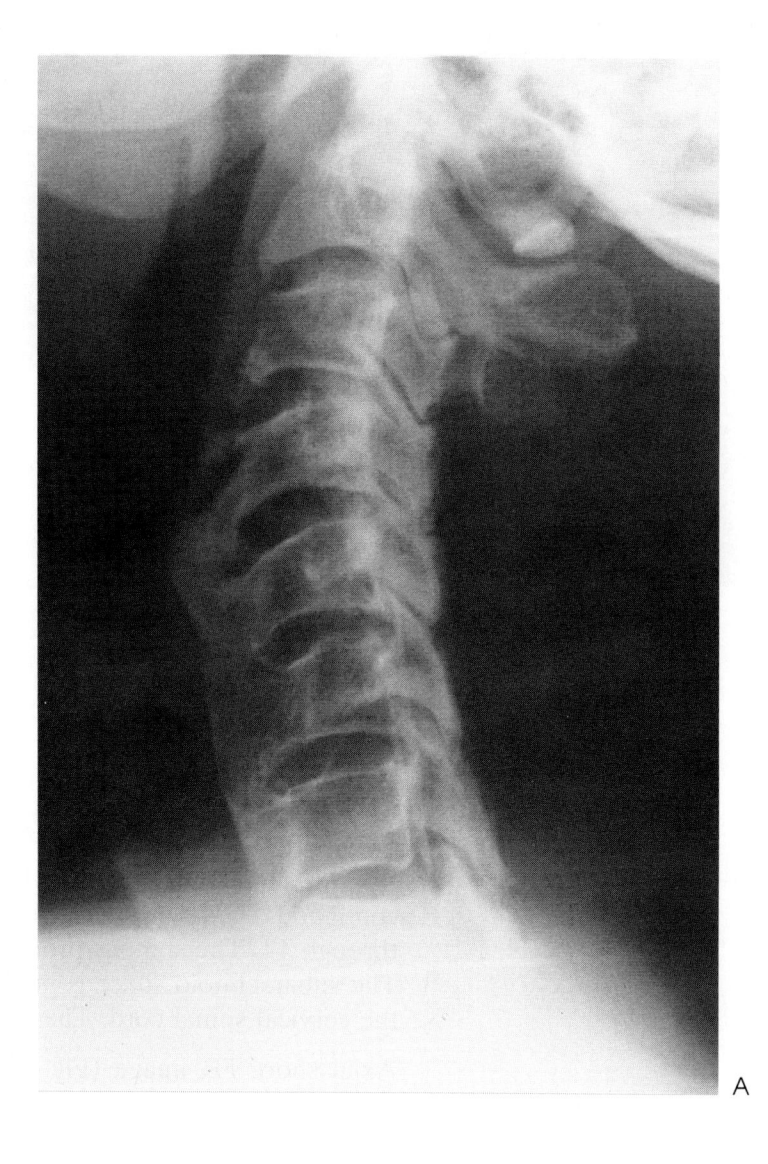

A

Radiologic Findings

Lateral view of the cervical spine (Fig. A) reveals large anterior osteophytes that extend from C 4 through T1. Vertebral body height and intervertebral disc space height are well preserved. There had been an extensive laminectomy, and the spinous processes are surgically absent from C4 through T1.

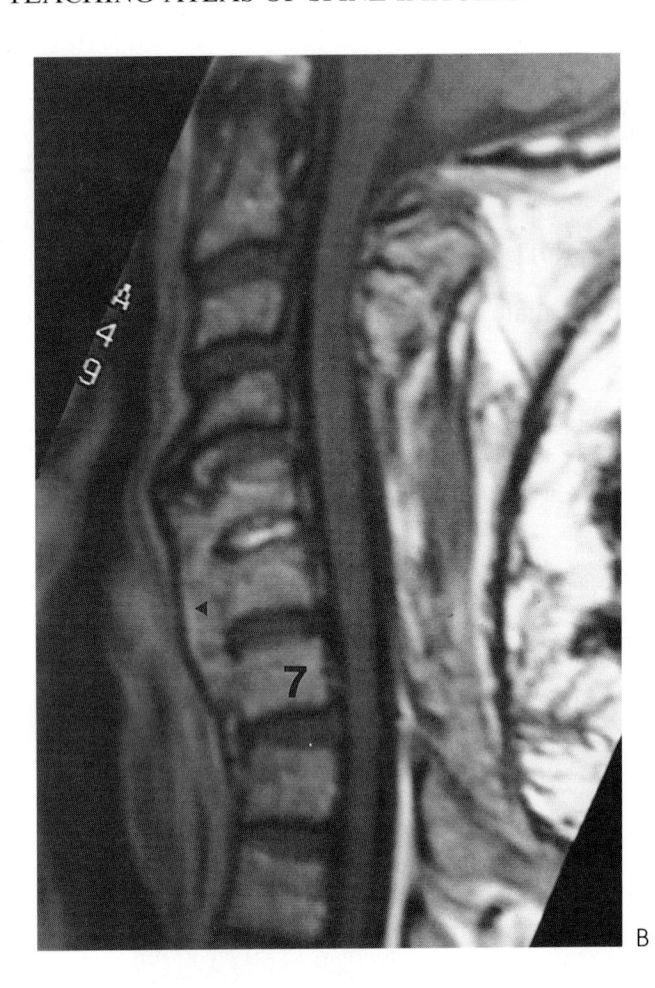

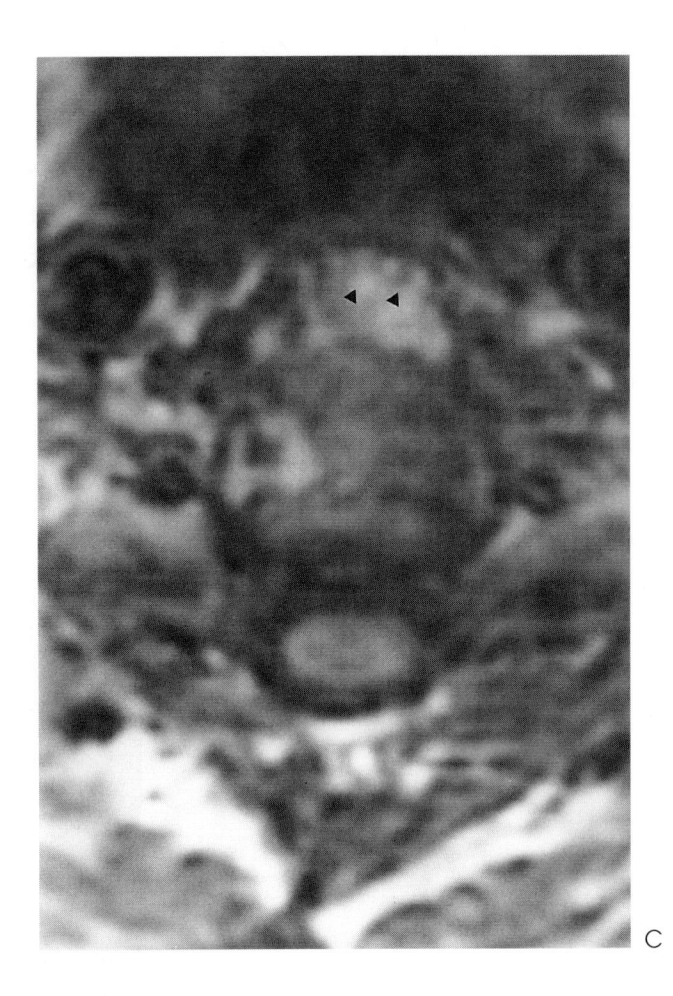

Radiologic Findings (continued)

Sagittal short TR image of the cervical spine (Fig. B) reveals the large, contiguous, anterior osteophytes (*arrowhead*), which extend from C4 through T1. The spinous processes of C4 through T1 are surgically absent. The subarachnoid space is preserved, and there is no encroachment upon the cervical spinal cord. The C7 vertebral body is identified with 7.

Axial short TR image (Fig. C) reveals the marrow filled, large anterior osteophyte (*arrowheads*) at the C6 level.

Diagnosis

Diffuse idiopathic skeletal hyperostosis (DISH).

Differential Diagnosis

- DISH
- degenerative osteophytes

CERVICAL DISC DISEASE

PEARL
- These changes may actually be related to degenerative changes although studies suggest that DISH may actually be a separate disease.

PITFALL
- Severe degenerative changes with osteophyte formation may have a similar appearance but do not meet these diagnostic criteria.

Discussion

The definition of DISH includes three specific criteria:

1. Calcification and ossification anteriorly and laterally extending over a minimum of four contiguous vertebral bodies with or without pointed excrescences at the intervening vertebral body-intervertebral disc junctions.

2. Preservation of intervertebral disc height and relative absence of degenerative disc disease.

3. Absence of apophyseal joint bony ankylosis and sacroiliac erosion, sclerosis or intra-articular osseous fusion.

These criteria have been chosen to eliminate other diagnostic considerations. Some believe that DISH may actually be extensive degenerative changes, and some patients with DISH may also have degenerative changes in the spine. DISH may also involve other bony structures, but the exact nature of these other changes has not yet been elucidated. In general, these patients are elderly and do not complain of pain in association with the abnormality.

Suggested Readings

Brown, BM, Schwartz RH, Frank E, Blank NK. Preoperative evaluation of cervical radiculopathy and myelopathy by surface-coil MR imaging. *AJNR*. 1988;9:859–866.

Czervionke LF, Daniels DL, Wehrli FW, et al. Magnetic susceptibility artifacts in gradient-recalled echo MR imaging. *AJNR*. 1988;9:1149–1155.

Enzmann DR, Rubin JB. Cervical spine: MR imaging with a partial flip angle, gradient-refocused pulse sequence. *Radiology*. 1988;166:467–472.

Enzmann DR, Rubin JB, Wright A. Cervical spine MR imaging: generating high-signal CSF in sagittal and axial images. *Radiology*. 1987;163:233–238.

Karasick MV, Schweitzer ME, Vaccaro AR. Complications of cervical spine fusion: imaging features. *AJR*. 1997;169:869.

Kulkarni MV, Narayana PA, McArdle CB, et al. Cervical spine MR imaging using multislice gradient echo imaging: comparison with cardiac gated spin echo. *Magn Reson Imaging*. 1988;6:517–525.

Luetkehans TJ, Coughlin BF, Weinstein MA. Ossification of the posterior longitudinal ligament diagnosed by MR. *AJNR*. 1987;8:924–925.

McAfee PC, Regan JJ, Bohlman HH. Cervical cord compression from ossification of the posterior longitudinal ligament in non-orientals. *J Bone Joint Surg (Br)*. 1987;69:569–575.

Modic MT, Masaryk TJ, Mulopulos GP, Bundschuh C, Hans JS, Bohlman H. Cervical radiculopathy: prospective evaluation with surface coil MR imaging, CT with metrizamide, and metrizamide myelography. *Radiology*. 1986;161:573–579.

Modic MT, Masaryk TJ, Ross JS, et al. Cervical radiculopathy: value of oblique MR imaging. *Radiology*. 1987;163:227–231.

Resnick D, Niwayama G. *Diagnosis of Bone and Joint Disorders*. 2nd ed. Philadelphia, Pa: W.B. Saunders Company; 1988.

Tsuruda JS, Norman D, Dillon W, et al. Three-dimensional graident-recalled MR imaging as a screening tool for the diagnosis of cervical radiculopathy. *AJNR*. 1989;10:1263–1271.

Tsuruda JS, Remley K. Effects of magnetic susceptibility artifacts and motion in evaluating the cervical neural foramina on 3DFT gradient-echo MR imaging. *AJNR*. 1991;12:237–241.

Widder DJ. MR imaging of ossification of the posterior longitudinal ligament. *AJR*. 1989;153:194–195.

Yamashita Y, Takahashi M, Matsuno Y, et al. Spinal cord compression due to ossification of ligaments: MR imaging. *Radiology*. 1990;175:843–848.

Yousem DM, Atlas SW, Goldberg HI, et al. Degenerative narrowing of the cervical spine neural foramina: evaluation with high-resolution 3DFT gradient-echo MR imaging. *AJNR*. 1991;12:229–236.

Section IX

Thoracic Spine

THORACIC SPINE

Case 1

Clinical Presentation

The patient is a 54-year-old male with severe midthoracic spine pain.

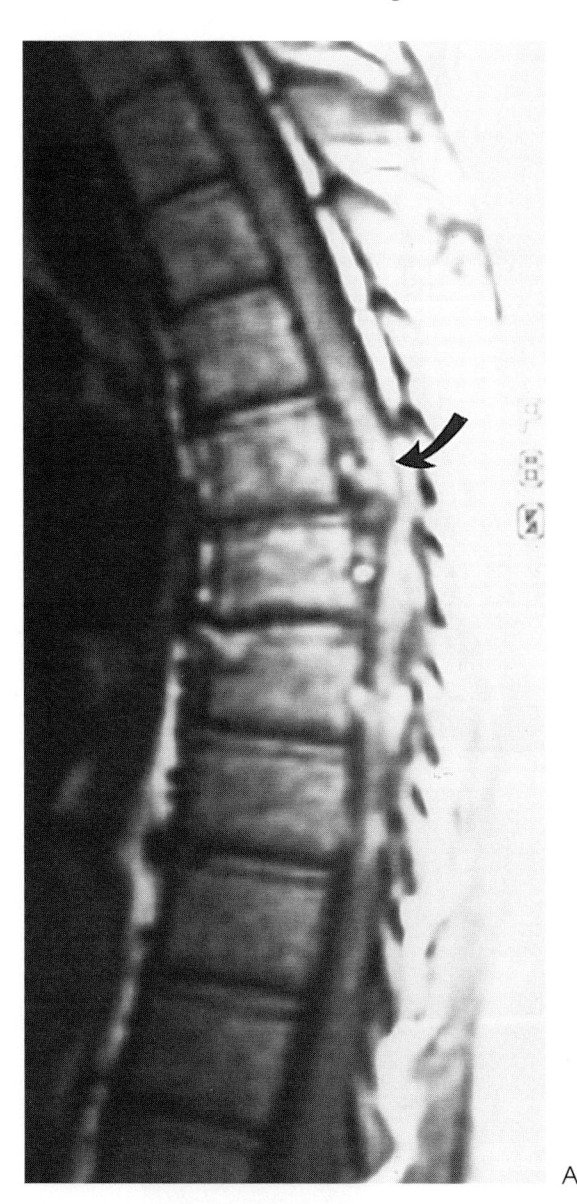

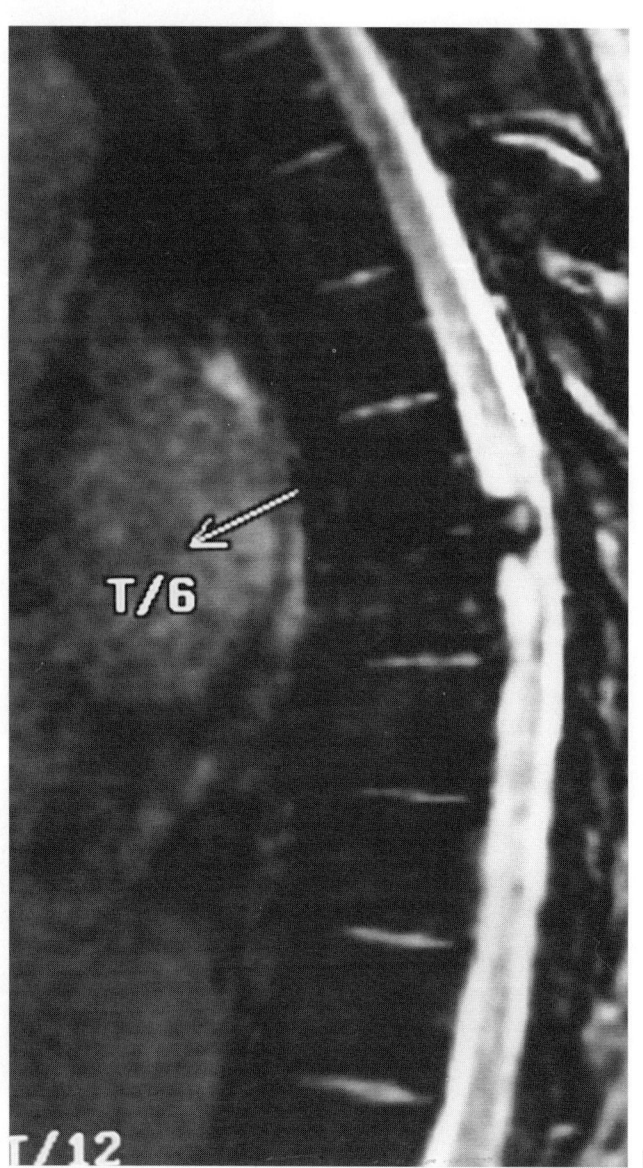

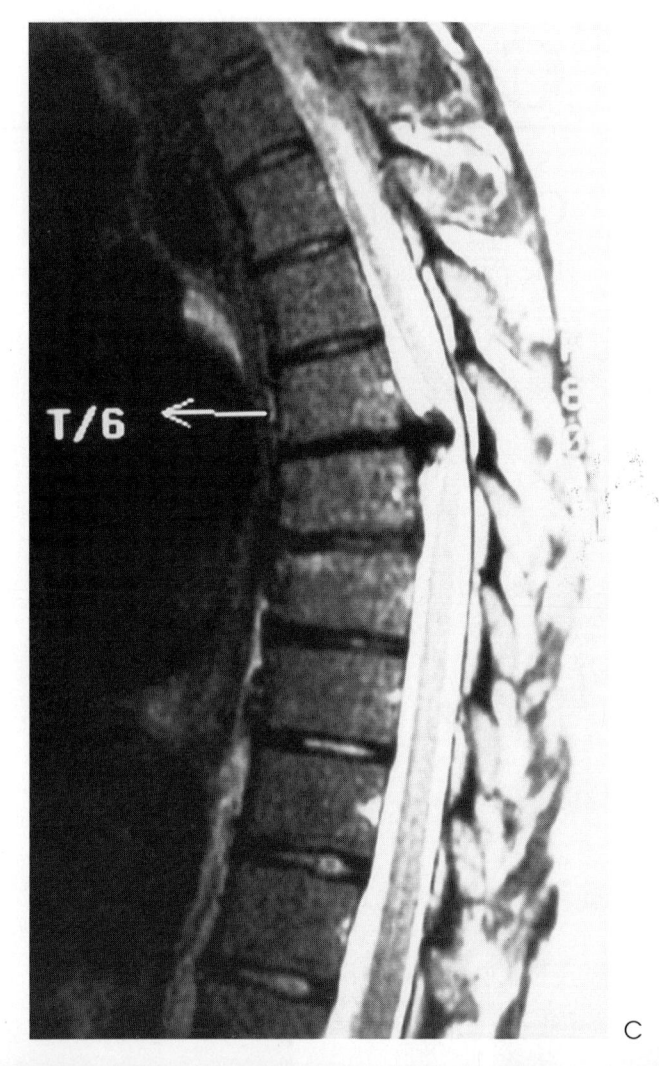

TEACHING ATLAS OF SPINE IMAGING

C

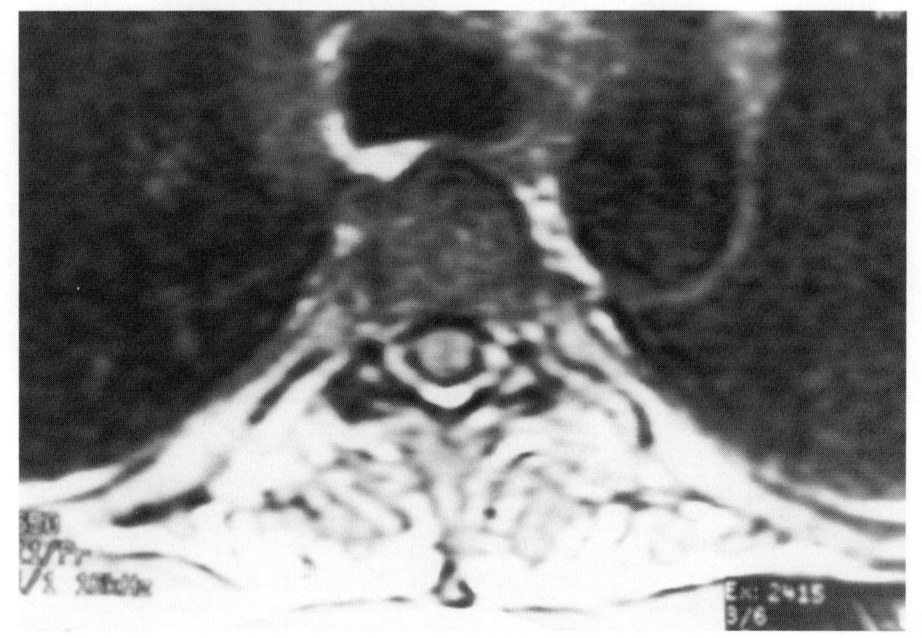

D

THORACIC SPINE

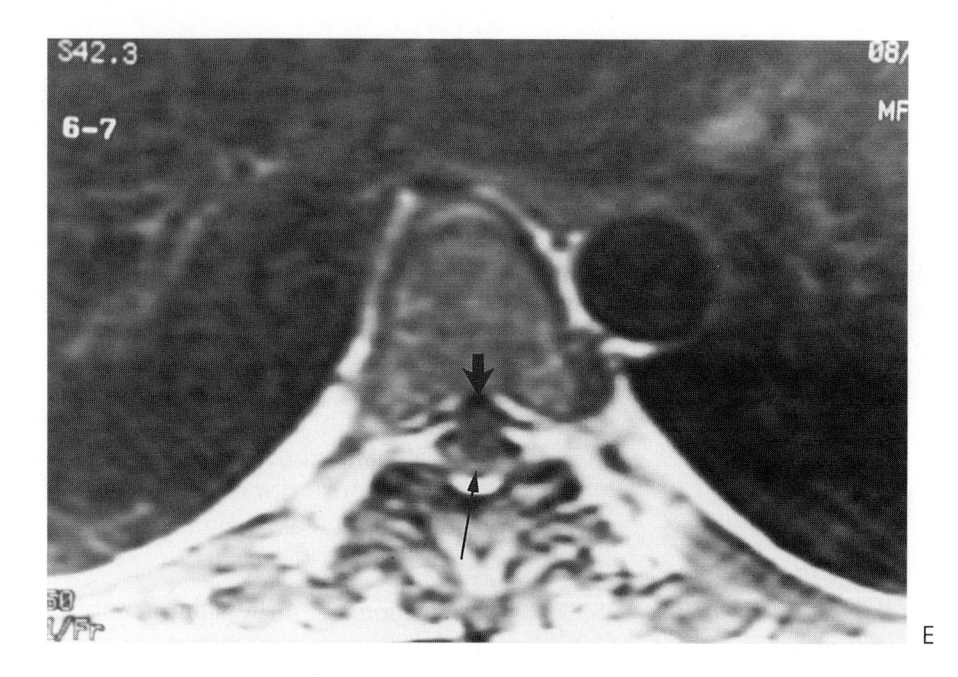

Radiologic Findings

Midsagittal short TR image of the thoracic spine (Fig. A) reveals an acute kyphosis of the thoracic spine. At the T6-7 level, there is intervertebral disc space narrowing and a ventral soft tissue mass anterior to the spinal cord that displaces the spinal cord posteriorly. Widening of the subarachnoid space is visible above and below the soft tissue mass. There is a questionable increase in signal intensity within the spinal cord just above the level of the soft tissue mass (*arrow*).

Midsagittal long TR image (Fig. B) reveals a very low signal intensity, mushroom-shaped mass arising at the T6-7 level which projects posteriorly into the vertebral canal. The spinal cord is displaced posteriorly and reveals a long area of increased signal intensity that extends multiple segments above and below the soft tissue mass. The T6 vertebral body is identified with T/6.

Slight parasagittal long TR image (Fig. C) reveals the decreased signal intensity mass projecting into the vertebral canal. The T6 vertebral body is identified with T/6.

Axial short TR image at the level of T5-6 (Fig. D) reveals the normal spinal cord with a normal circumferential ring of decreased signal intensity cerebrospinal fluid.

Axial short TR image at the T6-7 level (Fig. E) reveals the decreased signal intensity mass anterior to the spinal cord (*wide black arrow*) which displaces the spinal cord posteriorly and compresses it in a curvilinear fashion (*thin arrow*).

Diagnosis

Herniated intervertebral disc at the T6-7 level.

PEARL
- Computed tomographic scanning might be useful in this case to evaluate the presence of calcification in the intervertebral disc at the T6-7 level. Nonetheless, even if the disc is calcified, this probably would not change the surgical treatment or approach.

PITFALL
- Great care must be taken to identify the exact level of the abnormal disc so that surgery of the appropriate level can be planned.

Differential Diagnosis
- herniated disc
- meningioma
- Schwannoma

Discussion

The markedly decreased signal intensity of the herniated disc is consistent with a calcified disc. Herniated thoracic discs are typically calcified. There is marked posterior displacement of the thoracic spinal cord by the herniated disc. The increased signal intensity within the spinal cord is secondary to edema within the cord.

The widening of the subarachnoid space suggests that this mass is actually an intradural rather than an extradural mass. However, because of the appearance of an intradural process, meningioma certainly could be a strong diagnostic consideration. A schwannoma is also a consideration as schwannomas may be solitary lesions. Schwannomas may also be hemorrhagic and so could result in this low signal intensity appearance.

However, the fact that the lesion is centered at the level of the intervertebral disc and has a mushroomlike appearance arising from the level of the intervertebral disc makes meningioma and schwannoma less likely diagnostic considerations. Note also the marked disc space narrowing and decreased signal intensity of the intervertebral disc at the T6-7 level which would be consistent with a herniated disc. Note also accentuation of the dorsal kyphosis at the level of the herniated disc.

THORACIC SPINE

Case 2

Clinical Presentation

The patient is a 57-year-old male with a history of left-sided chest pain in the midthoracic region.

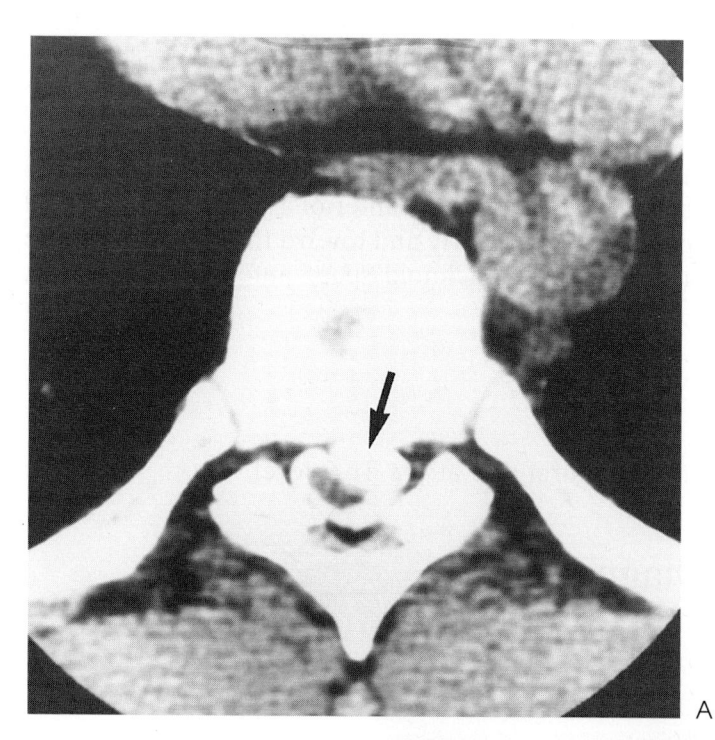

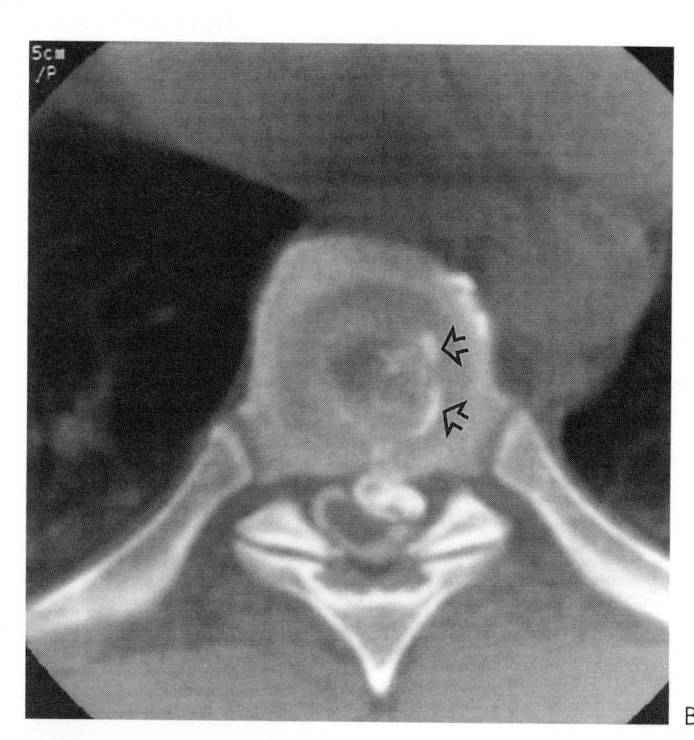

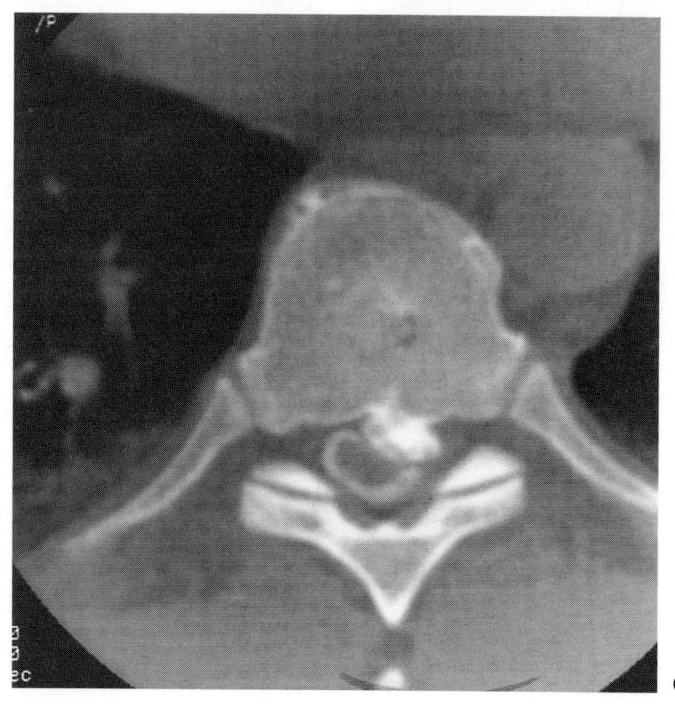

TEACHING ATLAS OF SPINE IMAGING

Radiologic Findings

Axial computed tomographic (CT) scan at the T6-7 level using soft tissue window widths after a thoracic myelogram (Fig. A) reveals an oval-shaped high density mass in the left side of the vertebral canal (arrow). The spinal cord is compressed, displaced posteriorly, and rotated away from the left side. The subarachnoid space is compressed.

Axial CT scan at the T6-7 level using bone window width technique (Fig. B) reveals calcification of the intervertebral disc at the T6-7 level (*arrows*). There is an umbilicated, oval, high density mass anteriorly on the left side. There is compression of the subarachnoid space, and the spinal cord is compressed, rotated away, and displaced to the right.

Axial CT scan taken just below the level of Figure B again (Fig. C) reveals the umbilicated, oval high density mass in the anterior aspect of the vertebral canal displacing the spinal cord posteriorly and toward the right side. There is complete obliteration of the subarachnoid space anteriorly on the left side at this level.

Diagnosis

Calcified, herniated intervertebral disc at the T6-7 level.

Differential Diagnosis

- herniated disc
- meningioma
- osteochondroma

Discussion

The appearance is typical of a calcified, herniated intervertebral disc. Note that there are patchy areas of increased density in the posterior aspect of the lung on the right side consistent with a patchy pneumonia.

In the absence of calcification within the intervertebral disc, diagnostic considerations would also include meningioma or osteochondroma.

PEARLS

- This mass arises at the level of the intervertebral disc and is associated with a calcified intervertebral disc, which strongly favors the diagnosis of a calcified herniated disc.

- Index images should be obtained such that the exact level of the abnormality can be identified.

PITFALL

- A calcified meningioma might be a diagnostic consideration in this patient; however, this mass is extradural rather than intradural, and this does not favor a meningioma.

THORACIC SPINE

Case 3

Clinical Presentation

The patient is a 54-year-old female with adenocarcinoma of unknown primary with new onset of weakness of the lower extremities.

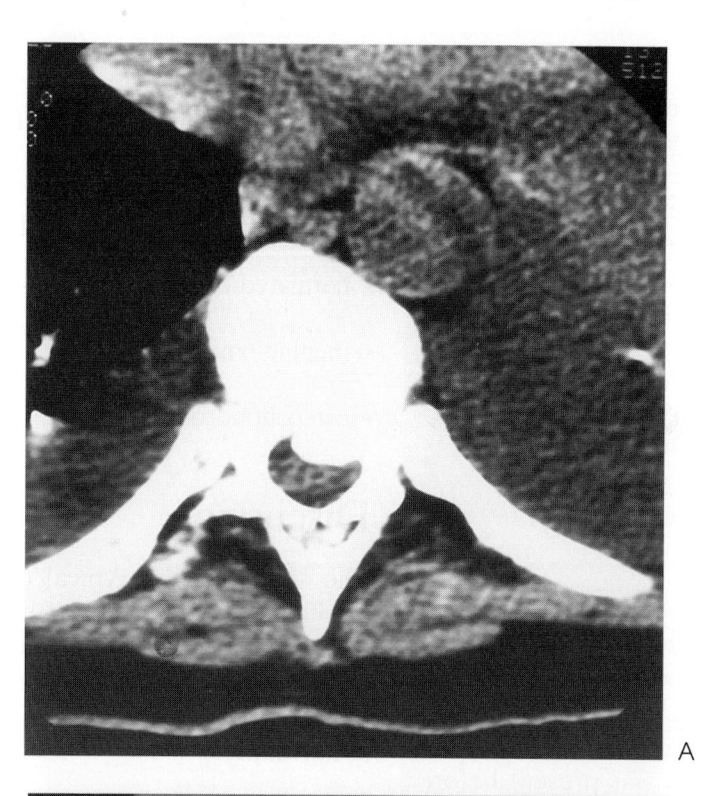

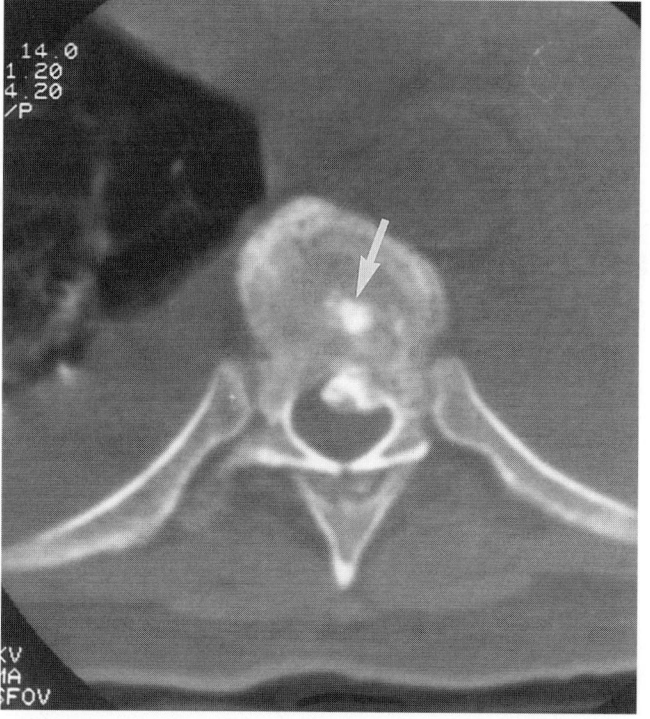

A

B

593

Radiologic Findings

Axial computed tomographic (CT) image at the T8-9 (Fig. A) reveals an oval area of increased density to the left of the midline ventral to the spinal cord. The spinal cord is displaced posteriorly and compressed on the left side. Axial CT image at the T8-9 level with bone window width technique (Fig. B) reveals calcification of the intervertebral disc (*arrow*). The high density mass seen in Figure A is again seen anterior to the spinal cord.

Diagnosis

Herniated, calcified intervertebral disc at the T8-9 level.

Differential Diagnosis

- herniated disc
- meningioma
- osteochondroma

Discussion

The appearance is typical of that seen with a herniated disc. The disc is calcified, and a portion of the nucleus pulposus is displaced posteriorly in the left side of the vertebral canal. Meningioma or osteochondroma could be diagnostic considerations; however, they are unlikely because of the presence of calcification within the intervertebral disc and the level of the abnormality.

If the herniated disc is lateralized, the side of the abnormality should be clearly identified so that if surgical removal is planned the correct side can be approached.

Note also that there are large pleural effusions bilaterally. Although the study is directed toward the vertebral column, it is important to evaluate the areas adjacent to the vertebral column within the field of view so that lung masses or abnormalities such as the pleural effusion seen in this patient will not be overlooked.

PEARLS

- The herniated disc is the obvious finding in this case; however, evaluation of the more peripheral portions of the images reveals the large pleural effusion.

- Great care must be taken to determine the exact level of the abnormality so that the correct level may be approached surgically.

PITFALL

- The surgical approach to such a densely calcified disc may be difficult and may result in a more pronounced neurological deficit than was present before surgery.

THORACIC SPINE

Case 4

Clinical Presentation

The patient is a 13-year-old male with midthoracic pain and mild lower extremity weakness.

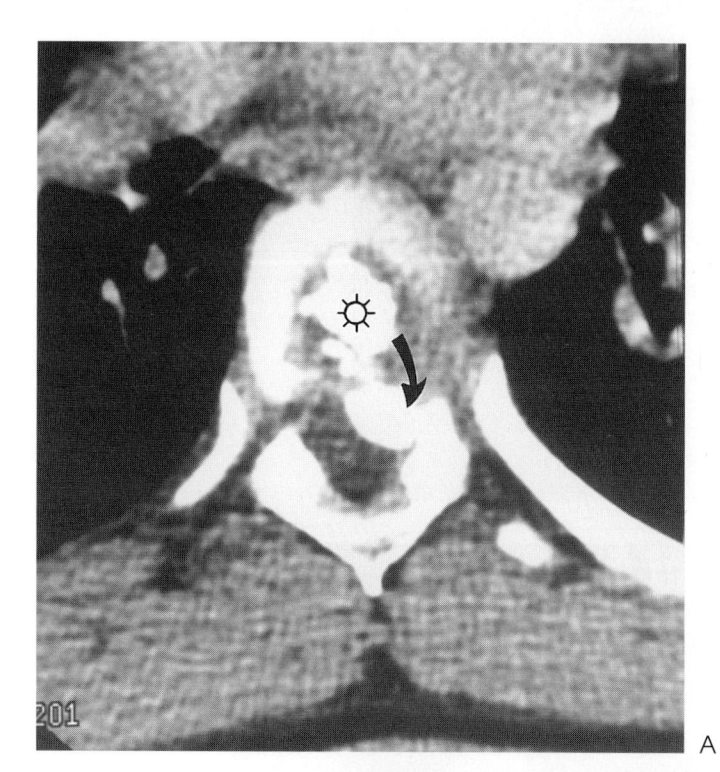

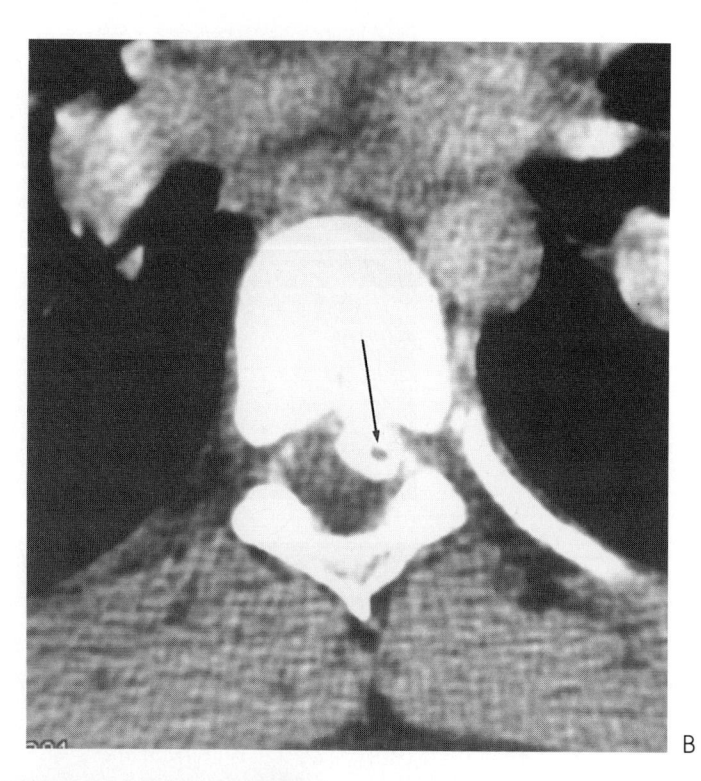

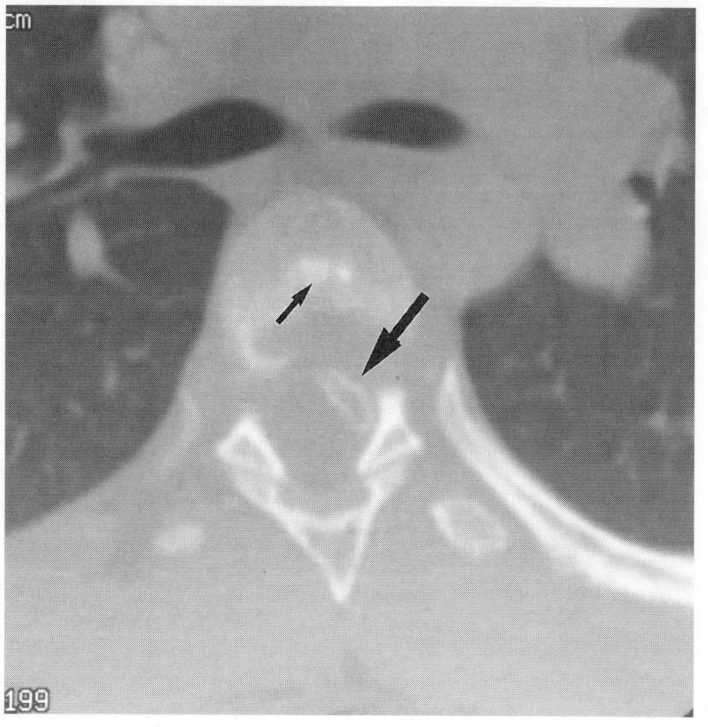

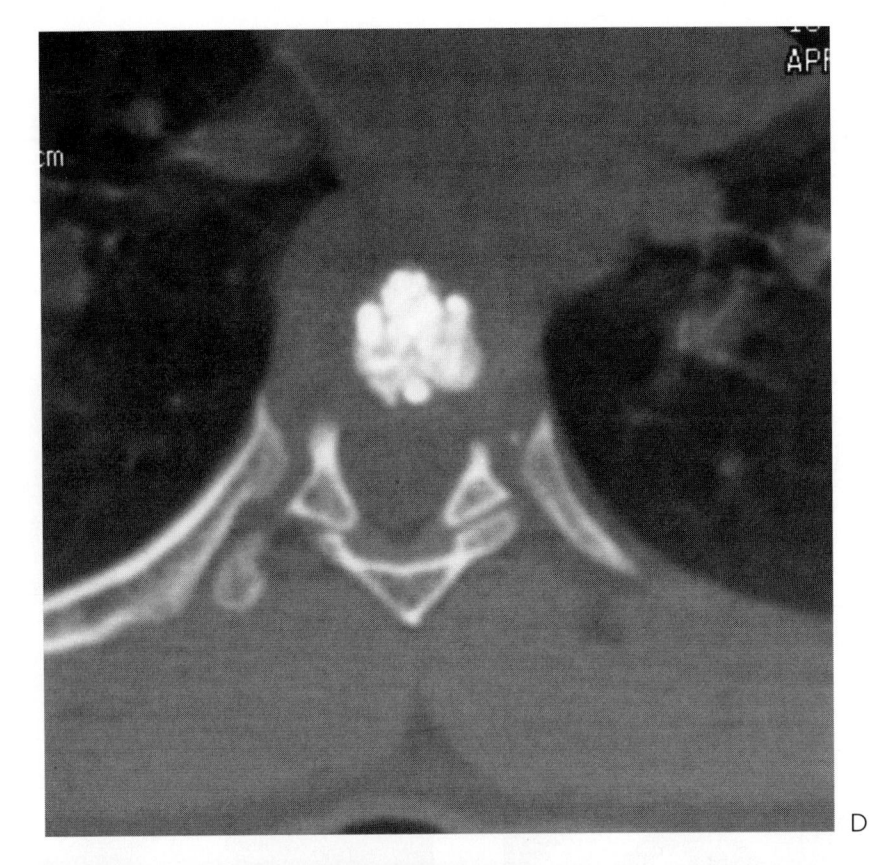

TEACHING ATLAS OF SPINE IMAGING

D

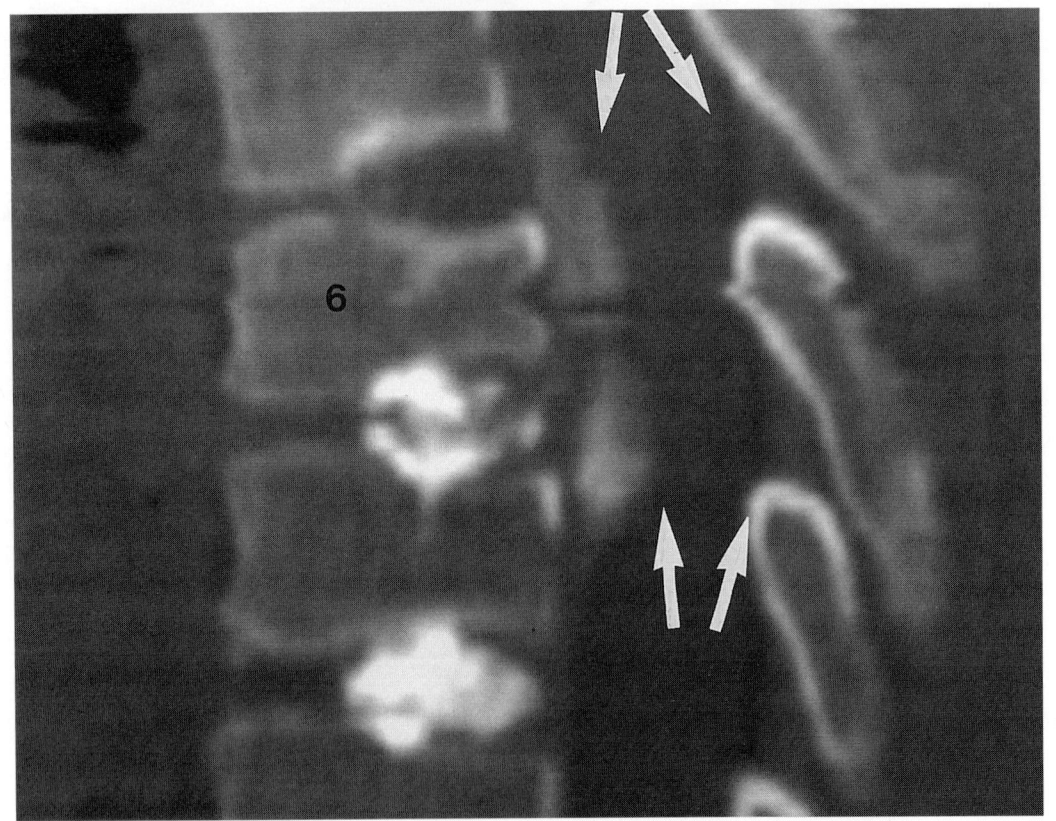

E

THORACIC SPINE

F

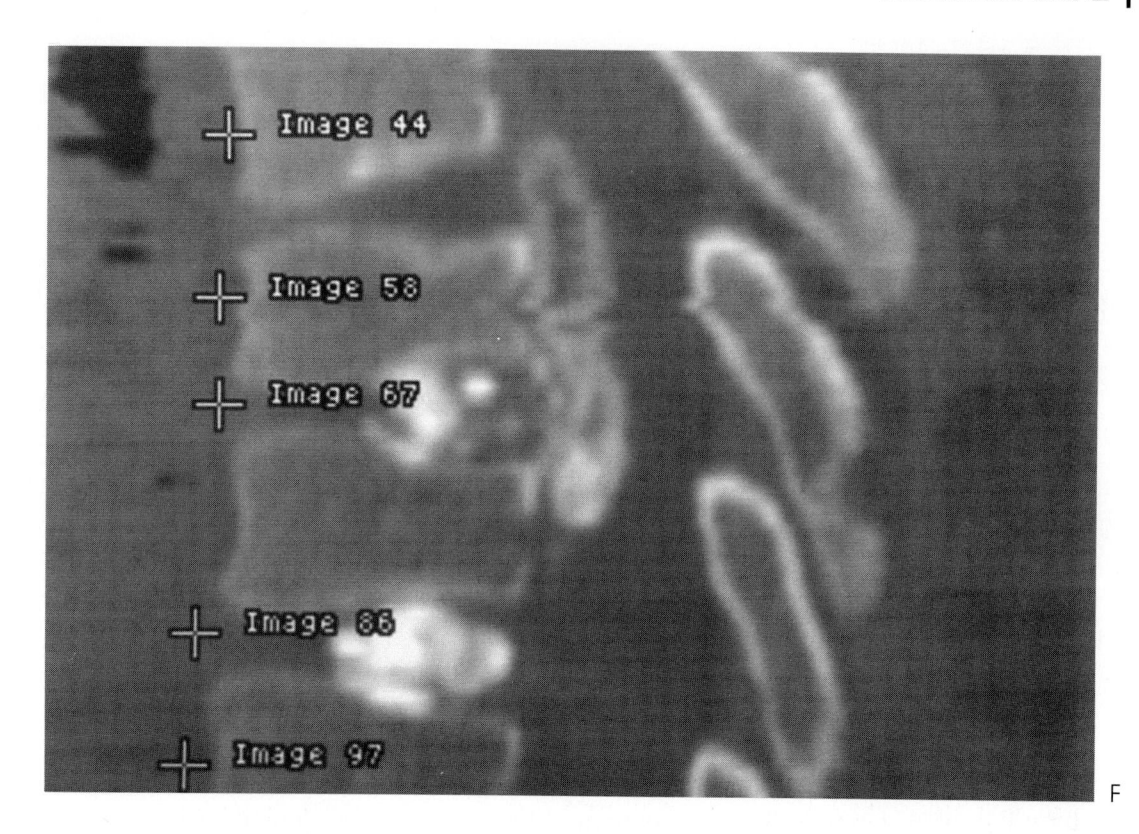

Radiologic Findings

Axial computed tomographic (CT) slice at the level of the C6-7 intervertebral disc (Fig. A) reveals dense, slightly irregularly marginated calcification of the intervertebral disc in the region of the nucleus pulposus (*). The calcification extends posteriorly in the midline and then off to the left side (*arrow*) into the intervertebral canal in the epidural space.

Axial CT scan at the level of the superior end plate of the C7 vertebral body (Fig. B) reveals a rounded area of increased density projecting in the anterior left side of the vertebral canal. There is a small internal area of low density (*arrow*).

Axial CT scan using bone window widths at the same level as Figure B (Fig. C) reveals the oval area of high density in the anterior lateral portion of the vertebral canal with a central area of low density (*large arrow*). There is faint calcification in the midportion of the intervertebral disc (*small arrow*).

Axial CT scan using bone window widths at the level of the T7-8 intervertebral disc (Fig. D) reveals dense amorphous calcification of the intervertebral disc.

Midsagittal reconstruction image of the thoracic spine using bone window widths (Fig. E) reveals dense calcification of the intervertebral discs at both of these levels. In addition, there is an area of dense, slightly inhomogeneous calcification that extends from the level of the intervertebral body of T5-6 through the level of the midbody of the T7 vertebral body. There is moderately severe narrowing of the vertebral canal. The anticipated position of the thecal sac is displaced posteriorly (*arrows*). The T6 vertebral body is identified with 6.

Left parasagittal reconstruction of the spine with bone window widths (Fig. F) identifies by number the levels of the individual CT images as they were obtained in the axial plane. The dense inhomogeneous calcification is again seen projecting posterior to the vertebral bodies at T5, T6, and T7. The calcification is slightly denser along the peripheral margin.

Diagnosis

Calcified, herniated intervertebral disc at the T6-7 level with compromise of the vertebral canal in the midline and on the left side.

Differential Diagnosis

- herniated disc

- ochronosis

Discussion

The appearance of dense intervertebral disc calcification is unusual in a patient of 13 years of age. Calcified intervertebral discs are common in older patients, and calcification is a typical end result of a degenerated thoracic disc. The thoracic vertebral canal is the narrowest portion of the vertebral canal, and encroachment upon the vertebral canal typically causes symptoms because the spinal cord is confined in this small space. The spinal cord is approximately 1.0 cm in size; therefore, narrowing of the vertebral canal below this size results in spinal cord compromise.

Note that there is narrowing of the intervertebral disc space at the T6-7 level because the nucleus pulposus has migrated out of the intervertebral disc space and into the vertebral canal.

Although this patient had lower extremity weakness, it was elected to follow rather than operate on this herniated disc. Over time, the herniated portion of the disc has gradually decreased in size and become compressed against the posterior margin of the vertebral bodies.

Ochronosis (alkaptonuria) may result in calcification of the intervertebral discs; however, there was no history of ochronosis in this individual. Alkaptonouria is an inherited disease which results in the excretion of homogentisic acid in the urine which subsequently turns very dark after standing for a period of time. The darkened mesenchmyal tissues in middle age appear blue through the skin, and degenerative joint changes occur. In the spine, this results in intervertebral disc calcification and large osteophyte formation. However, these changes typically occur in middle age.

PEARL
- The spine should also be evaluated for the presence or absence of the normal number of vertebral bodies as well as for the presence of transitional vertebrae.

PITFALL
- Digital localization images in both the anteroposterior and lateral projections will allow the best localization of these abnormal discs. These images should be clearly labeled as the to level of the slices so that the correct level can be identified.

THORACIC SPINE

Case 5

Clinical Presentation

The patient is a 17-year-old female with an elevated hematocrit and recent onset of an unsteady gait.

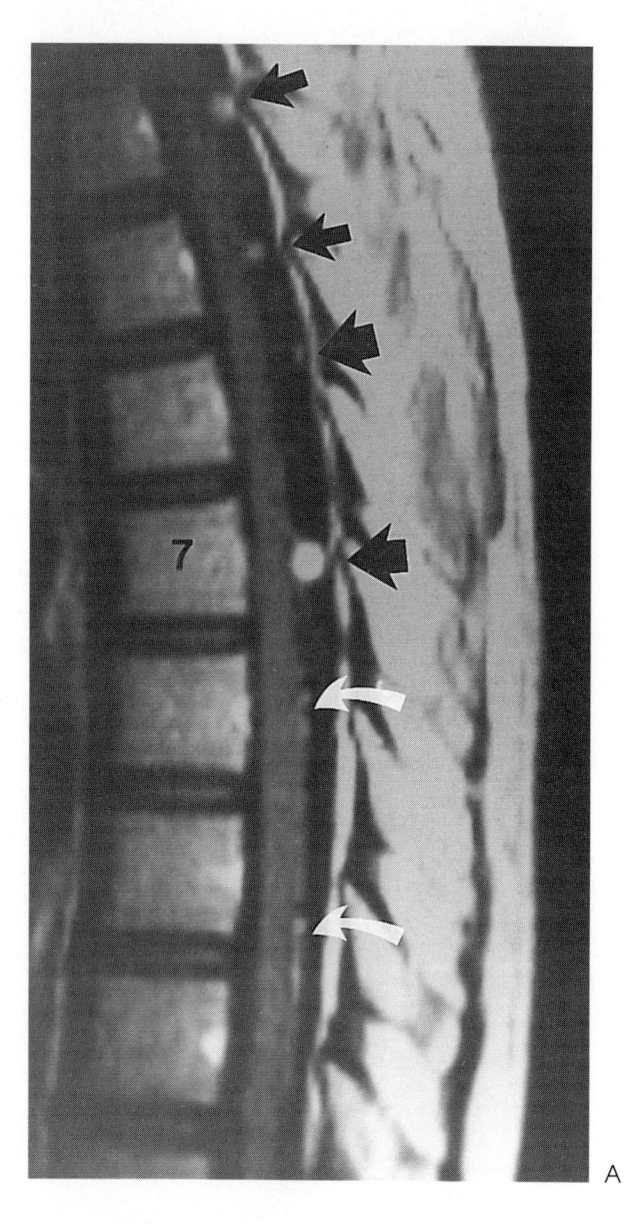

Radiologic Findings

Postcontrast sagittal short TR image (Fig. A) reveals multiple rounded, densely enhancing lesions in the subarachnoid space dorsal to the spinal cord (*black arrows*). There is also faint serpiginous areas of enhancement along the dorsal aspect of the thoracic spinal cord (*white arrows*). The spinal cord is displaced anteriorly and flattened slightly at the T7 level (*7*).

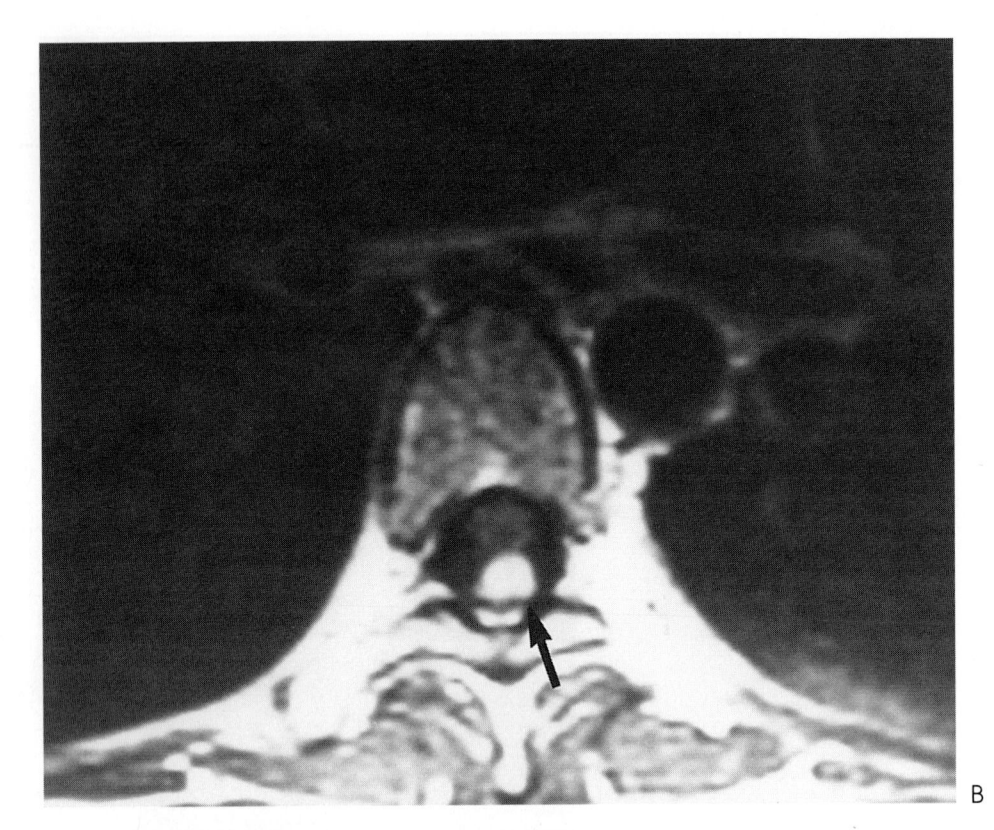

TEACHING ATLAS OF SPINE IMAGING

B

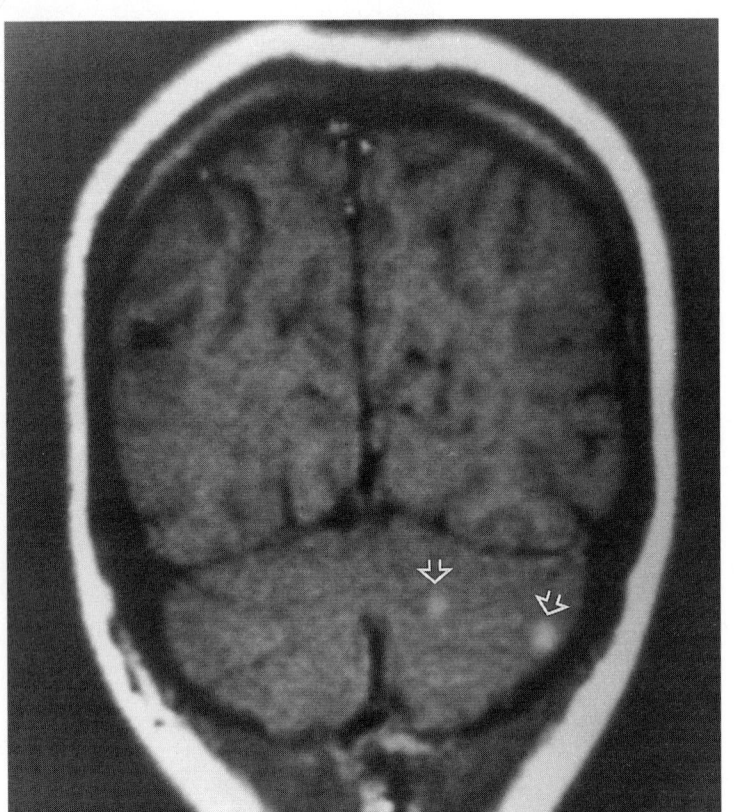

C

Radiologic Findings (continued)

Axial short TR image in the axial plane at the level of the T7 vertebral body (Fig. B) reveals a round, densely enhancing lesion in the subarachnoid space dorsal to the spinal cord (*arrow*).

Coronal short TR image of the brain (Fig. C) reveals two small, rounded areas of enhancement in the left cerebellar hemisphere (*arrows*).

Diagnosis

Von Hippel-Lindau disease with multiple cerebellar hemangioblastomas and spinal cord hemangioblastomas.

Differential Diagnosis

- multiple hemangioblastomas
- multiple abscesses
- metastases

Discussion

The imaging findings and clinical presentation are typical of von Hippel-Lindau disease. The densely enhancing lesions are multiple hemangioblastomas of the cerebellum and the spinal cord. These spinal cord hemangioblastomas are most common in the thoracic spine. Hemangioblastomas of the spinal cord may be intramedullary or extramedullary, in which case the tumor has a pial attachment. These tumors are very vascular and will reveal a dense blush when evaluated with angiography.

The differential diagnosis would include the possibility of multiple metastases to the cerebellum and the spinal subarachnoid space. Primary tumors would include malignant melanoma, lung cancer, or lymphoma. However, the clinical presentation with an elevated serum hematocrit strongly favors the diagnosis of von Hippel-Lindau disease and multiple hemangioblastomas. Presentation is uncommon in the first two decades of life. Von Hippel-Lindau disease is one of the neurocutaneous diseases; therefore, patients may also have retinal angiomas.

Multiple vascular metastases could also have a similar appearance but are less likely in this clinical setting.

PEARLS

- Angiography reveals a densely enhancing mass with enlarged draining veins. The cerebellar hemangioblastomas are typically cystic with a densely enhancing solid component. Angiography may mimic the appearance of an arteriovenous malformation.
- This disease is also associated with renal cell carcinomas.

PITFALLS

- Because of the multiplicity of lesions, successful surgical treatment may not be possible.
- These tumors may have a cystic component and may mimic the appearance of a cystic spinal cord tumor such as astrocytoma.

TEACHING ATLAS OF SPINE IMAGING

Case 6

Clinical Presentation

The patient is a 73-year-old male with a history of bilateral lower extremity paralysis following aortic aneurysm repair.

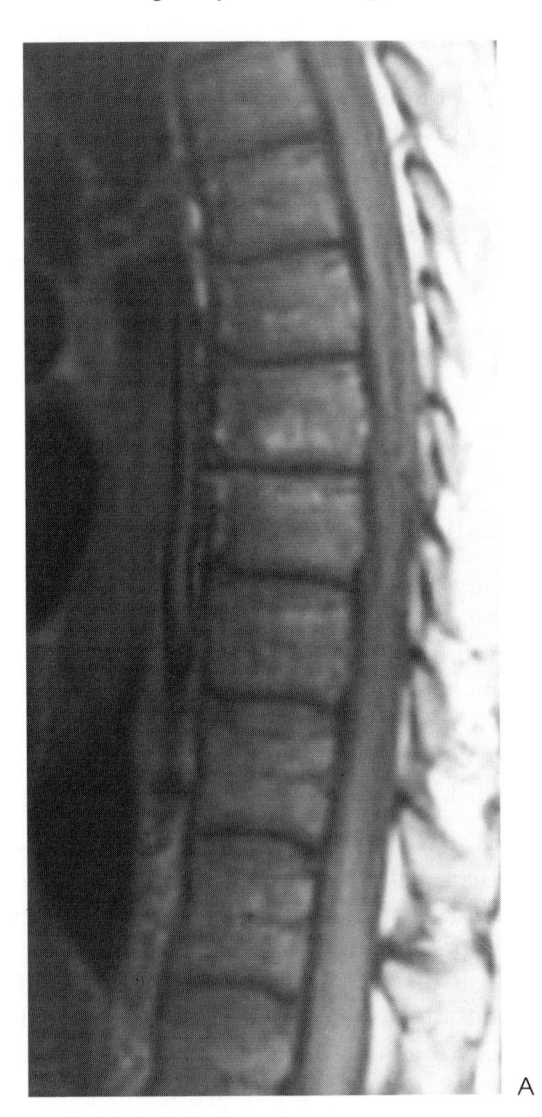

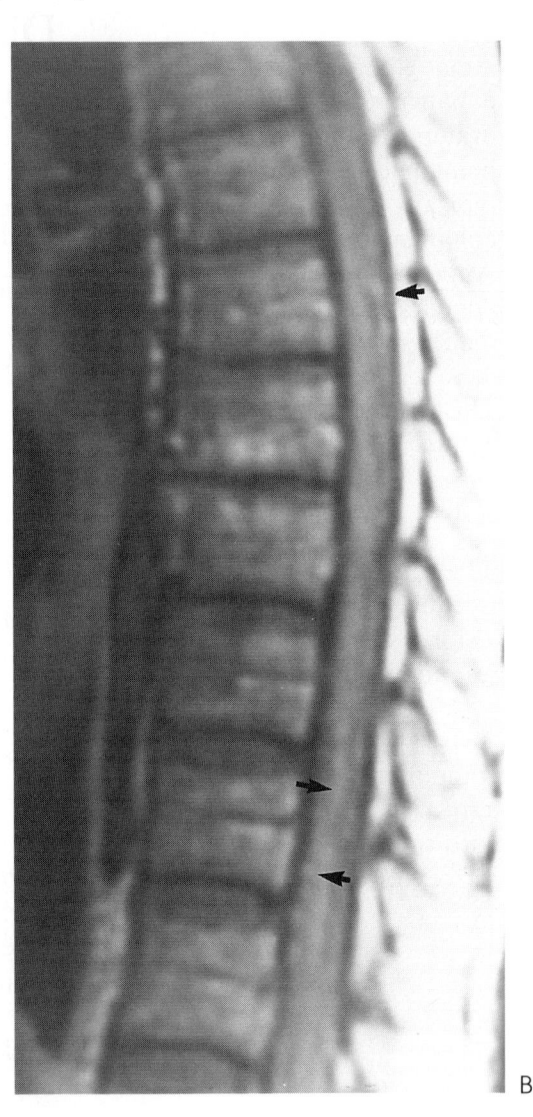

Radiologic Findings

The patient had a normal magnetic resonance study of the thoracic spinal cord immediately after the onset of symptoms, 3 days prior to the present study.

Precontrast sagittal short TR image (Fig. A) reveals diffuse increase in the size of the thoracic spinal cord. The thoracic subarachnoid space is almost completely obliterated. There is diffuse mottling of the marrow within the vertebral bodies at multiple levels with small focal areas of increased signal intensity.

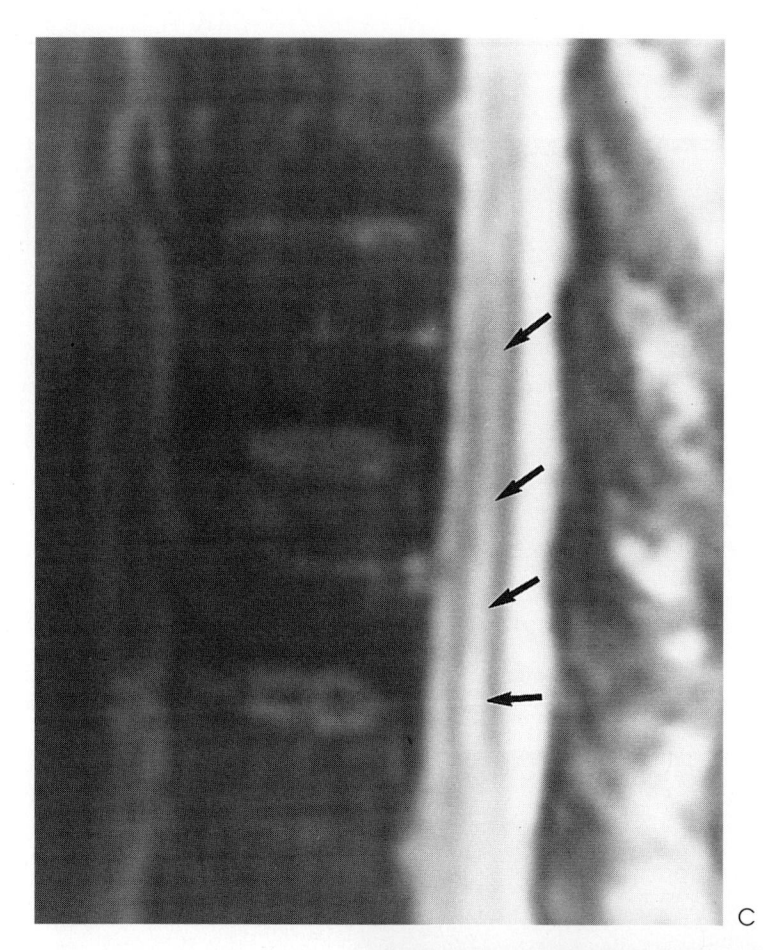

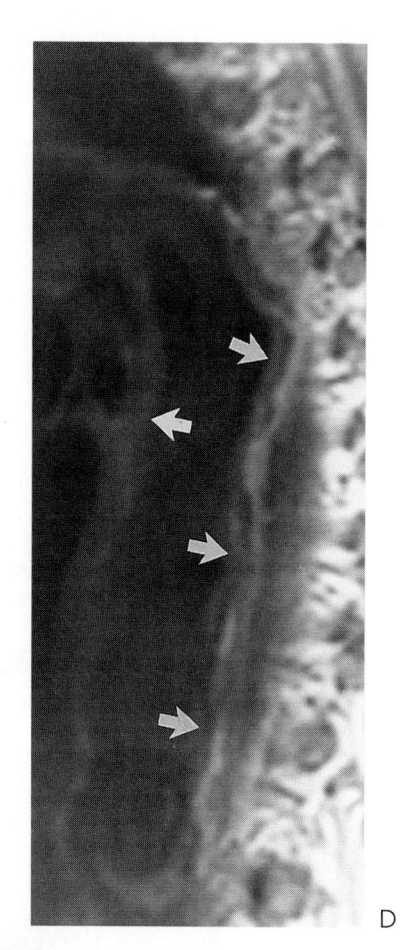

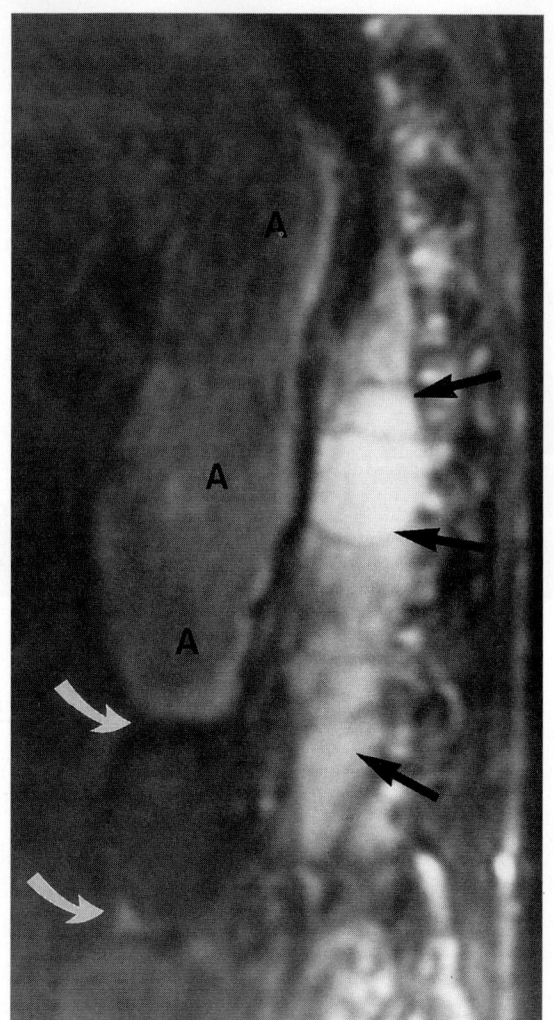

C

D

E

603

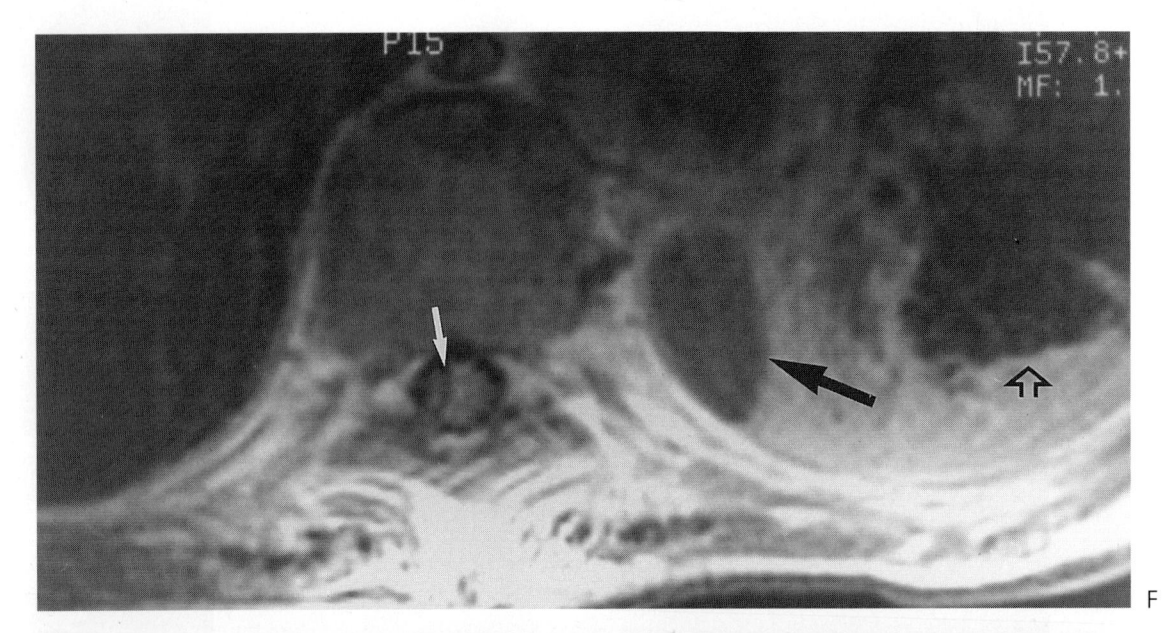

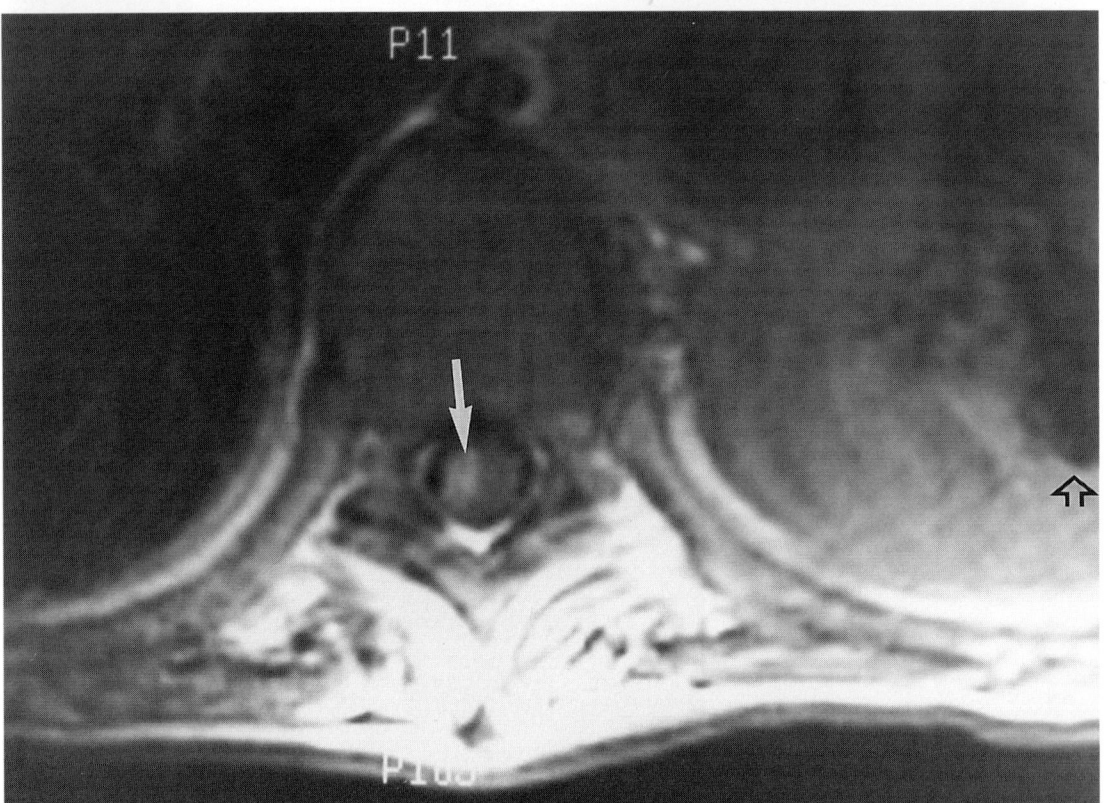

Radiologic Findings (continued)

Postcontrast sagittal short TR image (Fig. B) reveals questionable patchy areas of enhancement (*arrows*), but no large focal area of enhancement.

Sagittal long TR image in the lower thoracic region (Fig. C) reveals a longitudinal, multilevel area of increased signal intensity within the central portion of the distal thoracic spinal cord (*arrows*).

Left parasagittal short TR image (Fig. D) reveals that the thoracic aorta is enlarged in size and demonstrates a lobulated, thickened wall (*arrows*).

THORACIC SPINE

Radiologic Findings (continued)

Left parasagittal long TR image (Fig. E) reveals variable signal intensity within the dilated thoracic aorta (*A*). There are also focal areas of relative narrowing in the lower thoracic aorta (*curved arrows*). There is also a loculated area of variably increased signal intensity adjacent to the thoracic spine (*black arrows*).

Axial short TR image at the level of T7 (Fig. F) reveals an area of decreased signal intensity in the right side of the spinal cord (*white arrow*). There is a left-sided pleural effusion (*open arrow*) and an oval area of decreased signal intensity in the left paraspinal region (*black arrow*), as well as a variable signal intensity soft tissue mass that extends lateral to the spine on the left side. The dilated aorta projects anterior and to the left of the vertebral column.

Postcontrast axial short TR image (Fig. G) reveals an oval area of enhancement within the right side of the thoracic spinal cord (*white arrow*). The left-sided pleural effusion is again seen (*open arrow*).

PEARL
- Because the initial scan may be normal, repeat magnetic resonance scanning may be necessary for complete evaluation in a patient who has sudden onset of symptoms.

PITFALL
- Transverse myelopathy (myelitis) would be a diagnostic consideration in another clinical setting.

Diagnosis

Thoracic spinal cord ischemia and presumed infarction.

Differential Diagnosis

- aneurysm
- ischemia
- transverse myelopathy

Discussion

The blood supply of the distal spinal cord arises from the artery of Adamkewicz, which typically originates from the left ninth intercostal artery, although it may arise higher or lower and may arise from the right side. This arterial blood supply to the spinal cord may be interrupted at the time of aneurysm repair; it may also be interrupted with aortic dissection or even atherosclerosis of the aorta.

The fact that the imaging was normal immediately following the onset of symptoms and is abnormal 3 days later favors the diagnosis of an ischemic event. The enhancement is similar to that seen in the brain when there is an infarct.

When there is surgery for an aortic aneurysm, there may be interruption of the arterial trunk which supplies the spinal cord. This results in ischemic changes to the spinal cord. If there is not sufficient collateral circulation from other sources, this may result in infarction of the spinal cord. This has occurred in this case. The occurrence of spinal cord infarction is very dependent upon the existing blood supply to the cord and the ability to establish collateral blood supply. In the older patient, there is frequently existing atherosclerotic or arteriosclerotic changes in the blood vessels, which obviously compromises the blood supply to the spinal cord. Elderly patients may experience transient ischemic events involving the spinal cord in the same way that patients may have transient ischemic events of the brain.

Spinal cord ischemia and resulting infarction may also occur in patients who have a dissection of the aorta. Cord ischemia occurs because there is abrupt interruption of the blood supply to the spinal cord as a result of the dissection.

This patient has a thoracic aortic aneurysm that exhibits a thickened and irregular wall. There is a left-sided pleural effusion (*open arrow* in F and G), probably secondary to both fluid and hemorrhage, combined with postoperative changes. The left paraspinal fluid collection (*black arrow* in F) is consistent with a loculated collection of fluid.

In the absence of a history of aortic aneurysm dissection or recent surgery, the diagnosis of spinal cord infarction is less obvious. In these cases, the diagnosis of infarction or ischemic changes in the spinal cord becomes a diagnosis of exclusion. The imaging appearance may mimic transverse myelopathy (myelitis).

The variable signal intensity seen within the aorta in Figures C and D is secondary to flow-related enhancement because of turbulent flow of the blood within the aneurysm.

The mottled signal intensity within the vertebral bodies is secondary to osteoporosis and focal areas of fat deposition.

THORACIC SPINE

Case 7

Clinical Presentation

The patient is an 81-year-old male with a history of intermittent gait disturbance and sudden onset of lower extremity weakness.

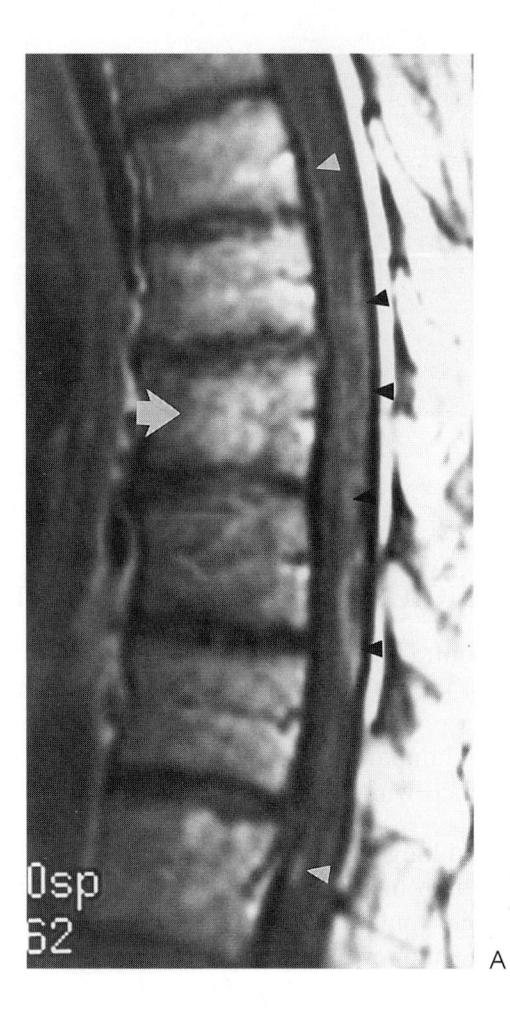

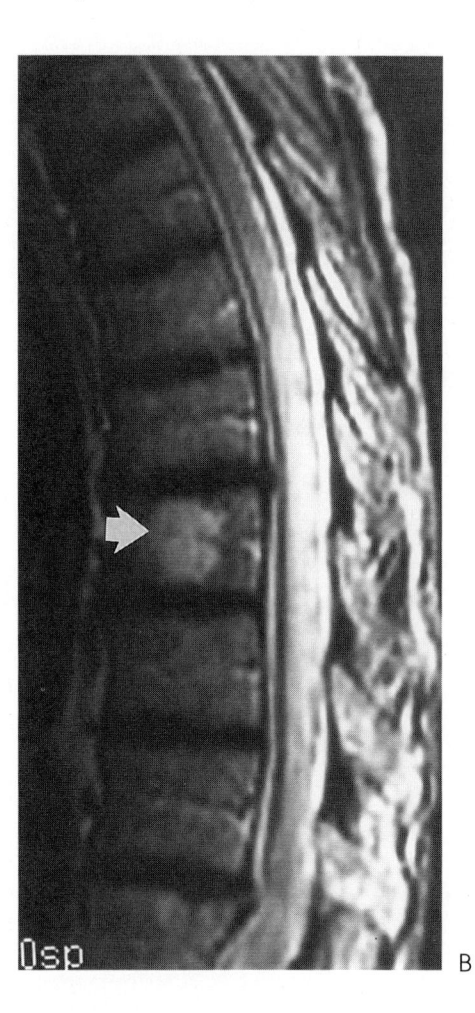

Radiologic Findings

Postcontrast sagittal short TR image in the lower thoracic region (Fig. A) reveals multiple irregular linear areas of enhancement in the lower thoracic spine (*small black and white arrows*). The spinal cord is mildly enlarged throughout its visualized course. There is a faint, rounded area of increased signal intensity within the vertebral body of T9 (*large white arrow*). The precontrast images revealed a mildly enlarged spinal cord.

Sagittal long TR image (Fig. B) reveals a large area of increased signal intensity within the central portion of the thoracic spinal cord. The area of increased signal intensity within the T9 vertebral body is better seen on the long TR image (*arrow*).

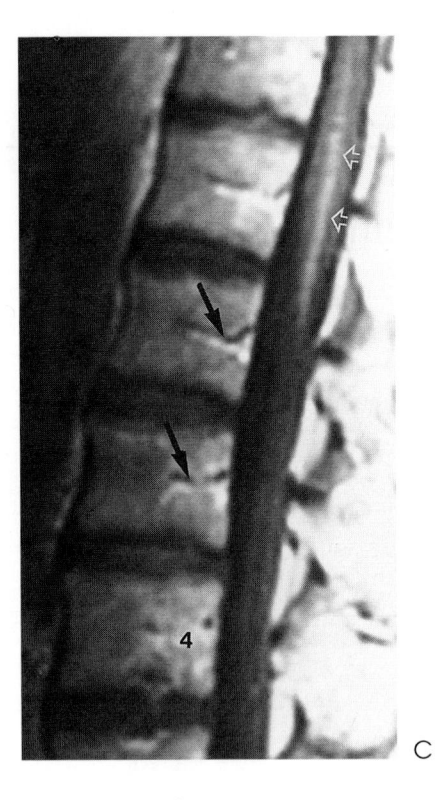

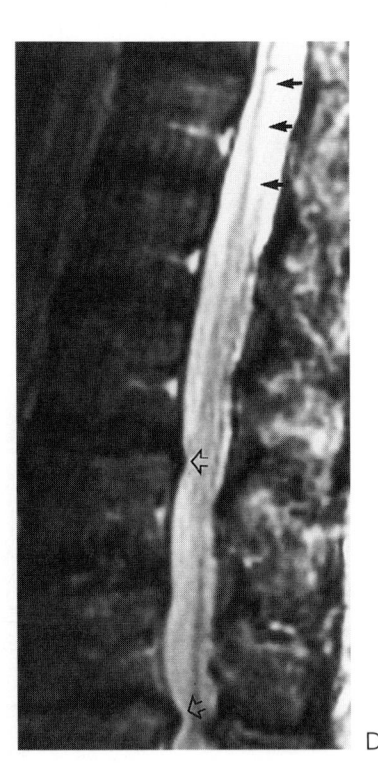

Radiologic Findings (continued)

Postcontrast sagittal short TR image at the level of the conus medullaris (Fig. C) reveals a central area of enhancement in the distal spinal cord (*open arrows*). There are also areas of enhancement within the central portions of the lumbar vertebral bodies (*black arrows*). The L4 vertebral body is identified with 4.

Sagittal long TR image at the level of the conus medullaris (Fig. D) reveals an area of increased signal intensity within the central portion of the distal thoracic spinal cord (*solid arrows*). Incidentally noted is minimal bulging of the intervertebral discs at the L3-4 and L5-S1 levels (*open arrows*).

Diagnosis

Probable spinal cord ischemia with areas of enhancement.

Differential Diagnosis

- spinal cord ischemia
- transverse myelopathy
- spinal cord tumor
- intramedullary inflammatory process

THORACIC SPINE

PEARL
- The imaging finding should also be correlated with the evaluation of the cerebrospinal fluid. This would reveal an elevated protein and decreased glucose in the presence of infection.

PITFALLS
- There is no known treatment for transverse myelopathy or for ischemic changes within the spinal cord.

- Follow-up scans might be helpful for more complete evaluation, particularly if the diagnosis is in doubt at the time of initial evaluation.

Discussion

The patient is an elderly patient with intermittent symptoms followed by sudden onset of more definite symptoms. The abnormal areas within the distal spinal cord most likely represent areas of ischemia with areas of enhancement. Transverse myelopathy (myelitis) could also have a similar appearance and is a diagnostic consideration.

The area of increased signal intensity within the vertebral body of T9 is a hemangioma. The enhancement within the vertebral bodies is enhancement of the basivertebral venous plexus, which is part of Batson's plexus (*black arrows* in Fig. C).

Spinal cord tumor is not a likely diagnosis because of the pattern of diffuse enhancement. An intramedullary inflammatory process could have a similar appearance, and should be correlated with the analysis of the cerebrospinal fluid.

TEACHING ATLAS OF SPINE IMAGING

Case 8

Clinical Presentation

The patient is a healthy 16-year-old male who experienced the sudden onset of paraplegia.

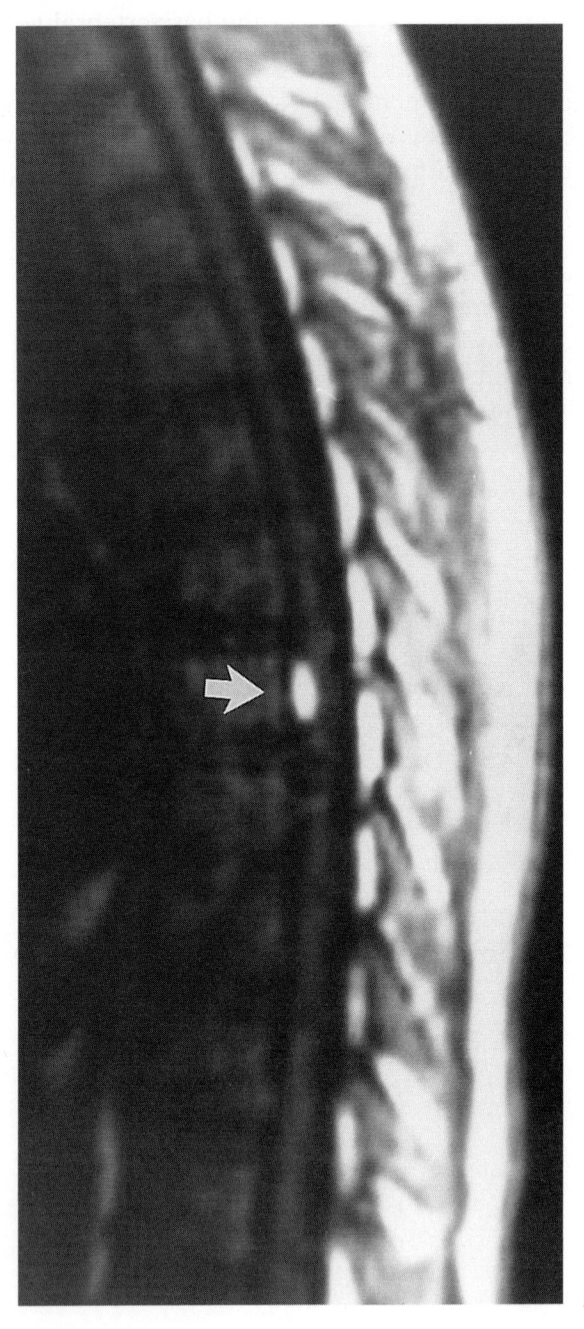

A

THORACIC SPINE

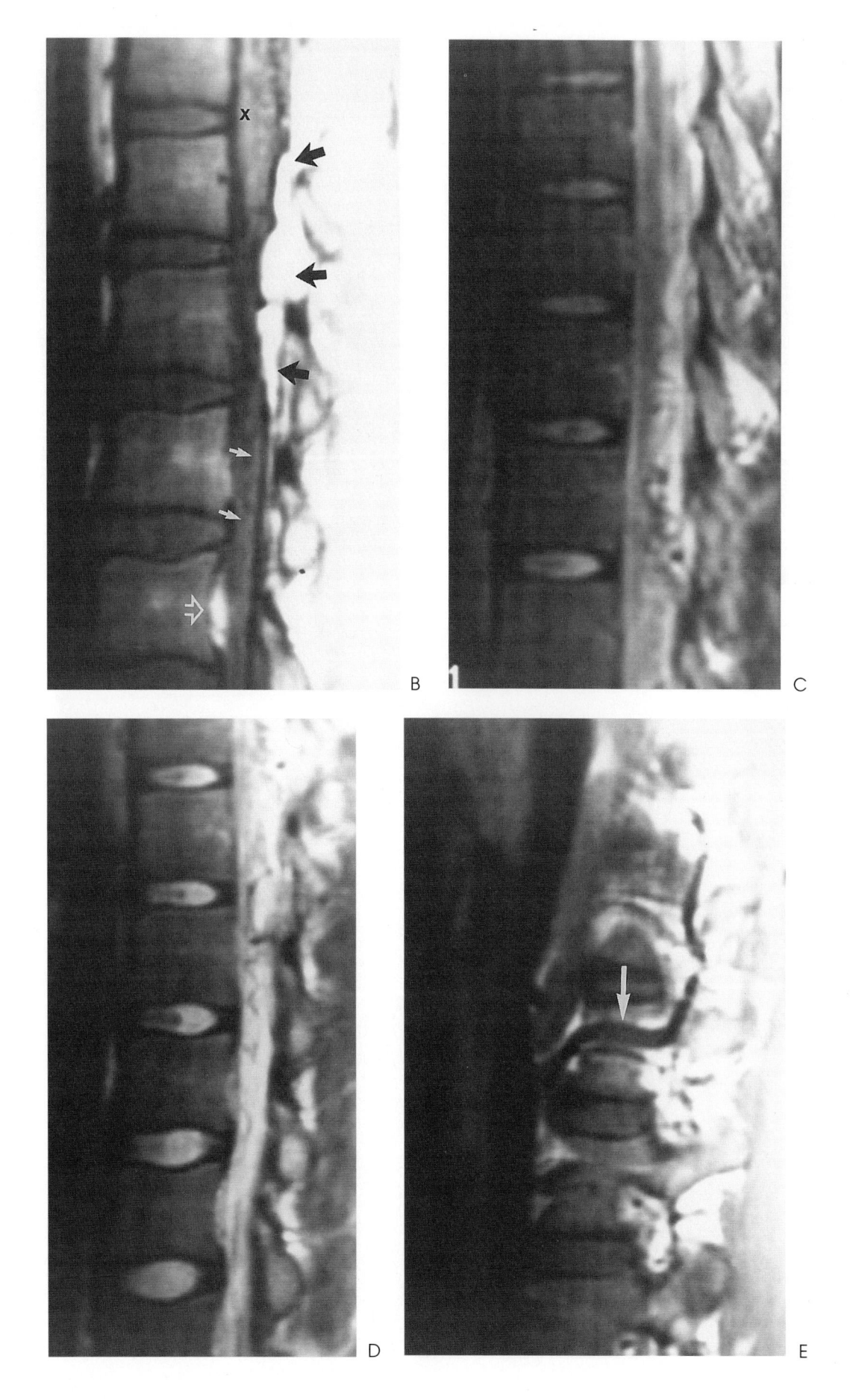

TEACHING ATLAS OF SPINE IMAGING

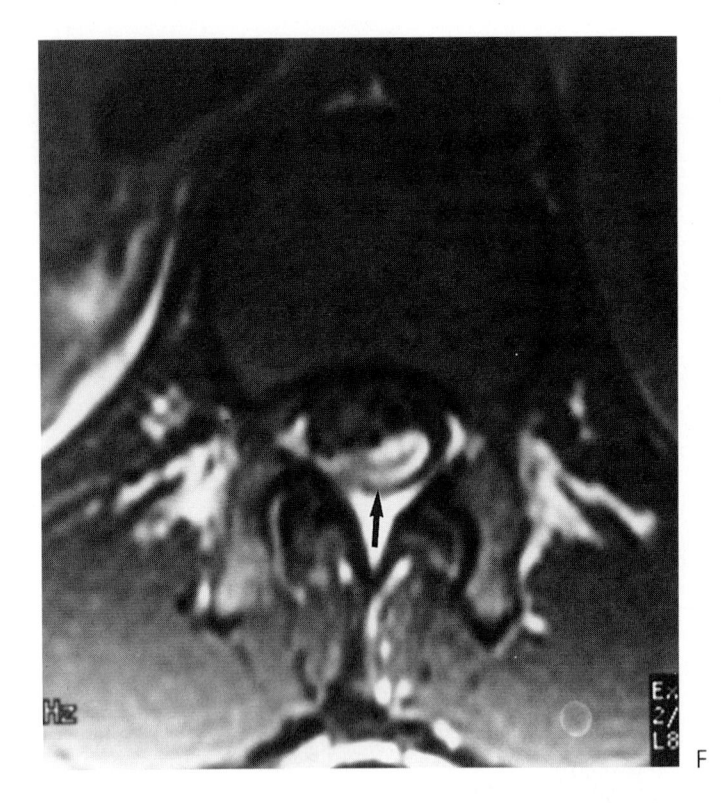

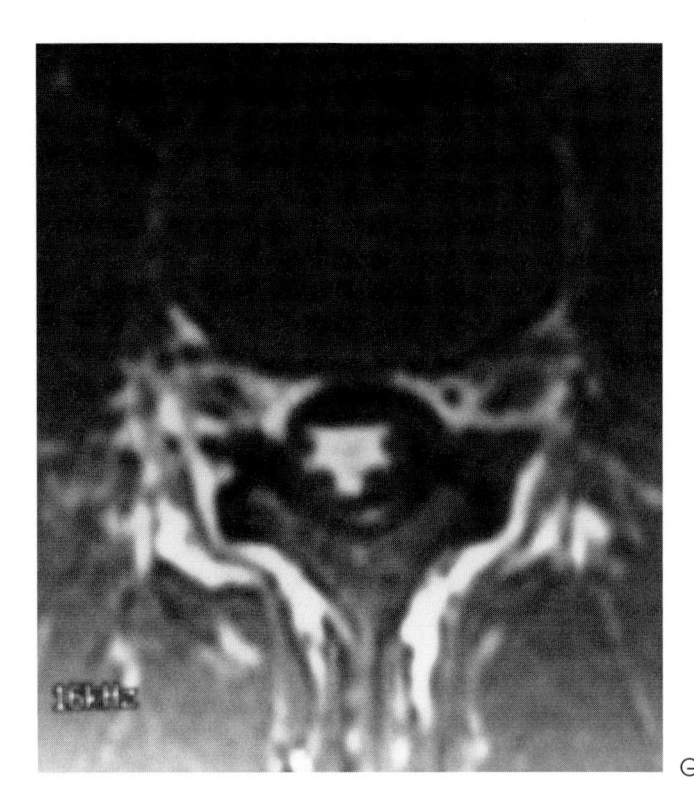

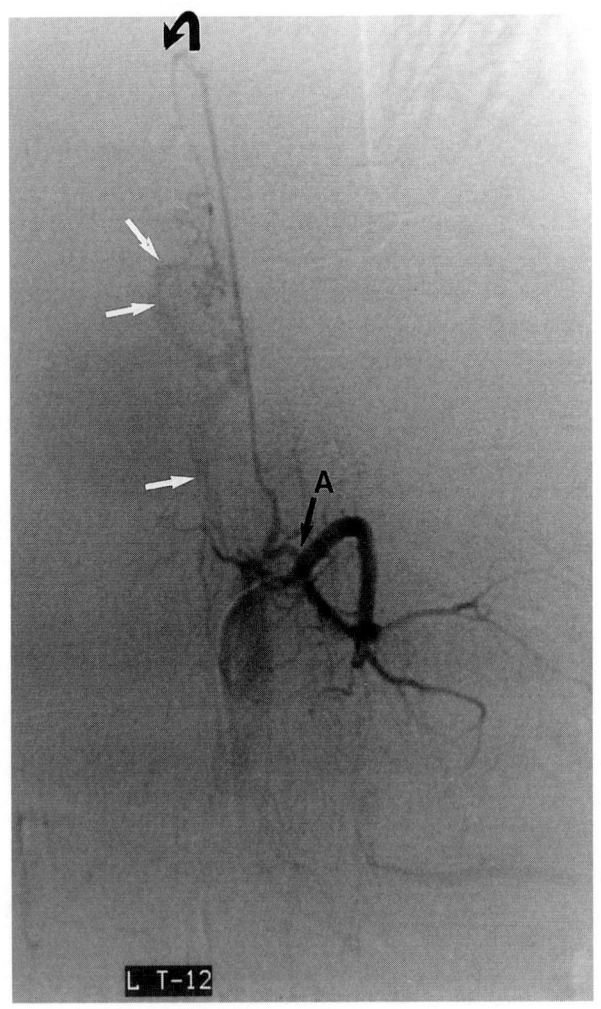

THORACIC SPINE

Radiologic Findings

Sagittal short TR image in the midthoracic spine (Fig. A) reveals a 1.2-cm oval area of increased signal intensity that projects posterior to the midbody of the T7 vertebral body (*arrow*).

Sagittal short TR image in the lower thoracic, upper lumbar region (Fig. B) reveals widening of the distal spinal cord at the level of the conus. The signal cord exhibits mottled signal intensity with multiple small dotlike areas of increased signal intensity with a faint halo of decreased signal intensity surrounding (*X*) them. There is a lobulated area of increased signal intensity dorsal to the thecal sac in the lower thoracic and upper lumbar region. This mass encroaches upon the distal thoracic and upper lumbar vertebral canal (*black arrows*). There is also a small, elongated, slightly lobulated area of increased signal intensity behind the vertebral body of L4 (*open arrow*) and patchy areas of illdefined increased signal intensity within the thecal sac (*white arrows*).

Midsagittal and parasagittal long TR images in the lower thoracic and upper lumbar regions (Figs. C and D) reveal variable increased and decreased signal intensity areas within the entire visualized vertebral canal. In addition, there are multiple internal areas of serpiginous decreased signal intensity.

Parasagittal short TR image in the upper lumbar region (Fig. E) reveals a dilated curvilinear vascular structure adjacent to the vertebral body (*arrow*).

Axial short TR image at the level of T12 (Fig. F) reveals a crescentic shaped area of increased signal intensity with a central area of decreased signal intensity dorsal to the spinal cord and within the thecal sac (*arrow*). The spinal cord is compressed and flattened and displaced anteriorly.

Axial short TR image at the level of L3 (Fig. G) reveals a stellate-shaped area of increased signal intensity within the central portion of lumbar thecal sac. The nerve roots of the cauda equina are displaced laterally around this area of increased signal intensity.

Digital angiogram of the left T12 intercostal artery (Fig. H) reveals an elongated arterial vessel (*A-arrow*) that initially courses cephalad, and then makes a sharp reversal of course (*curved black arrow*) to flow inferiorly. This vessel supplies an area of blush and is accompanied by an enlarged early draining venous structure (*white arrows*).

Diagnosis

Spinal cord arteriovenous malformation with subarachnoid hemorrhage and spinal cord ischemia.

Differential Diagnosis

- hemorrhagic tumor (unlikely)

- post-traumatic hemorrhage (unlikely)

PEARLS
- The artery of Adamkewicz typically arises from the intercostal artery on the left side at approximately the T9 level, but may arise from the midthoracic region through the lower lumbar region. Therefore, angiography may need to be performed of the entire length of the spinal cord if necessary to identify the blood supply to a vascular malformation.

- Magnetic resonance angiography has been attempted in the evaluation of the presence of a vascular malformation; however, angiography is necessary for complete evaluation.

TEACHING ATLAS OF SPINE IMAGING

> **PITFALL**
> - Angiography of multiple vessels is necessary for complete evaluation in these patients. Care must be taken at the time of angiography that the catheter tip does not occlude the entire blood vessel and result in an ischemia of the distal spinal cord.

Discussion

The catastrophic clinical presentation in this patient favors a vascular event such as hemorrhage. There is a small focal area of blood that projects anterior to the spinal cord in the midthoracic region. This blood is in the metabolic phase of methemoglobin and is therefore increased signal intensity on the short TR images. The entire distal thoracic and lumbar vertebral canal is filled with blood in varying stages of metabolism from deoxyhemoglobin to methemoglobin. The serpiginous areas of decreased signal intensity seen in Figures C and D are dilated draining veins flowing away from the malformation. The parasagittal image in Figure E reveals an enlarged draining vein flowing away from the malformation.

The artery supplying the arteriovenous malformation in this case arises from the left intercostal artery; it is the artery of Adamkewicz, which is the major vascular supply to the distal spinal cord.

Treatment of these patients includes direct surgical intervention with identification and occlusion of the supplying artery to the arteriovenous malformation. Occlusion of this supplying vessel may also be via interventional techniques with coils or glue to occlude the vessel that supplies the arteriovenous malformation.

The appearance and clinical presentation are typical of an arteriovenous malformation of the spinal cord.

Suggested Readings

Alvarez O, Roque CT, Pampati M. Multilevel thoracic disc herniations: CT and MR studies. *J Comput Assist Tomogr.* 1988;12:650.

Andersen NE, Willoughby EW. Infarction of the conus medullaris. *Ann Neurol.* 1987;21:470–474.

Berenstein A, Lasjaunias P. Endovascular treatment of spine and spinal cord lesions. In: *Surgical Neuro-Angiography.* Berlin: Springer-Verlag; 1992;5:1–85.

Bhole R, Gilmer RE. Two-level thoracic disc herniation. *Clin Orthop.* 1984;190:130.

Blumbergs PC, Byrne E. Hypotensive central infarction of the spinal cord. *J Neurol Neurosurg Psychiatry.* 1980;43:751–753.

Bowen BC, DePrima S, Pattany PM, et al. MR angiography of normal intradural vessels of the thoracolumbar spine. *AJNR.* 1996;17:483.

Cogen P, Stein BM. Spinal cord arteriovenous malformations with significant intramedullary component. *J Neurosurg.* 1983;59:471–478.

Djindjian R. Clinical symptomatology and natural history of arteriovenous malformation of the spinal cord: a study of the clinical aspects and prognosis, based on 150 cases. In: Pia HW, Djindjian R, eds. *Spinal Angiomas: Advances in Diagnosis and Therapy.* New York, NY: Springer-Verlag; 1978:48–83.

Djindjian R. Neuroradiological examination of spinal cord angiomas. In: Vinken PJ, Bruyn GW, eds. *Vascular Diseases of the Nervous System, Part II. Handbook of Clinical Neurology.* Vol. 12. Amsterdam: North-Holland; 1972, 631–643.

Djindjian R. *Angiographie de la Moelle Épinière.* Paris: Masson Edit.; 1970.

Dommisse GF. The arteries, arterioles, and capillaries of the spinal cord. Surgical guidelines in the prevention of postoperative paraplegia. *Ann R Coll Surg Engl.* 1980;62:369–376.

Dommisse GF. The blood supply of the spinal cord. *J Bone Joint Surg (Br).* 1974;56B:225–235.

Doppman JL, Di Chiro G, Ommaya AK. *Selective Arteriography of the Spinal Cord.* St. Louis, Missouri: Warren H. Green; 1969.

Dormont D, Gelbert F, Assouline E, et al. MR imaging of spinal cord arteriovenous malformations at 0.5T: study of 34 cases. *AJNR.* 1988;9:933–838.

Elliott JP, Szilogyi DE, Hageman JH, et al. Spinal cord ischemia: secondary to surgery of the abdominal aorta. In: Bernard VM, Towne JB, eds. *Complications in Vascular Surgery.* New York, NY: Grune & Stratton; 1985; 241–310.

Francavilla TL, Powers A, Dina T, Hugo V. MR imaging of thoracic disc herniations. *J Comput Assist Tomogr.* 1987;11:1063–1064.

Gueguen B, Merland JJ, Riche MC, Rey A. Vascular malformation of the spinal cord: intrathecal perimedullary arteriovenous fistulas fed by medullary arteries. *Neurology.* 1987;37:969–979.

Hurth M, Houdart R, Djindjian R, Rey A, Djindjian M. Arteriovenous malformations of the spinal cord. *Prog Neurol Surg.* 1978;9:238–266.

Kendall DE, Logue V. Spinal epidural angiomatous malformations draining into intrathecal veins. *Neuroradiol.* 1977;13:181–189.

Kulkarni MV, Burks DD, Price AC, et al. Diagnosis of spinal arteriovenous malformation in a pregnant patient by MR imaging. *J Comput Assist Tomogr.* 1985;9:171–173.

Masaryk TJ, Ross JS, Modic MT, Ruff RL, Selman WR, Ratcheson RA. Radiculomeningeal vascular malformations of the spine: MR imaging. *Radiology.* 1987;164:845–849.

Mascalchi M, Bianchi MC, Quilici N, et al. MR angiography of spinal vascular malformations. *AJNR.* 1995;16:289–297.

Merland JJ, Reizine D, Laurent A, et al. Embolization of the spinal cord vascular lesions. In: Viñuela F, Halbach VV, Dion JE, eds. *Interventional Neuroradiology: Endovascular Therapy of the Central Nervous System.* New York, NY: Raven Press; 1992:153–167.

Parizel PM, Rodesch G, Balériaux D, et al. Gd-DPTA-enhanced MR in thoracic disc herniations. *Neuroradiol.* 1989;31:75–79.

Provenzale JM, Tien RD, Felsberg GJ, Hacien-Bey L. Spinal dural arteriovenous fistula: demonstration using phase contrast MR an

Reagan TJ, Thomas JE, Colby MY. Chronic progressive radiation myelopathy. *JAMA.* 1968;203:128–132.

Resnick D, Niwayama G. Intravertebral disc herniations: cartilaginous (Schmorl's) nodes. *Radiology.* 1978;126:57–65.

Riche MC, Reizine D, Melki JP, Merland JJ. Classification of spinal cord malformations. *Radiat Med.* 1985;3:17–24.

Rosemblum B, Oldfield EH, Doppman JL, Di Chiro G. Spinal arteriovenous malformations: a comparison of dural arteriovenous fistula and intradual AVMs in 81 patients. *J Neurosurg.* 1987;67:795–802.

Ryan RW, Lally JF, Kozic Z. Asymptomatic calcified herniated thoracic discs: CT recognition. *AJNR.* 1988;9:364–365.

Terwey B, Becker H, Thron AK, Vahldiek G. Gadolinium-DPTA enhanced MR imaging of spinal dural arteriovenous fistulas. *J Comput Assist Tomogr.* 1989;13:30–37.

Van Duym FC van A, van Wiechen PJ. Herniation of calcified nucleus pulposus in the thoracic spine. *J Comput Assist Tomogr.* 1983;7:1123.

Section X

Lumbar Discs

Section X

Lumbar Discs

LUMBAR DISCS

Case 1

Clinical Presentation

The patient is a 37-year-old female with a clinical history of back pain, extremity pain, and numbness.

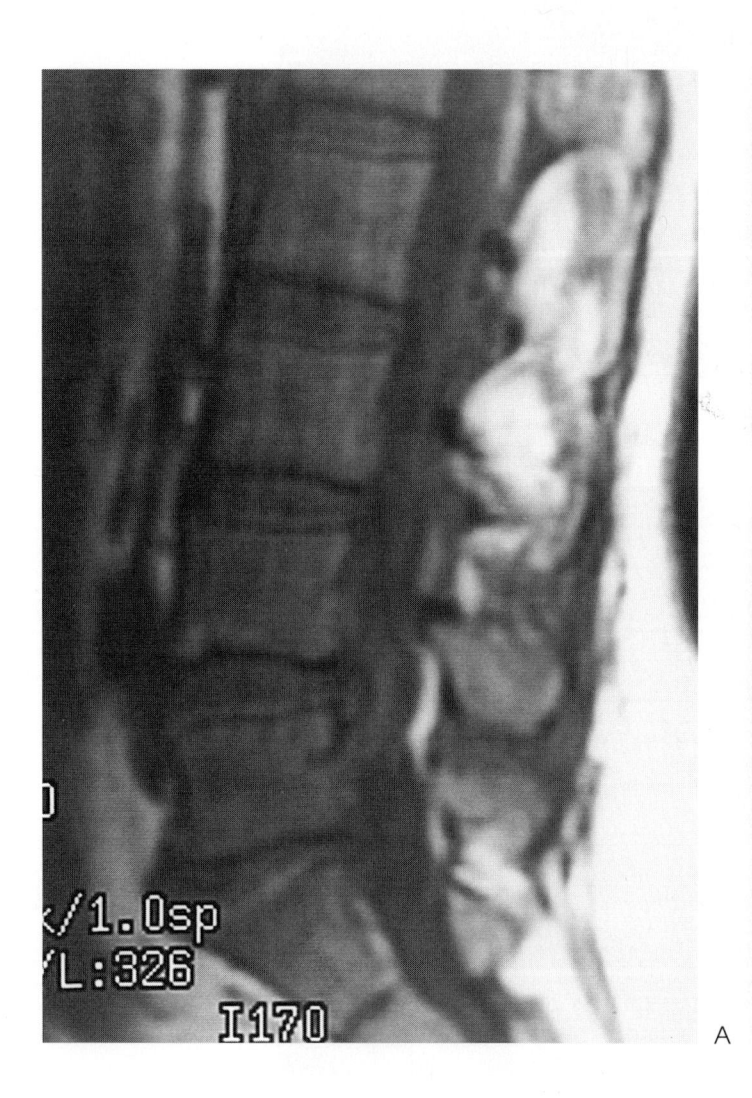

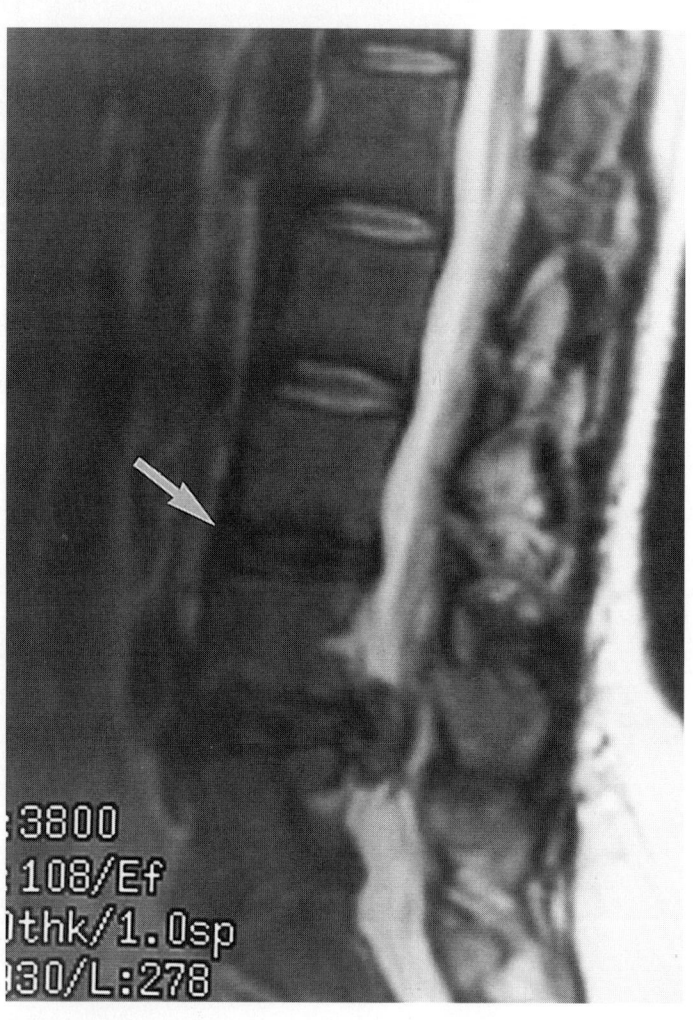

Radiologic Findings

Sagittal short TR image (Fig. A) reveals what appears to be a moderately large soft tissue mass projecting behind the intervertebral disc at the L4-5 level.

Sagittal long TR image (Fig. B) reveals that the soft tissue fragment is much larger than is apparent on the short TR image. There is essentially complete obliteration of the subarachnoid space at this level. In addition, there is decreased signal intensity of the intervertebral discs at L3-4 (*arrow*).

TEACHING ATLAS OF SPINE IMAGING

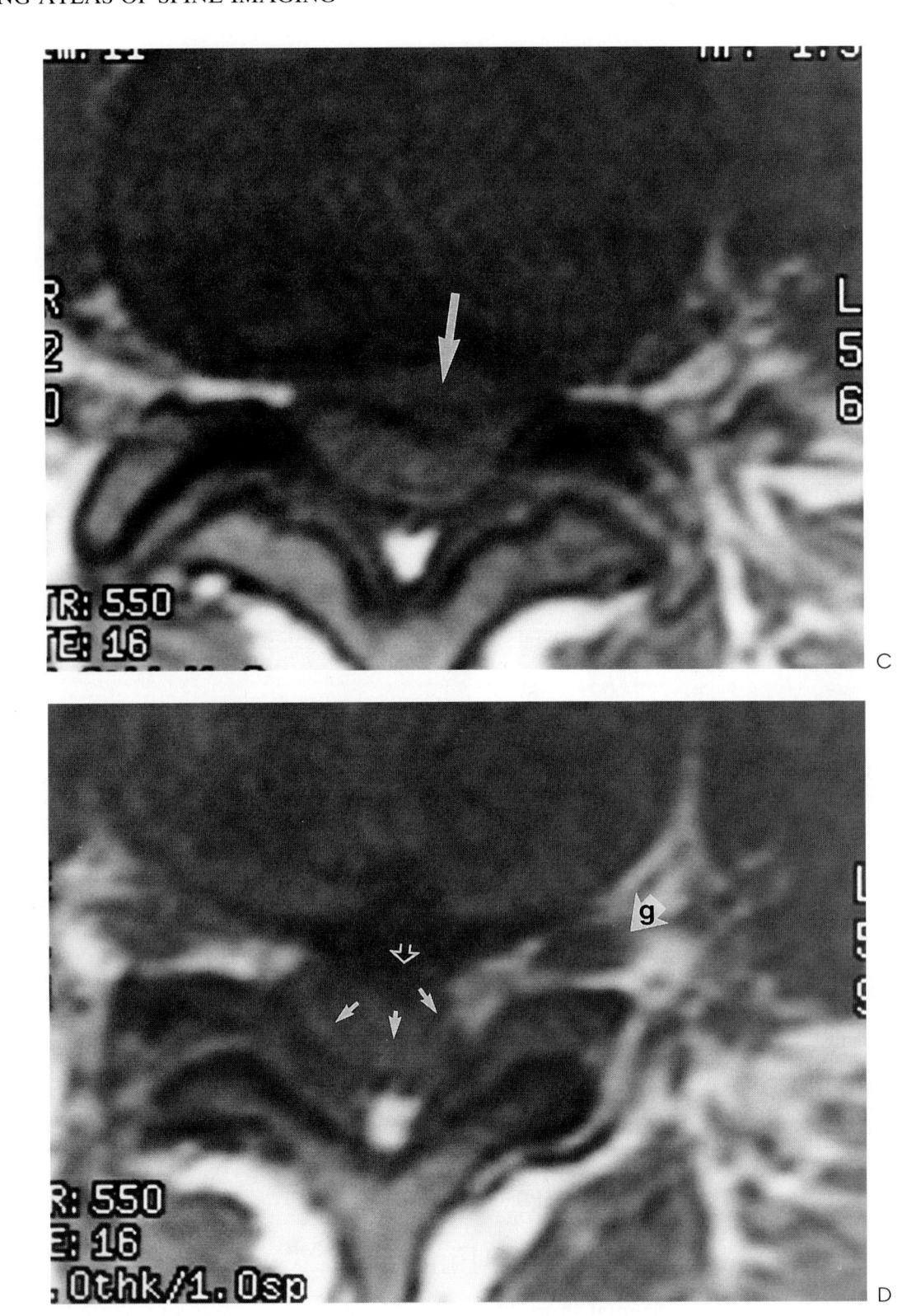

LUMBAR DISCS

PEARLS

- The evaluation of degenerative disc disease should include the use of long TR images. The long TR images duplicate the lateral view of the myelogram with the cerebrospinal fluid now appearing increased signal intensity on the MR images and high density on the myelogram images. The long TR images also allow the identification of decreased signal intensity discs which may be the source of back pain even in the patient who does not have a herniated disc.

- Because of the posterior longitudinal ligament, herniated discs occur only rarely in the midline; herniations occur more commonly off to the right or left side.

PITFALLS

- CT better demonstrates the area of bone fracture from the vertebral body if this is present.

- With CT imaging, a very large herniated disc may completely obliterate the vertebral canal. The resulting homogeneous density of the disc may mimic the appearance of the normal thecal sac and result in the failure to appreciate the presence of a large herniated disc.

Radiologic Findings (continued)

Axial short TR image at the level of the intervertebral disc (Fig. C) reveals a midline and slight left paracentral herniated disc (*arrow*) which causes curvilinear distortion of the thecal sac.

Axial short TR image just below the level of the intervertebral disc (Fig. D) reveals the large herniated disc which has an area of lower signal intensity just behind the vertebral body (*arrowhead*) and a larger component which extends posteriorly into the vertebral canal (*small arrows*) and essentially obliterates the vertebral canal. The thecal sac is compressed posteriorly into a crescentic configuration. The dorsal root ganglion is seen in the intervertebral foramen (*arrow-g*).

Diagnosis

Large herniated disc at the L4-5 level. Degenerated discs at the L3-4 and L5-S1 levels.

Differential Diagnosis

- herniated disc

Discussion

The herniated portion of the disc can be seen projecting behind the posterior margins of the vertebral bodies of L4 and L5. In Figure D, the decreased signal intensity midline and slightly paracentral mass is caused by a small avulsion fracture from the posterior margin of the vertebral body. This fracture occurs from the force of the herniation which is located adjacent to the posterior margin of the vertebral body. This fracture fragment is easily demonstrated by computed tomographic (CT) scanning, which is sensitive to bone density, but is difficult to demonstrate with certainty by magnetic resonance (MR) scanning.

The decreased signal intensity of the L3-4, L4-5, and L5-S1 intervertebral discs is consistent with degeneration and dehydration of these discs. Patchy areas of decreased signal intensity within the intervertebral discs area consistent with vacuum degenerative change or areas of calcification of the disc.

Case 2

Clinical Presentation

The patient is a 35-year-old male with sudden onset of low back and right leg pain.

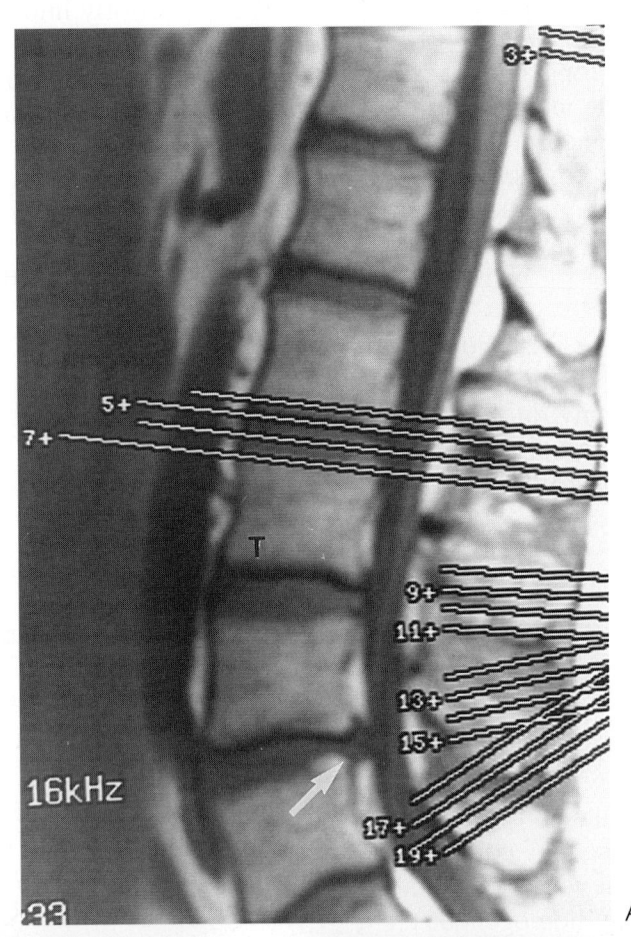

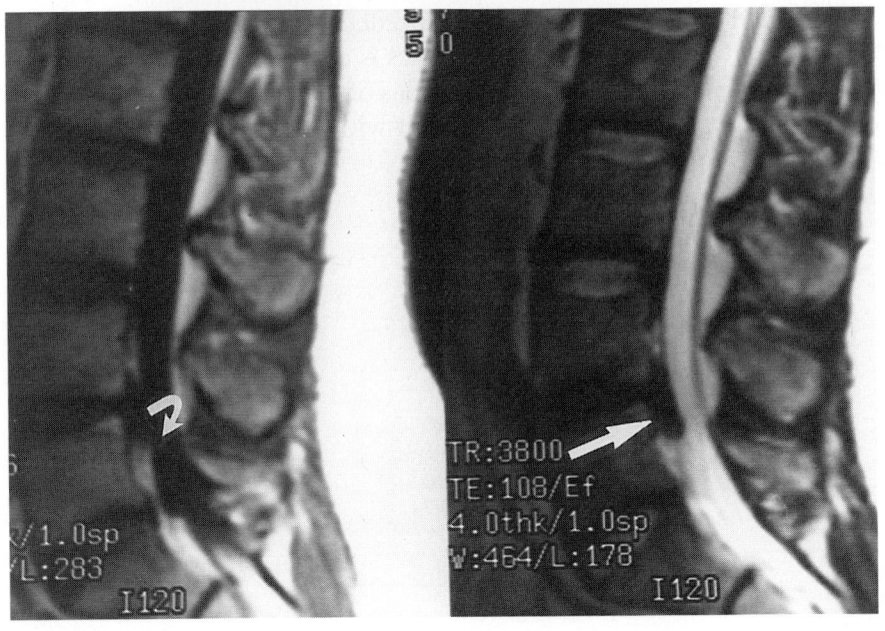

LUMBAR DISCS

C

D

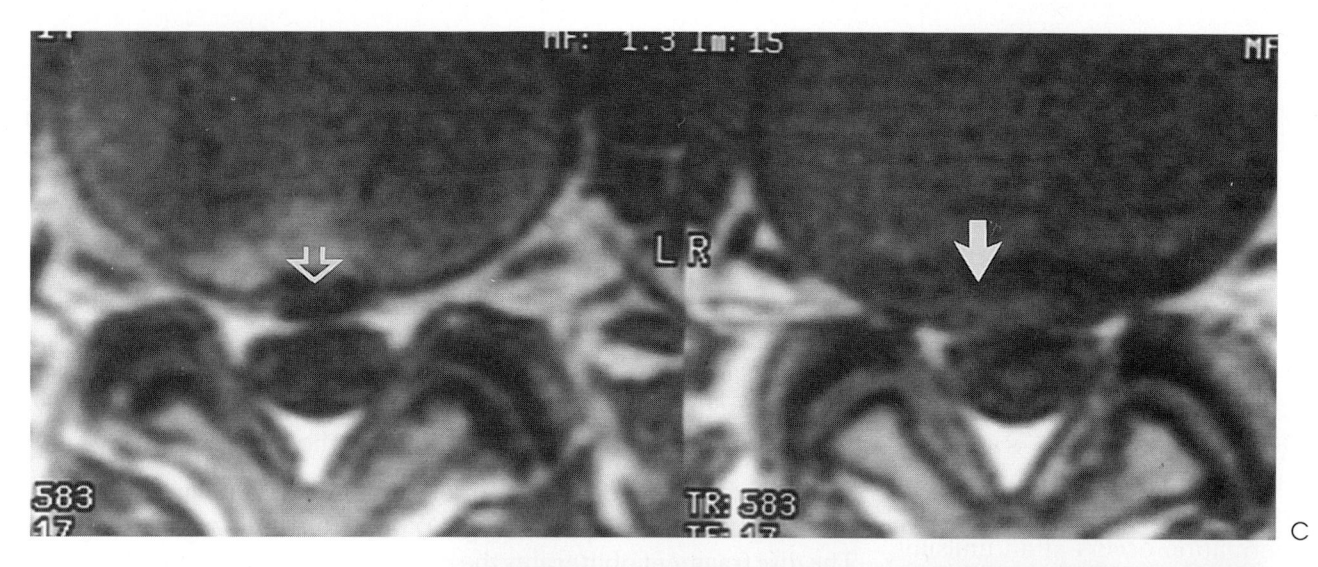

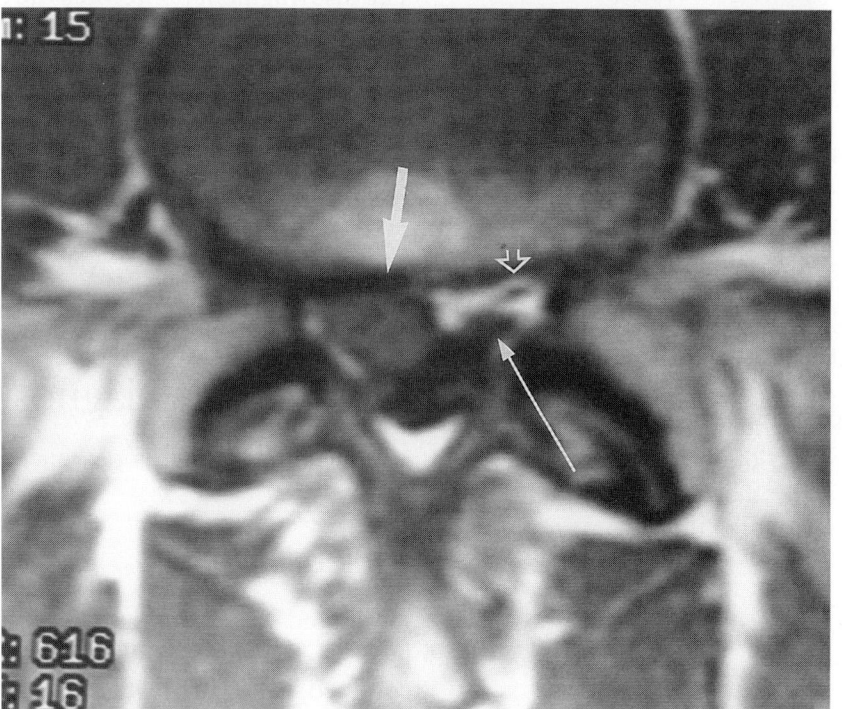

Radiologic Findings

Multiangle images for evaluation of the lumbar intervertebral discs (Fig. A). Multiangle slices are obtained in addition to routine parallel slices through the lumbar spine. These slices should include the symptomatic levels and/or the lowest three intervertebral disc levels, as well as any other abnormal appearing level.

There is a soft tissue prominence at the L4-5 level (*arrow*). The third lumbar vertebral body is identified with T.

Sagittal short (Fig. B, *left*) and long (Fig. B, *right*) TR images reveal a herniated disc at the L4-5 level. The short TR image reveals that the disc has herniated and extruded below the level of the disc at the L4-5 level.

Radiologic Findings (continued)

The curvilinear arrow (*left*) identifies the direction of the disc as it herniates below the disc level. The long TR image on the right reveals the herniated disc as decreased signal intensity and projecting below the level of the intervertebral disc (*arrow*).

Axial short TR images just above (Fig. C, *left*) and at the level of the intervertebral disc level (Fig. C, *right*) reveal the herniated midline disc projecting just above the level of the disc (*left, open arrow*) and in the midline and slightly off toward the right (*right, arrow*). The herniated disc obliterates the anterior epidural increased signal intensity fat (*arrow on right*) and extends beyond the margin of the vertebral body.

Just below the level of the intervertebral disc, a large fragment of the herniated nucleus pulposus (Fig. D) projects on the right side (*thick arrow*). The disc fragment obliterates the epidural fat, displaces the thecal sac posteriorly, and compresses it. The disc also encroaches upon the normal nerve root in the lateral recess. The normal nerve root sleeve can be seen on the left side (*thin arrow*). A small rounded area of decreased signal intensity projects just posterior to the vertebral body (*open arrow*).

Diagnosis

Herniated, extruded disc.

Differential Diagnosis

- herniated disc: The appearance is typical of a herniated disc.

Discussion

Herniated discs can migrate superior to or, more commonly, inferior to the level of the intervertebral disc. Therefore, imaging slices should not be confined just to the level of the intervertebral disc, but should extend above and below the level of the disc. A good rule to follow for imaging is to include the levels from one vertebral pedicle to the next. In general, imaging should include parallel contiguous slices beginning at the level of the midbody of L3 and extending inferiorly to the level of the midbody of S1. These images are accompanied by angled slices that extend through the individual intervertebral discs. These should be angled in such a way that the slices parallel the angle of the intervertebral disc. This is illustrated in Figure A.

The small area of decreased signal intensity posterior to the vertebral body in Figure D is the flow void of the anterior, internal vertebral view.

The more recent addition of helical computed tomographic (CT) scanning allows more rapid evaluation of the spine than was previously possible. Because of this, imaging of the spine may now conveniently include all of the intervertebral discs in the lumbar region. This is particularly helpful in cases of spinal stenosis, where it is recommended that all lumbar intervertebral discs should be evaluated.

PEARLS

- Herniated discs may occur at any level of the vertebral column. However, when a disc herniation occurs at an unusual level such as the lower thoracic or upper lumbar region or at an unusual location such as medial to the vertebral pedicle, the disc may be mistaken for a schwannoma or even a metastatic deposit.

- Although unusual, discs may even migrate to a location dorsal to the thecal sac.

- Rarely, a herniated disc may pierce the dura and rest inside of the thecal sac. Such an intrathecal disc is unusual, but when present, mimics the appearance of a schwannoma, neurofibroma, or even a meningioma or drop metastasis.

PITFALL

- If a herniated, sequestered disc is closely applied to the posterior margin of the vertebral body, it may be difficult to identify. In a patient with positive signs and symptoms it is helpful to perform both MR and CT. It may be necessary to perform CT after the instillation of contrast material in the subarachnoid space.

LUMBAR DISCS

Case 3

Clinical Presentation

The patient is a 38-year-old male with sudden onset of left leg pain and low back pain.

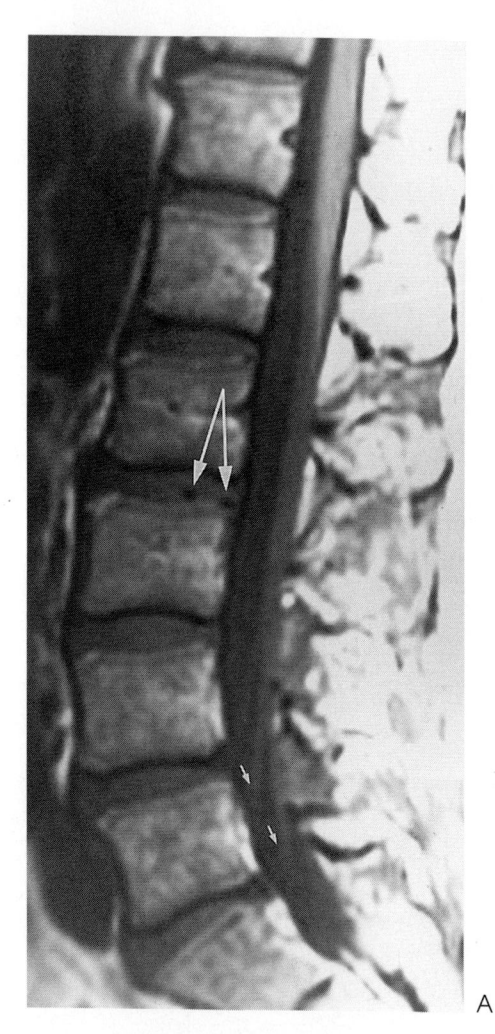

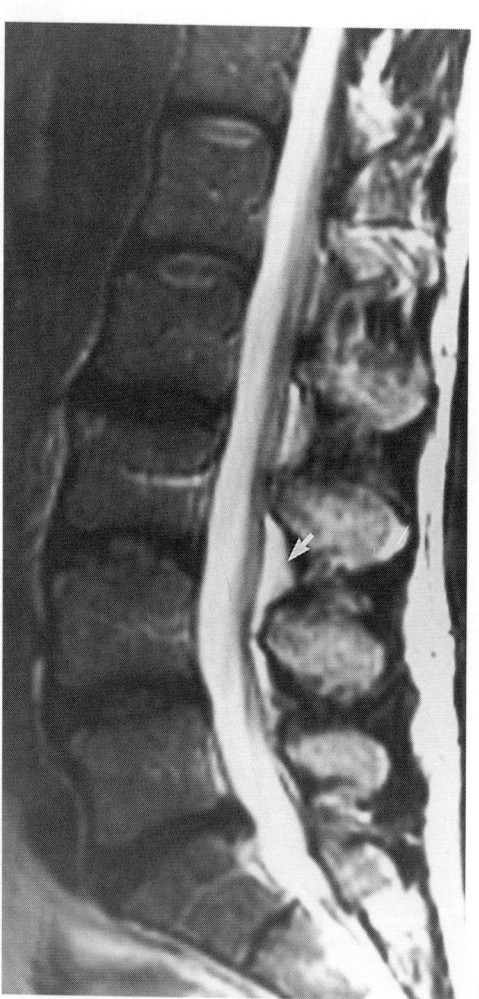

Radiologic Findings

Sagittal short TR image (Fig. A) reveals two small areas of decreased signal intensity in the posterior portions of the intervertebral disc at the L2-3 level (*long arrows*). There is a slight retrolisthesis of L5 on S1. There is slight disc space narrowing at the L5-S1 level. The individual nerves of the cauda equina appear as stringlike areas of intermediate signal intensity surrounded by decreased signal intensity cerebrospinal fluid (*short arrows*).

Sagittal long TR image (Fig. B) reveals decreased signal intensity of the lowest four lumbar intervertebral discs. There is a prominent soft tissue density mass at the L5-S1 level which protrudes into the vertebral canal. The normal high signal intensity epidural fat appears as a triangular shaped area of increased signal intensity (*arrow*).

TEACHING ATLAS OF SPINE IMAGING

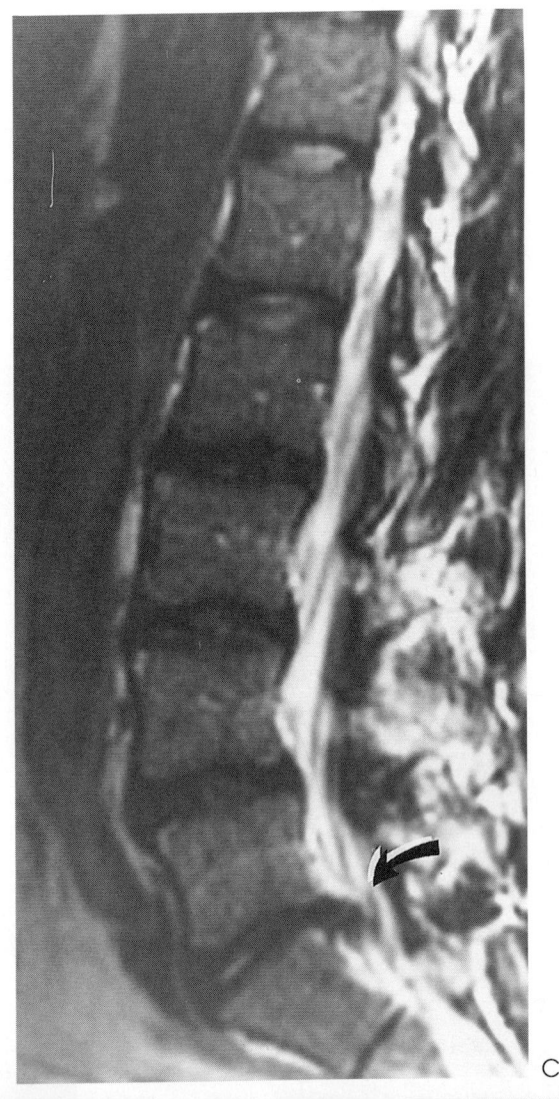

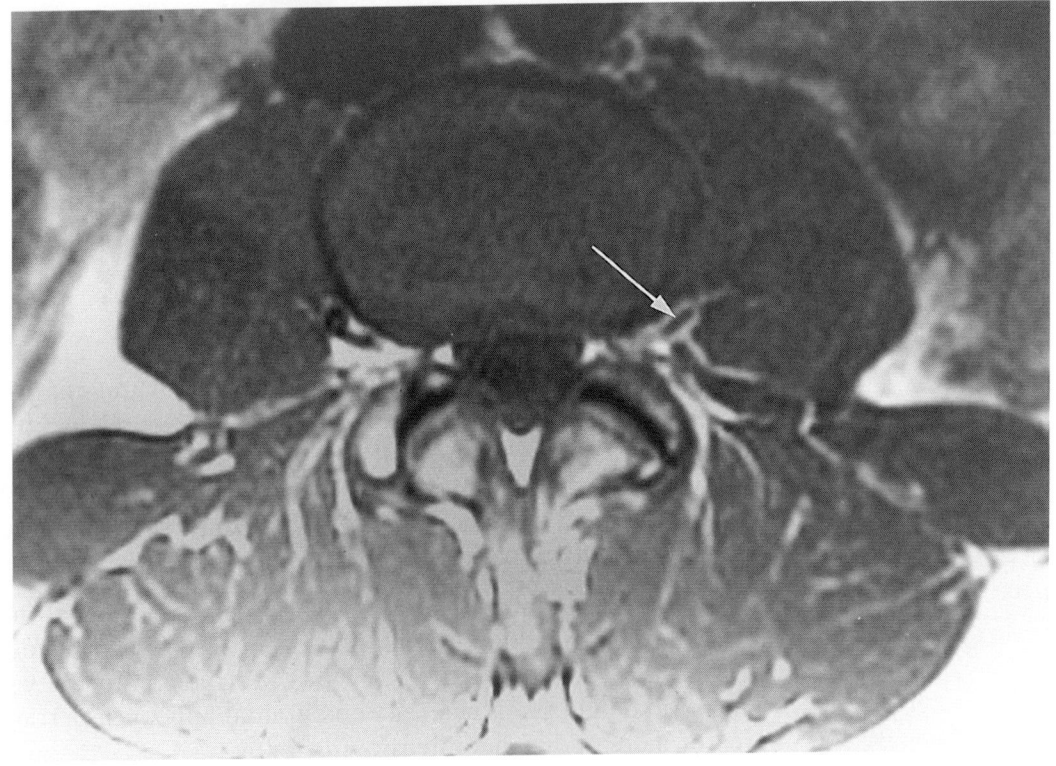

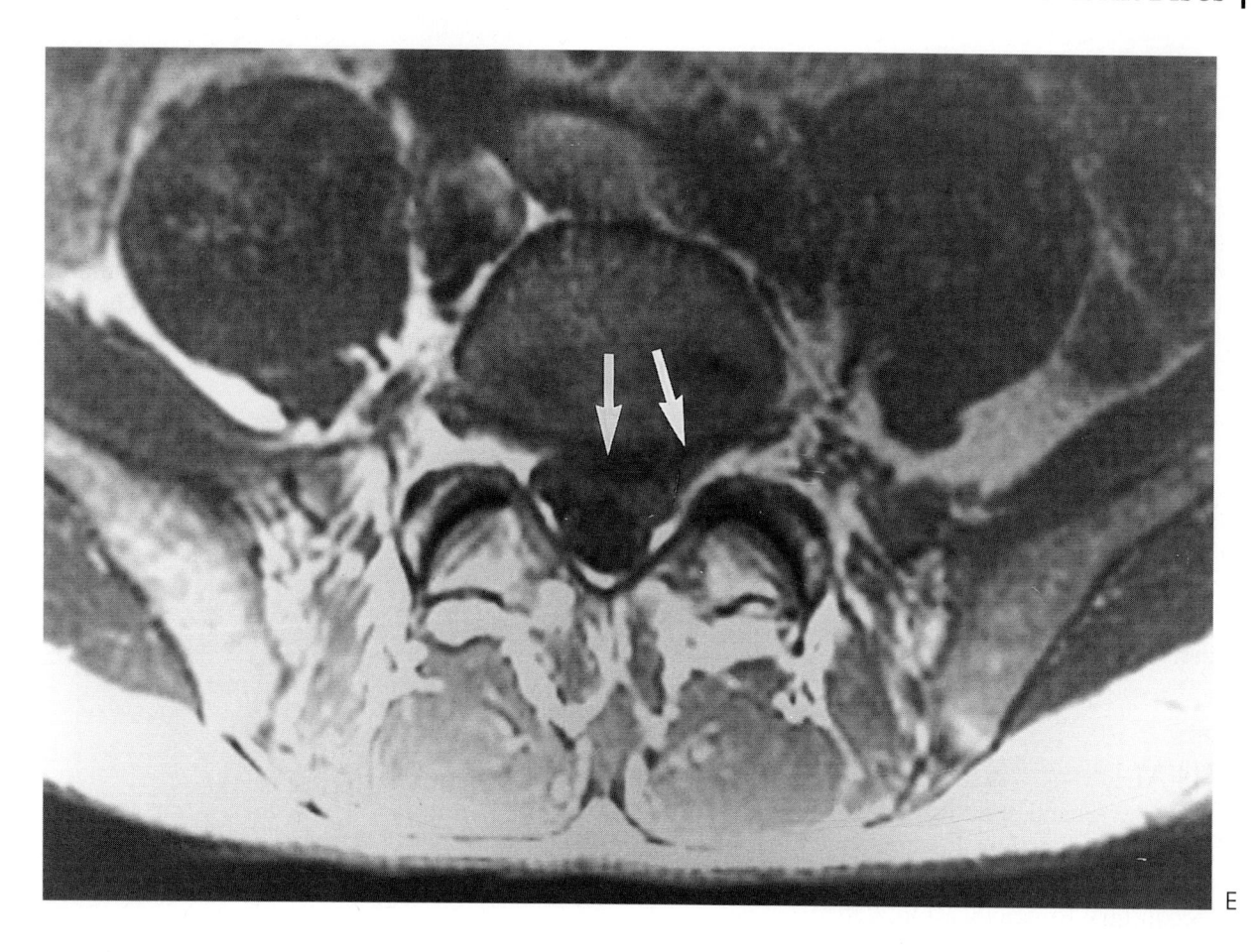

LUMBAR DISCS

E

Radiologic Findings (continued)

Parasagittal long TR image (Fig. C) reveals that the soft tissue mass at the L5-S1 level appears more prominent laterally than in the midline. The nerve root of the cauda equina appears as a stringlike area of decreased signal intensity which follows a curvilinear course around the soft tissue mass at the L5-S1 level (*curved arrow*).

Axial short TR image (Fig. D) reveals a normal appearing intervertebral disc configuration at the L3-4 level. The normal nerve can be seen surrounded by high signal intensity perineural fat (*arrow*).

Axial short TR image (Fig. E) reveals a soft tissue mass that obliterates the normal high signal intensity epidural fat at the L5-S1 level in the midline and off toward the left side (*arrows*).

Diagnosis

Laterally herniated disc at the L5-S1 level.

Differential Diagnosis

- herniated disc: The appearance is typical of a herniated disc.

TEACHING ATLAS OF SPINE IMAGING

PEARLS

- In this patient, the conspicuity of the disc is much greater on the long TR images than in the short TR images. In addition, the intervertebral disc appears relatively normal on the short TR images but reveals definite decreased signal intensity on the long TR images reflecting the presence of loss of hydration of the disc and early degenerative changes.

- Long TR images should be obtained in patients being evaluated for a possible herniated disc.

PITFALL

- The decreased signal intensity of the intervertebral disc at the L2-3 level could also be secondary to calcification. CT (computed tomography) is much more sensitive to the presence of calcification than magnetic resonance. CT also allows more ready differentiation between calcification and vacuum degenerative changes.

Discussion

In addition to a large herniated disc at the L5-S1 level, there are degenerated discs at all four of the lowest intervertebral disc levels. This is reflected as decreased signal intensity of the intervertebral disc on the long TR images because of loss of fluid. The small areas of decreased signal intensity in the intervertebral disc at the L2-3 level (Fig A) represent small areas of vacuum degenerative change within the intervertebral disc. The posterior displacement of the nerve root seen in Figure C is similar to that which would be seen myelographically.

LUMBAR DISCS

Case 4

Clinical Presentation

The patient is a 29-year-old male with severe low back and left leg pain.

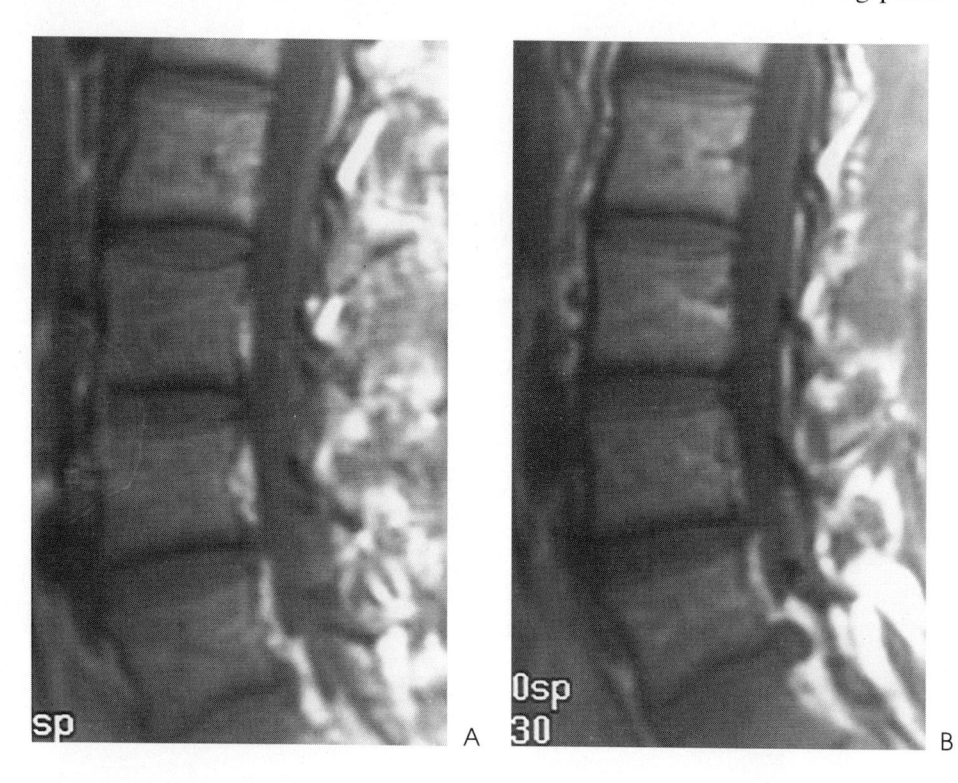

Radiologic Findings

Right parasagittal short TR image of the lumbar spine (Fig. A) reveals minimal prominence of the intervertebral disc at the L5-S1 level but is otherwise normal.

Left parasagittal short TR image (Fig. B) reveals an intermediate signal intensity, soft tissue mass at the L5-S1 level. The mass is laterally positioned and is surrounded by increased signal intensity perineural fat. There is also a mild prominence of the intervertebral disc at the L4-5 level.

TEACHING ATLAS OF SPINE IMAGING

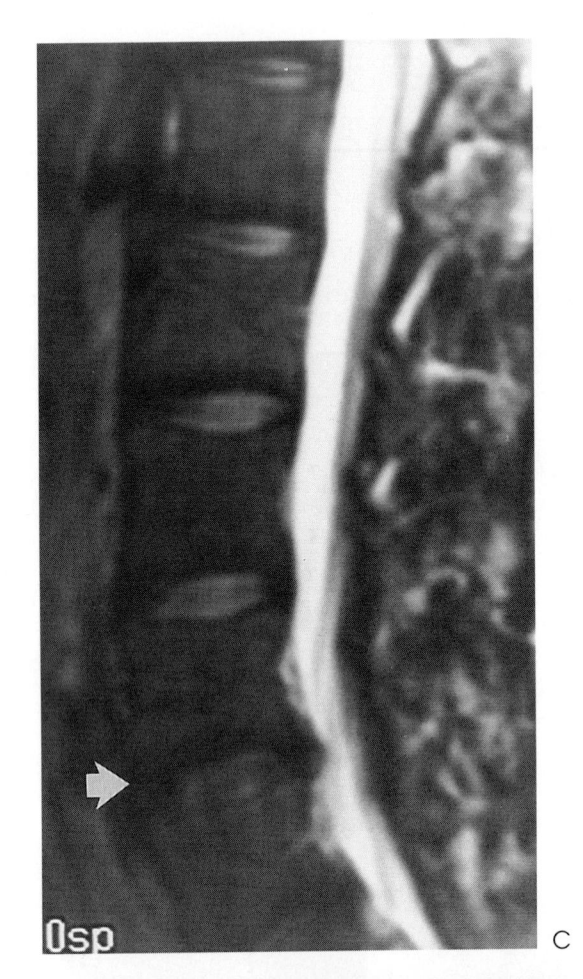

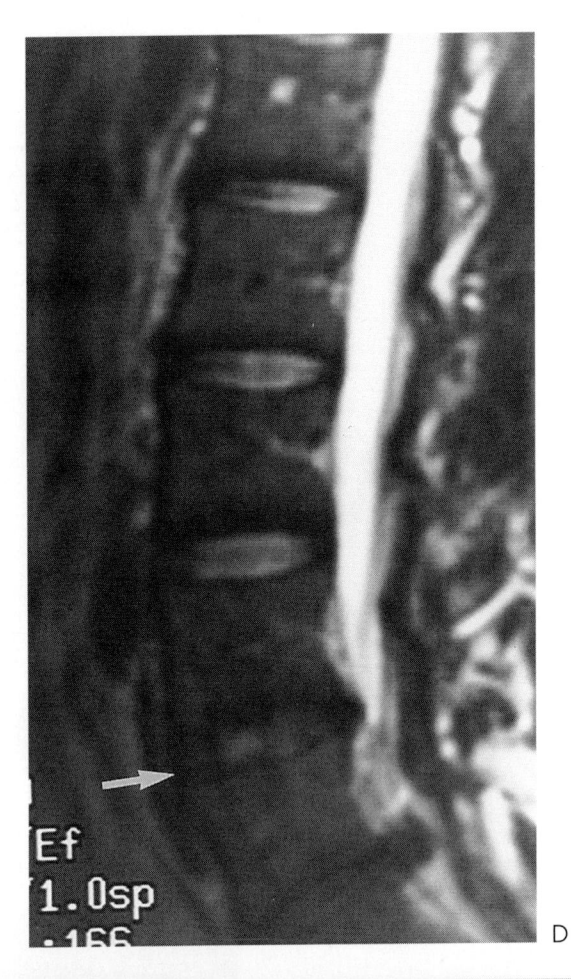

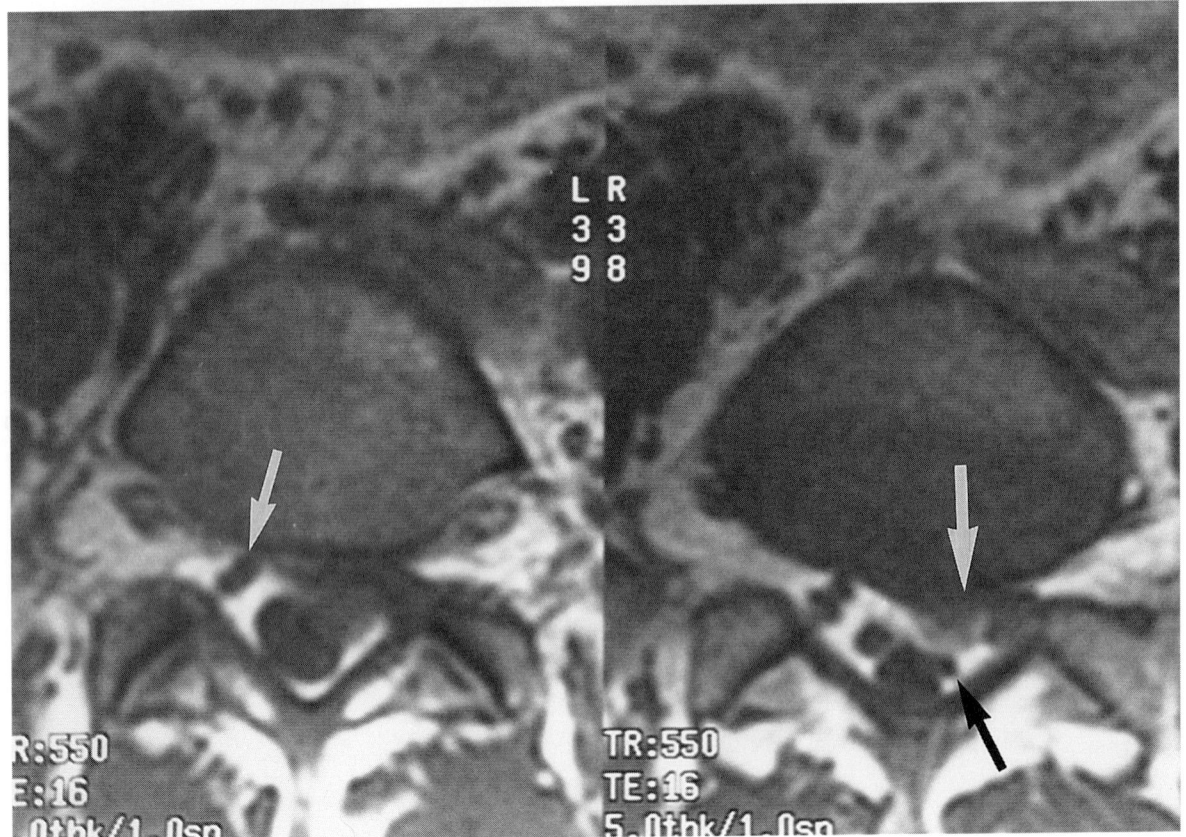

LUMBAR DISCS

Radiologic Findings (continued)

Midsagittal long TR image with fast spin echo technique (Fig. C) reveals that the intervertebral disc at the L4-5 level appears decreased signal intensity (*arrow*). There is narrowing of the intervertebral disc at the L5-S1 level.

Left parasagittal long TR image with fast spin echo technique (Fig. D) reveals the moderate sized disc at the L4-5 level (*arrow*) and the large soft tissue mass at the L5-S1 level. There is disc space narrowing at and decreased signal intensity of the L4-5 and L5-S1 intervertebral discs.

Axial short TR images just above (Fig. E, *left*) and at the level of the intervertebral disc of L5-S1 (Fig. E, *right*) reveal the left lateral soft tissue mass. There is obliteration of the normal nerve root and high signal intensity epidural fat on the left side by a large soft tissue mass (*white arrow, right image*). The normal right nerve root sleeve is identified on the right and is surrounded by high signal intensity perineural fat (*white arrow, left image*). At the level of the intervertebral disc (*right*), the normal root can be seen on the right side. There is a soft tissue density mass on the left side which obliterates the normal epidural high signal intensity fat (*right image, white arrow*). On the left side, the nerve root can be seen to be compressed and displaced posteriorly (*right image, black arrow*). Note the normal lemon shape of the L-5 vertebral body.

Diagnosis

Large left paracentral herniated disc at L5-S1 and a moderately sized disc at the L4-5 level.

Differential Diagnosis

- herniated disc: The appearance is typical of a herniated disc

Discussion

Herniated discs are most common at the L 4-5 and L5-S1 levels. In this patient, there are abnormal discs at both of these levels. The magnetic resonance (MR) findings of effacement of the thecal sac, compression of the nerve root sleeve, and posterior displacement of the nerve root reflect the findings that are seen by myelography.

PEARLS

- The normal perineural and epidural increased signal intensity fat provides an excellent contrast material in MRI. By computed tomographic (CT) evaluation, the fat is low density and is also useful for diagnosis; however, MR provides more contrast than CT, and the conspicuity of the epidural fat signal intensity is more readily demonstrated by MR than by CT.

- Note that when using the long TR fast spin echo technique the normally high signal remains high signal intensity, whereas when using the standard, routine long TR images, the normal high signal intensity fat becomes lower in signal intensity.

PITFALLS

- It is important to determine the laterality of a herniated disc so that a proper surgical approach can be planned.

- If there are abnormal discs at two or more levels, they should be clearly reported so that surgery may be performed at all levels of involvement.

TEACHING ATLAS OF SPINE IMAGING

C

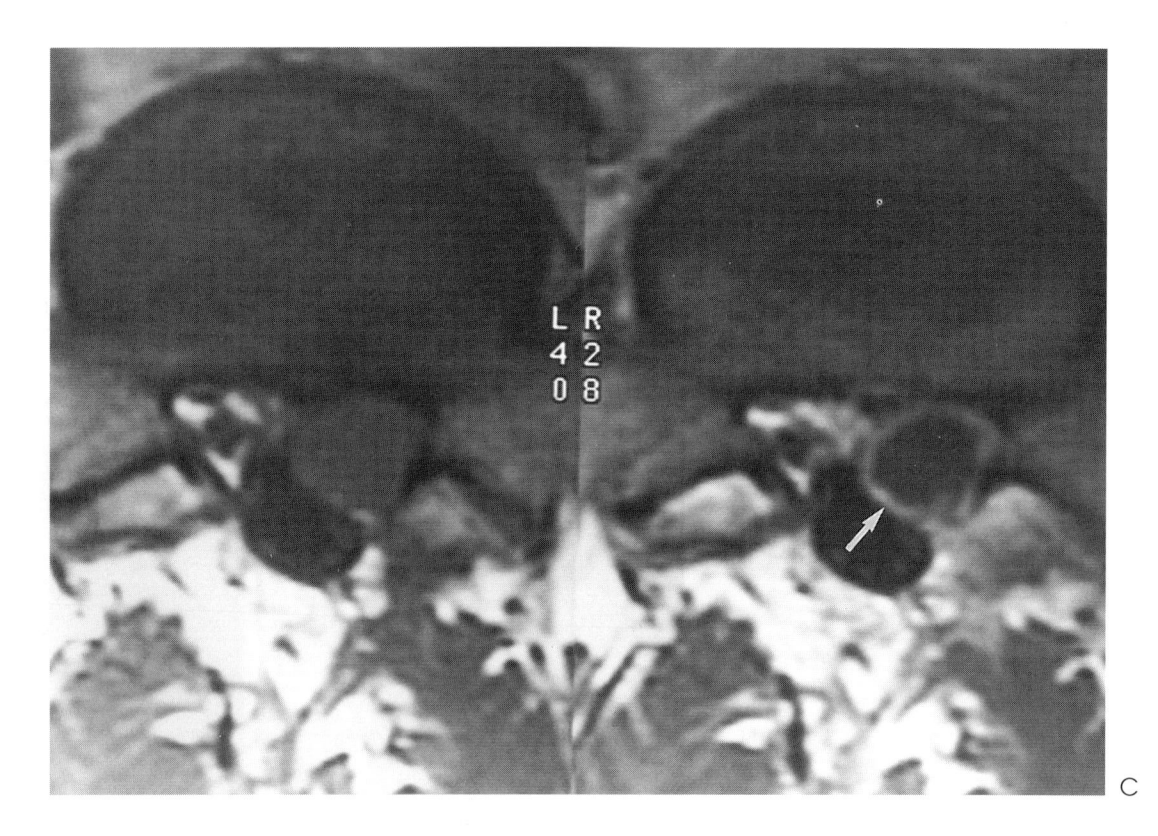

PEARLS

- The use of contrast enhancement allows better definition of the extent of the disc herniation. The enhancement is thought to be secondary to granulation tissue which surrounds the herniated disc and develops because of reaction to the disc.

- Magnetic resonance is the ideal method for follow-up of patients with recurrent herniated discs.

- If arachnoiditis is a clinical consideration in the postoperative patient, contrast material should be used. The study may reveal clumping of the nerve roots of the cauda equina or adherence of the nerve roots to the peripheral margins of the thecal sac. These areas may occasionally reveal enhancement postcontrast.

Radiologic Findings

Sagittal short (Fig. A, *left*) and long (Fig. A, *right*) TR images reveal a very large, intermediate signal intensity, soft tissue mass the L5-S1 level. The mass can be seen extruding posteriorly into the vertebral canal (*arrows*). There is disc space narrowing at this level and slightly decreased signal intensity on the adjacent vertebral body end plates. There is posterior bulging of the posterior margin of the thecal sac because there is a postoperative pseudomeningocele. High signal intensity fat (F) secondary to the previous surgery is seen dorsally at the L5 level (*right, arrows*).

Pre- (Fig. B, *left*) and postcontrast (Fig. B, *right*) sagittal short TR images reveal a rim of enhancement around the peripheral margin of the soft tissue mass.

Pre- (Fig. C, *left*) and postcontrast (Fig. C, *right*) axial short TR images reveal the large soft tissue mass which extends posteriorly into the vertebral canal. There is compression of the cerebrospinal fluid containing thecal sac and complete obliteration of the epidural fat at this level. There has been a bilateral complete laminectomy; therefore, the lamina of the vertebral body is not seen on either side. On postcontrast enhancement (*right*), a well-defined peripheral rim of enhancement can be seen outlining the large soft tissue mass (*arrow*). It is the absence of the vertebral lamina that allows the dura to bulge posteriorly and creates the pseudomeningocele.

Diagnosis

Large recurrent herniated disc fragment with peripheral enhancement.

LUMBAR DISCS

> **PITFALLS**
> - In a chronically herniated disc, the capillary ingrowth may extend through the herniated fragment and result in homogeneous enhancement. This homogeneous enhancement may then have the appearance of scar tissue rather than a herniated disc. Scar tissue enhances homogeneously in most cases. Occasionally, when there is a chronic retracted scar, there may be only peripheral enhancement of the scar. Therefore, clinical history and clinical correlation are very important for diagnosis.
>
> - A final combination is that of a herniated disc plus the presence of scar formation with any possible enhancement pattern.

Differential Diagnosis

- large recurrent herniated disc: A large recurrent disc herniation is uncommon following surgery because a large portion of the nucleus pulposus is removed at the time of surgery.

Discussion

In general, contrast material is not used in the diagnosis of a herniated disc. However, when contrast material is used, it may help to better define the margin of the herniated disc. As in this case, the peripheral rim of enhancement defines the outer margin of the herniated disc and defines the separation between the disc and the thecal sac. In general, only the peripheral margin of a disc exhibits enhancement. When there is scar tissue present following surgery, there is generally homogeneous enhancement of the scar tissue. Thus, contrast enhancement is recommended in all cases where there has been previous surgery.

The decreased signal intensity of the vertebral body end plates adjacent to the intervertebral disc is secondary to edema of the bone marrow. This therefore becomes increased signal intensity on the long TR images. On the axial images (Fig. C), there is increased signal intensity soft tissue dorsally to the thecal sac; this occurs because at surgery the epidural space is filled with fat.

TEACHING ATLAS OF SPINE IMAGING

Case 7

Clinical Presentation

The patient is a 31-year-old female with low back pain radiating to the left leg and into the left foot. The patient is status post lumbar laminectomy.

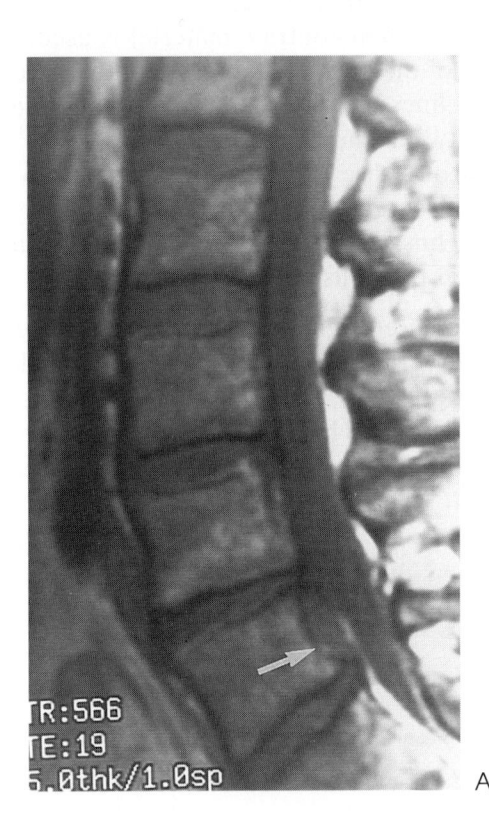

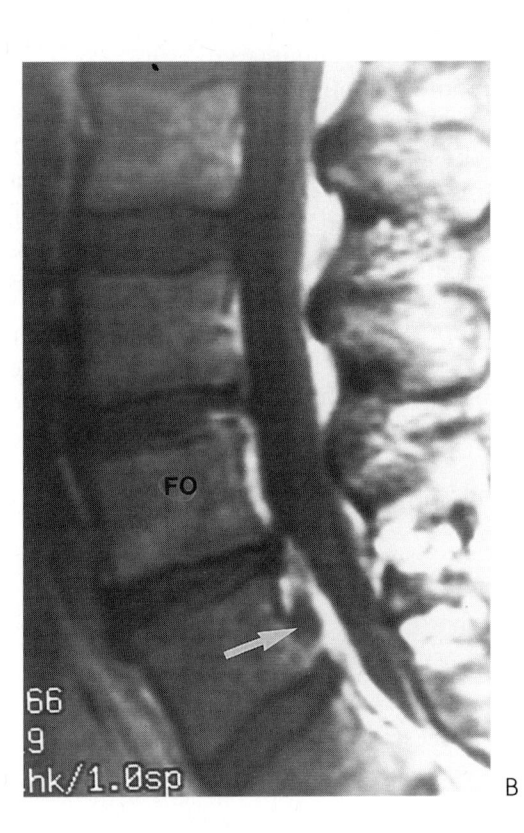

Radiologic Findings

Sagittal short TR image of the lumbar spine (Fig. A) reveals a soft tissue density mass that projects behind the L5 vertebral body (*arrow*).

Sagittal short TR image postcontrast (Fig. B) reveals a curvilinear line of enhancement surrounding the soft tissue density mass (*arrow*). The L4 vertebral body is identified with FO.

LUMBAR DISCS

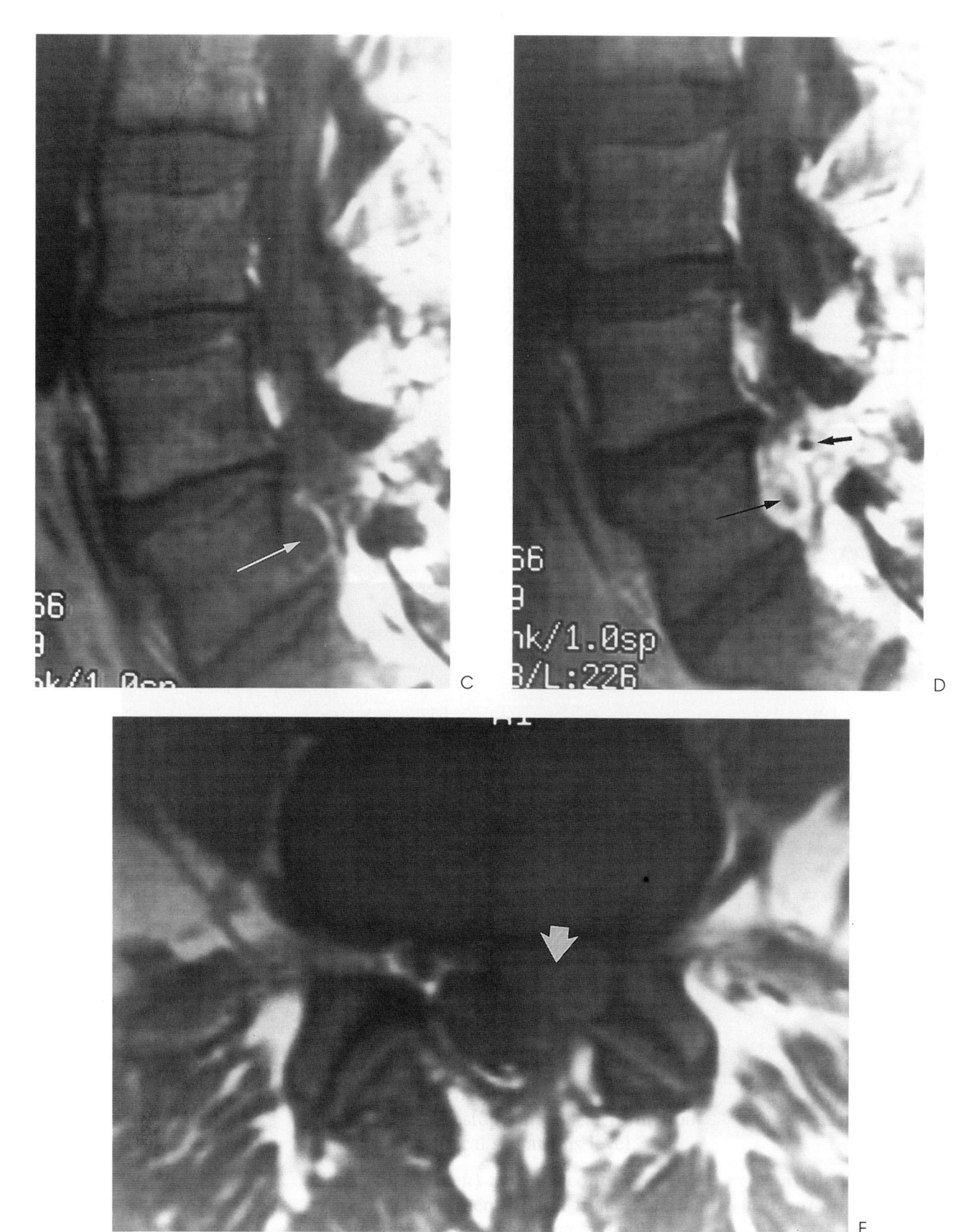

641

PEARLS

- An accurate description of this type of migrated disc should be provided so that an adequate surgical approach may be planned, the disc fragment identified at the level of the vertebral pedicle and removed.

- Patients with laterally herniated discs typically have severe radicular pain because the disc compresses the nerve root in the region of the lateral recess (in this case) or in the region of the intervertebral foramen.

PITFALL

- A synovial cyst could have a similar appearance, but these are typically associated with interfacet degenerative changes and are positioned more posteriorly and laterally. The absence of interfacet degenerative changes is also not in favor of the diagnosis of synovial cyst.

Radiologic Findings

Sagittal long TR image (Fig. A) reveals a rounded soft tissue density mass on the right side which appears decreased signal intensity (*white arrow*). The mass is at the anticipated level of the pedicle of the vertebral body of L3. There is slight disc space narrowing at the intervertebral disc level of L2-3.

Axial short TR image at the level of the L2-3 intervertebral disc (Fig. B) reveals a normal appearing disc (*left*). The nerve root can be seen just posterolateral to the disc surrounded by high signal intensity fat on the right side (*small arrow, left image*). The next image (*right*) is obtained just below the disc level and reveals a faint area of slightly increased signal intensity just medial to the pedicle and superior articulating facet on the right side in the region of the lateral recess (*long white arrow, right image*). There is obliteration of the epidural fat. Note the faint cleavage plane between the cerebrospinal fluid in the thecal sac and the soft tissue mass (*open arrow*).

Diagnosis

Herniated disc, probably arising from the L2-3 level. Surgically proved.

Differential Diagnosis

- schwannoma or neurofibroma: A schwannoma or neurofibroma could have a similar appearance.

Discussion

The herniated disc fragment has migrated inferiorly to rest in the region of the lateral recess. The disc fragment is "sequestered" from the main portion of the disc. A postcontrast study could be helpful in a case such as this and would potentially reveal enhancement around the peripheral margin of the disc. A schwannoma or neurofibroma would be expected to reveal homogeneous enhancement postcontrast. The location is somewhat difficult to approach at the time of surgery.

LUMBAR DISCS

Case 9

Clinical Presentation

The patient is a 40-year-old male who developed low back and severe right leg pain upon lifting a heavy object.

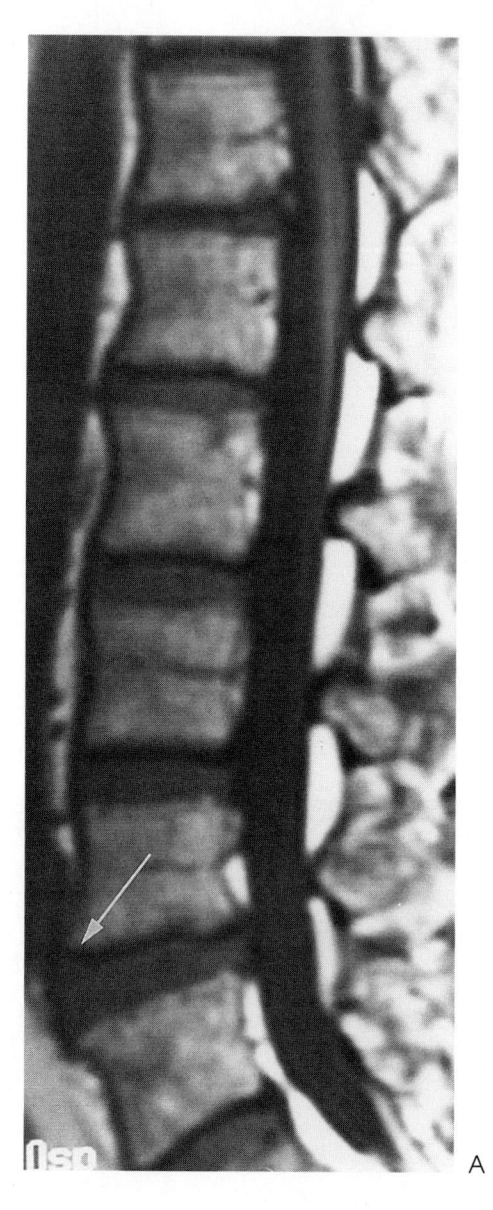

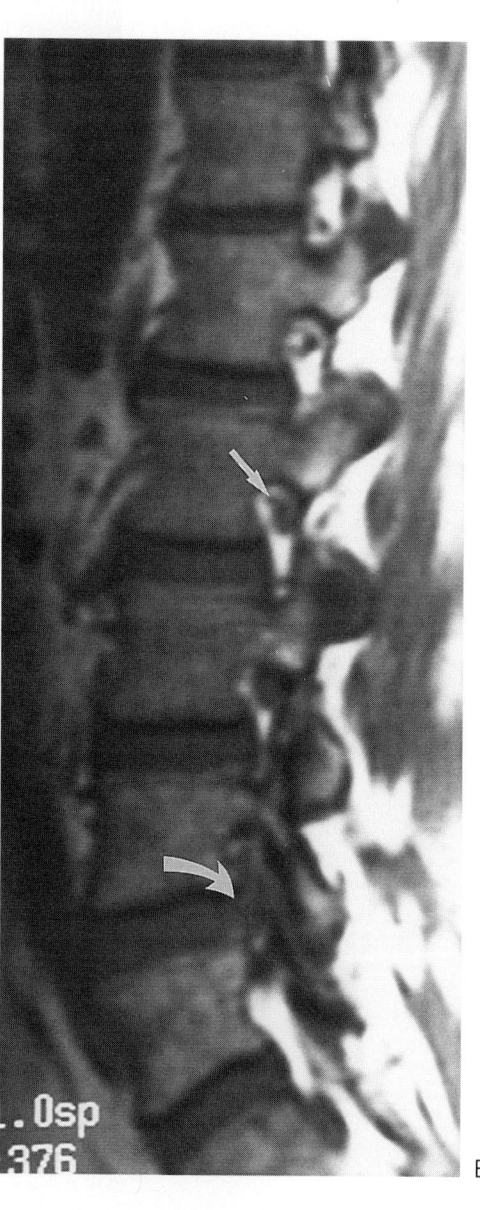

A

B

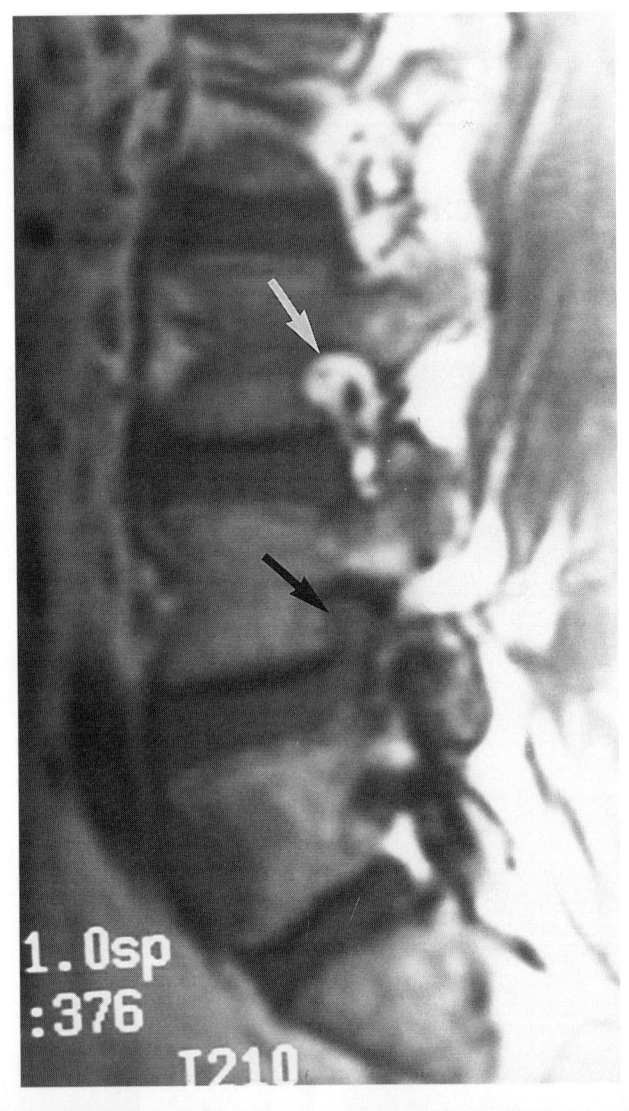

TEACHING ATLAS OF SPINE IMAGING

C

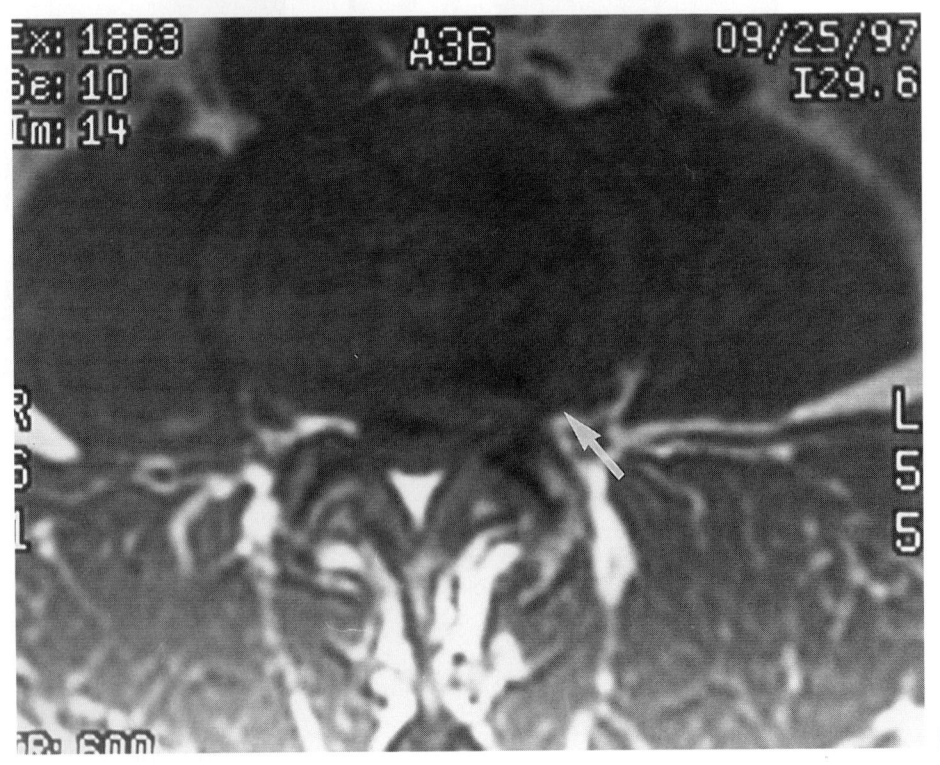

D

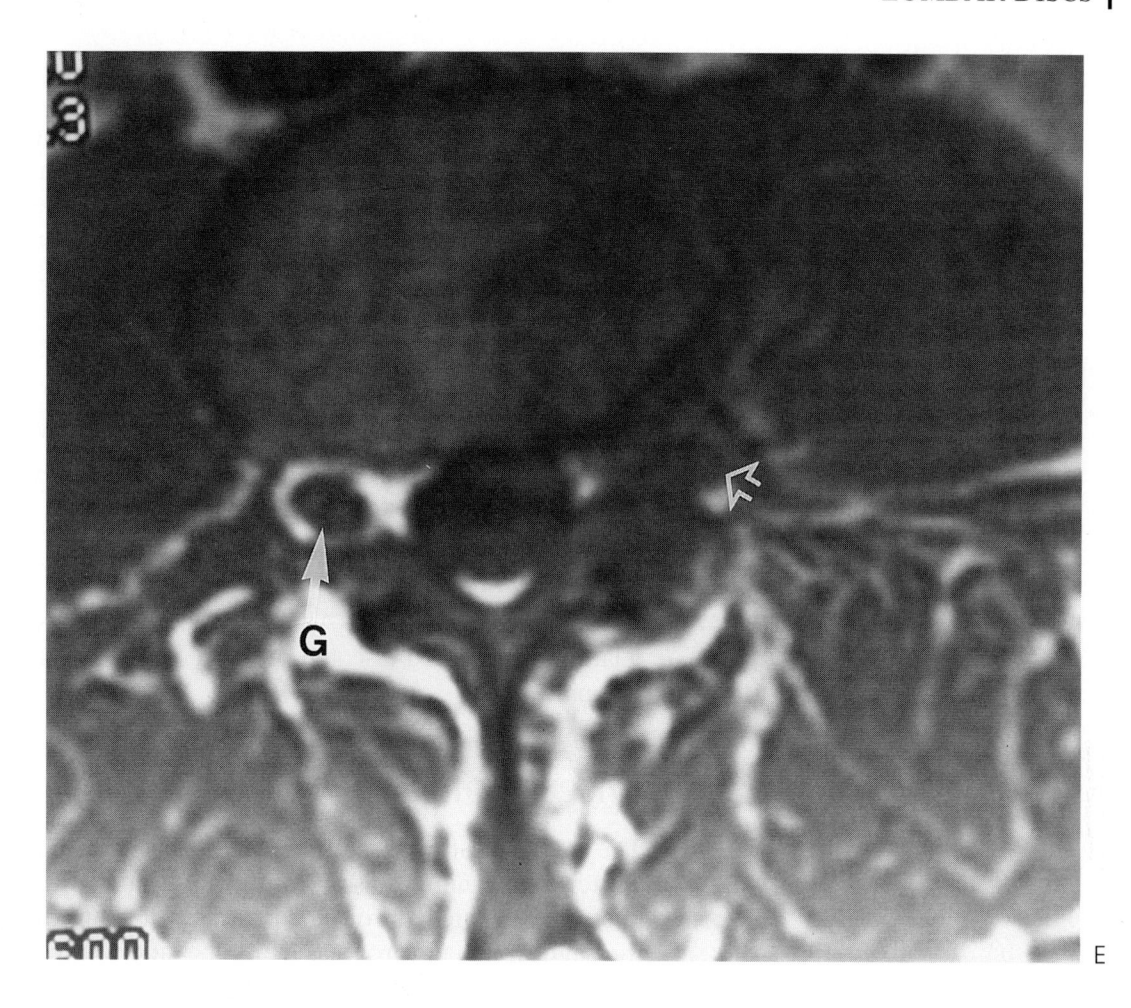

Radiologic Findings

Sagittal short TR image (Fig. A) reveals a bulging disc at the L4-5 level which interrupts the normal anterior, epidural, increased signal intensity adipose tissue. The anterior margin of the disc is also prominent and projects anterior to the vertebral bodies (*arrow*).

Left parasagittal short TR image at the level of the intervertebral foramenae (Fig. B) reveals that there is obliteration of the normally increased signal fat in the intervertebral foramen at the L4-5 level (*curved arrow*). The normal intermediate signal intensity dorsal root ganglion is seen projecting below the vertebral pedicle at the L2 level (*arrow*).

Magnified short TR image of the intervertebral foramen at the L4-5 level (Fig. C) reveals complete obliteration of the foramen secondary to an intermediate signal intensity mass (*black arrow*). At the L3-4 level, the normal high signal intensity adipose tissue surrounds the intermediate signal intensity of the dorsal root ganglion (*white arrow*). Other smaller rounded areas of decreased signal intensity are flow void of small vessels and nerves.

Axial short TR image at the level of the intervertebral disc (Fig. D) reveals what appears to be bulging of the intervertebral disc which is slightly more prominent off toward the left side. There is obliteration of the normal high signal intensity fat surrounding the nerve on the left side (*arrow*).

TEACHING ATLAS OF SPINE IMAGING

Radiologic Findings (continued)

Axial short TR image just below the level of the intervertebral disc (Fig. E) reveals the normal dorsal root ganglion on the right side (*white arrow-G*). On the left side, there is obliteration of the normal increased signal intensity fat surrounding the nerve root ganglion and compression of the ganglion into an oval-shaped mass (*open arrow*).

Diagnosis

Left laterally herniated disc at the L4-5 level with encroachment on the intervertebral foramen.

Differential Diagnosis

- laterally herniated disc: Although the appearance is typical of a far laterally herniated disc, the presence of such a disc may not be appreciated.

Discussion

The midsagittal images may appear deceptively normal in the presence of a laterally herniated disc. Close evaluation of the intervertebral foramen is necessary to rule in or out the presence of a laterally herniated disc. Because the sagittal images progress from one side to the other, the laterality of the herniated disc can be determined. The side-to-side progression of the sagittal slices is determined by the manufacturer of the equipment and can be used to predict the side of an abnormality.

In the presence of a herniated disc, the myelographic signs of a herniated disc are:

1. Posterior displacement of the nerve root.

2. Interruption of nerve root sleeve filling. These myelographic changes are reflected in the magnetic resonance (MR) scan as posterior displacement of the nerve root (as seen on the right in Fig. B) and interruption of nerve root sleeve filling (as seen on the left in Fig. B).

3. There is nerve root compression, also seen in Figure B where the nerve is compressed by the herniated disc.

4. Another myelographic sign is curvilinear deviation or compression of the thecal sac. This is seen by MR on the left in Figures B and D where the thecal sac is effaced and compressed along the left side by the large herniated disc.

There are also other findings in this case. On the right side at the L5-S1 level, there appear to be two conjoined nerve roots exiting together. These are seen together on the left side in Figure B and as two individual rounded low signal intensity structures on the right in Figure B. The dorsal root ganglion is also seen more laterally and is surrounded by perineural high signal intensity fat.

PEARLS

- Clinical evaluation is particularly important in these patients because they generally have severe radicular pain.

- Myelography may not reveal these laterally herniated discs because the herniated portion of the disc is sufficiently lateral that it does not lead to deformity of the thecal sac.

PITFALL

- Far laterally herniated discs may be difficult to appreciate, particularly if the parasagittal images at the level of the intervertebral foramen are not examined closely. The axial images may not clearly depict laterally herniated discs, and these laterally positioned discs are easily overlooked because they are relatively distant from the vertebral canal.

LUMBAR DISCS

Case 10

Clinical Presentation

The patient is a 74-year-old male with chronic low back pain with recent exacerbation of the back pain.

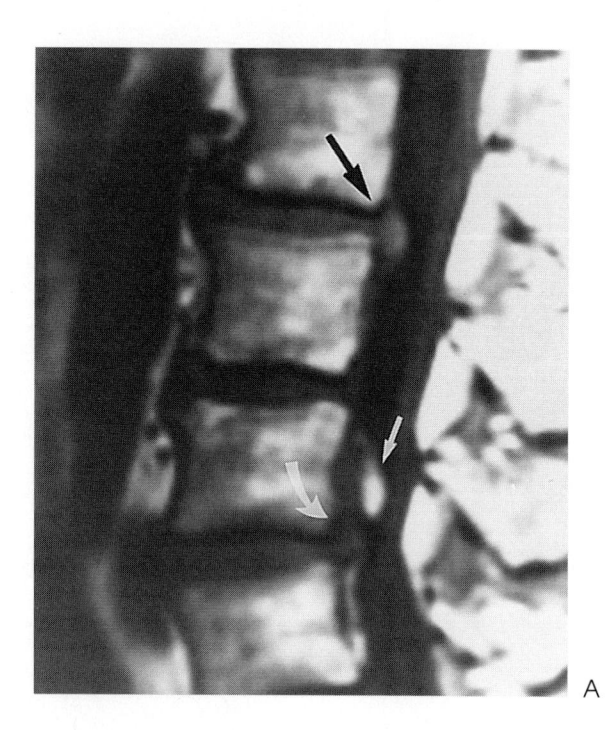

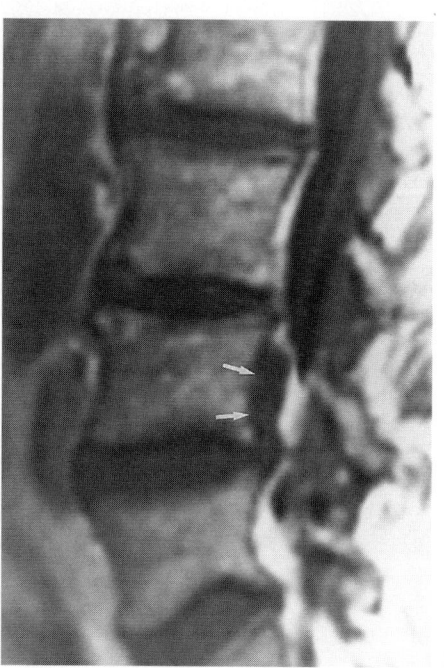

Radiologic Findings

Sagittal short TR image of the lumbar spine (Fig. A) reveals prominence of the intervertebral disc at the L2-3 level (*black arrow*). There is also prominence of the disc at the L4-5 level (*curved white arrow*) and an oval-shaped area of increased signal intensity that projects behind the vertebral body of L4 (*straight white arrow*).

Right parasagittal short TR image (Fig. B) reveals that there is a slightly lobulated area of decreased signal intensity behind the vertebral body of L4 (*arrows*).

TEACHING ATLAS OF SPINE IMAGING

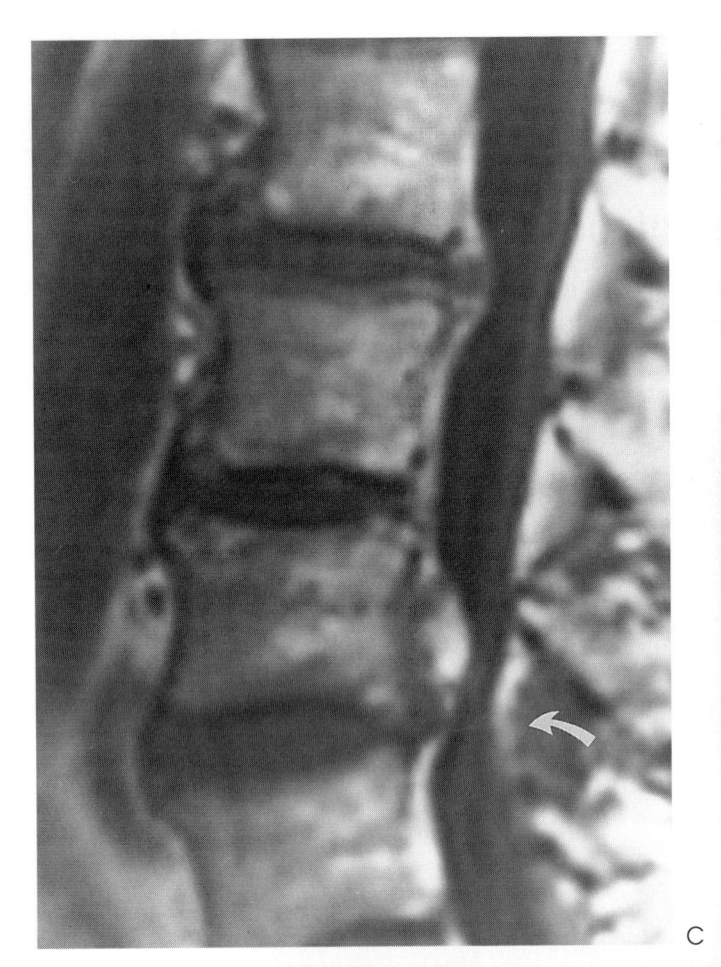

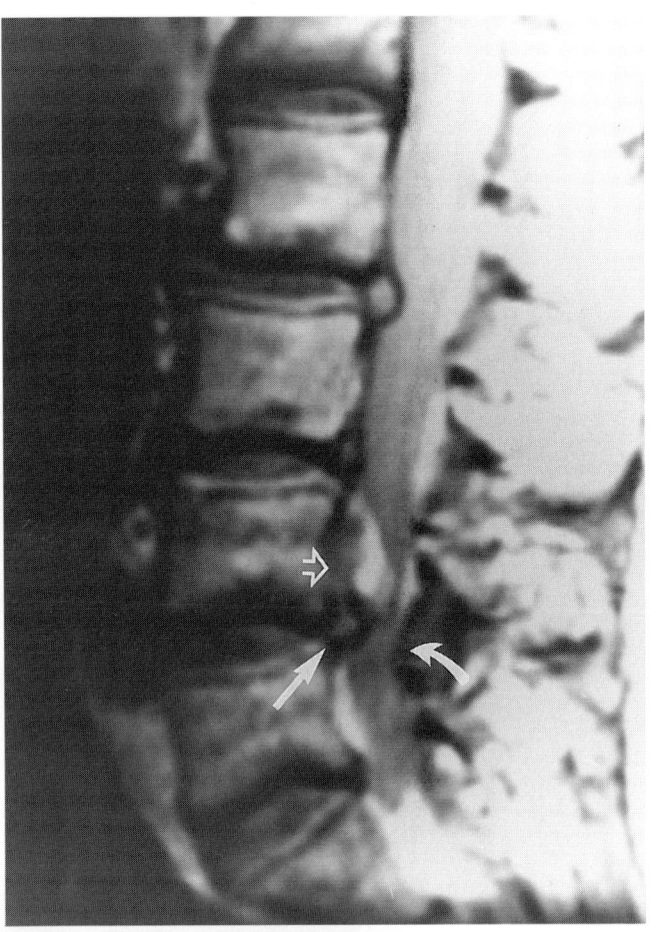

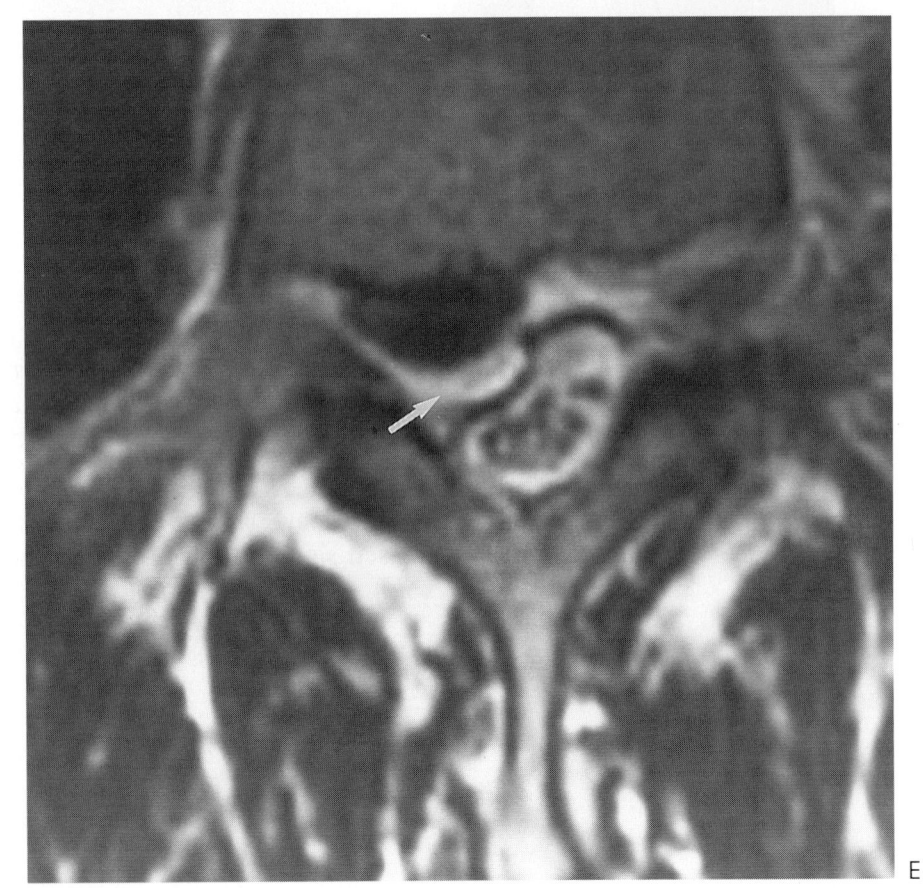

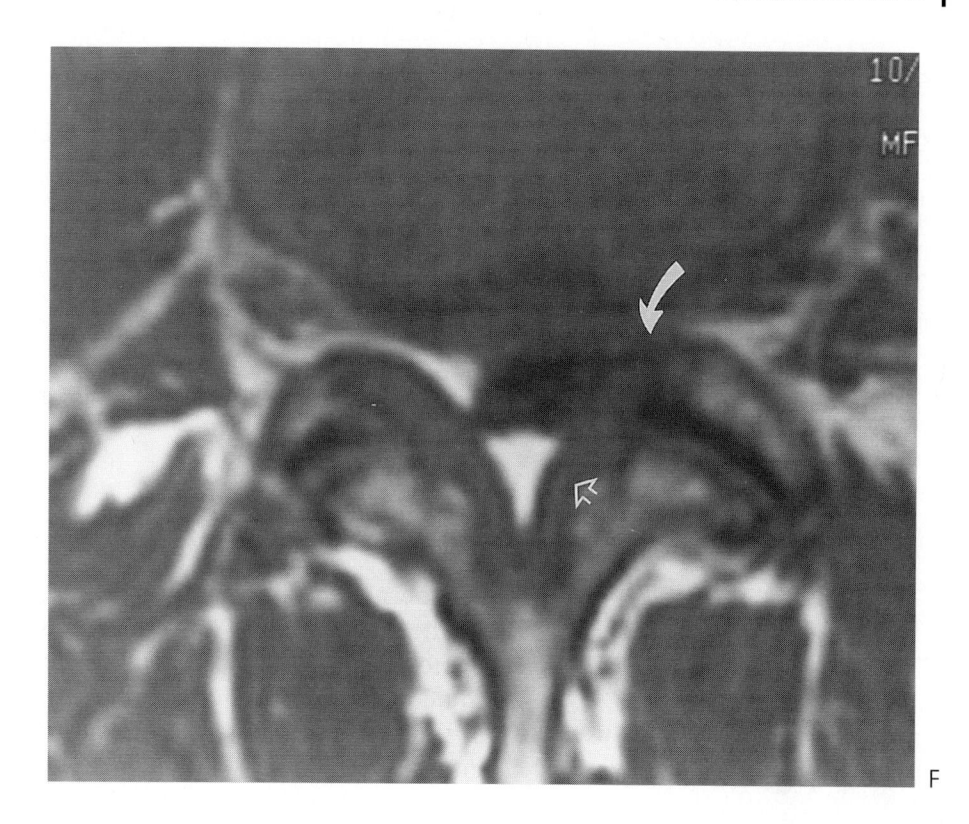

Radiologic Findings (continued)

Left parasagittal short TR image (Fig. C) reveals an oval-shaped area of increased signal intensity that projects behind the vertebral body of L4. There is also dorsal encroachment upon the thecal sac by a soft tissue mass (*curved arrow*).

Sagittal intermediate TR image of the lumbar spine (Fig. D) reveals prominence of the intervertebral disc at the L4-5 level (*white arrow*) and an area of variable signal intensity projecting posterior to the vertebral body of L4 (*open arrow*). The intervertebral disc at L2-3 protrudes into the vertebral canal. There is a decreased signal intensity soft tissue mass that encroaches upon the dorsal aspect of the thecal sac at the L4-5 level (*curved arrow*).

Axial long TR image at the level of the midbody of L4 (Fig. E) reveals a mushroom-shaped area of decreased signal intensity that projects behind the vertebral body of L4. This is capped by a crescentic area of increased signal intensity (*arrow*). The thecal sac is compressed posteriorly and toward the left side. The nerve roots of the cauda equina can be seen within the thecal sac.

Axial short TR image at the L2-3 level (Fig. F) reveals a midline and left paracentral prominence of the disc that encroaches upon the intervertebral foramen on the left side (*curved arrow*). There is slight prominence of the ligamentum flavum bilaterally (*open arrow on left side*).

TEACHING ATLAS OF SPINE IMAGING

PEARLS
- The ligamentum flavum does not actually "hypertrophy." Rather, the ligamentum flavum is normally stretched between the laminae of the vertebral bodies and therefore thinned. However, when there is disc space narrowing and degenerative changes of the interfacet joints, this results in closer approximation of the laminae and increased fullness of the ligamentum flavum.

- The appearance is unusual for a herniated disc, which is not usually associated with hemorrhage.

- If surgery is not performed early in the course of the patient's illness, a follow-up scan may be helpful for more complete evaluation.

PITFALL
- Hemorrhage is unusual in association with a herniated disc.

Diagnosis
Midline herniated disc at the L2-3 level; large extruded herniated disc with a sequestered fragment at the L4-5.

Differential Diagnosis
- hematoma: A hematoma from any source could have a similar appearance.

- metastatic disease: Metastatic disease could also be a consideration but is less likely.

Discussion
The herniated disc at the L4-5 level has extruded superiorly from the level of the intervertebral disc. There is an area of increased signal intensity hemorrhage along the dorsal aspect of the herniated disc. There continues to be evidence of a herniated disc at the L4-5 level; however, the majority of the nucleus pulposus has been extruded superiorly. The decreased signal intensity structure seen in Figure D is the ligamentum flavum which is "hypertrophied" and encroaches upon the dorsal aspect of the thecal sac. There is marked compression of the thecal sac at this level resulting in a spinal stenosis.

There is also a herniated disc at the L2-3 level. The disc is predominantly in the midline; however, a portion of the disc extends laterally into the left intervertebral foramen.

LUMBAR DISCS

Case 11

Clinical Presentation

The patient is a 19-year-old male with low back pain.

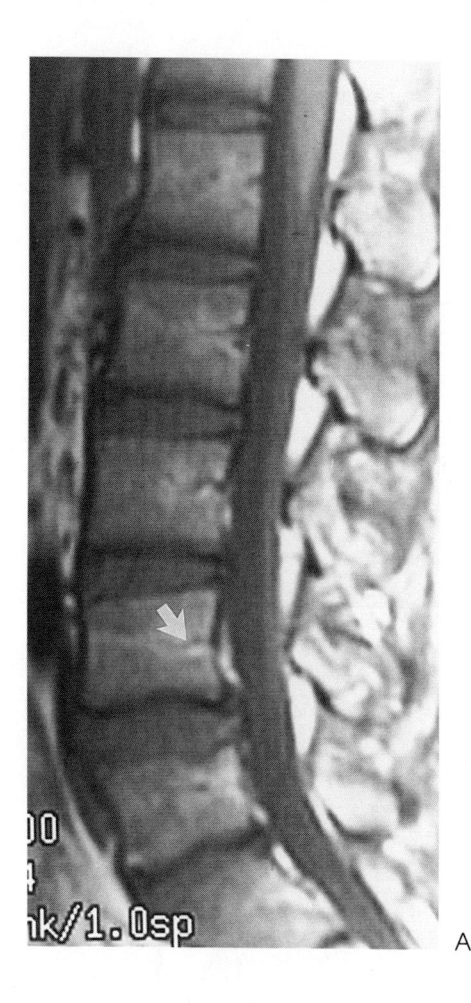

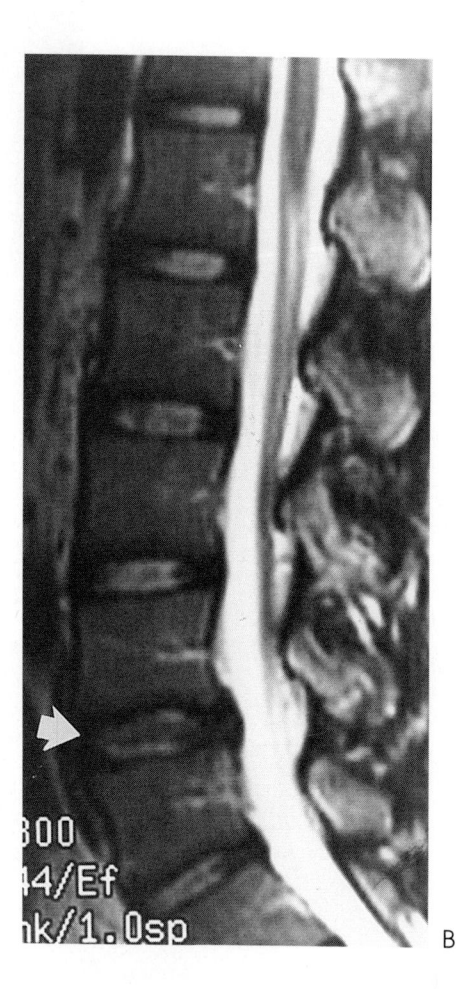

Radiologic Findings

Sagittal short TR image of the lumbar spine (Fig. A) reveals a minimal forward displacement of L4 on L5, a grade 1 spondylolisthesis. There is bulging of the disc at the L4-5 level. The normal basivertebral venous plexus is seen in the midportion of the lumbar vertebral body (*arrow*).

Sagittal long TR image of the lumbar spine (Fig. B) reveals slight decrease in signal intensity of the L4-5 intervertebral disc (*arrow*). There is also slight decrease in the signal intensity of the intervertebral disc at the L4-5 level.

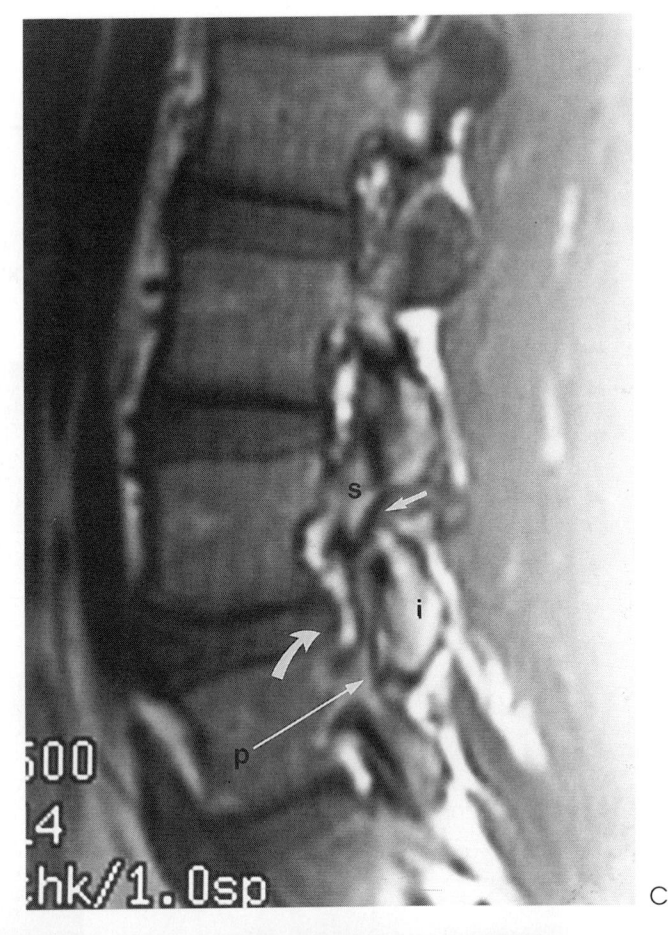

TEACHING ATLAS OF SPINE IMAGING

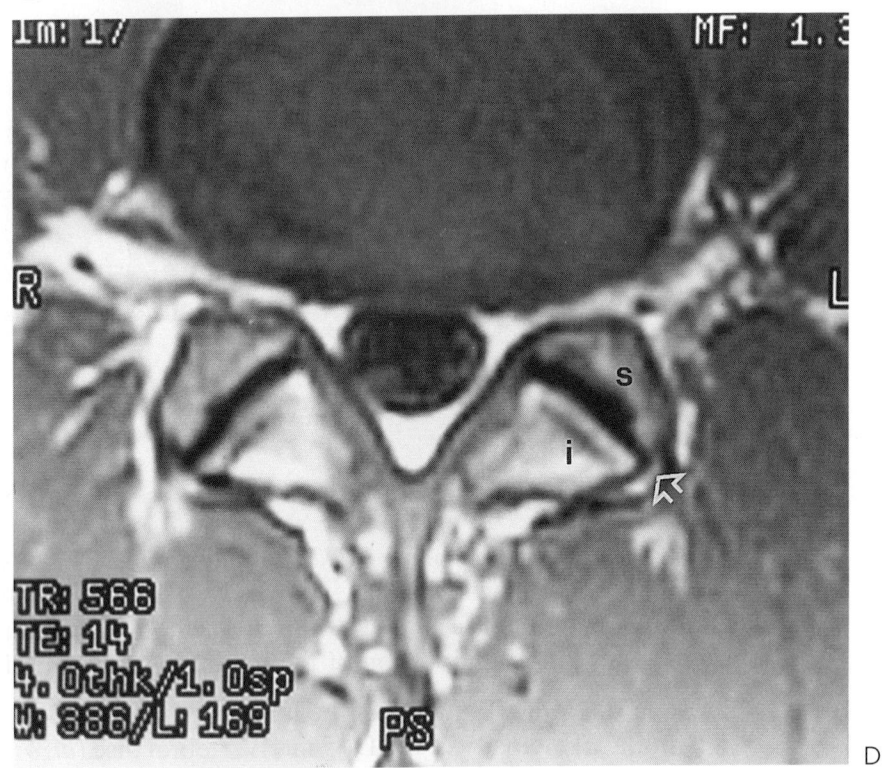

C

D

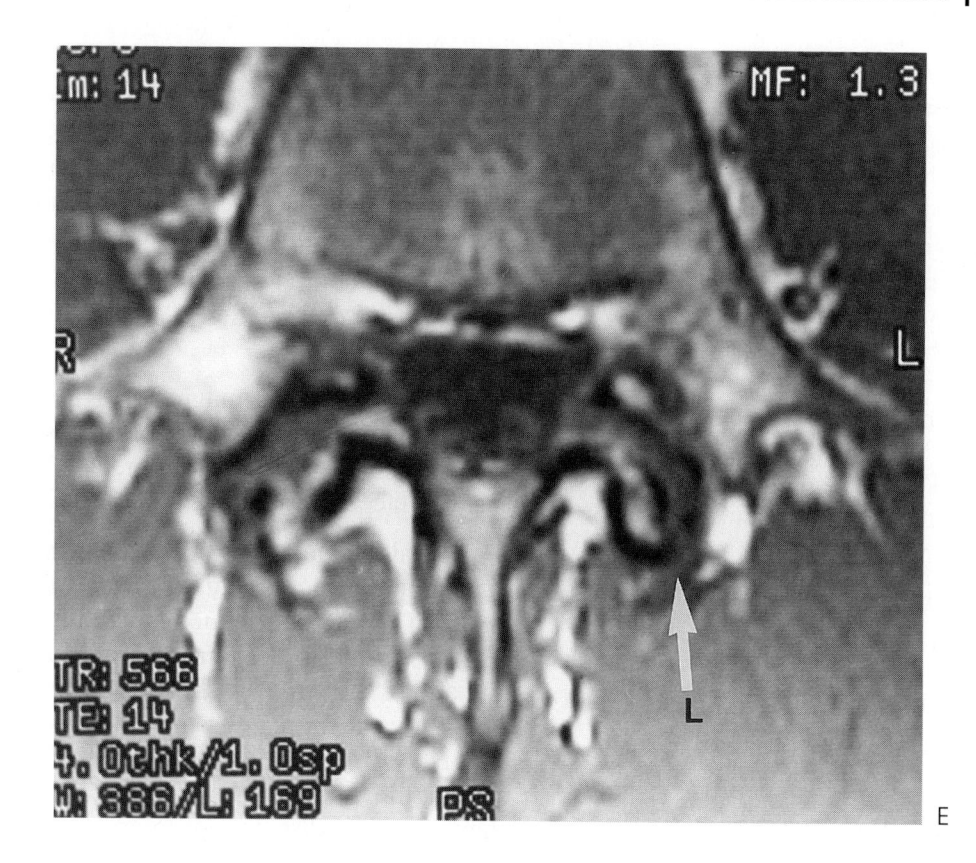

Radiologic Findings (continued)

Parasagittal short TR image (Fig. C) reveals an interruption of the pars interarticularis (*short arrow*). The superior articulating facet is seen above the level of the break (*s*) and the inferior articulating facet (*i*) is seen below the level of the break. There is bulging of the L4-5 disc which encroaches on the inferior aspect of the intervertebral foramen at the L4-5 level (*curved arrow*). The normal pars interarticularis (*p*) is seen at the L5 level (*long arrow*).

Axial short TR image (Fig. D) at the L3-4 level through the normal intervertebral disc. The interfacet joint is normal (*open arrow*). The superior articulating facet (*s*) is in normal apposition with the normal inferior articulating facet (*i*).

Axial short TR image at the L4-5 level (Fig. E) reveals irregularity of the bony structures. There is widening of the space between the bony structures (*arrow-L*).

Diagnosis

Grade 1 spondylolisthesis secondary to bilateral spondylolysis at the L4-5 level.

TEACHING ATLAS OF SPINE IMAGING

PEARLS

- Spondylolysis is generally more common in younger patients. In the older patient, the changes of spondylolisthesis are generally secondary to interfacet degenerative changes without a spondylolysis. In many patients, it is not possible to identify the spondylolysis on the MR images.

- The sagittal MR images are ideal for the identification of small degrees of spondylolisthesis.

PITFALLS

- Attempts may be made to stabilize the amount of forward or reverse slipping by utilizing metallic fixating devices to maintain the relationship between the vertebral bodies.

- CT scanning or plain spine films may reveal the spondylolysis if it is not visible by MR imaging.

Differential Diagnosis

- spondylolisthesis: A spondylolisthesis may be present even without a spondylolysis; however, if there is no spondylolysis, there are typically interfacet degenerative changes. Common in older patients, interfacet degenerative changes are unusual in a young patient.

Discussion

Magnetic resonance imaging (MRI) is the ideal method for evaluation of subtle changes related to spondylolisthesis. In this patient, there is slight but definite forward displacement of L4 on L5. Therefore, the reason for this displacement must be identified.

The axial image (Fig. D) reveals the normal interfacet joint, while the axial image (Fig. E) actually reveals the pars interarticularis, and the space between the bone fragments actually represents the spondylolysis (*arrow-L*). This break in the pars interarticularis results in instability of the spine and allows the vertebral body to slide forward on the vertebral body below. This forward slippage is the spondylolisthesis. The instability of the spine results in distortion of the intervertebral disc and creates a pseudobulging disc at the L4-5 level. However, these changes cause mild degenerative changes in the disc, loss of hydration, and decreased signal intensity. When there is a spondylolisthesis, the interfacet joints and the pars interarticularis should be evaluated very closely. The pars interarticularis may be seen on plain film evaluation, on computed tomographic scans, and with careful evaluation of this anatomic area on parasagittal images.

The combination of these changes and the bulging disc results in intervertebral foramenal narrowing with encroachment upon the lower aspect of the intervertebral foramen by the bulging disc. MR is an excellent method of evaluating this change because the increased signal intensity fat in the intervertebral foramen is an excellent contrast material.

In general, the interfacet joint is positioned at approximately a 45 degree angle, while the pars interarticularis defect is at an almost horizontal projection. However, in some cases, particularly when there is more marked forward displacement of one vertebral body on the next, the interfacet joint and the defect in the pars interarticularis may be almost superimposed. Therefore, careful evaluation must be made of the images in multiple planes.

LUMBAR DISCS

Case 12

Clinical Presentation

The patient is a 44-year-old male with a history of pain in left buttock which radiates down the left leg.

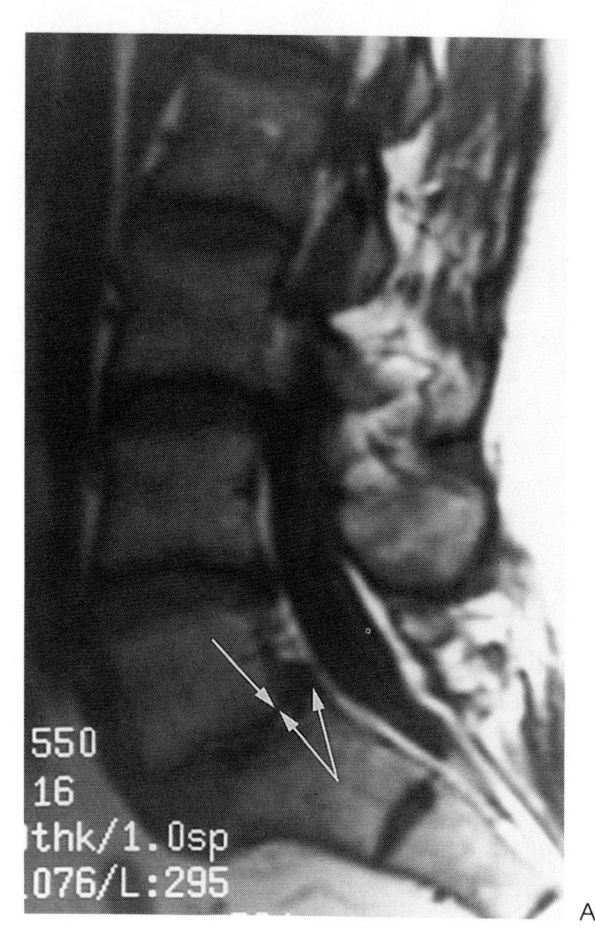

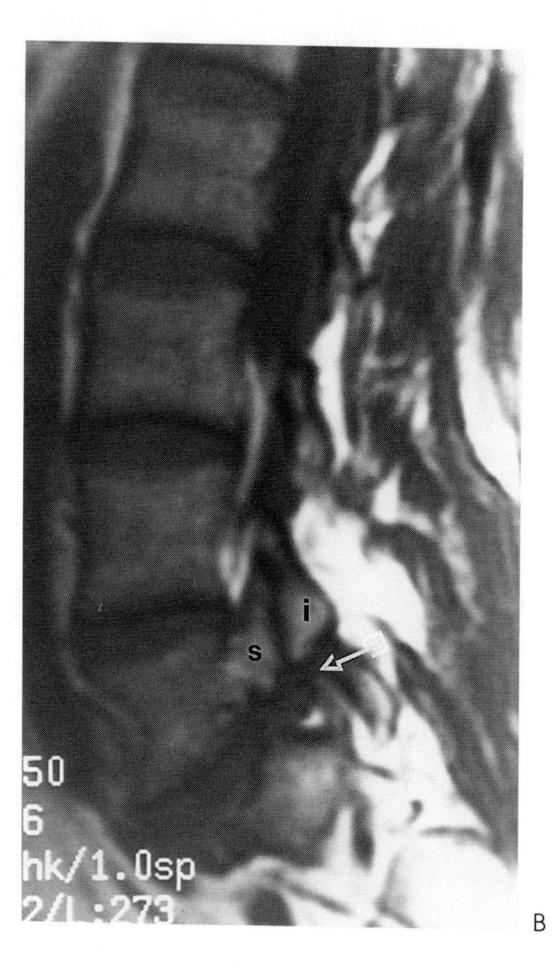

A

B

Radiologic Findings

Sagittal short TR image (Fig. A) reveals forward displacement of L5 on S1. The single arrow identifies the posterior inferior corner of the L5 vertebral body. The two arrows identify the amount of forward displacement of L5 on S1 which is approximately 8 mm. There is widening of the epidural space behind the vertebral body of L 5. This widened epidural space is filled with increased signal intensity fat. There is also a bulging disc at the L4-5 level. There is marked prominence of the disc at the L5-S1 level. The L5 vertebral body is identified.

Parasagittal short TR image at the level of the interfacet joints (Fig. B) reveals an interruption in the pars interarticularis at the L5 level (*open arrow*). The inferior articulating facet of the L4 vertebral body (*i*) projects dorsal to the superior articulating facet of the L5 vertebral body (*s*). There

TEACHING ATLAS OF SPINE IMAGING

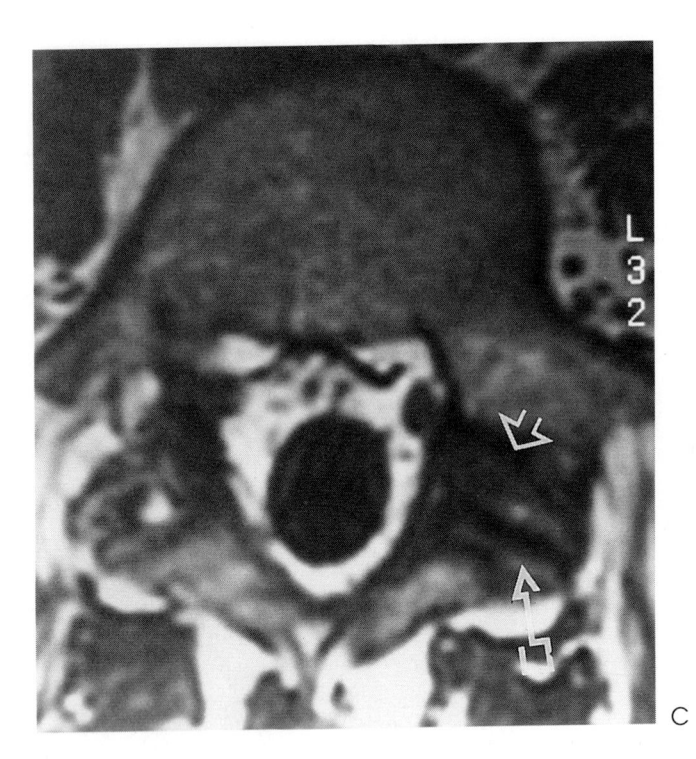

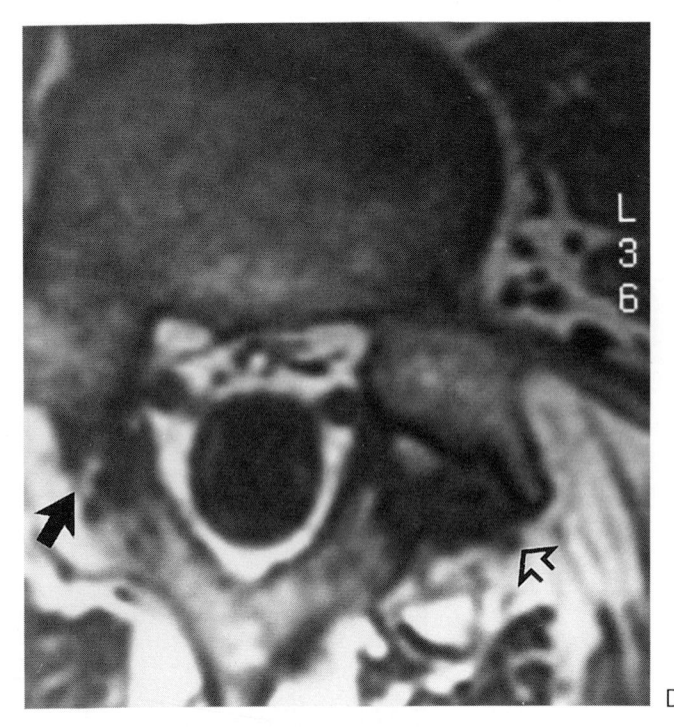

Radiologic Findings (continued)

is discontinuity between the superior articulating facet of L5 and the inferior articulating facet of L5.

Axial short TR image at the level of the pars defect (Fig. C) reveals sclerosis of the adjacent vertebral bodies which appear as decreased signal intensity. The superior articulating facet projects anterior (*open arrow*), while the inferior articulating facet projects posteriorly (*open arrow with box*).

Axial short TR image at the level of the interfacet joint (Fig. D) reveals bony sclerosis and resulting decreased signal intensity of the inferior articulating facet on the left side (*open arrow*). The area of the spondylolysis is seen on the right side (*black arrow*) on the same image and also reveals sclerosis with resulting decreased signal intensity surrounding the bones structures. Note that the interfacet joint is wider than the area of the pars interarticularis defect. In some cases the appearance of these two areas is very similar.

Diagnosis

Bilateral spondylolysis and grade 1 spondylolisthesis.

Differential Diagnosis

- spondylolysis and spondylolisthesis: The appearance is typical of a spondylolysis with spondylolisthesis.

PEARLS

- When there is spondylolysis, close evaluation should be made for the presence of spondylolysis. It may be necessary to perform a computed tomographic scan or plain spine images if further evaluation is needed.

- There is not typically a herniated disc in these patients, but rather a "pseudobulging" disc because the spondylolisthesis distorts the normal appearance of the intervertebral disc.

PITFALL

- It is not always possible to identify the presence of spondylolysis on magnetic resonance imaging. However, when there is a spondylolisthesis, a spondylolysis should be ruled in or out. Therefore, correlation should be made with plain film evaluation or CT scanning.

Discussion

The cause of spondylolysis is unknown, but it is thought to be related to trauma in some cases. The break, or "lysis," of the pars interarticularis results in forward displacement of one vertebral body upon the next. The dura of the thecal sac is firm and does not adhere to the posterior margin of the vertebral body but remains posteriorly placed. This results in an enlarged epidural space anterior to the thecal sac. This enlarged space fills with adipose tissue which appears increased signal intensity. The intervertebral disc appears prominent because the anterior displacement of one vertebral body on the next results in a "pseudobulging" disc as the disc is unable to remain normal in contour.

A practical method of grading spondylolisthesis is to consider a forward slip of one vertebral body on the other of 25% or less of the width of the vertebral body as grade I, 25 to 50% slippage of one vertebral body on the next as grade 2, 50 to 75% slippage of one vertebral body on the next as grade 3, and greater that 75% slippage as grade 4. Although there are other methods, this one is practical and easily used on a day-to-day basis. The slippage may be either forward (anterolisthesis) or posterior (retrolysthesis).

Because there is interruption of the pars interarticularis, the posterior elements of the vertebral body are independent from the anterior structures. Therefore, there is not forward displacement of the posterior elements.

There is usually disc space narrowing in association with spondylolysis and spondylolisthesis because the facet instability results in weakening of the disc and ultimately loss of disc height.

Case 13

Clinical Presentation

The patient is a 32-year-old male with a history of many years of low back pain.

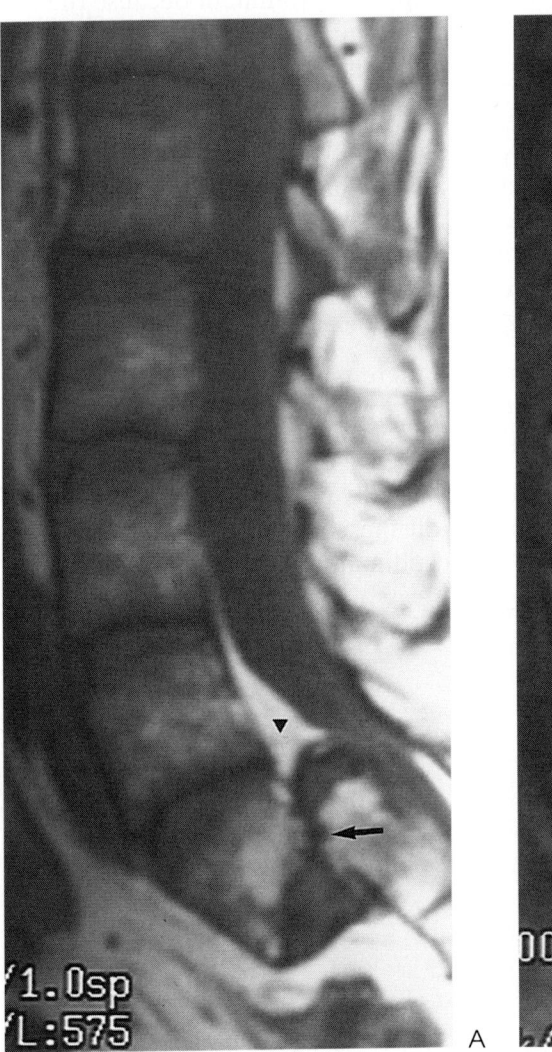

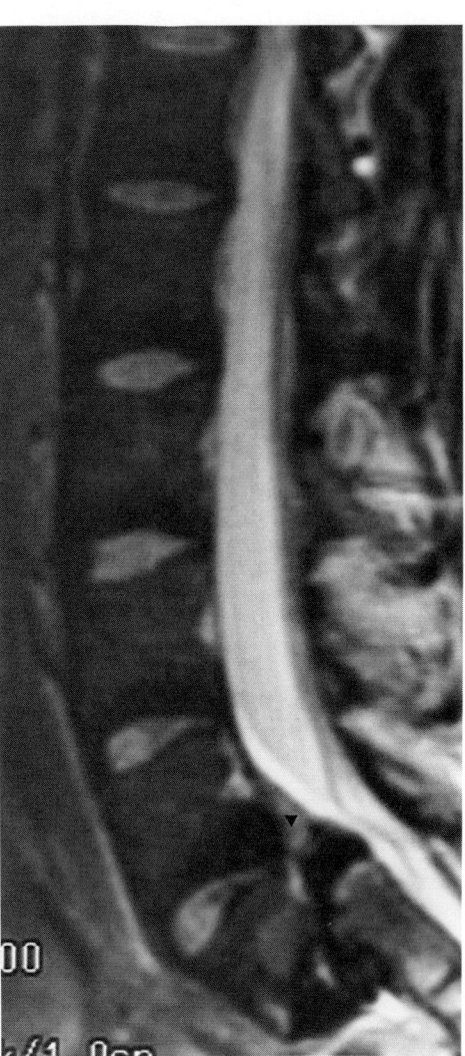

Radiologic Findings

Sagittal short TR image (Fig. A) reveals marked forward displacement of the L5 vertebral body relative to the S1 vertebral body. The posterior inferior corner of the L5 vertebral body is displaced anterior to the anterior superior corner of the S1 vertebral body (*arrow*). The S1 vertebrae is deformed, and the superior end plate is rounded. The intervertebral disc is markedly abnormal with both anterior and posterior prominence of the disc. The epidural fat is markedly widened behind the vertebral body of L4 and L5 (*arrowhead*).

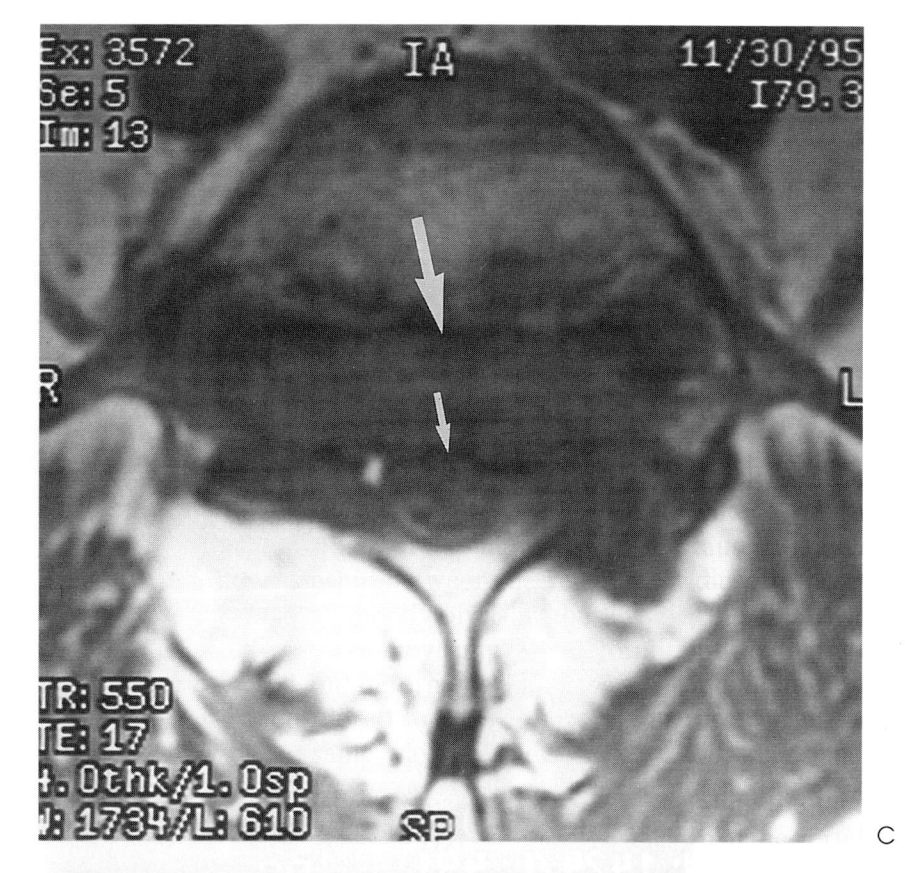

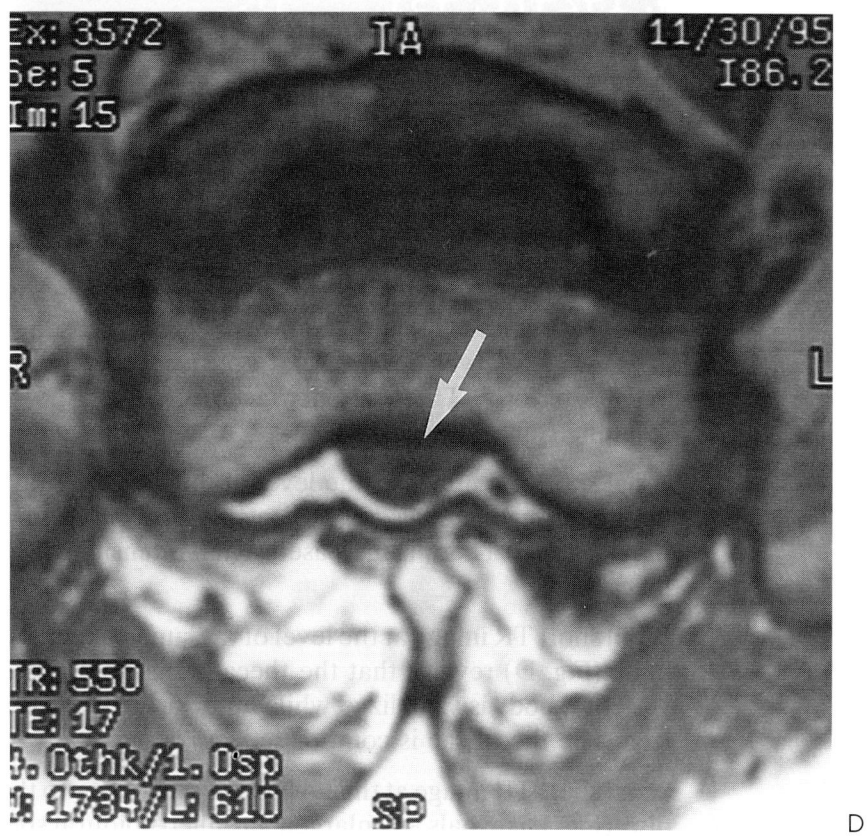

LUMBAR DISCS

C

D

663

Case 15

Clinical Presentation

The patient is a 73-year-old male with a clinical history of previous surgery for a lumbar disc.

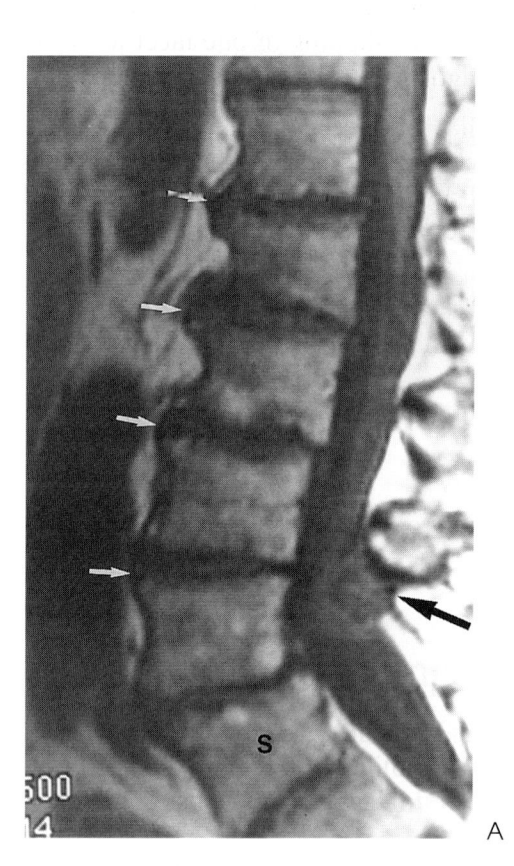

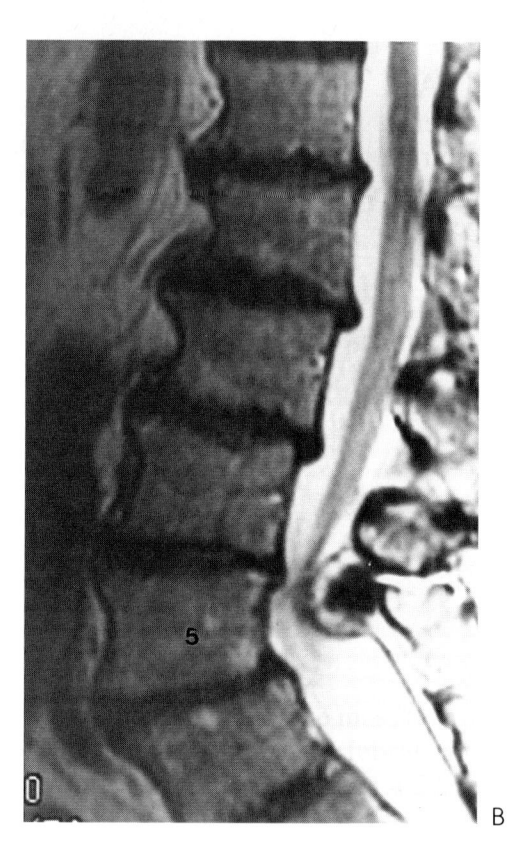

Radiologic Findings

Sagittal short TR image (Fig. A) reveals a grade 1 anterolisthesis (anterior spondylolisthesis) with forward displacement of L5 on S1. There is also disc space narrowing at the L5-S1 level. There is retrolisthesis (posterior spondylolisthesis) with posterior displacement of L2 on L3 and L1 on L2. The normal dorsal epidural fat at the L4 level (*arrow*) is obliterated, and a rounded, intermediate soft tissue mass projects into the vertebral canal and the thecal sac at the L4-5 level. There are anterior osteophytes at multiple levels (*short white arrows*). The S 1 vertebral body is identified with S.

LUMBAR DISCS

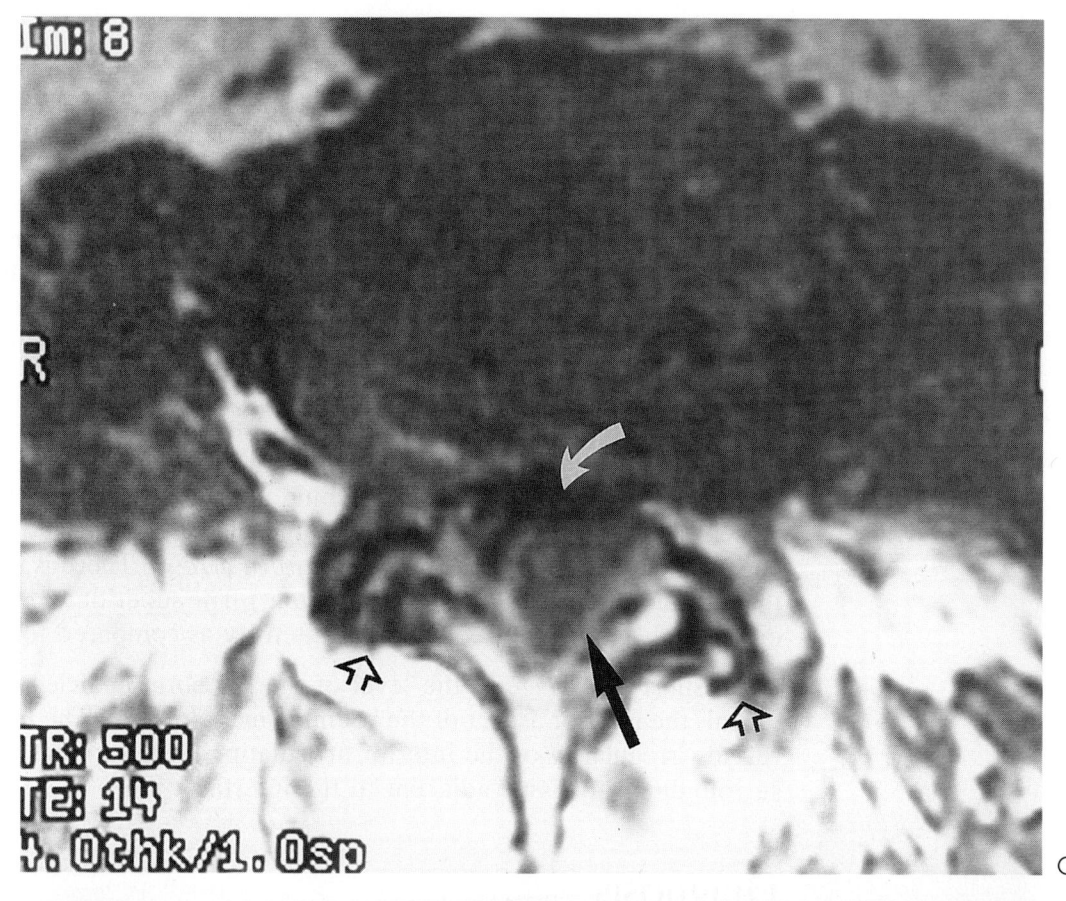

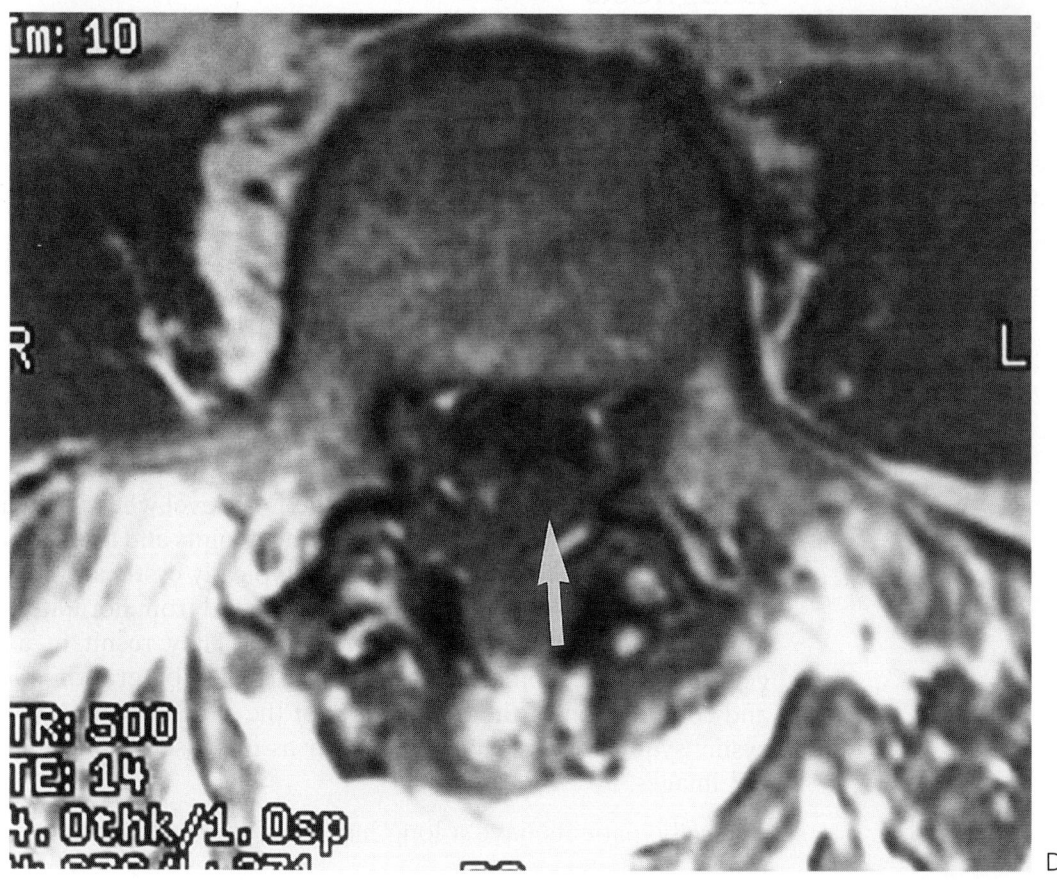

TEACHING ATLAS OF SPINE IMAGING

Radiologic Findings (continued)

Sagittal long TR image (Fig. B) again reveals the soft tissue mass which now appears as decreased signal intensity with an increased signal intensity rim and a peripheral surrounding rim of decreased signal intensity. The nerve roots of the cauda equina are displaced anteriorly by this mass. There is near complete obliteration of the thecal sac at this level. There are bulging discs at T12-L1, L1-2, and L2-3 with encroachment upon the high signal intensity cerebrospinal fluid. The L 5 vertebral body is identified with 5. There is decreased signal intensity of all of the visualized intervertebral discs. The patient had a previous laminectomy at the L4 and L5 level; the spinous processes are not seen.

Axial short TR image at the level of the L3-4 intervertebral disc (Fig. C) reveals the soft tissue mass encroaching upon the left dorsal aspect of the vertebral canal (*straight arrow*). The thecal sac is displaced forward and compressed in a curvilinear fashion (*curved arrow*). There is irregularity of the interfacet joint bilaterally (*open arrows*). The superior and inferior facets on the right are decreased in signal intensity as compared to the left side.

Axial short TR image at the level of the vertebral pedicle at L4 (Fig. D) reveals the inferior aspect of the rounded mass (*arrow*). The interfacet joint reveals irregularity of the inferior articulating facet and an increase in the surrounding soft tissue adjacent to the interfacet joint.

PEARL
- Synovial cysts may occasionally appear bright on short TR images because of hemorrhage. They may also calcify; calcification is best seen by computed tomographic scanning.

PITFALL
- Attempts have been made obliterate these cysts by aspirating the fluid within the cyst. This has met with varying degrees of success. Generally these cysts are treated surgically with total removal.

Diagnosis

Synovial cyst arising from the left interfacet joint at the L3-4 level.

Differential Diagnosis

- dense scar formation secondary to the previous surgery.
- an epidermoid.
- tissue introduced into the vertebral canal by a spinal tap.

Discussion

Synovial cysts are most common at the L4-5 level where they are associated with degenerative changes of the interfacet joints and arise from the synovial lining of the interfacet joint. They are typically cystic and may occasionally be hemorrhagic. They are easily differentiated from herniated discs because they arise dorsally rather than ventrally. They result in a variable, but generally severe, spinal stenosis with variable obliteration of the thecal sac and compression of the nerve roots of the cauda equina. Because they are cystic, synovial cysts typically appear as increased signal intensity on long TR images.

Typically, patients have a long history of low back pain.

LUMBAR DISCS

Case 16

Clinical Presentation

The patient is an 80-year-old man with weakness in the legs and numbness in the feet.

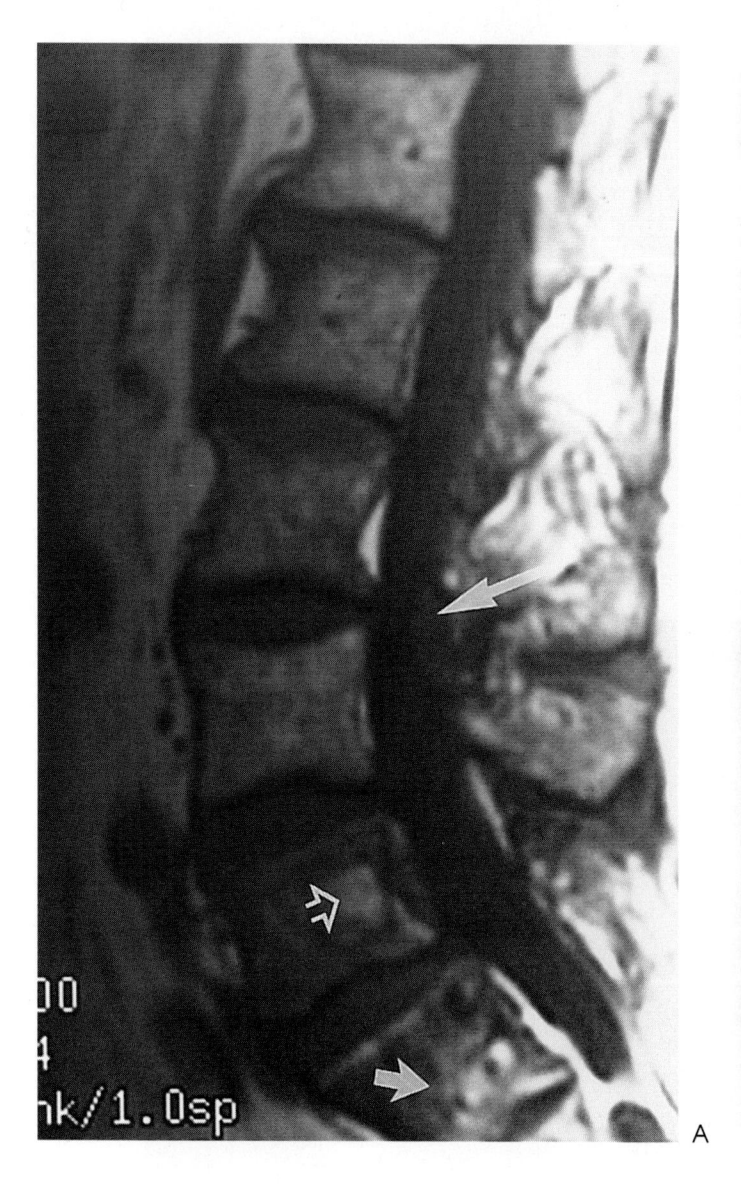

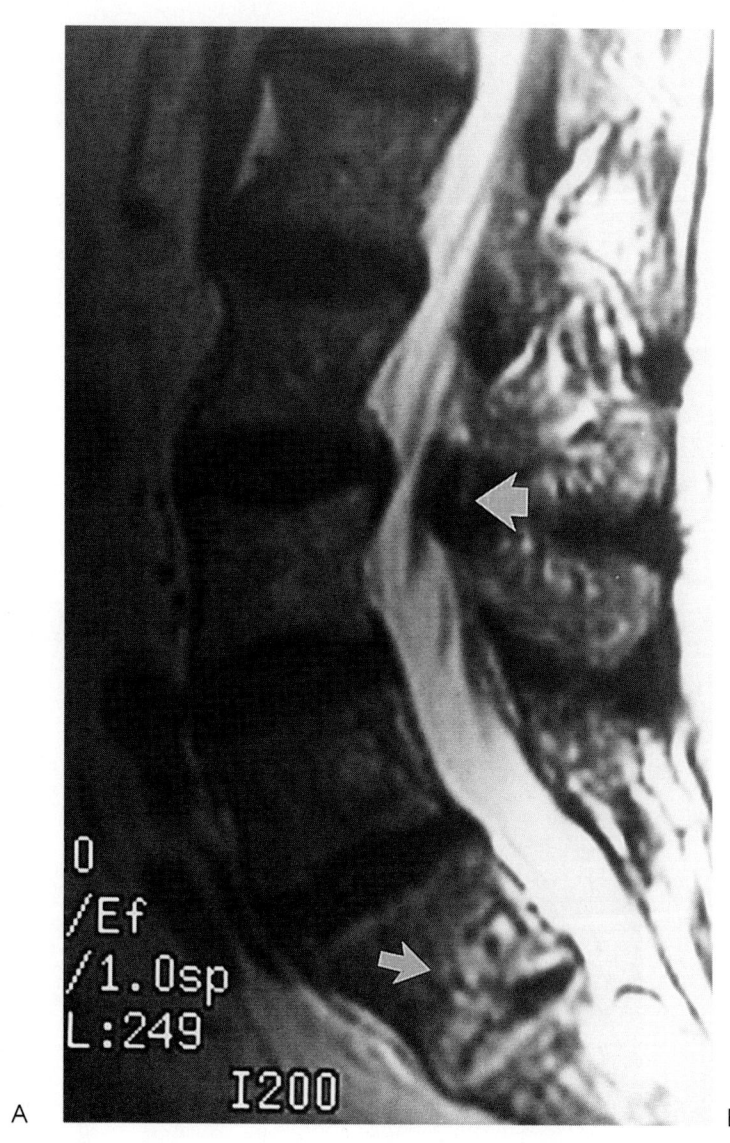

TEACHING ATLAS OF SPINE IMAGING

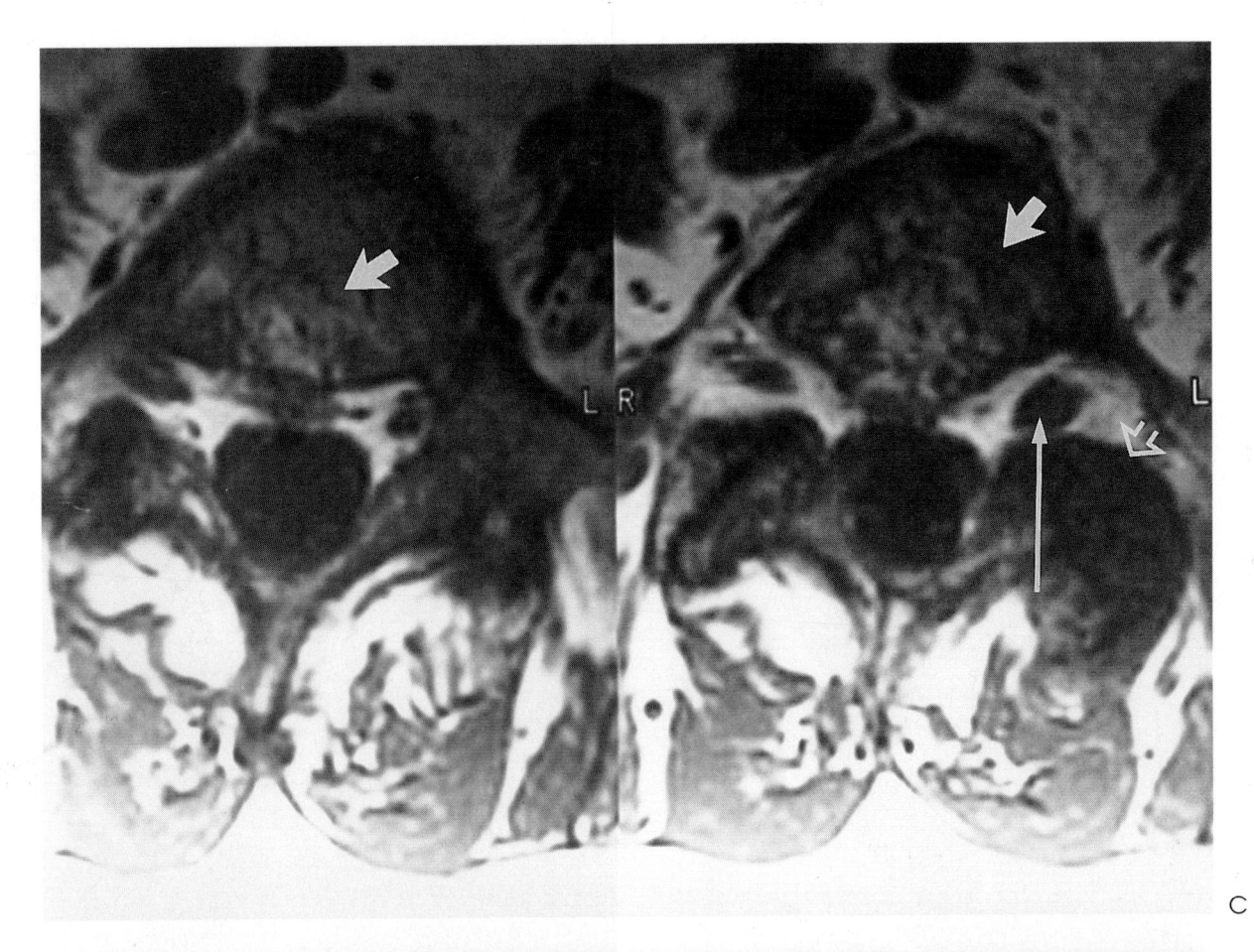

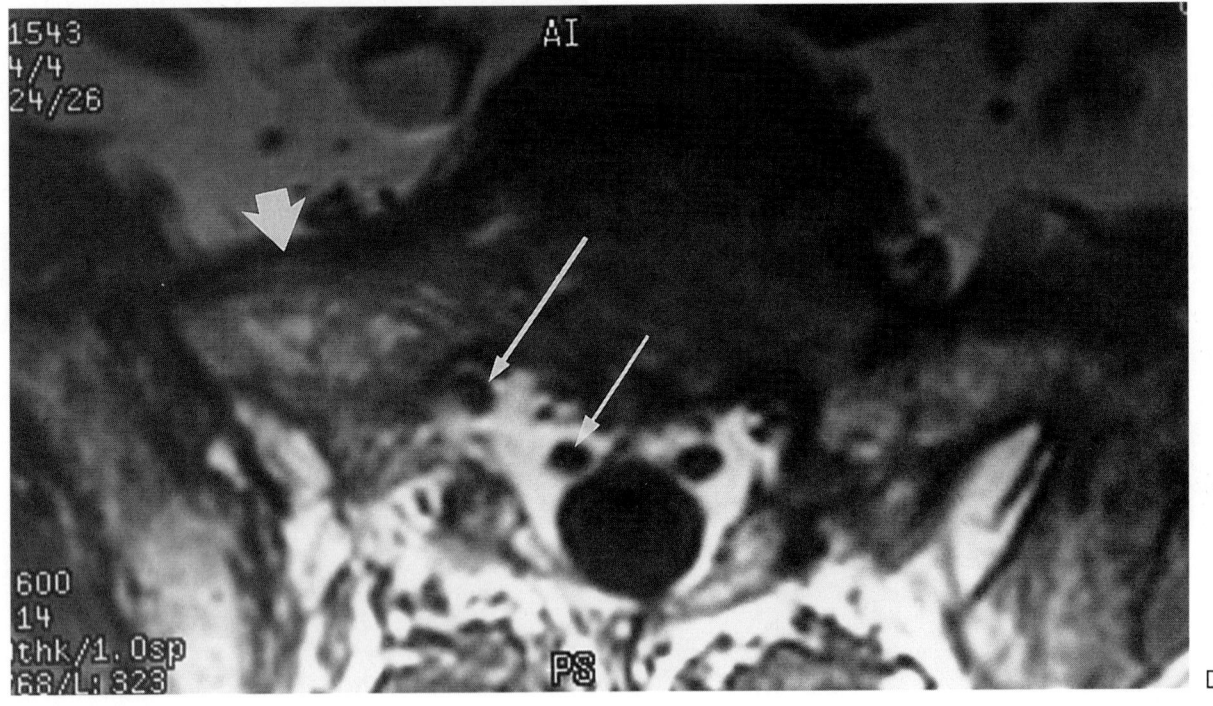

Radiologic Findings

Sagittal short TR image of the lumbar spine (Fig. A) reveals a very faint soft tissue signal intensity mass that projects into the dorsal aspect of the thecal sac at the L3-4 level (*long arrow*). There is a slight compression fracture of the superior end plate of the L3 vertebral body. There is mottled signal intensity involving the L5 (*open arrow*), S1 (*white arrow*) and S2 vertebral bodies.

Sagittal long TR image (Fig. B) reveals a decreased signal intensity soft tissue mass that encroaches upon the dorsal aspect of the thecal sac at the L3-4 level (*upper arrow*). There is also bulging of the intervertebral disc at the L3-4 level which encroaches upon the vertebral canal and the thecal sac. The mottled signal intensity is apparent in the L5 and S1 (*lower arrow*) and S2 vertebral bodies. There is an increase in the trabecular markings of the bone marrow.

Consecutive axial short TR images at the level of the L5 vertebral body (Fig. C) reveal an increase in the trabecular pattern within the bone marrow of the L5 vertebral body (*solid short arrow*). There are bilateral interfacet degenerative changes (*open arrow*); worse on the left side where there is complete loss of the joint space. The dorsal root ganglion is surrounded by high signal intensity fat (*long, solid arrow*).

Axial short TR image at the level of the S1 vertebral body (Fig. D) reveals an increase in the trabecular pattern of the vertebral marrow of the sacral alae (*short arrow*) as well as the iliac crests bilaterally. The normal nerve roots are seen surrounded by high signal intensity fat (*long arrows*).

PEARLS

- Radionuclide bone scanning is very useful in the evaluation of Paget's disease and reveals increased activity in the involved bony structures.

- A radiograph of the pelvis reveals increased density of the pelvic inlet with Paget's disease.

- Plain films of the spine reveal a typical appearance of Paget's disease.

Diagnosis

Spinal stenosis at the L3-4 level secondary to hypertrophy of the ligamentum flavum and encroachment upon the dorsal aspect of the vertebral canal. Incidental Paget's disease of the lumbar spine at the L5, S1, and S2 levels, as well as the sacral alae and the iliac crests.

Differential Diagnosis

- bone infarcts

- areas of focal fibrosis

- metastatic disease is a remote possibility

Discussion

Ligamentum flavum "hypertrophy" is related to and associated with interfacet degenerative changes. This results in narrowing of the interfacet joints and settling of one vertebral body upon the next. As a result of this, the normally tense ligamentum flavum, which stretches from one vertebral body lamina to the next, is no longer stretched and appears plump or "hypertro-

PITFALL

- Paget's disease may have a wide variety of appearances and may be mistaken for metastatic disease. Therefore, comparison should be made with the plain films as well as the radionuclide scans.

phied." This change results in encroachment upon the central canal and a central canal spinal stenosis.

Paget's disease is of unknown cause. Paget's disease results in an increase in the trabecular pattern of the bone marrow and may affect any bony structure. Typically, Paget's disease results in enlargement of the affected bony structure and the lumbar vertebrae, and increased density of the peripheral margin of the vertebral body, the "picture window" effect.

Although there is an increase in the trabecular pattern of the bony structures with Paget's disease, the bone is actually weaker than normal, and compression fractures, as seen in Figure A, may occur in these patients.

Routine radiographs of the spine or pelvis may reveal the typical appearance of Paget's disease and allow the diagnosis to be made.

LUMBAR DISCS

Case 17

Clinical Presentation

The patient is a 55-year-old female with 6-week history of right leg pain.

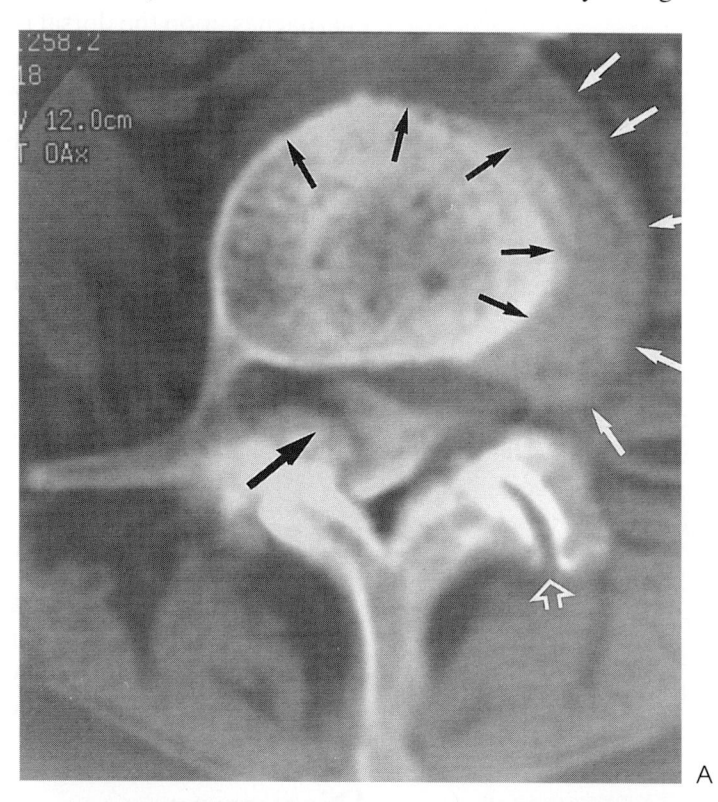

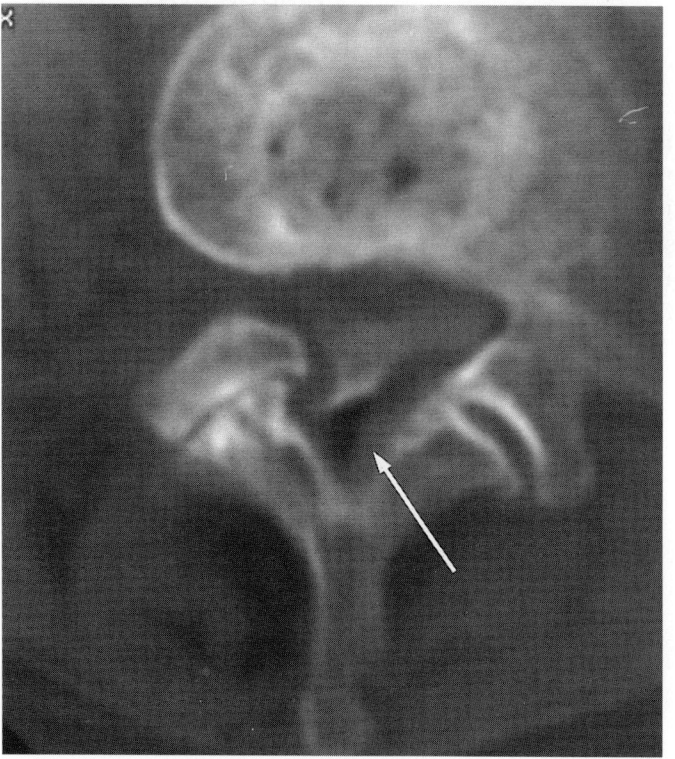

A

B

TEACHING ATLAS OF SPINE IMAGING

Radiologic Findings

Axial computed tomographic (CT) scan at the level of L4-5 performed postmyelogram with the bone window width technique (Fig. A) reveals a diffusely bulging disc that extends anterior to the vertebral body and toward the left side (*white arrows*). The small black arrows mark the margin of the vertebral body. There is a large osteophyte arising from the superior articulating facet on the right side (*large black arrow*). This osteophyte encroaches upon the dorsal right side of the vertebral canal. There is marked compression of the thecal sac at this level. On the left side, there is slight widening of the interfacet joint (*open arrow*) with fluid in the joint space.

Axial CT scan (Fig. B) using bone window width technique at a level slightly below the level in Figure A. There is slight prominence of the ligamentum flavum on the left side at the L4-5 level (*arrow*). There is resulting curvilinear encroachment upon the contrast-filled thecal sac on the left side.

PEARLS
- CT is more sensitive for the evaluation of bony osteophytes, while MR can readily diagnosis the compromise of the lateral recess and central spinal canal.

- Areas of stenosis are always associated with loss of epidural fat, and MR is excellent in the identification of epidural fat.

PITFALL
- MR may not identify areas of vertebral canal encroachment and may not be able to differentiate between bony versus soft tissue or areas of calcification. CT scanning is very sensitive to areas of bone formation or areas of calcification.

Diagnosis

Diffusely bulging disc, largest on the left side; lateral recess stenosis on the right side.

Differential Diagnosis

- degenerative changes: The appearance is typical of degenerative changes with degenerative changes in the intervertebral disc and hypertrophic bone formation. CT scanning may reveal small bony osteophytes that are not visible by magnetic resonance (MR) scanning.

Discussion

The lateral recess is a portion of the subarticular canal. The location of the lateral recess is between the superior articulating facet and the posterior margin of the vertebral body. When osteophytes arise from the articulating facet, they encroach upon the lateral recess of the vertebral canal. The nerve of the cauda equina arises from the thecal sac and courses through the lateral recess just before it exits via the intervertebral canal. Therefore, the nerve can be compressed by an osteophyte at the level of the lateral recess; this results in severe radicular pain. The enlargement of the ligamentum flavum results in encroachment upon the dorsal aspect of the vertebral canal and a central spinal canal stenosis. There is narrowing of the interfacet joint on the right side with small degenerative cysts in the inferior articulating facet as well as increased density within the facets secondary to bony sclerosis. The small oval areas of decreased density in the intervertebral disc are secondary to small areas of vacuum degenerative changes.

There is also encroachment upon the intervertebral foramen on the left side by the bulging disc which results in intervertebral foramenal stenosis.

MISCELLANEOUS

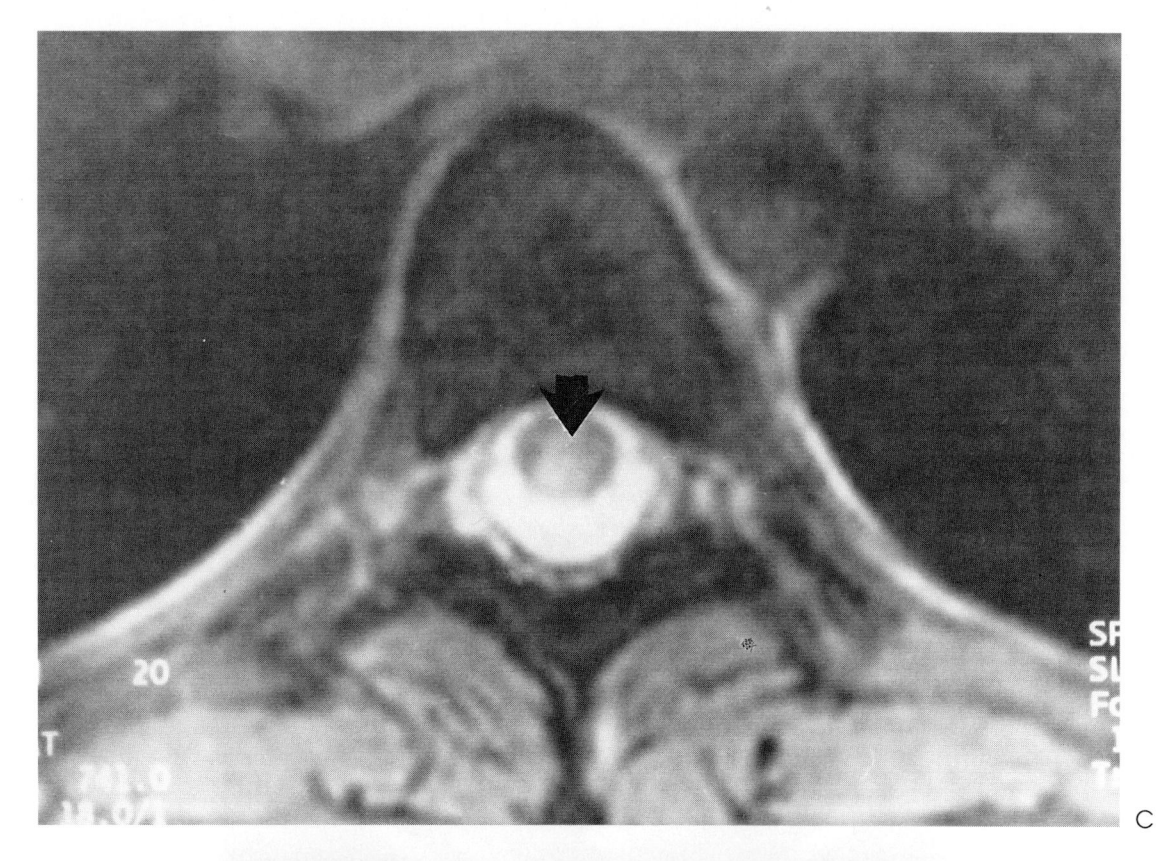

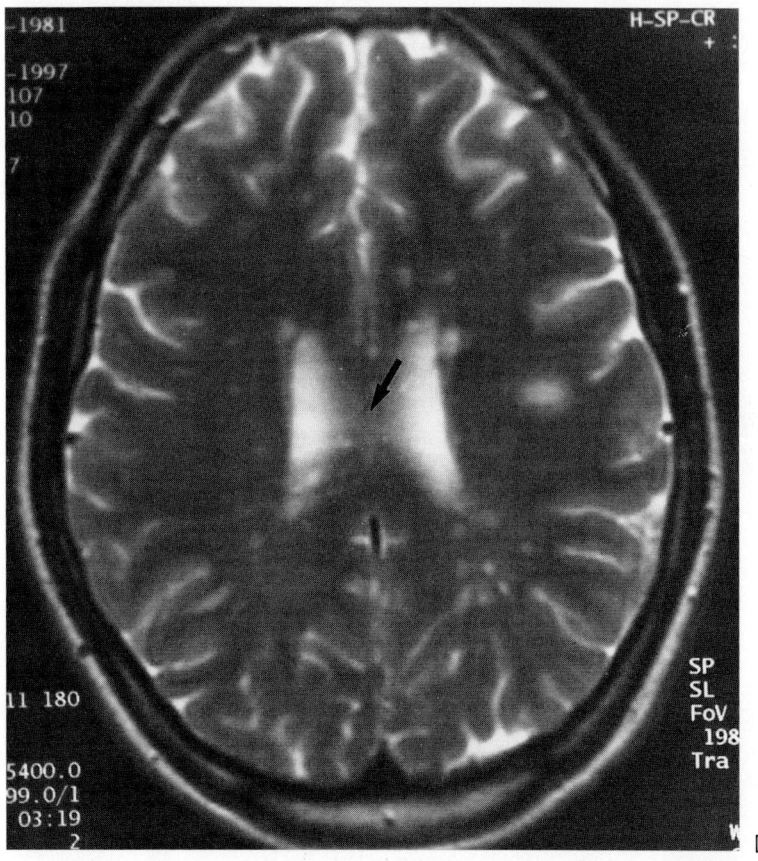

695

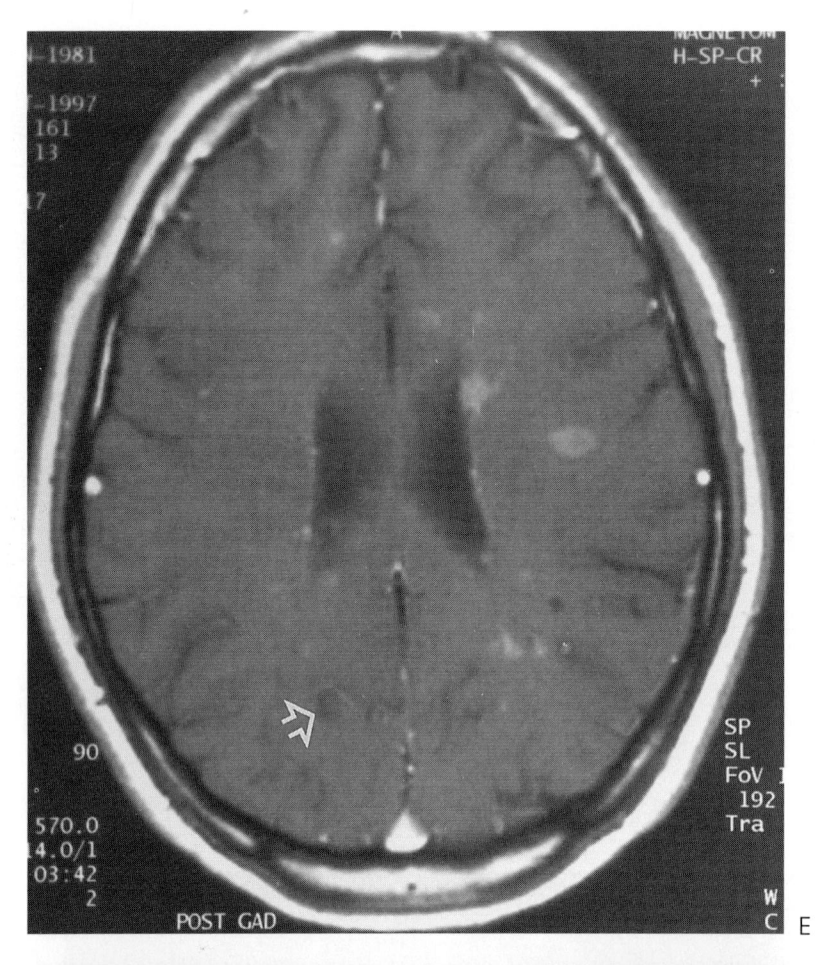

TEACHING ATLAS OF SPINE IMAGING

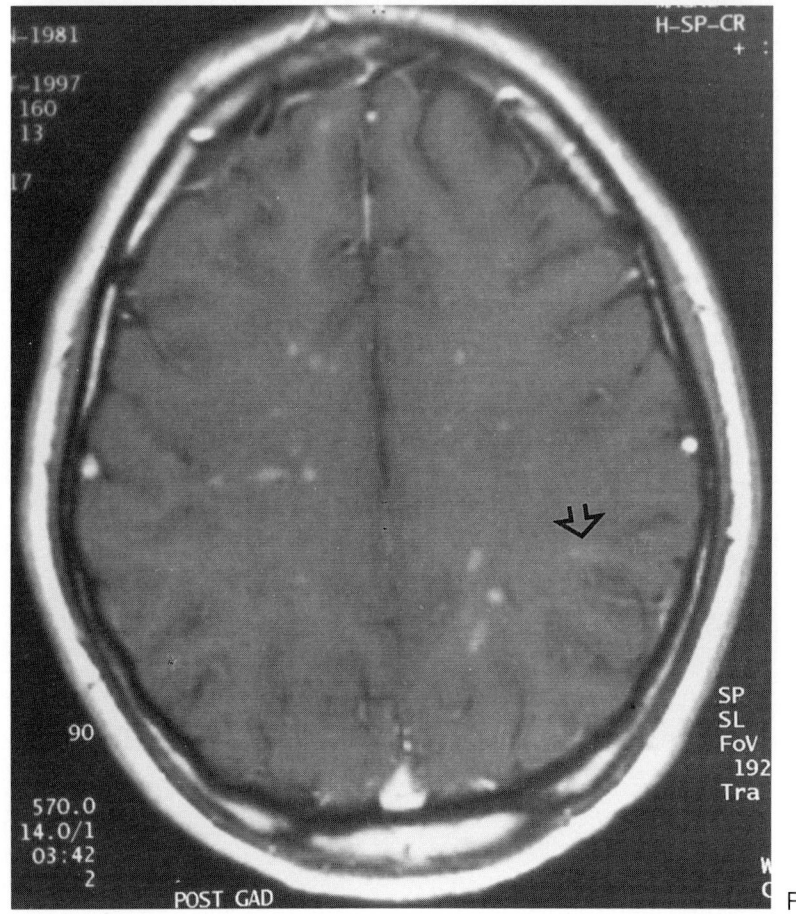

E

F

MISCELLANEOUS

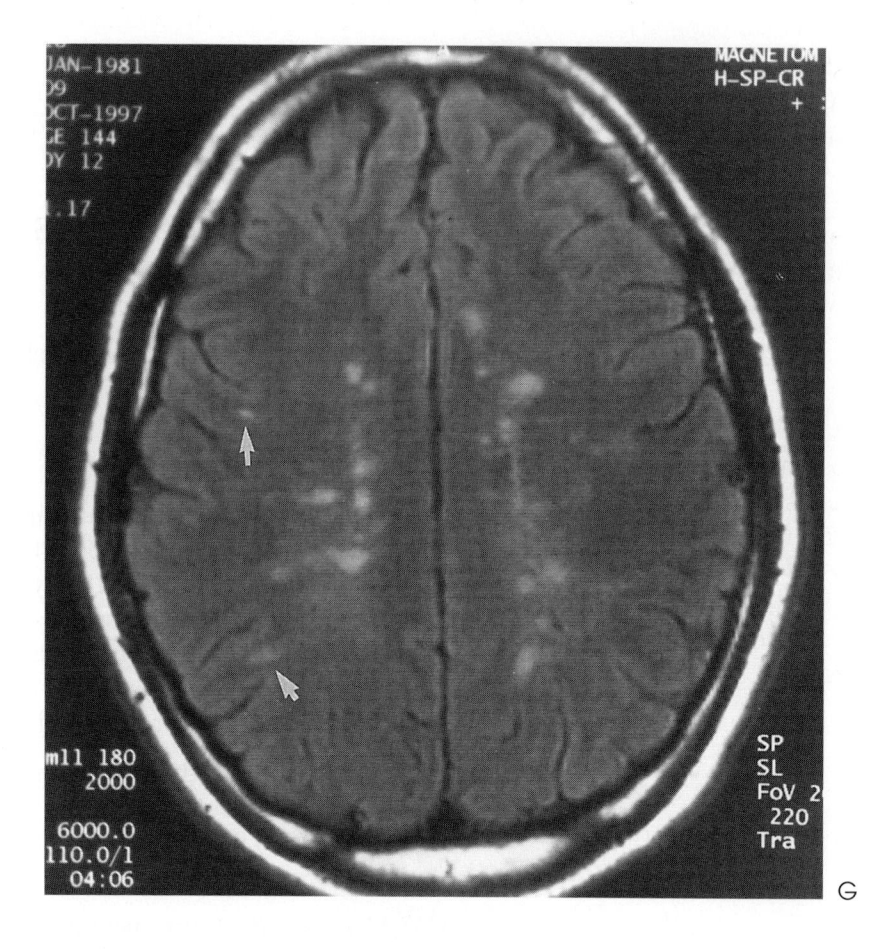

Radiologic Findings (continued)

Sagittal long TR image (Fig. B) reveals multiple patchy areas of increased signal intensity throughout the visualized spinal cord (*straight arrows*). Curvilinear areas of decreased signal intensity are seen in the subarachnoid fluid dorsal to the spinal cord (*curved arrows*).

Axial long TR image (Fig. C) reveals an area of increased signal intensity in the central spinal cord extending to the dorsal aspect of the spinal cord (*arrow*).

Axial long TR image of the brain at the level of the bodies of the lateral ventricles (Fig. D) reveals multiple rounded and oval areas of increased signal intensity surrounding the ventricles. There are streaky areas of increased signal intensity that involve the corpus callosum (*arrow*).

Axial short TR images postcontrast (Figs. E and F) reveal multiple areas of enhancement in the periventricular distribution. A faint area of enhancement is seen in the anticipated location of the arcuate or subcortical "U" fiber (Fig. F, *open arrow*). There is also a rounded area of decreased signal in the right parietal area (Fig. E, *open arrow*).

Axial FLAIR (fluid attenuated inversion recovery) image (Fig. G) reveals multiple periventricular and deep white matter areas of increased signal intensity. Areas of increased signal intensity deep to the sulci are presumably areas of involvement of the subcortical arcuate or "U" fibers (*arrows*).

PEARLS

- Correlation should be performed with cerebrospinal fluid evaluation.

- Follow-up would be helpful for evaluation for progression or regression of the abnormality.

PITFALL

- Occasionally multiple metastases may have a similar appearance. The diagnosis of metastases would be unlikely in a 16-year-old patient but could be a consideration in an older patient.

Diagnosis

Multiple sclerosis of the brain and spinal cord.

Differential Diagnosis

- multiple sclerosis

- acute disseminated encephalomyelitis (ADEM)

Discussion

The magnetic resonance imaging appearance of the brain is typical of multiple sclerosis, although the age of 16 years is unusually young. The involvement of the corpus callosum is typical and strongly favors a diagnosis of multiple sclerosis. Multiple sclerosis affects the white matter of the central nervous system, and the white matter is also present in the arcuate fibers, which are white matter tracts that extend from one gyrus to the next. These plaques of multiple sclerosis result in demyelination of the fibers.

The areas of decreased signal intensity seen in the subarachnoid space dorsal to the spinal cord are secondary to areas of flow-related enhancement, which are secondary to flow of cerebrospinal fluid in the subarachnoid space (Fig. B, *curved black arrows*).

ADEM (post-infectious encephalomyelitis) is also a strong diagnostic consideration in this patient because multiple sclerosis is uncommon in a patient as young as 16 years of age. If ADEM is a consideration, follow-up scans are necessary for complete evaluation.

MISCELLANEOUS

Case 3

Clinical Presentation

The patient is a 37-year-old female with paralyzed lower extremities and a history of optic neuritis.

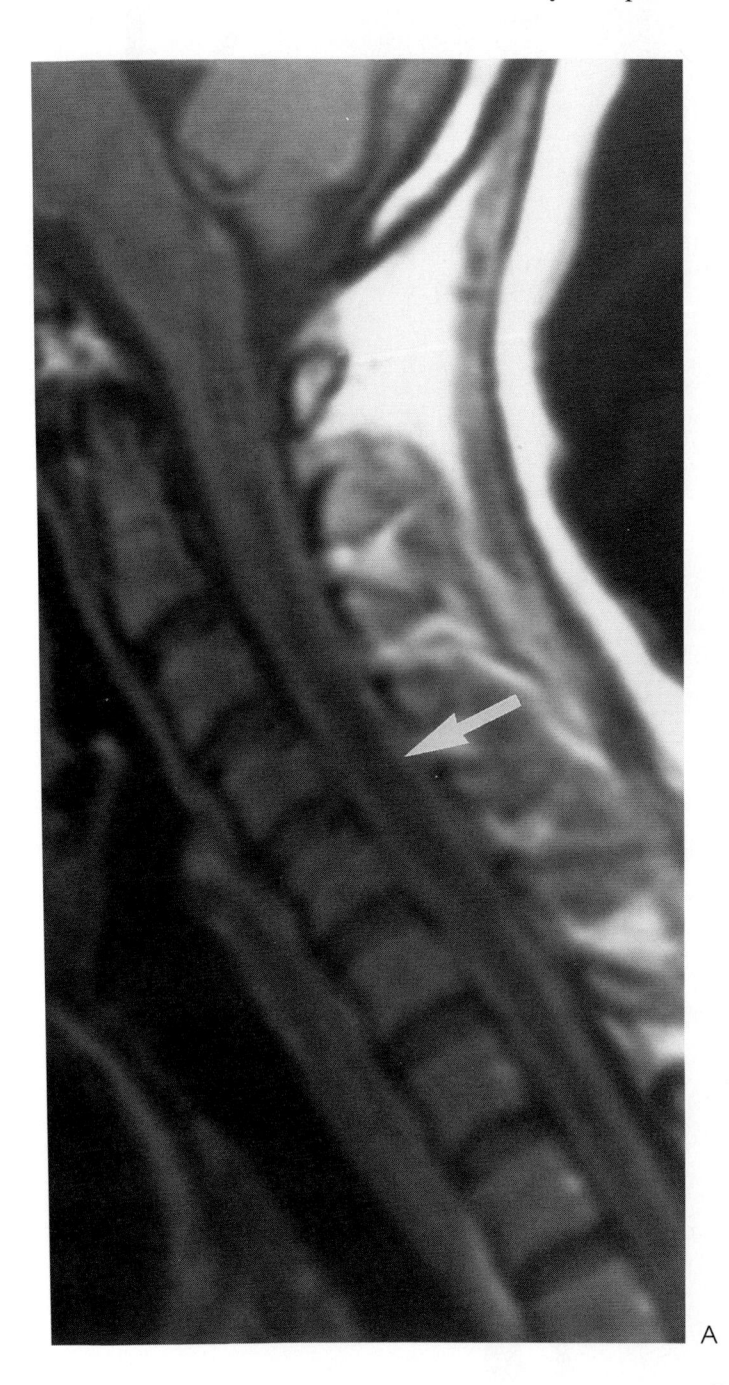

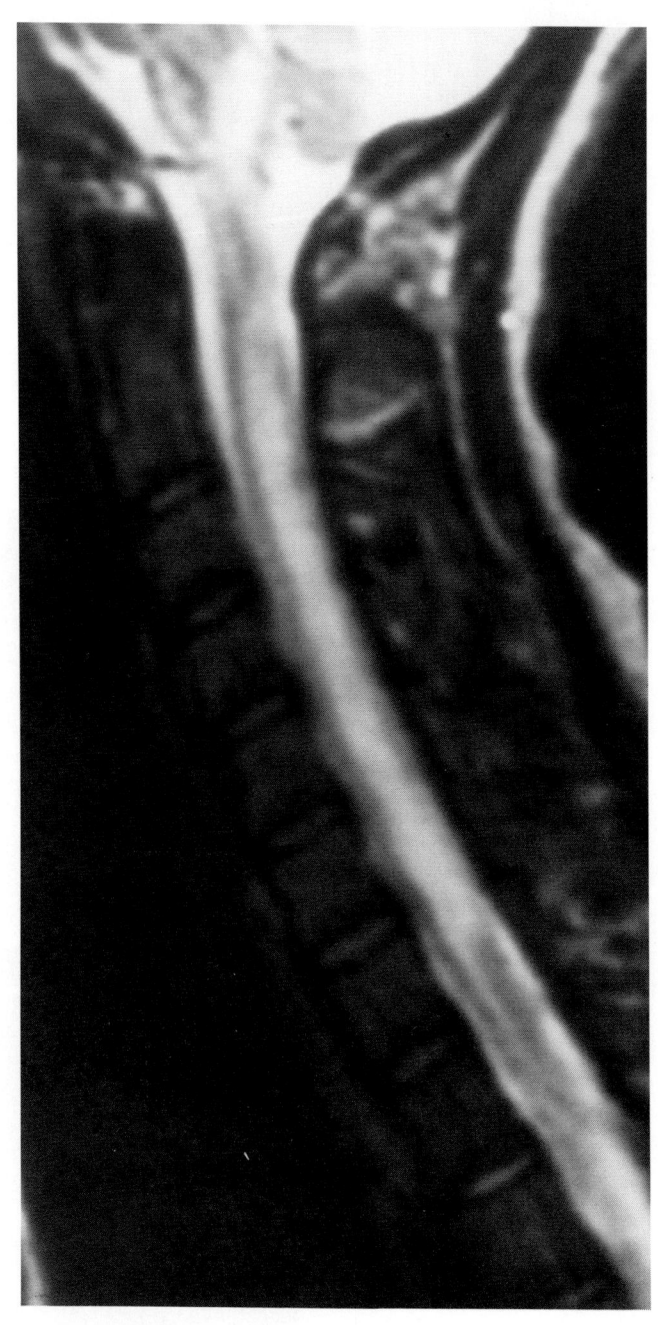

A

B

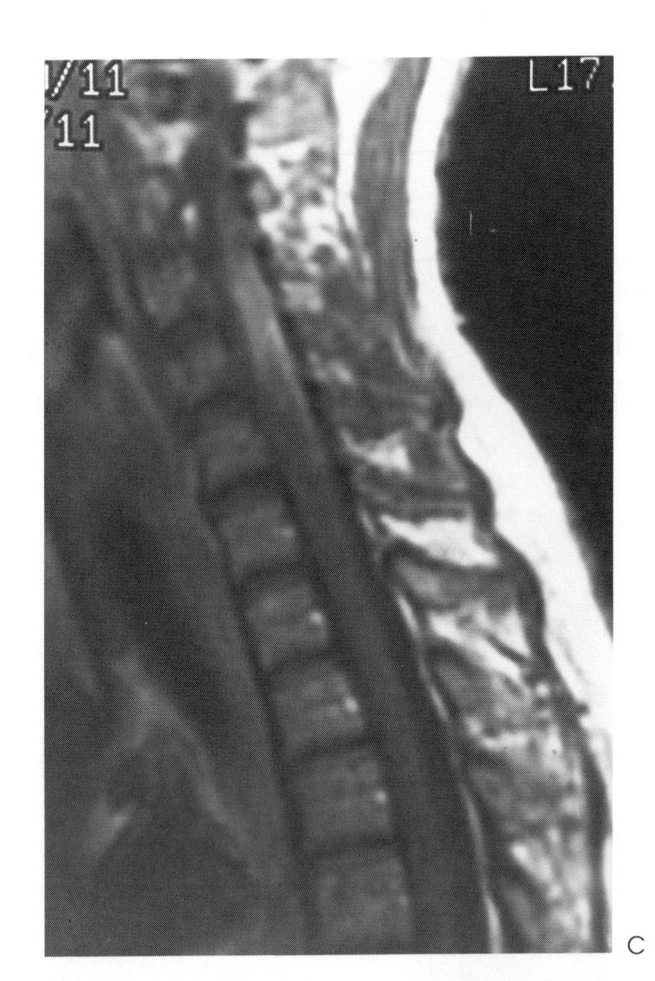

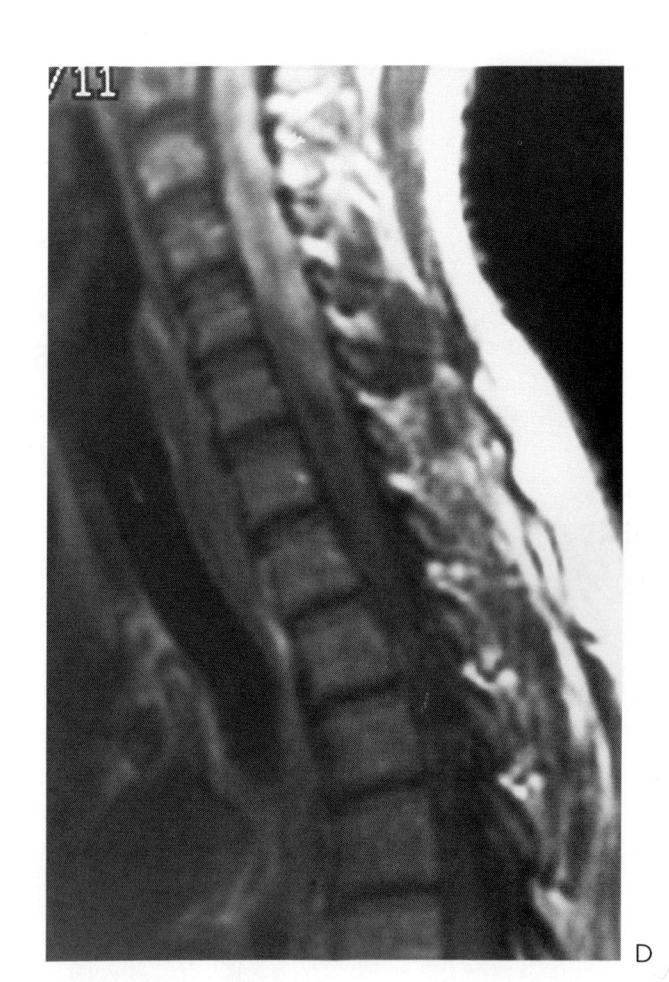

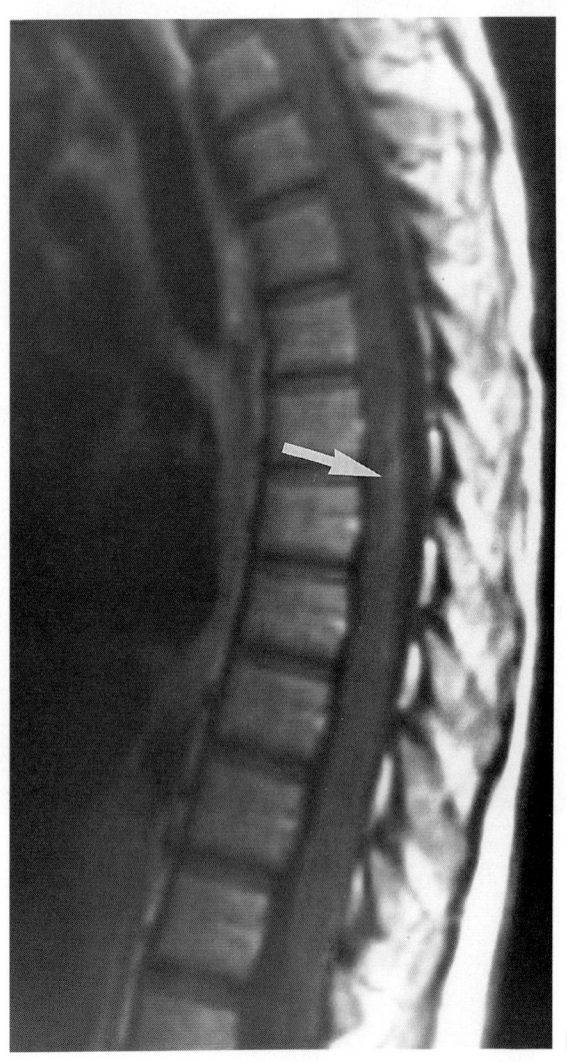

C

D

E

MISCELLANEOUS

F

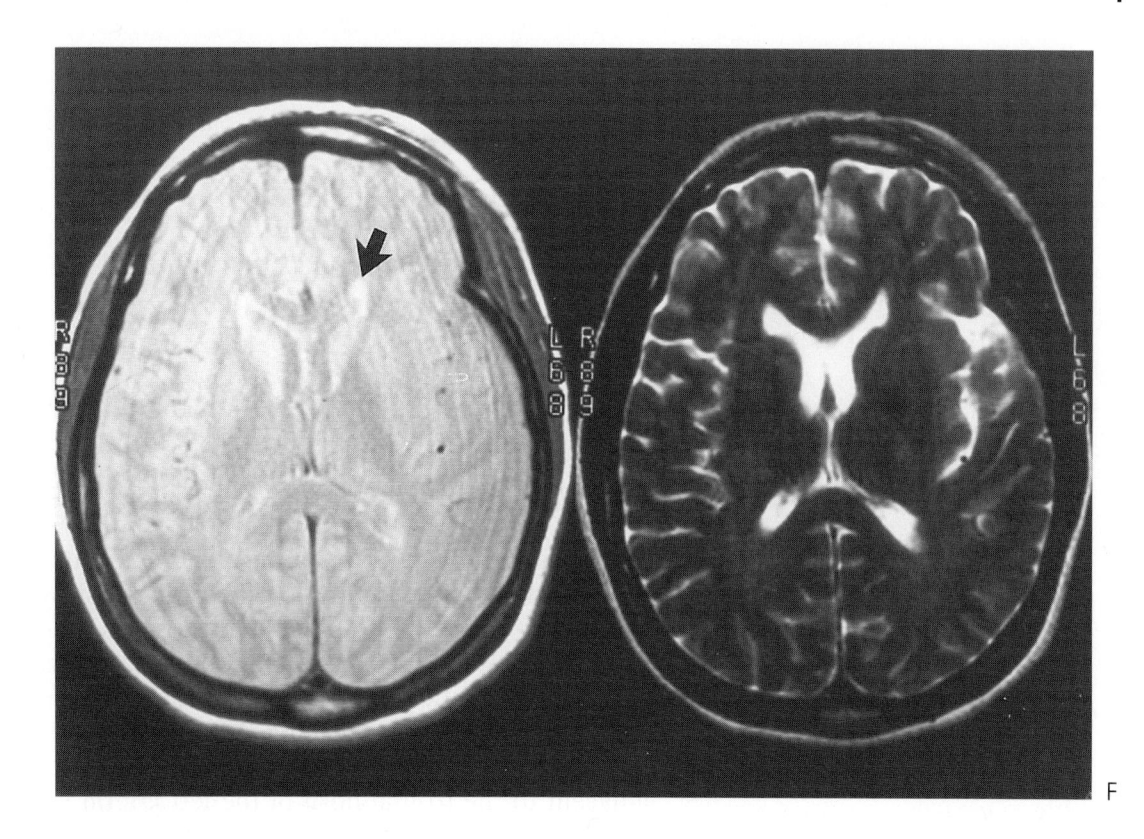

Radiologic Findings

Sagittal short TR image of the cervical spine (Fig. A) reveals that the cervical spinal cord is enlarged throughout its length. The central portion of the spinal cord appears as decreased signal intensity (*arrow*).

Sagittal long TR image (Fig. B) reveals a multisegmented area of increased signal intensity throughout the cervical spinal cord extending from the level of C1 through the level of C7.

Sagittal short TR images in the mid- and upper cervical region (Fig. C), lower cervical region (Fig. D), and thoracic region (Fig. E) reveal patchy areas of enhancement at multiple levels in the spinal cord (Fig. E, *arrow*).

Axial intermediate (Fig. F, *left*) and long (Fig. F, *right*) TR images reveal evidence of a small area of increased signal intensity adjacent to the frontal horn of the left lateral ventricle (*left, arrow*).

Diagnosis

Probable multiple sclerosis.

TEACHING ATLAS OF SPINE IMAGING

PEARLS

- Multiple sclerosis is more common in women than men, favoring the diagnosis of multiple sclerosis in this patient.

- Follow-up examination would be very helpful for complete evaluation of this patient.

- MRI of the brain would also be helpful because the presence of the typical areas of increased signal intensity in a periventricular and deep white matter distribution strongly favors the diagnosis of multiple sclerosis.

- Correlation should also be made with analysis of the cerebrospinal fluid.

PITFALLS

- Because the treatment may be different depending upon the diagnosis, it is important to attempt to make an accurate diagnosis in a case such as this.

- Biopsy of the spinal cord may make the patient clinically worse, so it is prudent to follow the patient with MRI with contrast enhancement to evaluate the progression of the disease.

Differential Diagnosis

- multiple sclerosis
- acute disseminated encephalomyelitis (ADEM)
- idiopathic transverse myelopathy
- Devic's disease
- syrinx cavity

Discussion

Based on the imaging appearance and clinical correlation with other tests, multiple sclerosis is the most likely diagnosis; other possibilities such as ADEM or idiopathic transverse myelopathy are considerations. Follow-up examinations and further evaluation of the clinical course are necessary for complete evaluation. The patient was diagnosed with multiple sclerosis based on magnetic resonance imaging (MRI) evaluation, cerebrospinal fluid analysis, and visual-evoked responses. The area of increased signal intensity adjacent to the frontal horn of the left lateral ventricle is thought to be an area of plaque formation secondary to multiple sclerosis.

Devic's disease (neuromyelitis optica), a possible diagnosis in this case, is thought to be a subtype of multiple sclerosis that presents with optic neuritis and spinal cord involvement.

The marked edema of the spinal cord is remotely similar in appearance to that seen with a syrinx cavity; however, the patchy-streaky pattern of enhancement rules out syrinx cavity as a diagnosis.

MISCELLANEOUS

Case 4

Clinical Presentation

The patient is a 26-year-old female with a clinical history of right arm pain and leg numbness.

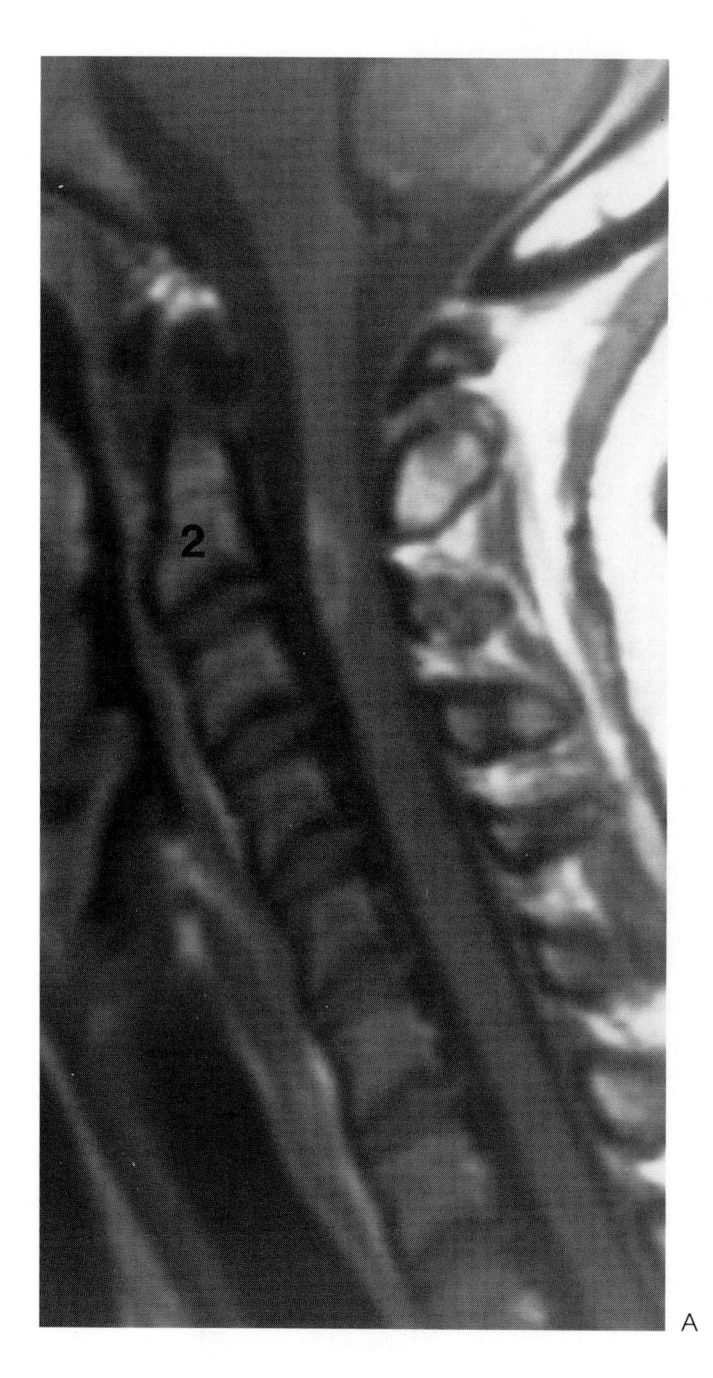

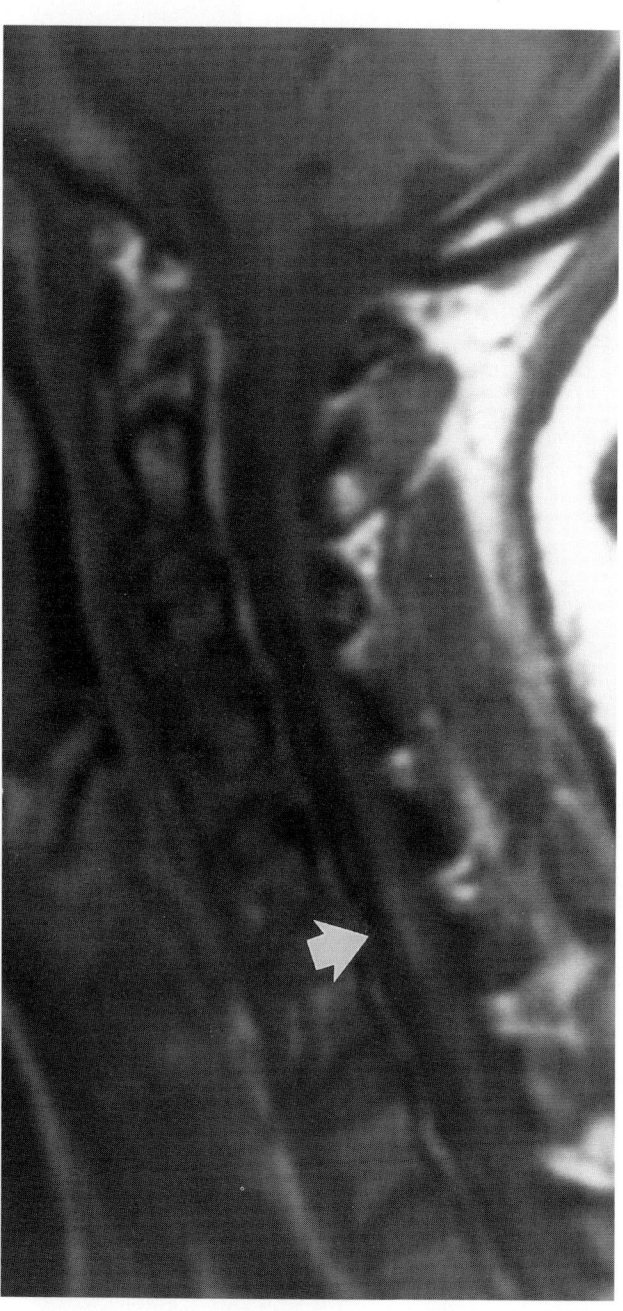

TEACHING ATLAS OF SPINE IMAGING

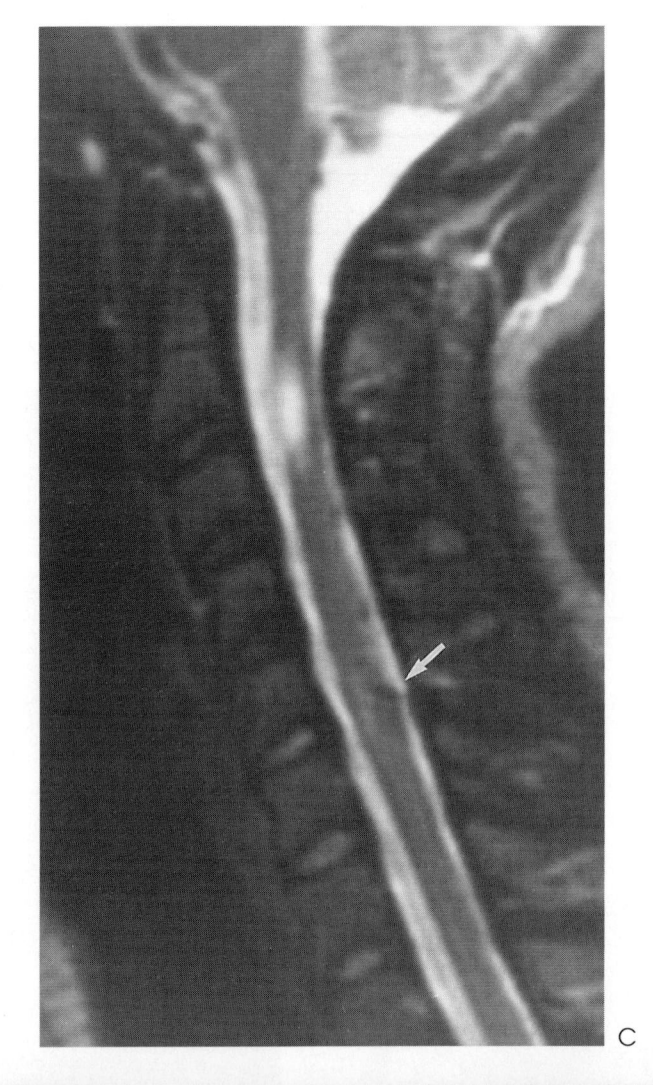

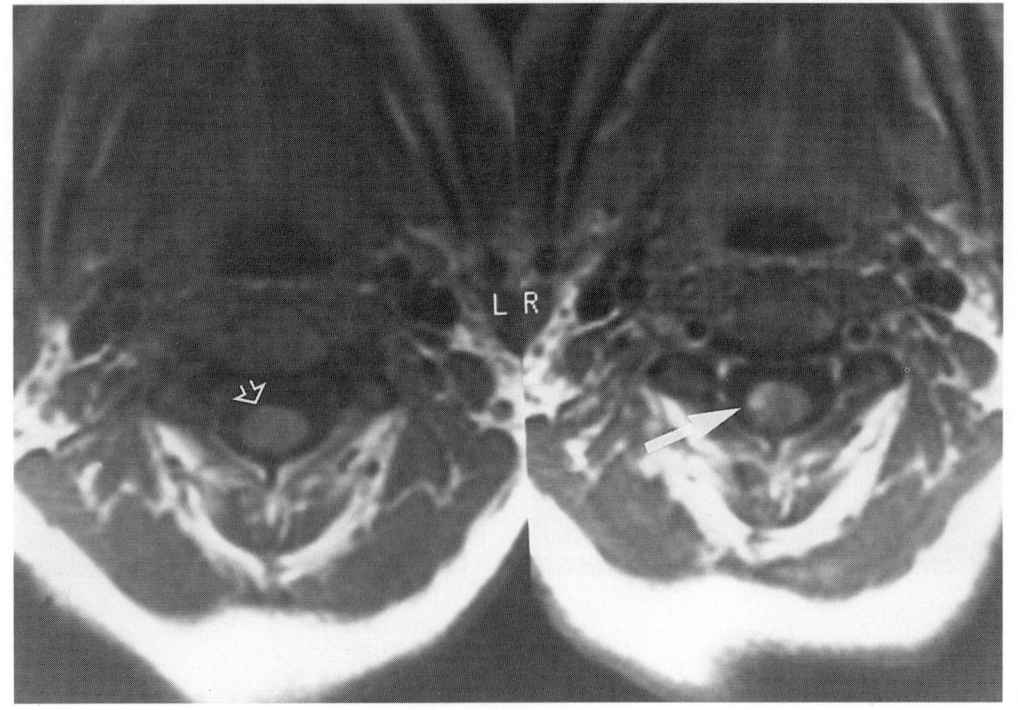

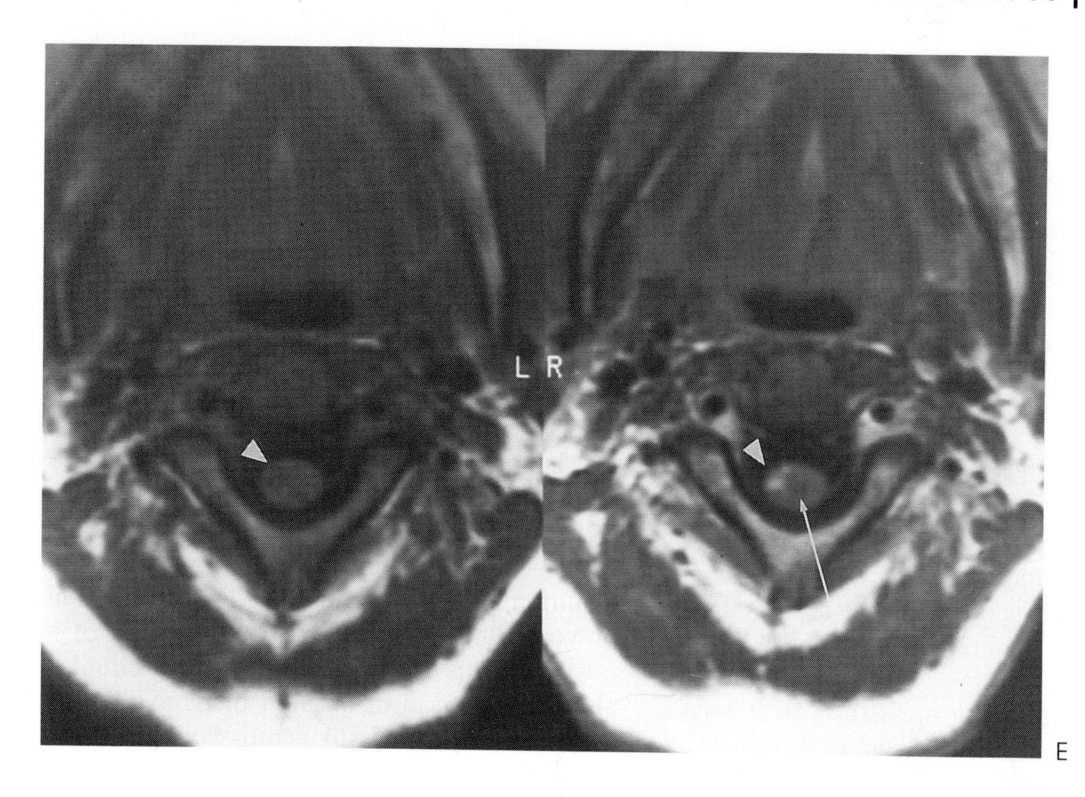

Radiologic Findings

Sagittal short TR image postcontrast (Fig. A) reveals an area of enhancement in the ventral aspect of the spinal cord at the C2-3 level. Note that the enhancement exhibits an elongated ring or oval-shaped appearance. The C2 vertebral body is identified with 2.

Sagittal short TR image postcontrast (Fig. B) reveals a second area of enhancement at the level of C5-6 (*arrow*).

Sagittal long TR image (Fig. C) reveals an oval area of increased signal intensity in the ventral aspect of the spinal cord at the C2-3 level. The linear area of decreased signal intensity dorsally at the C5 level is an artifact (*arrow*).

Pre- (Fig. D, *left*) and postcontrast (Fig. D, *right*) axial short TR images at the C2-3 level reveal an area of slight prominence of the ventral aspect of the spinal cord on the right side (*left, open arrow*). This area exhibits faint hypointensity. After the infusion of contrast, there is enhancement of the area of low signal intensity (*right, arrow*).

Axial short TR image (Fig. E) reveals a rounded area of decreased signal intensity on the right side of the cervical spinal cord (*arrowhead*). There is a bilobed area of enhancement in this same area after the infusion of contrast material (*right, arrow*).

Diagnosis

Multiple sclerosis of the spinal cord.

TEACHING ATLAS OF SPINE IMAGING

PEARLS

- Magnetic resonance imaging (MRI) evaluation of the brain would be very helpful.

- If there are areas of increased signal intensity typical of multiple sclerosis plaques, this would confirm the diagnosis.

PITFALLS

- Biopsy is rarely performed in cases such as this, so the diagnosis generally is made based on clinical presentation and imaging findings.

- Sarcoidosis of the spinal cord could also have a similar appearance. Therefore, the MR appearance should be correlated with cerebrospinal fluid evaluation.

Differential Diagnosis

- multiple sclerosis

- postinfectious encephalomyelitis

- syrinx cavity

Discussion

The lateral location of the areas of enhancement in the spinal cord are consistent with lesions of the white matter. The gray matter forms the central portion of the spinal cord and can be seen as an X-shaped area of decreased signal intensity. This is best seen on the right image of Figure E (*arrow*). The age of the patient is compatible with multiple sclerosis, which is more common in women than men. The lack of a history of previous vaccination or viral illness also favors the diagnosis of multiple sclerosis rather than postinfectious encephalomyelitis. The circular/oval area of enhancement is also more typical of an area of demyelination, while a spinal cord tumor would be more masslike and would not be confined to a white matter distribution. The marked edema of the spinal cord almost has the appearance of a syrinx cavity.

MISCELLANEOUS

Case 5

Clinical Presentation

The patient is a 22-year-old female with blurred vision and upper extremity tingling.

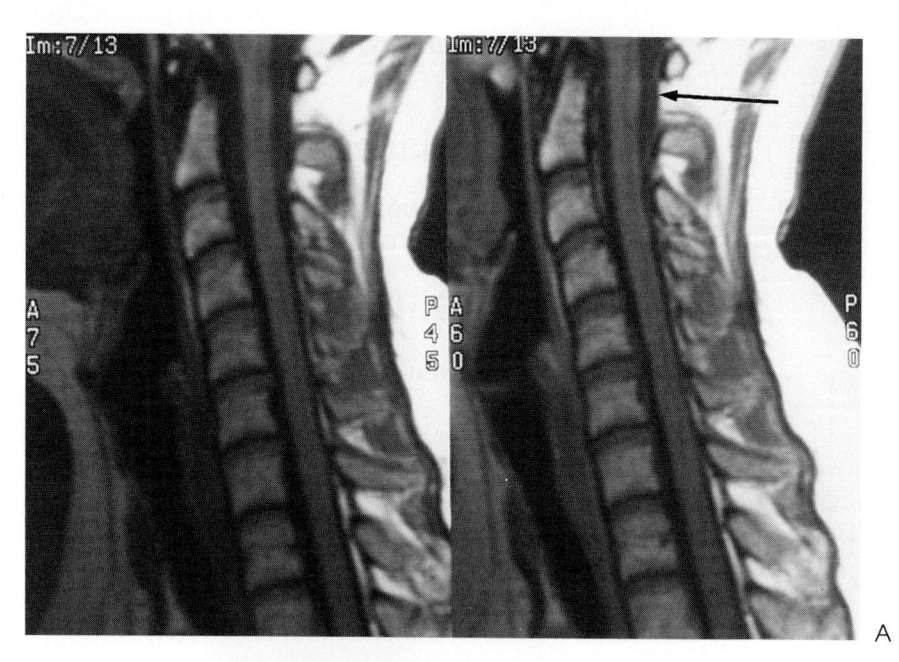

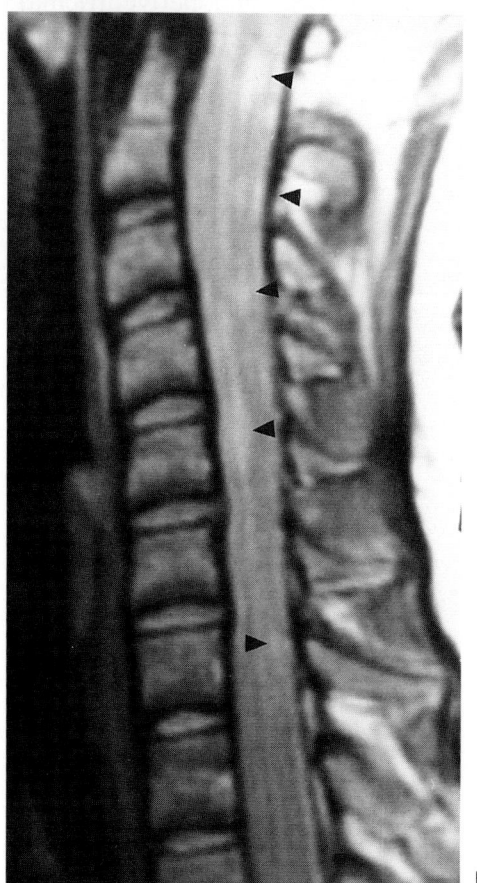

A

B

TEACHING ATLAS OF SPINE IMAGING

PEARLS
- Not all plaques of multiple sclerosis exhibit enhancement on the postcontrast study.

- The clinical history of blurred vision is significant in this patient because multiple sclerosis commonly affects the visual pathways.

- The patchy enhancement is not in favor of the diagnosis of a spinal cord tumor, but rather is a more typical finding in transverse myelopathy (myelitis).

PITFALL
- MRI of the brain should be performed to aid in better substantiating the diagnosis of multiple sclerosis.

Radiologic Findings

Sagittal short TR images in the cervical region pre- (Fig. A, *left*) and postcontrast (Fig. A, *right*) reveal that the precontrast study appears within normal limits. There is a questionable area of enhancement in the dorsal aspect of the spinal cord at the C2 level (*right, arrow*). The study otherwise appears within normal limits.

Sagittal intermediate TR image (Fig. B) reveals multiple patchy areas of increased signal intensity throughout the cervical spinal cord region (*arrowheads*).

Diagnosis

Multiple sclerosis of the spinal cord.

Differential Diagnosis

- multiple sclerosis

- acute disseminated encephalomyelitis (ADEM)

Discussion

The patient was known to have a diagnosis of multiple sclerosis, and magnetic resonance imaging (MRI) of the brain reveals multiple deep white matter and periventricular areas of increased signal consistent with the typical demyelinating plaques of multiple sclerosis. The appearance of the spinal cord is typical of the plaques of multiple sclerosis. No enhancement is seen in this patient; however, the plaques are seen as areas of increased signal intensity on the longer TR images.

In another setting, ADEM (postinfectious encephalomyelitis) should be considered as a possible diagnosis.

MISCELLANEOUS

Case 6

Clinical Presentation

The patient is a 48-year-old female with upper extremity proximal weakness and back and shoulder pain.

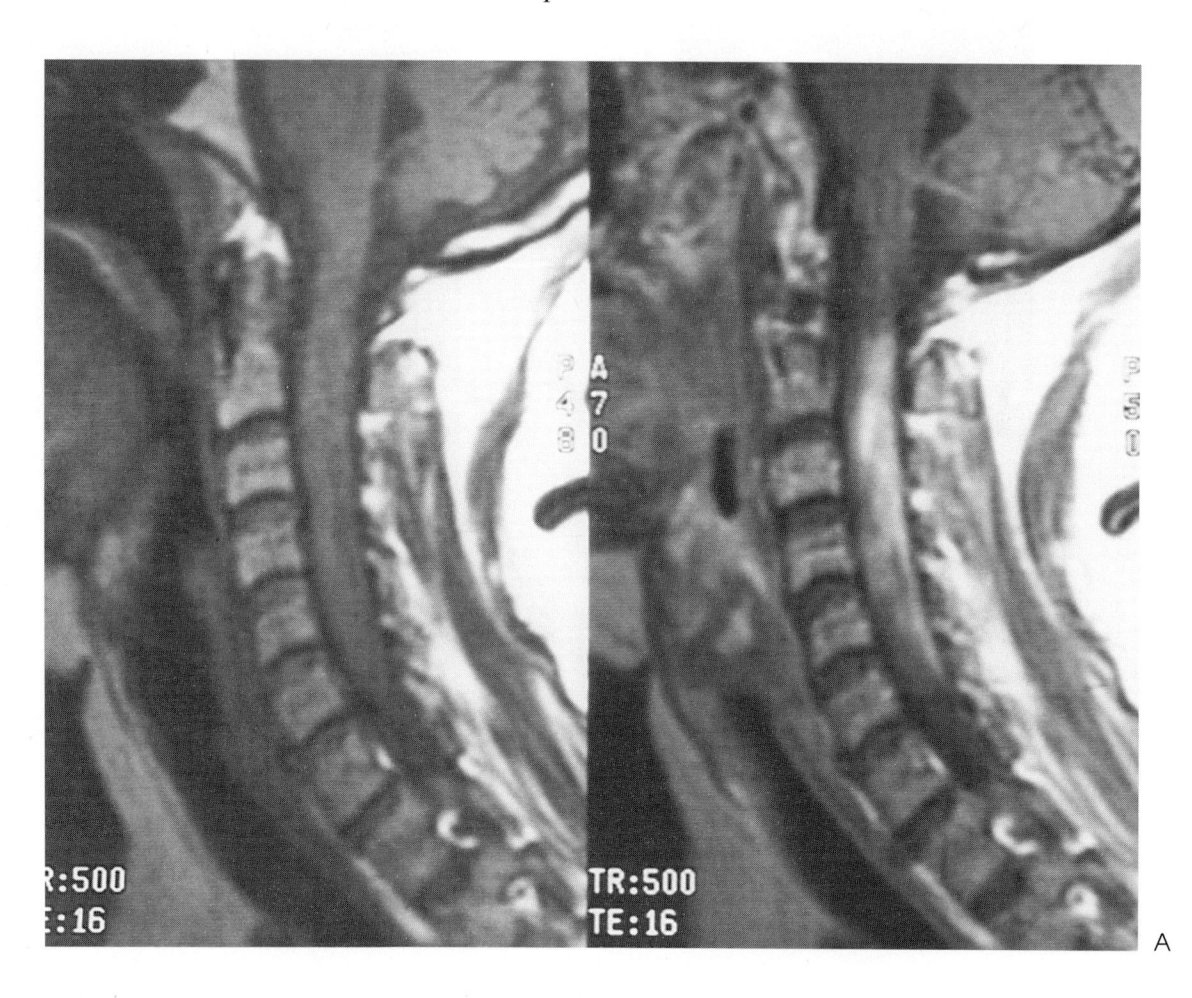

Radiologic Findings

Pre- (Fig. A, *left*) and postcontrast (Fig. A, *right*) sagittal short TR images reveal that the cervical spinal cord is diffusely enlarged throughout its visualized length. In addition, there is a streaklike area of low signal intensity within the central portion of the spinal cord that begins at the level of the midbody of C2 and extends inferiorly through C4. After the infusion of contrast (*right*), there is dense, irregular, and inhomogeneous enhancement throughout the cervical spinal cord.

TEACHING ATLAS OF SPINE IMAGING

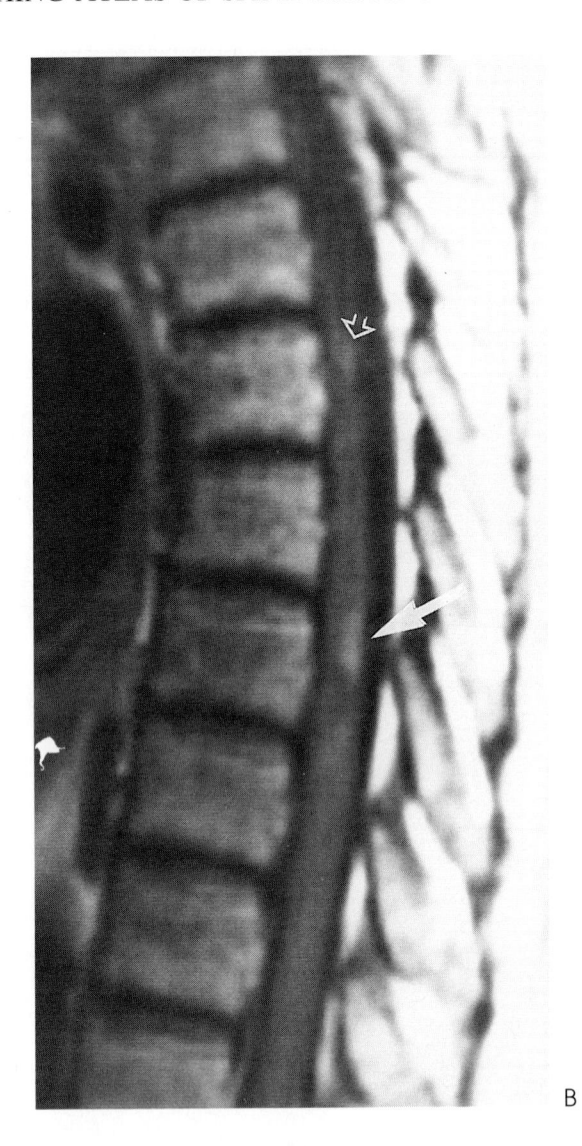

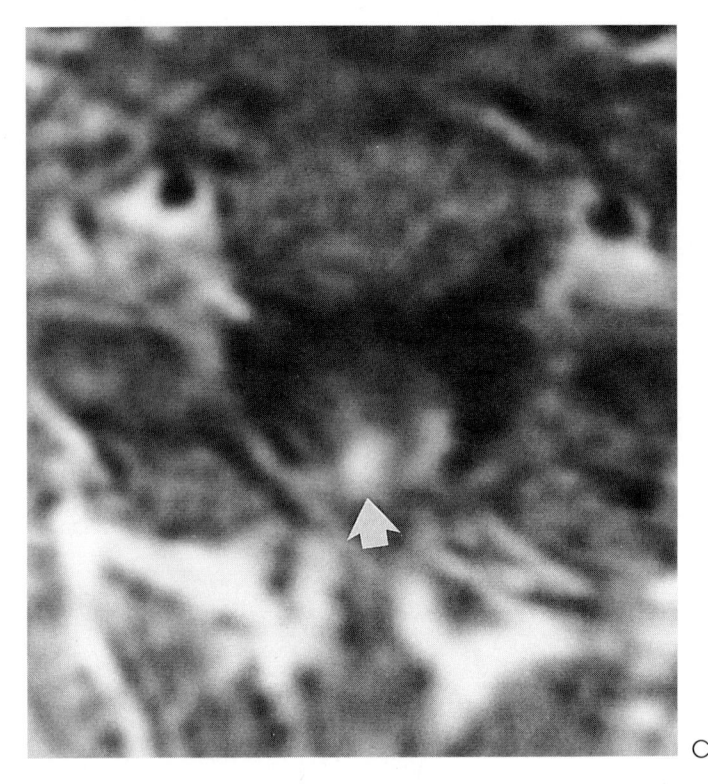

Radiologic Findings (continued)

Sagittal short TR image postcontrast in the thoracic region (Fig. B) reveals a small area of enhancement in the dorsal aspect of the spinal cord at the level of T8 (*solid arrow*). A small and less distinct area of enhancement is more superiorly placed (*open arrow*).

Axial short TR image postcontrast (Fig. C) reveals a dense patchy enhancement in the dorsal aspect of the spinal cord (*arrow*) in the midline, extending off to the left side.

Diagnosis

Transverse myelitis of unknown cause.

PEARL

- Multiple sclerosis may present with an appearance similar to idiopathic transverse myelitis. An MR scan of the brain may be helpful in these cases; when the typical appearance of multiple sclerosis is identified in the brain, the diagnosis of multiple sclerosis involvement of the spinal cord is more secure.

PITFALL

- Biopsy of a spinal cord lesion may result in an increased neurologic deficit, so a conservative management course is usually followed with evaluation with additional MR scans following a suitable period of medical management or when there is a sudden change in the clinical condition of the patient.

Differential Diagnosis

- transverse myelitis
- paraneoplastic syndrome
- spinal cord tumor
- intramedullary metastases

Discussion

The patient also had a history of multiple sclerosis; however, the brain magnetic resonance (MR) scan was within normal limits. Demyelinating plaques may be seen in the spinal cord in patients with multiple sclerosis when the brain scan is normal. However, it is much more common to have an abnormal brain MR scan when the spinal cord is abnormal. Patients may also have signs and symptoms of a spinal cord myelopathy and have a normal MR scan of the spinal cord.

Paraneoplastic syndrome may also present with the appearance of transverse myelopathy/myelitis. Spinal cord tumor is unlikely in this case because the patchy nature of the enhancement is not in favor of the diagnosis of tumor. Also, tumor is unlikely to reveal areas of intervening normal spinal cord tissue.

The possibility of intramedullary metastases from a primary tumor outside the central nervous system (e.g., breast or lung cancer or melanoma) or from within the central nervous system (e.g., from a pinealoma or ependymoma of the brain or spinal cord) are also considerations because of the multiple lesions but are actually uncommon and are therefore less likely.

TEACHING ATLAS OF SPINE IMAGING

Case 7

Clinical Presentation

The patient is a 43-year-old previously healthy male who presented with a 1-week history of progressive upper extremity weakness and lack of coordination. The patient also had neck pain. Two weeks prior to onset of symptoms, the patient had received a vaccination for hepatitis B.

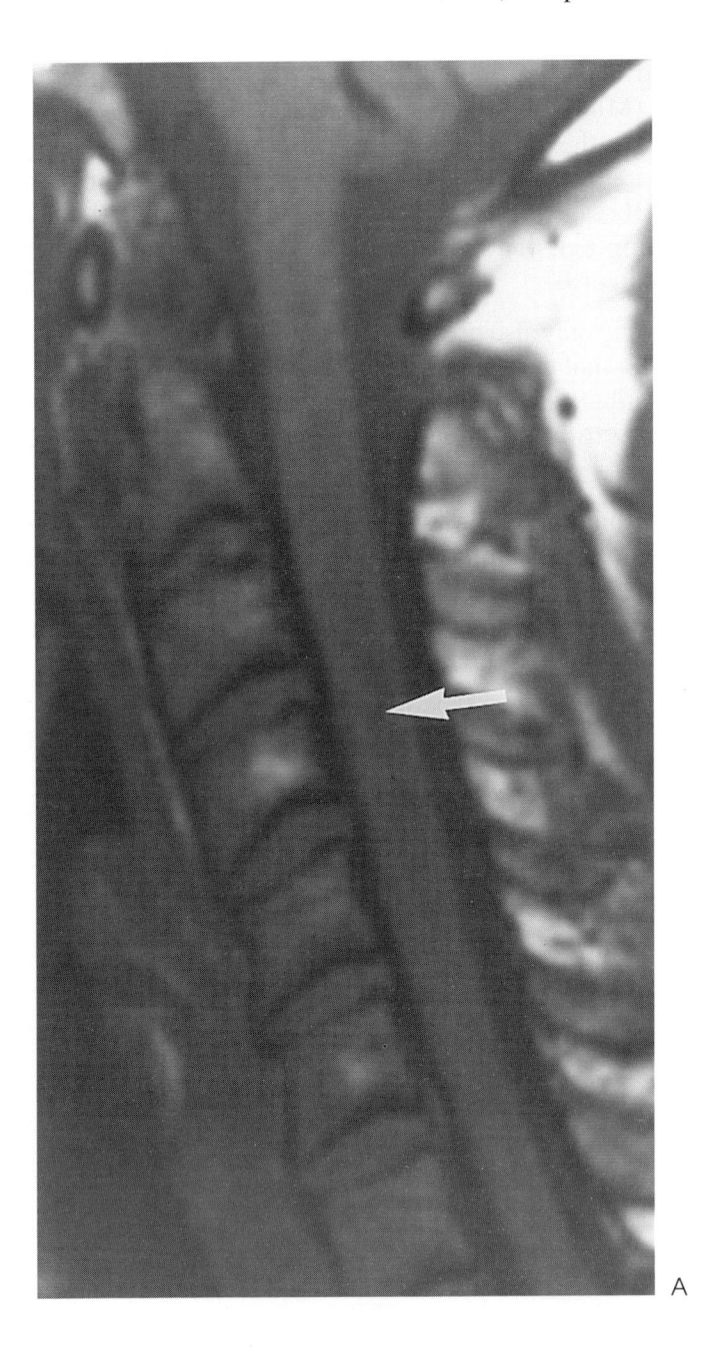

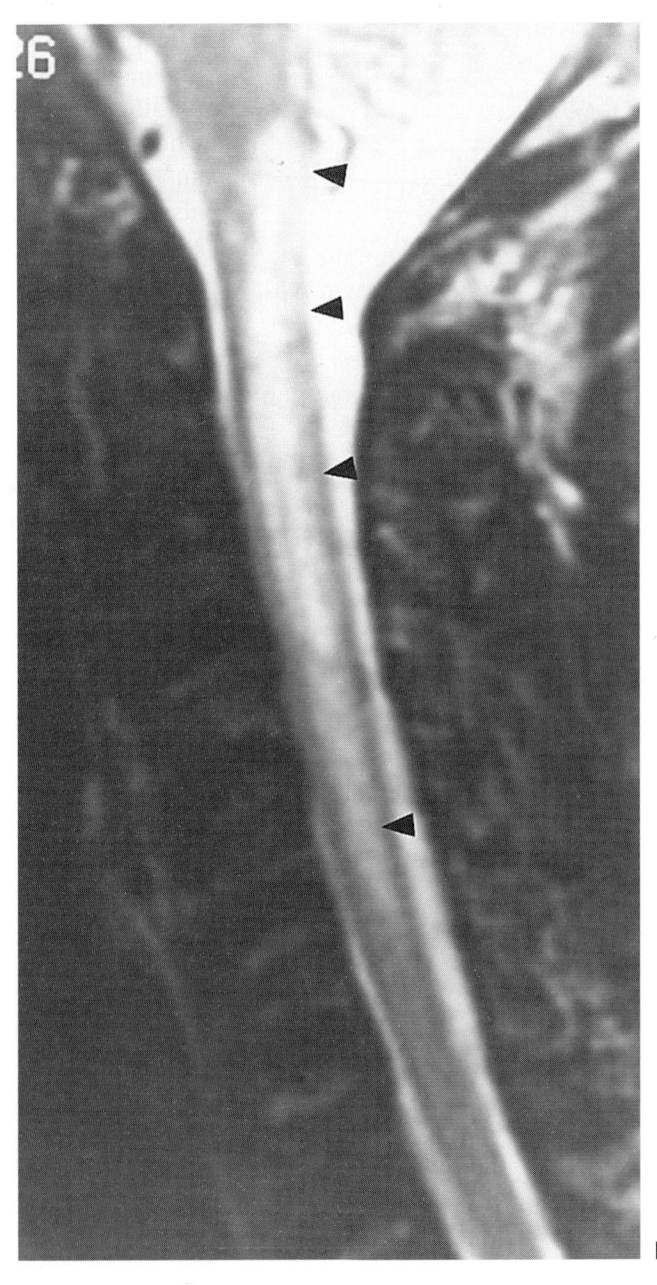

A

B

MISCELLANEOUS

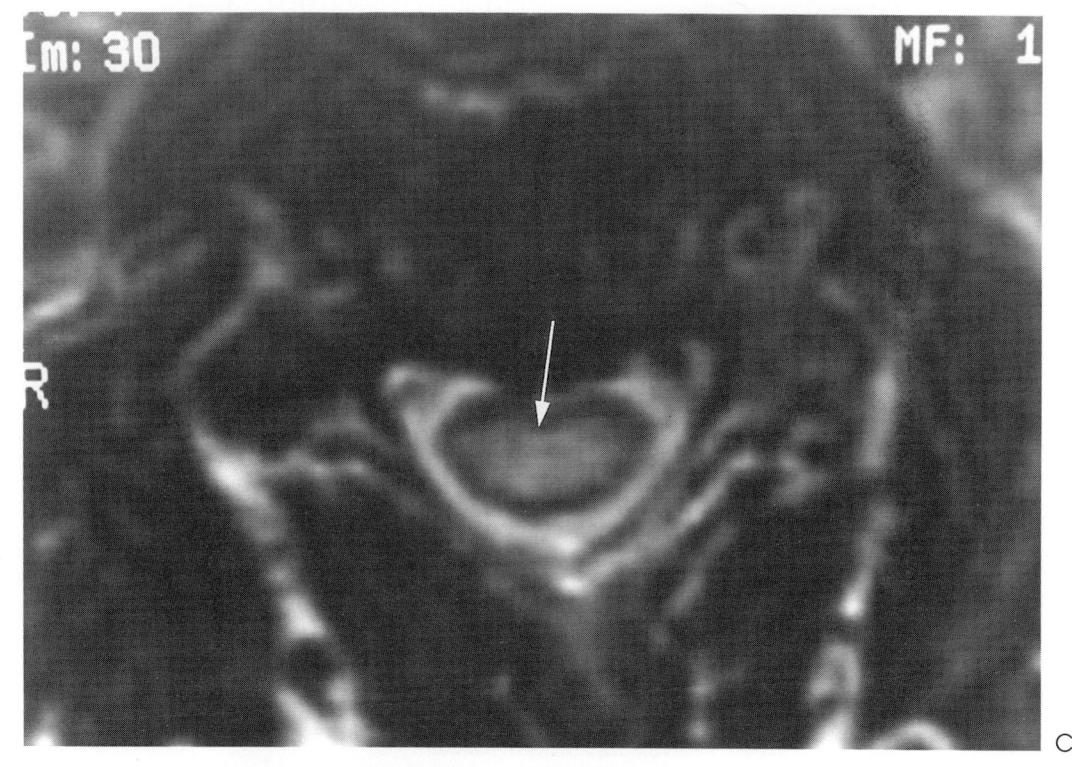

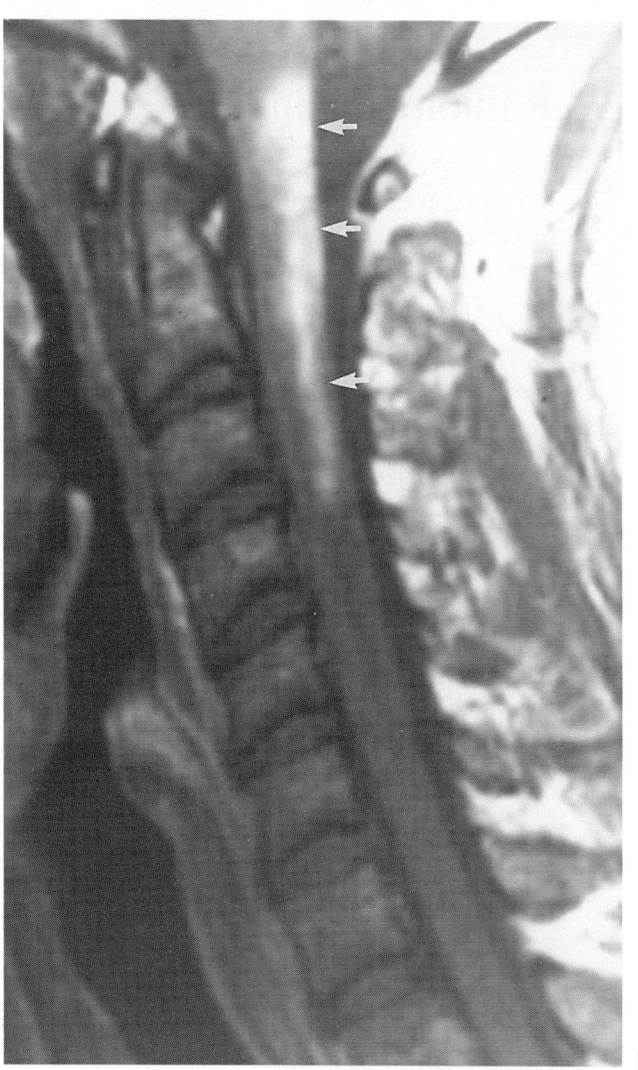

C

D

713

TEACHING ATLAS OF SPINE IMAGING

E

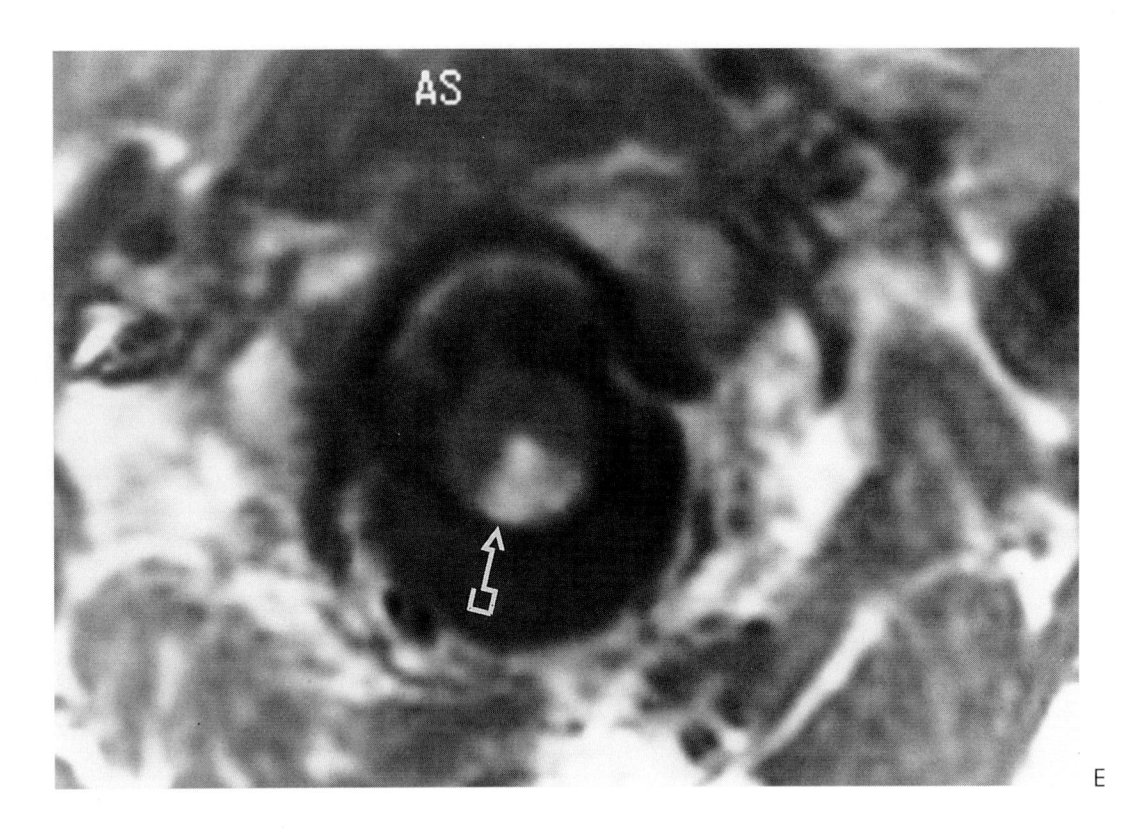

Radiologic Findings

Sagittal short TR image (Fig. A) reveals a central area of decreased signal intensity in the central portion of the spinal cord that extends from the level of C2 through the level of C5 (*arrow at C3-4*). The spinal cord is normal in size throughout its length.

Sagittal long TR image (Fig. B) reveals an area of increased signal intensity that extends from the medulla inferiorly through the level of C5-6 (*arrowheads*).

Axial long TR image (Fig. C) reveals a central area of increased signal intensity (*arrow*).

Sagittal short TR image postcontrast (Fig. D) reveals a dense area of enhancement in the dorsal aspect of the spinal cord that extends from the lower medulla through the level of C3-4 (*arrows*). The margin of the area of enhancement reveals an irregular edge.

Axial short TR image postcontrast (Fig. E) reveals a wedge-shaped area of enhancement in the dorsal aspect of the spinal cord. The area of enhancement extends slightly more toward the left than toward the right side (*arrow*).

Diagnosis

Postimmunization transverse myelopathy ("myelitis").

Differential Diagnosis

- transverse myelopathy

PEARLS

- The clinical history of a vaccination or viral illness is vital for accurate evaluation of the images.

- Spinal cord infarct with enhancement is a consideration in this patient; however, infarction is more typically seen in older age group patients and is often seen in association with congestive heart failure.

PITFALL

- This illness may also mimic the presentation of multiple sclerosis and the patient should be evaluated for this possibility. Magnetic resonance imaging of the brain would be helpful for more complete evaluation.

Discussion

This disease is also known as acute disseminated encephalomyelopathy (ADEM). Transverse myelopathy following immunization is rare. Similar changes may occur in the brain where it is called acute disseminated encephalomyelitis. These changes are not truly an inflammatory process but are secondary to an antibody-antigen reaction. The body makes antibodies against the antigen of the hepatitis immunization product; however, the antibody mistakes the normal myelin in the brain and spinal cord for the antigen, and demyelination results. The clinical presentation is approximately 2 weeks following the immunization. This process may also occur following viral illness such as an upper respiratory infection or the common cold. Therefore, the clinical history should include inquiry about these possibilities.

The areas of enhancement are thought to be secondary to acute demyelination.

The clinical course in this illness is highly variable. Recovery may occur; however, this illness may also progress to severe neurological deficit or even death.

Idiopathic transverse myelopathy would also have a similar appearance, and while quadriplegia may occur following immunization for hepatitis B virus, it is very rare.

The patchy, irregularly marginated areas of increased signal intensity within the vertebral bodies of C4 and C6 are secondary to areas of fat deposition within the marrow of the vertebral body and are of no clinical significance.

Case 8

Clinical Presentation

The patient is a 53-year-old female who developed lower extremity weakness 2 weeks following a second vaccination against hepatitis B virus.

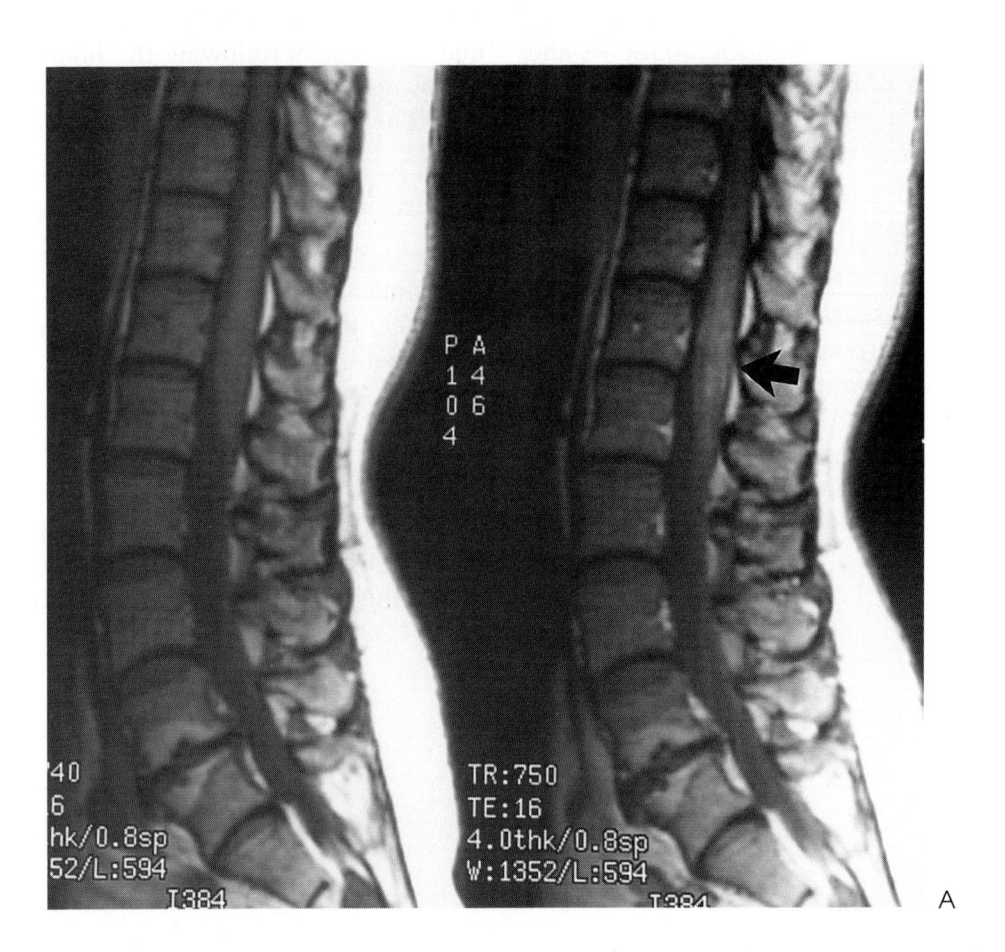

A

Radiologic Findings

Pre- (Fig. A, *left*) and postcontrast (Fig. A, *right*) sagittal short TR images reveal enlargement of the distal end of the spinal cord. There is also increased signal intensity within the enlarged portion of the spinal cord on the postcontrast study (*right, arrow*). Incidentally noted is disc space narrowing at the L5-S1 level with Schmorl's nodule deformities in the adjacent vertebral body end plates. There is also increased signal intensity in the vertebral bodies adjacent to the degenerated disc. Posterior osteophytes are encroaching upon the vertebral canal, indenting the thecal sac, and widening the epidural fat above and below the bulging disc at L5-S1.

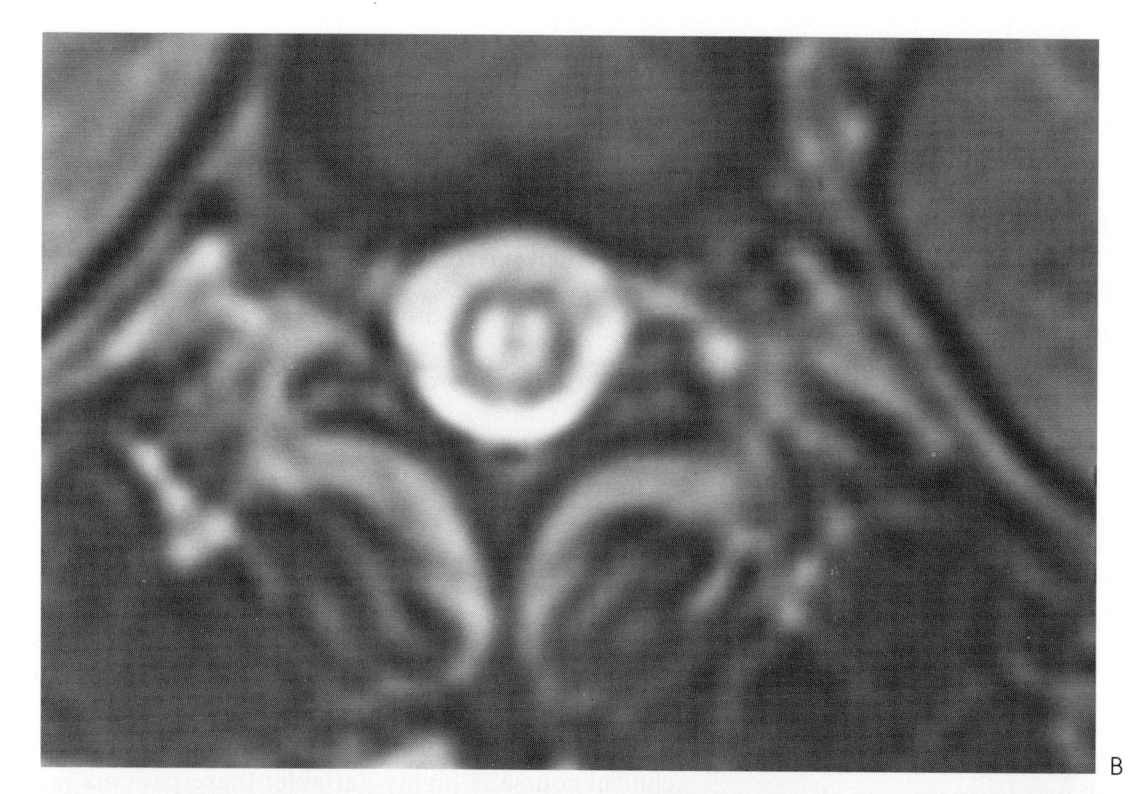

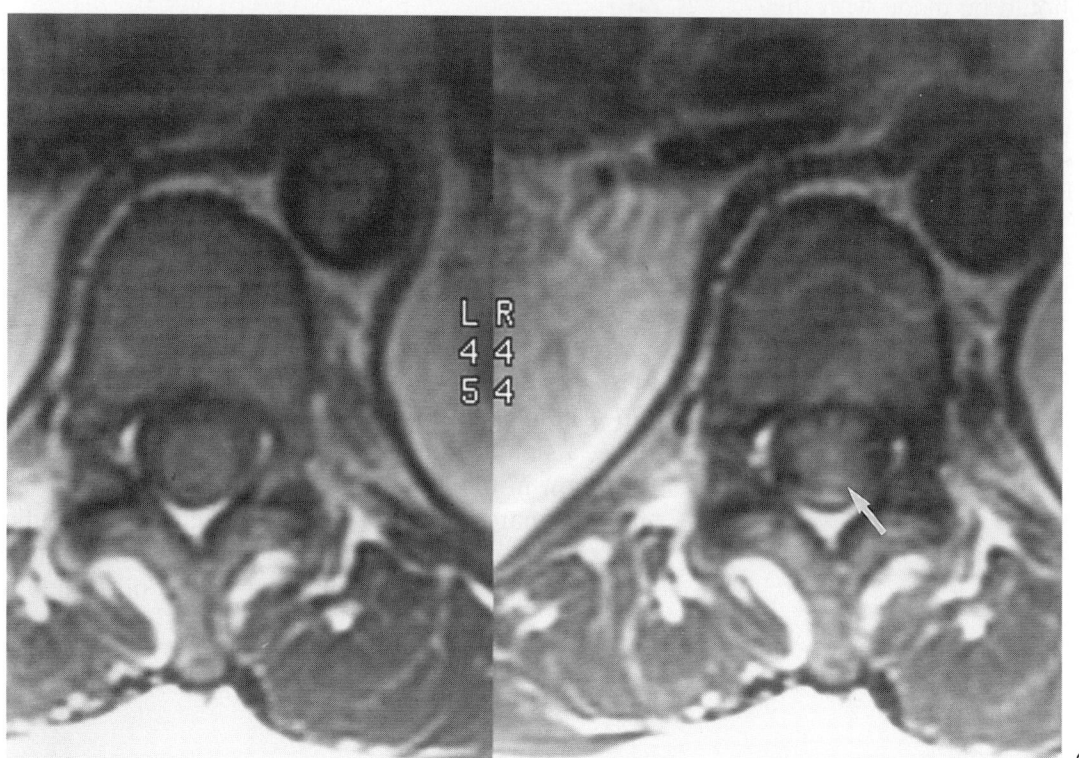

Radiologic Findings (continued)

Axial long TR image (Fig. B) reveals increased signal intensity within the central portion of the spinal cord.

Pre- (Fig. C, *left*) and postcontrast (Fig. C, *right*) axial short TR images reveal patchy enhancement in the spinal cord (*right, arrow*).

PEARLS

- The term *myelitis* should be replaced with the term *myelopathy*.

- Follow-up evaluation with magnetic resonance imaging is helpful and is the ideal noninvasive method to follow the response to treatment.

PITFALLS

- Follow-up is necessary for complete evaluation of this patient.

- The administration of steroids may decrease the enhancement that is seen postinfusion, so correlation of the images should be made with the clinical treatment.

Diagnosis

Postvaccination encephalomyelopathy (acute disseminated encephalomyelopathy) secondary to vaccination.

Differential Diagnosis

- transverse myelopathy

- primary spinal cord tumor

- spinal cord infarction

Discussion

The patient received a vaccination for hepatitis B and experienced no symptoms. The patient received a second vaccination approximately 2 weeks prior to this study, following which she developed lower extremity weakness. This history is typical of patients with transverse myelopathy associated with a viral illness such as an upper respiratory illness or after vaccination. The clinical course is highly variable; these patients may do well, or they may progress to permanent neurological deficit or even death.

Transverse myelopathy (myelitis) following vaccination is actually an antibody-antigen reaction. Following vaccination with a foreign antigen, the patient develops antibodies against the foreign antigen. The antibodies "mistake" the normal nervous system tissue for the foreign antigen. This results in an antibody-antigen reaction in the patient, resulting in symptoms.

The increased signal intensity in the vertebral body end plates is secondary to transformation of the bone marrow from red marrow to fatty white marrow. This is seen adjacent to degenerated intervertebral discs.

The differential diagnosis includes a primary spinal cord tumor. A follow-up scan may aid to differentiate this diagnosis. Spinal cord infarction could have a similar imaging appearance, although the clinical history would be different in the case of cord infarct. Spinal cord infarcts are typically seen in older patients who have arteriosclerotic vascular disease or in patients who have had surgery for abdominal aortic aneurysm or aortic dissection in which there is interruption of the blood supply to the spinal cord.

MISCELLANEOUS

Case 9

Clinical Presentation

The patient is a 58-year-old female with a history of bilateral lower extremity weakness and numbness. The patient also has a history of optic neuritis.

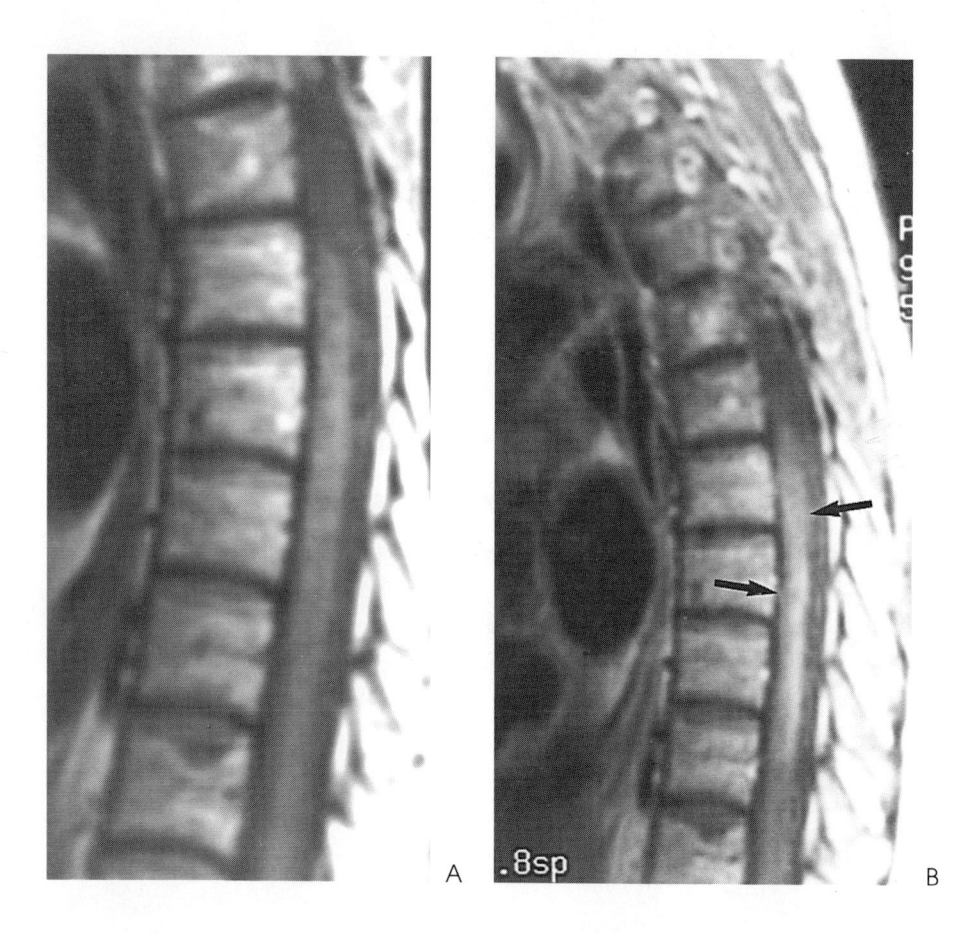

Radiologic Findings

Sagittal short TR image precontrast (Fig. A) reveals that the thoracic spinal cord in the midthoracic region appears larger than normal in size.

Short TR image postcontrast (Fig. B) reveals patchy enhancement of the midthoracic spinal cord extending over approximately four vertebral body levels (*arrows*).

TEACHING ATLAS OF SPINE IMAGING

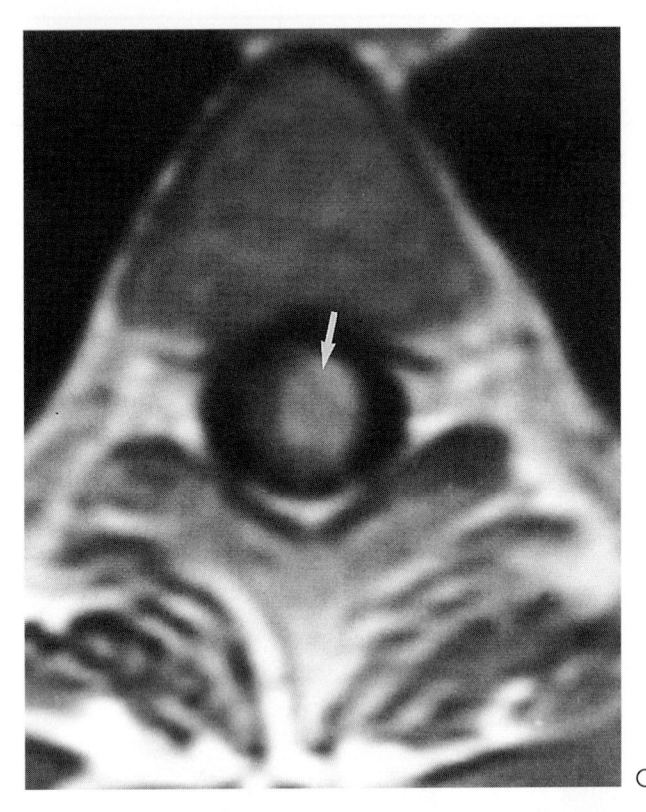

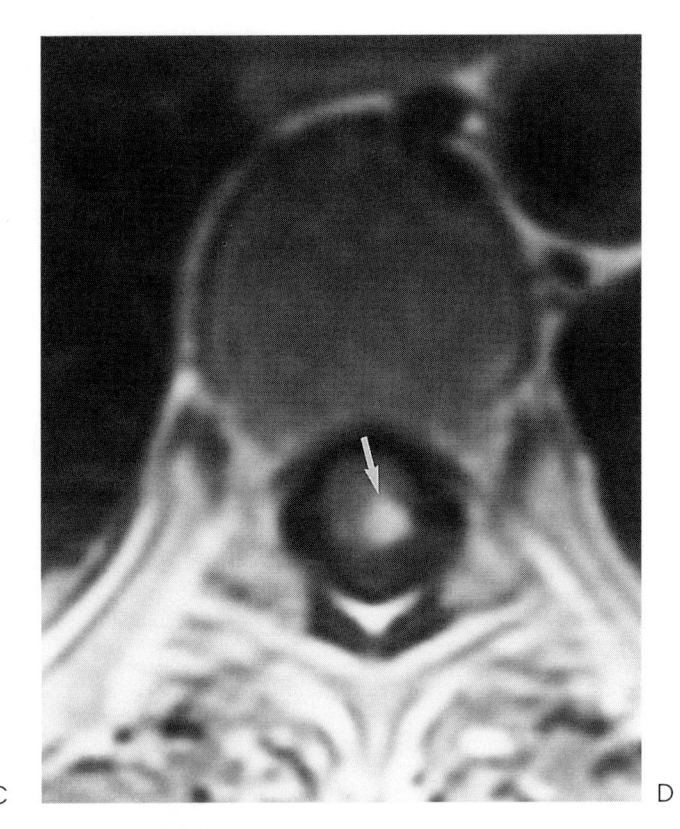

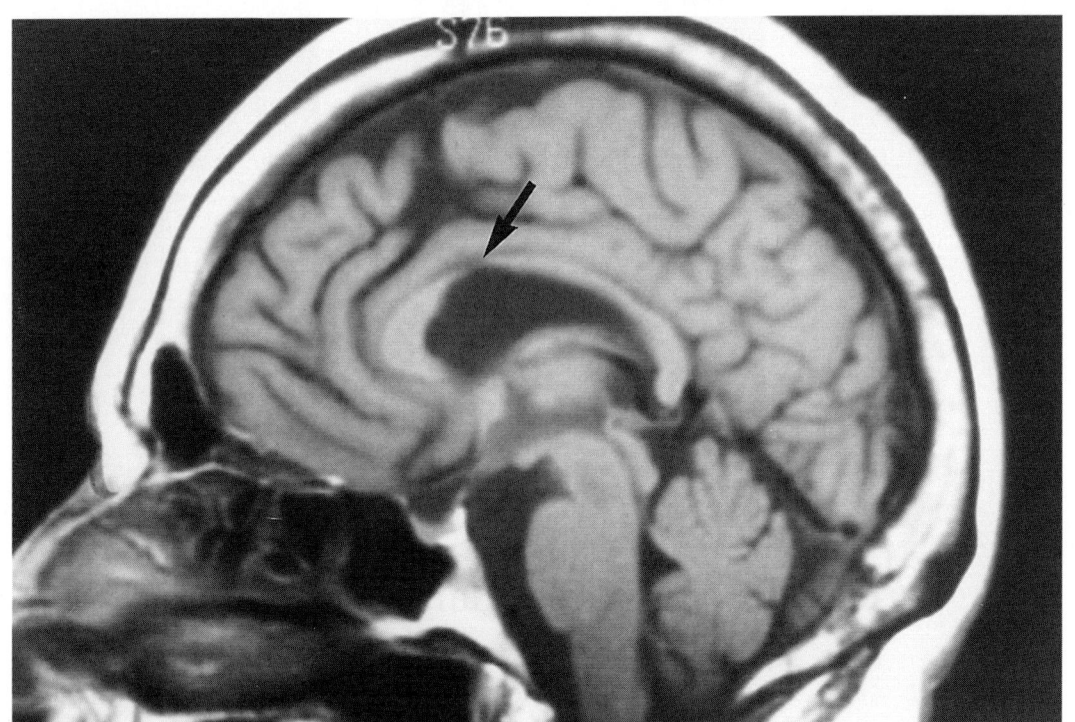

MISCELLANEOUS

Radiologic Findings (continued)

Axial short TR image postcontrast (Fig. C) reveals a slightly irregularly marginated, very thick rimmed, rounded area of enhancement in the left side of the thoracic spinal cord (*arrow*).

Axial short TR image of the spinal cord at the lower end of the area of enhancement (Fig. D) reveals a rounded area of dense enhancement in the dorsal left side of the spinal cord (*arrow*).

Sagittal short TR image of the brain (Fig. E) reveals a defect in the cerebral cortex and an accompanying defect in the corpus callosum (*arrow*).

Diagnosis

Transverse myelitis, most likely secondary to multiple sclerosis.

Differential Diagnosis

- multiple sclerosis
- spinal cord tumor
- idiopathic transverse myelopathy

Discussion

A spinal cord tumor could have similar appearance. However, the abnormal appearance of the brain is more in favor of the diagnosis of multiple sclerosis. The remainder of the brain images reveal additional areas of increased signal intensity in the brain. The anatomic location of the area of enhancement in the dorsal aspect of the spinal cord definitely favors a demyelinating process. Idiopathic transverse myelopathy might also be a consideration. Transverse myelitis has many causes, including multiple sclerosis, sarcoidosis, and paraneoplastic syndrome. Transverse myelitis may also occur following a viral illness or vaccination.

PEARLS

- Correlation with brain imaging is very helpful for more complete evaluation and to confirm the diagnosis of multiple sclerosis.

- The clinical history is significant in this patient because of the presence of optic neuritis, which is a common presenting complaint in patients with multiple sclerosis.

PITFALL

- Follow-up may be necessary in a patient such as this. Biopsy is often not performed because biopsy may make the patient's symptoms worse.

TEACHING ATLAS OF SPINE IMAGING

Case 10

Clinical Presentation

The patient is a 15-year-old previously healthy male with a 6-month history of chronic leg weakness. The patient is now wheelchair-bound.

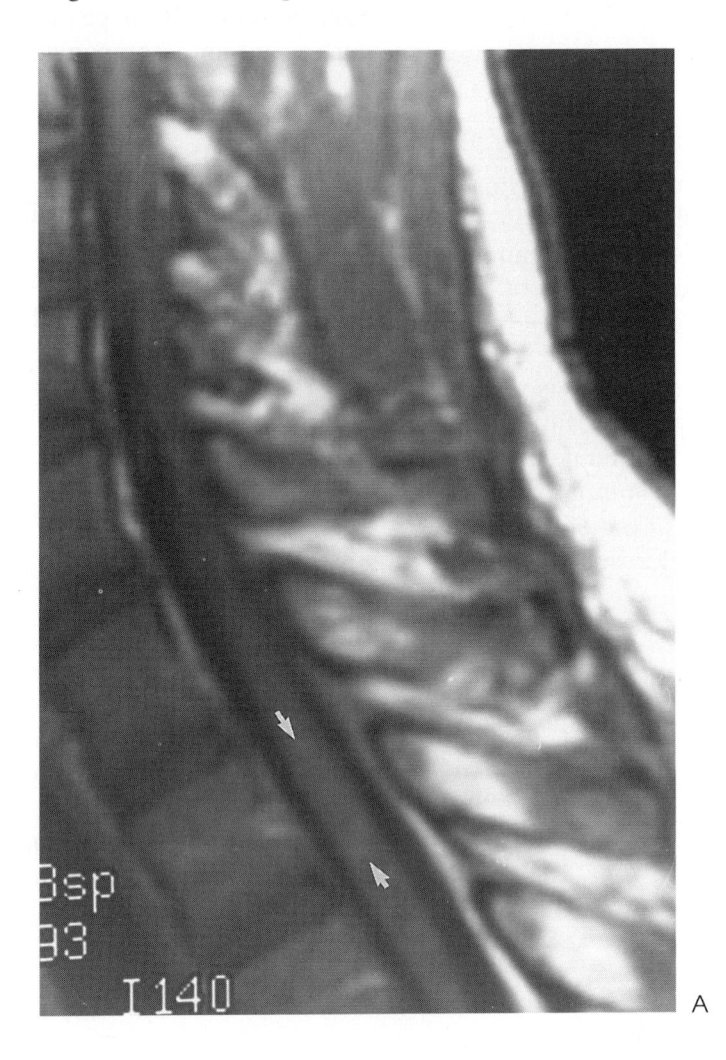

Radiologic Findings

Sagittal short TR postcontrast image (Fig. A) reveals faint patchy areas of enhancement of the upper thoracic spinal cord (*arrows*). The spinal cord is otherwise normal in size and configuration.

Sagittal long TR image (Fig. B) reveals a long area of increased signal intensity within the central portion of the lower cervical and upper thoracic spinal cord (*arrow*).

Follow-up image with smaller field of view (Fig. C) reveals the definite enhancement of the lower cervical and upper thoracic spinal cord (*arrow*). The cord is otherwise of normal size.

MISCELLANEOUS

B

C

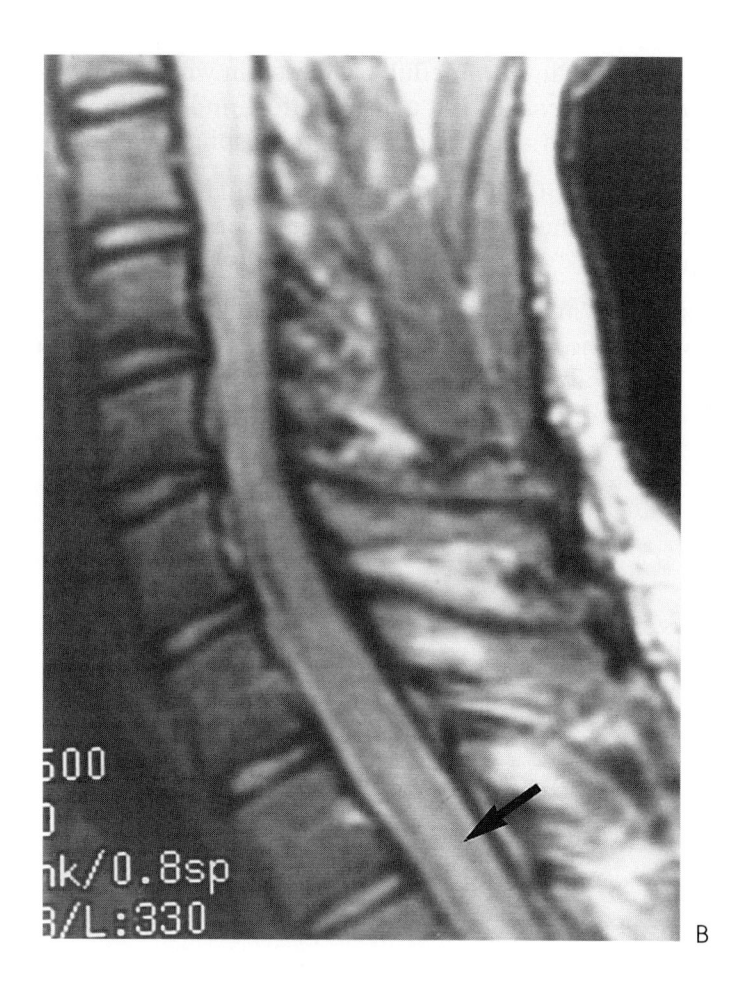

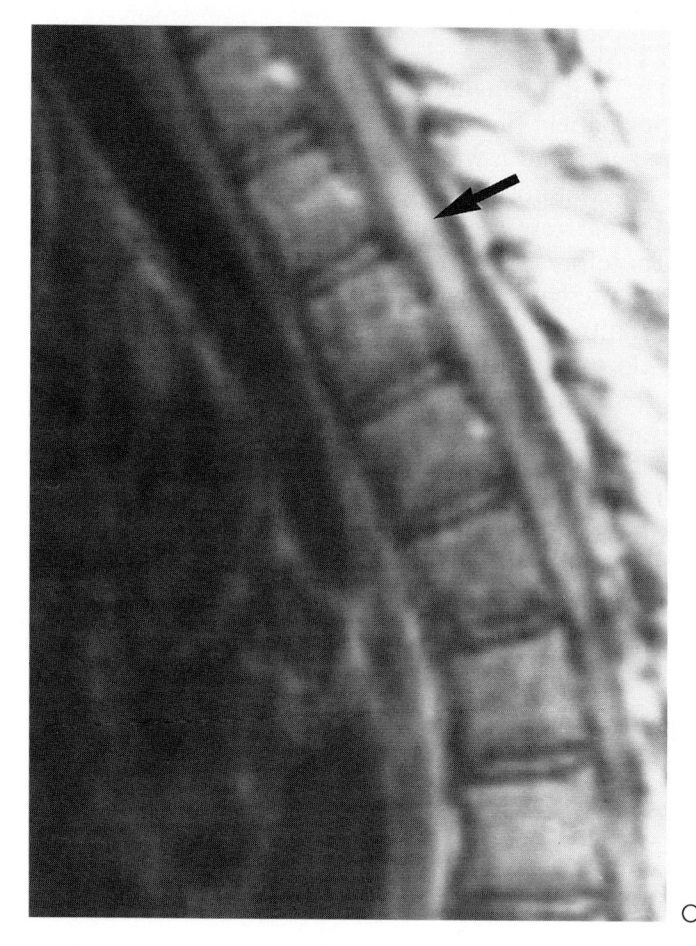

PEARL
- Transverse myelitis may be idiopathic, secondary to multiple sclerosis, part of the paraneoplastic syndrome, or a manifestation of acute disseminated encephalomyelitis

Diagnosis

Transverse "myelitis," cause unknown.

Differential Diagnosis

- multiple sclerosis

- intramedullary infection

- spinal cord infarct

- acute disseminated transverse myelitis

Discussion

These changes could be related to multiple sclerosis, but there was no history of cerebral symptoms, and the brain magnetic resonance study was normal. Although this does not rule out multiple sclerosis, it makes the diagnosis less likely.

TEACHING ATLAS OF SPINE IMAGING

PITFALLS

- The initial imaging findings in this patient, using body coil imaging and a wide field of view, did not initially demonstrate the abnormality. Therefore, in a patient with definite clinical symptoms, additional imaging with a small field of view directed at the area of interest is certainly warranted.

- The administration of systemic steroids may decrease the amount of visible enhancement, so imaging findings should be correlated with the clinical treatment.

Although rare, the possibility of an intramedullary infection with an organism such as *Mycobacterium tuberculosis* is a consideration, and the imaging findings should be correlated with analysis of the cerebrospinal fluid.

In an older patient, the diagnosis of spinal cord infarct should be considered, particularly in the presence of other symptoms of atherosclerotic or arteriosclerotic vascular disease.

Acute disseminated transverse myelitis is also a strong diagnostic consideration in this patient, even in the absence of a history of recent vaccination or viral illness.

MISCELLANEOUS

Case 11

Clinical Presentation

The patient is a 53-year-old male with a history of esophageal cancer who was previously treated with radiation therapy. The patient has a 2-week history of increased tingling in the lower thoracic area.

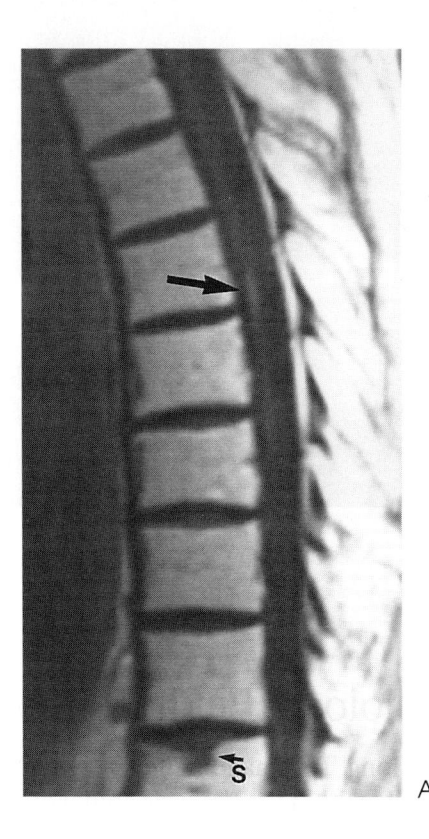

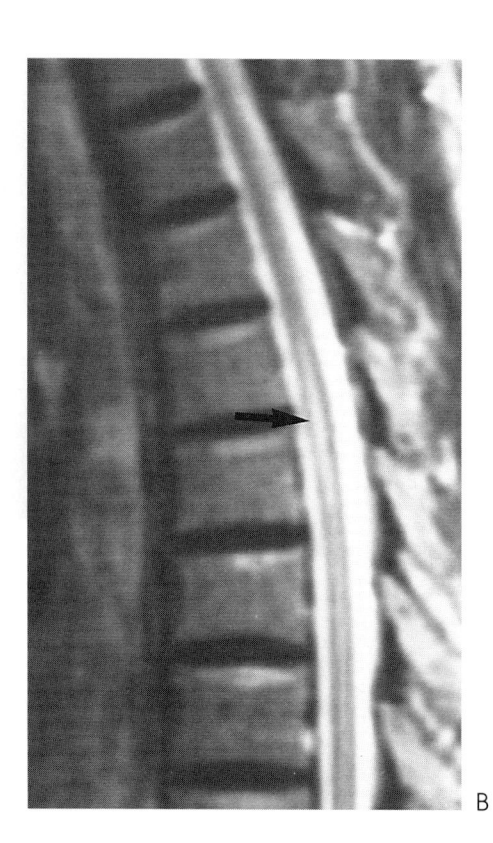

A

B

Radiologic Findings

Sagittal short TR postcontrast image (Fig. A) reveals an approximately 1-cm oval area of enhancement in the midthoracic spinal cord (*arrow*). There is no deformity of the cord. All the vertebral bodies are diffusely increased in signal intensity secondary to previous radiation therapy to a mediastinal mass. There is a Schmorl's nodule deformity in the superior end plate of one of the lower thoracic vertebral bodies (*S*).

Sagittal long TR image (Fig. B) reveals an area of increased signal intensity in the midthoracic region (*arrow*) that extends over approximately two vertebral body segments. This area is at the level of the previous area of enhancement.

TEACHING ATLAS OF SPINE IMAGING

Case 12

Clinical Presentation

The patient is a 53-year-old female who received previous thoracic radiation for hilar lymphadenopathy because of metastases.

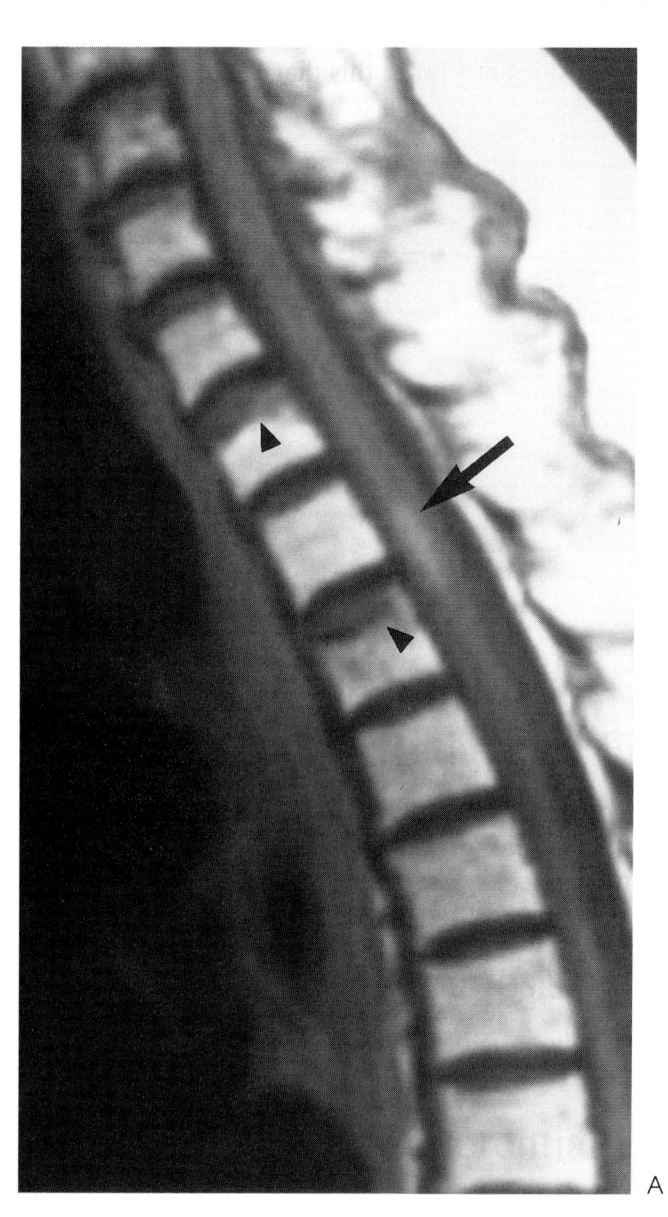

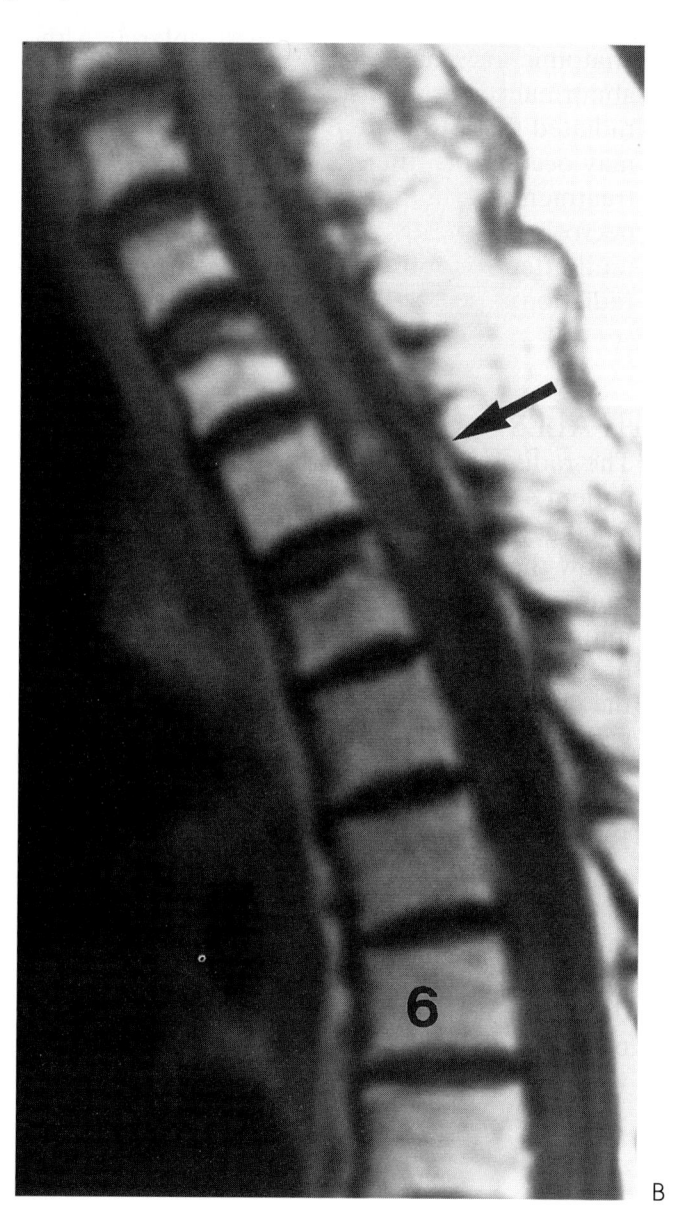

Radiologic Findings

Sagittal short TR image precontrast infusion (Fig. A) reveals an area of increased signal intensity within the spinal cord at the T2-3 level (*arrow*). There are superior end plate compression fractures of T1 and T3 (*arrowheads*). The marrow within the visualized thoracic vertebral bodies appears diffusely increased in signal intensity.

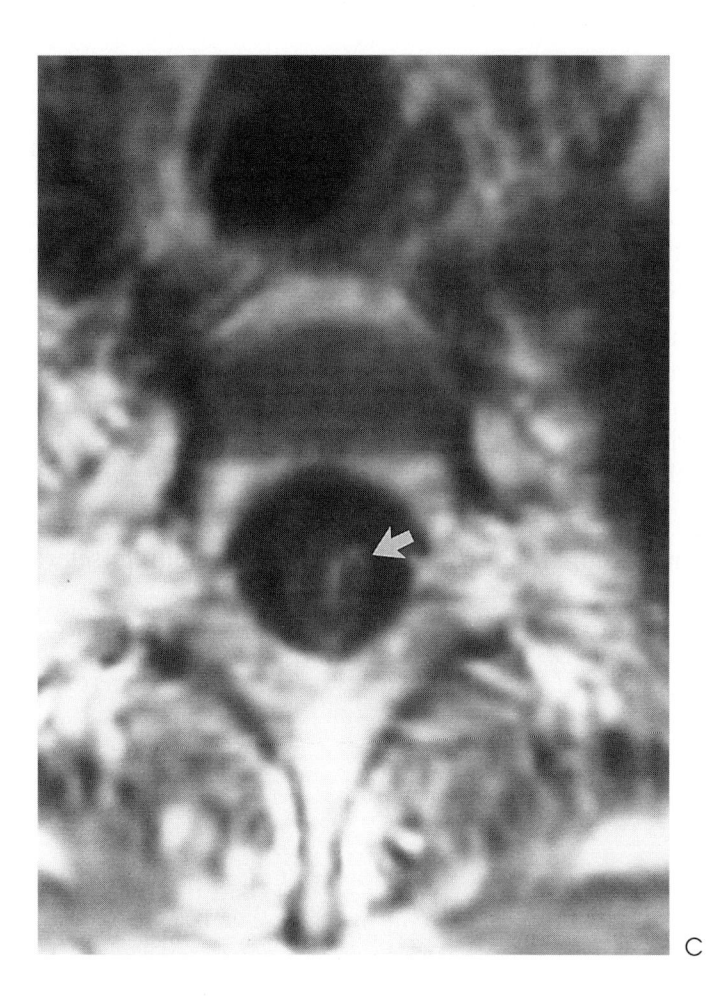

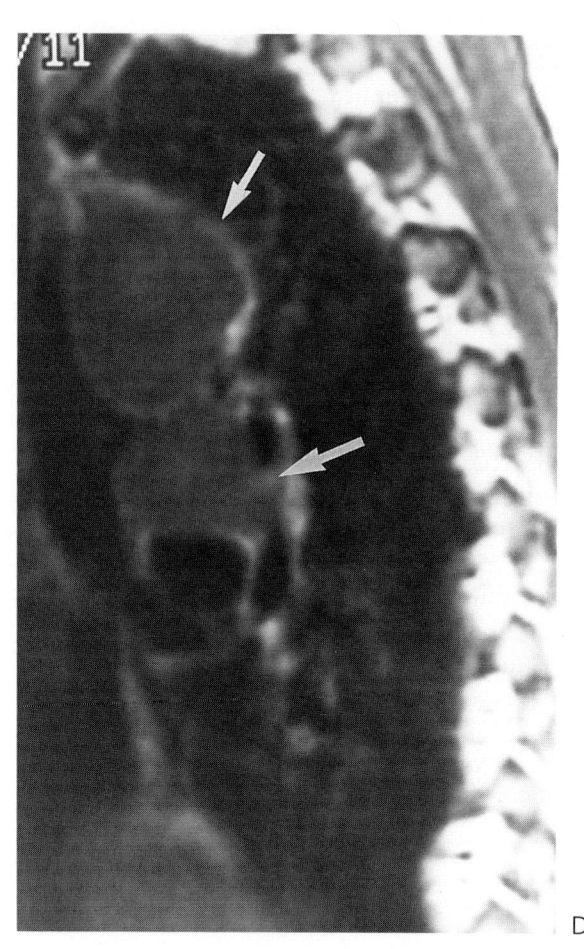

Radiologic Findings (continued)

Sagittal short TR image postcontrast (Fig. B) reveals an oval area of enhancement at the level of, and surrounding the area of, increased signal seen in Figure A (*arrow*). The T6 vertebral body is identified with 6.

Axial short TR image postcontrast (Fig. C) reveals a ring of enhancement within the ventral lateral aspect of the spinal cord at the T2-3 level (*arrow*).

Parasagittal short TR image at the level of the hilum (Fig. D) reveals a bilobed mass in hilar above the level of the tracheal bifurcation (*arrows*).

Diagnosis

Postradiation change with enhancement of the spinal cord.

Differential Diagnosis

- radiation change
- multiple sclerosis
- paraneoplastic syndrome with transverse "myelitis"

TEACHING ATLAS OF SPINE IMAGING

PEARLS
- The enhancement in the white matter of the spinal cord favors a demyelinating process rather than a spinal cord tumor.

- The lack of mass effect is strongly in favor of a demyelinating process.

PITFALLS
- Follow-up may be necessary for complete evaluation.

- Correlation should also be made with cerebrospinal fluid evaluation to rule out the presence of oligoclonal bands, which may be seen in multiple sclerosis.

Discussion

The mass in the hilar region is a primary lung cancer. Within the radiation treatment field, there is radiation effect upon the spinal cord with demyelination and consequent enhancement. The enhancement is presumed to be secondary to the advancing margin of demyelination of the white matter secondary to radiation effect even in the absence of radiation necrosis.

The previous radiation treatment has resulted in an increased amount of fat within the marrow of the vertebral bodies, and consequently they appear as increased signal intensity. The vertebral bodies are weakened because of the radiation change, and this has resulted in multiple compression fractures secondary to this osteoporosis.

Multiple sclerosis would have a similar appearance on imaging. However, the history is not compatible with the diagnosis of multiple sclerosis.

MISCELLANEOUS

Case 13

Clinical Presentation

The patient is a 46-year-old diabetic male with non-Hodgkin's lymphoma with possible meningeal carcinomatosis.

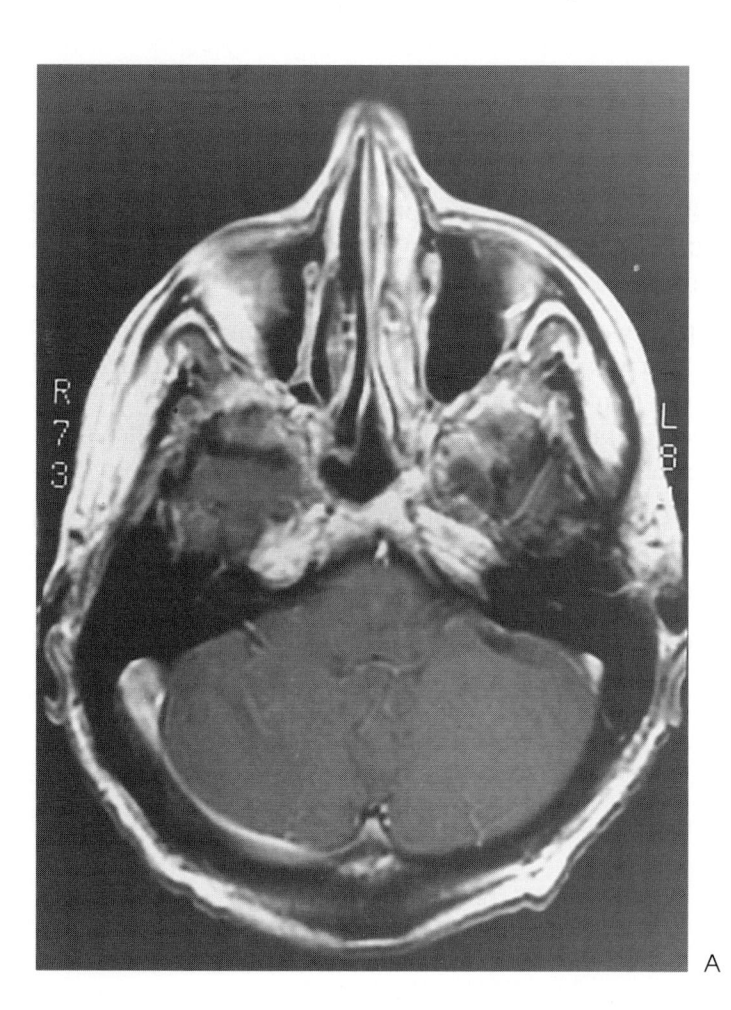

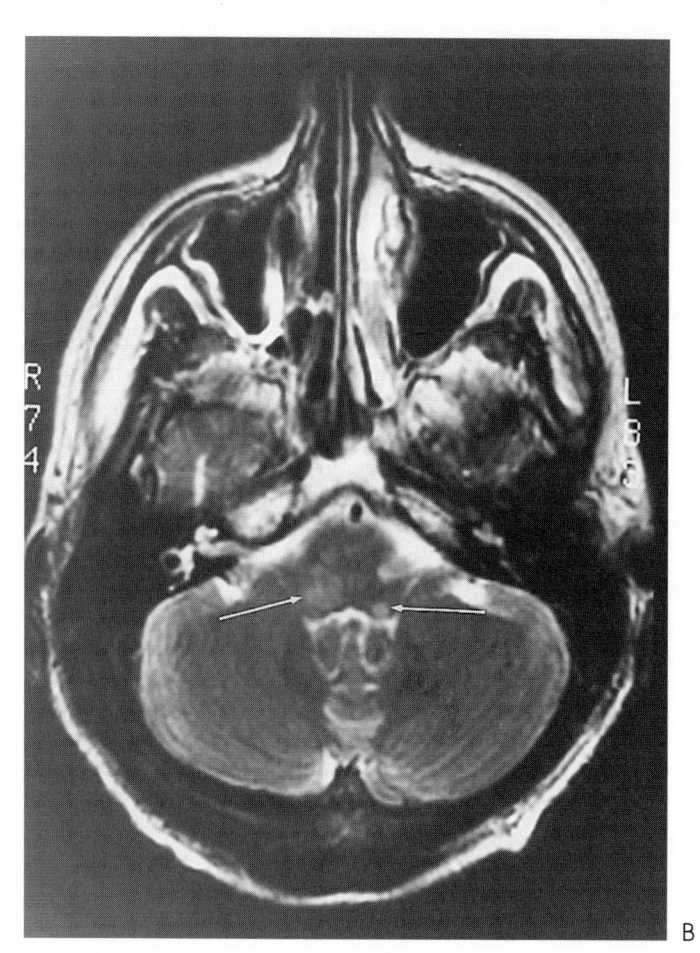

Radiologic Findings

Axial short TR image postcontrast at the level of the pontomedullary junction (Fig. A) appears within normal limits. There are no abnormal areas of enhancement.

Long TR image at the level of the junction between the lower pons and the medulla (Fig. B) reveals multiple, variable sized areas of increased signal intensity in the medulla (*arrows*). The scan is otherwise normal.

PEARLS

- The history of mantle radiation is important in this patient. In addition, the time from treatment to symptoms would be compatible with the diagnosis of "radiation effect" in the absence of radiation necrosis.

- The imaging findings in this patient are very subtle and close evaluation to the lowest slices is important for complete evaluation.

PITFALL

- Other diseases, such as spinal cord infarction, could have a similar appearance. Multiple sclerosis could also have a similar appearance; however, the clinical history is not in favor of this diagnosis. Radiation effect is a diagnosis of exclusion, and other diagnostic considerations should be ruled out. Follow-up is also helpful for more complete evaluation.

Diagnosis

Postradiation change.

Differential Diagnosis

- postradiation change
- metastases

Discussion

This patient with non-Hodgkin's lymphoma had received radiation of the neck, chest, and axillary nodes. The symptoms began approximately 9 months after treatment. The areas of abnormal signal intensity are presumably areas of demyelination secondary to the patient's radiation treatment.

Meningeal carcinomatosis would be anticipated to show areas of enhancement of the meninges; this was not present in this patient. Intraparenchymal areas of metastases from non-Hodgkin's or Hodgkin's lymphoma are rare but may occur. However, metastases generally exhibit areas of enhancement; no enhancement was seen in this patient.

Although the patient is diabetic, a condition that results in small vessel infarcts, the magnetic resonance pattern of increased signal intensity is not typical for vascular lesion.

The history of diabetes is non-contributory in this patient relative to the imaging findings.

MISCELLANEOUS

Case 14

Clinical Presentation

The patient is a 73-year-old female with weight loss and tenderness of the lumbar spine. There was left leg weakness with decreased sensation.

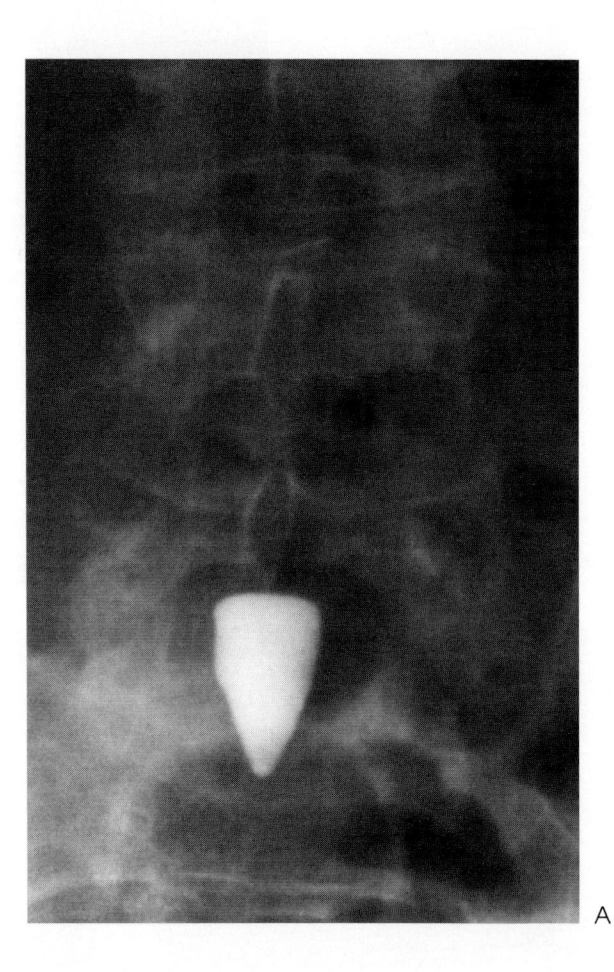

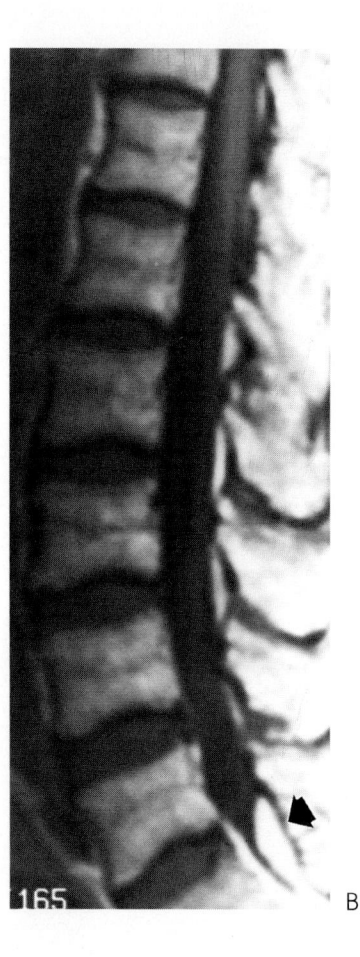

Radiologic Findings

Anteroposterior view of the lumber spine (Fig. A) reveals a small amount of retained pantopaque in the very distal end of the thecal sac, which appears as increased density and exhibits a fluid level.

Sagittal short TR image (Fig. B) reveals that the retained pantopaque appears as an area of increased signal intensity in the lower end of the distal thecal sac (*arrow*).

TEACHING ATLAS OF SPINE IMAGING

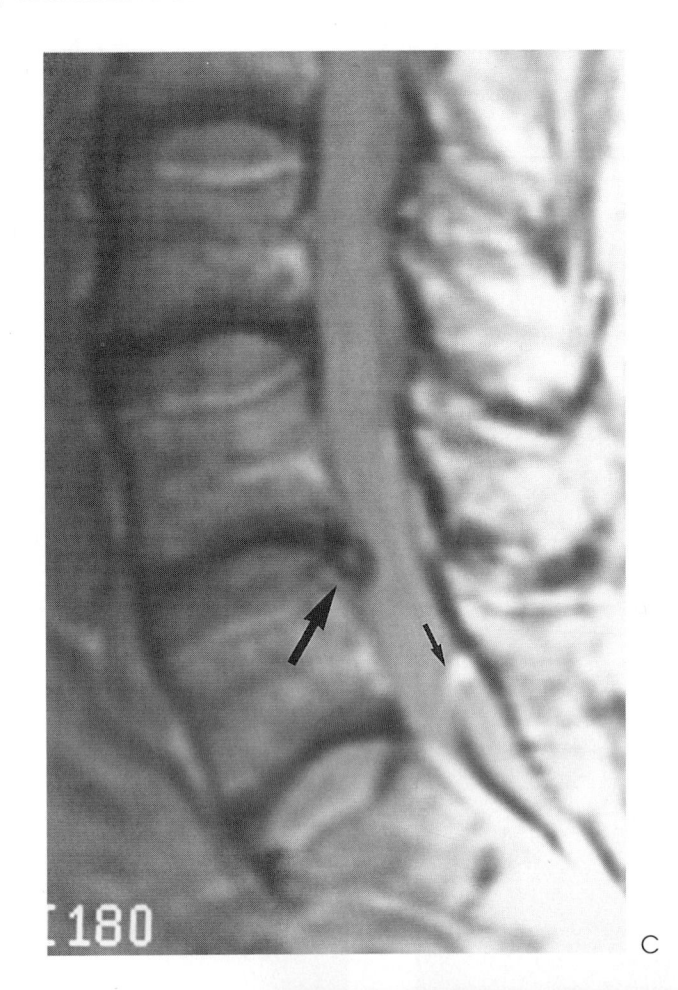

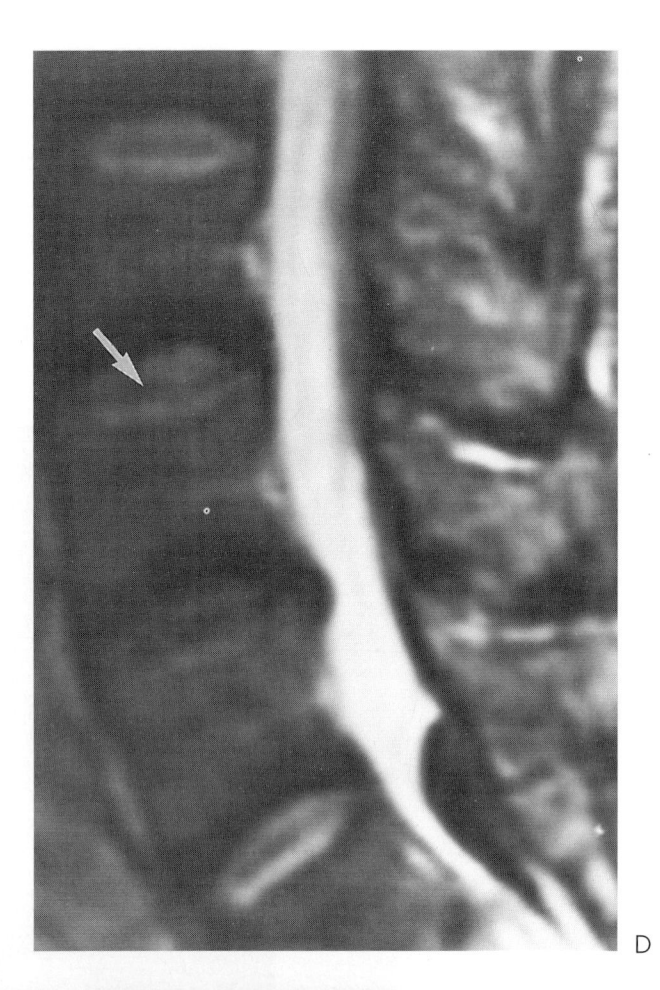

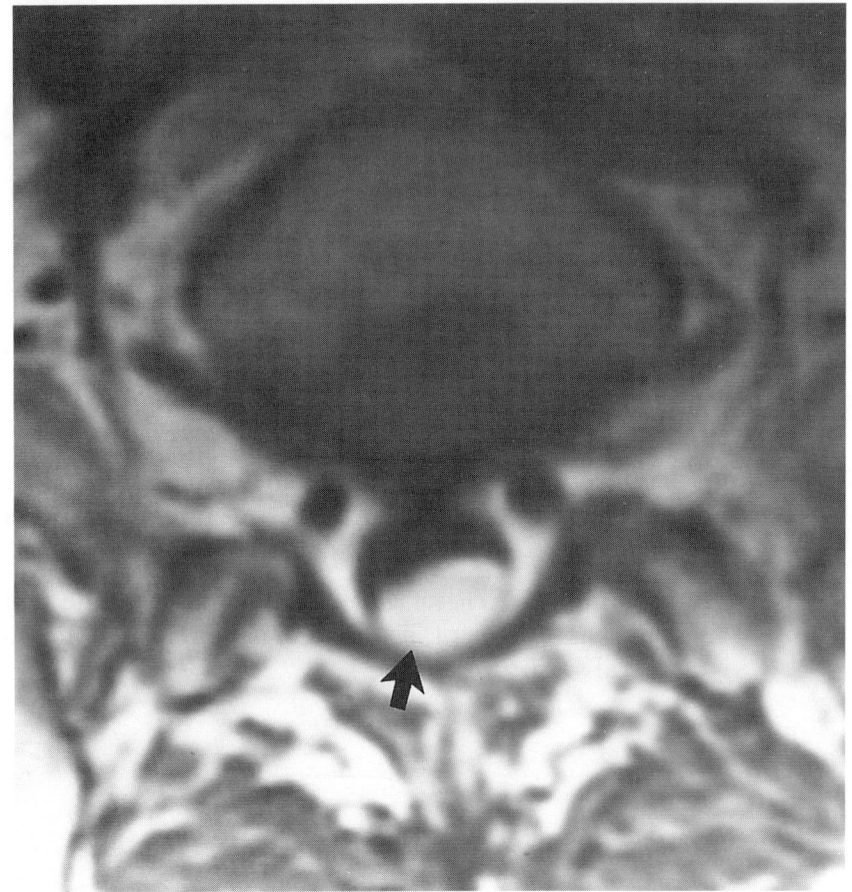

MISCELLANEOUS

Radiologic Findings (continued)

Sagittal intermediate TR image (Fig. C) reveals chemical shift artifact surrounding the retained pantopaque. There is a halo of increased signal superior to the pantopaque (*small arrow*) and a streak of decreased signal anterior to the pantopaque. Also present is a herniated disc at the L4-L5 level (*large arrow*).

Sagittal long TR image (Fig. D) reveals that the retained pantopaque appears as decreased signal intensity. The herniated disc at the L4-5 level is well demonstrated. There is slight encroachment upon the high signal intensity cerebrospinal fluid. Note the normal decreased signal intensity cleft within the intervertebral discs at the normal levels (*arrow*).

Axial short TR image (Fig. E) reveals the retained pantopaque in the dependent portion of the lumbar thecal sac (*arrow*). The nerve root sleeves can also be identified lateral to the thecal sac and surrounded by increased signal intensity perineural fat.

Diagnosis

Retained pantopaque; herniated disc at L4-5.

Differential Diagnosis

- retained pantopaque

Discussion

Reports have been published that link pantopaque with arachnoiditis—especially when there is associated hemorrhage or blood in the subarachnoid space. However, no direct cause and effect has been conclusively proven, and essentially all of these patients with pantopaque myelograms have also had spinal surgery. Pantopaque, an oil-based contrast material, appears as increased signal intensity on short TR images and decreased signal intensity on long TR images.

PEARL

- Plain spine films will usually demonstrate areas of retained pantopaque. There may also be retained droplets of pantopaque within the cranial vault. The use of pantopaque has been discontinued since the development of water soluble contrast material.

PITFALL

- Increased-signal-intensity-retained oily pantopaque can be mistaken for blood in the methemoglobin phase of metabolism. However, pantopaque will become decreased signal intensity on long TR images, while methemoglobin will appear as increased signal intensity on long TR images.

Case 15

Clinical Presentation

The patient is a 49-year-old male with a history of previous surgery for spinal cord ependymoma.

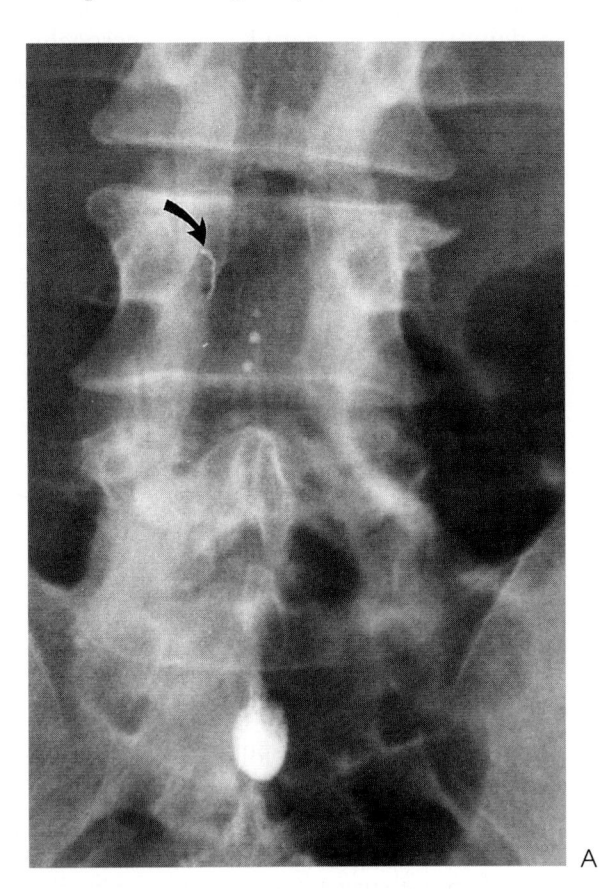

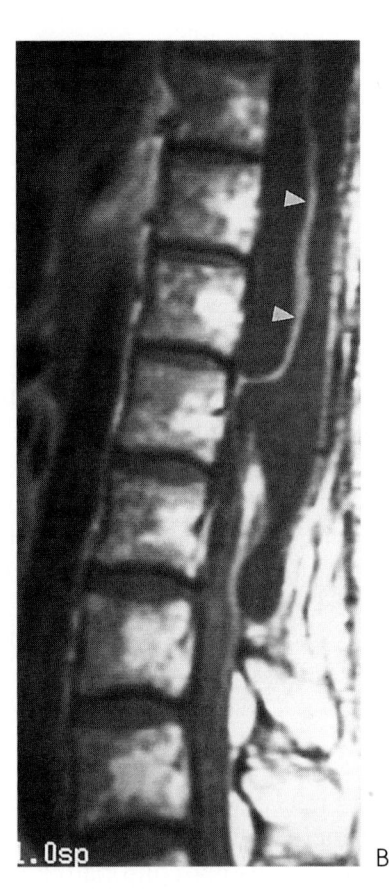

Radiologic Findings

Anteroposterior view of the lower lumbar regions (Fig. A) reveals laminectomy changes at the L3 and L4 levels. There is a metallic suture projecting just medial to the right pedicle at the L4 level (*arrow*). There are multiple small droplets of high density pantopaque contrast material and one large droplet in the lower end of the thecal sac.

Sagittal short TR image (Fig. B) reveals a long laminectomy that extends from L2 superiorly through the thoracic region. There is no normal appearing spinal cord remaining. The spinal cord remnant is a thin irregular strand of neural tissue (*arrowheads*) that floats in the dilated thecal sac. In the lower lumbar region, the nerve roots of the cauda equina are thickened and matted together. There is a streaklike area of increased signal intensity within these nerve roots.

Radiologic Findings (continued)

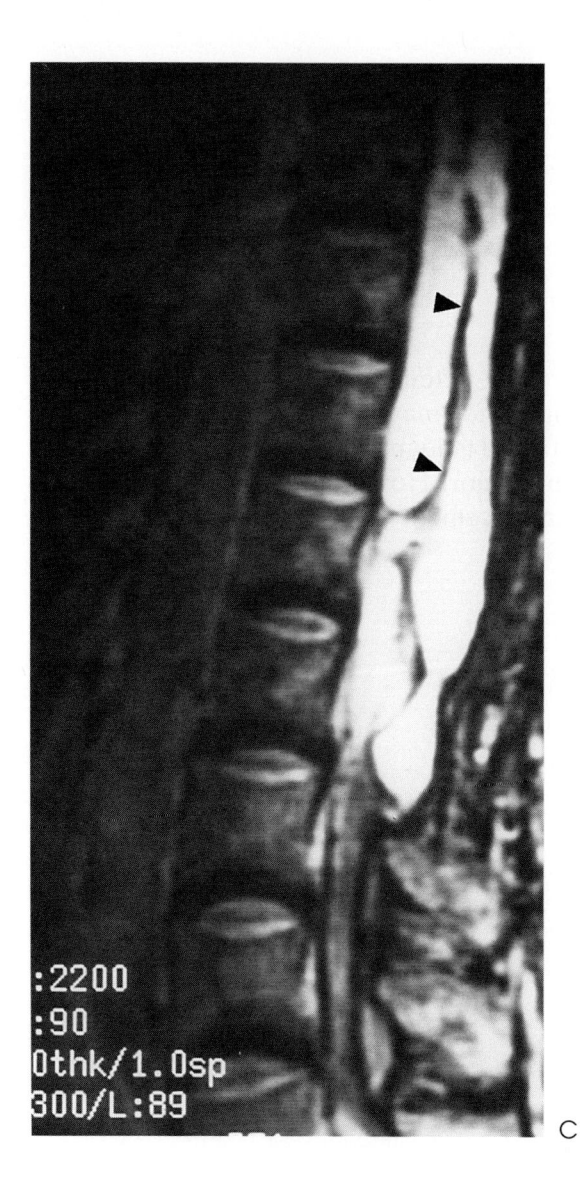

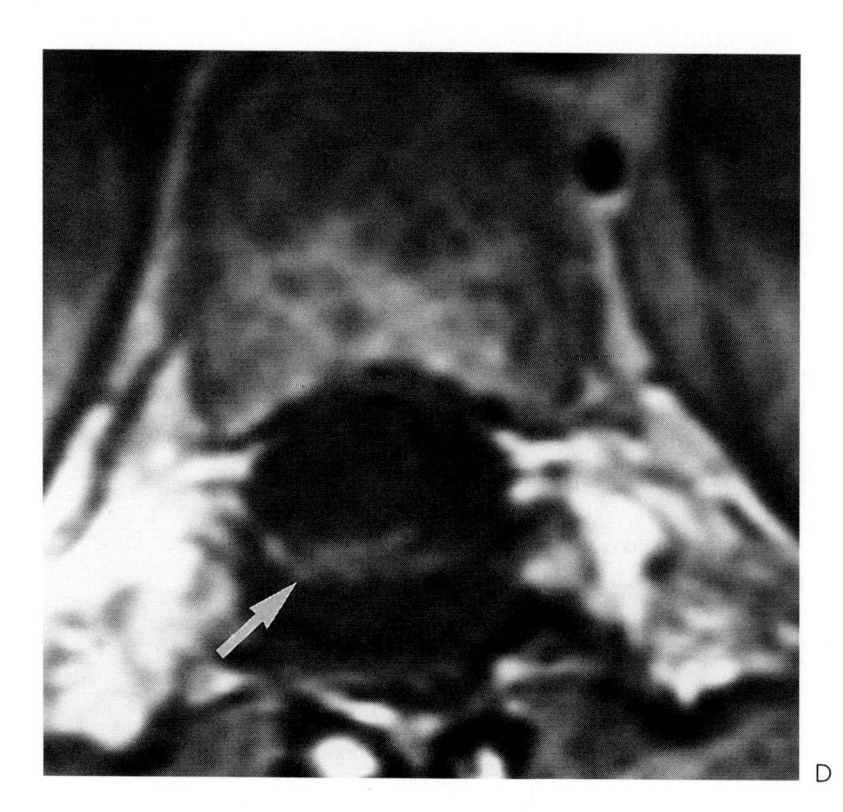

Sagittal long TR image (Fig. C) reveals the dilated thecal sac in the lower thoracic region secondary to surgery and the development of a postoperative pseudomeningocele with outpouching of the dorsal aspect of the thecal sac into the laminectomy site. The remaining strands of neural tissue appear as irregular bands of decreased signal. The matted nerve rootlets of the cauda equina are seen as a cordlike structure in the lower lumbar thecal sac.

Axial short TR image (Fig. D) reveals the flattened, scarred, matted nerve rootlets of the cauda equina (*arrow*).

Diagnosis

Extensive postoperative changes with scarring and adhesions of the nerve roots of the cauda equina.

PEARLS

- Follow-up studies may be helpful for complete evaluation; tumor would be expected to progress, while arachnoiditis would remain stable.

- Although no mass lesions are seen, rather streaky areas more consistent with scar formation are visible.

PITFALL

- While attempts have been made to surgically release adhesions, these attempts are generally unsuccessful and are not recommended. In a patient with such severe distortion of the normal anatomy, a follow-up examination is certainly warranted for more complete evaluation, particularly as there is no known treatment for arachnoiditis.

Differential Diagnosis

- postoperative changes

- arachnoiditis

Discussion

In cases such as this where there are extensive postsurgical changes, the presence or absence of remaining tumor may be impossible to determine. Postcontrast images should be obtained to identify any areas of enhancement as this would indicate a recurrent tumor. However, areas of arachnoiditis may also show enhancement. Enhancement in areas of arachnoiditis are highly variable.

MISCELLANEOUS

Case 16

Clinical Presentation

The patient is a 67-year-old male with severe low back pain.

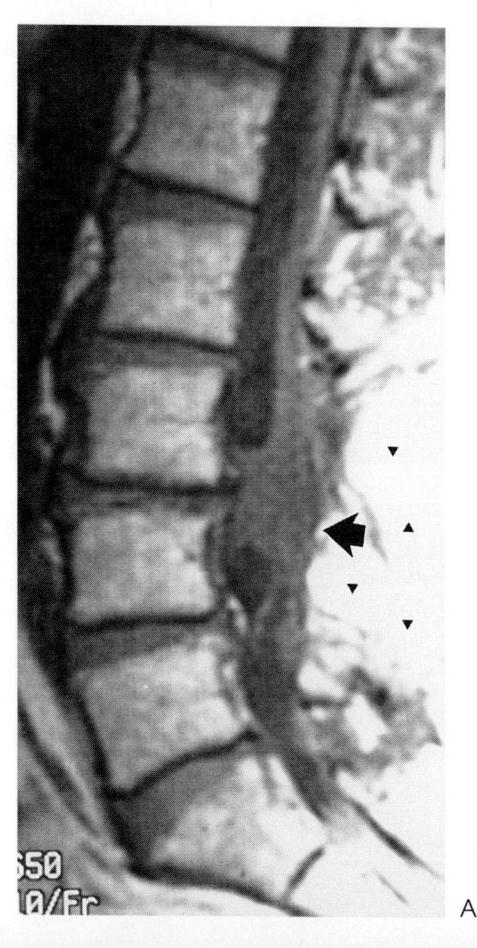

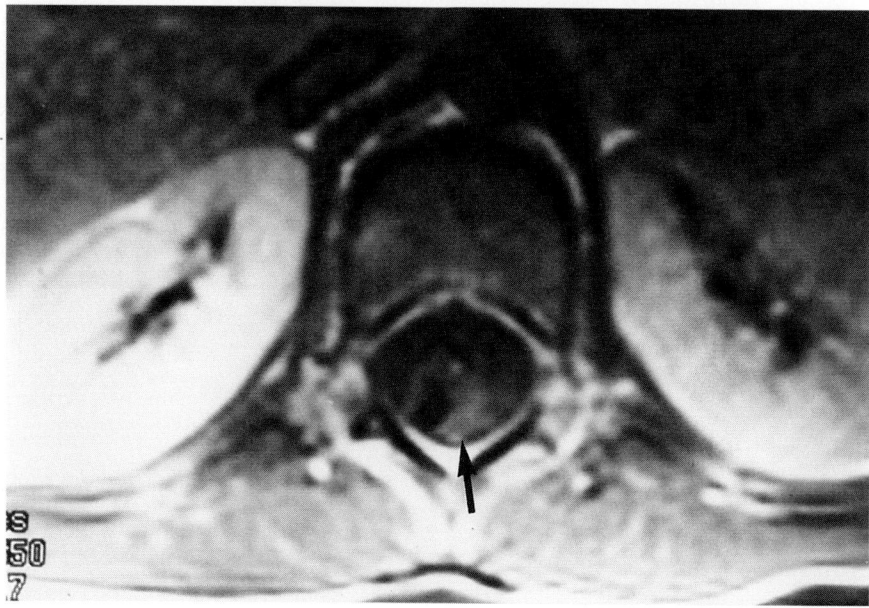

TEACHING ATLAS OF SPINE IMAGING

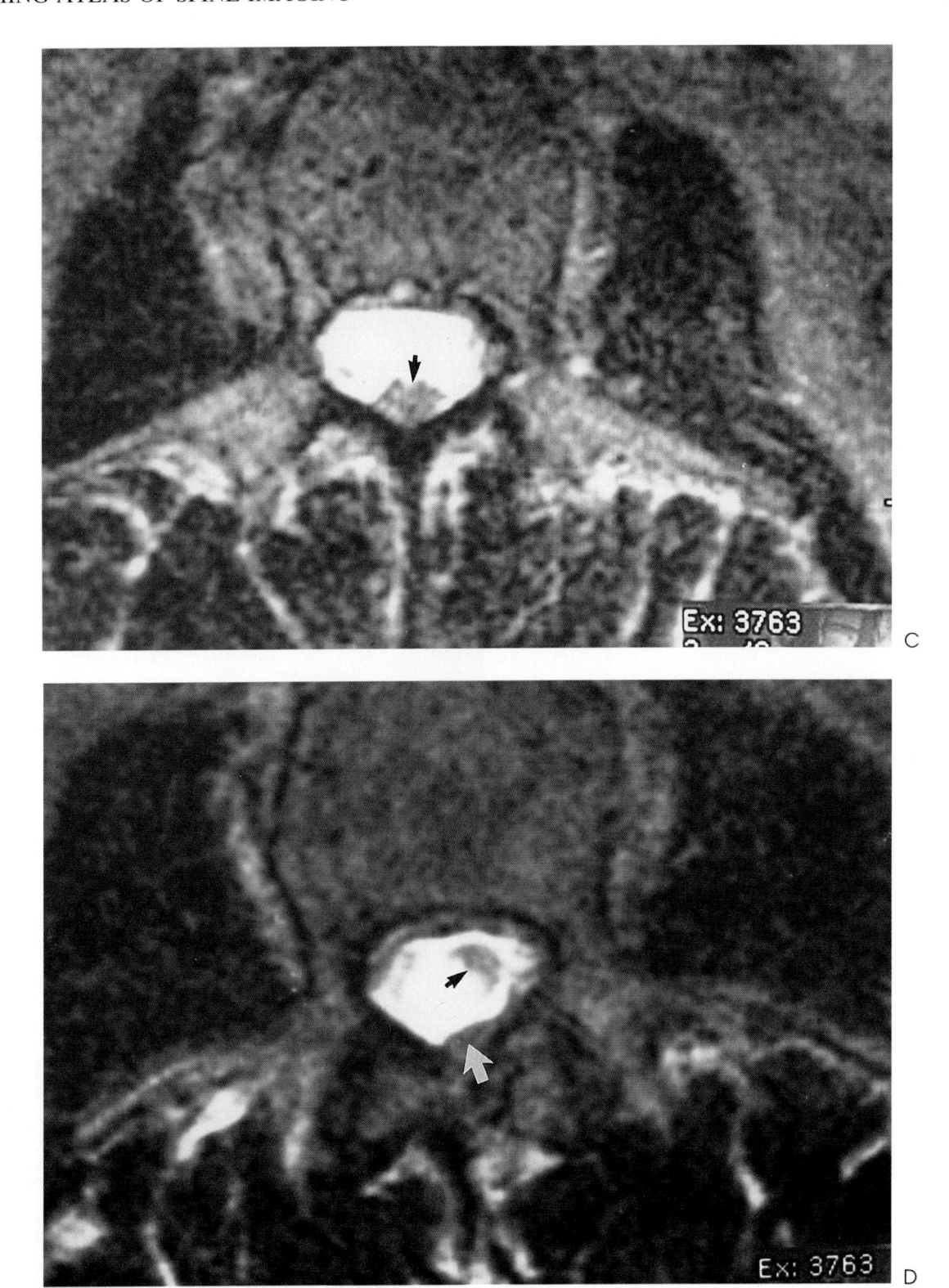

PEARLS

- A postcontrast scan may also be performed and may occasionally reveal areas of enhancement with adhesions within the area of scar formation.

- In patients in whom the area of nerve root adhesion is masslike, the possibility of drop metastases is a consideration. However, this is less likely when there are postoperative changes and no history of a primary tumor.

PITFALLS

- The changes related to arachnoiditis may be very subtle in some patients, so careful evaluation of the scans must be performed.

- In rare cases, the magnetic resonance scan may be entirely normal even when there is arachnoiditis present. In these patients, a repeat myelogram with postmyelogram computed tomographic scanning may be necessary for complete evaluation and demonstration of the typical changes seen with adhesive arachnoiditis.

Radiologic Findings

Sagittal short TR image (Fig. A) reveals total laminectomy at L3 and L4 and a partial laminectomy at the L5 level. The spinous processes have been replaced by increased signal intensity fat (*arrowheads*). The spinal cord appears as a solid structure extending to the level of L3. At the L3 level, the nerve roots of the cauda equina are matted and distorted. There is a large, plaquelike area of matted, distorted nerve rootlets filling the distal thecal sac (*arrow*). The anterior, irregular extensions of the nerve material is presumed to be areas where the neural structures are adherent to the anterior margin of the thecal sac. The nerve rootlets of the cauda equina are also tethered posteriorly in the lumbar region from L3 inferiorly.

Axial short TR image at the level of the kidneys (Fig. B) reveals the distorted neural tissue in the thecal sac (*arrow*).

Axial long TR image in the upper lumbar region (Fig. C) reveals the irregularly marginated spinal cord positioned posteriorly in the thecal sac and adherent to the posterior margin of the thecal sac (*arrow*).

Axial long TR image at the level of the cauda equina (Fig. D) reveals that the nerve roots are matted together and displaced anteriorly and toward the left side (*black arrow*). In addition, there are multiple nerve roots matted together and adherent to the posterior margin of the thecal sac (*white arrow*).

Diagnosis

Postoperative adhesive arachnoiditis.

Differential Diagnosis

- arachnoiditis

- drop metastases

- meningeal carcinomatosis

Discussion

The remote possibility of drop metastases or meningeal carcinomatosis is a consideration. However, there is no history of a primary tumor either within or outside of the central nervous system. The history of previous surgery and the evidence of a laminectomy are strongly in favor of arachnoiditis. Arachnoiditis seems to be related to the presence of blood in the subarachnoid space and may occur in any patient who has had surgery. Surgery has been attempted to lyse adhesions; however, surgery is not found to be successful for treatment of arachnoid adhesions.

Adhesive arachnoiditis may also appear as an "empty tube" with all the nerve roots of the cauda equina adherent to the walls of the thecal sac; therefore, they are no longer visible within the thecal sac.

Case 17

Clinical Presentation

The patient is a 36-year-old female who complained of severe headache and back pain following spinal anesthesia for childbirth. A blood patch had been attempted without success.

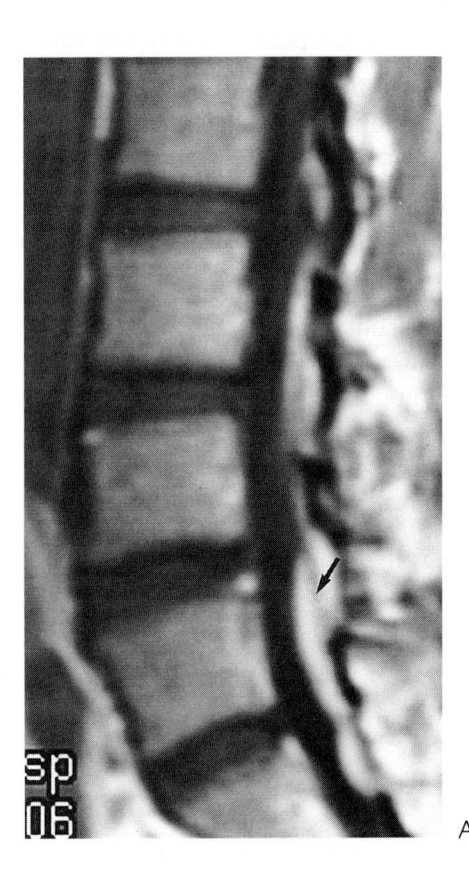

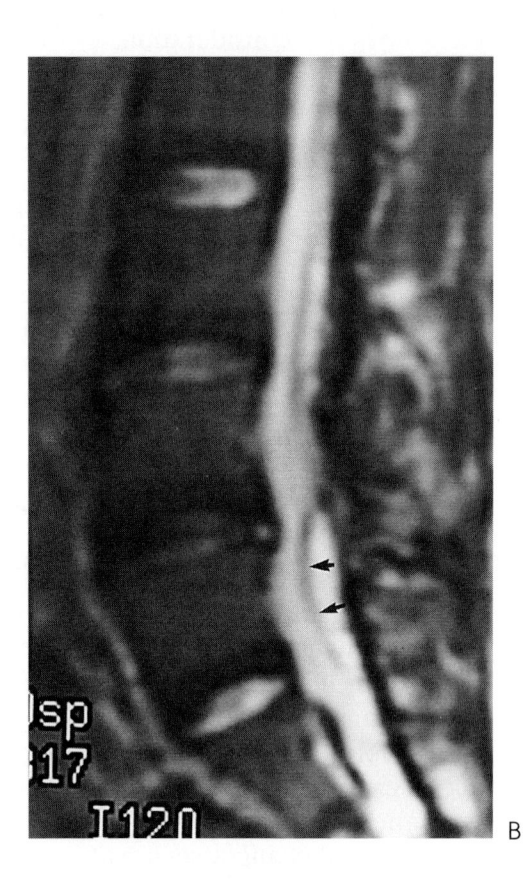

Radiologic Findings

Sagittal short TR image in the lumbar region (Fig. A) reveals an elongated area of increased signal intensity dorsal to the thecal sac in the lower lumbar region (*arrow*).

Sagittal long TR image (Fig. B) reveals a thin black line (*arrows*) along the anterior margin of the area of increased signal intensity seen in Figure A. This area remains increased signal intensity on the long TR image.

Axial short TR image at the level of L5 (Fig. C) reveals a semilunar area of increased signal intensity in the dorsal left side of the thecal sac (*arrow*).

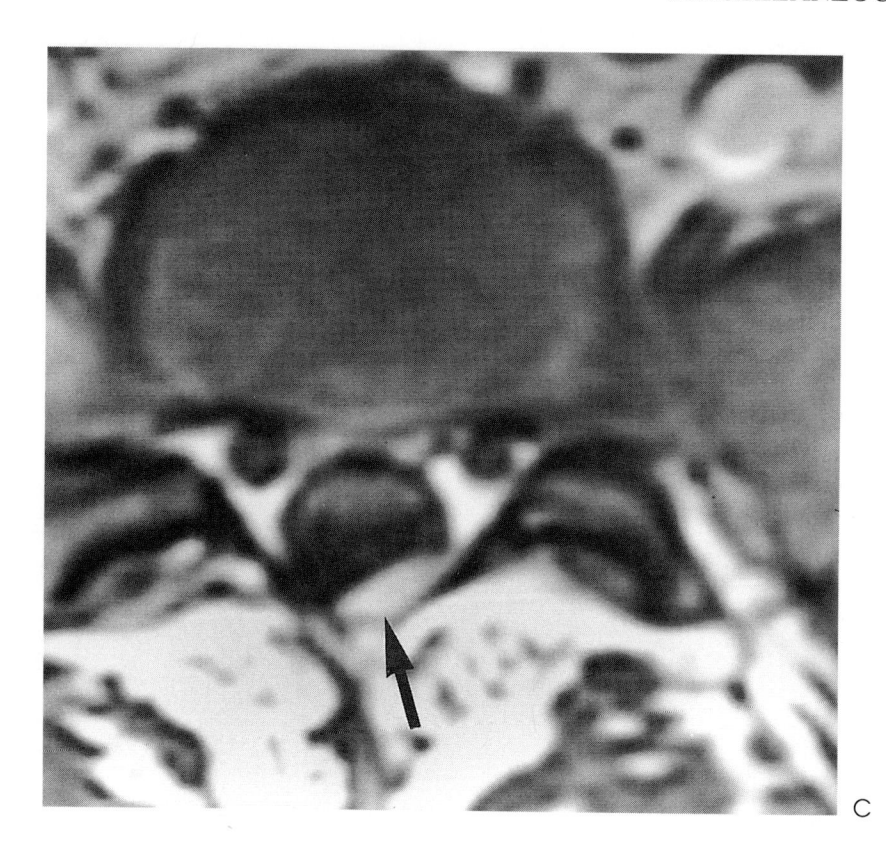

MISCELLANEOUS

C

PEARLS
- Magnetic resonance imaging (MRI) is the procedure of choice for the evaluation of areas of hemorrhage and can be used both for diagnosis and follow-up.

- If surgery is contemplated, the surgical approach can be planned based on the MR images because they accurately reflect the clinical situation.

PITFALL
- Pantopaque retained following myelography could have a similar appearance. However, pantopaque would be expected to accumulate in the dependent portion of the thecal sac. The history is also helpful for evaluation of this patient.

Diagnosis

Epidural hematoma.

Differential Diagnosis

- epidural hematoma
- epidural lipoma

Discussion

It is uncertain if the epidural hematoma is secondary to the initial spinal anesthesia, epidural anesthesia, or blood patching procedure, as either could lead to this appearance. The black line seen in Figure B is the anteriorly displaced posterior margin of the dura. There is also decreased signal intensity on the intervertebral disc at the L4-5 level and a small herniation of the disc into the vertebral canal.

The differential diagnosis based on the short TR images could also suggest an epidural lipoma; however, the clinical setting and the increased signal intensity of the mass on the long TR image is more consistent with an epidural hematoma.

TEACHING ATLAS OF SPINE IMAGING

Case 18

Clinical Presentation

The patient is a 32-year-old male with AIDS (acquired immunodeficiency syndrome) who now presents with lower extremity loss of reflex, decreased sensation, and loss of movement. The patient experienced an episode of *Pneumocystis carinii* pneumonia 6 months prior to this admission.

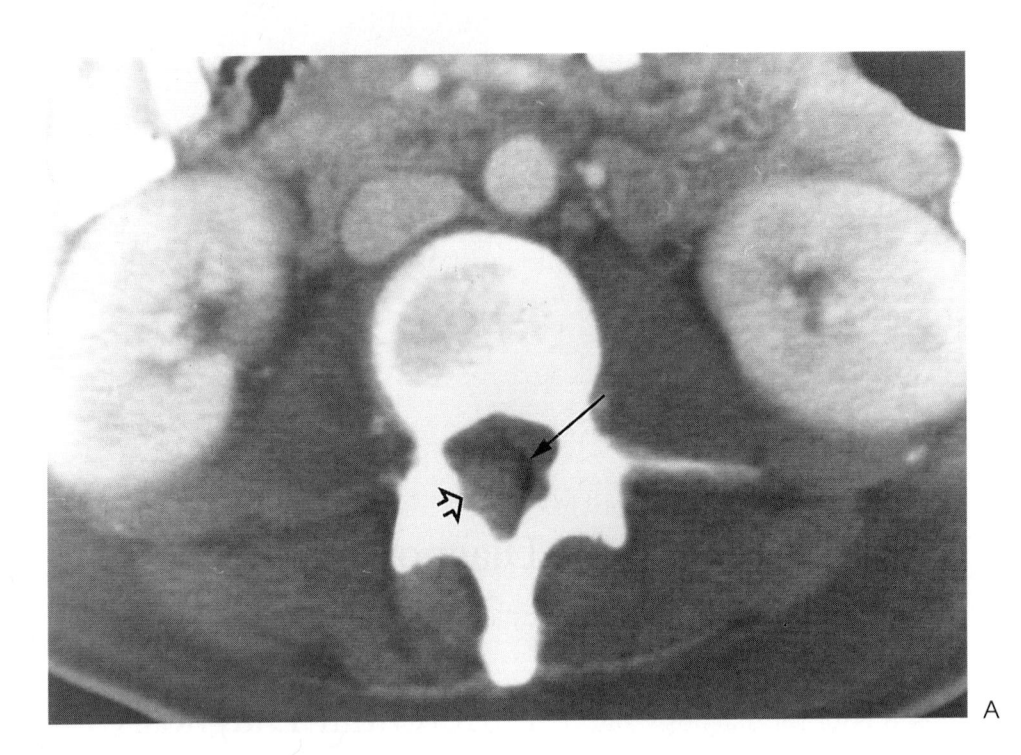

Radiologic Findings

Axial postinfusion computed tomographic (CT) image through the upper lumbar region (Fig. A) reveals a high-density rounded mass in the right dorsal aspect of the vertebral canal (*open arrow*). The low-density thecal sac is compressed and deformed to a semilunar configuration (*solid arrow*).

Radiologic Findings (continued)

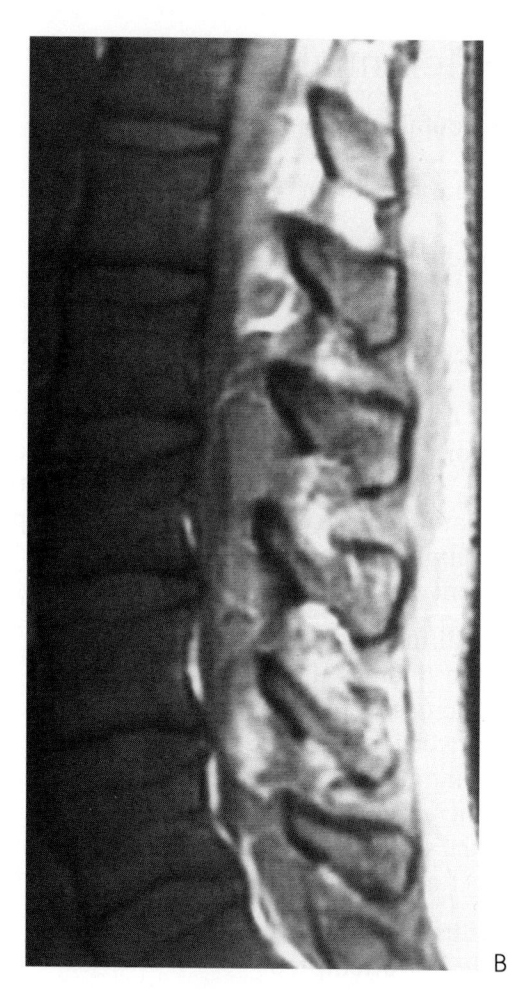

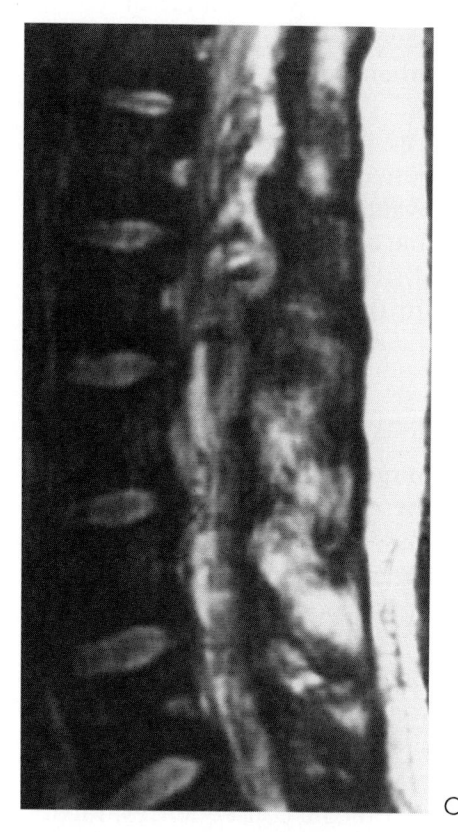

Sagittal short TR image of the lumbar spine (Fig. B) reveals numerous curvilinear areas of increased signal intensity interspersed with intermediate and slightly decreased signal intensity soft tissue material throughout the lumbar vertebral canal. The thecal sac is displaced anteriorly and markedly compressed. The nerve roots of the cauda equina cannot be seen. The marrow within the vertebral bodies is diffusely decreased in signal intensity.

Sagittal long TR image (Fig. C) reveals that the material within the vertebral canal appears variably increased and decreased in signal intensity.

Diagnosis

Multilevel epidural hematoma in the lumbar region.

TEACHING ATLAS OF SPINE IMAGING

PEARLS

- Epidural hematoma may also occur spontaneously in patients who are taking coumadin or have bleeding dyscrasias for other reasons.

- The presence of an epidural hematoma is difficult to evaluate on CT images, and magnetic resonance imaging (MRI) is much more accurate for this type of evaluation.

PITFALLS

- Surgery may be attempted in these patients; however, blood may also accumulate in the thecal sac, and removal may not be possible.

- Because prolonged spinal cord compression from a process such as an epidural hematoma may result in devastating neurologic consequences, rapid evaluation with MRI is necessary for evaluation. Treatment may be performed based upon the MR images.

Differential Diagnosis

- epidural hematoma
- metastatic tumor
- epidural empyema

Discussion

The CT evaluation is nonspecific and could be consistent with metastatic tumor or epidural empyema; a chloroma could also have a similar appearance. The mottled signal intensity within the vertebral canal is consistent with hematoma of varying ages. The normal epidural increased signal intensity fat is completely obliterated in this patient. The cause of the hematoma in this patient was not known.

The diffuse low density of the marrow within the vertebral bodies is typical of the findings that may be seen in the AIDS patient and is secondary to an increased amount of iron deposition. This is a result of more rapid cell turnover in the AIDS patient. This low density marrow may also be seen in patients who have had multiple blood transfusions, which also result in an increased cell turnover and increased iron deposition in the reticuloendothelial system of the bone marrow. The increased iron creates a paramagnetic effect and the resulting decreased signal intensity.

Evaluation should be made of the entire spine if surgical removal is contemplated or attempted.

MISCELLANEOUS

Case 19

Clinical Presentation

The patient is a 37-year-old female with upper extremity weakness.

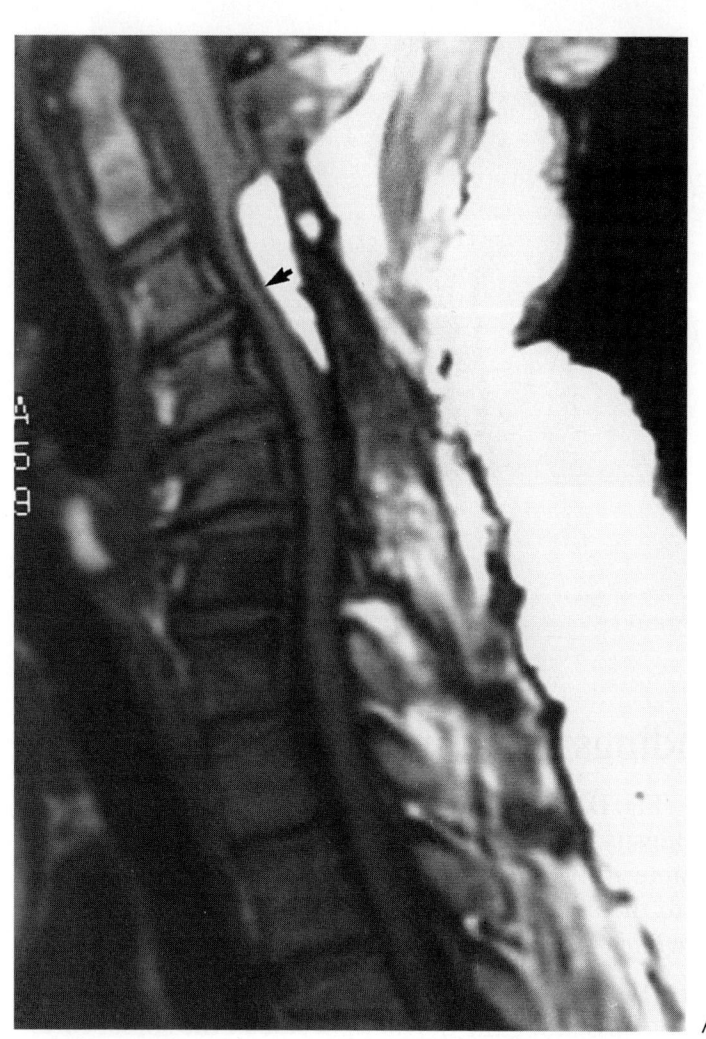

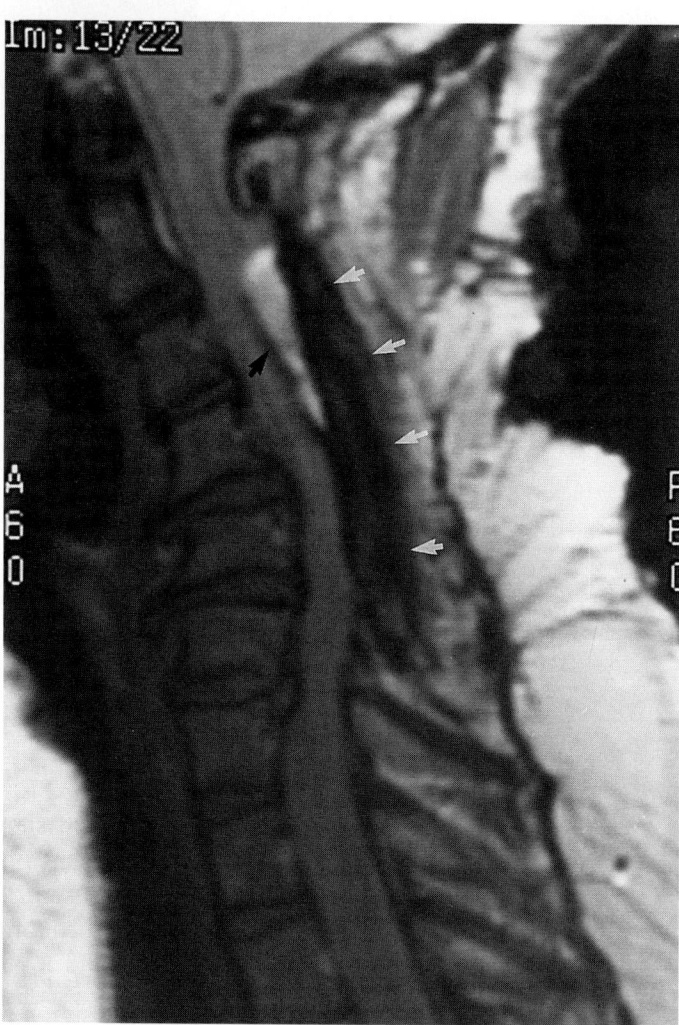

A

B

Radiologic Findings

Sagittal short TR image (Fig. A) reveals an elongated, triangular shaped, increased signal intensity mass along the dorsal aspect of the spinal cord. The mass extends from the superior end plate of C3 to the inferior endplate of C4. The normal lordotic curve of the cervical spine and the spinal cord is reversed. There is a faint decreased signal intensity line along the anterior margin of the mass (*black arrow*). There had been a previous laminectomy. Incidentally noted are moderately severe degenerative changes with both anterior and posterior osteophytes at multiple levels in the cervical spine. There is decreased signal intensity within the marrow of the C6 vertebral body.

TEACHING ATLAS OF SPINE IMAGING

Radiologic Findings (continued)

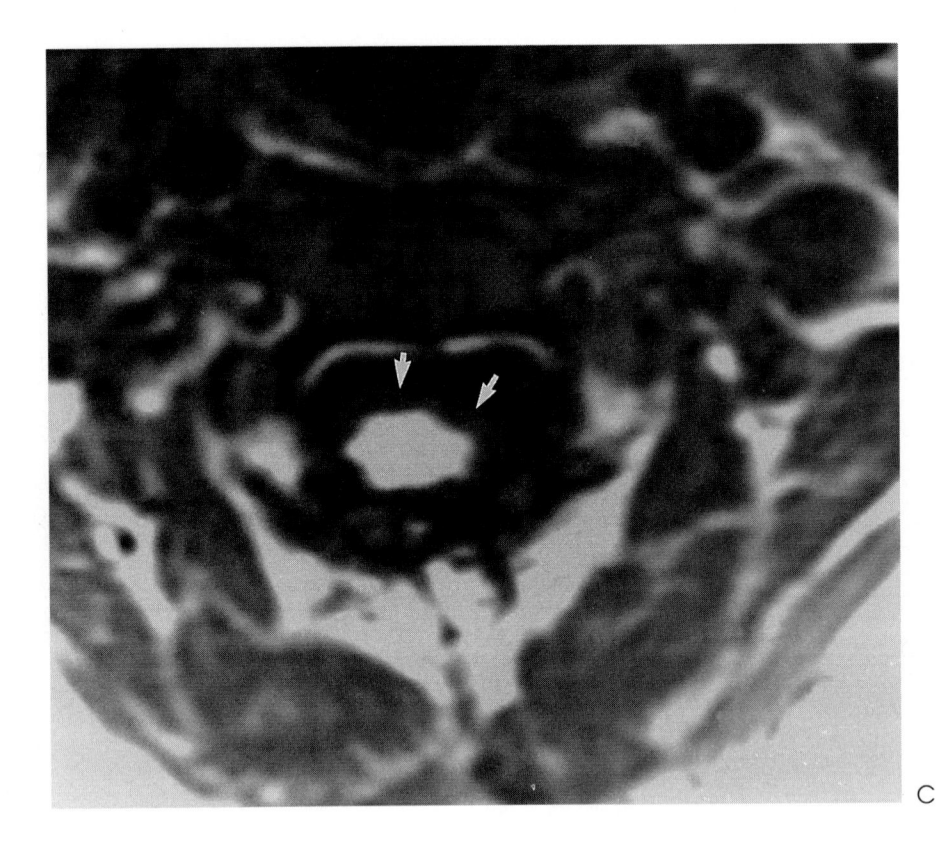

Sagittal long TR image (Fig. B) reveals that the mass now appears relatively decreased in signal intensity. The mass continues to exhibit a decreased signal intensity border anteriorly (*black arrow*). There is an area of decreased signal intensity dorsal to the area of increased signal intensity that extends from C2 through C7 (*white arrows*).

Axial short TR image (Fig. C) reveals a slightly irregularly marginated increased signal intensity mass along the dorsal right side of the spinal cord. The cord is curved around the anterior margin of the mass (*white arrows*). The midline decreased signal intensity defect in the muscle of the dorsal spine area is secondary to the previous laminectomy.

Diagnosis

Spinal cord lipoma.

Differential Diagnosis

- spinal cord lipoma
- spinal cord tumor

MISCELLANEOUS

PEARLS
- The possibility of the increased signal intensity being secondary to methemoglobin is a consideration; however, methemoglobin would become increased signal intensity on the long TR images. In addition, chemical shift artifact is typically associated with adipose tissue and not with a hematoma.

- Fat suppression images may also be obtained to demonstrate that the signal intensity becomes decreased when using this technique.

PITFALL
- Clinical history is important in a case such as this where hemorrhage could also be a diagnostic consideration. The long history in this patient is not in favor of hematoma, as patients with hemorrhage exhibit a catastrophic presentation.

Discussion

In addition to the lipoma of the spinal cord, there are postsurgical changes in the cervical spine and the incidental findings of degenerative changes in the spine. The lipoma itself is congenital. The appearance of decreased signal intensity in the longer TR image is consistent with lipoma. Note that the linear decreased signal intensity border along the anterior aspect of the lipoma is secondary to chemical shift artifact. Lipomas are more common in the lumbar region and are typically seen in the clinical setting of the Chiari malformation. However, small lipomas may occur in the filum terminale and be seen even in asymptomatic patients.

The parient had a previous laminectomy with partial removal of the mass. The decreased signal intensity area dorsal to the lipoma (Fig. B) is secondary to scar formation. Complete removal of a lipoma that is intimately associated with the spinal cord is usually not possible. The reversal of the curve of the spine may occur following a wide laminectomy.

A spinal cord tumor is not likely because tumors are not elongated, and the increased signal intensity would reflect the presence of extensive hemorrhage, in which case the patient would present with devastating clinical symptoms, which were not present in this patient.

Case 20

Clinical Presentation

The patient is an obese 55-year-old female who presents with low back pain.

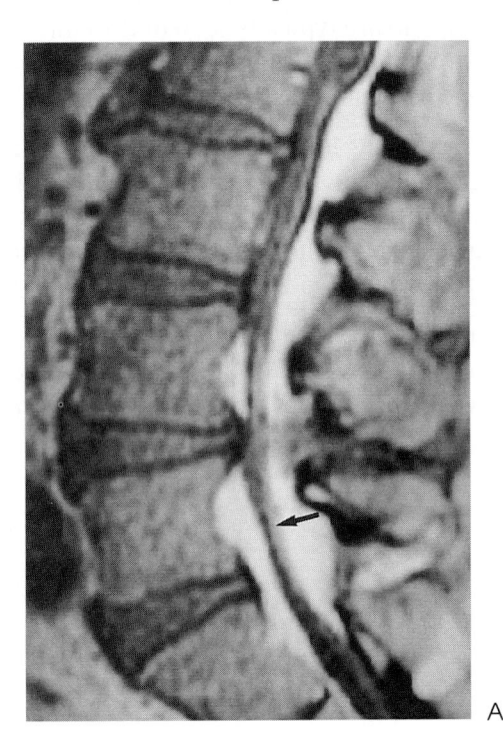

A

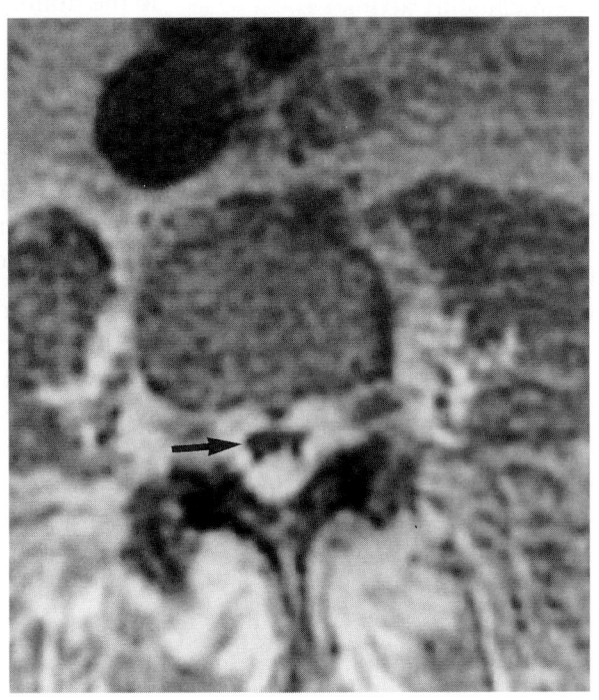

B

Radiologic Findings

Sagittal short TR image (Fig. A) reveals diffuse increased signal intensity soft tissue dorsally throughout the lumbar spine and anteriorly at the L4-S1 levels. There is diffuse encroachment upon the thecal sac, which is compressed (*arrow at L5*). Incidentally noted are anteriorly bulging discs at multiple levels; there are small posterior bulges of the discs.

Axial short TR image (Fig. B) reveals a marked increase in the amount of epidural fat surrounding compressing the thecal sac (*arrow*).

Diagnosis

Epidural lipomatosis.

Differential Diagnosis

- epidural lipomatosis
- epidural hematoma

PEARLS

- The clinical history was helpful in this patient because it further substantiated a diagnosis of epidural lipomatosis. However, even in the absence of a history of steroid treatment, the diagnosis would remain the same.

- MRI with use of a fat suppression technique would also aid in making the identification of fat because the adipose tissue will then appear as decreased signal intensity, while blood will remain as increased signal intensity.

PITFALL
- An epidural hematoma could have a similar appearance because blood in the methemoglobin phase appears as increased signal intensity. However, there was no history of trauma or blood dyscrasia in this patient. Surgery can be attempted in patients with epidural lipomatosis; however, the degree of success is variable.

Discussion

Epidural lipomatosis has a variety of causes. Additional history reveals that this patient had been on long-term steroid treatment, which has been shown to result in epidural lipomatosis. Other causes of idiopathic epidural lipomatosis are exogenous obesity and Cushing's disease, which results in increased endogenous steroid production. Magnetic resonance imaging (MRI) provides an ideal method of evaluation of this condition because fat is an excellent contrast material. Because epidural lipomatosis may involve multiple levels, magnetic resonance imaging (MRI) is an ideal method of evaluation.

Epidural hematoma could also have a similar appearance. However, in patients with hemorrhage, the clinical history is of a catastrophic presentation rather than prolonged back pain.

TEACHING ATLAS OF SPINE IMAGING

Case 21

Clinical Presentation

The patient is a 56-year-old male with known thalassemia and new weakness in the right arm and numbness in the right leg.

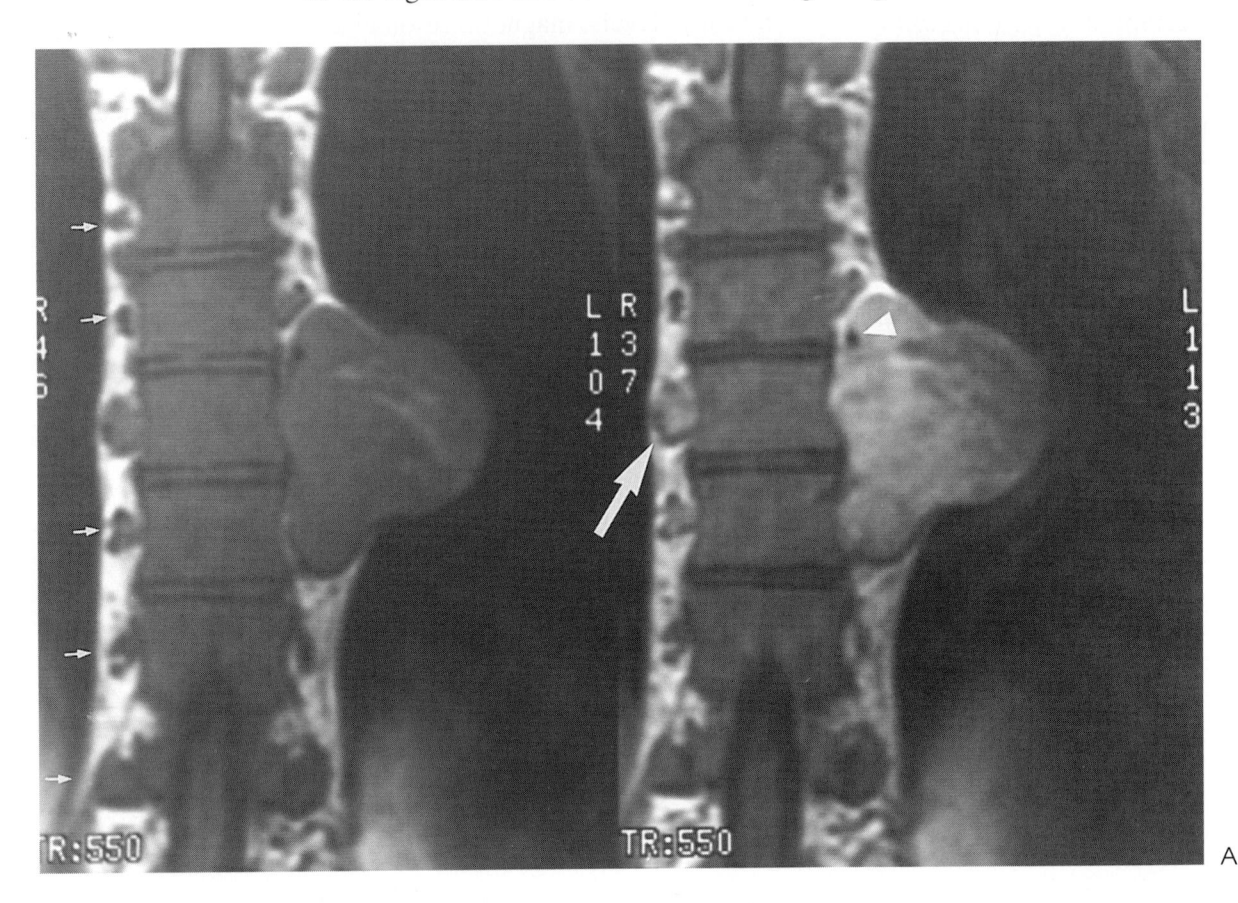

Radiologic Findings

Pre- (Fig. A, *left*) and postcontrast (Fig. A, *right*) coronal short TR images reveal a smoothly marginated paraspinal mass projecting along the left side of the spine in the midthoracic region. There is an intermediate-sized soft tissue mass opposite the larger left-sided mass (*right, arrow*). There are also multiple smaller soft tissue masses along the right side of the spine in the paraspinal region (*left, arrows*). All these areas exhibit mild enhancement postcontrast (*right*). There is a small rounded area of decreased signal intensity within the upper portion of the mass on the left side (*right, arrowhead*).

MISCELLANEOUS

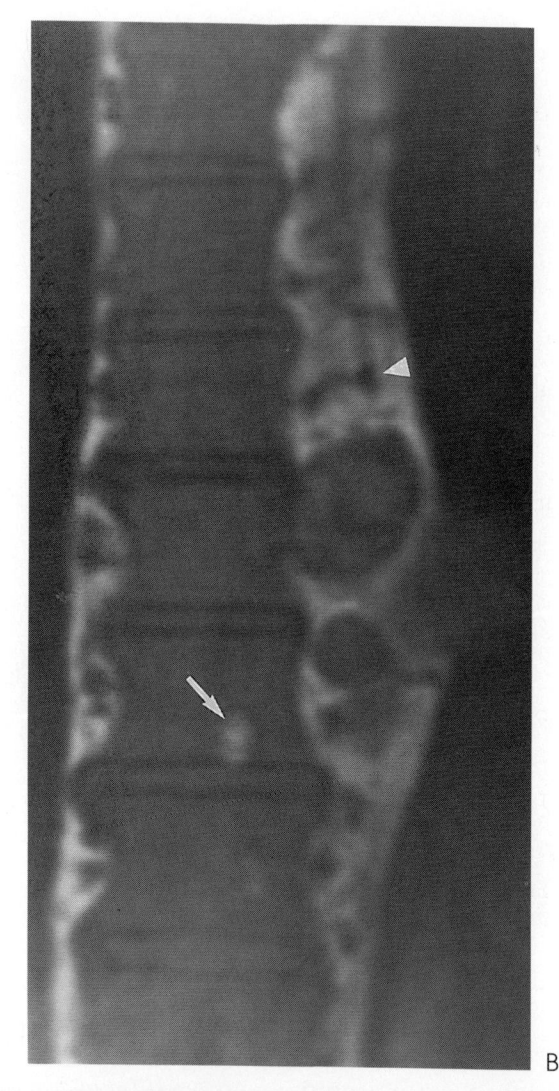

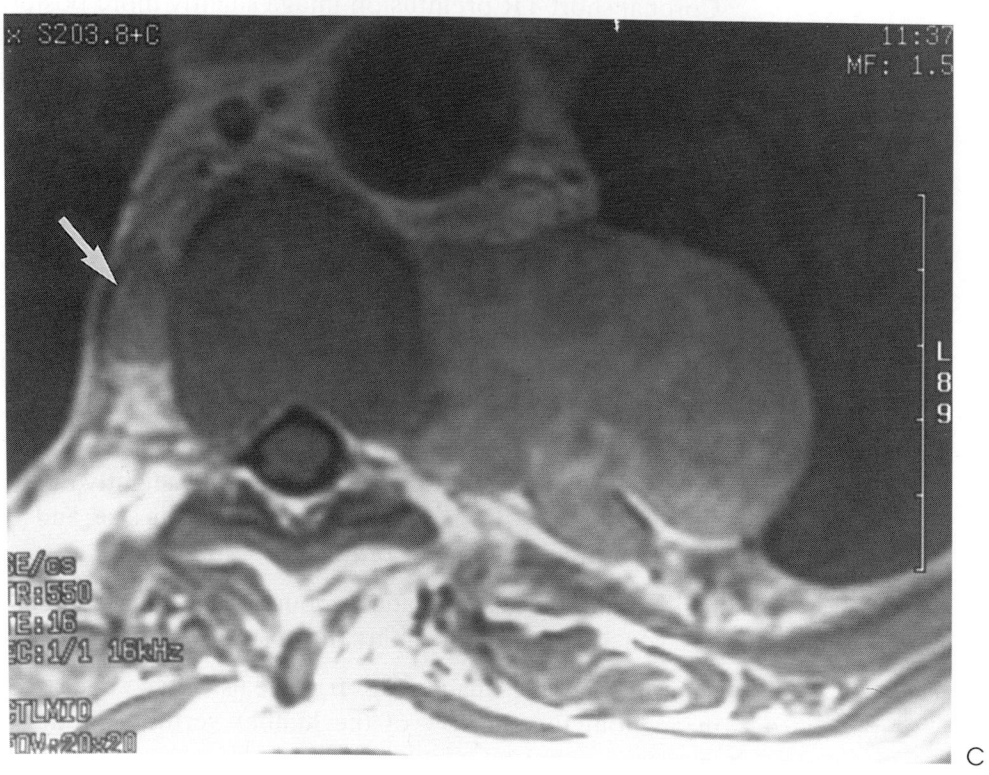

B

C

753

TEACHING ATLAS OF SPINE IMAGING

Radiologic Findings (continued)

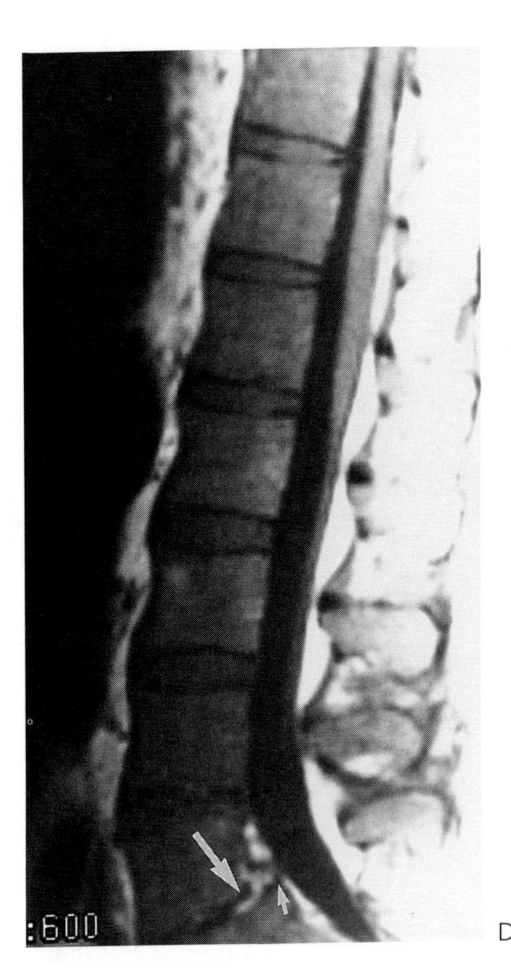

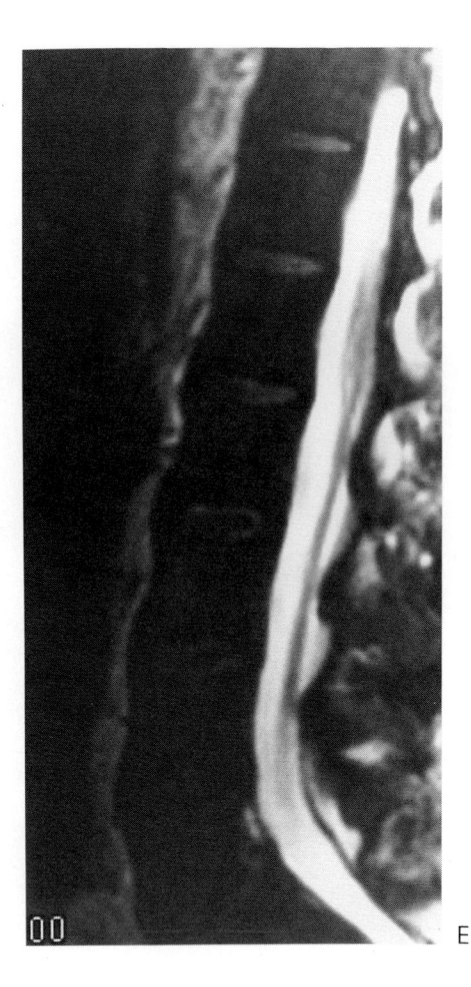

Coronal short TR preinfusion image slightly more posterior than Figure A (Fig. B) reveals multiple additional rounded areas of intermediate signal intensity on the left side of the spine. The pleural margin is displaced laterally in a curvilinear fashion around these masses. There is a rounded area of decreased signal intensity (*arrowhead*) that projects above the mass. A small oval area of increased signal intensity is visible at the level of the inferior end plate of one of the lower thoracic vertebral bodies (*arrow*).

Axial short TR image postcontrast (Fig. C) reveals a large lobulated, smoothly marginated mass on the left side. The smaller right-sided area of enhancement is again seen (*arrow*). Both exhibit mild, inhomogeneous enhancement. There is no encroachment upon the spinal cord or vertebral canal.

Sagittal short TR image in the lumbar region (Fig. D) reveals that the marrow of the vertebral bodies is uniformly slightly decreased signal intensity. Otherwise, the spinal cord is normal in size and configuration, and there is no encroachment on the vertebral canal.

Incidentally there is a grade I spondylolisthesis with forward displacement of L5 on S1 (*white arrows* mark the posterior margins of the vertebral bodies).

Sagittal long TR image (Fig. E) reveals diffuse decreased signal intensity throughout the marrow of the lumbar vertebral bodies without areas of increased signal intensity.

PEARLS
- The clinical history is important in making a diagnosis of extramedullary hematopoiesis.

- The magnetic resonance appearance of multiple rounded areas of soft tissue masses adjacent to the spine is pathognomonic of the diagnosis of extramedullary hematopoiesis.

PITFALL
- Without a history, diagnostic considerations would include multiple metastases or possibly multiple neurofibromas or schwannomas. Other diagnostic considerations are very unlikely in this clinical setting and with this typical imaging appearance.

Diagnosis

Extramedullary hematopoiesis.

Differential Diagnosis

- extramedullary hematopoiesis
- metastases

Discussion

The multiple paraspinal soft tissue masses represent areas of extramedullary hematopoiesis. This appearance is typical and pathognomonic of the appearance of extramedullary hematopoiesis. This is seen typically in patients with thalassemia and occasionally in patients with sickle cell anemia. There was no evidence of cord compression in this patient, so the cause of the patient's symptoms is unknown. The rounded areas of decreased signal intensity are areas of flow void because of blood vessels. Multiple metastases might be a clinical consideration in this patient; however, the patient was not known to have a primary tumor. In addition, there is no evidence of bony destructive change.

In the lumbar region, the marrow appears as decreased signal intensity because there is increased deposition of iron in the marrow secondary to rapid cell turnover because of the patient's underlying disease. Therefore, the marrow remains as decreased signal intensity on the long TR images. The decreased signal intensity is secondary to paramagnetic effect.

TEACHING ATLAS OF SPINE IMAGING

Case 22

Clinical Presentation

The patient is a 25-year-old male presenting with low back pain who is being evaluated to rule out osteomyelitis. The patient has a prosthetic left hip made from titanium.

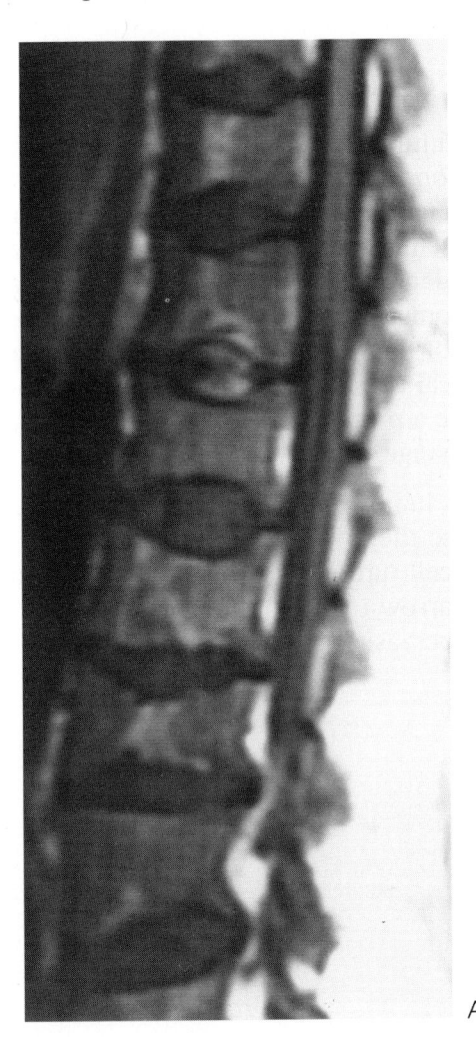

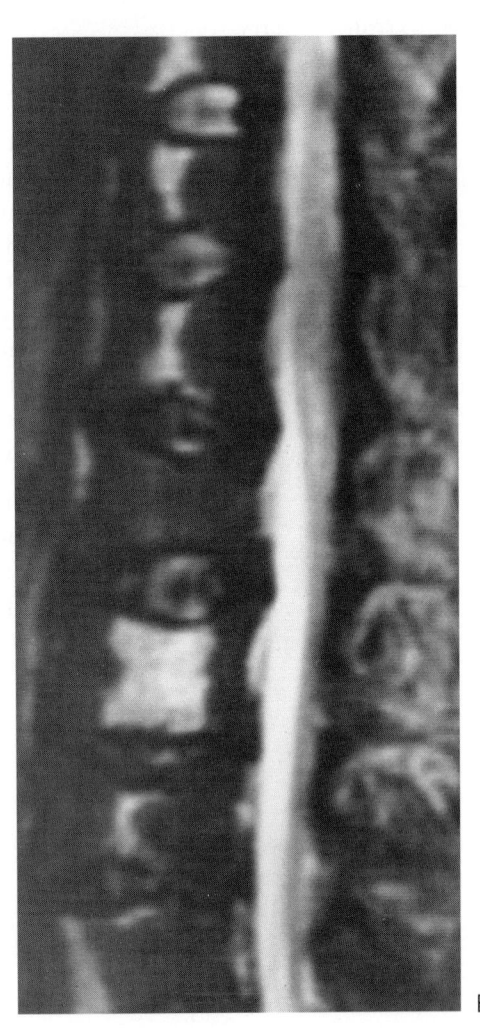

A

B

Radiologic Findings

Sagittal short TR image in the lumbar region (Fig. A) reveals a biconcave appearance of multiple vertebral bodies. There are also varying degrees of compression fractures involving multiple vertebral bodies. The marrow of the vertebral bodies exhibits mottled areas of increased and decreased signal intensity.

Sagittal long TR image (Fig. B) reveals expansion of the intervertebral discs because of the biconcave deformity of the vertebral bodies. There are multiple vertical areas of increased signal intensity of varying size involving multiple vertebral bodies.

Diagnosis

Sickle cell anemia with multiple bone infarcts.

Differential Diagnosis

- sickle cell anemia
- myelofibrosis
- metastatic disease

Discussion

Sickle cell anemia typically results in the biconcave deformity of the vertebral bodies seen in this patient. Bone infarcts, which appear as areas of decreased and increased signal intensity within the marrow of the vertebrae, are common in patients with sickle cell anemia. The areas of infarction may be associated with an increase in fat deposition, and this appears as increased signal intensity. There may also be deposition of iron, which appears as decreased signal intensity. The edema resulting from either the compression fractures or the infarcts appears as increased signal intensity on the long TR images.

Infections are more common in patients with sickle cell anemia than the general population, although this patient does not exhibit evidence of an inflammatory process.

The patient had a hip replacement because of infarction of the femoral head related to the sickle cell anemia. The metallic hip prosthesis is not a contraindication to magnetic resonance imaging (MRI). The MR images that include the prosthesis may be degraded by artifact; however, the images obtained distant from the metallic prosthesis will not be degraded.

Sickle cell anemia is an inherited gene for abnormal α-globin chain subunit of adult hemoglobin. Sickle cell anemia may be homozygous or heterozygous. The disease is seen in black persons of African or African-American ancestry. The disease results in a sickle-shaped red blood cell. The heterozygous state for hemoglobin S (sickle cell trait) apparently confers a biologic advantage against infection with falciparum malaria.

Areas of myelofibrosis could result in a similar imaging appearance; however, myelofibrosis would not result in the biconcave appearance of the vertebral bodies.

PEARLS

- Patients with metallic hip, shoulder, or other joint prostheses may be safely evaluated with MRI.

- Although images may be degraded in one imaging plane, they are often satisfactory in another imaging plane. The choice of scanning sequence is also significant. Gradient echo images are most susceptible to magnetic susceptibility artifact, followed by fast spin echo long TR images, routine long TR images, and short TR images. Imaging should be planned accordingly.

PITFALL

- MRI of metallic devices results in mild heating of the metal of any metallic prosthesis. However, the heating is not sufficient to cause tissue damage, and the heat is rapidly dissipated from the metallic device.

TEACHING ATLAS OF SPINE IMAGING

Case 23

Clinical Presentation

The patient is a 58-year-old male who complains of left hand weakness. The patient has end stage renal disease with an abnormal protein electrophoresis.

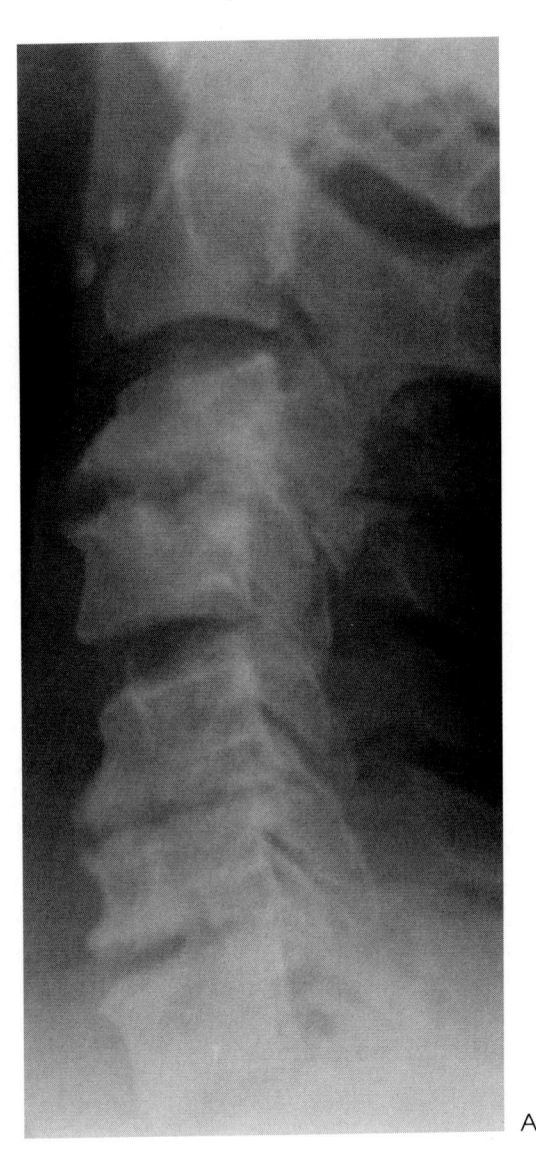

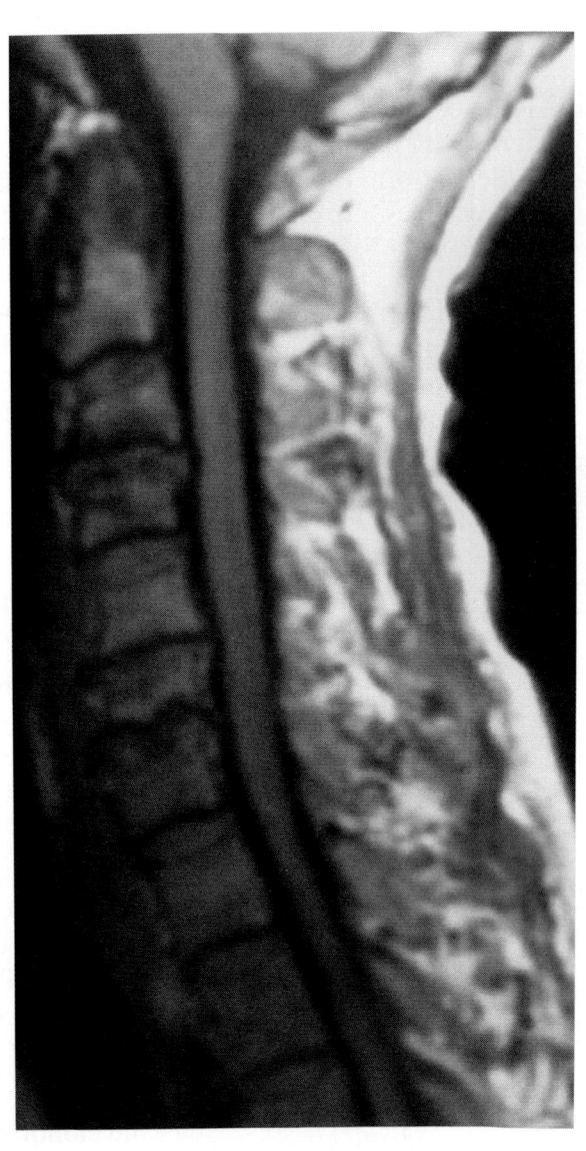

A

B

Radiologic Findings

Lateral plain spine radiograph (Fig. A) reveals hypertrophic spurs at multiple levels of the cervical spine. The degenerative changes are disproportionately severe for a patient of 58 years of age. There is slight retrolisthesis of C3 on C4. There is disc space narrowing at C3-4, C5-6, and C6-7.

MISCELLANEOUS

Radiologic Findings (continued)

Sagittal short TR image of the cervical spine in the same patient (Fig. B) reveals disc space narrowing with a bulging disc at the C3-4 level that indents the subarachnoid space. There is also disc space narrowing at C5-6 and C6-7. There is irregularity of the end plates adjacent to the narrowed discs. Posterior osteophytes result in mild encroachment upon the subarachnoid space.

Diagnosis

Amyloidosis secondary to chronic renal failure with β_2 microglobulinemia.

Differential Diagnosis

- chronic renal failure
- multiple myeloma

Discussion

Amyloidosis with increase in β_2 microglobulin results in acceleration of the degenerative changes in the cervical spine. Amyloidosis may also occur in patients with multiple myeloma. Amyloidosis is progressive, and although treatment is supportive, it is usually ineffective.

The clinical history is vital to accurate diagnosis because without an appropriate clinical history, the changes could be attributed to simply degenerative changes.

PEARLS

- Clinical history here is very helpful for diagnosis.
- Amyloid deposition may also be seen in patients with chronic multiple myeloma.

PITFALL

- In the absence of a history of amyloidosis with β_2 microglobulinemia, degenerative changes secondary to osteoarthritis could have a similar appearance.

TEACHING ATLAS OF SPINE IMAGING

Case 24

Clinical Presentation

The patient is a 67-year-old male with a history of polio as a child, long-term back pain, and gradually progressive scoliosis and proximal muscle weakness.

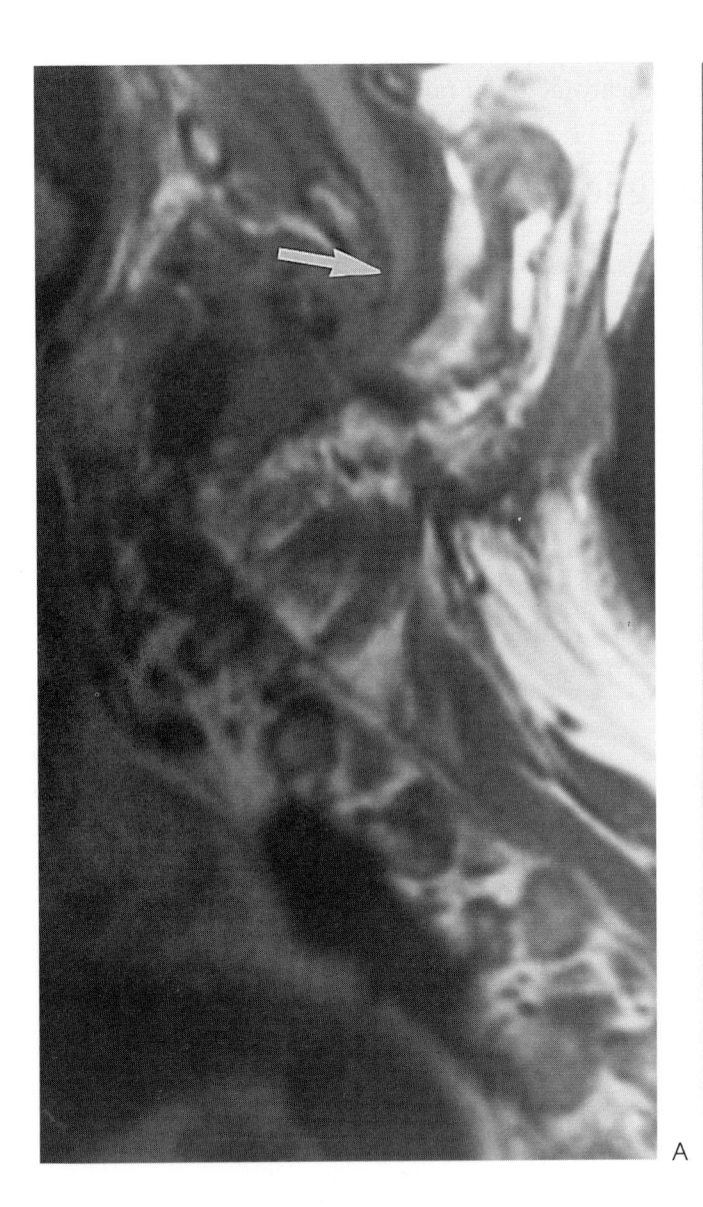

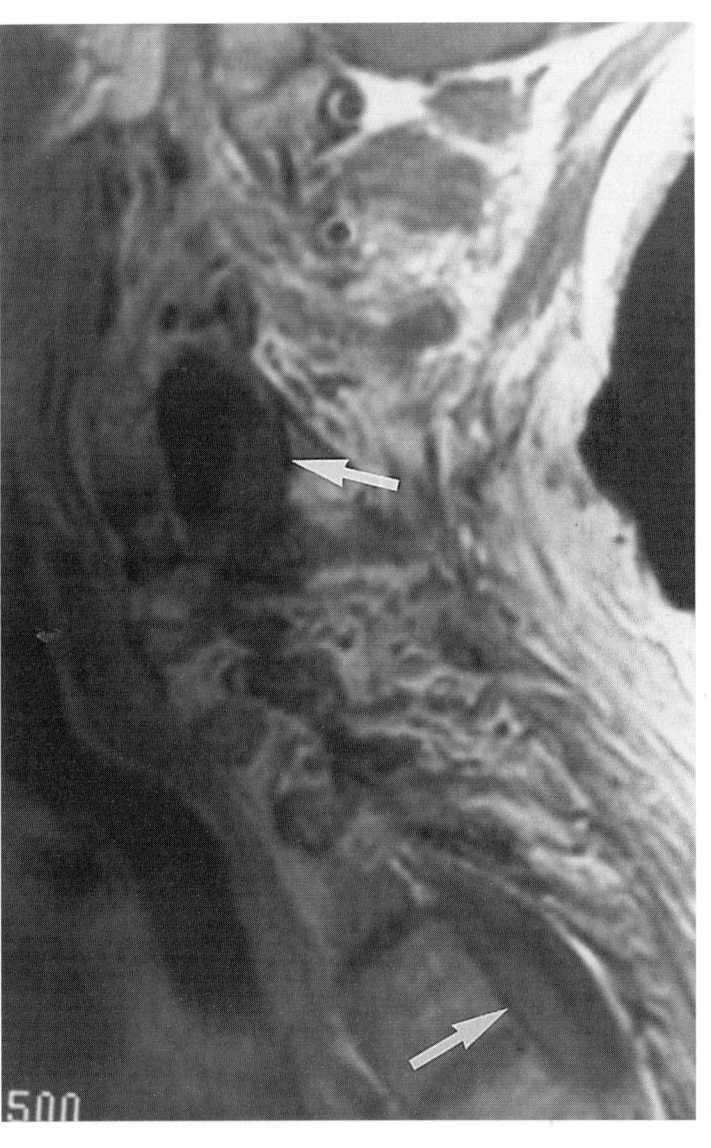

MISCELLANEOUS

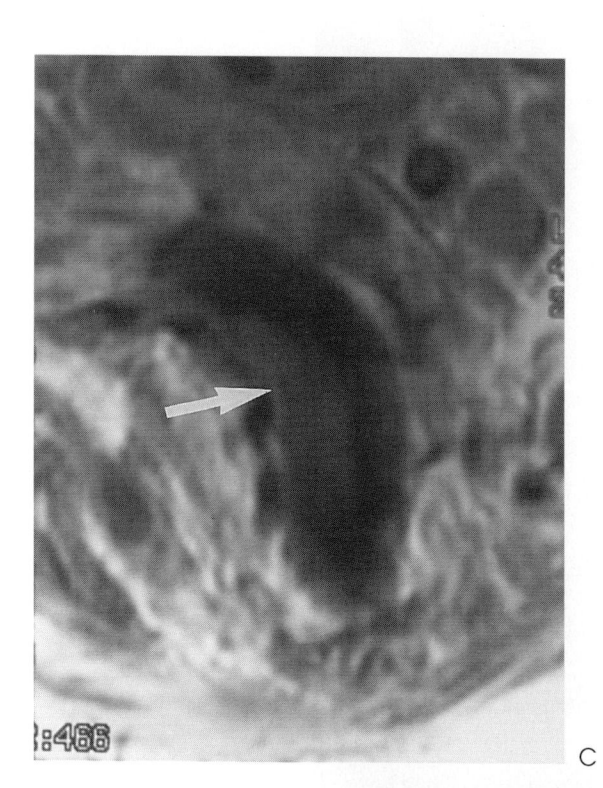

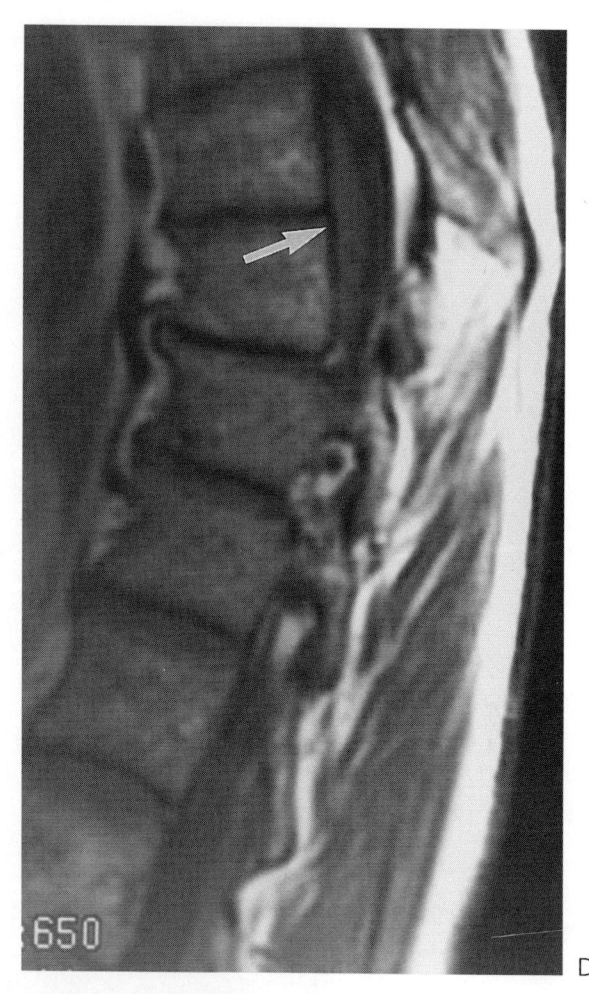

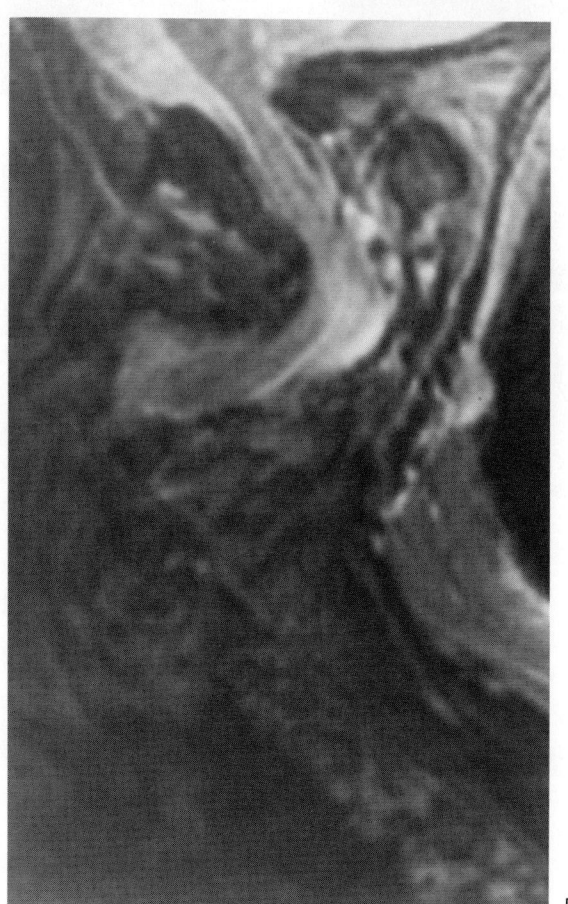

C

D

E

761

TEACHING ATLAS OF SPINE IMAGING

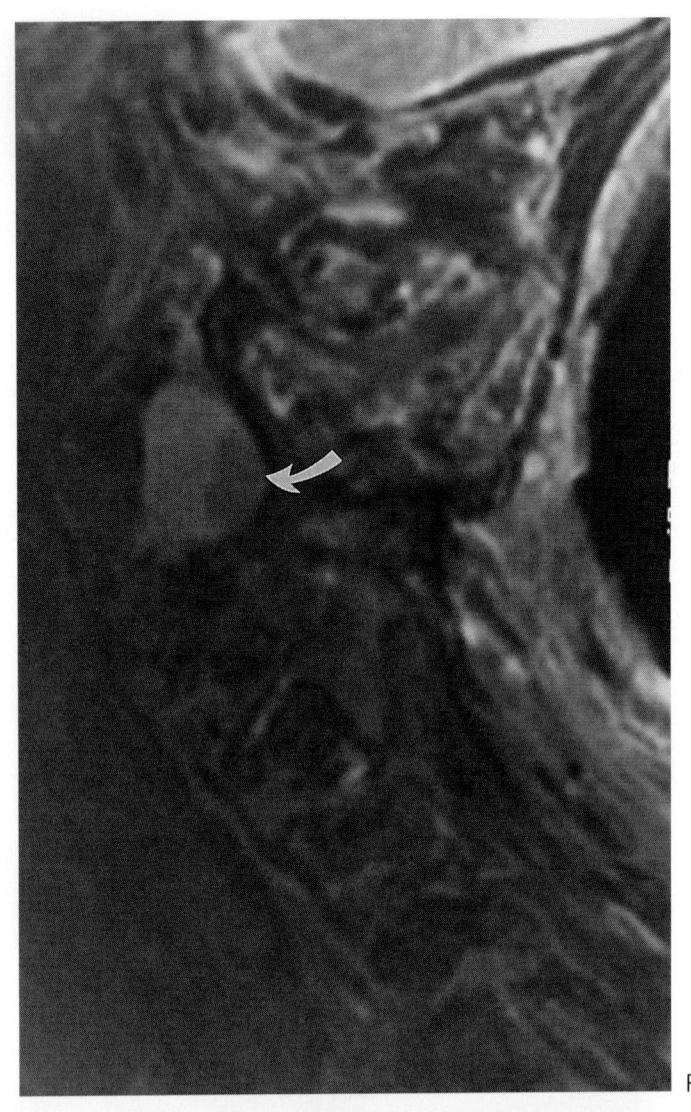

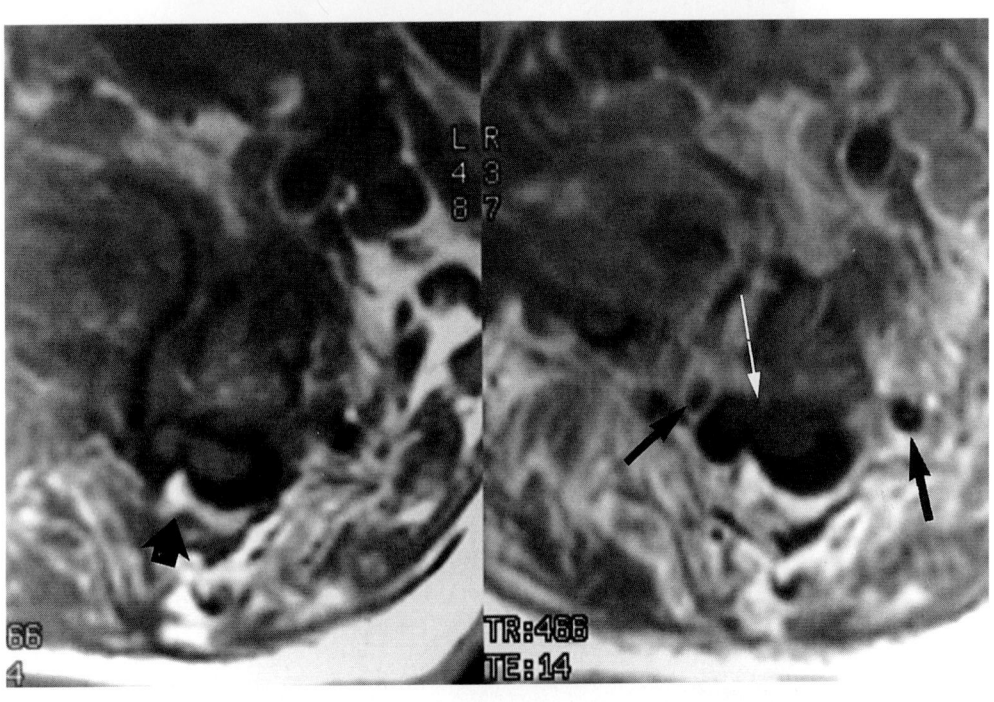

MISCELLANEOUS

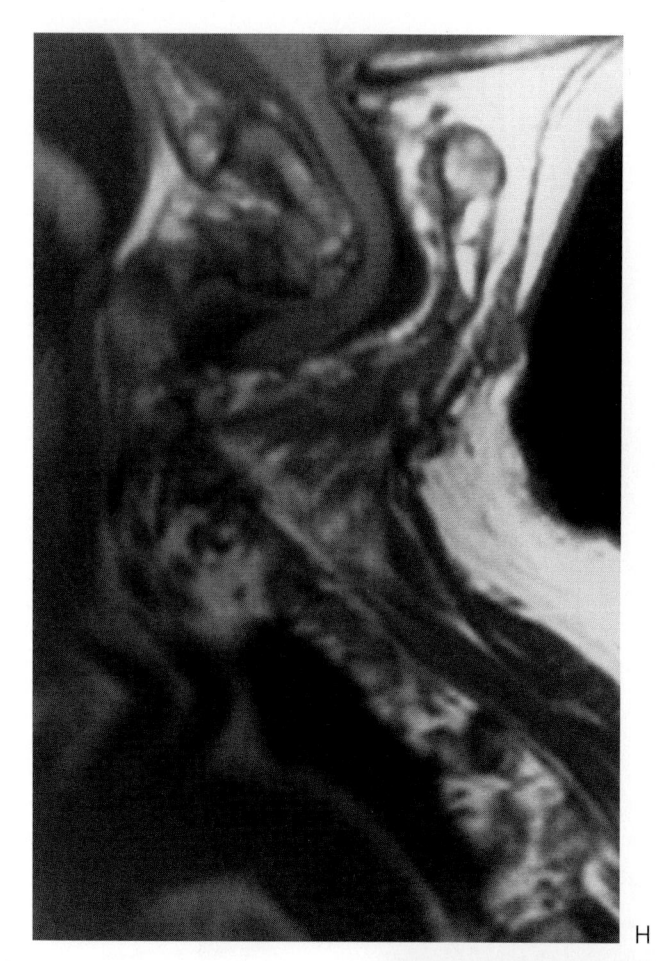

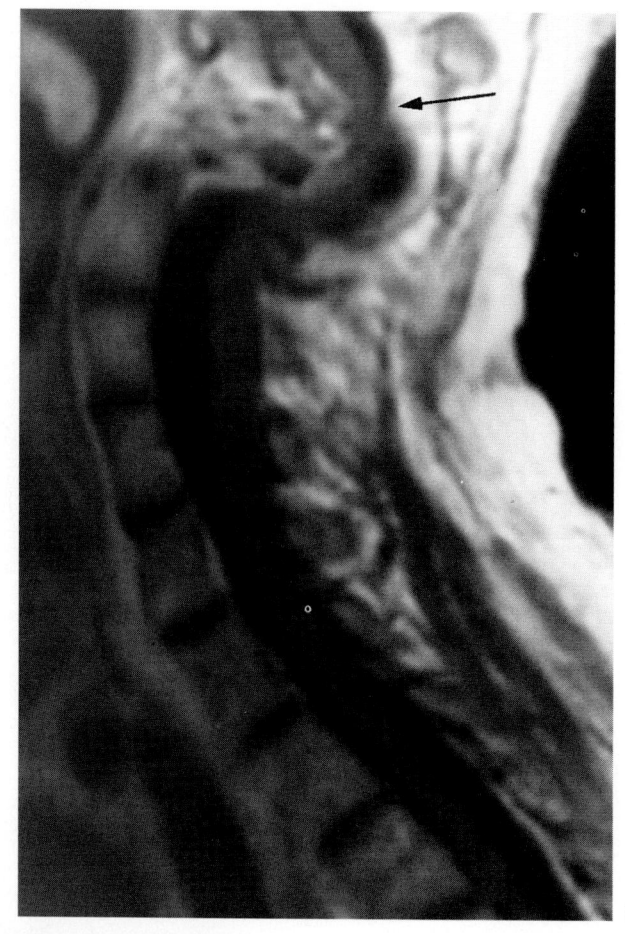

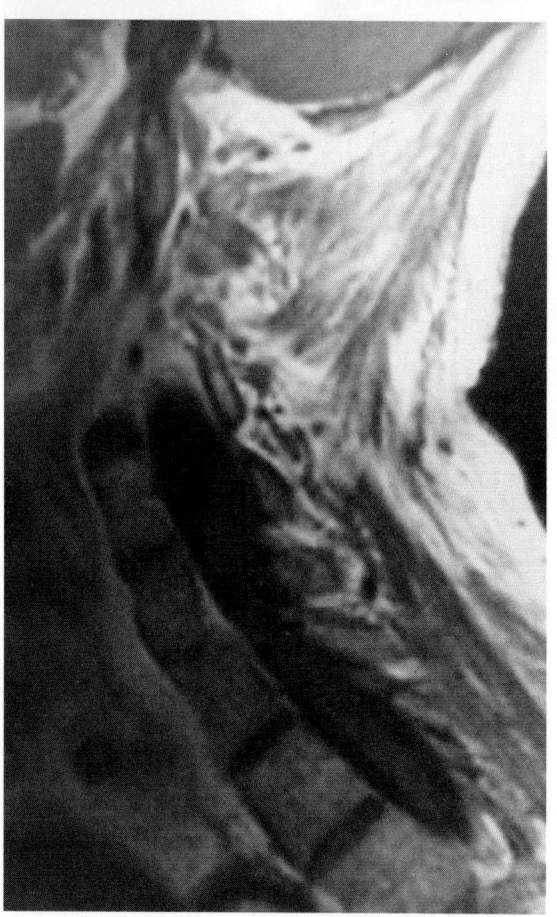

763

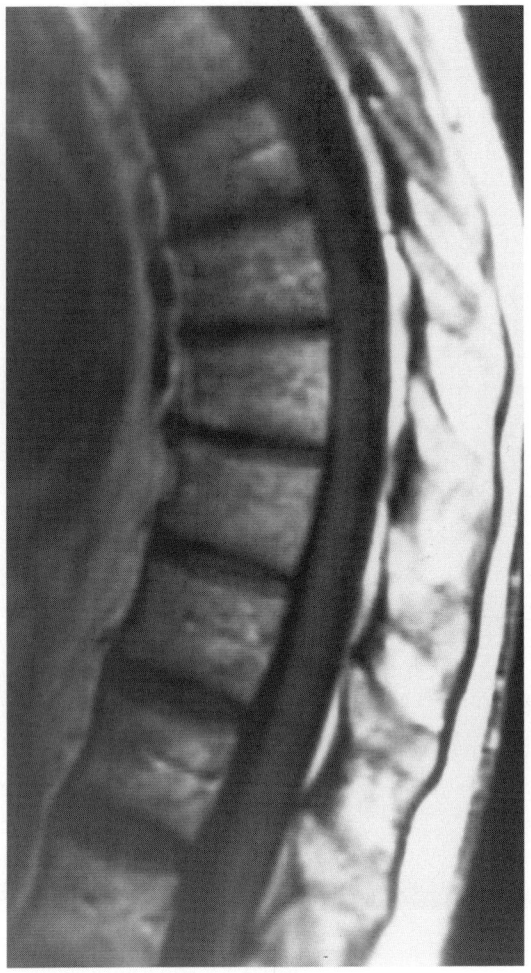

K

Radiologic Findings

Sagittal short TR images of the upper cervical (Fig. A), midcervical (Fig. B), lower cervical (Fig. C), and upper thoracic (Fig. D) regions reveal that because of a very severe scoliosis, there is visualization of the spinal cord in only very short segments (*arrows*). It is impossible to confirm or rule out the presence of a spinal cord tumor or encroachment upon the spinal cord.

Sagittal long TR image at the level of the cervicomedullary junction (Fig. E) reveals the spinal cord at the level of the foramen magnum. There is marked curvilinear deformity of the spinal cord at all levels; as a consequence, the spinal cord is never well demonstrated.

Sagittal long TR image at the midcervical region (Fig. F) reveals that a short segment of the spinal cord is seen in the deformed vertebral canal (*arrow*).

Axial short TR images (Fig. G) reveal a bone spur that arises from the lateral masses or facet joints and encroaches upon the dorsal aspect of the vertebral canal and compresses the spinal cord (*left, arrow*). There is also anterior encroachment upon the spinal cord (*right, white arrow*). The vertebral arteries appear as areas of flow void (*right, black arrows*).

Sagittal short TR images utilizing the spine straightening program (Figs. H–K) allow the images to be reformed, so the vertebral bodies and spinal cord appear to have a normal relationship to one another. Although there

MISCELLANEOUS

Radiologic Findings (continued)

is still evidence of a minor scoliosis of the spine, the spinal cord is readily identified. There is still demonstrable evidence of encroachment on the spinal cord in the upper cervical region in Figure 1 (*arrow*).

Diagnosis

Scoliosis with dorsal encroachment secondary to degenerative changes, no tumor. Secondary to poliomyelitis; postpolio syndrome.

Differential Diagnosis

- idiopathic scolioses

Discussion

When there is a severe scoliosis, exact evaluation of the spinal cord and the surrounding structures cannot be performed. The scoliosis correction program allows reformatting of the images and allows ready evaluation of the spinal cord. This program modifies the original images via a computer reformatting program to eliminate the appearance of a scoliosis.

Poliomyelitis (acute anterior poliomyelitis) is a disease that destroys the motor neurons of the spinal cord (anterior horn cells). It is a viral illness that is acquired orally. Previously common, it is now rare and has been almost completely eradicated by vaccination. The disease attacks specific neuronal populations, and the affected cells undergo sequential degenerative change followed by cell death. The disease preferentially affects the motor neuron cells of the lower brain stem and the spinal cord. The muscles supplied by these neurons subsequently become flaccid because of lack of enervation and atrophy with fatty replacement of the muscles, which occurs rapidly and is not reversible.

The postpolio syndrome is characterized by progressive weakness of the muscles many years after the initial infection. This initial infection may be subclinical. Therefore, imaging is usually performed on a patient older than 45 years of age and most likely in patients in their 50s to 70s. Patients with such severe atrophy are generally presumed to have had polio and are not presenting in the clinical setting of the postpolio syndrome. This syndrome is often associated with back pain.

PEARL
- In institutions where a reformatting program is not available, multiplanar imaging may allow demonstration of the spinal cord in a sufficient fashion that cord compression can be ruled out.

PITFALL
- Myelography with postmyelography computed tomography (CT) may also be used for better evaluation of the patient with scoliosis. However, even CT may not allow exact evaluation of the distorted anatomy.

TEACHING ATLAS OF SPINE IMAGING

Case 25

Clinical Presentation

The patient is a 66-year-old female with back pain and progressive scoliosis.

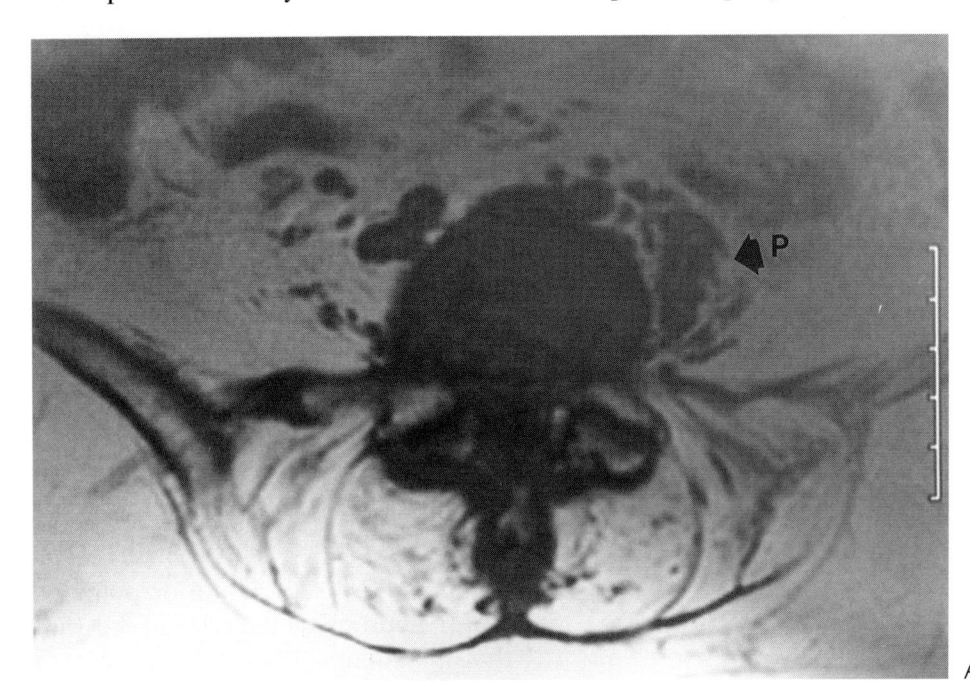

A

Radiologic Findings

Axial short TR image at the L4 level (Fig. A) reveals that all the paraspinal muscles of the back have been replaced by increased signal intensity fat. There is no normal appearing muscle remaining. The left psoas muscle is markedly atrophic (*black arrow-p*). The right psoas muscle is not seen. The gluteal muscles are also absent and replaced by increased signal intensity fat. There are also degenerative changes involving the interfacet joints bilaterally. The changes are worse on the right than on the left.

PEARL
- The changes of fatty muscle infiltration are very marked in this patient but occur in varying degrees in different patients.

Diagnosis

Postpolio syndrome.

Discussion

Clinical history revealed that the patient had polio as a child. The patient was experiencing increasing back pain and a progressive scoliosis, a history

MISCELLANEOUS

PITFALL
- In any older patient, an attempt should be made to elicit a history of polio in childhood. However, even in the absence of a positive history of polio, the magnetic resonance imaging appearance in this patient is typical of the postpolio patient, and the disease is then presumed to have been subclinical.

typical of the postpolio syndrome. There is almost complete absence of the muscles at the level visualized. Extensive fatty infiltration of the muscles occurs because of the lack of enervation. This denervation is secondary to loss of the anterior horn cells related to the polio virus. The degenerative changes in the spine are related to the scoliosis and additional stress on the interfacet joints. In occasional cases, inactivity and prolonged bed rest may result in some muscle atrophy, but the changes are not as extensive as those seen in this patient.

The imaging appearance is typical for the postpolio syndrome; however, the changes are usually not as severe as seen in this patient. In some patients, the atrophy may be very subtle, and it is frequently asymmetric and occasionally affects only one side.

Radiologic Findings

Sagittal short TR image of the thoracic spinal cord (Fig. A) reveals an area of focal atrophy of the spinal cord at the level of previous surgery (*white arrow*). The spinous processes of the spine are surgically absent. The other two arrows identify the T1 and T6 vertebral bodies.

Sagittal long TR image of the thoracic spine (Fig. B) reveals a V-shaped area of variable signal intensity at the level of previous surgery in the dorsal aspect of the thoracic subarachnoid space; this extends to the level of focal cord atrophy. The T1 vertebral body (*long arrow*) is identified with T-1.

Axial short TR image at the level of focal cord atrophy (Fig. C) reveals that the spinal cord is triangular in shape and displaced anteriorly adjacent to the anterior margin of the subarachnoid space (*arrow*). The spinous processes are surgically absent at this level, and there is increased signal intensity fat dorsal to the thecal sac.

Axial postmyelogram computed tomographic (CT) image at the same level as Figure C (Fig. D) reveals the irregular spinal cord configuration with close approximation of the spinal cord to the posterior margin of the vertebral body (*black arrow*). A high density surgical clip is present dorsally on the left side of the spine (*white arrow*). The spinous process is absent at this level.

Lateral reconstruction image of the thoracic spine (Fig. E) mimics the appearance of the short TR magnetic resonance (MR) image with focal narrowing of the thoracic spinal cord (*arrow*). The spinous processes are surgically absent. There is slight dilatation of the thecal sac at this level with outward bulging into the laminectomy site.

Diagnosis

Postoperative change with focal atrophy of the spinal cord and anterior tethering of the cord to the posterior margin of the vertebral body.

Differential Diagnosis

- postoperative change

Discussion

This patient presumably had a dorsal arachnoid cyst removed at the time of the previous surgery. There is now an area of focal atrophy of the spinal cord, probably secondary to vascular compromise or direct cord trauma related to the surgery. It is also possible that the patient had a spinal cord tumor removed rather than a cyst. The triangular shaped area of variable signal intensity seen in Figure B is probably a thin area of scarring and prominence of the arachnoid layer related to the surgery. The decreased signal intensity areas are related to deposition hemosiderin related to the previous surgery. Note that the MR scan is remarkably similar to the postmyelogram CT scan. However, MRI is noninvasive and allows convenient multiplanar imaging. MRI is the procedure of choice for evaluation in a patient such as this.

PEARLS

- Pre- and postcontrast multiplanar imaging with MRI should be performed in a patient with this history to rule out tumor or "cyst" recurrence. If tumor is present, areas of enhancement would be anticipated.

- If the diagnosis of postoperative change with scarring is in doubt, a follow-up examination will be helpful for complete evaluation.

PITFALL

- Without re-operation the exact nature of the triangular shaped area of variable signal intensity seen in Figure B cannot be absolutely evaluated. However, repeat surgery in a patient such as this risks causing the development of even greater symptoms.

MISCELLANEOUS

Case 27

Clinical Presentation

The patient is a 27-year-old male with back pain.

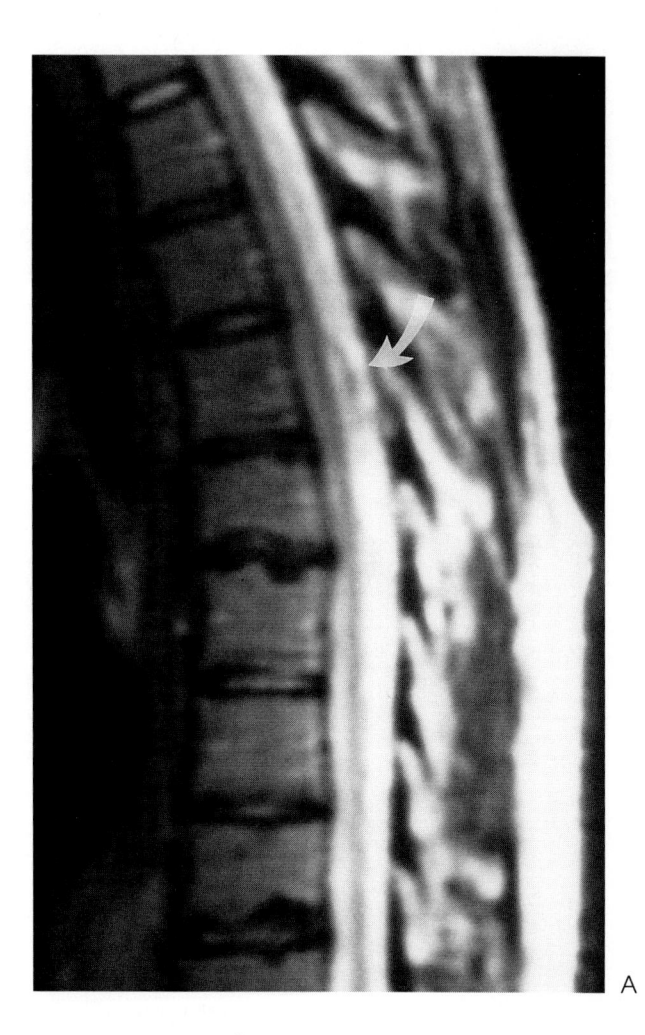

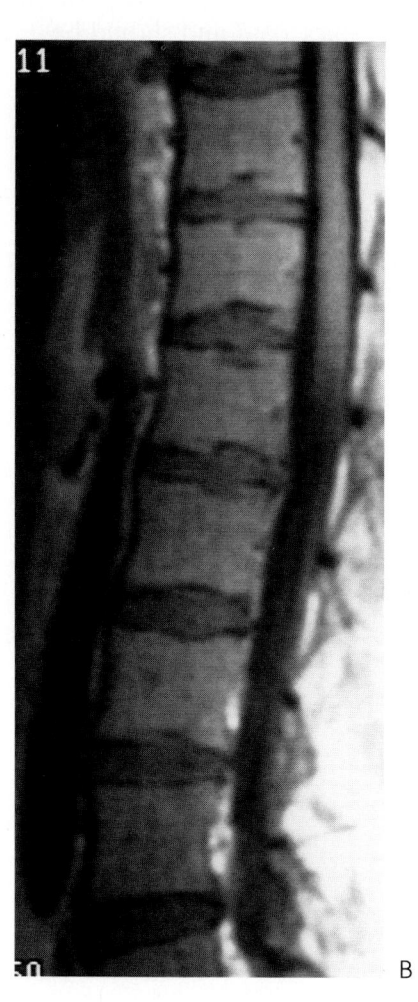

Radiologic Findings

Sagittal long TR image in the thoracic region (Fig. A) reveals multiple small curvilinear end plate deformities. There is slight accentuation of the normal dorsal kyphosis. Small curvilinear areas of decreased signal intensity in the cerebrospinal fluid dorsal to the spinal cord are visible in the midthoracic region (*arrow*).

Sagittal short TR image in the lumbar region also (Fig. B) reveals multiple curvilinear defects in the end plates of the vertebral bodies.

TEACHING ATLAS OF SPINE IMAGING

PEARLS
- These end plate herniations are typically seen in young patients, such as athletes, who sustain repeated axial loading injuries.

- While not of pathologic significance, these end plate herniations may be the source of back pain and should be reported when they are identified on plain films or other imaging studies.

PITFALLS
- These end plate disc herniations may be associated with such symptoms as back pain.

- The flow void of the cerebrospinal fluid should not be mistaken for a disease process such as an arteriovenous malformation.

Diagnosis

Multiple end plate herniations of the intervertebral discs, called Schmorl's node deformities.

Differential Diagnosis

- end plate herniations

Discussion

These curvilinear defects in the vertebral end plates are secondary to herniation of the intervertebral disc into the vertebral body. The disc herniates directly into the vertebral end plate rather than posteriorly into the vertebral canal through a tear in the annulus fibrosus. The appearance is very typical of a Schmorl's node deformity. Enhancement has been reported in association with these Schmorl's nodes.

The curvilinear areas of decreased signal intensity seen dorsal to the spinal cord in Figure A are areas of flow void secondary to moving cerebrospinal fluid.

MISCELLANEOUS

Case 28

Clinical Presentation

The patient is a 37-year-old male with a history of sudden onset of paraplegia that gradually cleared over the following 48 hours.

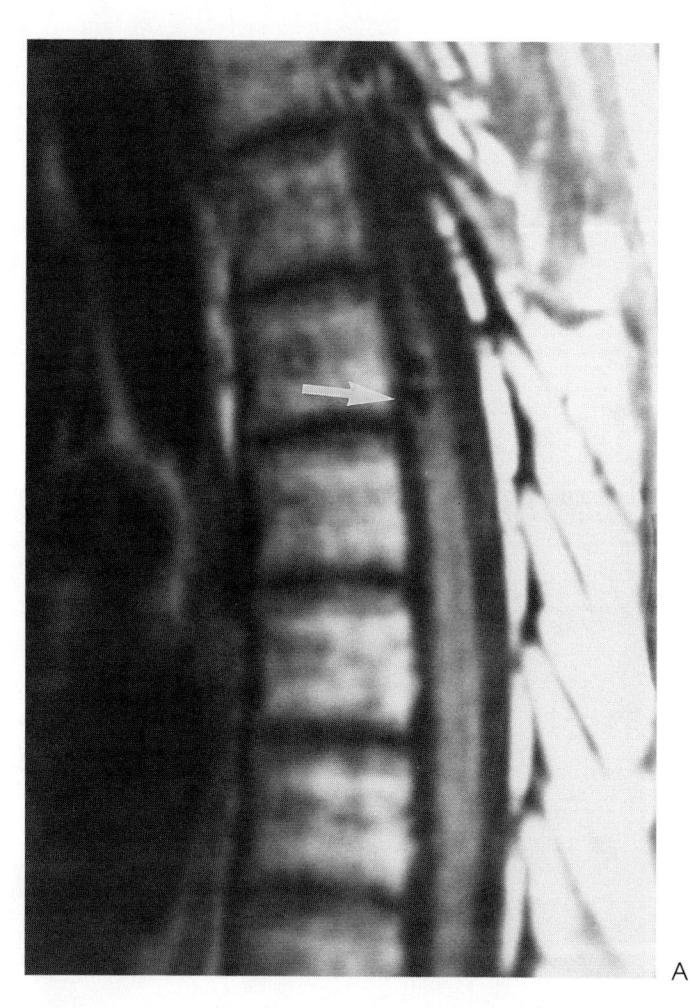

A

Radiologic Findings

Sagittal short TR image (Fig. A) reveals bilobed area of decreased signal intensity in the anterior aspect of the spinal cord in the mid-thoracic region (*arrow*).

TEACHING ATLAS OF SPINE IMAGING

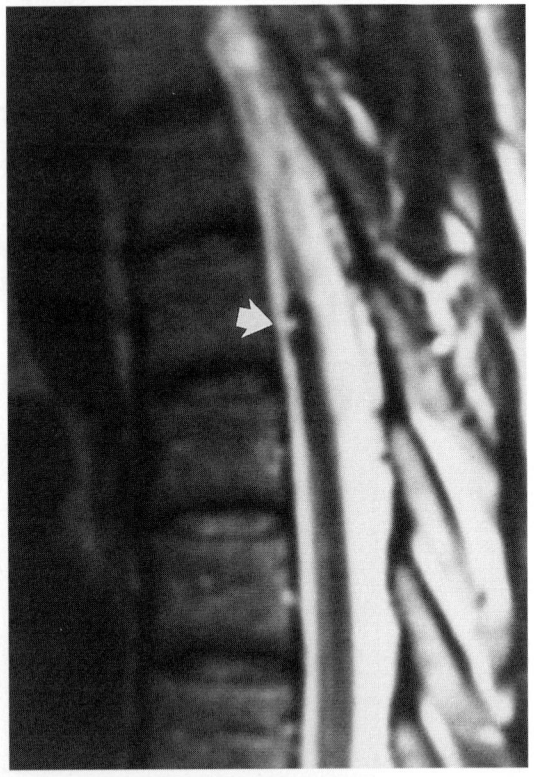

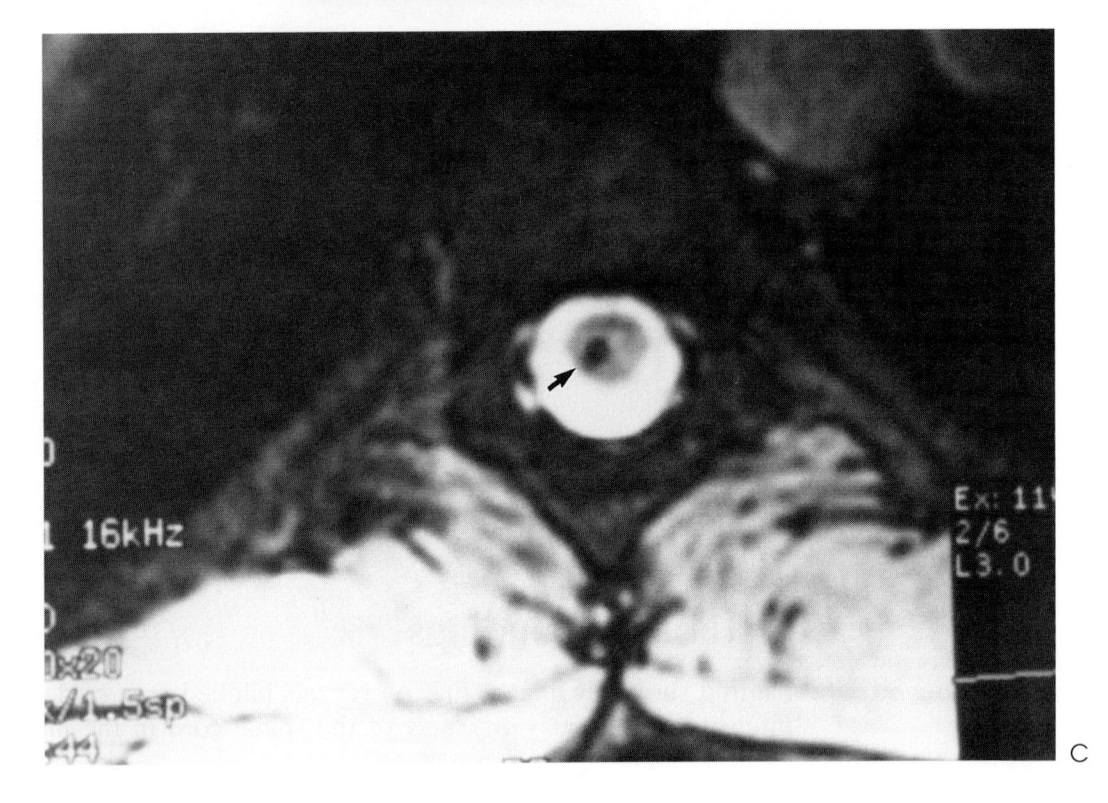

B

C

774

Radiologic Findings (continued)

Sagittal long TR image (Fig. B) reveals that the area of decreased signal intensity in the thoracic spinal cord appears more prominent than on the short TR image (*arrow*).

Axial long TR image (Fig. C) reveals a rounded area of decreased signal intensity in the right, dorsal, and lateral aspect of the spinal cord (*arrow*).

Diagnosis

Cavernous angioma of the spinal cord with hemorrhage.

Differential Diagnosis

- cavernous angioma
- spinal cord ependymoma
- hemorrhagic metastasis

Discussion

The history of acute onset of symptoms is consistent with a catastrophic event such as might occur with a vascular malformation. The areas of decreased signal intensity are consistent with areas of hemosiderin deposition. These areas are more prominent on the long TR images because the long TR images are more susceptible to magnetic susceptibility artifact. The appearance of the areas of hemosiderin deposition seen in association with cavernous angiomas is typically slightly irregularly marginated with a peripheral margin that fades into the normal tissues.

Spinal cord ependymoma may also be associated with areas of hemorrhage; however, in those cases, the hemorrhage is seen within a larger mass that typically shows areas of enhancement. In addition, the areas of hemosiderin deposition are generally amorphous with a better defined rim than that seen in patients with cavernous angiomas. Remote considerations could also include a hemorrhagic metastasis from a primary tumor such as malignant melanoma.

PEARLS

- The appearance is typical of a cavernous angioma. These lesions may be multiple and may also be seen in the brain.

- The clinical presentation is typically progressive with a spinal cord tumor, but onset is typically rapid and is associated with devastating neurologic symptoms in a patient with a cavernous angioma.

PITFALL

- Angiography would not reveal an abnormality in this patient as these lesions are angiographically occult.

Suggested Readings

Abdelaal MA, McGuinness FE, Sagar G. Case report: spinal extradural haematoma in haemophila-A-diagnosis not to be missed. *Clin Radiol.* 1994;49:573–575.

Adriani J, Naragi M. Paraplegia associated with epidural anesthesia. *Southern Med J.* 1986;79:1350–1355.

Boden G. Radiation myelitis of the cervical spinal cord. *Br J Radiol.* 1948;21:464–469.

Brown E, Virapongse C, Gregorios JB. MR imaging of cervical spinal cord infarction. *JCAT.* 1989;13:920–922.

Campi A, Filippi M, Comi G, et al. Acute transverse myelopathy: spinal and cranial MR study with clinical follow-up. *AJNR.* 1995;16:115–123.

Casselman JW, Jolie E, Dahaene I, Meeus L, St.-Jan AZ. Gadolinium-enhanced MR imaging of infarction of the anterior spinal cord. *AJNR.* 1991;12:561.

Castillo M, Carrier DA, Smith JK. Spinal cord infarction after solitary rib fracture. *Emergency Radiol.* 1995;2:105.

Chen CJ, Fang W, Chen CM, Nan YL. Spontaneous spinal epidural hematomas with repeated remission and relapse. *Neuroradiol* 1997;39:737–740.

Chen CJ, Ro LS. Central gadolinium enhancement of an acute spontaneous spinal epidural haematoma. *Neuroradiol.* 1996;38:S114–S116.

Choi KH, Lee KS, Chung SO, et al. Idiopathic transverse myelitis: MR characteristics. *AJNR.* 1996;17:1151–1160.

Dibbern DA, Jr, Loevner LA, Lieberman AP, et al. MR of thoracic cord compression caused by epidural extramedullary hematopoiesis in myelodysplastic syndrome. *AJNR.* 1997;18:363–366.

Doppman J. Epidural lipomatosis. *Radiology.* 1989;171:581–582.

Edwards MK, Farlow MR, Stevens JC. Cranial MR in spinal cord MS: diagnosing patients with isolated spinal cord symptoms. *ANJR.* 1986;7:1003–1005.

Fortuna A, Ferrante L, Acqui M, et al. Spinal cord ischemia diagnosed by MRI: case report and review of the literature. *J Neuroradiol.* 1995;22:115–122.

Fowler M, Williams R, Alba J, Byrd C. Extra-adrenal myelolipomas compared with extramedullary hematopoietic tumors. *Am J Surg Pathol.* 1982;6:363–374.

Gouliamos AD, Plataniotis GA, Michalopoulos ES, et al. Case report: magnetic resonance imaging of spinal cord compression in thalassaemia before and after radiation treatment. *Clin Radiol.* 1995;50:504–505.

Grossman RI, Gonzalez-Scarano F, Atlas SW, Faletta S, Silberberg DH. Multiple sclerosis: gadolinium enhancement in MR imaging. *Radiology.* 1986;161:721–725.

Hittmair K, Mallek R, Prayer D, et al. Spinal cord lesions in patients with multiple sclerosis: comparison of MR pulse sequences. *AJNR.* 1996;17:1555–1565.

Holtas S, Basibuyuk N, Fredriksson K. MRI in acute transverse myelopathy. *Neuroradiol.* 1993;35:221–226.

Holtas S, Heiling M, Lönntoft M. Spontaneous spinal epidural hematoma: findings at MR imaging and cinical correlation. *Radiology.* 1996;199:409–413.

Honig LS, Sheremata WA. Magnetic resonance imaging of spinal cord lesions in multiple sclerosis. *J Neurol Neurosurg Psychiatry.* 1989;52:459–466.

Johnson CE, Sze G. Benign lumbar arachnoiditis: MR imaging with gadopentetate dimeglumine. *AJNR.* 1990;11:763–770.

Kader S, Kalisher L, Schiller A. Extramedullary hematopoiesis in Paget's disease of bone. *AJR.* 1977;129:493–495.

Kornreich L, Dagan O, Grunebaum M. MRI in acute poliomyelitis. *Neuroradiol.* 1996;38:371–372.

Krag D, Reich S. Heterotopic bone marrow (myelolipoma) of the mediastinum. *Chest.* 1972;61:514–515.

Lau SK, Chan CK, Chow YY. Cord compression due to extramedullary hematopoiesis in a patient with thalassemia. *Spine.* 1994;19:2467–2470.

Liou RJ, Chen CY, Choul TY, et al. Hypoxic-ischaemic injury of the spinal cord in systemic shock: MRI. *Neuroradiol.* 1996;38:S181–S183.

Luyendijk W, et al. Spinal cord compression due to extramedullary hematopoiesis in homozygous thalassemia. *J Neurosurg.* 1975;42:212–216.

Lycklama à Nijeholt GJ, Barkhof F, Castelijns JA, et al. Comparison of two MR sequences for the detection of multiple sclerosis lesions in the spinal cord. *AJNR.* 1996;17:1533–1538.

Lycklama à Nijeholt GJ, Barkhof F, Scheltens P, et al. MR of the spinal cord in multiple sclerosis: relation to clinical subtype and disability. *AJNR.* 1997;18:1041–1048.

Mann KS, Yue CP, Chen KH, et al. Paraplegia due to extramedullary hematopoiesis in thalassemia. *J Neurosurg.* 1987;66:938–940.

Maravilla KR, Weinreb JC, Suss R, Nunnally RL. Magnetic resonance demonstration of multiple sclerosis plaques in the cervical cord. *AJR.* 1985;144:381–385.

Markus JB, Franchetto AA, Fairbrother J. Magnetic resonance imaging and computed tomography of hyperacute spinal epidural hematoma. *Canad Assoc Radiol J.* 1994;45:391.

Mulder DW, Rosenbaum RA, Layton DD. Late progression of poliomyelitis or forme fruste amytrophic lateral sclerosis? *Mayo Clin Proc.* 1972;47:756–761.

Papavasiliou C, Gouliamos A, Vlahos L, et al. CT and MRI of symptomatic spinal involvement by extramedullary hematopoiesis. *Clin Radiol.* 1990;42:91–92.

Suh DC, Kim SJ, Jung SM, et al. MRI in presumed cervical anterior spinal artery territory infarcts. *Neuroradiol.* 1996;38:56–58.

Sze G, Kawamura Y, Negishi C, et al. Fast spin-echo MR imaging of the cervical spine: influence of echo train length and echo spacing on image contrast and quality. *AJNR.* 1993;14:1203–1213.

Tartaglino LM, Croul SE, Flanders AE, et al. Idiopathic acute transverse myelitis: MR imaging findings. *Radiology.* 1996;201:661–669.

Tartagliano LM, Friedman DP, Flanders AE, Lublin FD, Knobler RL, Leim M. Multiple sclerosis in the spinal cord: MR appearance and correlation with clinical parameters. *Radiology.* 1995;195:725–732.

Tartaglino LM, Heiman-Patterson T, Friedman DP, et al. Multiple sclerosis in the spinal cord: MR appearance and correlation with clinical parameters. *Radiology.* 1995;195:725–732.

Tartaglino LM, Heiman-Patterson T, Friedman DP, et al. MR imaging in a case of postvaccination myelitis. *AJNR.* 1995;16:581–582.

Thielen KR, Miller GM. Multiple sclerosis of the spinal cord: magnetic resonance appearance. *JCAT.* 1996;20:434–438.

Thorpe JW, Kidd D, Moseley IF, et al. Serial gadolinium-enhanced MRI of the brain and spinal cord in early relapsing-remitting multiple sclerosis. *Neurology.* 1996;46:373–378.

Weinstock-Guttman B, Ross JS, Ransohoff RM. Unusual long-standing Gd-DPTA enhancement in a chronic progressive myelopathy. *JCAT.* 1995;19:649–651.

Wiebe S, Lee DH, Karlik SJ, et al. Serial cranial and spinal cord magnetic resonance imaging in multiple sclerosis. *Ann Neurol.* 1992;32:643–650.

Yuh WTC, Marsh EE, Wang AK, et al. MR of spinal cord and vertebral body infarction. *AJNR.* 1992;13:145–154.

TEACHING ATLAS OF SPINE IMAGING

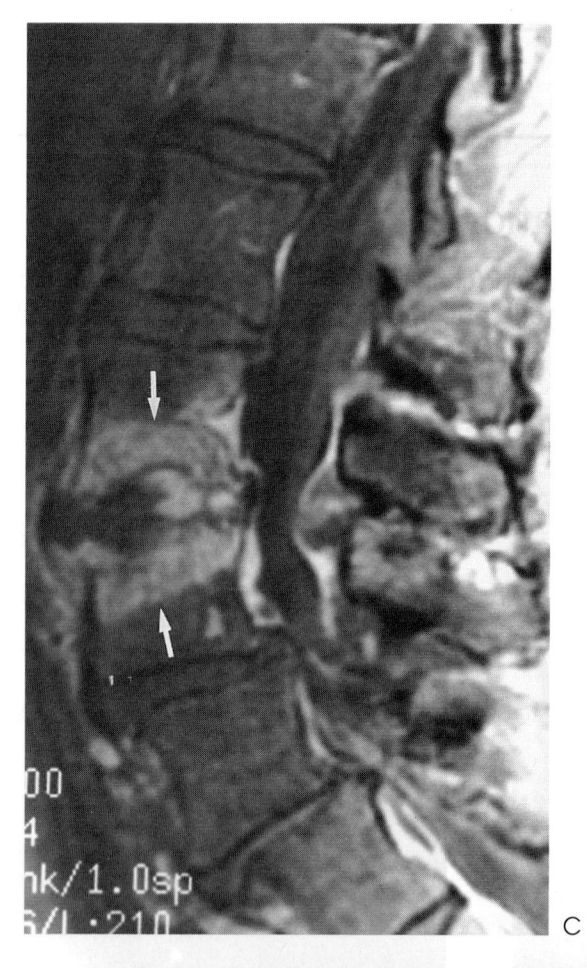

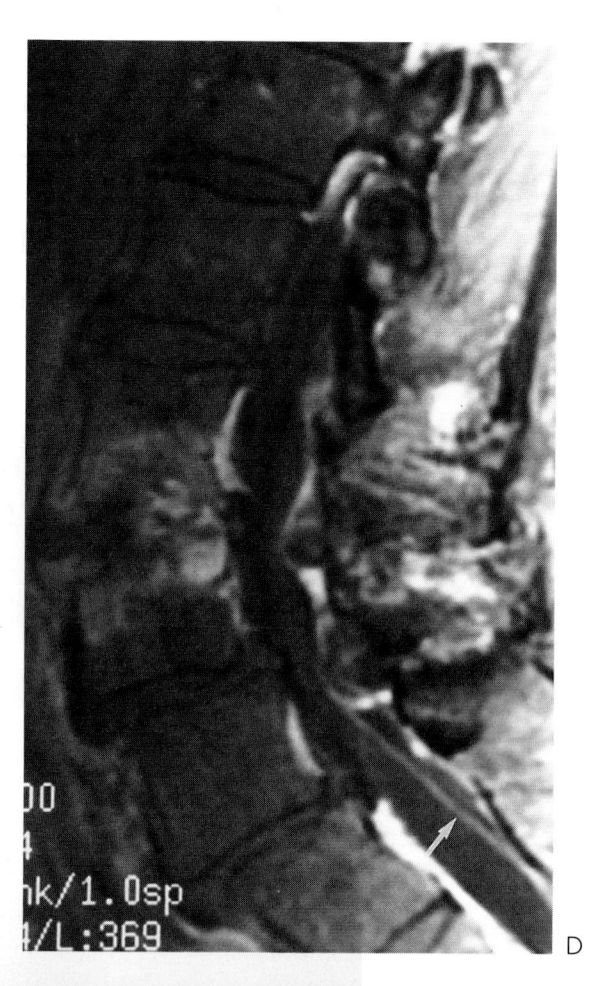

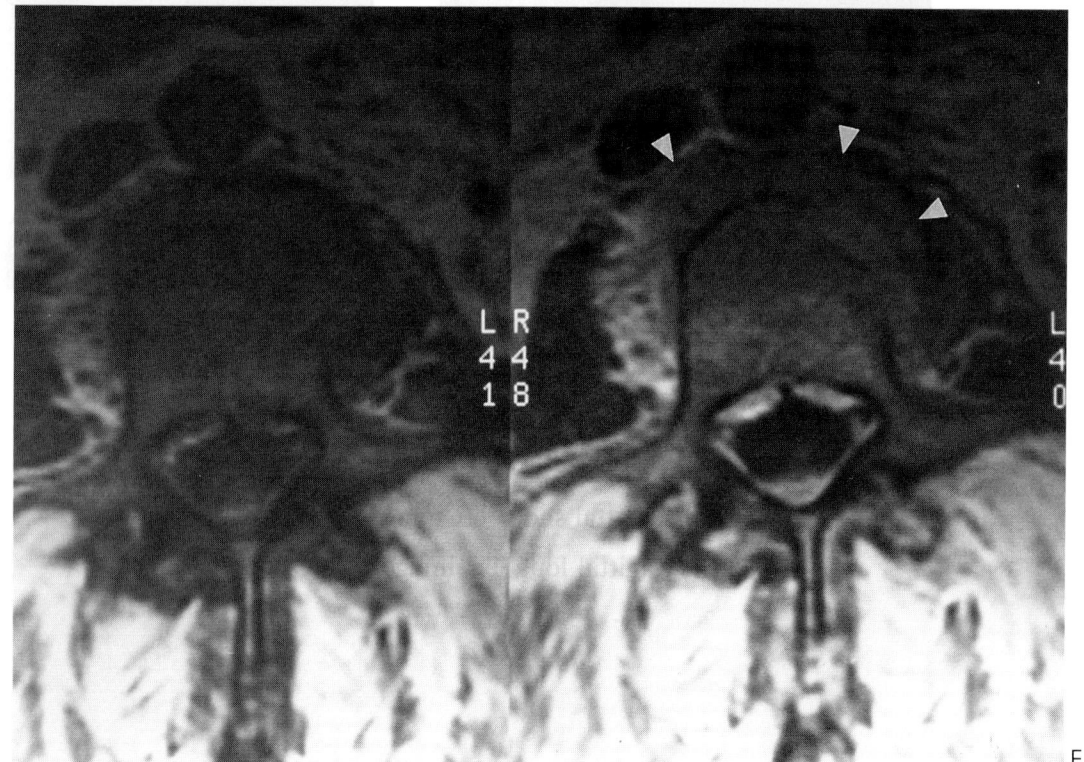

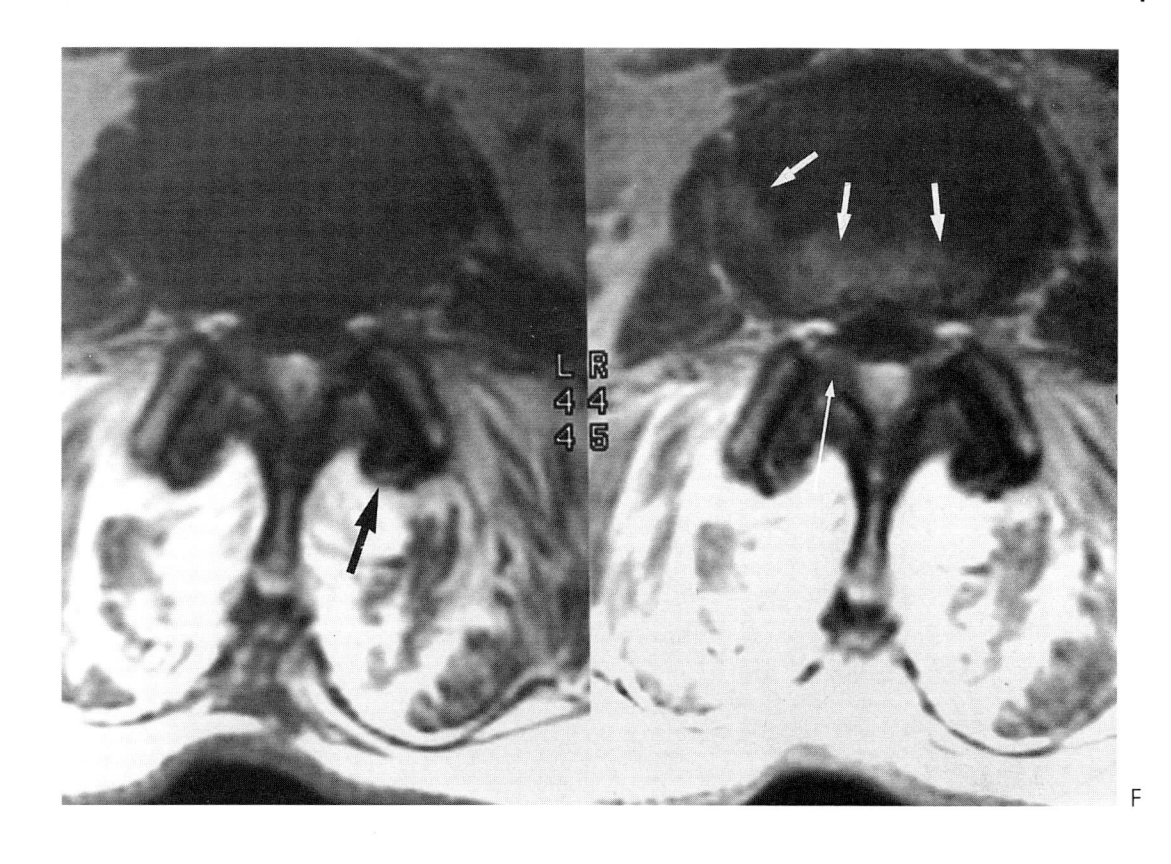

Radiologic Findings (continued)

(Fig. C) Sagittal short TR images postcontrast.

(Fig. D) Axial short TR image postcontrast at the L3 vertebral body level.

(Fig. E) Axial short TR images pre- (*left*) and postcontrast (*right*) at the level of the L3 vertebral body.

(Fig. F) Axial short TR images pre- (*left*) and postcontrast (*right*) at the intervertebral disc level of L3-4.

Diagnosis

Discitis with vertebral osteomyelitis at the L3-4 level and severe spinal stenosis.

Differential Diagnosis

- discitis
- degenerative changes
- metastatic disease

PEARLS

- In an older patient with spondylolisthesis, it is unlikely that the slippage is secondary to a spondylolysis, but rather is more likely secondary to interfacet degenerative changes. These interfacet degenerative changes often result in secondary loss of intervertebral disc height. Hypertrophy of the ligamentum flavum then results and consequently spinal stenosis.

- For confirmation of the diagnosis, a CT-guided biopsy is helpful.

PITFALLS

- A CT-guided biopsy may successfully yield a diagnosis of an inflammatory process; however, an organism may not be identified because these patients are frequently treated with antibiotics prior to the aspiration. However, the biopsy will identify inflammatory cells and rule out the presence of malignant cells.

- If contrast material had not been used in this patient, it might have been assumed that the loss of disc height was secondary to degenerative changes and not because of a discitis. The increased signal intensity within the disc is typical of an infected disc, but not typical of degenerative changes where, because of loss of hydration, the disc is generally decreased signal intensity on the long TR images.

Discussion

The sagittal short TR image (Fig. A) prior to the infusion of contrast material reveals that the intervertebral disc at the L3-4 level is indistinct and there is low signal intensity involving the lower half of L3 and upper half of L4 secondary to edema. There is also an anterolisthesis of L3 on L4 and L4 on L5. Increased signal intensity of the intervertebral disc is apparent at the L3-4 level. This appearance is typical of the changes seen in patients with discitis. There is dense enhancement of the intervertebral disc and adjacent vertebral bodies on the postinfusion studies (Figs. C to F). The arrows in Figure C define the limit of the area of enhancement. There is also enhancement of one of the nerve roots of the cauda equina as seen in Figure D (*arrow*). This enhancement represents an irritation of the nerve root because of a type of neuritis.

In Figure E, the anterior soft tissue component is seen to enhance (*right, arrowheads*). There is also a scalloped area of enhancement in the anterior epidural space behind the vertebral body of L3 which encroaches upon the thecal sac. This can also be seen in Figures C and D. In Figure F, the enhancement of the posterior portion of the intervertebral disc can be seen (*right, short white arrows*); the hypertrophied ligamentum flavum can also be seen (*right, long white arrow*). There are interfacet degenerative changes with cupping of one facet around another (*left, black arrow*).

The hypertrophied ligamentum flavum can be identified at the lowest three intervertebral disc levels as curvilinear areas of decreased signal intensity in Figure B. The curved arrow identifies the ligamentum flavum at the L3-4 level.

The involvement of the intervertebral disc and the two adjacent vertebral bodies is typical of a discitis. The decreased signal intensity and the enhancement reflect the fact that there is also involvement of the vertebral bodies with osteomyelitis. This can be confirmed with a CT-guided needle aspiration of the intervertebral disc space; this also may allow the identification of the organism that is causing the discitis. Thus, the appropriate antibiotic may be instituted.

There is multilevel spondylolisthesis in this patient secondary to multilevel interfacet degenerative changes. These interfacet degenerative changes result in forward slipping of one vertebra on the next with consequent "hypertrophy" of the ligamentum flavum. Hypertrophy is actually a misnomer, as the enlargement of the ligamentum flavum is secondary to the lack of traction and resulting stretching thinning of the normal ligamentum flavum.

Without the infusion of contrast material and the resulting enhancement, it is possible that the marked disc space narrowing and low signal intensity of the adjacent vertebral bodies could be secondary to degenerative changes. Therefore, if there is doubt regarding the diagnosis or if the patient has an elevated erythrocyte sedimentation rate or other signs of an inflammatory process, a postcontrast study is imperative.

Metastatic disease usually does not involve the intervertebral disc space, and therefore, metastases is not a likely diagnostic consideration in this patient.

UNKNOWNS

Case 2

Clinical Presentation

The patient is a 47-year-old female with paralysis of the extremities.

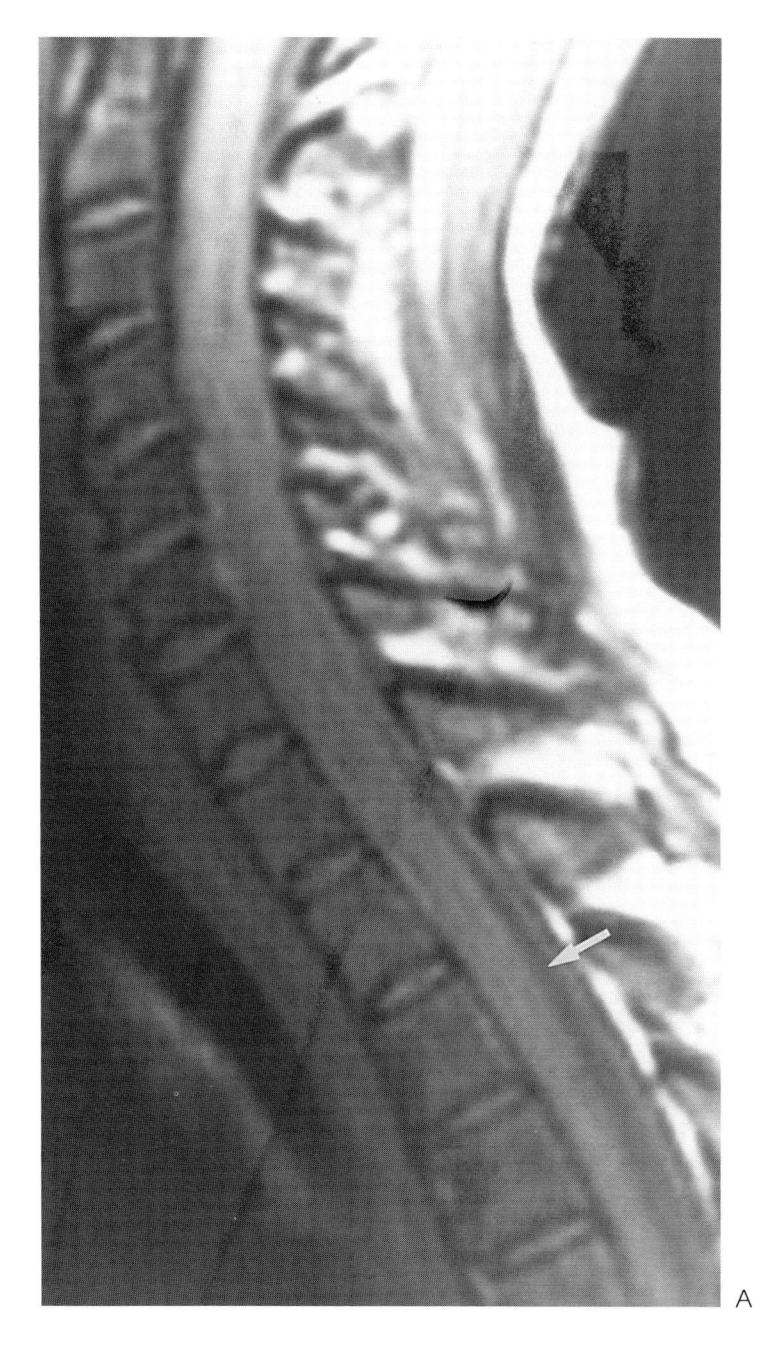

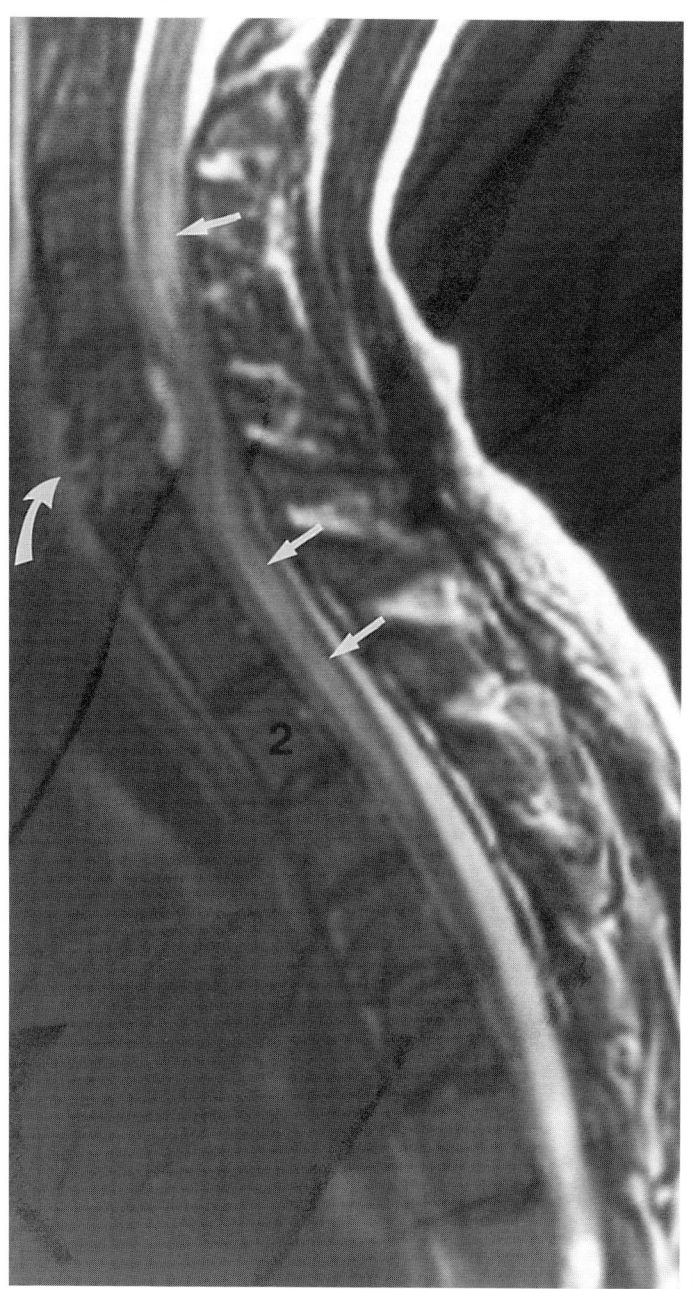

A

B

Radiologic Findings

(Fig. A) Sagittal intermediate signal intensity image of the cervical spine.
(Fig. B) Sagittal long TR image of the cervical spine.

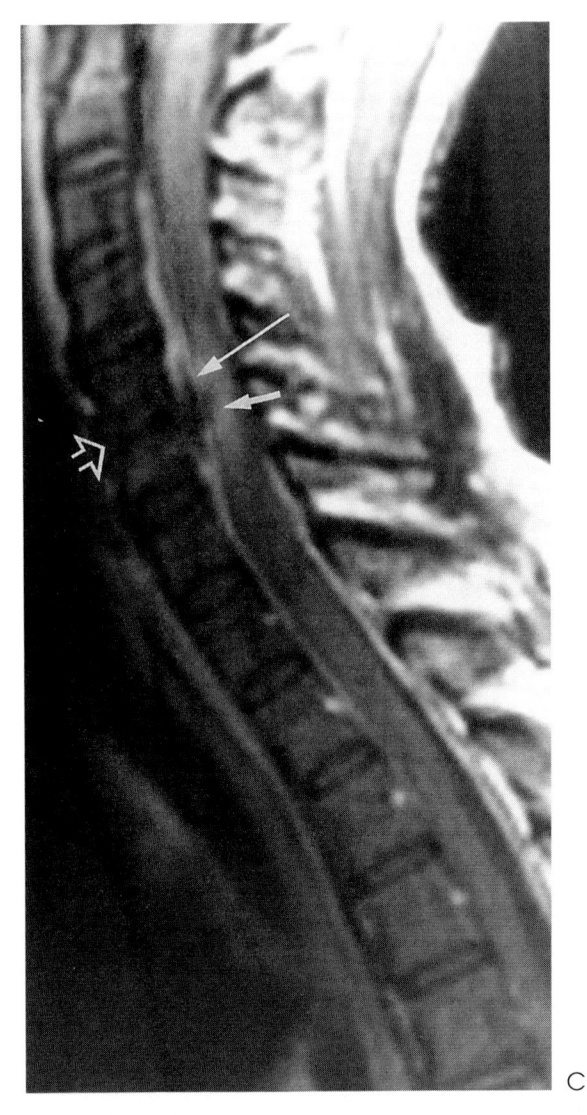

TEACHING ATLAS OF SPINE IMAGING

C

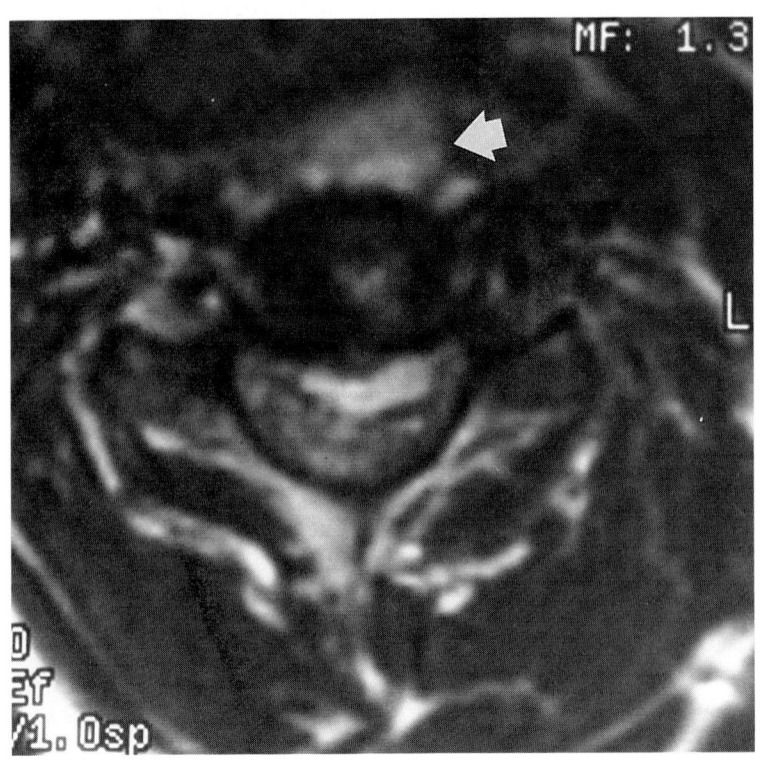

D

786

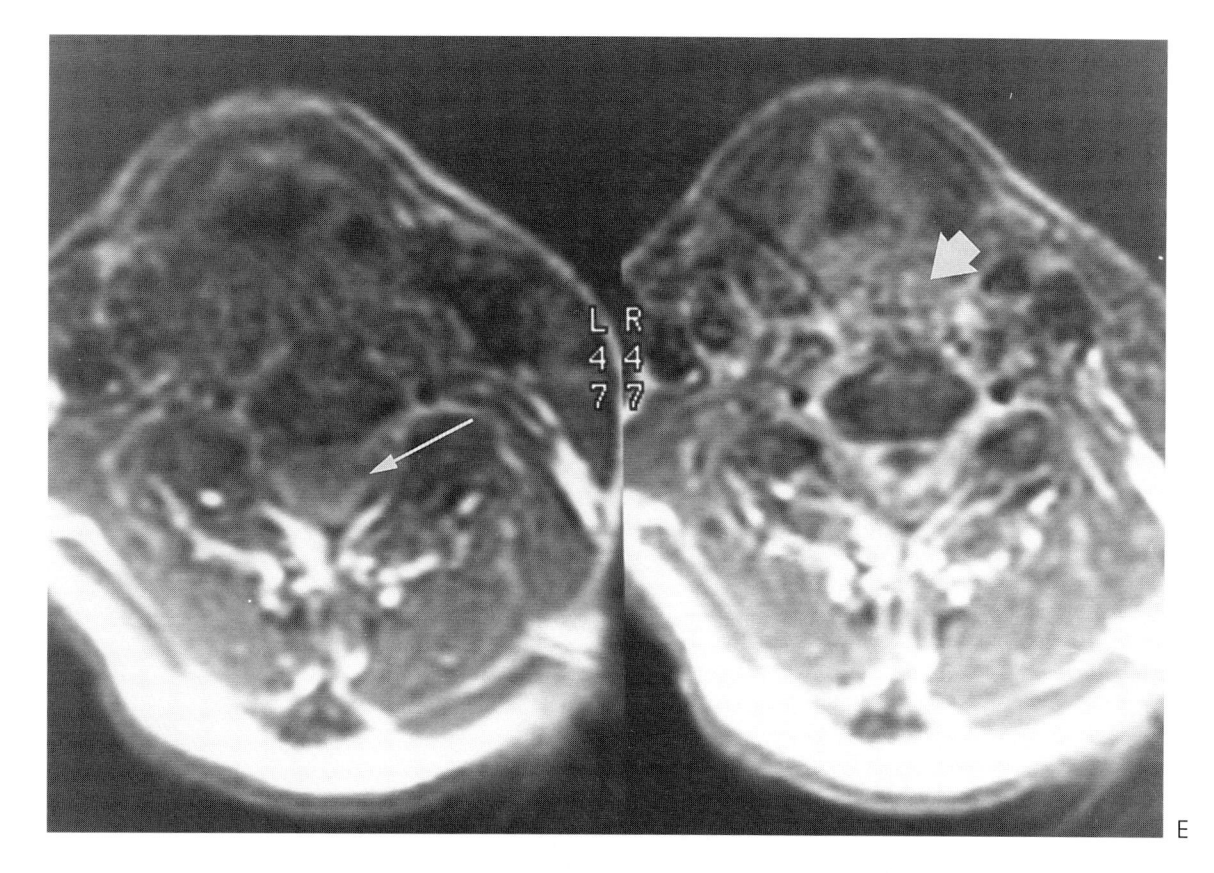

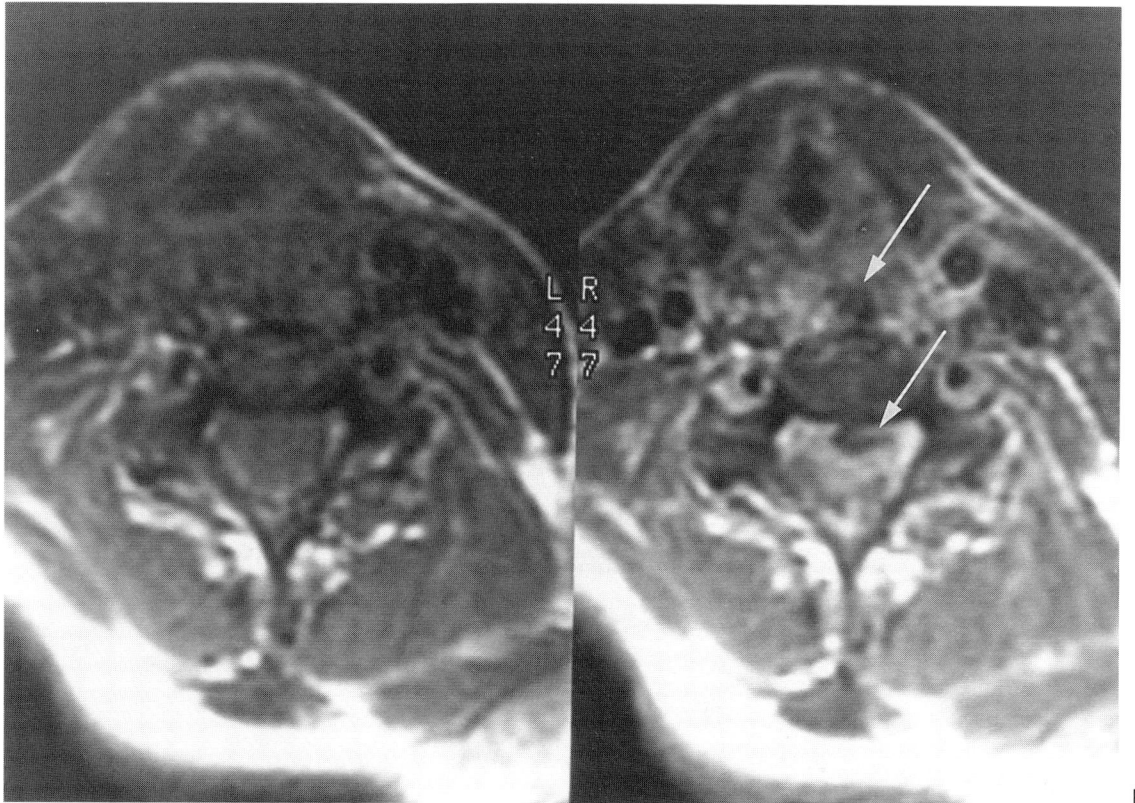

UNKNOWNS

E

F

Radiologic Findings (continued)

(Fig. C) Sagittal short TR image postcontrast.

(Fig. D) Axial long TR image.

(Fig. E) Pre- (*left*) and postcontrast (*right*) axial short TR image.

(Fig. F) Pre- (*left*) and postcontrast (*right*) axial short TR image.

Diagnosis

Epidural and prevertebral abscess.

Differential Diagnosis

- epidural and prevertebral abscess
- herniated disc

Discussion

The intermediate TR image (Fig. A) reveals slight disc space narrowing at the C4-5, C5-6, and C6-7 levels. There is also anterior disc prominence at both of these levels. The spinal cord is edematous and reveals a long area of increased signal intensity above and below the lesion (*straight white arrows* in Fig. B). The subarachnoid space is obliterated throughout the length of the cervical canal. The spinal cord is visible as distinct from the subarachnoid space in the upper thoracic region (*arrow*).

The long TR image (Fig. B) reveals a semilunar area of increased signal intensity posterior to the intervertebral disc at the C5-6 level. There is a concentric rim of decreased signal intensity surrounding this area and a semilunar area of increased signal intensity anterior to the disc at the C5-6 level (*curved arrow*). There is also a very long area of increased signal intensity within the spinal cord that extends superiorly to the level of C2 and inferiorly to the level of T3. The T2 vertebral body is identified with 2.

Postinfusion (Fig. C) there is an elongated oval-shaped area of enhancement posterior to the vertebral bodies at the C5-6 level (*short solid arrow*). The central area of decreased signal intensity (*long solid arrow*) is the abscess cavity and is secondary to pus and necrotic debris. The vertebral body endplates are indistinct at the C5-6 level (*open arrow*).

The long TR image in the axial plane (Fig. D) reveals similar findings with an area of increased signal intensity in the prevertebral space that extends into the vertebral canal posterior to the vertebral body. This area compresses the spinal cord posteriorly. There is also an oval-shaped abscess in the prevertebral space (*white arrow*).

The axial images reveal similar changes. In Figure E, the absence of the normal decreased signal intensity surrounding the thecal sac is also noted (*left, arrow*). There is enhancement in the prevertebral space (*right, arrow*). There is also peripheral enhancement surrounding an area of decreased

PEARLS
- Additional history in this patient revealed that there was a history of intravenous drug abuse.

- Spinal abscesses may also be seen in patients who are diabetic, immunosuppressed, or have autoimmunodeficiency syndrome (AIDS). In the AIDS patient, infection may occur with *Mycobacterium avium intracellularae*. An abscess may also be seen in any patient who has a septicemia from any source, such as bacterial endocarditis.

PITFALL
- A tumor such as a meningioma might be a remote consideration, but is less likely than an inflammatory process.

signal intensity anterior to the spinal cord similar to that seen in Figure C. The spinal cord is markedly compressed and displaced posteriorly.

In Figure F, the precontrast study (*left*) again reveals obliteration of the subarachnoid space, while the postcontrast study (*right*) reveals the decreased central portion of the abscess cavity (*lower arrow*) within the vertebral canal. There is also a decreased signal intensity cavity seen anterior to the vertebral body (*anterior arrow*).

Herniated disc is unlikely because the pattern of enhancement is typical of an abscess.

Radiologic Findings

(Figs. A and B) Pre- (*left*) and postcontrast (*right*) sagittal images of the lumbar spine. The L4 vertebral body is identified with 4 (Fig. A).

Diagnosis

Neurofibromatosis type 2 (NF2) with multiple schwannomas.

Differential Diagnosis

- NF2 with multiple schwannomas
- multiple metastases
- inflammatory process

Discussion

Additional history in this patient is the fact that she had a history of NF2. The slightly thickened nerve roots of the cauda equina can be seen in the lumbar thecal sac (Fig. A, *left, arrow*). There are multiple rounded and oval-shaped areas of enhancement which arise from the distal spinal cord and the nerve roots of the cauda equina (Figs. A and B, *right, white and black arrows*).

Also present is disc space narrowing at the L5-S1 level with areas of increased signal intensity involving the adjacent vertebral bodies. There is also a slight retrolisthesis of L5 on S1.

Incidentally, there is moderately severe disc space narrowing at the L4-5 intervertebral disc level. There is increased signal intensity of the vertebral marrow of the adjacent vertebral bodies because the marrow changes from red to "white" marrow. The white marrow contains an increased amount of adipose tissue and so appears as increased signal intensity. A herniated disc at the L4-5 level projects posteriorly into the vertebral canal.

Multiple metastases with "drop" metastases is a strong diagnostic consideration in this patient. Primary tumors of the central nervous system which develop drop metastases include pinealoma or glioblastoma in an adult, and medulloblastoma, ependymoma, or pinealoma in a child; primary tumors outside of the central nervous system include lung cancer, breast cancer, melanoma, and lymphoma. An inflammatory process is a possibility but unlikely, as these patients are very ill and typically have severe back pain.

PEARLS

- The clinical history is vital in this patient.

- An excellent method for remembering the abnormalities associated with NF2 is to use the mnemonic MISME: Multiple–Inherited–Schwannomas–Meningiomas–Ependymomas (spinal cord). (Attributed to James Smiriniotopoulus, M.D.)

- Correlation should be made with analysis of cerebrospinal fluid for more complete evaluation and to rule out the presence of malignant cells.

PITFALL

- An initial discovery of multiple schwannomas is highly unusual in a patient of 47 years of age. It should be noted that patients with neurofibromatosis may not have the typical clinical stigmata.

UNKNOWNS

Case 5

Clinical Presentation

The patient is a 48-year-old female with diffuse spine pain.

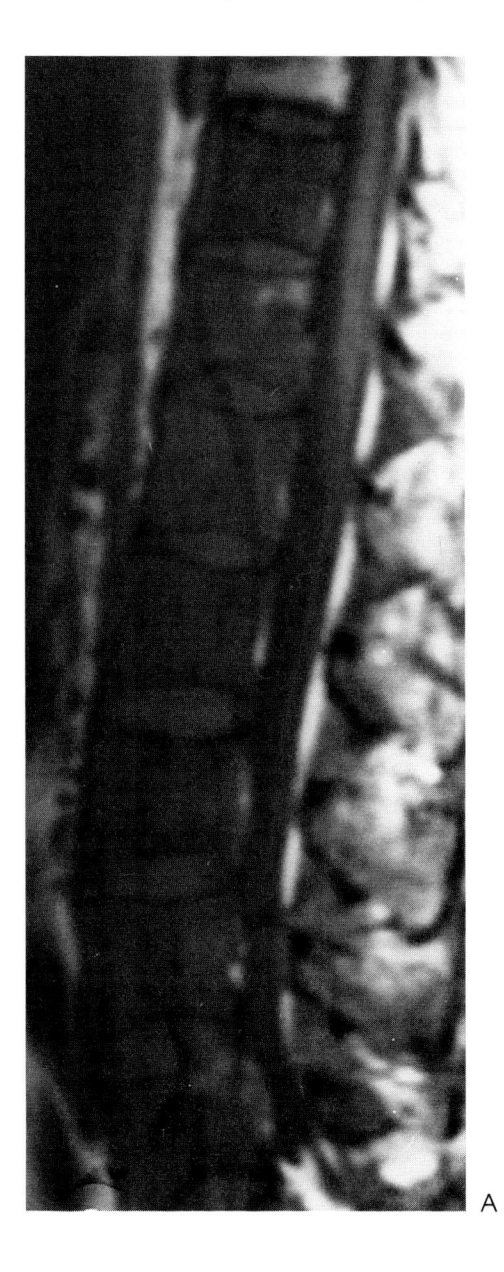

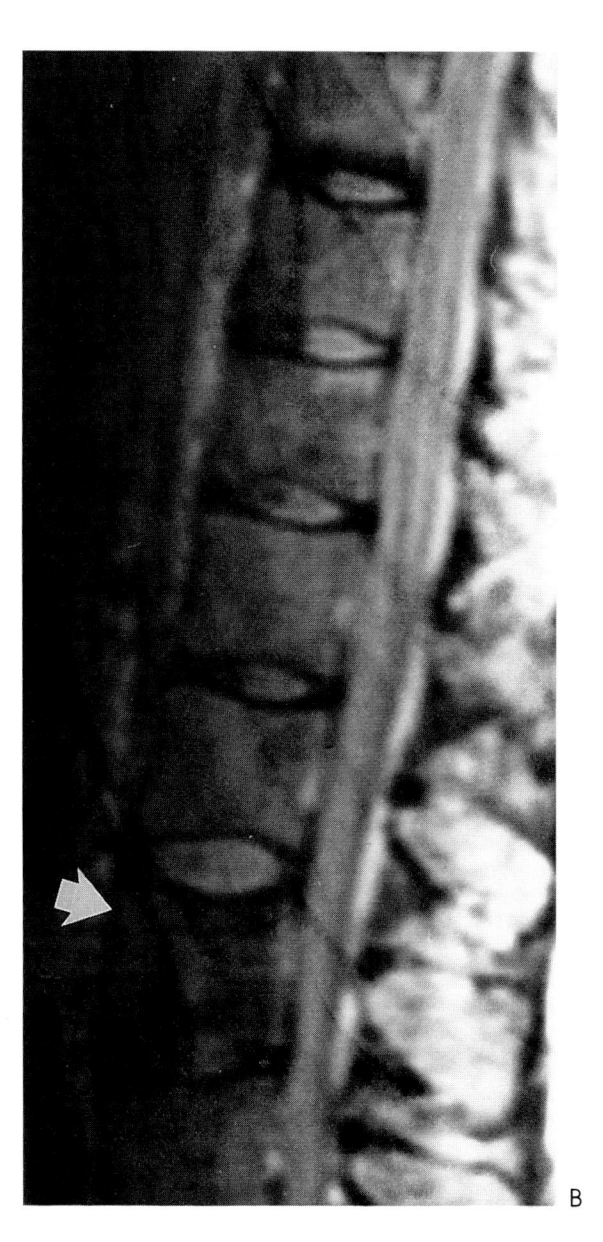

Radiologic Findings

(Fig. A) Sagittal short TR image of the lumbar spine.
(Fig. B) Sagittal long TR image of the lumber spine.

TEACHING ATLAS OF SPINE IMAGING

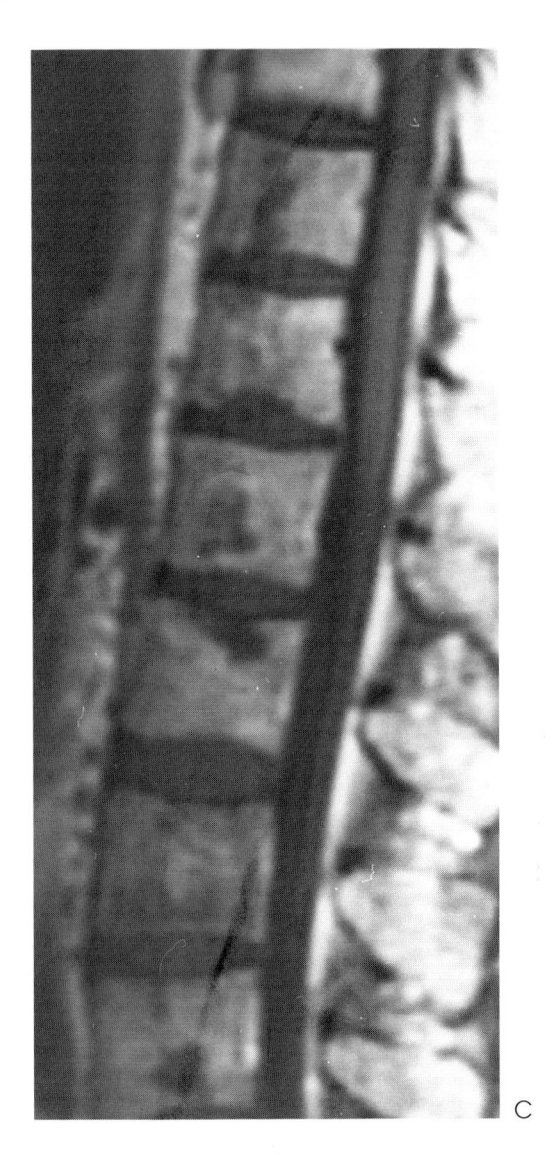

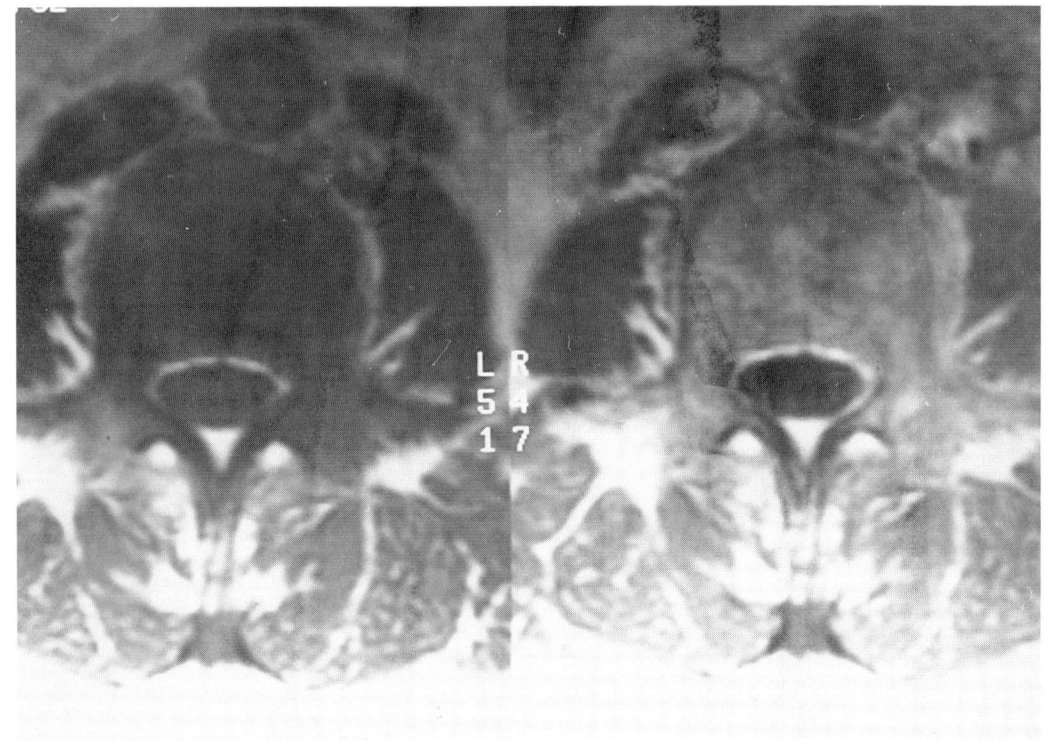

C

D

UNKNOWNS

Radiologic Findings (continued)

(Fig. C) Sagittal short TR image postcontrast enhancement.

(Fig. D) Pre- (*left*) and postcontrast (*right*) axial short TR images at the level of L3.

Diagnosis

Diffuse osteolytic and osteoblastic metastases involving all the visualized bony structures.

Differential Diagnosis

- metastases
- multiple myeloma
- sickle cell disease
- myelofibrosis

Discussion

The sagittal short TR image (Fig. A) reveals the "disc reversal" sign with the intervertebral disc appearing higher in signal intensity than the marrow in the vertebral body. This reflects the diffuse replacement of the normally high signal intensity fat-filled marrow with decreased signal intensity metastatic disease. The long TR image (Fig. B) reveals only faint areas of decreased signal intensity within the marrow of the vertebral bodies. The vertebral body of L3 (*arrow*) is slightly expanded.

The postcontrast sagittal image (Fig. C) reveals diffuse enhancement of the majority of the marrow with multiple patchy areas of irregularly marginated decreased signal intensity throughout multiple vertebral bodies. The axial short TR image (Fig. D) reveals diffuse decreased signal intensity preinfusion (*left*) and diffuse homogeneous enhancement postcontrast (*right*). Note that there is a circumferential rim of enhancement that surrounds the vertebral body and that the vertebral pedicles are decreased signal intensity preinfusion.

The spinous processes are mottled signal intensity in Figure A secondary to diffuse involvement with metastatic disease.

Care must be taken when evaluating a patient with diffuse homogeneous changes in the vertebral bodies. The scan in Figure A appears normal except for the disc reversal sign. Likewise, the long TR image appears almost normal except for subtle alterations in the marrow signal intensity. The postcontrast image (Fig. C) reveals that the osteolytic metastatic deposits enhance, while the osteoblastic metastatic deposits remain decreased signal intensity. The axial images reveal a thin rim of tumor extending outside

PEARLS

- It may be necessary to correlate these magnetic resonance findings with radionuclide bone scan results.

- For a final diagnosis, it may be necessary to perform a bone biopsy. This can be performed with computed tomographic guidance if necessary. If multiple myeloma is a diagnostic consideration, correlation should be made with results of serum protein electrophoresis.

PITFALL

- In a patient with diffuse bony involvement, a normal appearing vertebral body is not available for comparison. It may occasionally be necessary to perform a coronal image, which includes the femoral bones or ilium with normal bone marrow, so that a comparison can be made with the vertebral column. In addition, when there is a "disc reversal" sign, the vertebral body, which is normally higher in signal intensity than the intervertebral disc because of the fatty bone marrow, becomes lower in signal intensity. Therefore, the intervertebral disc becomes relatively increased signal intensity, and a "reversal" of the normal relationship between the two structures is seen.

of the vertebral body. Involvement of the vertebral pedicle is typical of metastatic disease.

A diffuse marrow process such as multiple myeloma could have a similar appearance, as could entities such as sickle cell disease with or without bone infarcts. Myelofibrosis is also a diagnostic consideration. However, the clinical presentation is generally very helpful in ruling in or out these various diagnostic considerations.

UNKNOWNS

Case 6

Clinical Presentation

The patient is an 81-year-old male who presented to the emergency room because he was unable to walk.

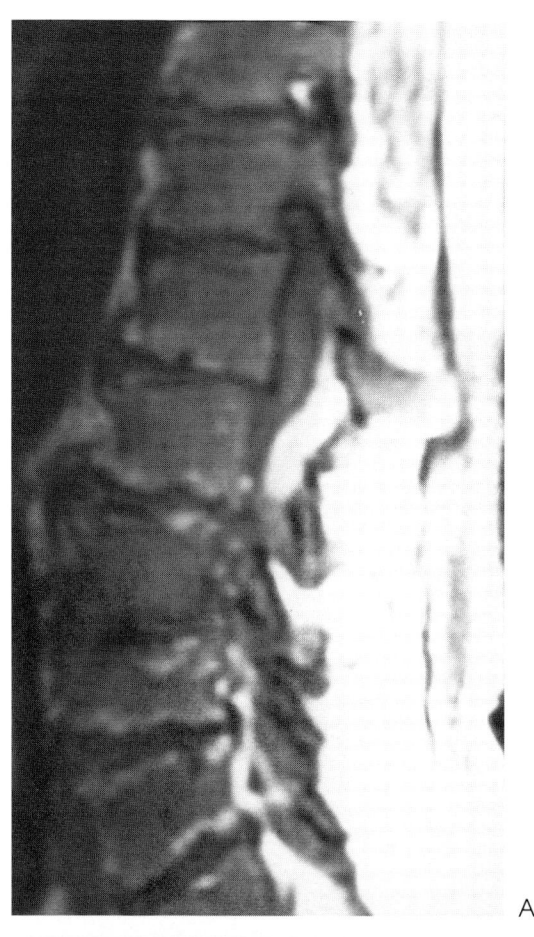

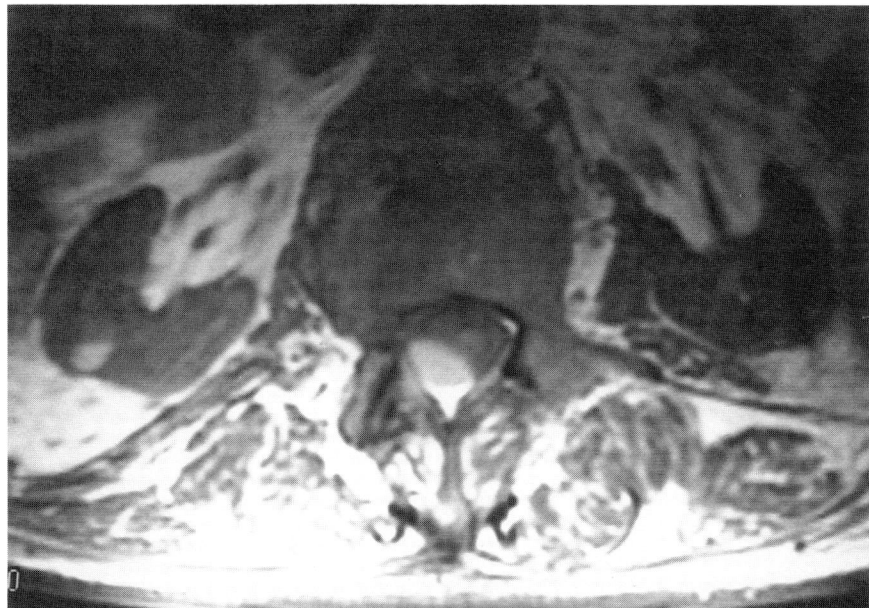

A

B

TEACHING ATLAS OF SPINE IMAGING

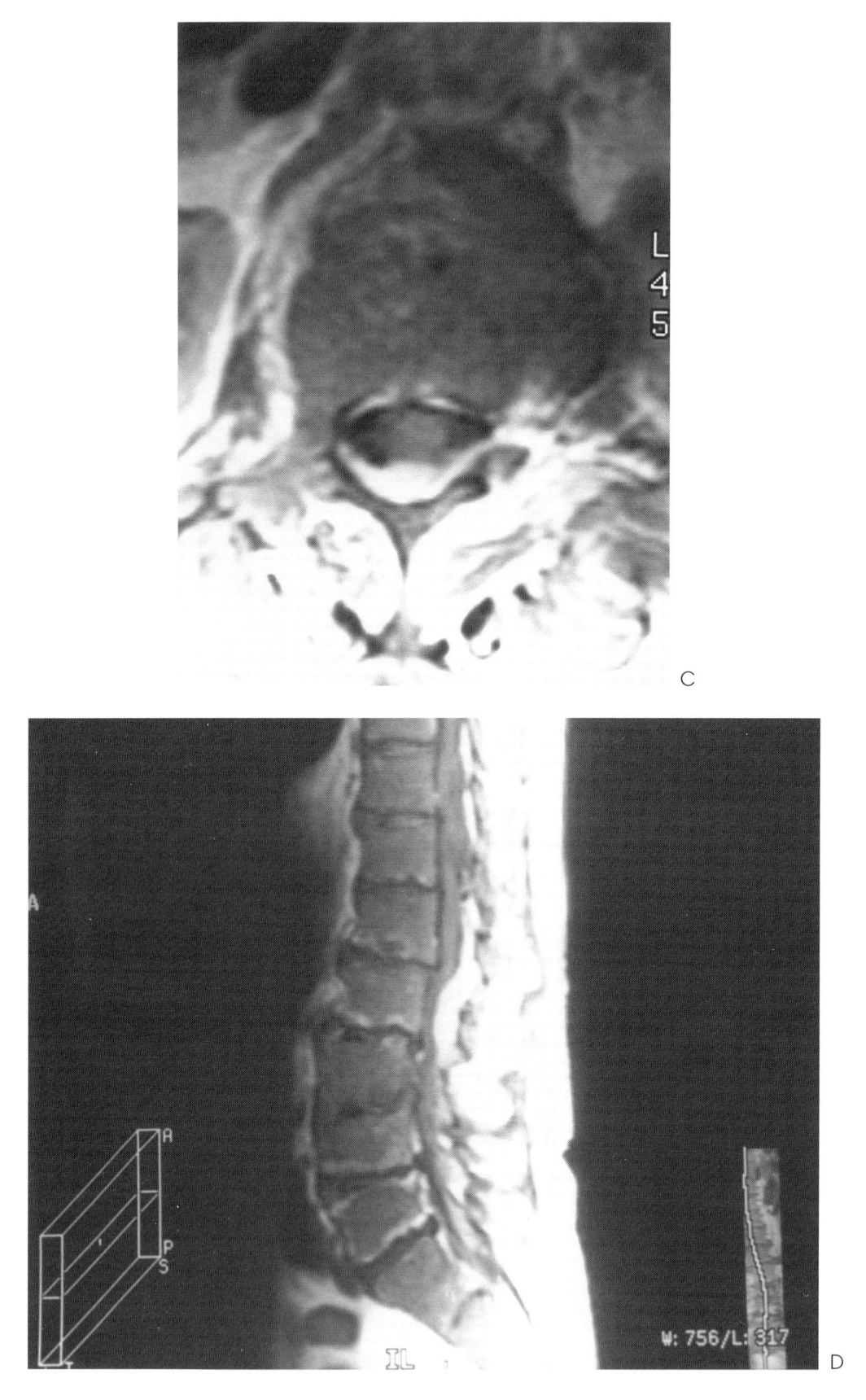

Radiologic Findings

(Fig. A) Sagittal short TR image of the lumbar spine.
(Fig. B) Axial short TR image of the lumbar spine.

(Fig. C) Axial short TR image of the spine.
(Fig. D) Sagittal short TR image of the spine after reformatting utilizing the spine straightening technique.

Diagnosis

Epidural hematoma, cause unknown.

Differential Diagnosis

- epidural hematoma
- lipoma
- chloroma
- posttraumatic hematoma

Discussion

An elongated area of increased signal intensity is dorsal to the thecal sac in the lumbar region extending from the level of L1 through the midbody of L3. The signal intensity is increased and is consistent with the presence of an area of subacute hematoma formation. A second area of intermediate signal intensity is superior to the area of increased signal intensity that extends from the level of the superior end plate of T11 through the inferior end plate of T12. The normal low signal intensity of the subarachnoid space is obliterated, and there is compression of the spinal cord from the level of the superior end plate of T11 through the midbody of L3. At surgery, these represented areas of hemorrhage. The more superior area is acute hemorrhage while the more inferior, increased signal intensity area is secondary to subacute hemorrhage.

The axial images (Figs. B and C) reveal a lentiform area of increased signal intensity dorsal to the thecal sac which compresses the thecal sac and the spinal cord. In Figure C, the area of increased signal intensity appears more crescentic in appearance. The image with straightening of the spine (Fig. D) reveals that the hematoma is actually larger than is apparent in the unstraightened sagittal image (Fig. A).

A large anterior osteophyte at the L2-3 level is seen on the sagittal images and also projects anteriorly and toward the left side on the axial image in Figure C.

Magnetic resonance imaging (MRI) is the procedure of choice for evaluation of the abnormality in this case because it rapidly and noninvasively identifies both the abnormality and the anatomic location of the lesion.

Although lipoma is a diagnostic consideration, the location is very uncommon in an older individual.

A focal area of accumulation of leukemic cells is a remote possibility.

A posttraumatic hematoma is also a consideration, and history should be obtained regarding the possibility of a spinal tap or steroid injection resulting in hematoma formation.

PEARLS

- The spine-straightening technique was helpful in this case to more accurately define the extent of the accumulation.

- The cause of bleeding in this patient must be determined. It is possible that the patient is medicated with anticoagulants or has a blood dyscrasia which results in abnormal areas of hemorrhage.

- MR is the procedure of choice for evaluation and should be obtained as an emergency. Emergent surgical evacuation of the hematoma is probably indicated in a case such as this.

PITFALL

- Computed tomographic (CT) scanning or myelography with the use of postmyelographic CT would not provide an accurate diagnosis of the abnormality in this case.

TEACHING ATLAS OF SPINE IMAGING

Case 7

Clinical Presentation

The patient is a 65-year-old male with a history of many years of low back pain.

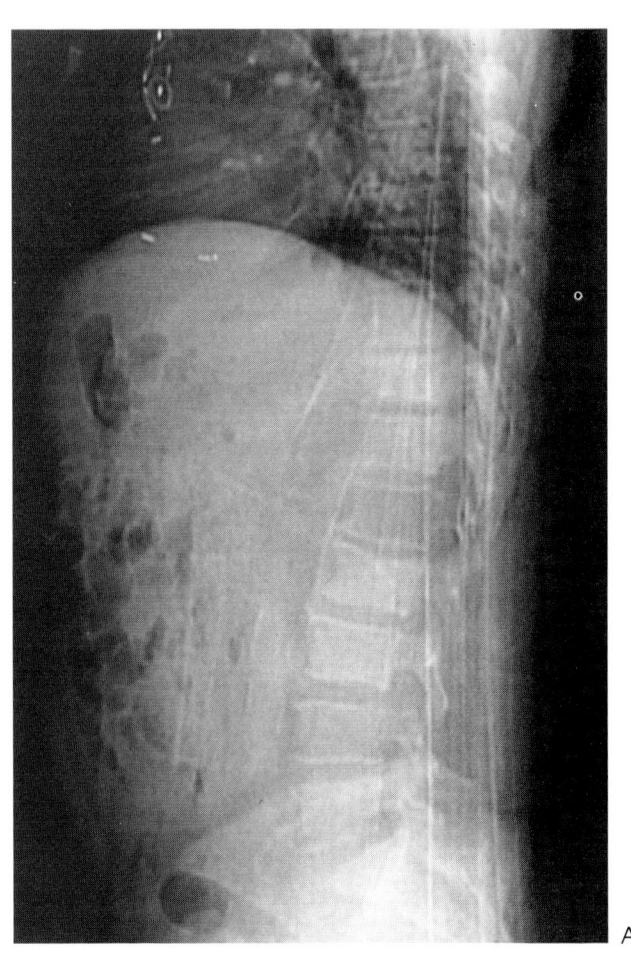

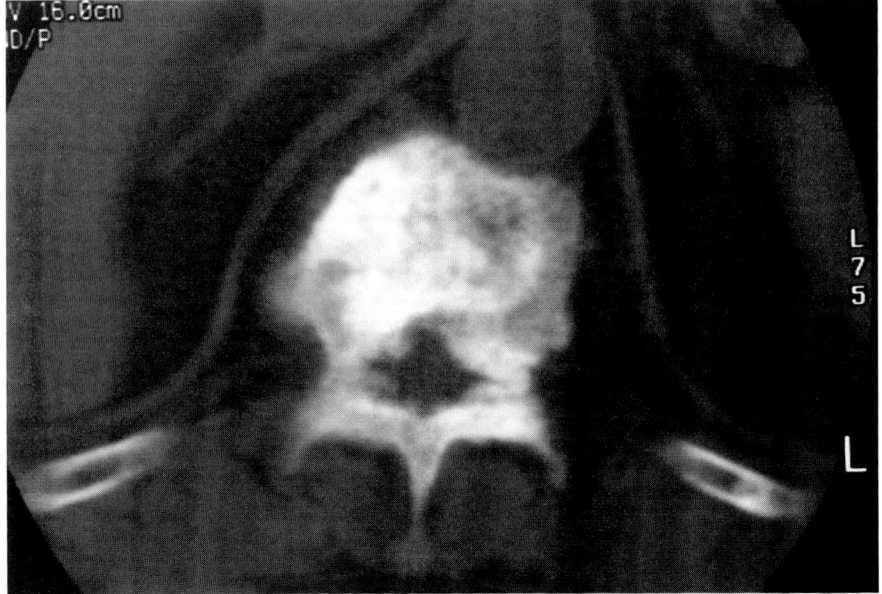

A

B

Radiologic Findings

(Fig. A) Lateral plain view of the thoracolumbar spine.

(Fig. B) Axial computed tomographic (CT) scan at the level of T11.

Diagnosis

Diffuse osteoblastic and osteolytic metastases from prostate cancer.

Differential Diagnosis

- metastases

- gastrointestinal tumors such as carcinoid tumors

- multiple myeloma in the clinical setting of POEMS (*P*olyneuropathy–*O*rganomegaly–*E*ndocrinopathy–*M*yeloma) (M-protein) and skin changes

Discussion

The most common primary tumor that leads to osteoblastic metastases is prostate cancer. The lateral view of the spinal column (Fig. A) reveals both osteoblastic as well as osteolytic metastases involving all of the vertebral bodies. Incidentally noted are surgical clips from a previous cardiac surgery.

The axial CT scan (Fig. B) reveals diffuse sclerosis of the T11 vertebral body. There is expansion of the vertebral body with bone formation and encroachment upon the vertebral canal and destruction of the cortex of the vertebral body.

Magnetic resonance (MR) is the procedure of choice for the evaluation of possible spinal cord compression because it provides the most accurate evaluation of the location, amount, and type of abnormality. However, it is generally not possible to differentiate osteoblastic from osteolytic metastases with MR imaging. This is because the marrow generally appears as increased signal intensity secondary to the presence of fat. Therefore, when this fatty marrow is replaced with tumor, the marrow appears as decreased signal intensity.

PEARL

- In an older male, metastatic prostate cancer is the most common metastatic lesion. It is not uncommon to find diffuse osteoblastic metastases even when there is no history of known prostate cancer.

PITFALL

- Because it is not possible to differentiate osteoblastic from osteolytic metastases with certainty, it may be necessary to obtain plain spine film and/or a CT scan to differentiate between the two.

TEACHING ATLAS OF SPINE IMAGING

Case 8

Clinical Presentation

The patient is a 25-year-old male with a history of known neurofibromatosis type 2.

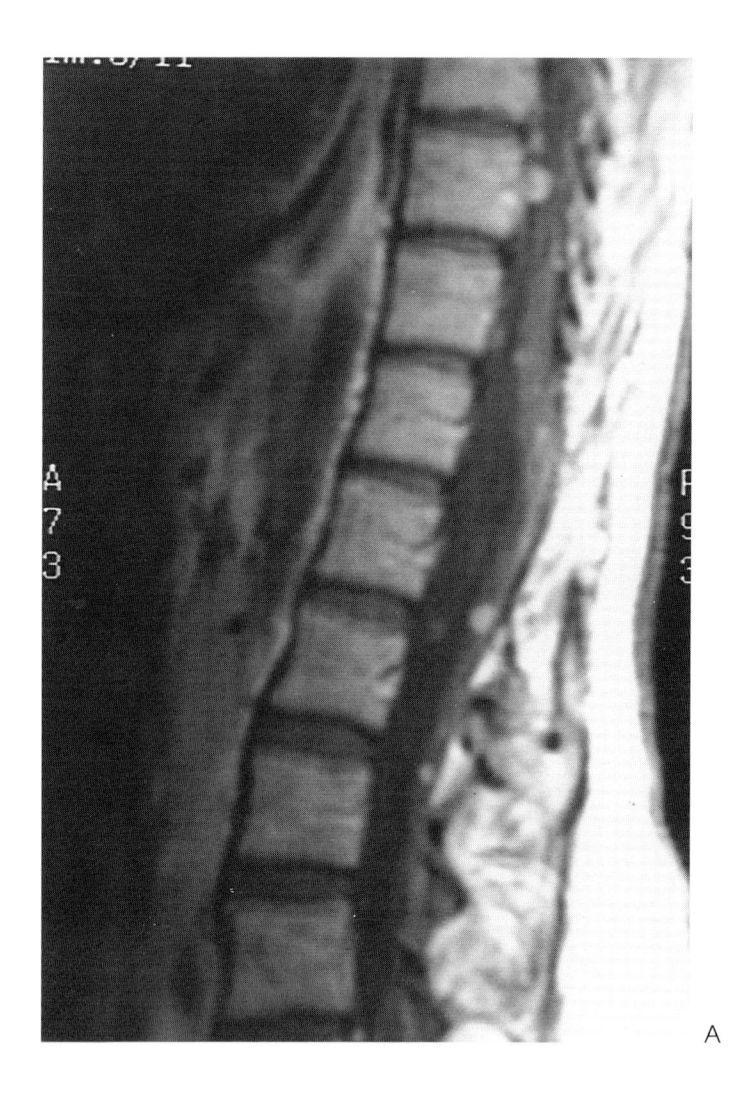

Radiologic Findings

(Fig. A) Sagittal short TR image postcontrast in the lumbar spine.

Diagnosis

Multiple schwannomas and postoperative changes with laminectomy and tethering of the spinal cord posteriorly at the T12-L1 level.

PEARL
- The patient who has been successfully operated for a spinal cord lesion may later develop recurrent symptoms because of dorsal tethering of the spinal cord by scar formation. This scar may form because when the dura is opened, scar develops and the spinal cord is pulled dorsally and becomes attached to the point where the dura is opened.

PITFALL
- If one abnormality is identified, in this case the multiple schwannomas, care should be taken to evaluate the presence of additional abnormalities at other levels. It is prudent to evaluate the entire vertebral column for complete evaluation.

Differential Diagnosis

- multiple schwannomas

- drop metastases: An additional diagnostic consideration includes drop metastases; however, in this clinical setting, this diagnostic consideration is unlikely.

Discussion

Patients with neurofibromatosis type 2 may have multiple spinal cord or cauda equina schwannomas. This patient had previous surgery for removal of a large schwannoma at the L1 level. Following this surgery, there is evidence of a laminectomy defect with surgical absence of multiple spinous processes from T11 through L2. In addition, the spinal cord is displaced posteriorly at the T12-L1 level and is attached to the dorsal aspect of the thecal sac secondary to scar formation.

TEACHING ATLAS OF SPINE IMAGING

Case 9

Clinical Presentation

The patient is a 14-year-old female who suffered a fall while skiing, and when evaluated in the emergency room because of neck pain, was found to have a palpable left neck mass.

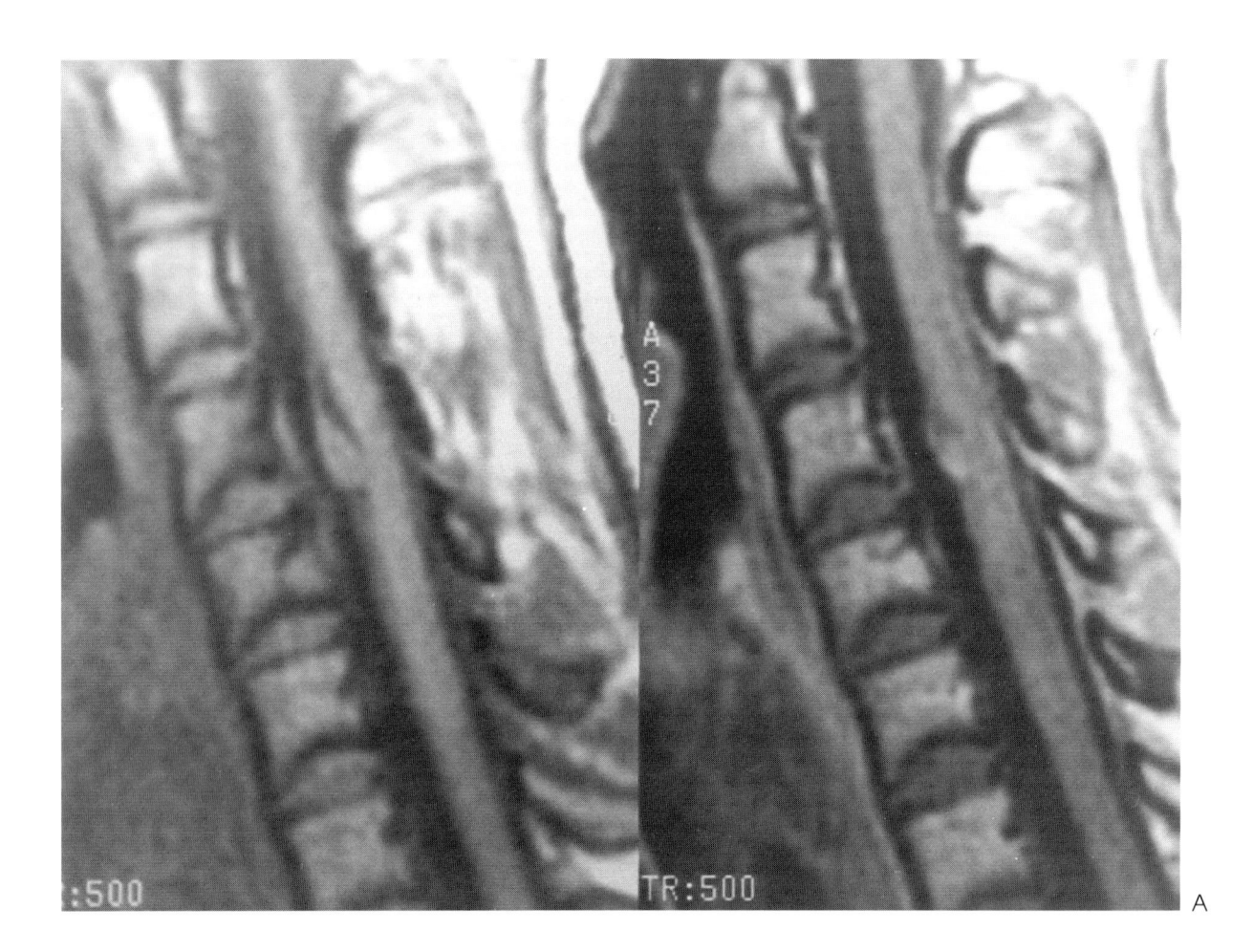

A

Radiologic Findings

(Fig. A) Pre- (*left*) and postcontrast (*right*) sagittal short TR images of the cervical spine.

(Fig. B) Parasagittal short TR image postcontrast.

(Fig. C) Pre- (*left*) and postcontrast (*right*) axial fat saturation images.

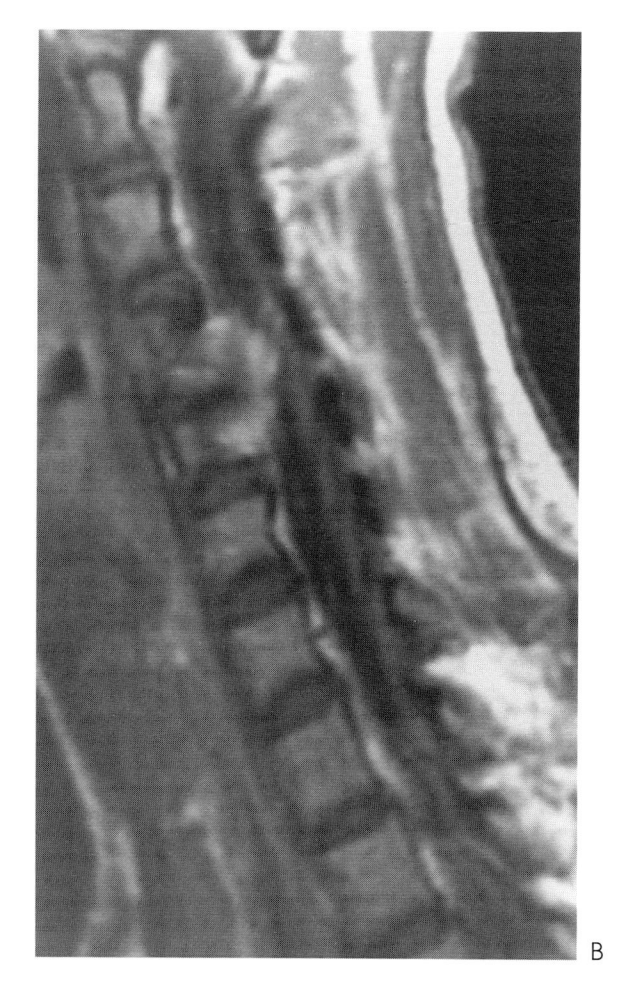

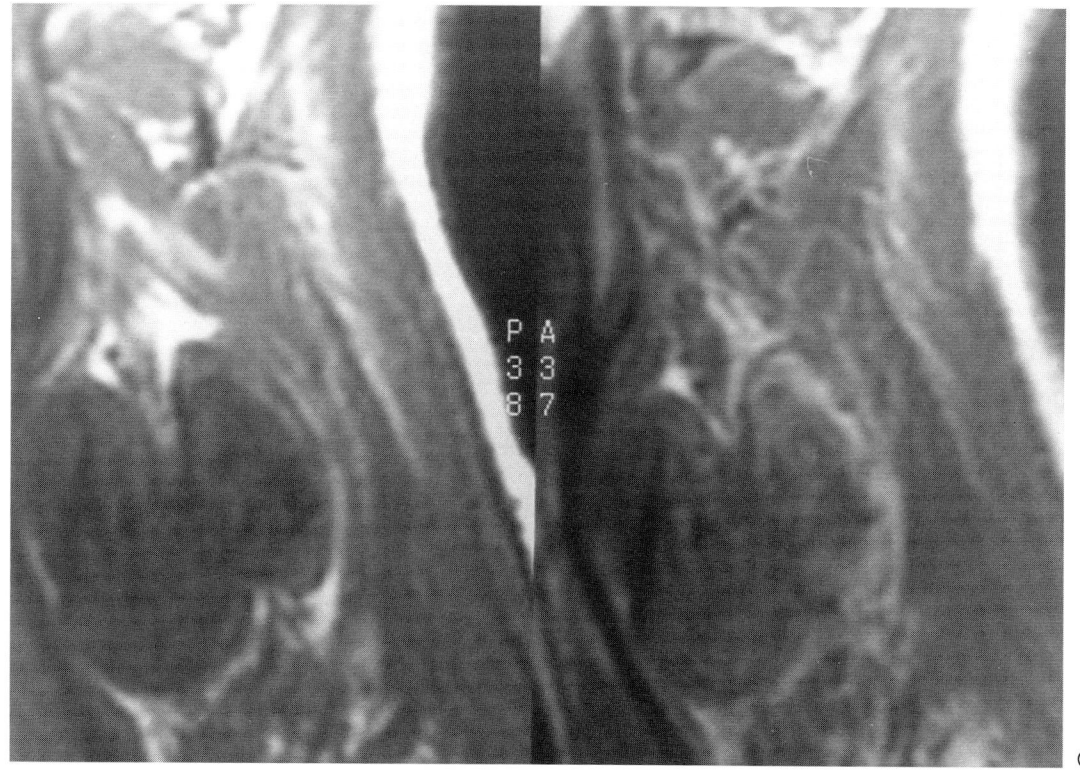

B

C

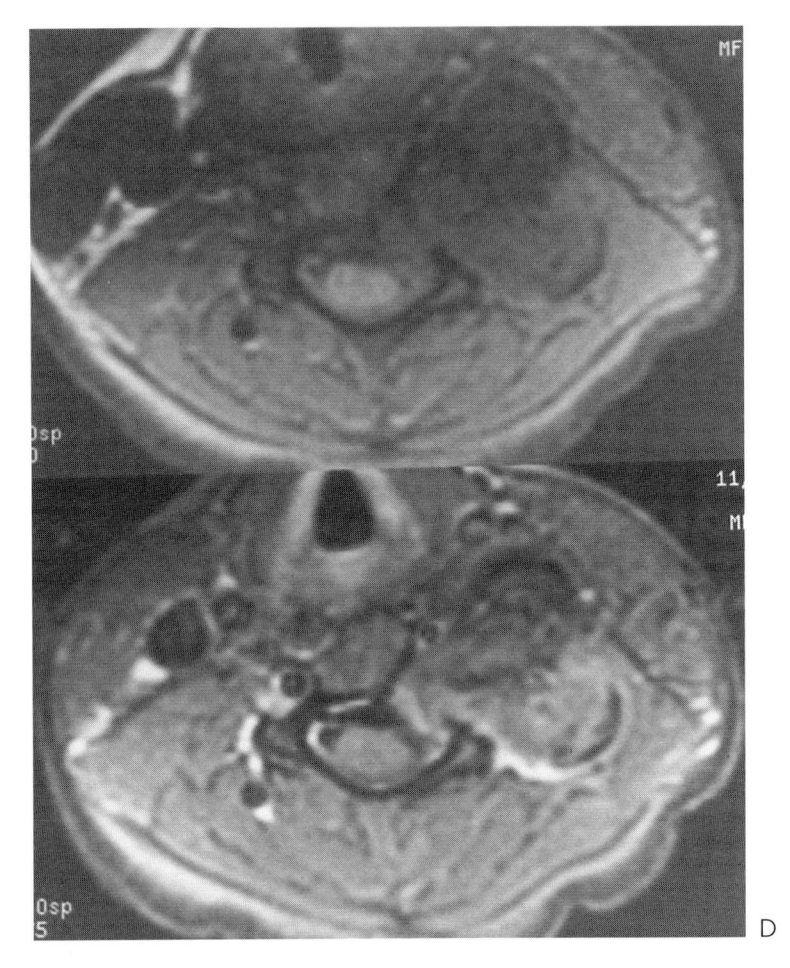

TEACHING ATLAS OF SPINE IMAGING

D

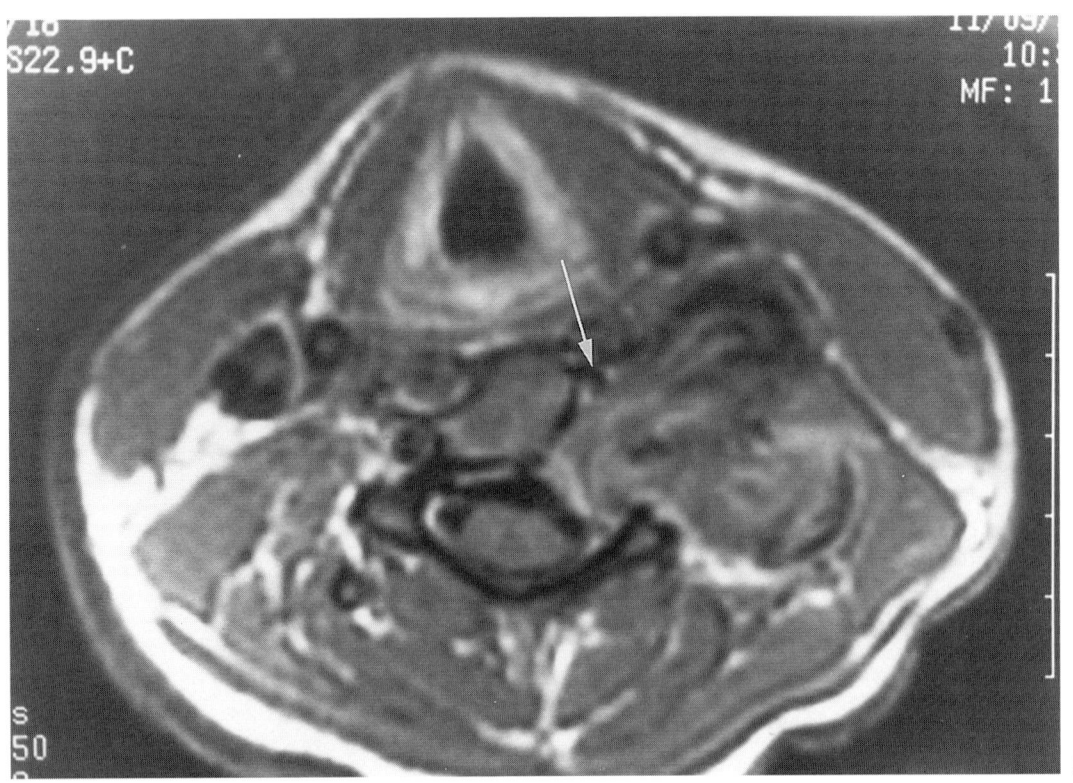

E

Radiologic Findings (continued)

(Fig. D) Pre- (*top*) and postcontrast (*bottom*) axial short TR images at the same level as Figure C.

(Fig. E) Pre- (*left*) and postcontrast (*right*) sagittal short TR images of the cervical spine at the level of the palpable mass.

Diagnosis

Desmoid tumor (unrelated to the recent trauma).

Differential Diagnosis

- desmoid tumor
- rhabdomyosarcoma
- hemorrhagic schwannoma
- lymphoma

Discussion

There is a lobulated mass in the left side of the neck which extends down to the level of the intervertebral foramen. This tumor was present prior to the recent trauma, but only became apparent at the time of examination. The decreased signal intensity of the mass seen in Figures C and E is related to the dense fibrous tissue. No hemorrhage was noted at the time of surgery. The mass expands the intervertebral foramen, as seen in Figure E, and extends to the level of the thecal sac. There is effacement of the left lateral, anterior margin of the thecal sac; there is pressure erosion of the posterior margin of the vertebral body secondary to the longstanding nature of this process.

The vertebral artery is seen as an area of flow void and is displaced anteriorly by the mass (Fig. E, *arrow*).

The diagnosis of desmoid (*fibrous tumor*) is unusual and could not be anticipated by the imaging appearance.

PEARLS

- Magnetic resonance imaging with multiplanar imaging and contrast enhancement is the procedure of choice for evaluation.

- Angiography may be necessary to evaluate the possibility to neovascularity and to determine the relationship of the tumor to the vascular bundle.

PITFALL

- The clinical history of trauma suggests the possibility that this lesion could represent an acute hematoma. However, the pressure erosion and expansion of the intervertebral foramen is not consistent with an acute lesion, but is consistent with a longstanding slow-growing lesion.

TEACHING ATLAS OF SPINE IMAGING

Case 10

Clinical Presentation

The patient is a 29-year-old male with a history of progressive upper and lower extremity weakness.

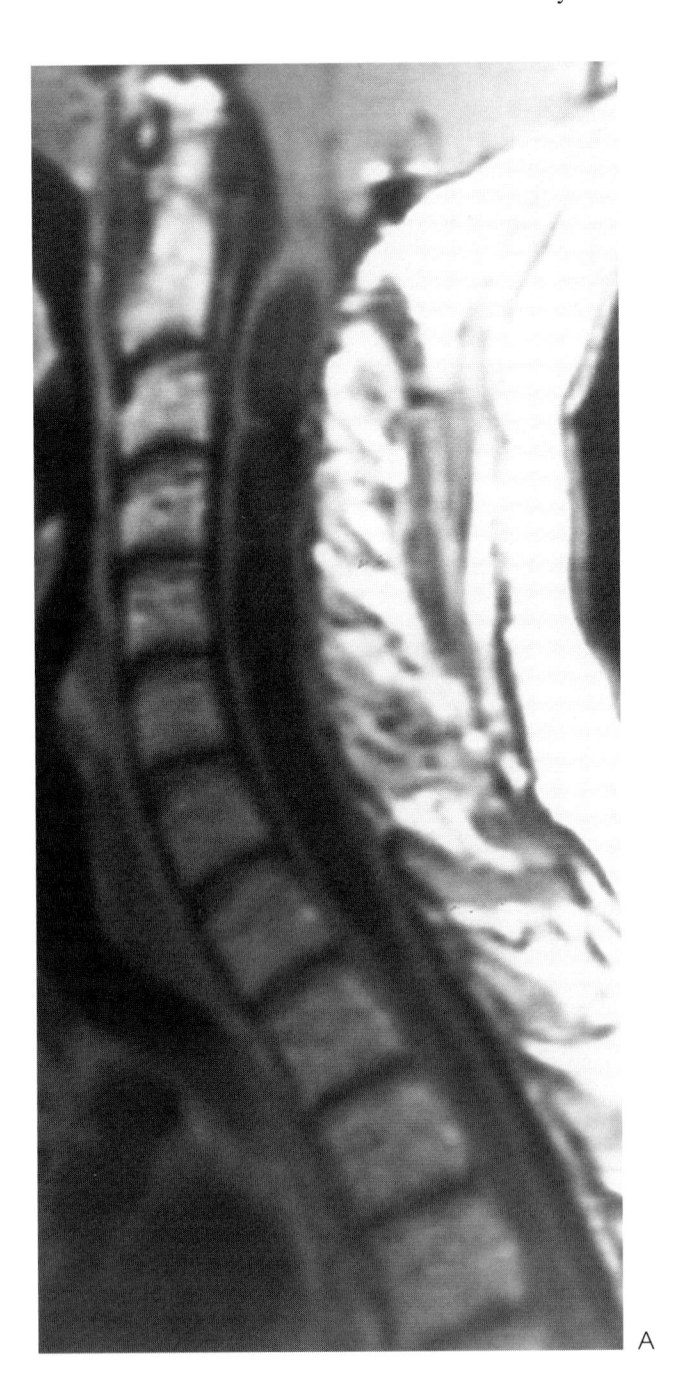

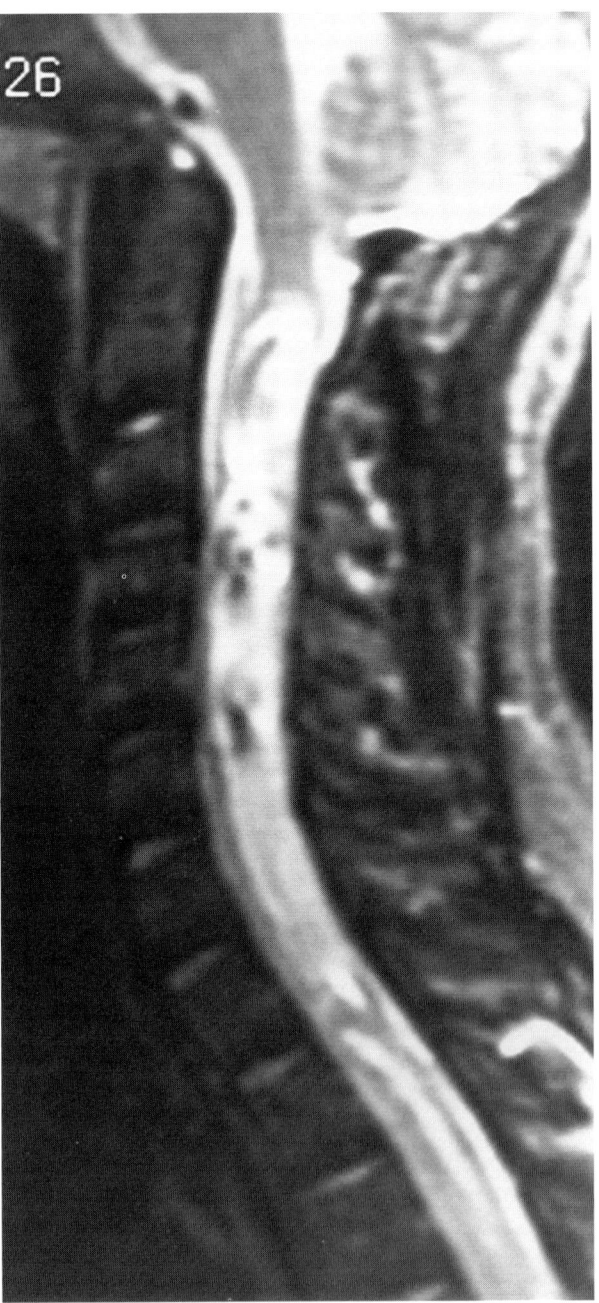

A

B

UNKNOWNS

(Fig. C) Axial short TR image.

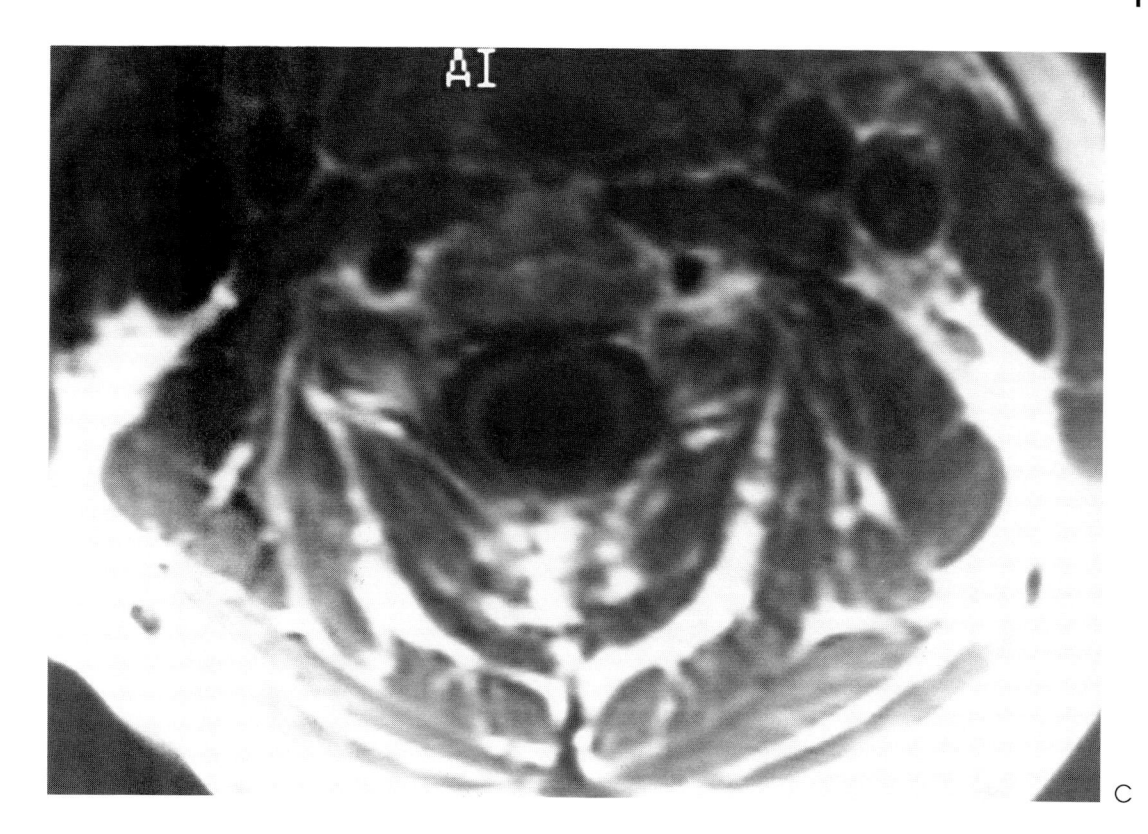

Radiologic Findings

(Fig. A) Sagittal short TR image.

(Fig. B) Sagittal long TR image.

(Fig. C) Axial short TR image.

Diagnosis

Chiari I malformation, postoperative changes in the posterior fossa, syrinx cavity.

Differential Diagnosis

- Chiari I malformation and postoperative changes
- cervical spinal cord tumor

Discussion

This patient had a previous decompression of the posterior fossa for relief of a Chiari I malformation. The patient initially did well, but then returned with increasing symptoms. The sagittal short (Fig. A) and long (Fig. B) TR images reveal a loculated syrinx cavity in the cervical spinal cord. This cavity extends into the upper thoracic region. There are postoperative changes in the posterior fossa with absence of the inferior portion of the occipital bone.

PEARLS
- The magnetic susceptibility artifact is slightly more prominent on the long TR image than on the other imaging sequences.

- If the possibility of an associated tumor is a diagnostic consideration, a postinfusion study should be obtained for complete evaluation. Most tumors enhance on the postinfusion study.

TEACHING ATLAS OF SPINE IMAGING

> **PITFALL**
> - The syrinx cavity is quite prominent; the postsurgical changes are subtle and therefore easily overlooked. A history of surgery would be helpful for better evaluation of the magnetic resonance images; however, careful evaluation will allow identification of the typical postsurgical changes.

There is also a magnetic susceptibility artifact at the level of the anticipated location of the posterior margin of the foramen magnum from a metallic surgical clip. The posterior arch of C1 has also been removed.

On the long TR image (Fig. B), rounded and curvilinear areas of decreased signal intensity appear within the cavity secondary to areas of flow void because of motion of the cerebrospinal fluid within the syrinx cavity. This appearance of internal areas of flow void has sometimes been used as a predictor that the patient will respond to shunting of the syrinx cavity. It is thought that these areas of flow void are secondary to transmitted heart beat and respiration from the fourth ventricle through the foramen of Magendie/opex of the fourth ventricle into the central canal of the spinal cord.

The spinal cord is enlarged throughout its length secondary to the syrinx cavity, and the normal subarachnoid space has been almost completely obliterated.

A cervical spinal cord tumor with an associated syrinx cavity is a diagnostic consideration; however, there is no evidence or history of a tumor.

UNKNOWNS

Case 11

Clinical Presentation

The patient is a 74-year-old male with a history of many years of upper and lower extremity discomfort.

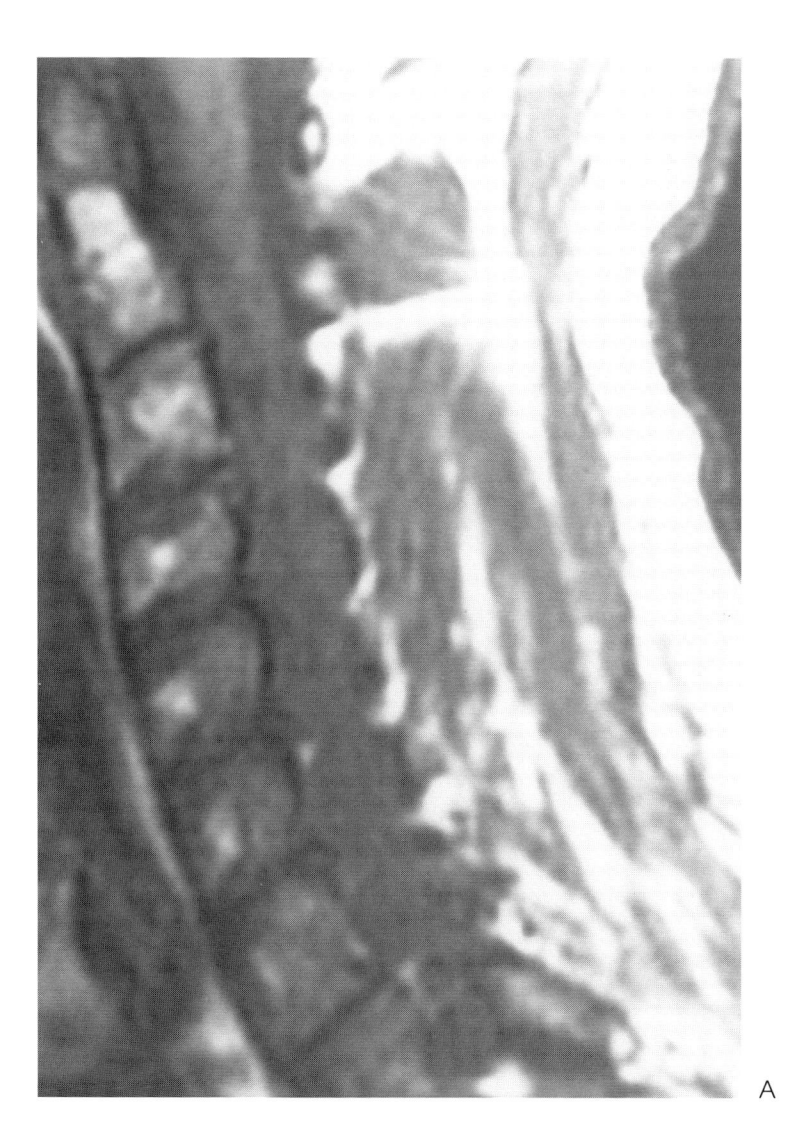

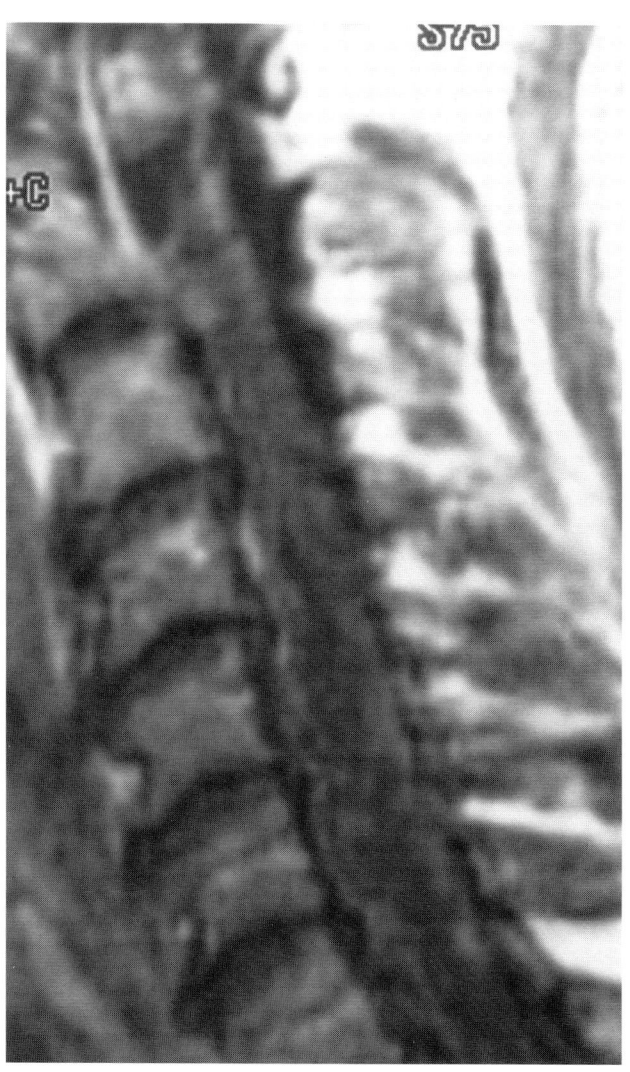

Radiologic Findings

(Fig. A) Sagittal short TR image.

(Fig. B) Midsagittal short TR image postinfusion.

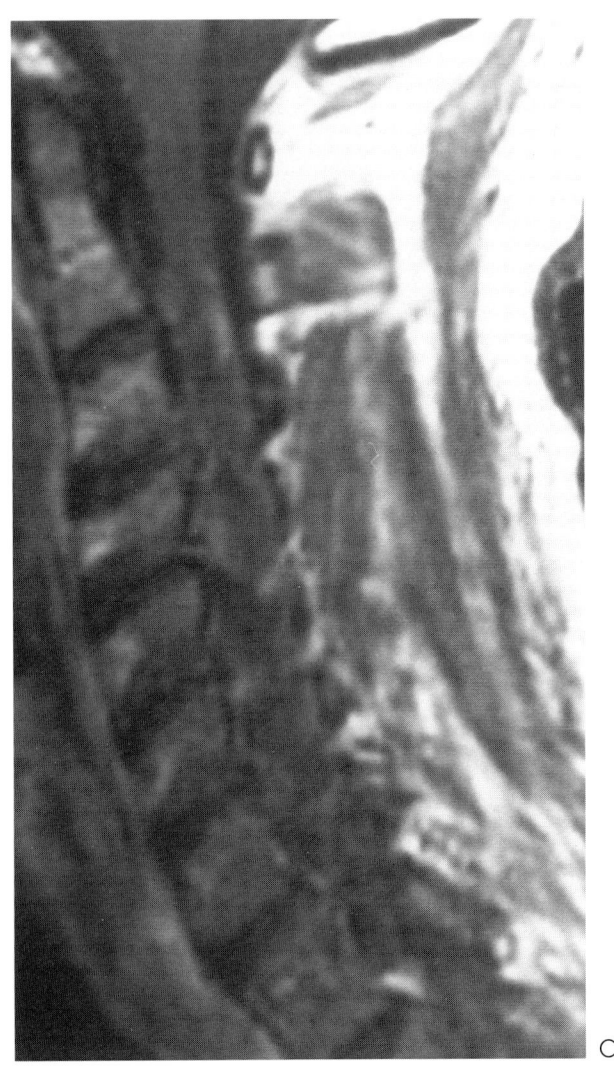

TEACHING ATLAS OF SPINE IMAGING

C

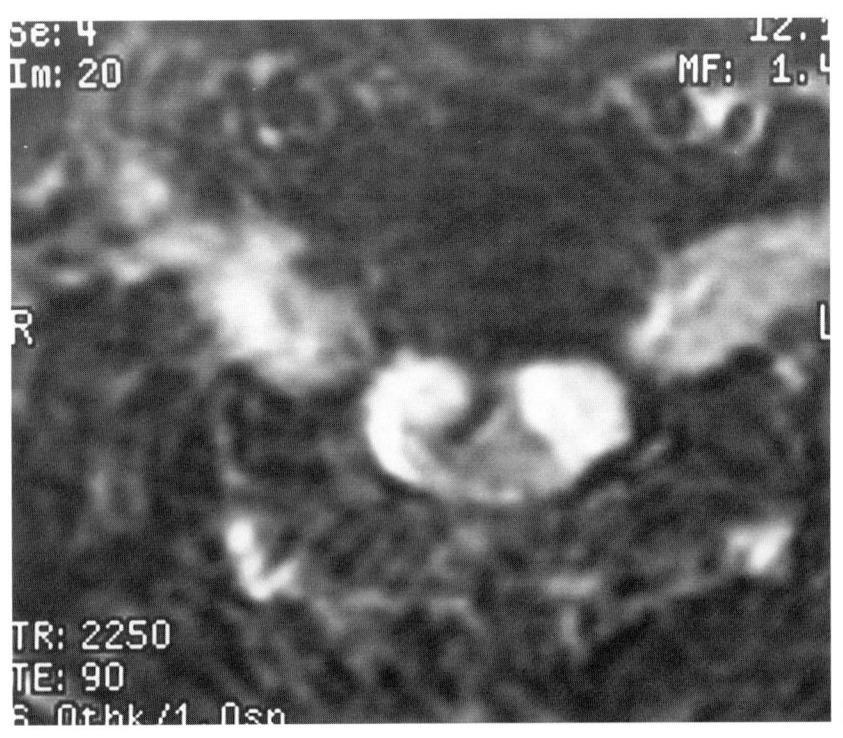

D

814

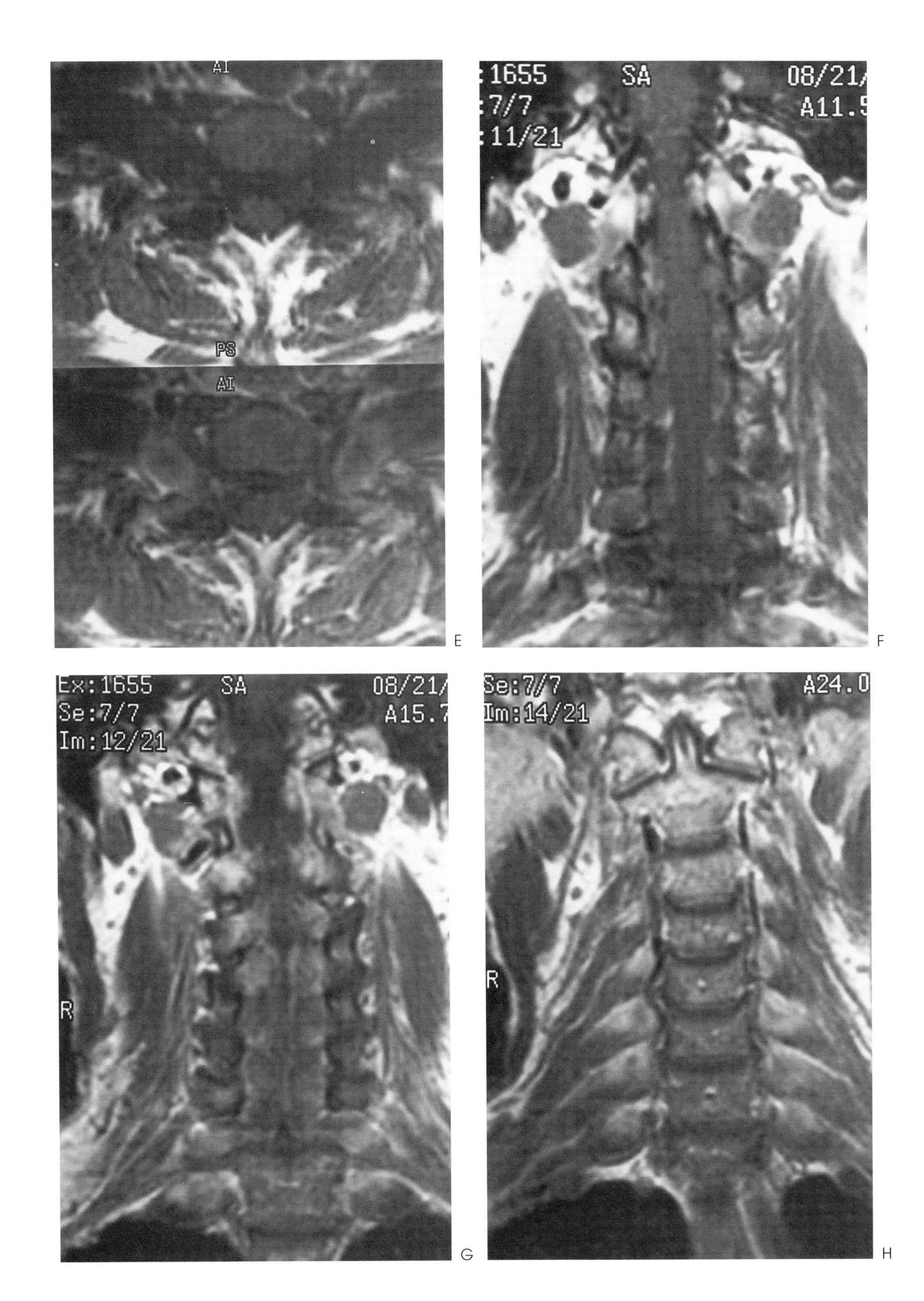

E

F

G

H

815

TEACHING ATLAS OF SPINE IMAGING

Radiologic Findings (continued)

(Fig. C) Parasagittal short TR image postinfusion.

(Fig. D) Axial long TR image at the level of C4-5.

(Fig. E) Pre- (*top*) and postcontrast (*bottom*) axial short TR images at C4-5.

(Fig. F) Postcontrast coronal short TR image of the cervical spine.

(Fig. G) Postcontrast coronal short TR image at the level of the lateral mass.

(Fig. H) Postcontrast coronal short TR image at the level of the vertebral artery.

Diagnosis

Neurofibromatosis type 1 with plexiform neurofibromata at all levels in the cervical spine.

Differential Diagnosis

- neurofibromatosis type 1 with plexiform neurofibromata
- diffuse metastases
- plexiform neurofibroma
- inflammatory process

Discussion

Additional history revealed that the patient was known to have neurofibromatosis type 1. The finding of such extensive changes of neurofibromatosis type 1 with multiple level plexiform neurofibromata is unusual in a patient of this age. In this patient, there is the spurious appearance of marked expansion of the cervical spinal cord on the sagittal short TR image (Fig. A). The midsagittal postcontrast image (Fig. B) demonstrates a mass with an intradural appearance behind the intervertebral disc space at the C1-2 level. There are also multiple additional ill-defined areas of enhancement at all levels in the vertebral canal. The parasagittal short TR image postcontrast (Fig. C) reveals multiple linear and patchy areas of enhancement. These areas of enhancement represent the enhancing peripheral portions of the bilateral plexiform neurofibromata.

In Figure D, the increased signal intensity neurofibromas are seen in the vertebral canal, compressing the cervical spinal cord into a triangular-shaped structure. There are also areas of increased signal intensity in the region of the nerve roots of the brachial plexus as they exit via the intervertebral foramen.

In Figure E, the neurofibromas appear to be isointense and to exhibit a thick wall of peripheral enhancement. No definite enhancement is seen surrounding the intracanalicular component of the tumors.

PEARL
- The multiplanar imaging ability of magnetic resonance allows the accurate evaluation of the changes seen in this patient. A single plane, such as the sagittal view, gives the appearance that there is diffuse enlargement of the spinal cord. However, the spinal cord is actually compressed, and the multiple dumbbell tumors compress the spinal cord and make it appear enlarged.

PITFALL
- In this case, the clinical history is very helpful in the evaluation of the images.

UNKNOWNS

The coronal postcontrast image at the level of the spinal cord (Fig. F) reveals rounded areas of enhancement at all levels of the spine at the origin of the nerve roots. The spinal cord is markedly compressed toward the midline. Multiple areas of enhancement along the lateral margins of the spinal cord are seen in Figure F, which was taken at the level of the ventral aspect of the spinal cord.

In Figure G, taken at the level of the vertebral artery, the plexiform neurofibromas can be seen just lateral to the vertebral column bilaterally. There is enhancement of all of these lesions. These multiple neurofibromata follow the course of the nerves of the brachial plexus and project between the anterior and middle scalenus muscles.

The sagittal images alone suggest that the diagnosis could be a process such as diffuse metastases.

However, the multiplanar imaging is much more in favor of the diagnosis of a plexiform neurofibroma.

An inflammatory process would be unlikely in this patient.

TEACHING ATLAS OF SPINE IMAGING

Case 12

Clinical Presentation

The patient is a 69-year-old male with a history of left groin pain.

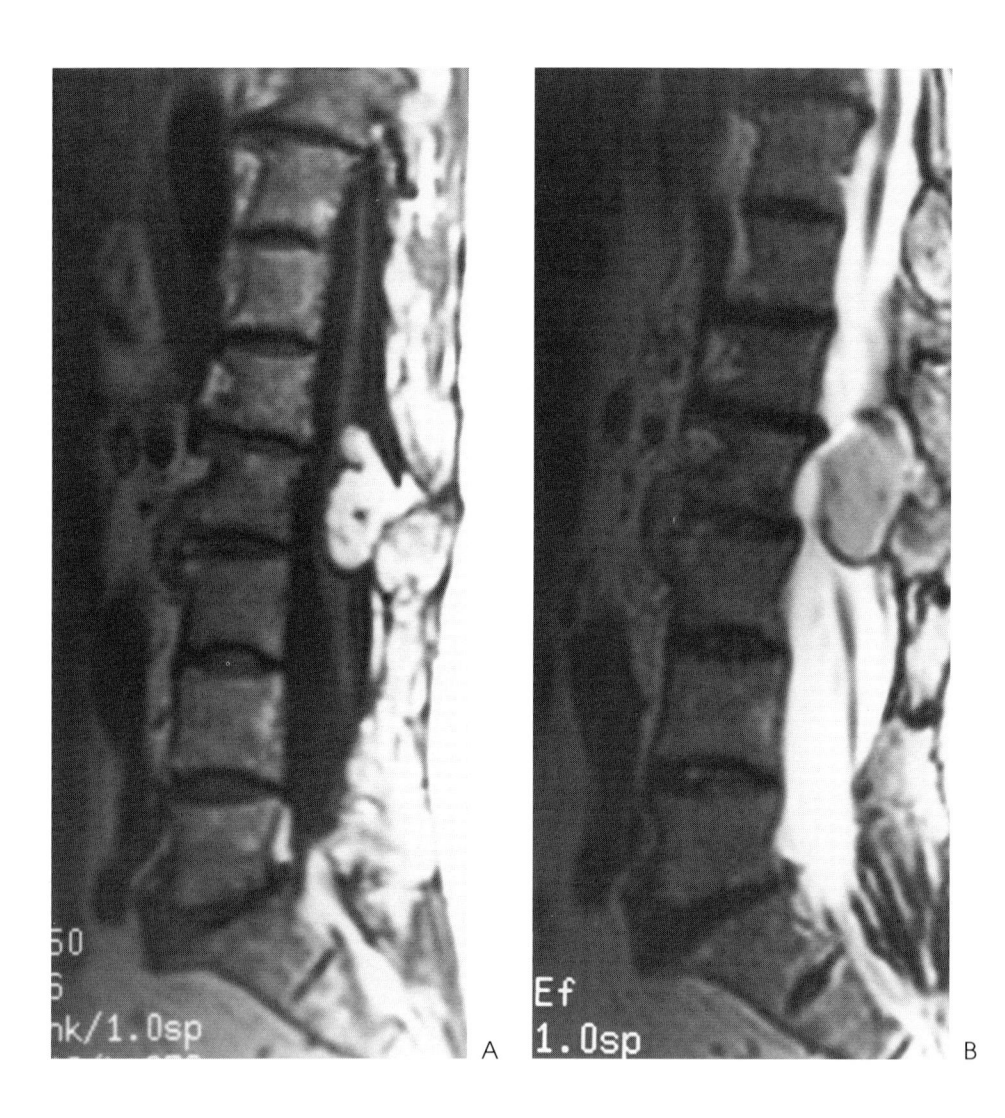

Radiologic Findings

(Fig. A) Sagittal short TR image of the lumbar spine.
(Fig. B) Midsagittal long TR image.

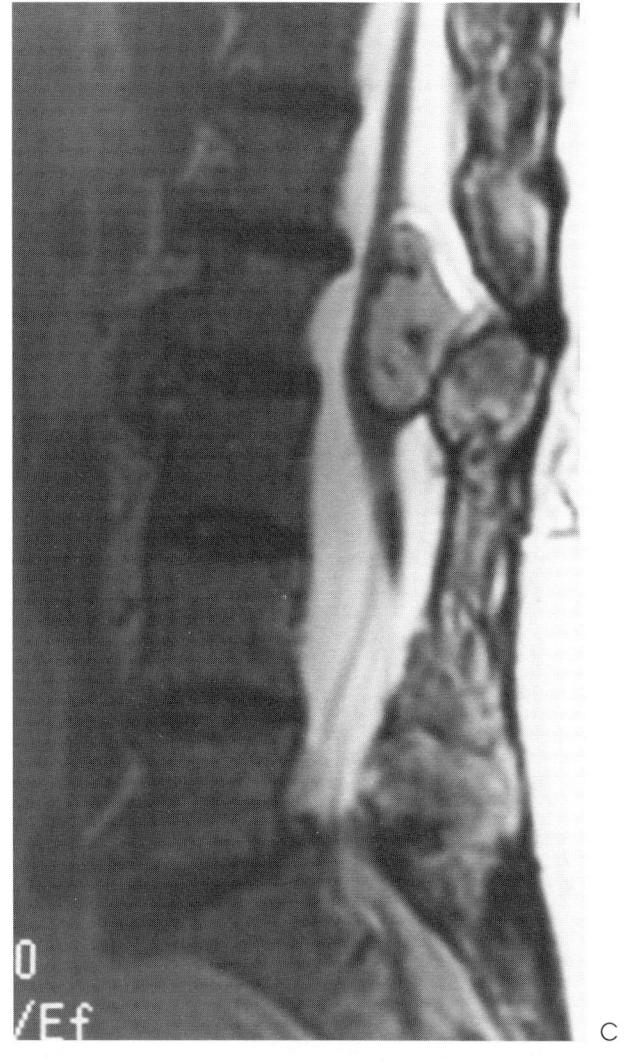

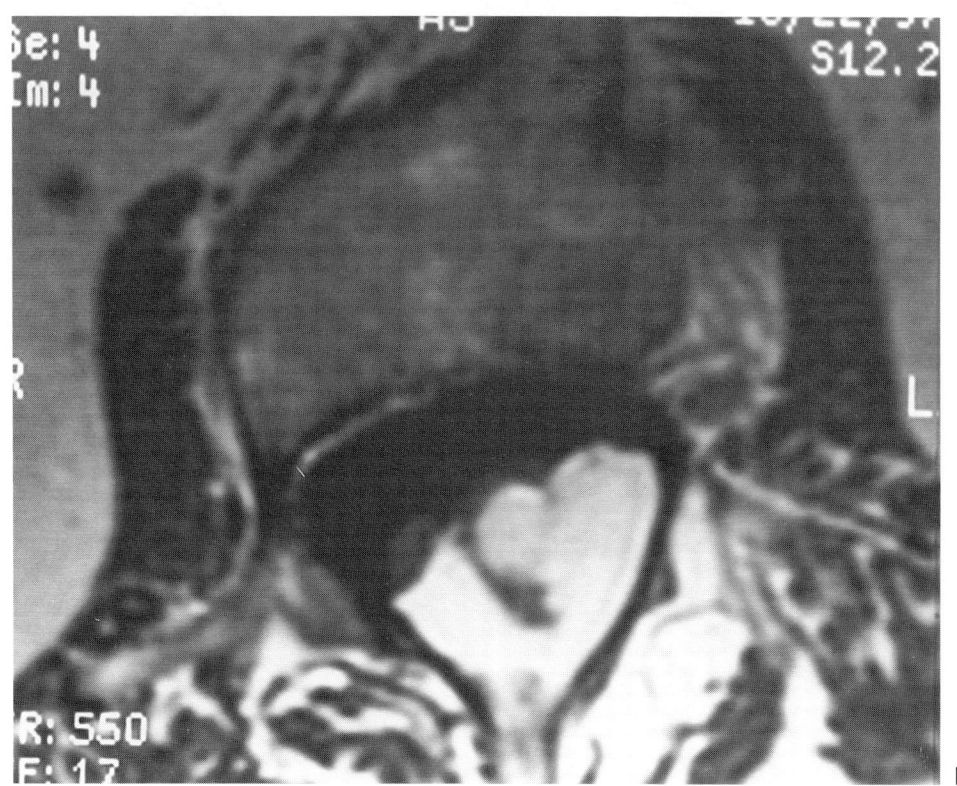

UNKNOWNS

C

D

TEACHING ATLAS OF SPINE IMAGING

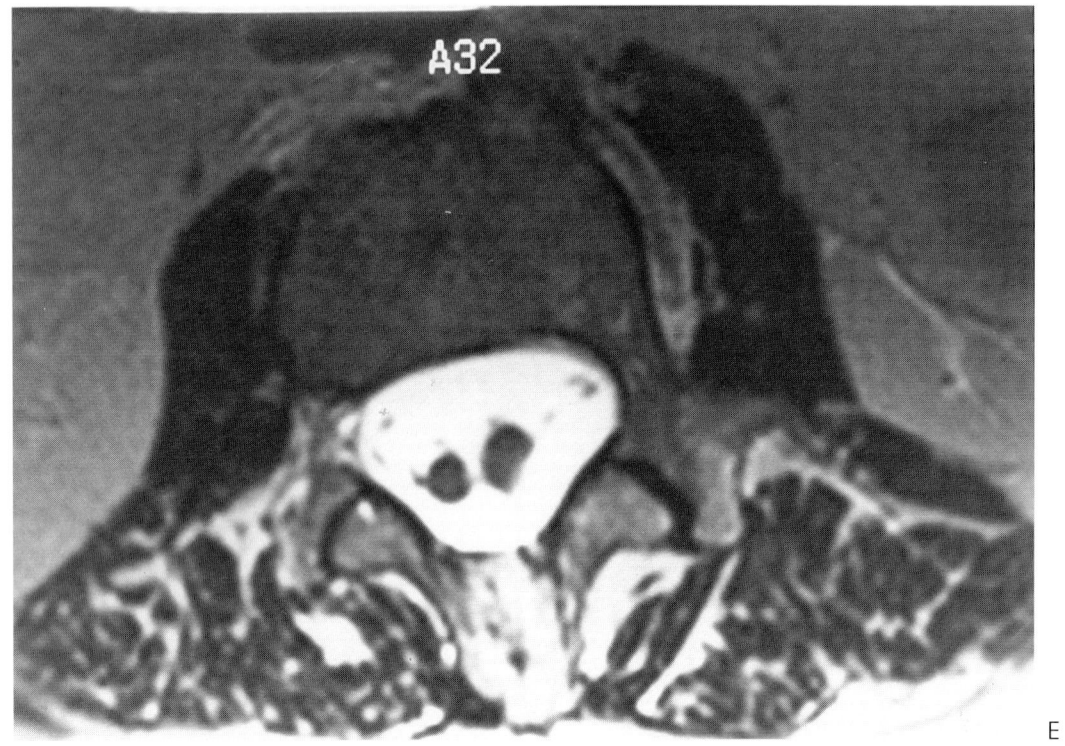

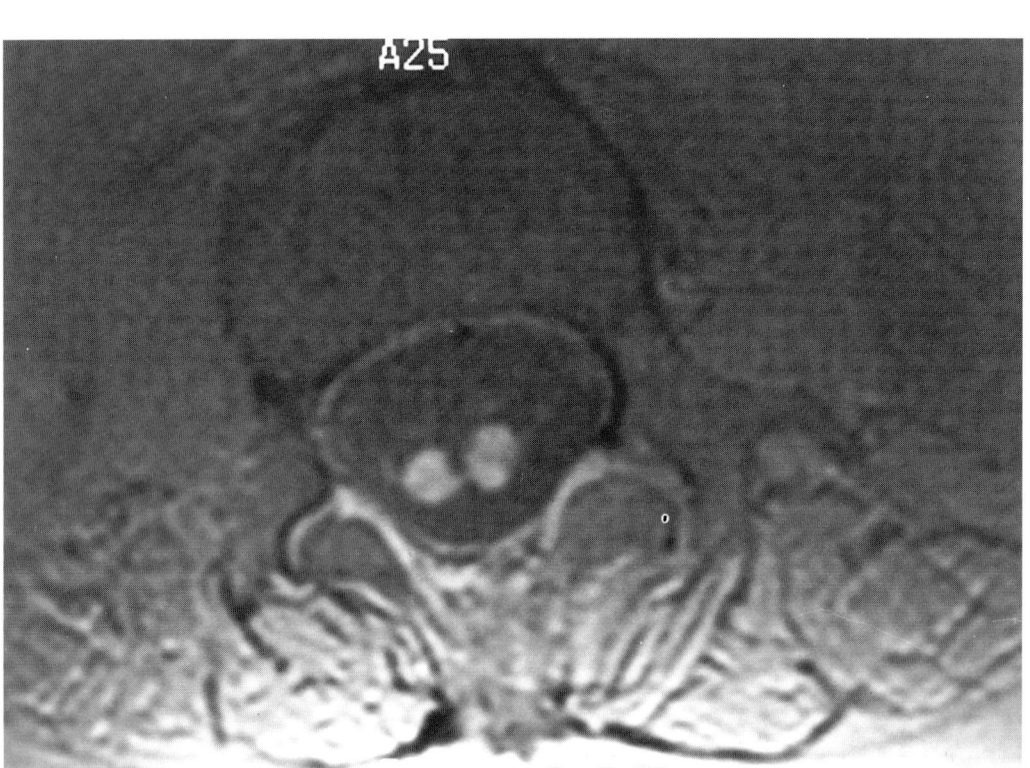

E

F

UNKNOWNS

G

Radiologic Findings (continued)

(Fig. C) Parasagittal long TR image.

(Fig. D) Axial short TR image at the level of L2.

(Fig. E) Axial long TR image at the level of L3.

(Fig. F) Axial fat saturation image at the level of L3.

(Fig. G) Axial fat saturation image at the level of L2 (same as Fig. D).

Diagnosis

Lipoma at the L2 level with tethered spinal cord and diastematomyelia.

Differential Diagnosis

- lipoma, tethered spinal cord, diastematomyelia

- hematoma

Discussion

There is a lobulated lipoma at the level of the L2 vertebral body. The spinal cord is pulled inferiorly and appears as a solid structure on the sagittal images (Figs. A to C); the split nature of the tethered cord is well demonstrated on

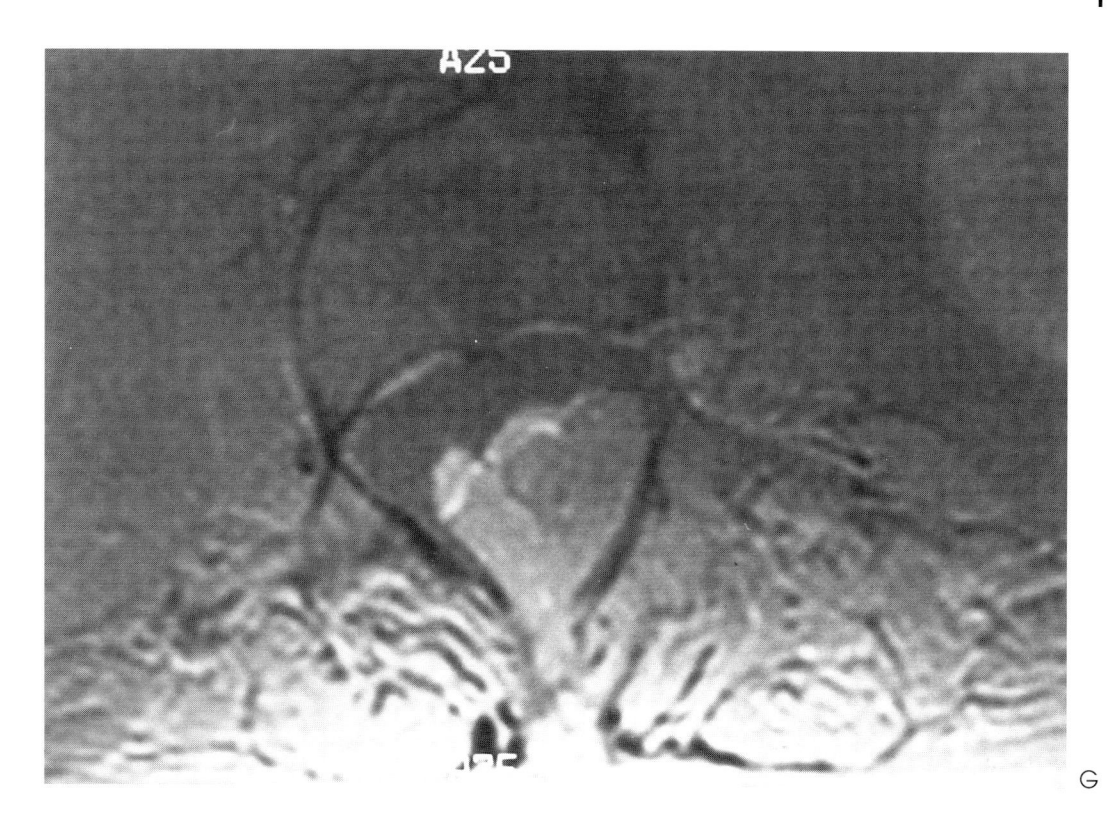

PEARLS

- In the absence of a split spinal cord, this lesion could be mistaken for a posttraumatic or spontaneous hematoma; therefore, a gradient echo imaging sequence should be used to differentiate between these two lesions.

- It is very unusual to identify this type of extensive congenital abnormality in a patient of 69 years of age. Magnetic resonance imaging is the ideal method to diagnose and evaluate the complex nature of this abnormality. No further diagnostic examinations are necessary in this patient.

PITFALLS

- There may also be an associated syrinx cavity with these patients, so evaluation should be performed of the entire length of the spinal cord.

- Other diagnostic procedures, such as myelography or computed tomographic scanning with or without myelography, would not provide an accurate diagnosis in this case. Myelography could potentially be dangerous in this patient because of the low-lying spinal cord.

the axial images (Figs. E, F). The findings of a lipoma, tethered spinal cord and split spinal cord is very unusual in a patient of this age. This finding would be anticipated in a newborn or young child. The normal spinal cord, ends at the level of the inferior end plate of L1 or superior end plate of L2. In this patient, the spinal cord extends down to the level of L4. The lipoma appears as increased signal intensity on the short TR images (Figs. A and D) and as decreased signal intensity on the long TR images (Figs. B and C) and on the fat suppression image (Fig. G).

The vertebral canal is expanded secondary to the longstanding nature of this process and because there is spinal dysraphism with incomplete spinous processes in the midlumbar region. These changes are best demonstrated in the axial images.

In Figure F, the spinal cord is actually a nodular area of tissue which is slightly higher in signal than the suppressed fat of the lipoma and is closely applied to the lipoma along its anterior margin.

Note that there is chemical shift artifact with a superior rim of increased signal intensity on the upper margin of the lipoma and a decreased signal intensity rim along the inferior margin of the mass. This chemical shift artifact occurs in the frequency encoding direction. The appearance is typical of that seen with a lipoma in any part of the body.

Hematoma is a possible diagnosis. However, the fat saturation reveals that the lipoma actually becomes decreased signal intensity; had this mass actually been a hematoma, it would have appeared increased signal intensity on the fat saturation images.

UNKNOWNS

Case 13

Clinical Presentation

The patient is an 18-year-old female with polycythemia and symptoms of visual disturbance with head shaking and poor responsiveness lasting a few minutes.

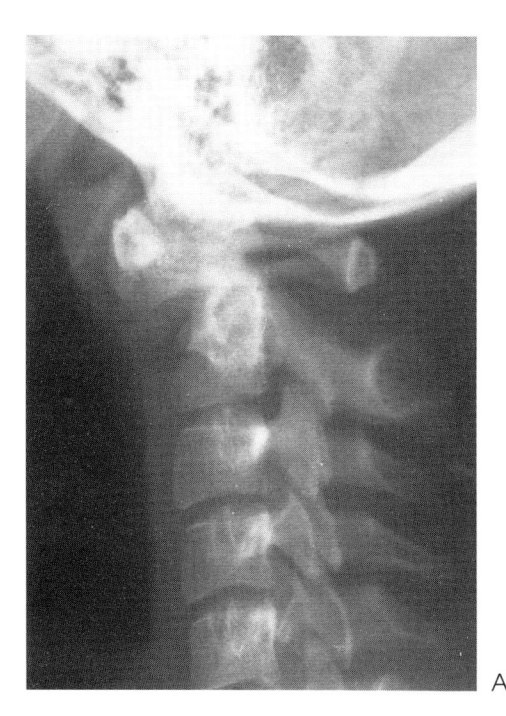

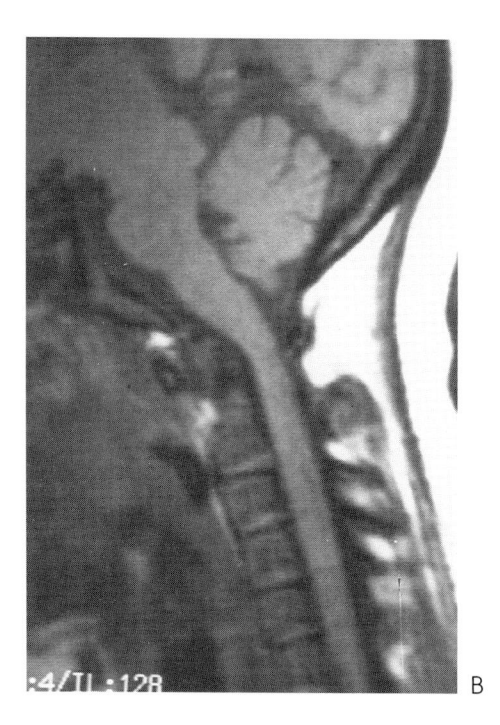

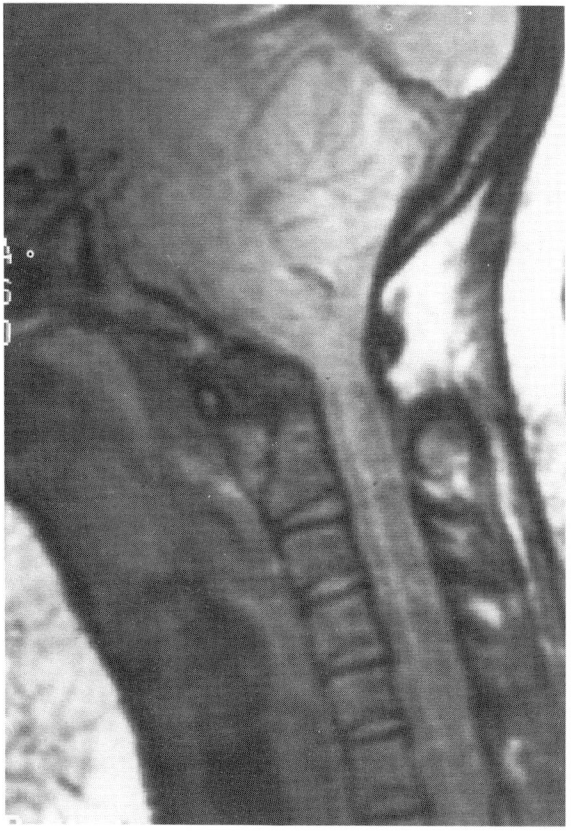

TEACHING ATLAS OF SPINE IMAGING

D

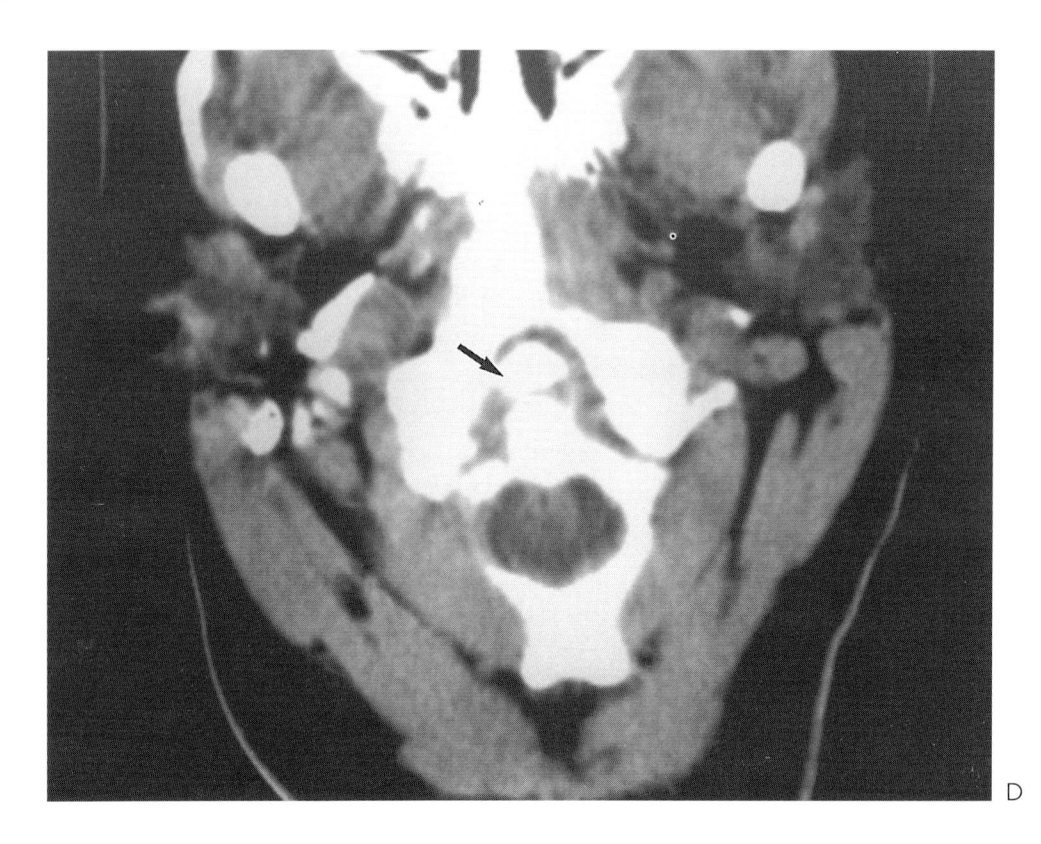

Radiologic Findings

(Fig. A) Lateral view of the upper cervical spine and the skull base.

(Fig. B) Sagittal short TR image of the posterior fossa and the upper cervical spine.

(Fig. C) Sagittal long TR image of the posterior fossa and the upper cervical spine.

(Fig. D) Axial computed tomographic (CT) scan at the level of the upper cervical spine and foramen magnum.

Diagnosis

C1-2 subluxation in association with Down syndrome.

Differential Diagnosis

- C1-2 subluxation
- posttraumatic dislocation

Discussion

The patient had polycythemia in association with cyanotic congenital heart disease; the typical abnormality is an atrial septal defect. The episodic shaking spells were thought to be secondary to seizures.

PEARLS

- Rheumatoid arthritis may also result in C1-2 subluxation; however, there is overgrowth of the pannus when the patient has rheumatoid arthritis.

- In some patients, C1-2 subluxation may be identified on the head CT scan; this abnormality should be sought when reviewing a head CT scan on a patient with Down syndrome.

PITFALL

- Care must be taken when manipulating the spine in patients so that no damage occurs to the spinal cord.

There is an association of C1-2 subluxation with Down syndrome. The subluxation is secondary to relaxation of the transverse and cruciate ligaments that transfix the odontoid process to the anterior arch of C1. This ligamentous laxity causes posterior and upward displacement of the odontoid process which results in widening of the space behind the anterior arch of C1. The posterior displacement of the odontoid process causes posterior displacement of the upper cervical spinal cord and compression of the spinal cord at the level of the C1 vertebral body.

The long TR image (Fig. C) better reveals the compromise of the subarachnoid space surrounding the upper cervical spinal cord. If spinal cord compression is present, the study may reveal increased signal intensity within the spinal cord on the long TR images. Magnetic resonance imaging (MRI) may also be obtained using short TR images with the patient in flexion and extension. These views are helpful because there may be cord compression in one position when none is seen in other position.

The CT scan at the level of the foramen magnum (Fig. D) reveals the rounded odontoid process as it projects superiorly into the foramen magnum (*arrow*).

Patients with Down syndrome may participate in athletic games such as the Special Olympics. It is prudent (and frequently required) to evaluate the upper cervical region prior to allowing participation in athletic games to determine if there is C1-2 subluxation. If there is C1-2 subluxation, injury to these individuals at the time of trauma can be life threatening.

A posttraumatic dislocation could be possible; however, there is no evidence of soft tissue swelling and no history of trauma in this patient.

Case 14

Clinical Presentation

The patient is a 53-year-old male with lower back pain and severe right-sided radicular pain. The patient also has a history of previous surgery for a herniated disc.

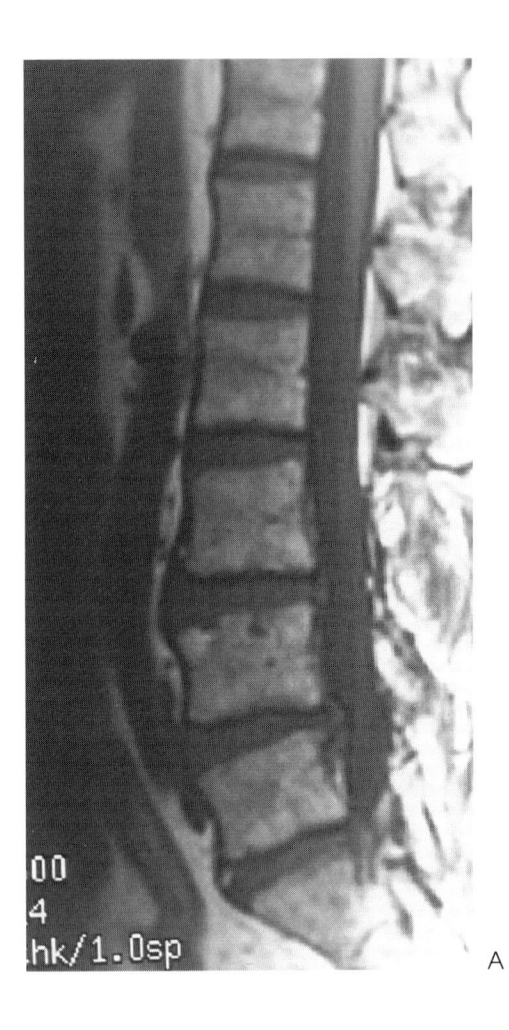

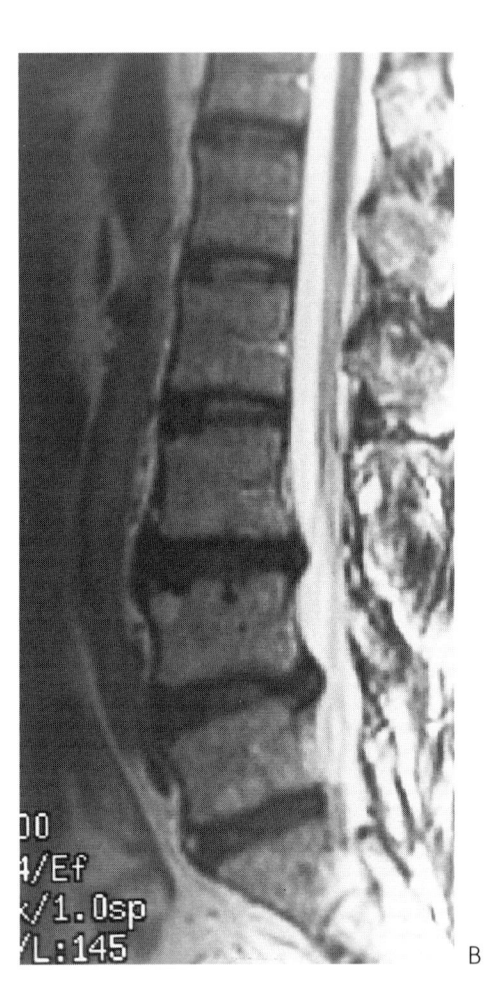

Radiologic Findings

(Fig. A) Sagittal short TR image.

(Fig. B) Sagittal long TR image.

(Fig. C) Right parasagittal short TR image.

(Fig. D) Left parasagittal short TR image.

(Fig. E) Pre- (*left*) and postcontrast (*right*) axial short TR images at the L2-3 level.

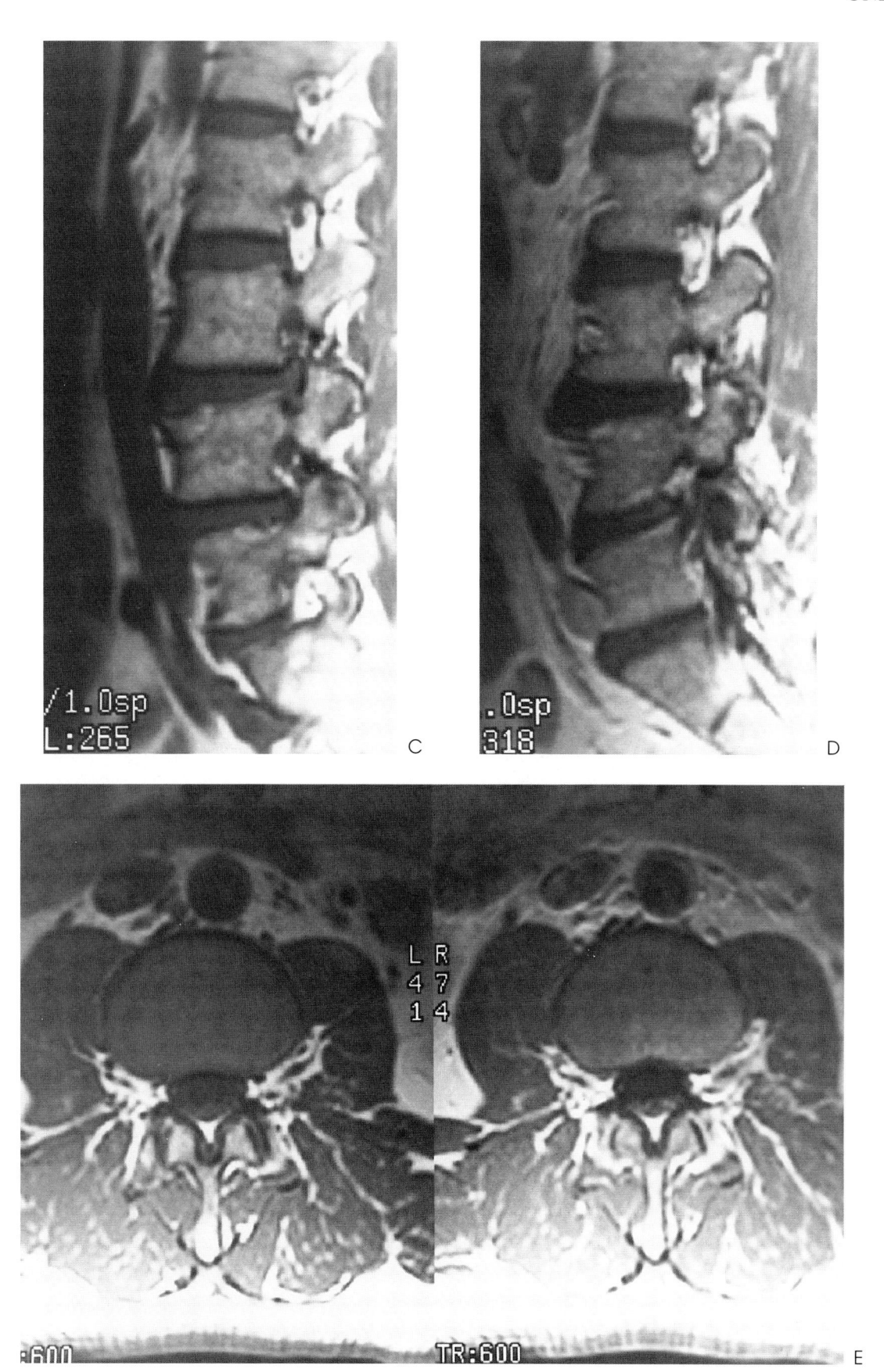

C

D

E

TEACHING ATLAS OF SPINE IMAGING

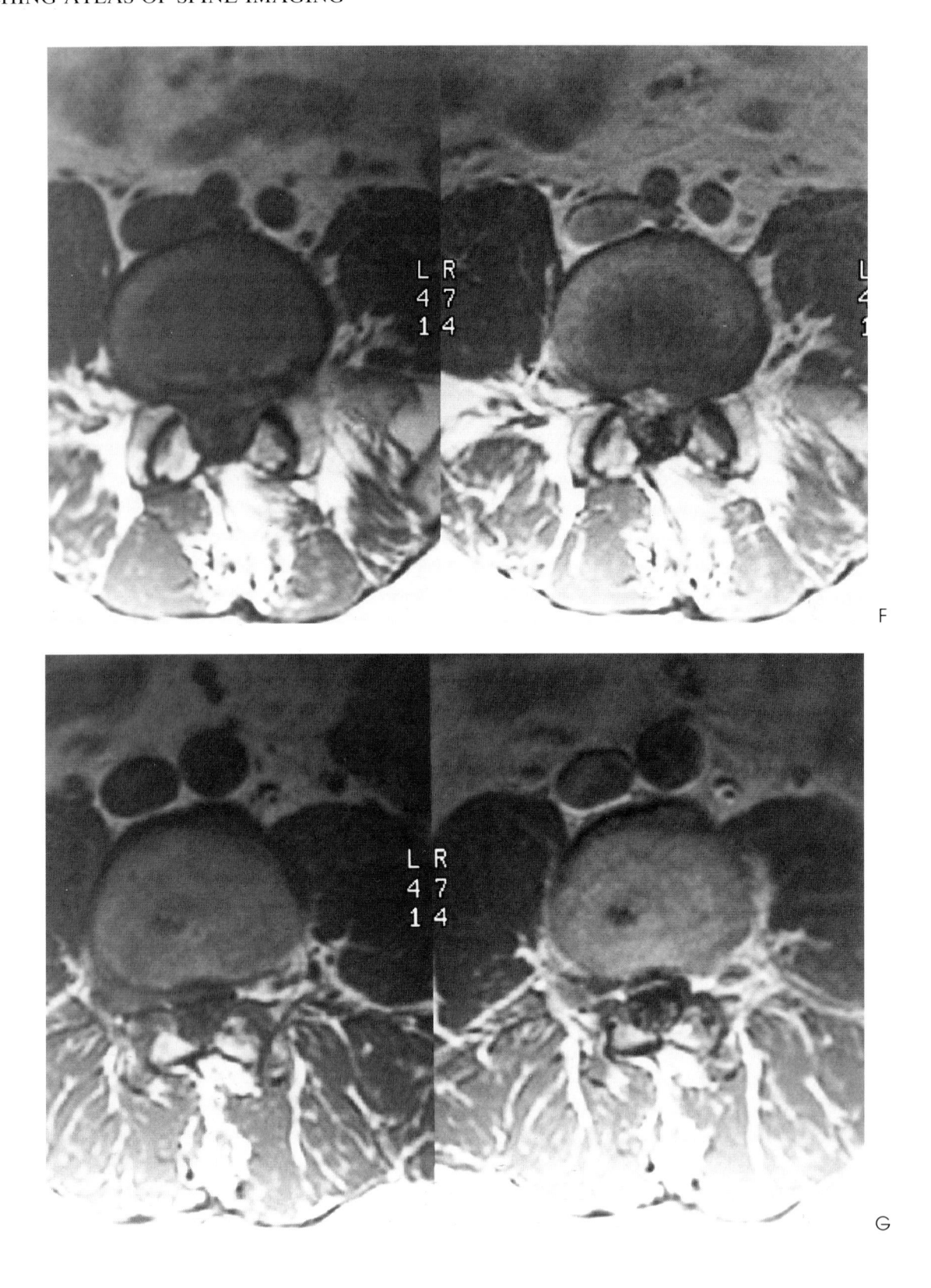

F

G

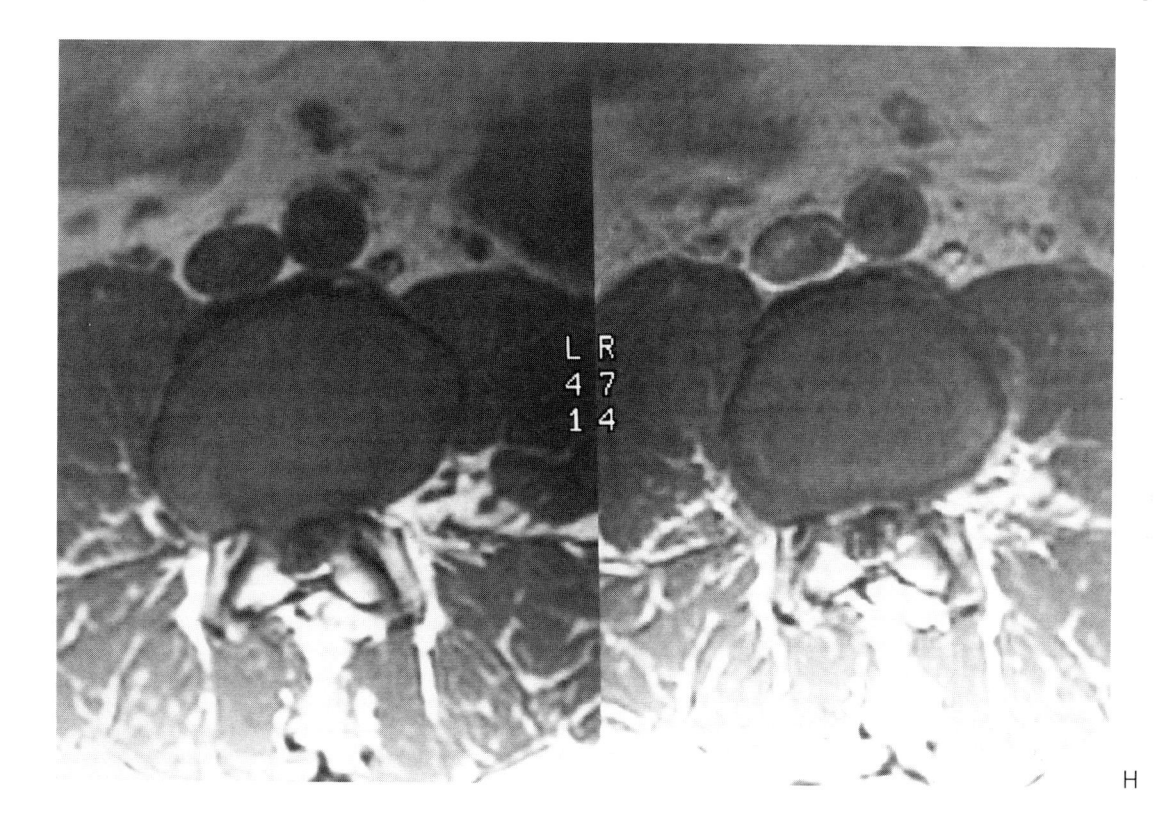

Radiologic Findings (continued)

(Fig. F) Pre- (*left*) and postcontrast (*right*) axial short TR images at the level of L3-4.

(Fig. G) Pre- (*left*) and postcontrast (*right*) axial short TR images at the level of L4, just above the L4-5 disc.

(Fig. H) Pre- (*left*) and postcontrast (*right*) axial short TR images at the level of L4-5.

Diagnosis

Large far laterally herniated disc at the L3-4 level; small midline herniated disc at L4-5 level.

Differential Diagnosis

- herniated disc

Discussion

The sagittal short TR images reveal a slight posterior prominence of the thecal sac in the low lumbar region secondary to the previous laminectomy. The lone TR image reveals the intervertebral disc prominence at the L3-4 and L4-5 levels. Significantly there is obliteration of the perineural fat in

PEARL

- The parasagittal images readily demonstrate the intervertebral foramen. When there is encroachment on the foramen by a herniated disc, there is obliteration of the high signal intensity fat in the lower portion of the foramen. This is seen in this patient in Figure C. Patients with laterally herniated discs typically have very severe radicular pain because the disc compresses the nerve at the level of the intervertebral foramen.

PITFALLS

- A note of caution: A far laterally herniated disc is easily overlooked at the time of interpretation. These patients generally have severe radicular pain because of nerve compression. The surgical approach to these laterally placed discs is occasionally difficult and sometimes requires a lateral approach.

- Because of the atypical location, a laterally herniated disc may occasionally be misdiagnosed as a schwannoma.

the lower portion of the intervertebral foramen at the L3-4 level on the right side; this is best demonstrated on the parasagittal short TR image (Fig. C).

The axial short TR images at the L2-3 level reveal a normal intervertebral disc with posterior concavity of the disc corresponding to the posterior margin of the vertebral body. The normal nerve can be seen surrounded by perineural fat in the region of the intervertebral foramen.

The short TR axial images at the L3-4 level (Figs. F and G) which are just above and at the level of the intervertebral disc reveal the far laterally herniated disc. The normal high signal intensity fat in the intervertebral foramen is obliterated. The nerve is displaced posteriorly and laterally by the herniated disc. There is effacement of the thecal sac along its right anterior margin. Far laterally herniated discs are uncommon and therefore these changes are also uncommon and may be easily overlooked.

At the L4-5 level (Fig. H), the short TR images reveal the midline herniated disc with indentation upon the thecal sac. There is also postoperative change with removal of the spinous process at this level.

The appearance is typical of a herniated disc, however, the far laterally herniated disc may not be appreciated unless proper attention is paid to the intervertebral foramenae.

UNKNOWNS

Case 15

Clinical Presentation

The patient is an 86-year-old-female with severe lower back and pelvic pain.

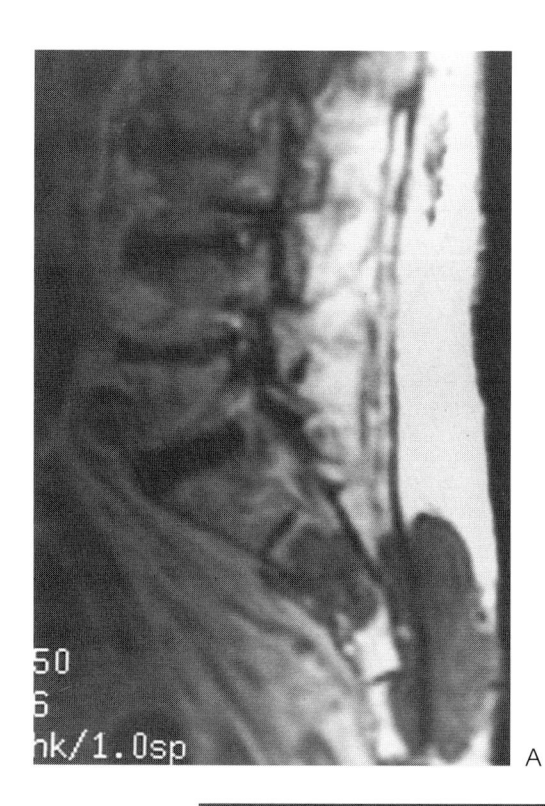

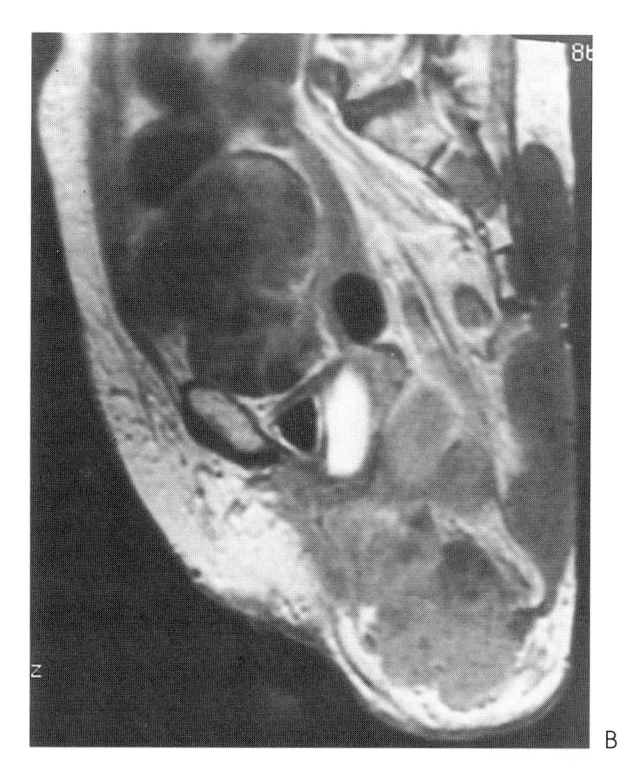

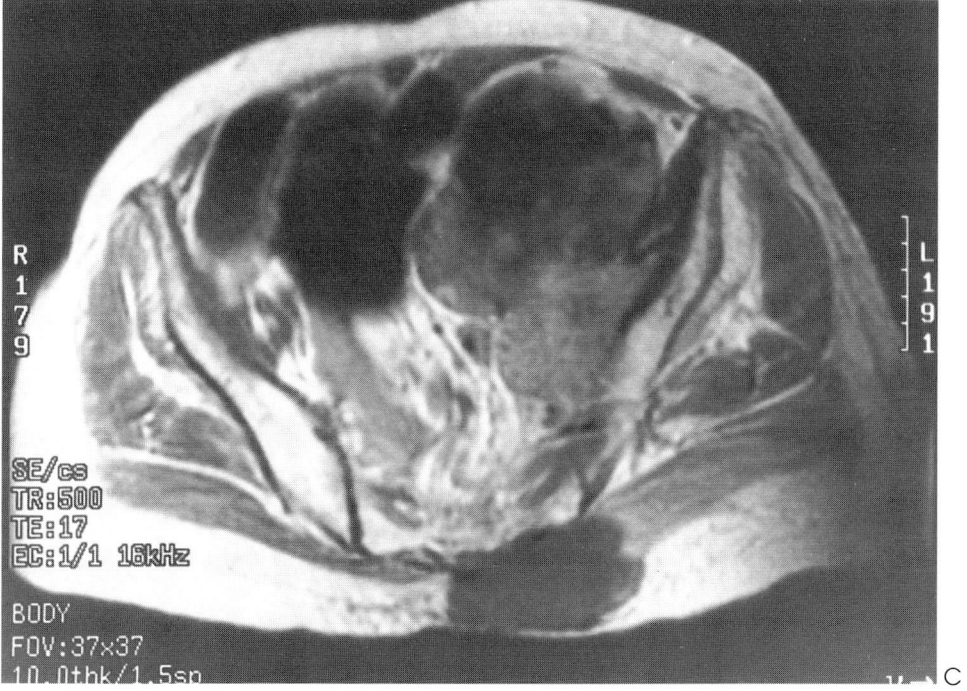

TEACHING ATLAS OF SPINE IMAGING

D

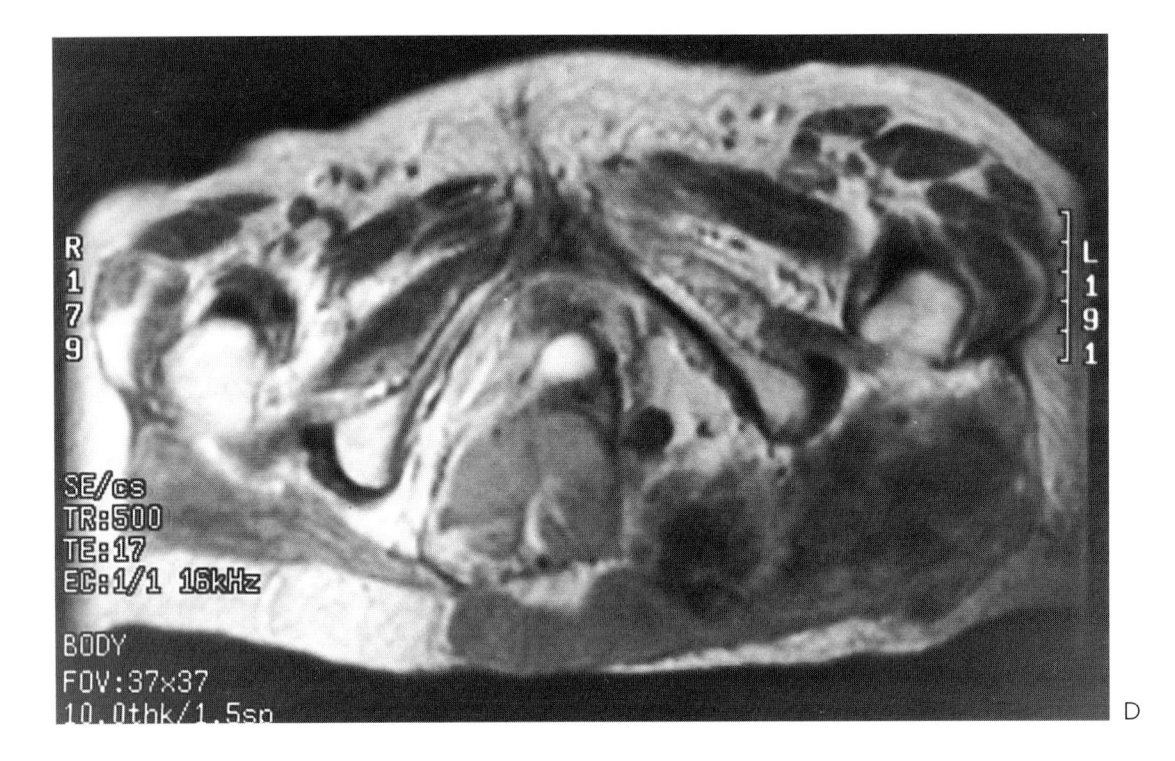

Radiologic Findings

(Fig. A) Sagittal short TR image of the lower lumbar spine, sacrum, and coccyx.

(Fig. B) Sagittal short TR image postcontrast of the sacrum and coccygeal area.

(Fig. C) Axial short TR image at the level of the pelvis.

(Fig. D) Axial short TR image at the level of the pubic symphysis.

Diagnosis

Chordoma of the distal lumbar spine, iliac crest, sacrum, and coccyx.

Differential Diagnosis

- chordoma
- sacral teratoma
- metastatic disease

Discussion

The short TR images in the sagittal plane (Figs. A and B) reveal a large decreased signal intensity mass that has invaded the sacrum at the level of C2 and has completely replaced the coccyx with decreased signal intensity tumor. The lowest two sacral/coccygeal segments reveal increased signal

PEARL
- magnetic resonance imaging (MRI) is the procedure of choice for evaluation. Multiplanar imaging is necessary, but may be the only imaging that is needed prior to treatment. MR is the ideal method for follow-up evaluation. The relationships between the vertebral column, the cauda equina, and the pelvic structures are readily identified.

UNKNOWNS

PITFALL
- If a lumbar spine MR scan is performed, the image may not extend sufficiently inferiorly to evaluate the sacrum and coccyx. Therefore, when low back pain is present, it is important to be aware of the level of the pain.

intensity and additional history revealed that the patient had previous radiation therapy for treatment of chordoma. The axial images (Figs. C and D) reveal a lobulated variable signal intensity mass that occupies the entire left side of the pelvis (Fig. C). At the level of the pubic symphisis, the study reveals a variable signal intensity lobulated mass that has replaced the entire left iliac bone and extends to the midline in the region of the spine.

In Figure B, there is irregular, inhomogeneous enhancement of the mass in the pelvis. The bladder is seen as an oval-shaped area of increased signal intensity because it is filled with gadolinium which settles in the dependent portion of the bladder because it is heavier than urine. The visualized loops of bowel are dilated, probably because of partial obstruction by the pelvic mass.

Sacral teratoma is a possibility in a child. Metastatic disease can be identified in an older patient even without a history of a known primary tumor; primary tumors include breast, lung, or renal cancers.

TEACHING ATLAS OF SPINE IMAGING

Case 16

Clinical Presentation

The patient is a 32-year-old female with upper and lower extremity weakness of sudden onset.

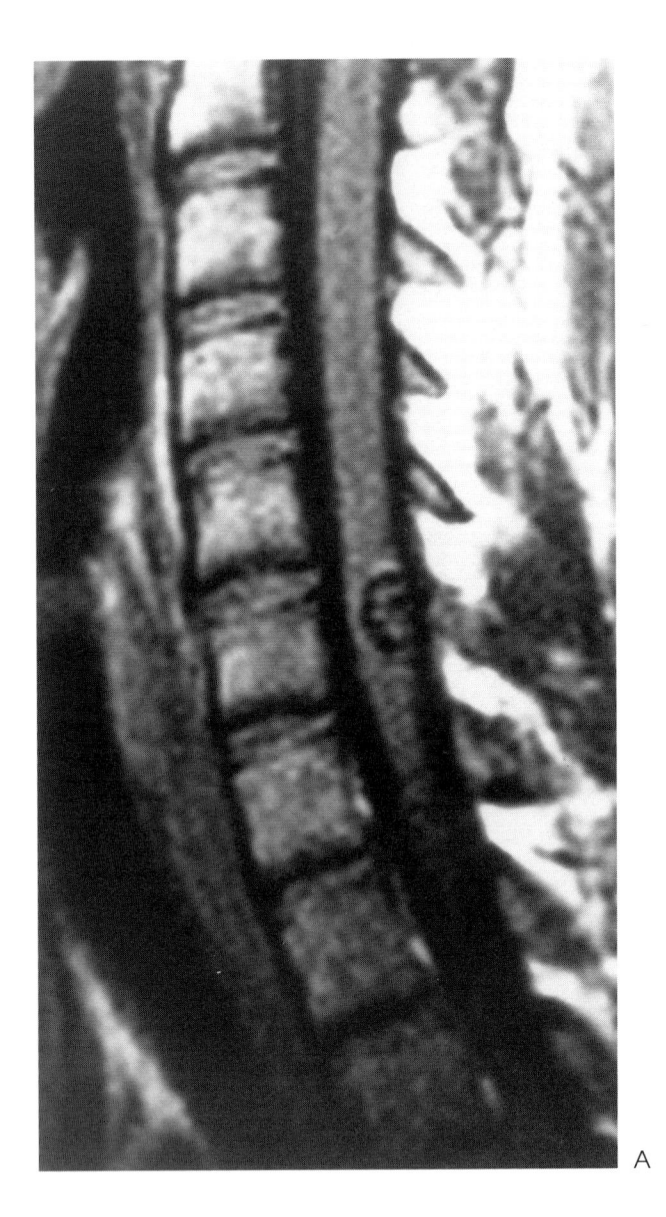

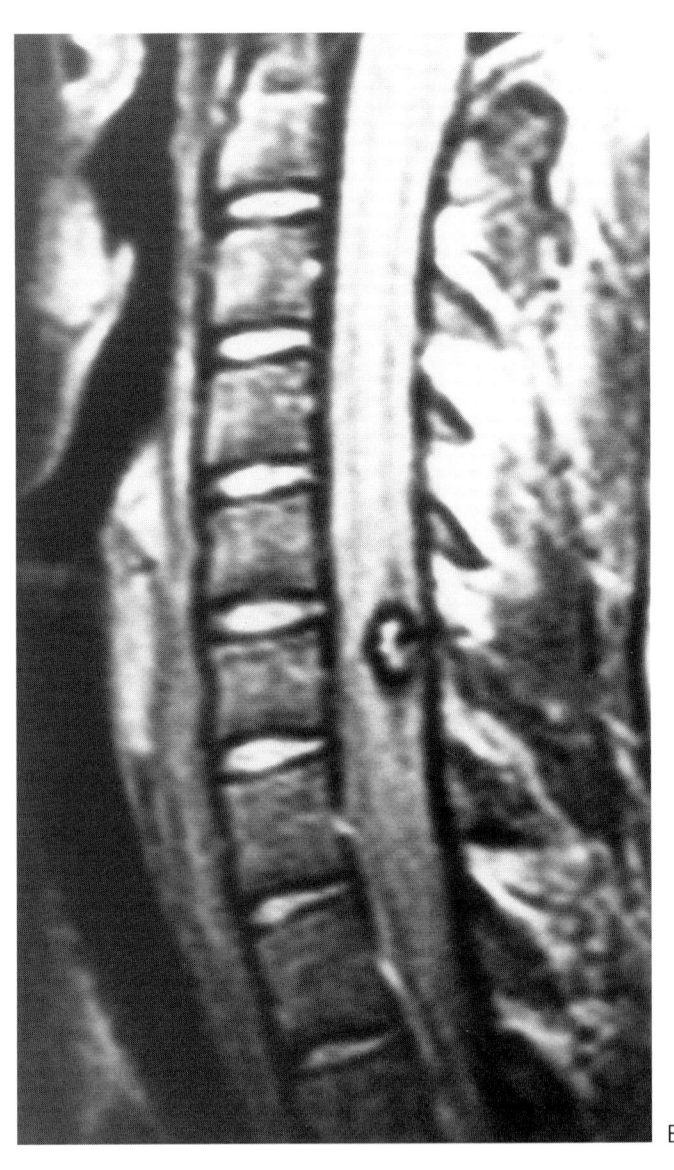

Radiologic Findings

(Fig. A) Sagittal short TR image of the cervical spine.

(Fig. B) Sagittal intermediate signal intensity image.

(Fig. C) Sagittal long TR image of the cervical spine.

(Fig. D) Axial short TR image of the cervical spine at the level of C6.

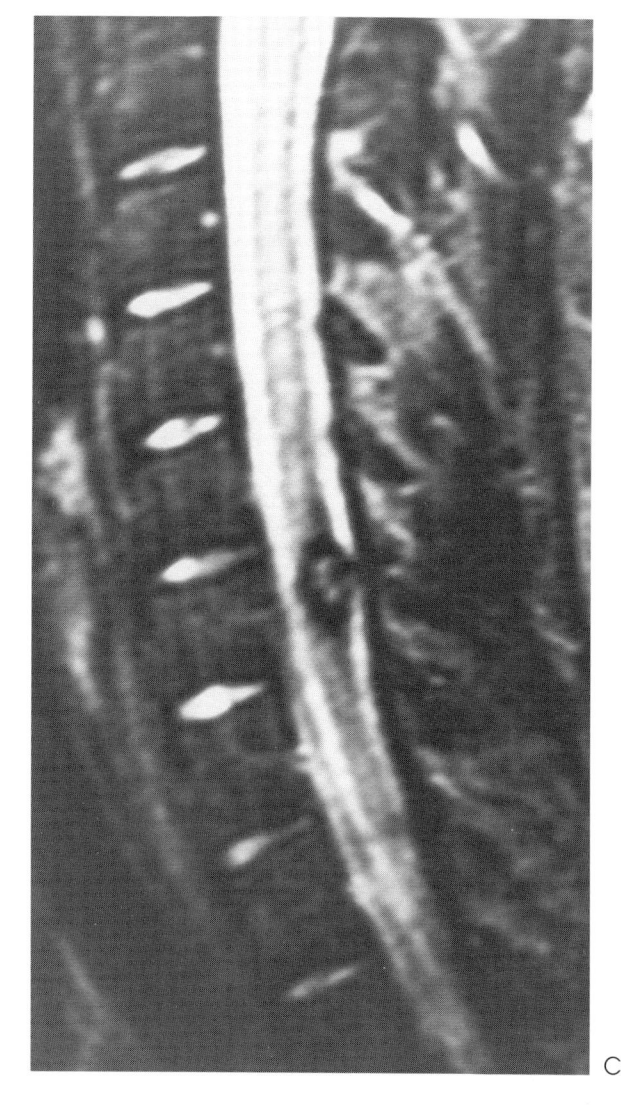

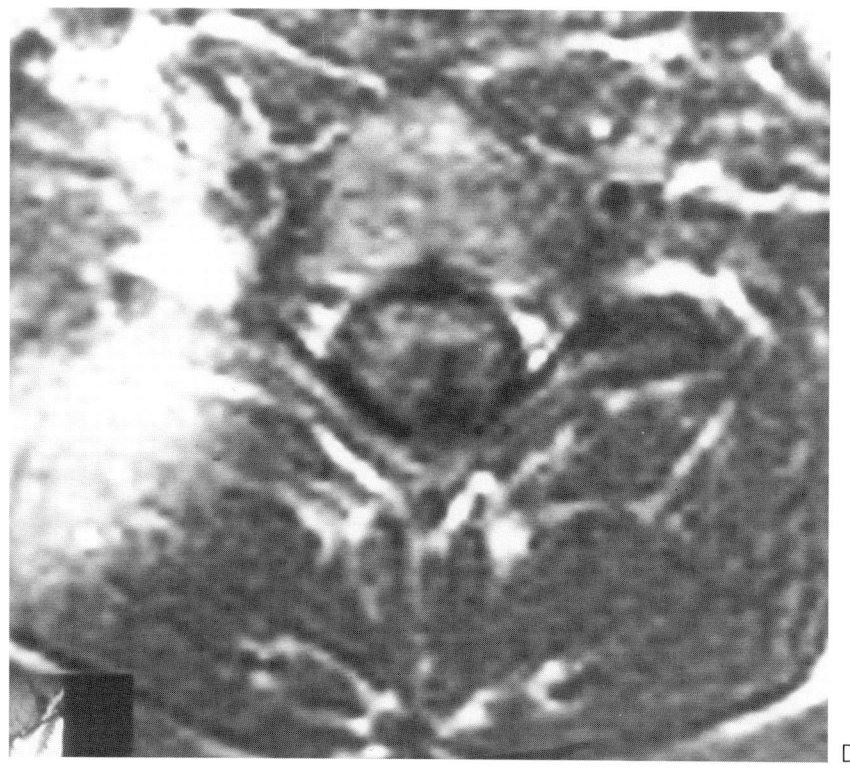

C

D

TEACHING ATLAS OF SPINE IMAGING

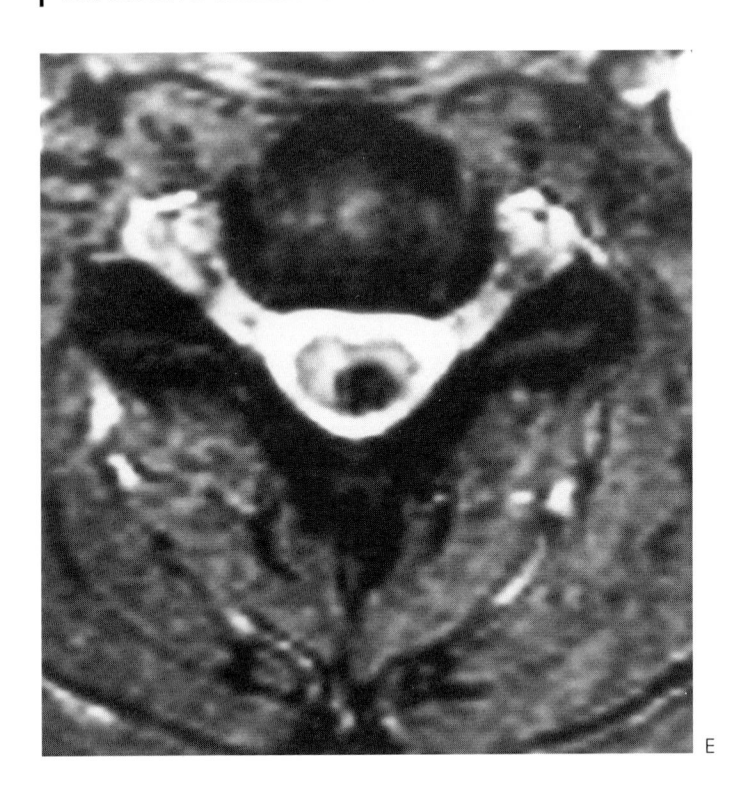

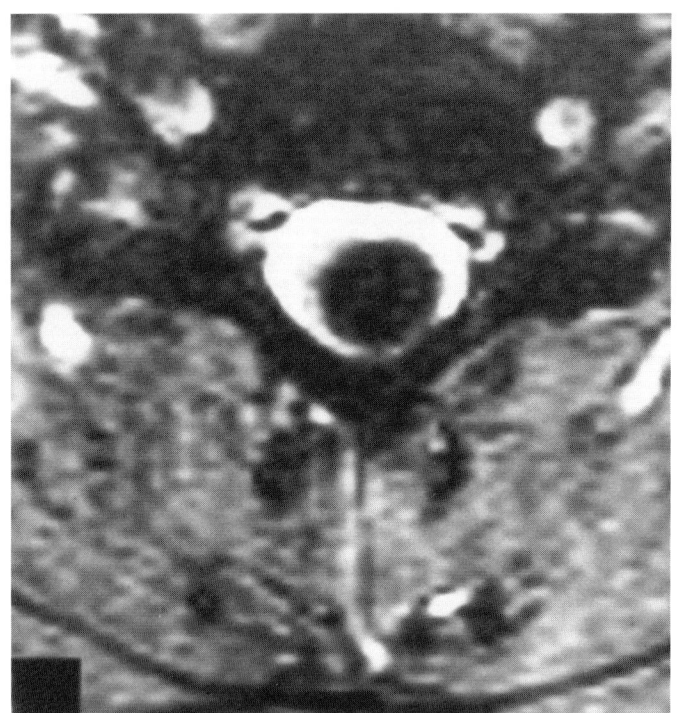

Radiologic Findings (continued)

(Fig. E) Axial long TR image at the level of C5-6.

(Fig. F) Axial gradient echo image at the level of C6.

Diagnosis

Cavernous angioma of the spinal cord.

Differential Diagnosis

- intramedullary hematoma
- ependymoma

Discussion

The short TR image in the sagittal plane (Fig. A) reveals an oval-shaped ring of decreased signal intensity in the central portion of the cervical spinal cord at the C6 level. The intermediate and long TR images (Figs. B and C) reveal that the lesion now appears as a rather thick-walled oval of decreased signal intensity with a small central area of decreased signal intensity along the dorsal margin. In addition, small streaks of decreased signal intensity extend superior and inferior to the mass.

PEARLS

- The appearance is very typical of a cavernous angioma, which exhibits a central appearance of increased signal intensity with a peripheral margin of decreased signal intensity that has a poorly defined outer margin. The decreased peripheral margin is thought to be secondary to subclinical areas of hemorrhage with resulting staining of the surrounding tissue with hemosiderin.

- Angiography will not reveal a vascular blush in cases of cavernous angioma as they are angiographically occult.

PITFALL

- When gradient echo imaging is used for evaluation, the magnetic susceptibility artifact will result in the spurious appearance of the lesion being larger than it actually is.

The axial short TR image reveals the mass in the dorsal aspect of the spinal cord (Fig. D). The spinal cord is slightly prominent and bulges dorsally at this level. At the C5-6 level (Fig. E), which is at the upper margin of the mass, it appears as a rounded area of decreased signal intensity in the left dorsal portion of the cord.

The axial gradient echo image at the level of C6 (Fig. F) reveals that the lesion again appears as decreased signal intensity but now appears to occupy the entire diameter of the spinal cord. This spuriously enlarged appearance is because the gradient echo images are more susceptible to the magnetic susceptibility artifact than the long TR images and the short TR images are the least susceptible to magnetic susceptibility artifact.

The appearance is typical of a cavernous angioma (previously called an occult vascular malformation). The decreased signal intensity areas are secondary to deposition of hemosiderin which is thought to arise from small hemorrhages or leakage of blood cells into the tissue. These lesions typically exhibit the increased signal intensity central portion which is seen here.

The lesion was successfully removed surgically.

Intramedullary hematoma is unlikely in the absence of an underlying lesion such as a cavernous angioma. Ependymomas of the spinal cord may be associated with areas of hemosiderin deposition and so may be a diagnositic consideration. However, ependymomas typically exhibit enhancement on the postinfusion study.

TEACHING ATLAS OF SPINE IMAGING

Case 17

Clinical Presentation

Metallic plate and postoperative change in the cervical spine.

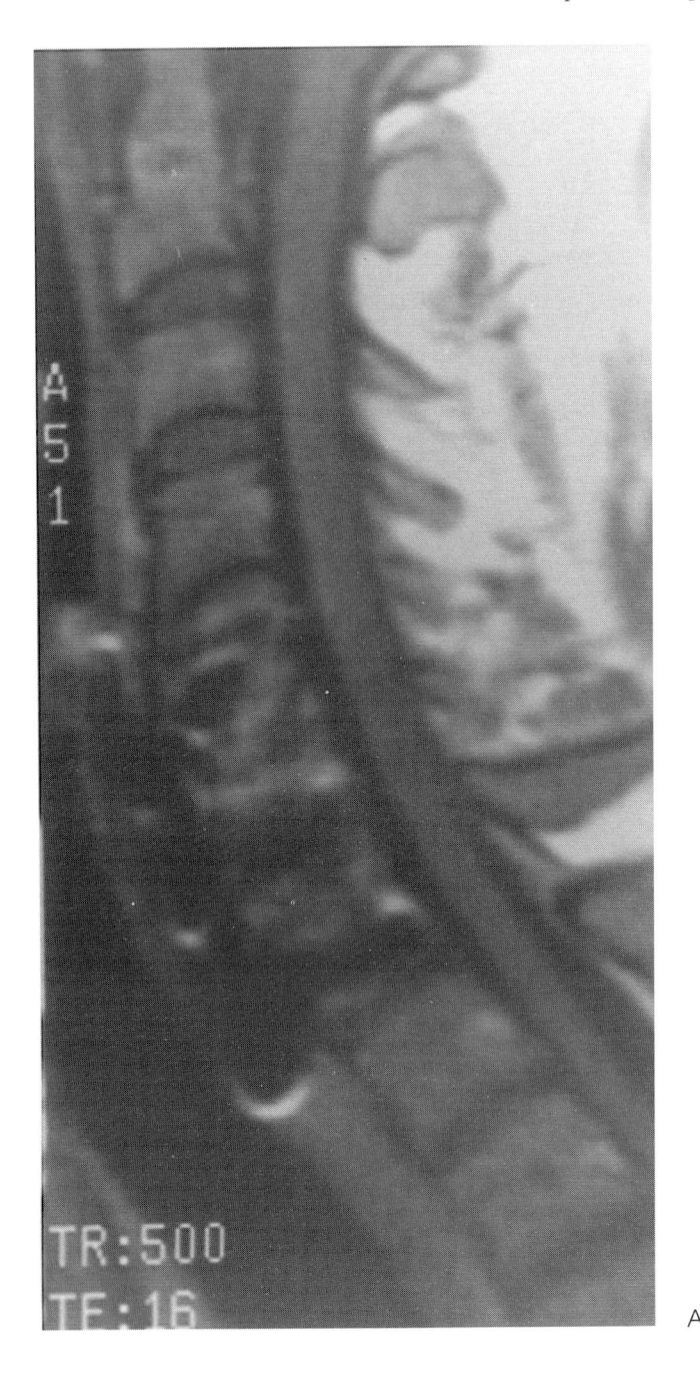

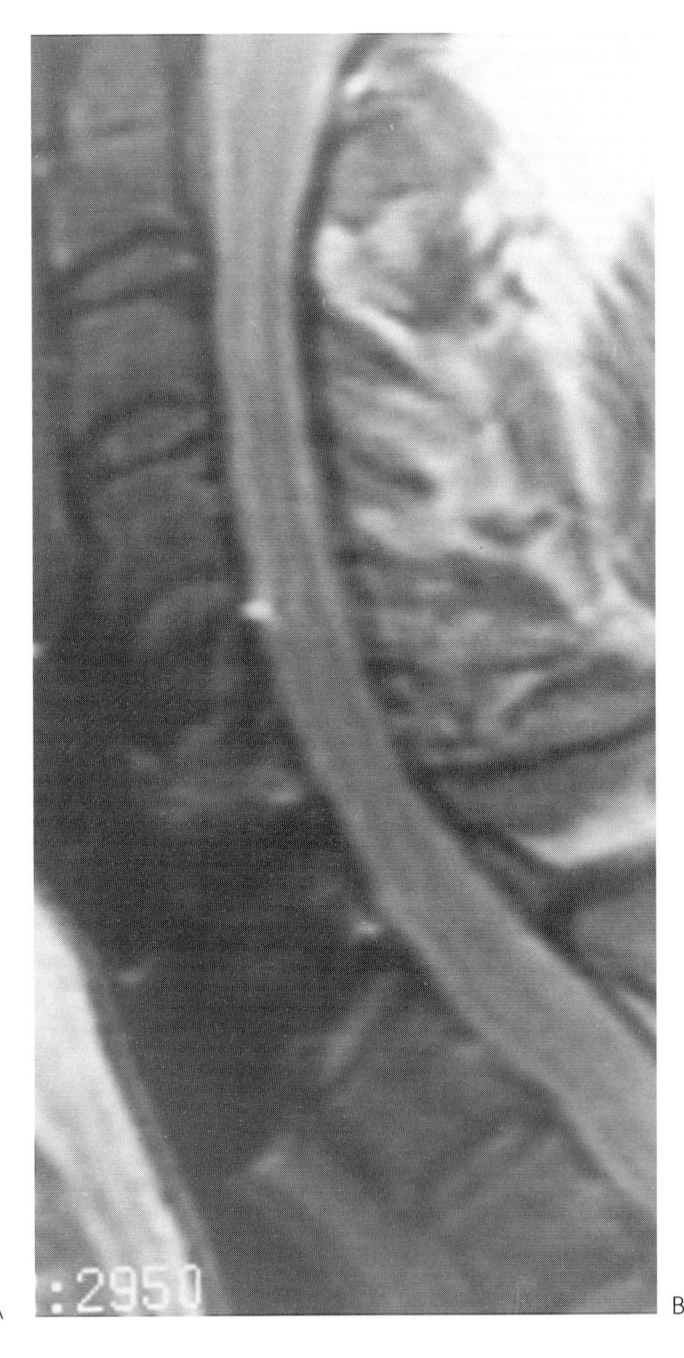

Radiologic Findings

(Fig. A) Sagittal short TR image of the cervical spine.
(Fig. B) Sagittal intermediate TR image of the cervical spine.

UNKNOWNS

C

D

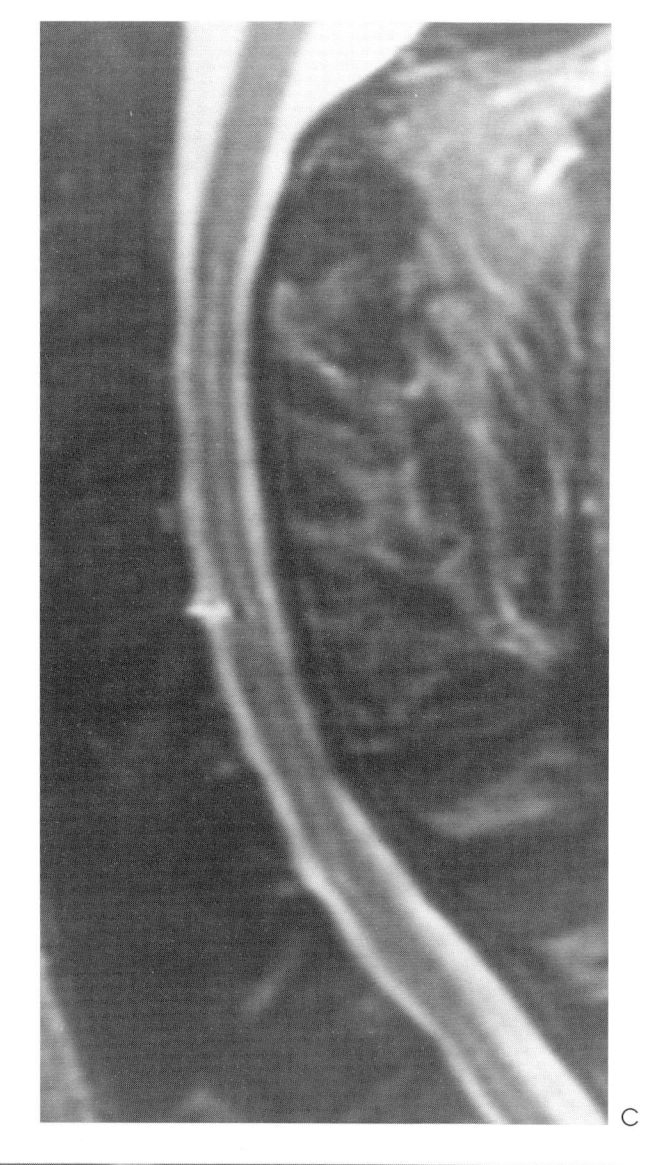

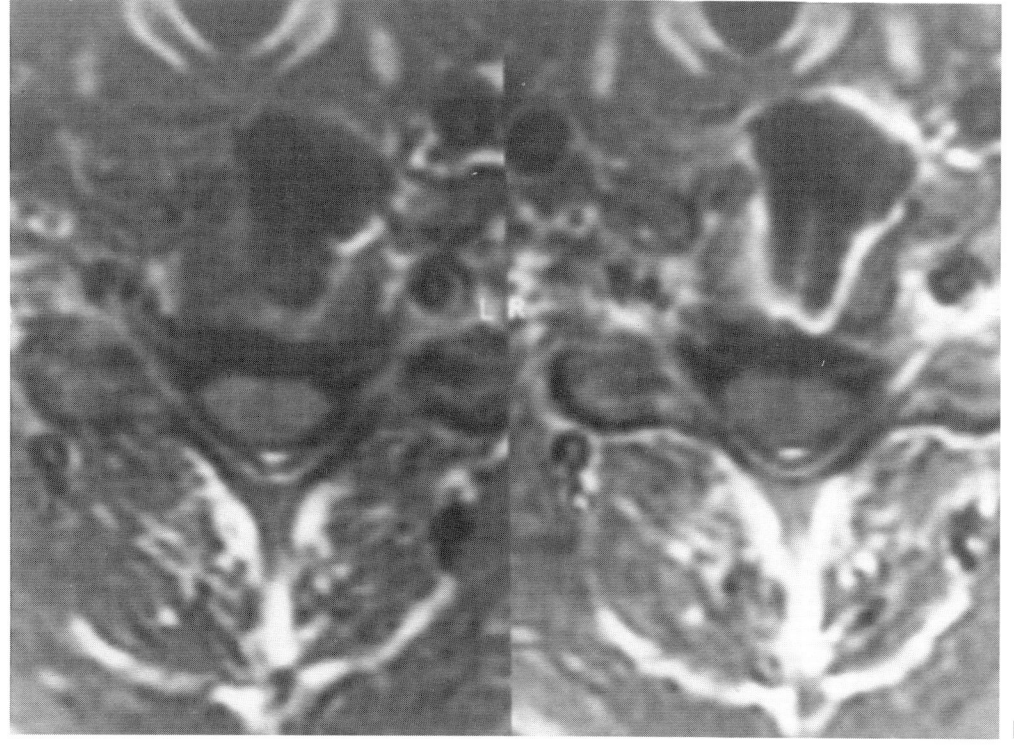

839

TEACHING ATLAS OF SPINE IMAGING

E

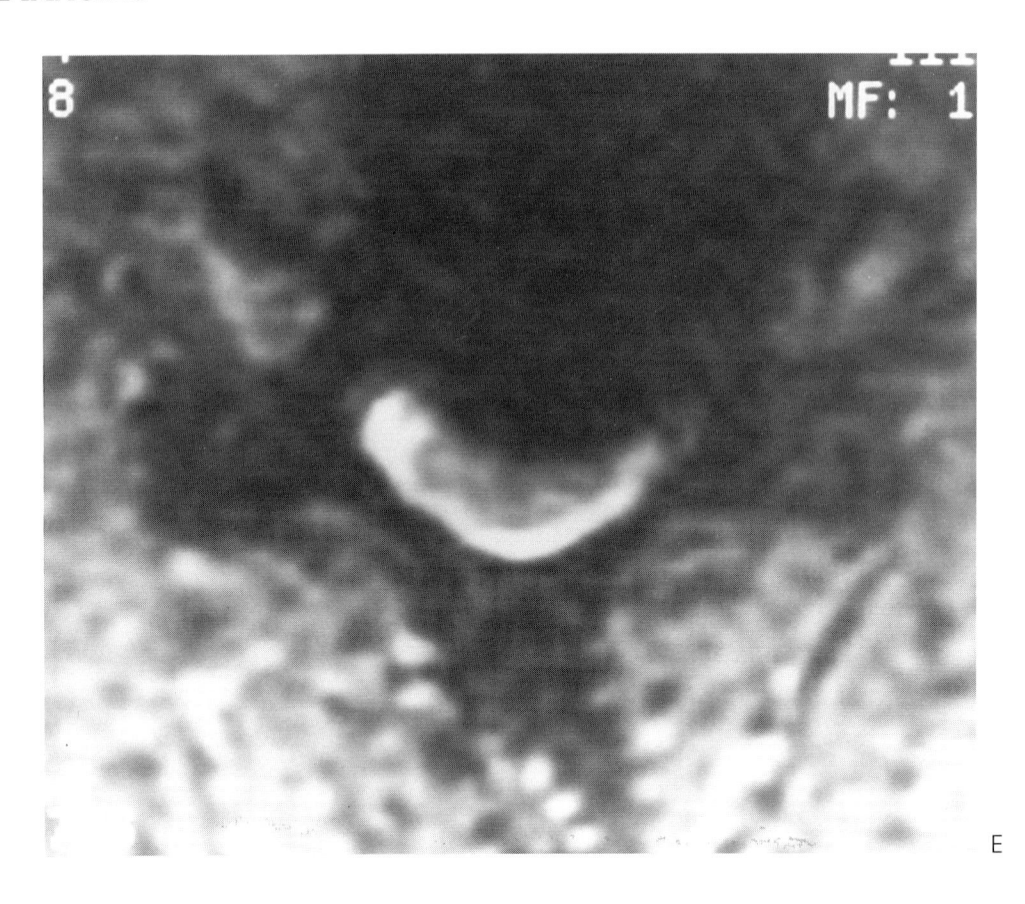

Radiologic Findings (continued)

(Fig. C) Sagittal long TR image of the cervical spine.

(Fig. D) Pre- (*left*) and postcontrast (*right*) axial short TR images of the cervical spine at the level of C6.

(Fig. E) Axial gradient echo image at the level of C6.

Diagnosis

Metallic fusion plate and fixating screws.

Differential Diagnosis

- metallic fixation device, with resulting artifacts

Discussion

The patient had previous surgery for removal of herniated discs at the C5-6 level and at the C6-7 level. At the time of surgery, fusion plugs were put in place, and a metallic fixating plate was utilized to hold the fusion plugs in place. The metallic plate caused magnetic susceptibility artifact. On the various sagittal images (Figs. A to C), there is progressively greater degradation of the images with the longer TR images.

PEARL
- Comparison with plain film evaluation would demonstrate the presence of the metallic fixating plate and confirm the diagnosis of these postoperative changes. Magnetic resonance imaging with its capability for multiplanar imaging will generally allow evaluation of the spinal cord and surrounding subarachnoid space. In this patient, the spinal cord and normal appearing subarachnoid space are well demonstrated in the short TR images in the sagittal (Fig. A) and axial (Fig. D) planes.

UNKNOWNS

PITFALL
- It is important to be aware of the artifacts generated by metallic devices so that these artifacts are not mistaken for a true abnormality.

The pre- and postcontrast axial short TR images (Fig. D) reveal a wedge-shaped area of decreased signal intensity anterior to the spine with a peripheral rim of increased signal intensity on the left side. After the infusion of contrast, the high signal intensity linear artifact surrounds the wedge-shaped artifact. The gradient echo image (Fig. E) is severely degraded by the susceptibility artifact and gives the spurious appearance of marked encroachment on the vertebral canal.

Dotlike areas of increased signal intensity in the anterior subarachnoid space on the sagittal intermediate and long TR images (Fig. B and C) are also artifactual.

The appearance is typical for postoperative changes with metallic fixating devices in place; however, various scanner artifacts may mimic a less marked metallic device artifact.

TEACHING ATLAS OF SPINE IMAGING

Case 18

Clinical Presentation

The patient is a 35-year-old female with a history of modified radical mastectomy, chemotherapy, and bone marrow transplant, now presenting with new onset of low back pain.

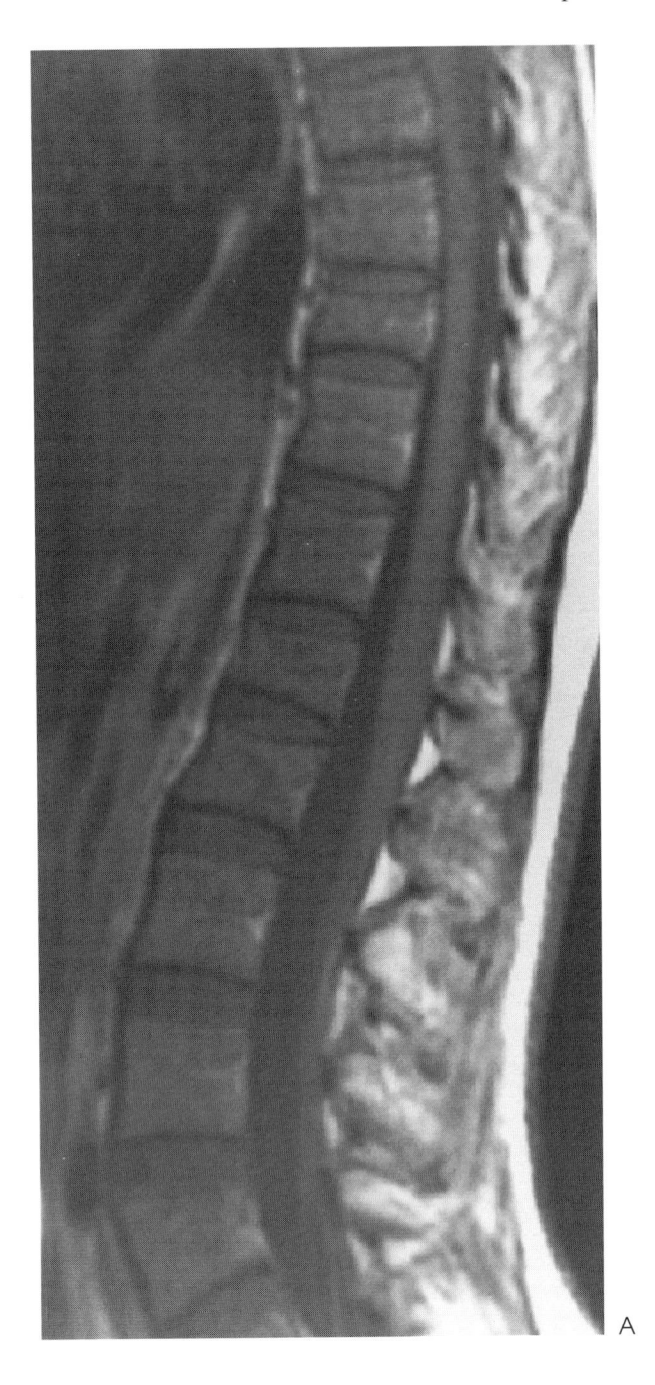

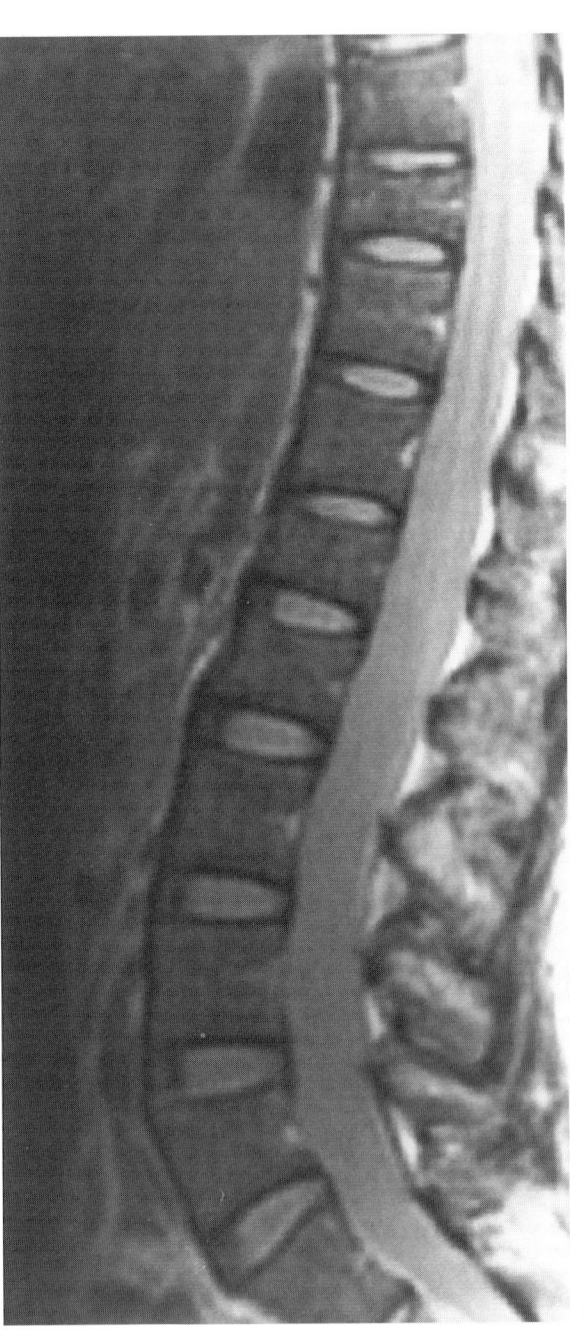

UNKNOWNS

C

D

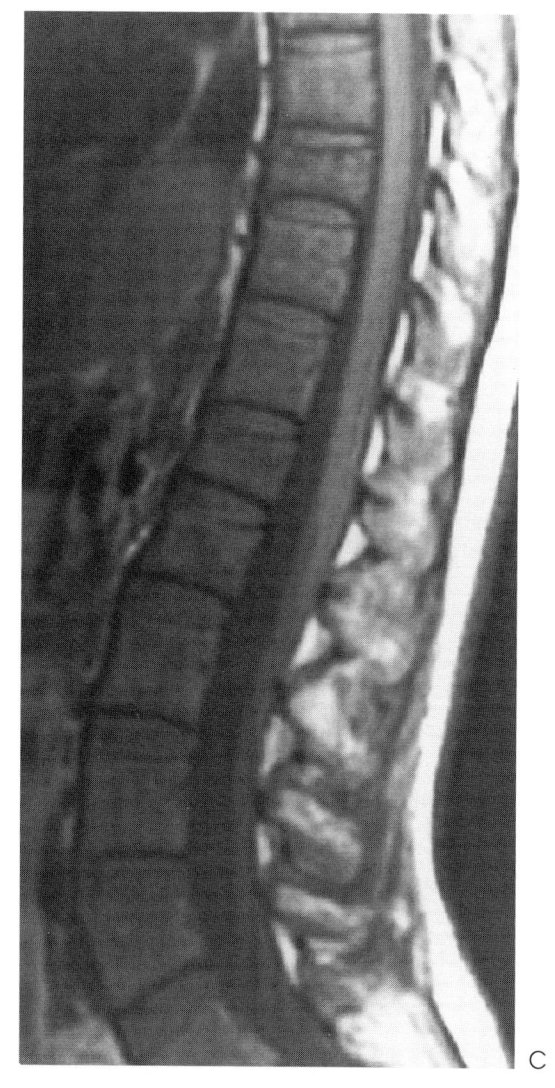

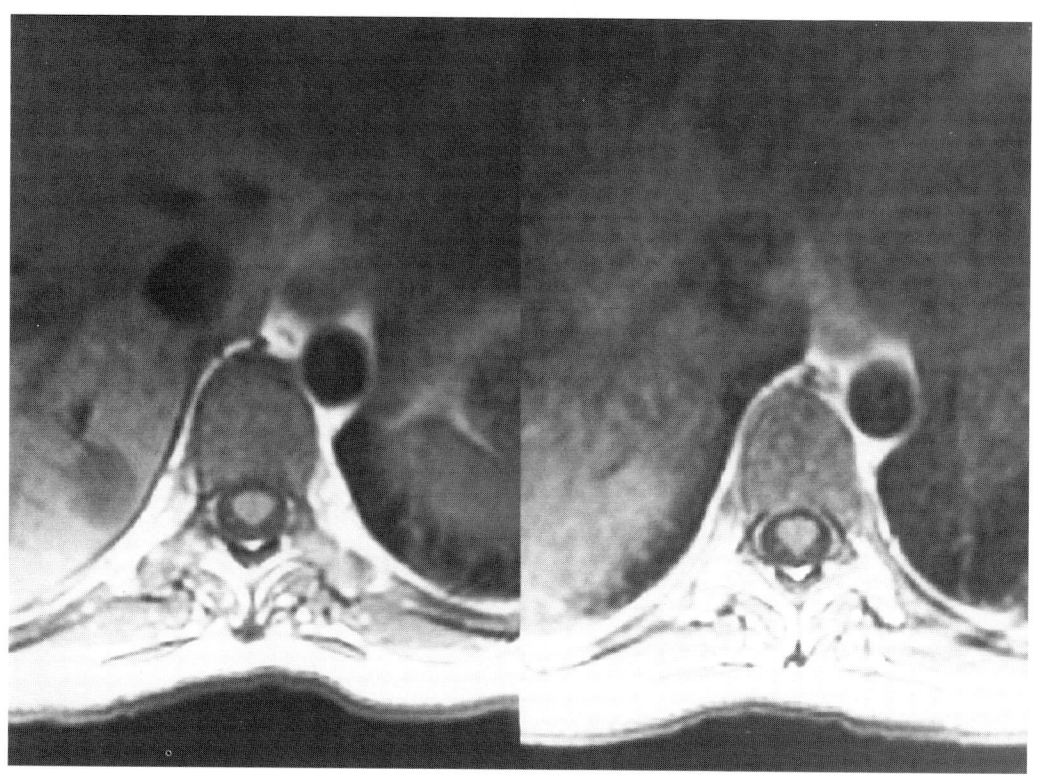

843

Radiologic Findings

(Fig. A) Sagittal short TR image.

(Fig. B) Sagittal intermediate TR image.

(Fig. C) Sagittal postcontrast image.

(Fig. D) Pre- (*left*) and postcontrast (*right*) axial short TR images.

Diagnosis

Diffuse bony metastases with pathologic fractures of T10, L1, and L2 and a metastatic deposit in the right lobe of the liver.

Differential Diagnosis

- diffuse metastases

Discussion

The abnormalities in this patient are subtle. Cursory evaluation would potentially overlook the abnormalities that are present. On the sagittal short (Fig. A) and intermediate (Fig. B) TR images, the compression fractures of the T10, L1, and L2 are apparent. In addition, on the postcontrast image (Fig. C), there is actually diffuse enhancement of the marrow of the vertebral bodies at all levels.

Close inspection of the T10, L1, and L2 vertebral bodies reveal that the pattern of enhancement is not homogeneous, but rather is somewhat heterogeneous, more so than in the remaining vertebral bodies. There is no encroachment on the vertebral canal. The axial short TR images through the level of the T10 vertebral body (Fig. D) reveal a rounded, approximately 1.8-cm rounded area of low density in the right lobe of the liver just lateral to the hemidiaphragm (*left*). On the left in Figure D, there is mottled signal intensity in the marrow of the vertebral body secondary to the metastases, and decreased signal intensity tumor in the pedicle of the vertebral bodies bilaterally. Involvement of the vertebral pedicle is typical of metastatic disease.

On the axial short TR images post contrast (*right*, in Fig. D), the T10 vertebral body also reveals the inhomogeneous pattern of enhancement within the marrow of the vertebral body secondary to the metastatic deposits. The linic metastases enhances and is no longer visible.

It is possible that this study could (inappropriately) be considered diffuse metastases from another tumor primary with metastases, such as multiple myeloma, which could have a similar appearance. However, metastases to the liver would be unusual with multiple myeloma.

PEARLS

- In a patient with known cancer, careful evaluation may reveal subtle abnormalities as seen in this case. Subtle compression fractures should not be ignored, but carefully correlated with other findings.

- Correlation with magnetic resonance findings with other imaging, such as body imaging for the evaluation of the liver, is helpful for arriving at a final diagnosis.

- Radionuclide bone scanning may be necessary for complete evaluation.

PITFALL

- When all the vertebral bodies are abnormal, there are no normal vertebral bodies available for comparison, and identification of abnormalities is difficult.

UNKNOWNS

Case 19

Clinical Presentation

The patient is a 65-year-old man with a history of recent onset of low back pain.

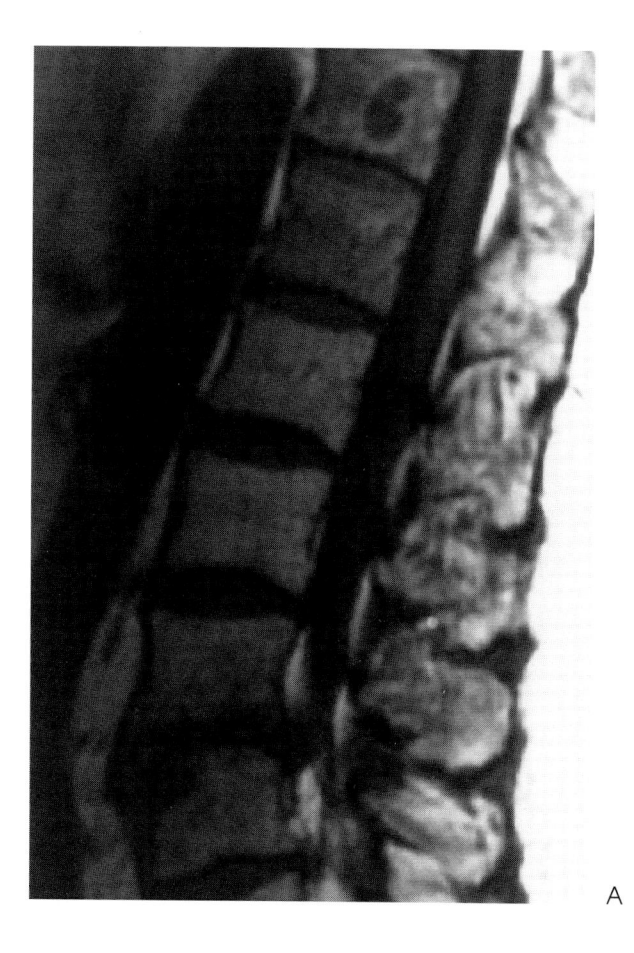

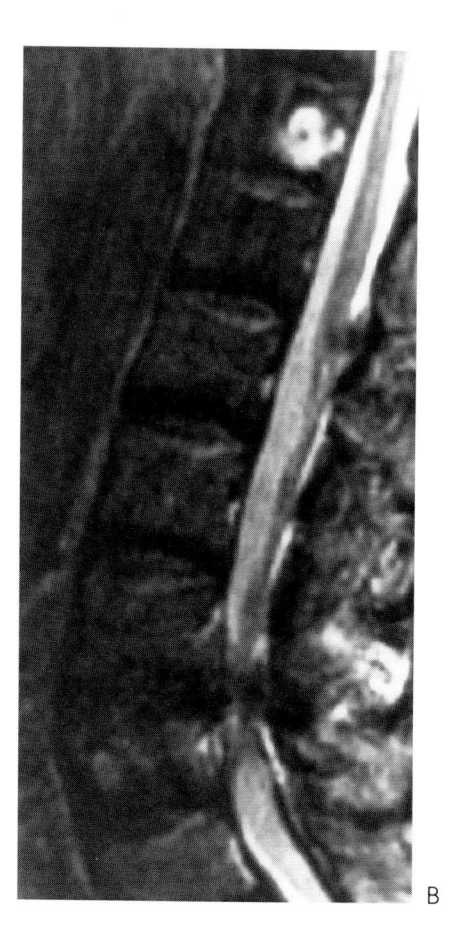

Radiologic Findings

(Fig. A) Sagittal short TR image.

(Fig. B) Sagittal long TR image.

(Fig. C) Sagittal short TR image postcontrast.

(Fig. D) Sagittal short TR image postcontrast with fat suppression technique.

TEACHING ATLAS OF SPINE IMAGING

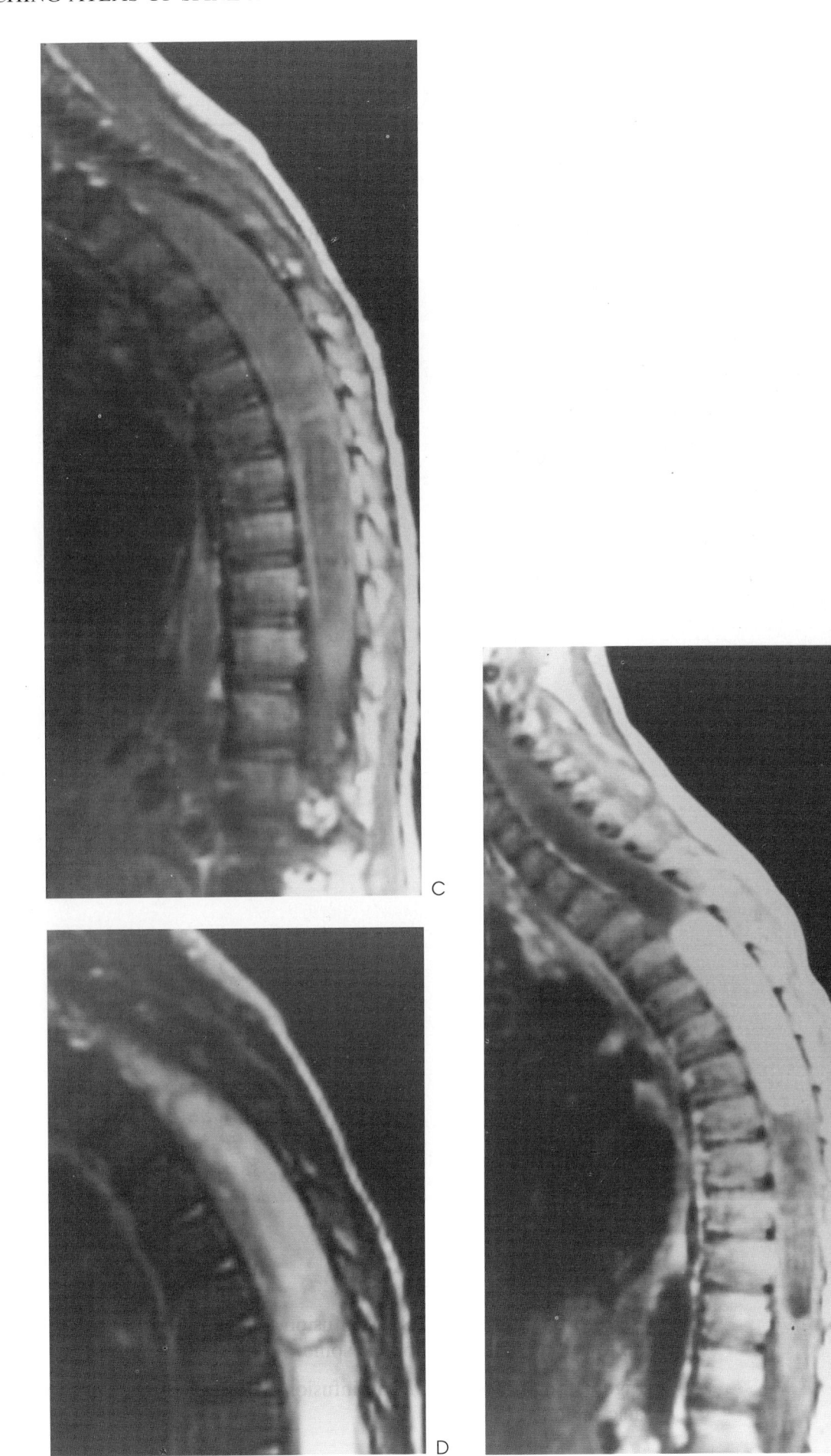

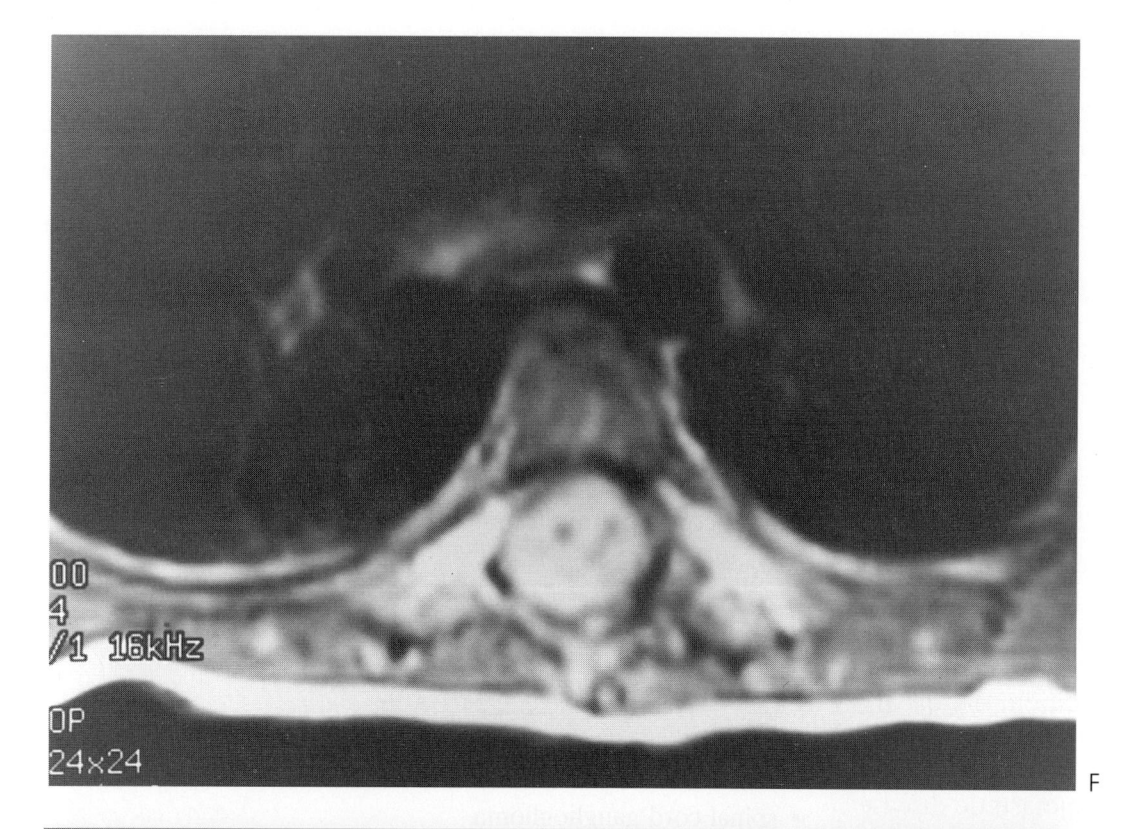

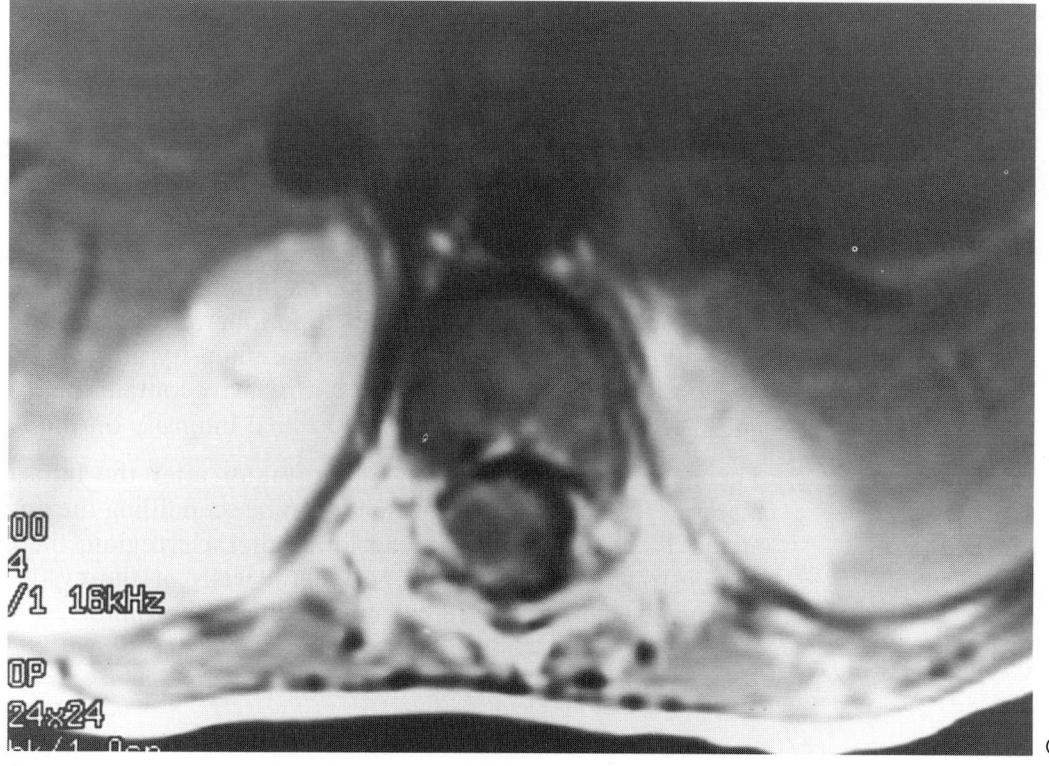

UNKNOWNS

F

G

851

Radiologic Findings (continued)

(Fig. C) Sagittal short TR preinfusion MR scan of the thoracic region.

(Fig. D) Sagittal long TR image in the upper thoracic region.

(Fig. E) Postcontrast sagittal short TR image of the lower cervical and thoracic spine.

(Fig. F) Postcontrast axial short TR image at the T4 level.

(Fig. G) Postcontrast axial short TR image at the T10 level.

Diagnosis

Spinal cord ependymoma with an associated syrinx cavity

Differential Diagnosis

- spinal cord astrocytoma
- spinal cord ependymoma
- spinal cord ganglioglioma

Discussion

There is a large, sausage-shaped mass in the mid- and upper thoracic region that is associated with a syrinx cavity above and below the mass. The syrinx cavity extends from the level of the C2 vertebra through the upper margin of the mass at the T2 level and is again visible from the inferior margin of the tumor at the T6 level and extends through the distal end of the spinal cord. The mass itself also exhibits a peripheral margin of decreased signal intensity. The areas of decreased signal intensity are consistent with areas of deposition of hemosiderin. The syrinx cavity contains high protein content and therefore appears as increased signal intensity on the long TR image.

There is dense enhancement of the tumor after the infusion of contrast material. The area of enhancement can be seen filling the entire spinal cord at the T4 level (Fig. F). In the lower thoracic region, the cystic cavity is demonstrated (Fig. G). The peripheral walls of the cystic cavity do not enhance because they are not involved with the tumor.

PEARLS

- The entire length of the spinal cord should be evaluated to determine the length of the tumor and the associated syrinx cavity. In addition, the distal lumbar thecal sac should be evaluated to rule out the presence of metastatic disease in the thecal sac.

- The presence of low signal intensity hemosiderin seen in the long TR images (Fig. D) within the tumor mass favors the diagnosis of ependymoma.

PITFALL

- Surgical removal of a lesion such as this is difficult because there is extensive involvement of the spinal cord and total removal is essentially impossible without creating severe neurologic deficit.

UNKNOWNS

Case 21

Clinical Presentation

The patient is a 52-year-old male with a clinical history of left-sided weakness; there also was a history of acute myeloid leukemia.

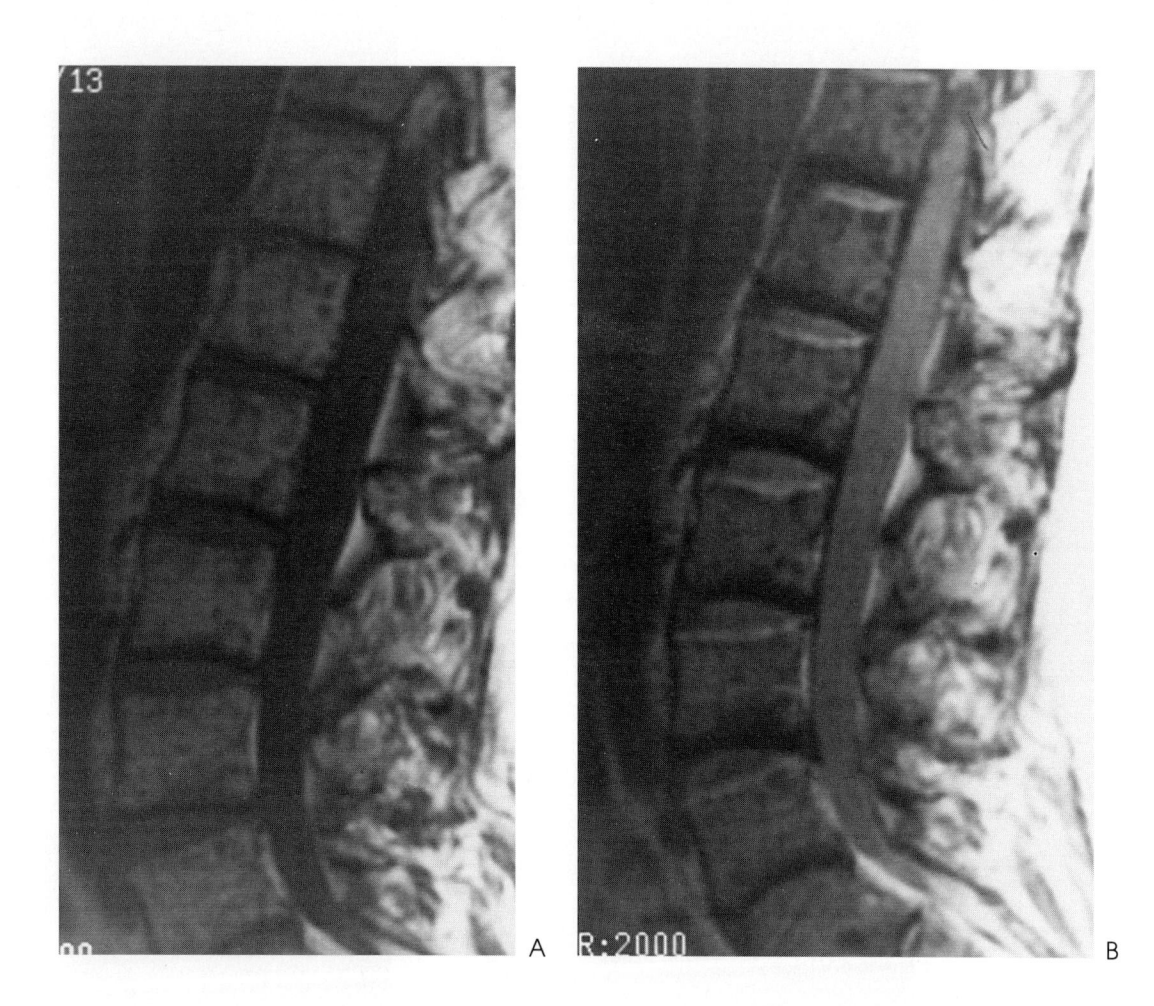

Radiologic Findings

(Fig. A) Sagittal short TR image in the lumbar spine.
(Fig. B) Sagittal intermediate TR image in the lumbar spine.

TEACHING ATLAS OF SPINE IMAGING

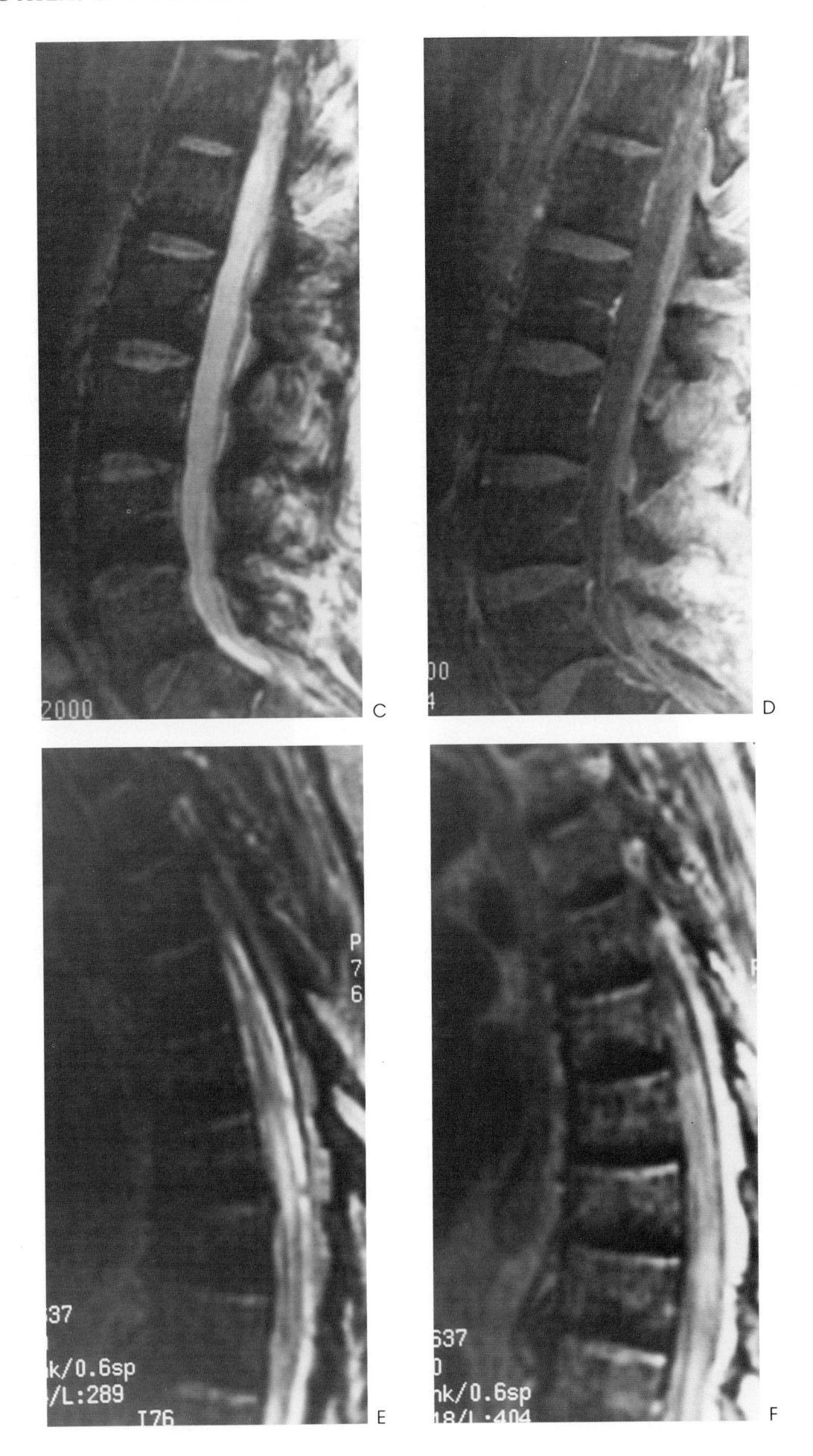

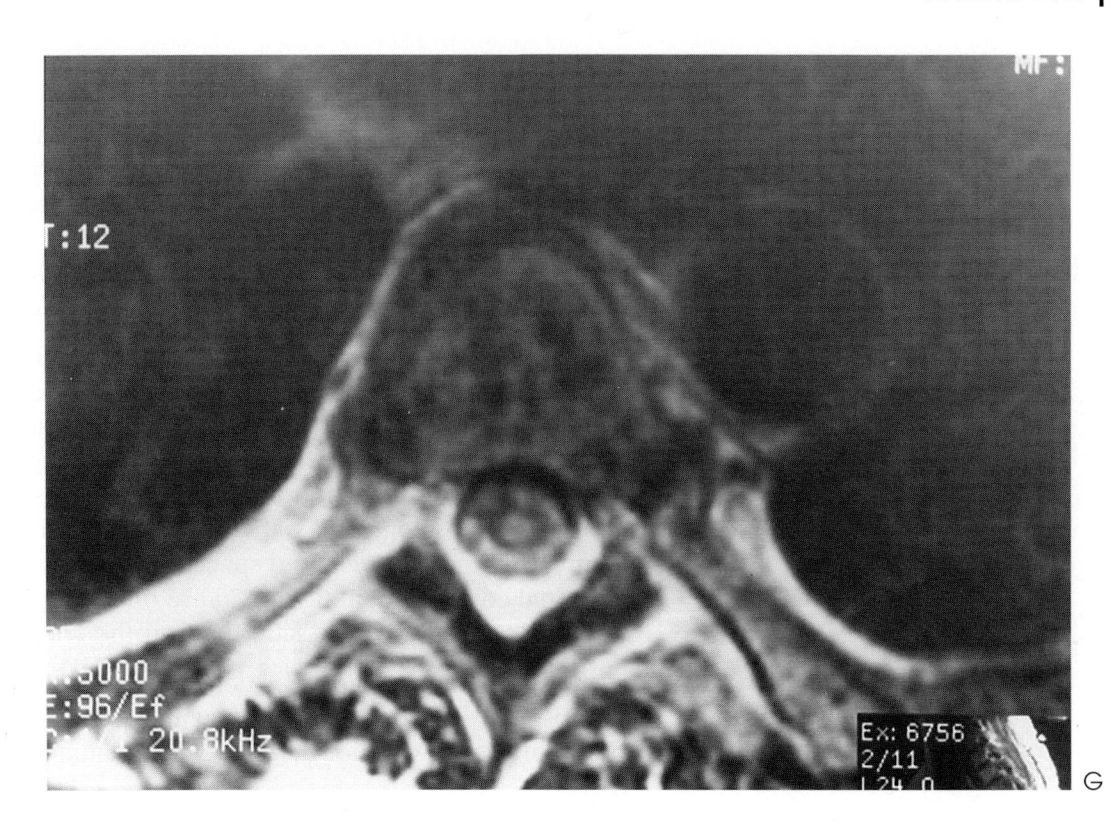

UNKNOWNS

Radiologic Findings (continued)

(Fig. C) Sagittal long TR image in the lumbar spine.

(Fig. D) Postcontrast sagittal fat suppression image in the lumbar spine.

(Fig. E) Sagittal long TR image of the thoracic spine.

(Fig. F) Postcontrast sagittal short TR image of the thoracic spine.

(Fig. G) Postcontrast axial short TR image of the thoracic spine.

Diagnosis

Leukemic infiltrate of the bone marrow; leptomeningeal carcinomatosis.

Differential Diagnosis

- multiple myeloma
- metastases from another primary

Discussion

The short (Fig. A) and intermediate (Fig. B) TR images reveal diffuse abnormal signal intensity throughout the marrow of the vertebral bodies with multiple small rounded areas of decreased signal intensity. The intermediate

TEACHING ATLAS OF SPINE IMAGING

PEARL
- Clinical history is very helpful in the evaluation of this patient.

PITFALL
- This patient has a rapid progression of symptoms and was imaged several times within a short period of time. The initial images did not reveal meningeal carcinomatosis, although the subsequent studies were grossly abnormal. The fat suppression images in this patient obliterated the presence of the bone lesions.

signal intensity sagittal images in the lumbar region (Fig. B) do not add significantly to the diagnosis; however, the long TR image reveals that the nerve roots of the cauda equina appear somewhat thickened in the midlumbar region (Fig. C). The fat-suppressed postcontrast image (Fig. D) reveals prominent enhancement of the distal spinal cord and the nerve roots of the cauda equina. The areas of abnormal signal intensity within the marrow are no longer visible and the areas within the vertebral bodies do not exhibit demonstrable enhancement postinfusion.

The sagittal long TR image of the thoracic region (Fig. E) reveals increased signal intensity within the central portion of the thoracic spinal cord. The postcontrast short sagittal TR image (Fig. F) at the same level reveals diffuse enhancement of the spinal cord and surrounding subarachnoid space. This finding is consistent with intramedullary cancer as well as meningeal carcinomatosis. The postcontrast axial short TR image (Fig. G) reveals the enhancement within the subarachnoid space as well as within the central portion of the spinal cord. Incidentally noted are bilateral pleural effusions, which are slightly larger on the right side than on the left.

Although fat suppression postcontrast images are helpful in this case to diagnose the presence of meningeal carcinomatosis and intramedullary spread of tumor, was not helpful in the evaluation of the bony metastases.

Metastases from another primary such as prostate carcinoma is unlikely because the meningeal component is not likely in a patient with prostate cancer.

UNKNOWNS

Case 22

Clinical Presentation

The patient is a 37-year-old male with progressive neurologic deficit.

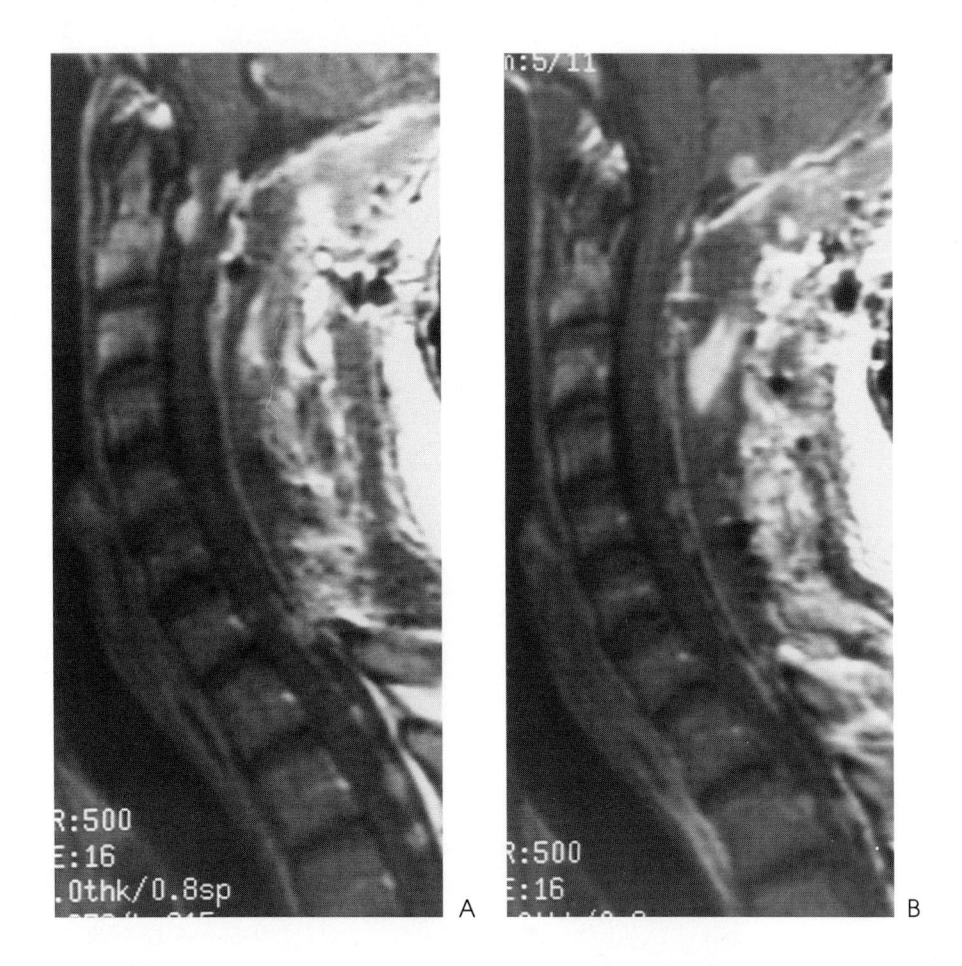

Radiologic Findings

(Fig. A) Postcontrast sagittal short TR image of the cervical spine.//
(Fig. B) Postcontrast parasagittal short TR image of the cervical spine.

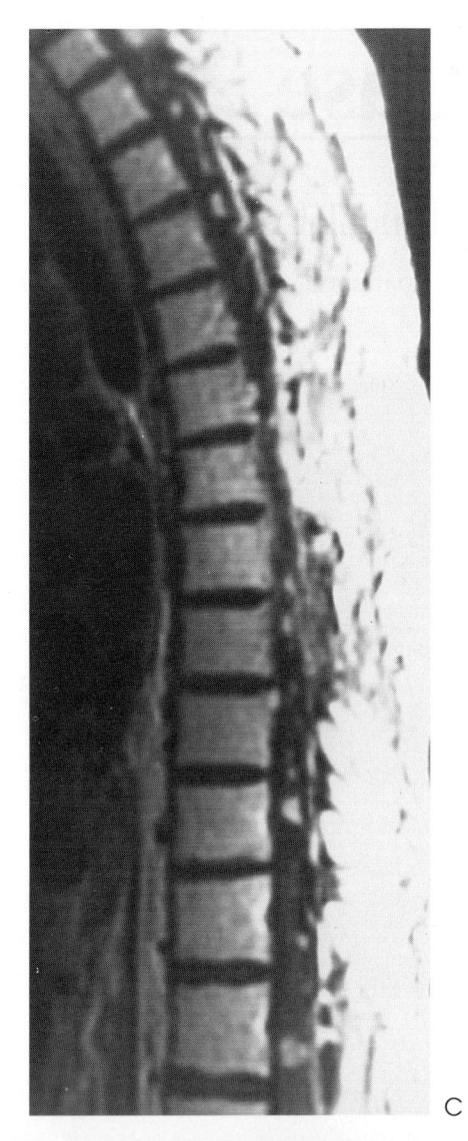

TEACHING ATLAS OF SPINE IMAGING

C

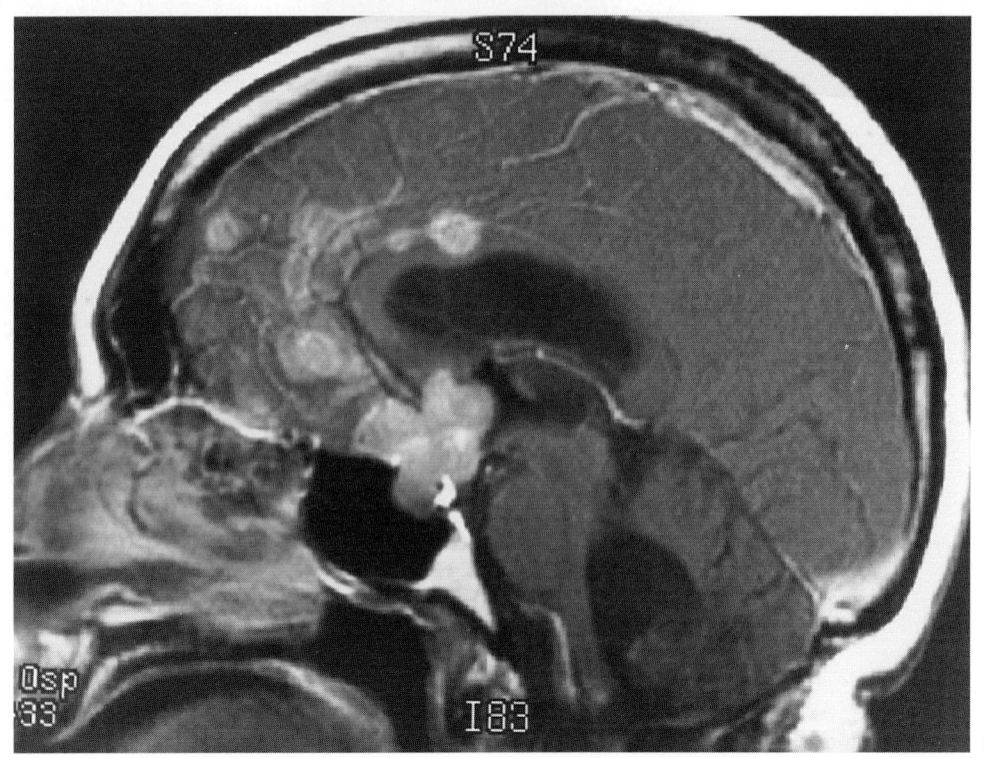

D

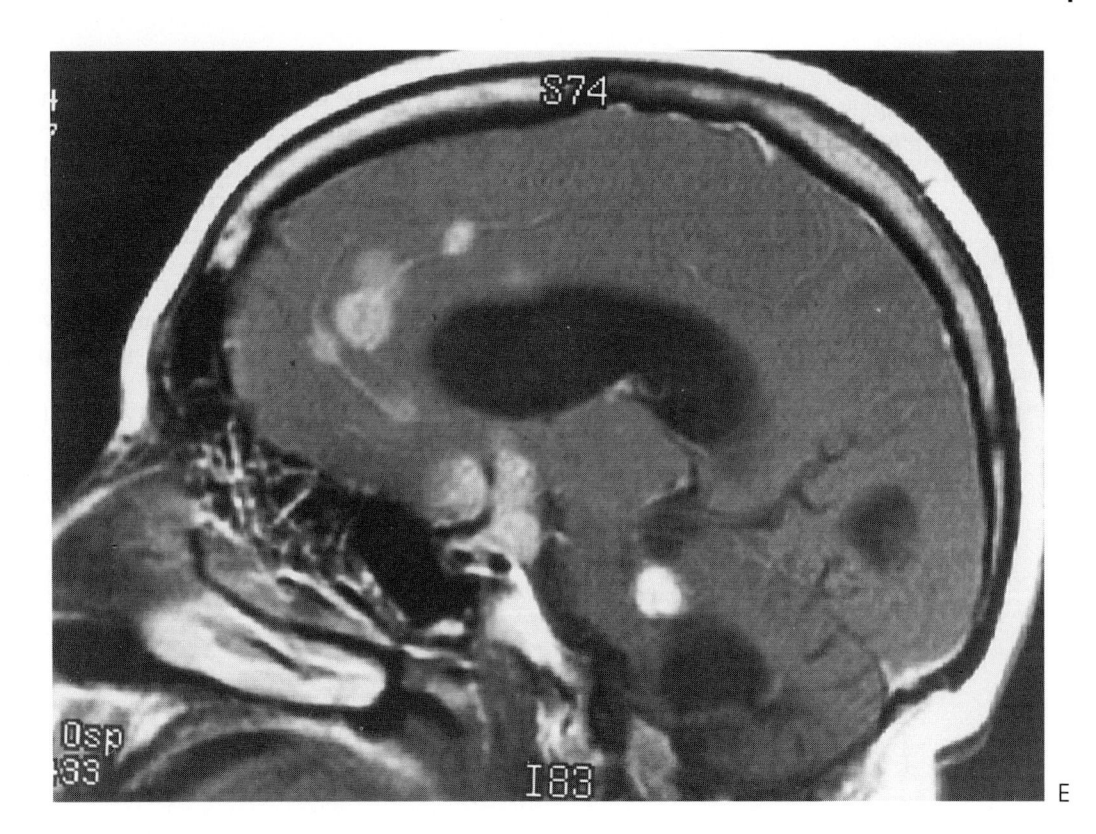

UNKNOWNS

Radiologic Findings (continued)

(Fig. C) Postcontrast sagittal short TR image of the thoracic spine.

(Fig. D) Postcontrast sagittal short TR image of the brain.

(Fig. E) Postcontrast parasagittal short TR image of the brain.

Diagnosis

von Hippel-Lindau syndrome with multiple spinal and cerebral hemangioblastomas.

Differential Diagnosis

- multiple hemangioblastoma (in the patient with von Hippel-Lindau disease)

- multiple schwannomas of the spine and multiple cerebral meningiomas (in the patient with neurofibromatosis type 2)

Discussion

The patient has multiple enhancing masses measuring less than 1 cm throughout the cervical and thoracic spinal cord. Postsurgical changes are visible

TEACHING ATLAS OF SPINE IMAGING

PEARL
- The clinical history is important in this patient.

PITFALL
- In the absence of sufficient history, it is important to evaluate the presence of postsurgical changes.

in both the cervical (Figs. A and B) and thoracic spine areas (Fig. C) where the patient previously underwent laminectomy. Areas of decreased signal intensity in the soft tissues dorsally in the cervical region are secondary to the magnetic susceptibility artifact that is seen following surgery. The patient previously underwent occipital craniectomy; the fourth ventricle is enlarged secondary to surgery in the posterior fossa for removal of a cerebellar hemangioblastoma.

The brain has multiple enhancing lesions of varying sizes (Figs. D and E), which are located in the region of the midbrain and the suprasellar cistern and along the interhemispheric falx.

UNKNOWNS

Case 23

Clinical Presentation

The patient is a 47-year-old female with acute myelogenous leukemia.

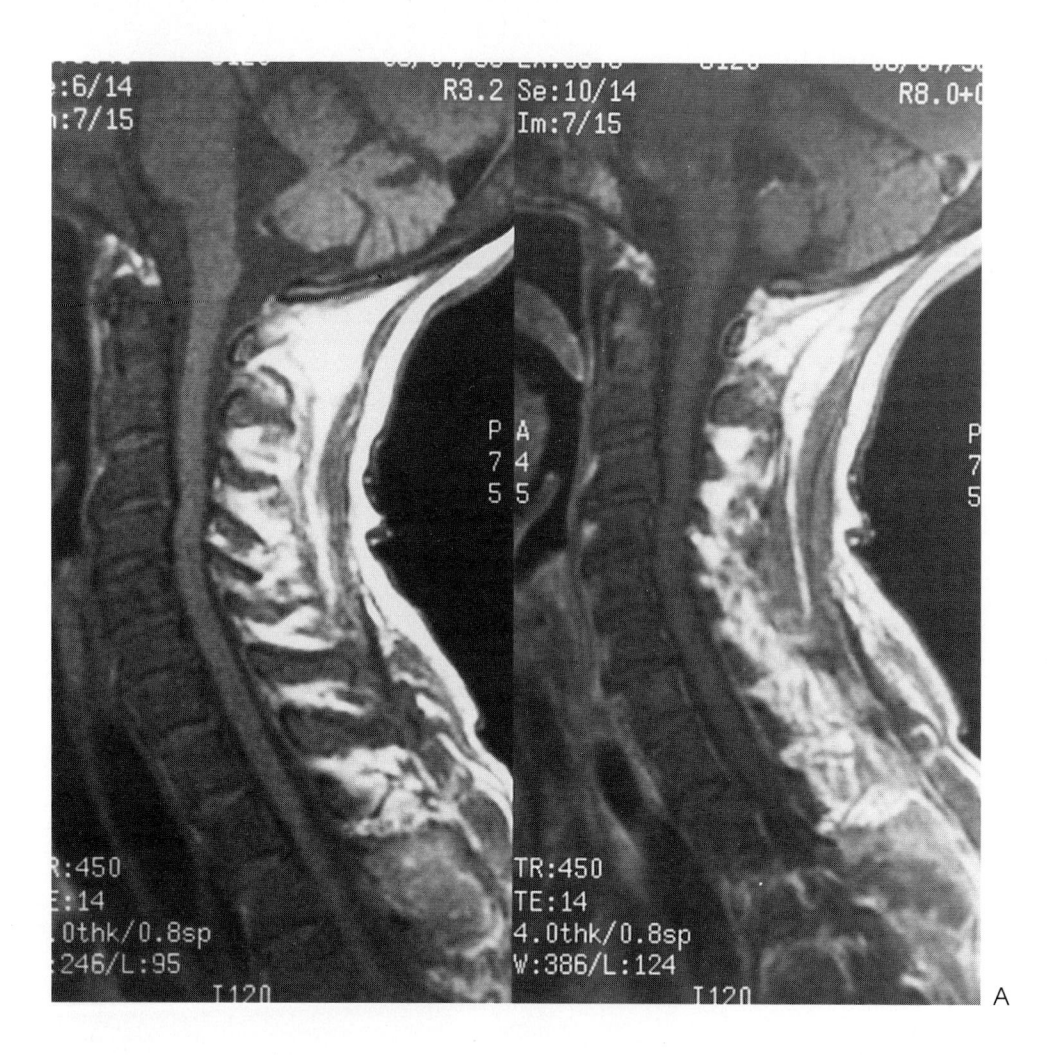

Radiologic Findings

(Fig. A) Pre- (*left*) and postcontrast (*right*) sagittal short TR images of the cervical spine.

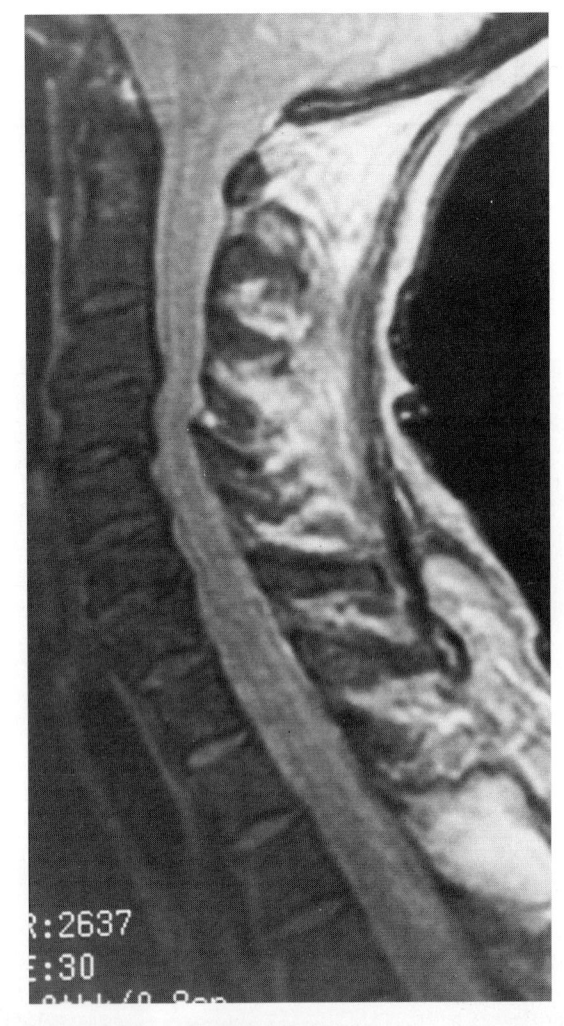

TEACHING ATLAS OF SPINE IMAGING

B

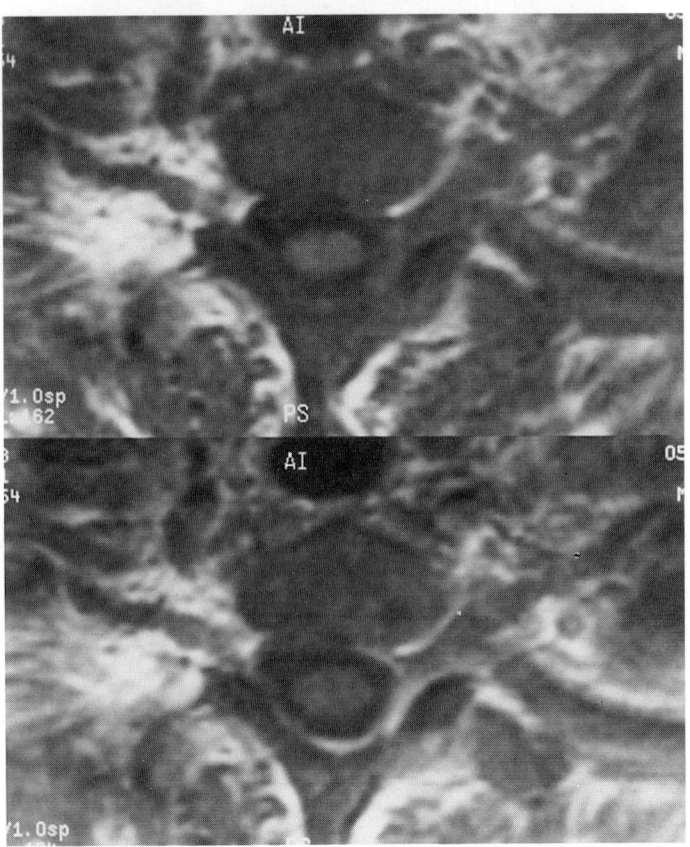

C

862

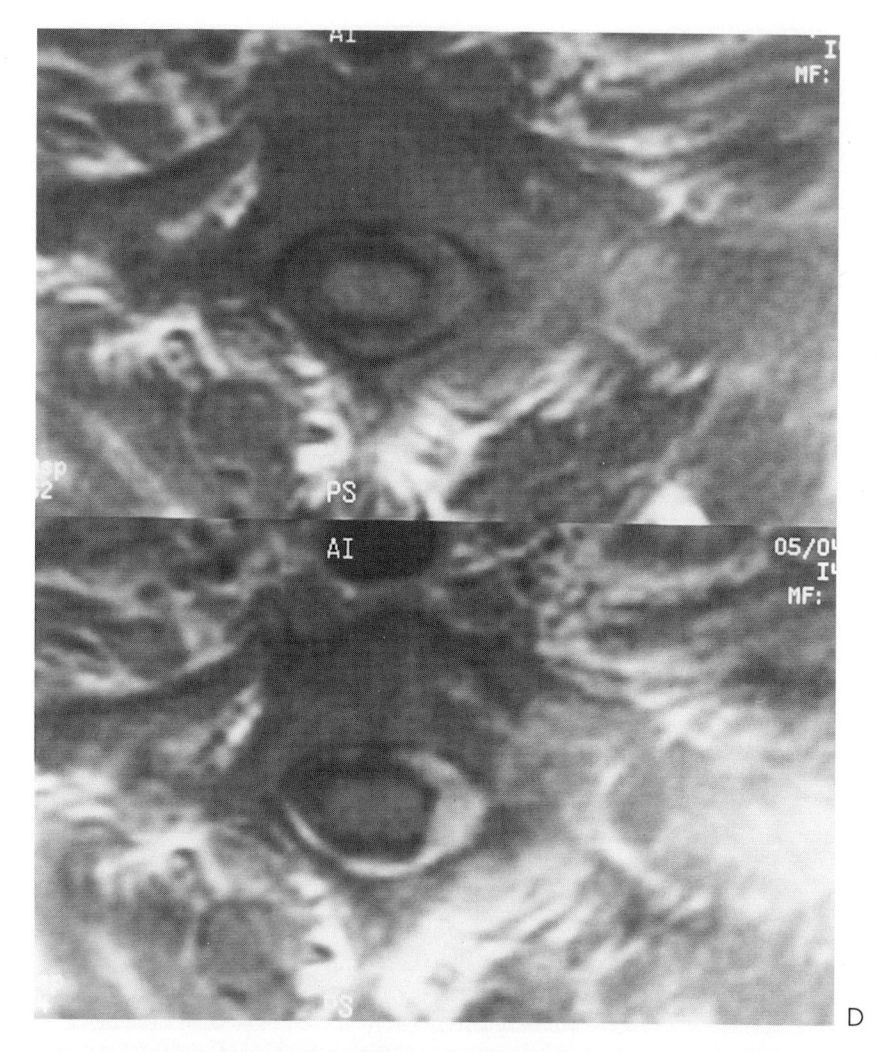

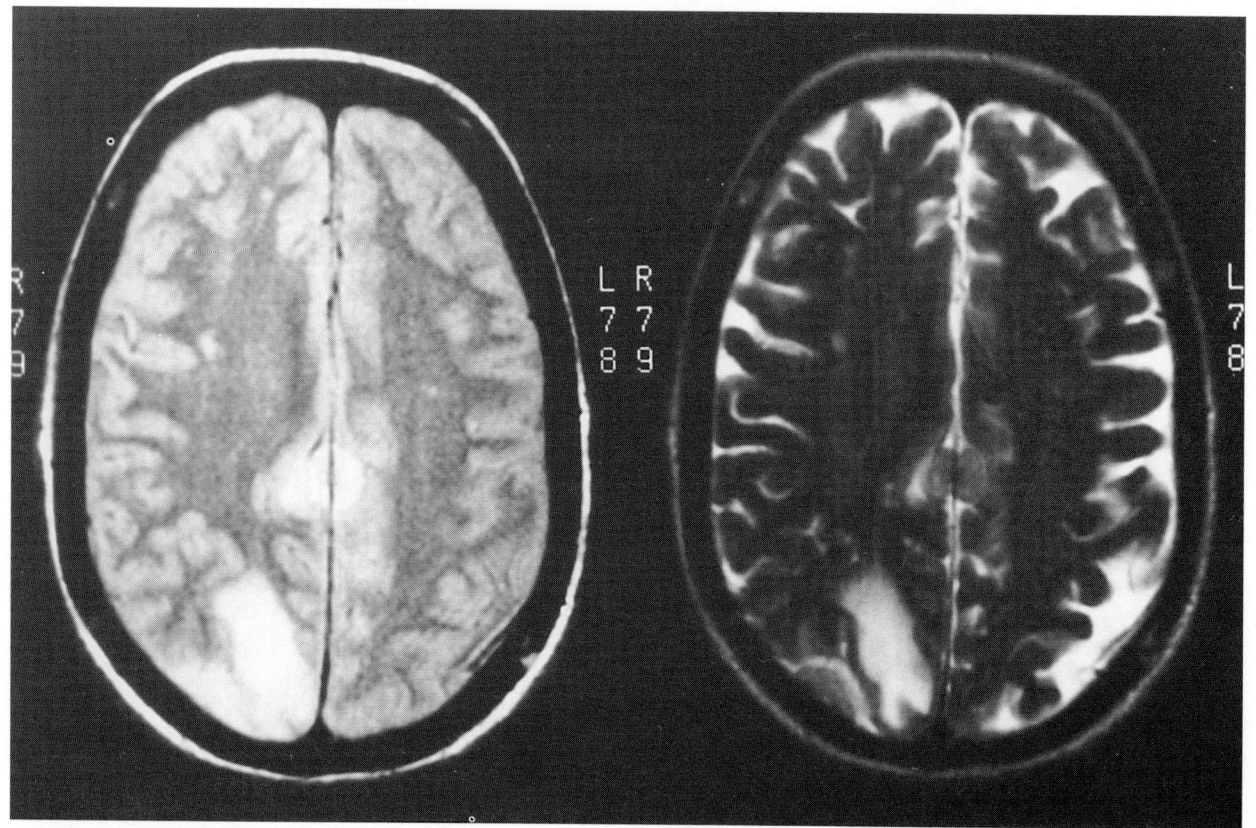

UNKNOWNS

D

E

863

TEACHING ATLAS OF SPINE IMAGING

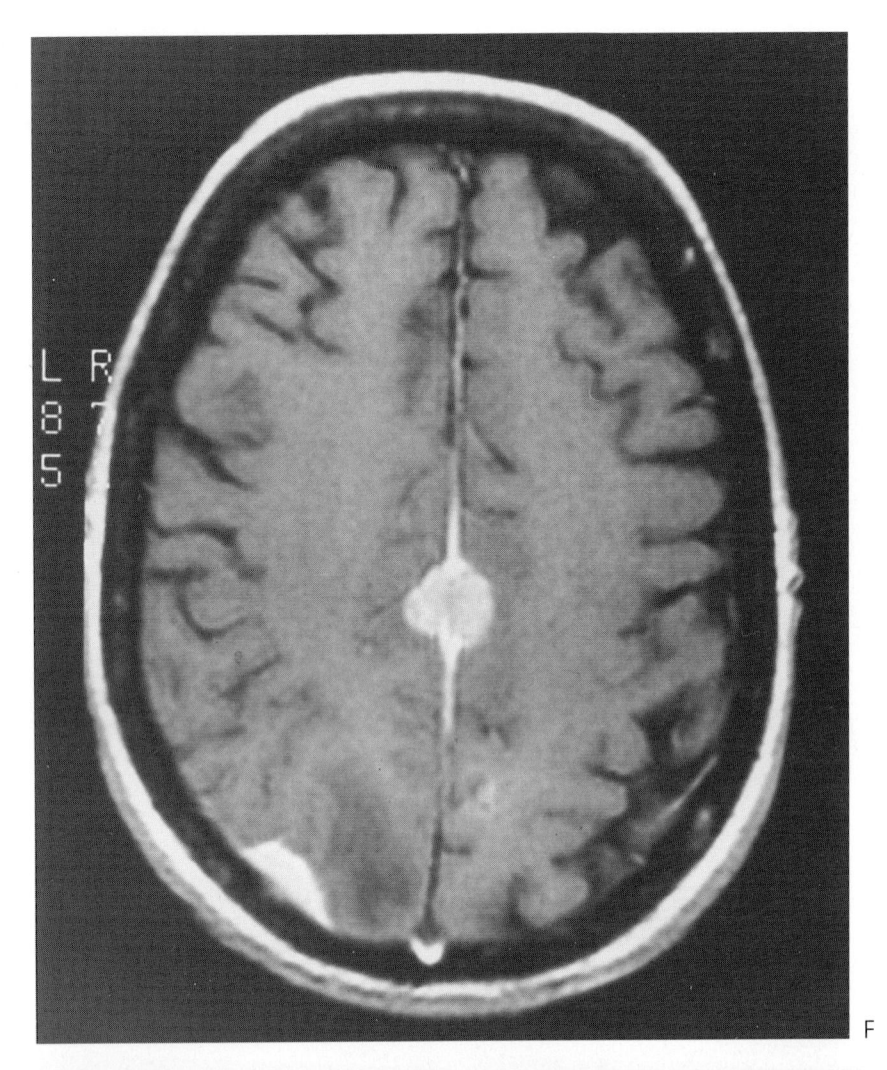

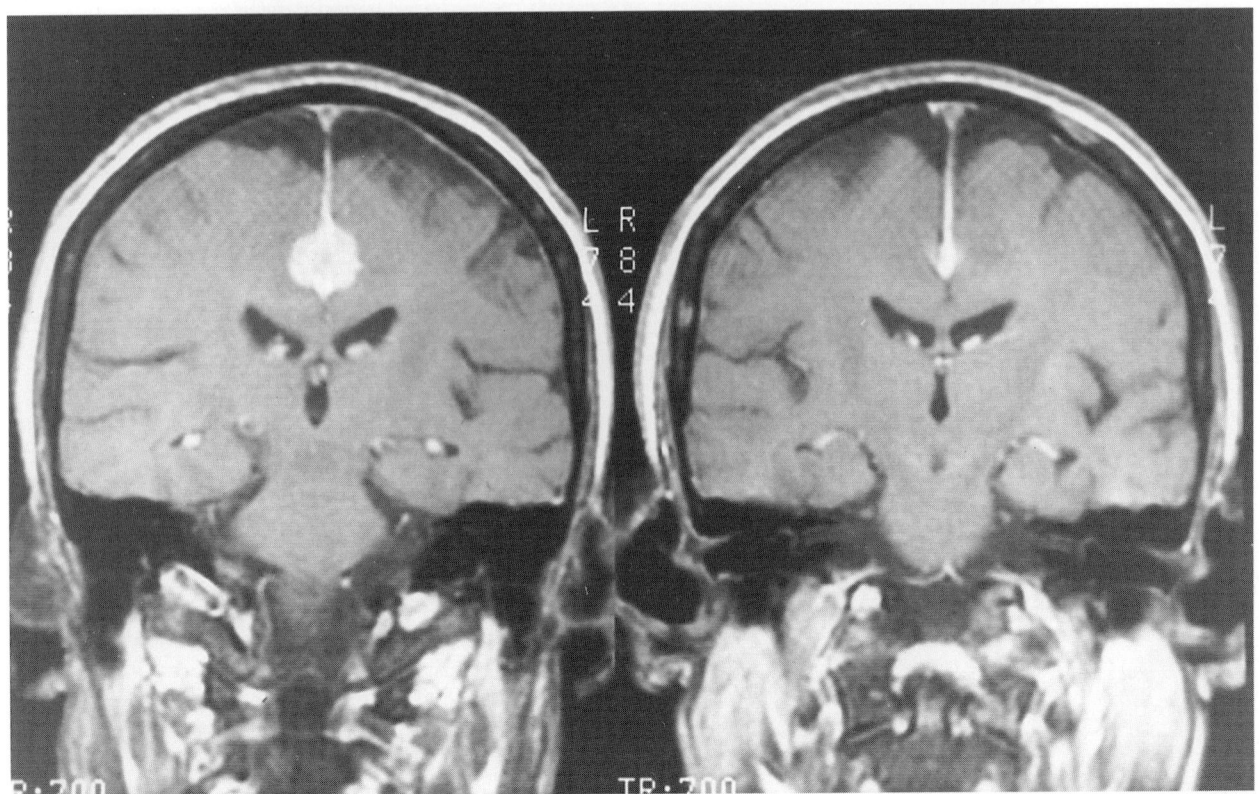

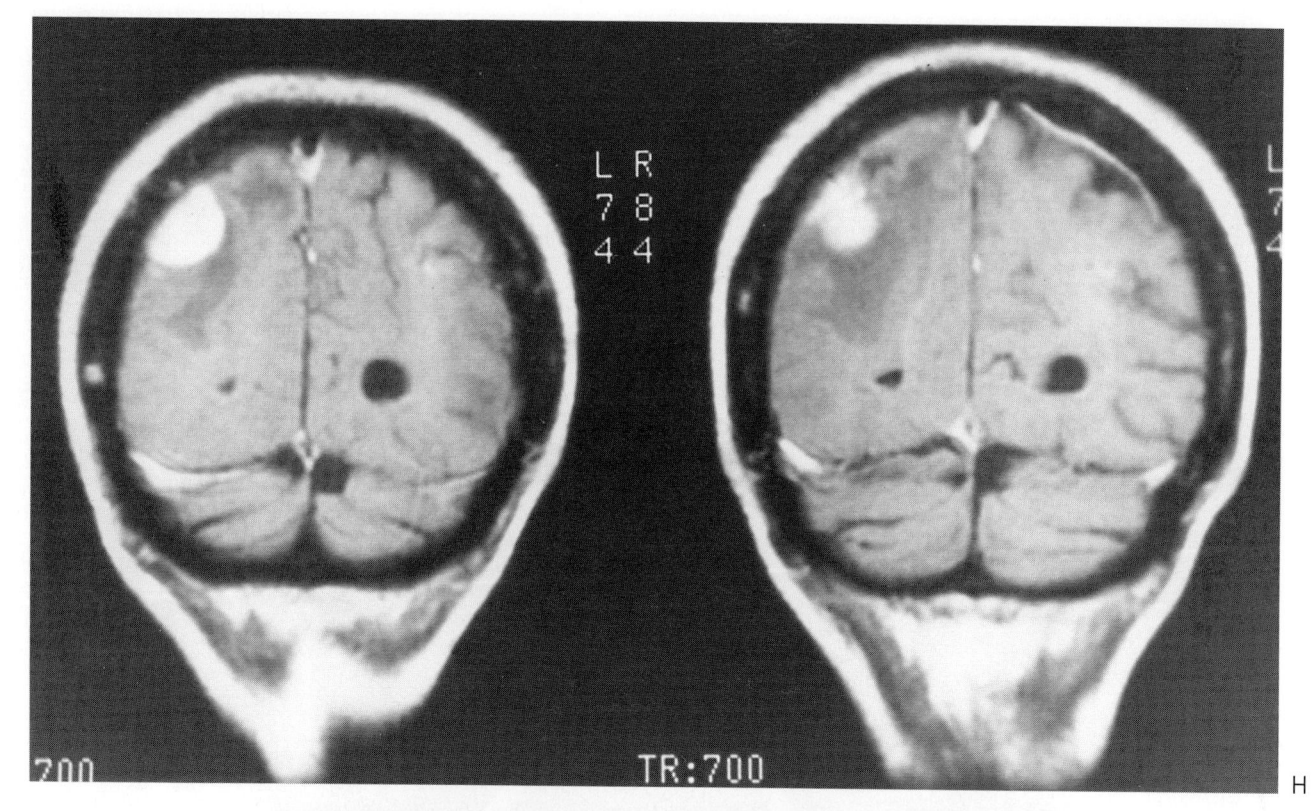

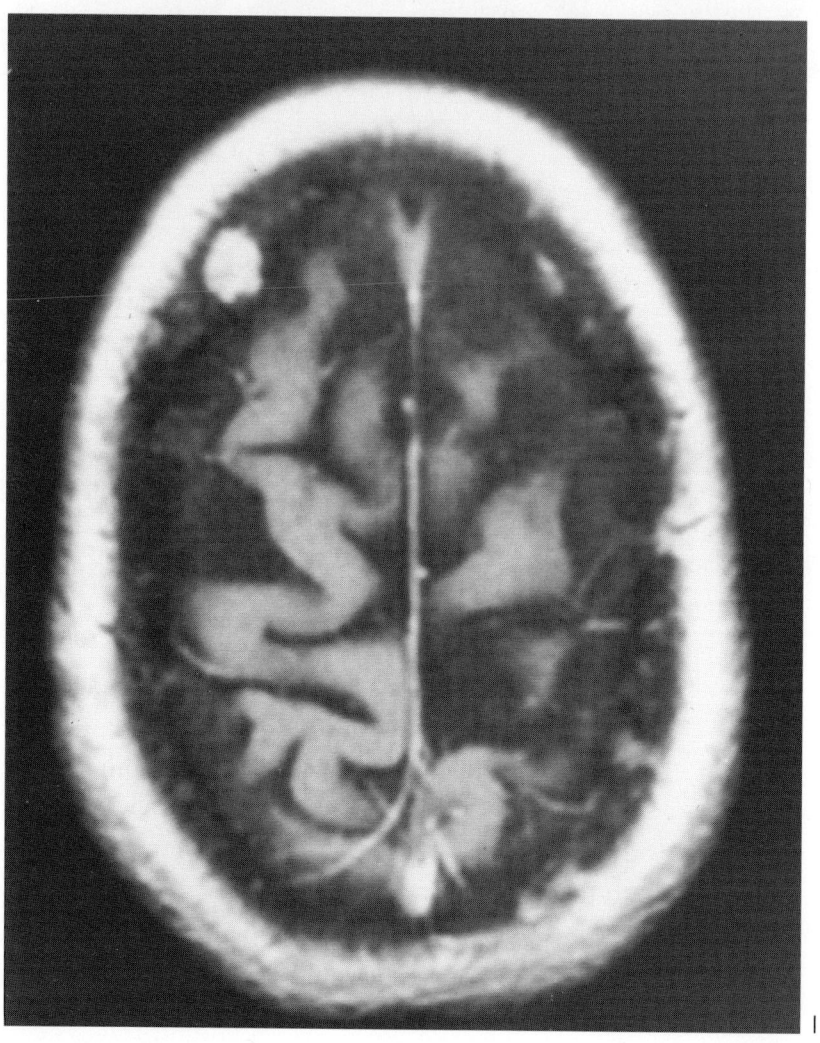

UNKNOWNS

865

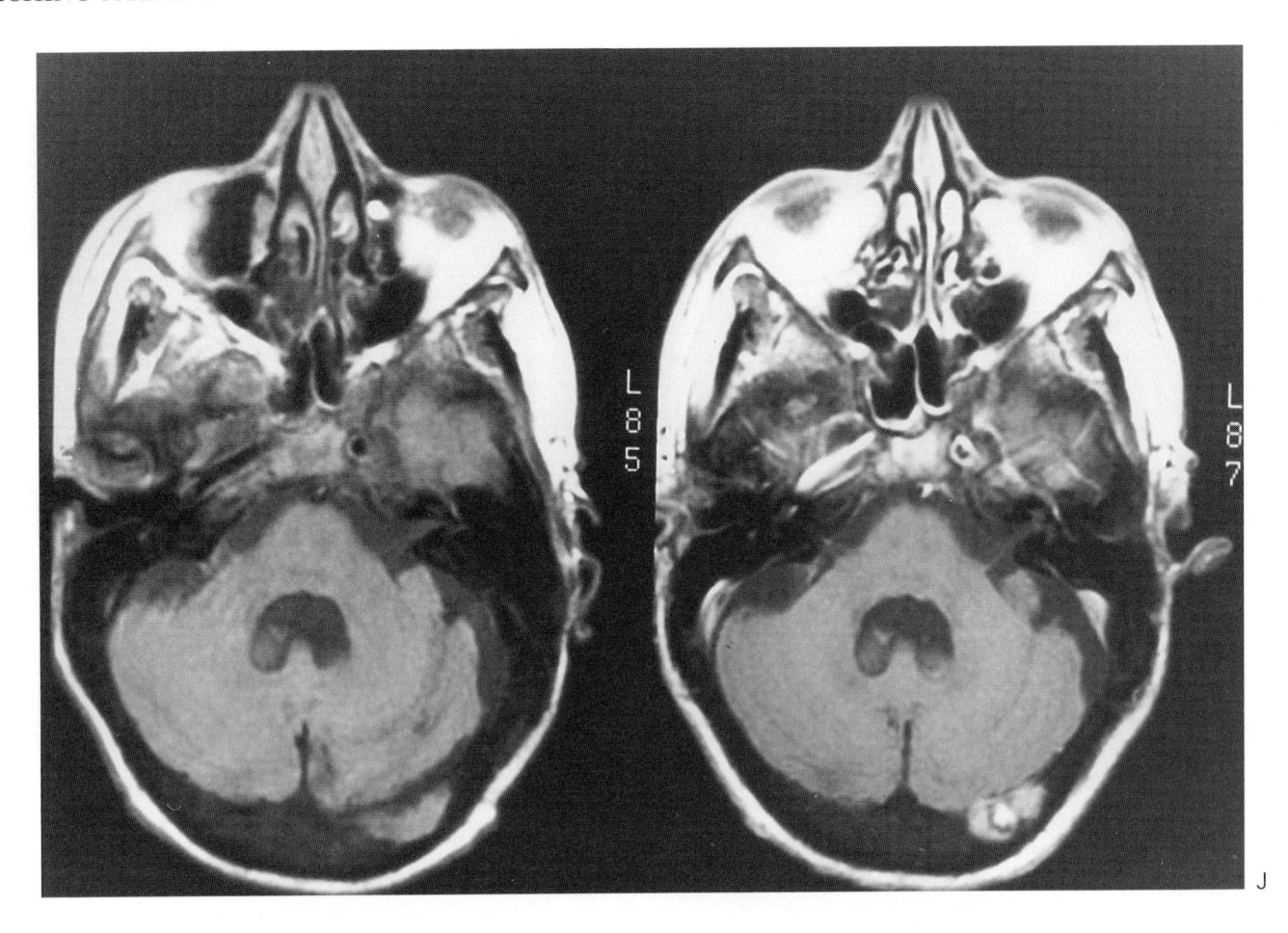

TEACHING ATLAS OF SPINE IMAGING

Radiologic Findings (continued)

(Fig. B) Sagittal intermediate TR image of the cervical spine.

(Fig. C) Pre- (*top*) and postcontrast (*bottom*) axial short TR images of the lower cervical spine.

(Fig. D) Pre- (*top*) and postcontrast (*bottom*) axial short TR images of the upper thoracic region.

(Fig. E) Axial intermediate (*left*) and long (*right*) TR images of the brain.

(Fig. F) Postcontrast axial short TR image of the brain.

(Fig. G) Postcontrast coronal short TR image of the brain at the level of the frontal horns of the lateral ventricles.

(Fig. H) Postcontrast coronal short TR image of the brain at the level of the occipital horns of the lateral ventricles.

(Fig. I) Axial postcontrast axial short TR image of the brain with attention to the bony calvarium.

(Fig. J) Axial pre- (*left*) and postcontrast (*right*) short TR image with attention to the bony calvarium.

INDEX

rheumatoid arthritis with herniated discs at C3-4, C4-5 levels *versus,* 548
Calvarium
  destruction in multiple myeloma, 390, 391, 396
  inner and outer table of
    cervical spine, 5
  metastases to, 861–867
  in multiple myeloma, 389–391
Carcinomatosis, spinal and cerebral meningeal, secondary to breast cancer, 429–432
Carotid artery flow void
  of external, 250–251
  in neurofibromatosis type 1, 219, 223
  plexiform neurofibromas and, 213, 215
Cauda equina nerve roots
  in anterior sacral myelomeningocele, 88
  axial CT image
    in dorsal aspect thecal sac, 57
    postmyelogram, 56
  axial long TR image, 49, 55
  long TR image of, 52
  lumbar
    MR myelogram, three-dimensional, 61
  postoperative changes with scarring and adhesions, 736–738
  in thecal sac
    parasagittal long TR image, 59
Caudal regression syndrome
  infant, 96
    sacrum and coccyx in, 97, 98
    sagittal short TR image, 98
    with tethered cord and vertebral anomalies, 97–99
  in neonate, 103
  with tethered cord and vertebral anomalies, 97–99
    anteroposterior and lateral plain film, 97
Cavernous angioma
  of cervical spinal cord, 834–837
    axial gradient echo image, C6, 836, 837
    axial long TR image, C5-6, 836, 837
    axial short TR image, C6, 834–835, 837
    hemosiderin deposition in, 837
    magnetic susceptibility artifact in, 837
    sagittal intermediate signal intensity image, cervical spine, 834
    sagittal long TR image, cervical spine, 834–835, 837
    sagittal short TR image, cervical spine, 834
    typical appearance of, 834–836
  ependymoma *versus,* 140
  of spinal cord, with hemorrhage, 773–775
    axial long TR image, 774–775
    sagittal long TR image, 774–775
    sagittal short TR image, 773
Cerebellar artery, in Chiari I malformation, 71
Cerebellar tonsils
  in Chiari II malformation
    in neonate, 79
  downward displacement of,
    in Chiari malformation, 67, 68, 70
    in Chiari I malformation, 71, 76
  herniation of
    in Chiari II malformation, 80–82
    in Chiari III malformation, 87
Cerebellum
  glioma of, 149–150
  pilocytic astrocytoma in, 155, 158, 159
Cerebrospinal fluid
  in Chiari malformation
    axial short TR image, 68–69
  in differentiation of metastatic from inflammatory disease, 359
  effect on
    of heart beat and respiration, 356
  L3-4
    long TR image, 53
  L5
    long TR image of, 52
  leak, with fracture dislocation L1-2 spinous process and dural tear, 282–283
  lumbar
    midsagittal long TR image, standard spin-echo technique, 33
  thoracic
    flow-related enhancement of
      on axial TR image, 23
    sagittal long TR image, 21, 22
    sagittal short TR image, 20

Cervical cancer
  postradiation changes in, 338–339
    axial short TR image, 339
    osteophytes at L2-3 level, 338–339
    sagittal short TR image L2 end plate through sacrum, 338–339
    Schmorl's node, L1 vertebral body, 338–339
Cervical disc herniation, 563–566
  C4-5
    with atlantoaxial fusion and Klippel-Feil anomaly, 549–552
  case 1: C5-6 level, right side
    axial gradient-echo images, C5-6, 529–530
    bulging disc in, C5-6, 527
    cervical spinal cord displacement in, 528, 530
    dura in, 529–530
    gradient-echo images in, rationale for, 530–531
    loss of cervical lordotic curve in, 528, 531
    narrowing of disc space in, 527
    obliteration of intervertebral foramen in, 529–530
    plain film readings and, 531
    right intermediate/long parasagittal TR images, 528, 530
    soft tissue encroachment on vertebral canal in, 528, 530
    spinal cord compression in, 529–530
    subarachnoid space compromise in, 528, 530
    vertebral canal compromise in, 528, 530
  case 2: C5-6 level, right side, 532–534
    axial gradient-echo image, C5-6 level, 533–534
    CT in conjunction with MR imaging for, 534
    lordotic curve loss in, 532, 534
    midsagittal short TR image, 532, 534
    plain film and, 534
    radicular pain with, 534
    right parasagittal long TR image, 533–534
    right parasagittal short TR image, 532, 534
    trauma to spinal cord and, 534
    vascular compromise and, 534
  case 4: C4-5 midline and left lateral
    cervical venous plexus in, 539
  case 4: C4-5 midline and left paracentral, 538–539
    axial CT image, postcontrast, 538
    subarachnoid space compromise in, 538
  C3-4 with posterior longitudinal ligament ossification, 553–556
    axial gradient echo images, 554–555
    displacement of spinal cord at C5, 554–555
    obliteration of subarachnoid space in, 554–555
    osteophytes in, 553, 555
    sagittal intermediate TR image, 553, 555
    sagittal long TR image, 554–555
    sagittal short TR image, 553, 555
    spinal cord compression in, C2-C6, 553, 554, 555
    subarachnoid space compromise in, 553, 554, 555
    T1 on T2 displacement, 553, 555
    vertebral canal narrowing in, 553, 555
  C4-5 level, 535–537
    anterior herniation at C5-6, 535, 537
    axial gradient-echo image, C4-5, C5-6, 536–537
    cervical spinal cord compression in, 536–537
    encroachment on subarachnoid space, 535, 536–537
    intervertebral disc height loss at C3-4, C4-5, C5-6, 535, 537
    midsagittal long TR image, 535, 537
    midsagittal short TR image, 535
    obliteration of epidural fat, 536–537
    parasagittal images for lateral herniation, 537
    parasagittal T2W image, 536–537
  C5-6 level
    commonality of, 530
    right side, 527–531, 532–534
  midline at C3-4 secondary to surgical fusion at C5-6 and C6-7, 563–566
    axial long TR image, 564–565, 566
    axial short TR images, 564, 565, 566
    encephalomalacia in, 564, 565
    mechanism in, 566
    myelomalacia in, 566
    sagittal long TR image, 564–565
    sagittal short TR image, 563
    spinal cord compression in, 564–565, 566
    spinal cord displacement in, 564–565
    syrinx formation in, 565, 566
  myelogram with postmyelogram CT scan *versus* MRI in, 534, 536, 539

radicular pain in
  cause of, 537
  in rheumatoid arthritis. *See under* Rheumatoid arthritis
Cervical spinal cord
  in Chiari malformation
    axial short TR image, 69
  edema of
    in sarcoidosis, 516–517
    in transverse myelopathy, 709
    with traumatic compression fracture, 271
  glioma of, 149–150
  in metastatic colon carcinoma, 202, 204
  in neurofibromatosis type 2 with astrocytoma, 167, 168, 170
  pilocytic astrocytoma in, 164–166
  post pilocytic astrocytoma removal, 159
  in sarcoidosis, 516–518
  syrinx in, 579–580
  tumor of
    cervical disc herniation *versus,* 530, 534
    Chiari I malformation with postoperative changes, syrinx cavity *versus,* 811
Cervical spine
  C1-2 dislocation
    in Down's syndrome, 133–134
  contrast material in, 3
  degenerative changes and post discectomy changes in, 570–573
    bony fusion plugs in, 570, 571, 572
    interspinous space in, 571–572, 573
    loss of lordotic curve in, 571–572, 573
    odontoid process in, posttraumatic, 571–572
    osteophyte in, 570, 571, 572, 573
    retrolisthesis in, C5-6, 571–572
    sagittal long TR image, 571–572
    sagittal short TR images, pre- and postsurgical, 570, 571, 572, 573
    sclerosis in, 570, 573
    subarachnoid space compromise in, 571, 572, 573
    truncation artifact in, 571–572
    vertebral canal compromise in, 571–572
  degenerative changes secondary to fusion at C4-5, 567–569
    changes with disc protrusion at C6-7 level, 567, 569
    myelomalacia, 567, 569
    osteophyte at C4-5 with subarachnoid space compromise, 567, 569
    retrolisthesis of C4 on C5, 567, 569
    sagittal long TR images, 568–569
    sagittal short TR images, 567, 569
    spinal cord compression , C3-C5, 567, 569
    subarachnoid space compromise in, 567, 569
  diffuse idiopathic skeletal hyperostosis of, 580–583
    axial short TR image, 582
    lateral plain film, 581
    osteophytes C4 through T1, 581, 582
    post laminectomy, 581–583
    sagittal short TR image, 582
  imaging sequences in, 3–4
  midsagittal short TR image, 9
  normal anatomy, 3–15
    axial, 8, 14, 15
    coronal, 7
    midsagittal, 9
    parasagittal, 11, 12
    sagittal, 5, 6, 10, 13
  nucleus pulposus herniation at C5-6 with myelomalacia, 574–578
    anterior herniation at C5-6, 575, 577
    axial gradient echo image, 576–577
    axial short TR images, 575, 576, 577
    encephalomyelitis and, disseminated with demyelination, 578
    lordotic curve reversal in, 574, 577
    MRI of brain in, 577
    myelomalacia in, 574, 577
    sagittal intermediate TR image, 575, 577
    sagittal short TR image, 576
    spinal cord compression, C5-6, 574, 575, 577
    syrinx cavity and, spinal cord tumor-related, 578
  post discectomy/surgical fusion changes
    axial gradient echo image at C6, 580
    cervical syrinx in, 579–580
    CT with myelography in, 580

Cervical spine (continued)
    osteophyte encroachment on vertebral foramen, 579–580
    sagittal short TR image, C5-6 through T1-2, 579–580
    postoperative changes C5-6 through T1-2
        post discectomy and surgical fusion, 579–580
    sagittal long TR image, 6
    sagittal short TR image, 5
    vertebral bodies of
        metastases to, 344–346
        postsurgical changes with metallic plate and screws, 344–346
Cervicomedullary junction
    in pilocystic astrocytoma, 164, 166
Chamberlain's line, 5
Chance fracture
    characterization of, 275
    compression fracture in auto accident versus, 275
Chemical shift artifact
    with lipoma, L2 level, 822
    with retained Pantopaque®, 734–735
    sagittal intermediate intensity lumbar image, 43
Chiari malformation
    axial short TR image
        cerebrospinal fluid in, 68–69
        cervical spinal cord in, 68–69
        foramen magnum in, 68–69
        with focal syrinx cavity, 67–70
        hydromyelia in, 70
        Lhermitte's sign in, 70
        spinal cord evaluation in, 73
        with syrinx cavity
            cervical and thoracic, 71–73
            evaluation of, 70
            focal, 67–70
            postoperative changes with shunt tube placement, 83–85
            thoracic, 74–76
    type 1
        and postcraniotomy meningitis with arachnoid adhesions, 503–506
Chiari I malformation
    defined, 10, 70
    diagnosis of
        MR imaging versus clinical, 70
    with focal syrinx
        axial short TR image, 68–69
        sagittal short TR image, 67
    forme fruste
        with deformity of posterior fossa, 122–124
    Klippel-Feil anomaly in, 112–114
    with lower cervical and thoracic syrinx
        axial short TR image, 72
        sagittal short TR image, 71–72
        surgical treatment of, 73
    postoperative changes in posterior fossa, 810–812
    and postoperative changes in posterior fossa, syrinx cavity, 810–812
        axial short TR image, 811
        cerebrospinal fluid flow void in, 810, 811, 812
        magnetic susceptibility artifact in, 811, 812
        sagittal long TR image, 810–811
        sagittal short TR image, 810–811
        spinal cord enlargement in, 812
        subarachnoid space obliteration in, 812
        syrinx cavity in, 810, 811, 812
    syringohydromyelia in, 79, 85
    with syrinx cavity
        postoperative, 810–812
    with syrinx cavity, C2-C6
        axial short TR image, 83, 85
        cerebellar tonsils in, 85
        post shunt tube placement, 83, 85
        sagittal long TR image, 84, 85
        sagittal short TR image, 83, 85
    with thoracic syrinx, 74–76
        axial short TR image, 75–76
        cerebrospinal fluid flow void in, 74–75
        cervical spinal cord evaluation and, 76
        sagittal long TR image, 74–75
        sagittal short TR image, 74–75
Chiari II malformation
    cerebellar tonsils in, 79
    defined, 79
    dysraphism in, 78, 79

epidural fat in, 78
in infant
    axial short TR image, 81–82
    cerebellar tonsillar herniation in, 80, 82
    lumbar vertebral canal in, 81–82
    meningomyelocele in, 81–82
    sagittal long TR image, 81–82
    sagittal short TR image, 80, 81, 82
    tethered cord in, 81–82
    vertebral malformation in, 81–82
meningocele in, 78, 79
with meningomyelocele, sacral agenesis, 77–79
with meningomyelocele and sacral agenesis
    sagittal short TR image, cervical spine, 77
meningomyelocele in, 78, 79
with multiple abnormalities, 80–82
platybasia of skull base, 77
tethered cord in, 78, 79
thoracic lumbar
    syrinx in, 77–78
vertebral canal in
    cervical, 77
    lumbar, 77, 78
Chiari III malformation, 86–87
    corpus callosum agenesis in, 87
    meningocele in, occipital, 87
    meningoencephalocele in, 87
    in neonate, 86–87
    syringohydromyelia in, 87
    syrinx cavity in
        cervical, 86
Child
    cytomegalovirus radiculitis in, 519–521
    diastematomyelia in, 115–118, 119–121
    glioma in, 149–150
    medulloblastoma in, 448–450, 507–508
    meningitis postcraniotomy with arachnoid adhesions in, 503–506
    meningocele/myelomeningocele in
        anterior sacral, 88–89
Child abuse, fall from couch, 289–291
Chloroma (granulocytic sarcoma)
    in brain, 379
    definition of, 379
    epidural hematoma versus, 801
    multiple myeloma versus, 403
    secondary to acute myelogenous leukemia, 377–379
        axial short TR image, T4, 378
        axial short TR image at L3, 378–379
        descending aorta, 378
        lumbar thecal sac in, 379
        parasagittal short TR images, 377–378
        paraspinal mass at L3, 379
        paraspinal masses, 378
        soft tissue mass at T3-T4 and T6-T8, 377–378
    of soft tissues of neck, 861–867
    in spinal cord, 379
Chordoma
    characterization of, 251
    distal lumbar spine, iliac crest, sacrum, coccyx, 831–833
        axial short TR image, pelvis, 831–832, 833
        axial short TR image, pubic symphysis, 832, 833
        at S2, 832
        sagittal short TR images, 831–832, 833
    within L3 vertebral body, 256–257
        ligamentum flavum hypertrophy in, 256
        osteophytes in, 256
        sagittal short TR image, L2-S1, 256
        sagittal short TR image with fat suppression technique, 256
        spinal stenosis in, L2-3, L3-4
    with postoperative changes, 249–252
    postoperative metastatic, 253–255
        axial short TR image, 254
        sagittal short TR image, 253–254
    recurrent postoperative, 249–252
        axial short TR image, 250–251
        jugular vein flow void in, 250–251
        sagittal intermediate TR image, 250–251
        sagittal short TR images, 249, 251
    sacral
        sacral myelomeningocele versus, 89
        sacral teratoma versus, infant, 262
Chronic renal failure
    secondary amyloidosis in, 758–759

Clivus, 5
    degenerative changes in postoperative, 249, 251
    fusion with odontoid process
        in chordoma, postoperative metastatic, 253–254
    midsagittal short TR image, 9
Coccygeal agenesis, in infant, 90–92
Coccyx
    chordoma involving, 831–833
    incomplete development of
        in caudal regression syndrome, 97, 98
Colon carcinoma
    metastatic, 201–205
        axial short TR images, 202, 204
        axial TR image, 204–205
        to medulla, 202, 204
        parasagittal TR images, 203, 205
        postcontrast scan for, 448
        sagittal long TR image, 202, 204
        sagittal short TR images, cervical, 201, 204
        to spinal cord, 202, 204
        spinal cord displacement in, 201, 204
        spinal cord in, 202, 204
        to subcutaneous tissue of forearms, 448
    metastatic in subarachnoid space, 447–448
        axial level short TR image, C2, 447–448
        correlation with cerebrospinal fluid analysis, 448
        sagittal short TR image, lumbar, 447–448
    metastatic to T12 with bone expansion and cord compression, 367–368
        axial short TR image, 367–368
        involvement of ribs and transverse process in, 367–368
        lumbar vertebral bodies in, 368
        sagittal short TR images, 367–368
        soft tissue mass, paraspinal area, 367–368
        spinal cord compression, 367–368
Comminuted fracture
    of T7 vertebral body, 278, 280
    vertebral body fragments at C2, 293, 296
Compression fracture(s)
    benign osteoporotic
        L3, L4, L5, 182–183
        multiple, 324–325
        T4 and T12, 320–321
    comminuted of T6 vertebral body, 278, 280
    L1 with distraction of interfacet joints, L1-2 level, 272–275
    L1 with spinal cord hematoma, 284–285
        axial short TR image, 284–285
        retropulsion L1 vertebral body into vertebral canal, 284–285
        sagittal long TR image, 284–285
        sagittal short TR image, 284–285
        spinal cord compression in, 284–285
    L3, L4, L5 vertebral bodies, 182–183
    lumbar spine, 272–275
    multiple, 322–323
    in multiple myeloma, 392–394
    secondary to osteoporosis
        sagittal short TR images, 320
        sagittal short TR images, lumbar/thoracic, 324
        T4, T6, T7, T10, 324–325
        T4, T10, T11, 322–323
        T4 and T12, 320–321
    traumatic
        axial short TR images, 270–271
        of L2 vertebral body, 269–271
        sagittal short and long TR images, 269
        with spinal cord edema, 269–271
    traumatic, L1, and distraction of L1-2 interfacet joints
        axial long TR images, 273–274
        parasagittal long TR image, 273–274
        sagittal long TR image, 272, 274
        sagittal short TR image, 272
Contrast enhancement, indications for, 29
Contrast material
    adipose tissue as, 29
    in cervical spine, 3
Corpus callosum agenesis, in Chiari III malformation, 87
Cortical bone destruction, CT sensitivity to, 366
Coumadin
    secondary epidural hematoma and bleeding dyscrasia with, 746
    secondary lumbar epidural hematoma and, 313–316

INDEX

C6 radiculopathy, pain, weakness, 527–531, 532–534
Cruciate ligaments, cervical, sagittal long TR image, 13
Cytomegalovirus (CMV) radiculitis, 519–521
   axial short TR image, postcontrast, 520–521
   cerebrospinal fluid analysis in, 521
   CT scan of brain, 520–521
   sagittal short TR image, postcontrast, 519
      lower thoracic/upper lumbar enhancement on, 519

D

Degenerative changes
   in chordoma, recurrent postoperative, 249, 251
   discitis with vertebral osteomyelitis, L3-4, and spinal stenosis *versus,* 781
   interfacet joint
      synovial, 670–672
      synovial cysts with, 669, 672
   in intervertebral disc
      L4-5 disc bulge with lateral recess stenosis *versus,* 678
Degenerative changes with osteophyte formation posttrauma
   axial gradient echo image, 541–542
   axial short TR images, 541–542
   cervical lordotic curve loss in, 540
   cervical subarachnoid space compromise, 541, 542
   disc herniation at C4-5, C5-6 and disc bulge at C6-7, C7-T1, 530
   encroachment on subarachnoid space, 541–542
   MRI evaluation of hematoma, 543
   myelomalacia in, 541–542, 543
   osteophyte projection in, 541–542
   sagittal long TR images, 540, 541–542
   sagittal short TR image, 540
   syrinx cavity in, 543
Degenerative disc disease
   changes in, 181–183
   discitis *versus,* 469
Deoxyhemoglobin, 311, 317, 319
Dermoid cyst, sacral myelomeningocele *versus,* 89
Dermoid tumor
   caudal regression syndrome with tethered cord and vertebral anomalies *versus,* 99
   characterization of, 264
   low spinal cord and, 263–265
   sagittal T1W image
      distal spinal cord at L2-3, 263–264
      soft tissue mass, 263–264
   spinal cord, 263–264
Desmoid tumor, 806–809
   in adolescent, 806–809
      angiography in, 809
      axial fat saturation images, pre- and postcontrast, 806–807
      axial short TR images, 808–809
      dense fibrous tissue in, 806, 807, 808
      versus hematoma, 809
      parasagittal short TR image, postcontrast, 806–807
      sagittal short TR images, cervical pre- and post contrast, 806, 808–809
      thecal sac effacement in, 809
      vertebral artery flow void in, 808, 809
Devic's disease, multiple sclerosis *versus,* 702
Diastematomyelia
   with atrophic spinal cord, asymmetric hemicords, syrinx cavity, Chiari I malformation, 115–118
   anteroposterior abdominal film, 122, 124
   with atrophic spinal cord and other anomalies, 122–124
   axial short TR image, lumbar, 120–121
   cerebellar tonsil displacement in, 121
   cerebral anomalies in, 121
   characterization of, 117
   in child, 119–121
      axial T1W image, 123–124
      coronal short TR image, 119, 121
      corpus callosum in, 121
      hemicords in, 121
      sagittal short TR image, 119, 121, 122
   hemicords in
      asymmetric, 123–124
      with lipoma, 818–822
   midsagittal short TR image, 120–121
   with scoliosis and vertebral body anomalies

      anteroposterior myelogram, 115, 117
      axial CT myelogram, 116–117
   in child, 115–118
      hemicords in, 115, 116–117
      thecal sac in, 115, 116, 117
   spinal cord in, 121
      atrophic asymmetric, 123–124
   syringomyelia with, 118
   thecal sac in, 121
   vertebral body, deformed T10 and T11, 123–124
Diffuse idiopathic skeletal hyperostosis (DISH), criteria for, 583
Diffuse metastases
   bony with pathologic fractures, T10, L1, and L2 post breast cancer treatment, 842–844
   leukemic infiltrate in bone marrow
      with granulocytic sarcoma (chloroma) of neck; dural meningeal metastases; bony calvarium metastases *versus,* 867
   neurofibromatosis type 1 with plexiform neurofibromas in cervical spine *versus,* 816, 817
Diplomyelia, *versus* hemicords, 117
Disc degeneration. *See also* Disc herniation
   discitis *versus,* 469
   evaluation of
      long TR images in, 621
      at L3-4 and L5-S1 levels, 619–621
   vacuum *versus* calcification
      CT differentiation of, 628
Disc disease. *See also* Disc herniation
   cervical
      imaging sequences in, 3
      long TR images in, 29
Discectomy
   C4-5 and C5-6 with bony fusion plugs, 561–562
      complications of, 562
      loss of lordosis with, 561–562
      postoperative evaluation of, 562
      recurrent herniated disc fragment following, 637–639
      sagittal short TR images, pre- and postcontrast, 561–562
Disc fragment
   recurrent migratory post lumbar laminectomy, 640–644
      axial short TR image, L5-S1, 641, 643
      axial short TR images, pre- and postcontrast, 642, 643
      disc herniation *versus* scar on postcontrast scan, 644
      magnetic susceptibility artifact in, 643, 644
      parasagittal short TR image, 641, 643
      sagittal short TR image, postcontrast, 641, 643
      sagittal short TR images, 640
      scar formation in, 642–643, 644
      soft tissue mass behind epidural space and, 643
      soft tissue mass behind L5 vertebral body, 640, 641, 643
      thecal sac displacement in, 641, 642, 643
   recurrent post discectomy, 637–639
      arachnoiditis and, 638
      axial short TR images, 638
      clinical correlation in, 639
      contrast enhancement in, 638
      edema of bone marrow in, 639
      MR imaging for, 638
      pseudomeningocele in, postoperative, 637, 638
      sagittal long TR image, 637–638
      sagittal short TR image, 637–638
      versus scar tissue, 639
      soft tissue mass at L5-S1, 637–638
      thecal sac bulging in, 637–638, 639
      thecal sac compression in, 638
      vertebral body endplates in, 637–638, 639
Disc height, lumbar, midsagittal short TR image, 30
Disc herniation. *See also* Disc degeneration; Disc disease
   calcification in, 592
   C2-C3 level
      in battered person, 294, 296, 297
      in hangman's fracture at C2-3, 292–297
   C3-4 level, 563–566
      and posterior longitudinal ligament ossification, 553–556
   C3-4 and C4-5 levels, 544–548
   C4-5 level
      left lateral, 535–537

      midline and left paracentral, 538–539
      right-sided, 549–552
   C5-6 level
      right side, 527–531, 532–534
      right-sided nucleus pulposus and myelomalacia, 574–578
   disc migration and imaging in, 624
   end plate, 771–772. *See also* Schmorl's node deformity
   epidural and prevertebral abscess *versus,* 788, 789
   with extrusion, 622–624
   at L5-S1 level
      lateral, 625–628
      left paracentral, 629–631
   intrathecal disc in, 624
   L2-3, 645–646
      midline, 651–654
   L3-4, 826–830
   L4-5, 619–621, 826–830
      lateral with encroachment on intervertebral foramen, 647–650
      midline, 828, 830
      Pantopaque® retention in, 733–735
      post epidural block, 306–307
   lateral
      caution in, 830
   lateral L3-4, 826–830
      sagittal short TR image, 828–829, 830
      thecal sac prominence in, 826, 829
   lateral L3-4 and midline L4-5, 826–830
      axial short TR images, L2-3 pre- and postcontrast, 826–827, 830
      axial short TR images, L3-4 pre- and postcontrast, 828–829
      axial short TR images, L4 pre- and postcontrast, 828–829
      axial short TR images, L4-5 pre- and postcontrast, 829
      left parasagittal short TR image, 826–827
      right parasagittal short TR image, 826–827
      sagittal long TR image, 826–827
      sagittal short TR image, 826–827
   myelographic signs of, 650
   nerve encroachment in, 38
   parasagittal short TR image, 38
   postlaminectomy, 826–830
   postoperative changes with fusion at C5-6 and C6-7 levels, 563–566
   recurrent with migration behind L5 vertebral body, 640–644
   synovial cyst *versus,* lumbar, 668, 669
   T6-7 level, 587–590
      with calcification, 591–592
      with calcification and vertebral canal compromise, 595–598
   T8-9 level
      with calcification, 593–594
   traumatic
      C4-5 level, 286–288
      C5-6 level, 302–305
   with traumatic anterolisthesis, C4 on C5, 286–288
Disc herniation fragment
   recurrent with peripheral enhancement, 637–639
   sequestered
      at L4-5 level, 651–654
      with nerve root enhancement, 632–636
Disc infection, postoperative wound infection with draining sinus tract and, 480–482
Discitis
   versus degenerative disc disease, 469
   and epidural and paraspinal abscesses
      aorta displacement in, 484–485
      axial short TR images, pre- and postcontrast, 484–485
      axial short TR images, T4, 484–485
      chest x-ray in, 486
      CT-guided aspiration biopsy in, 485
      in intravenous drug abuser with pulmonary tuberculosis, 483–486
      kyphosis at L3-4 level, 483
      loss of vertebral body height in, 483
      Mycobacterium tuberculosis-associated, 483–486
      paraspinal mass in, 484–485
      prevertebral soft tissue mass, C2-T6, 483, 484–485
      sagittal short TR images, T3-4 level, 483, 485
      thecal sac compression in, 484–485

Discitis (*continued*)
　in intravenous drug abuser, 477–479, 487–490
　with pulmonary tuberculosis, 483–486
　with L3-4 vertebral osteomyelitis and spinal stenosis, 781–784
　MR imaging *versus* plain film and CT evaluation of, 469
　organisms in, 489–490
　　Mycobacterium species in, 475, 479
　　Pseudomonas aeruginosa in, 475
　and osteomyelitis
　　cervical spine degenerative changes and post discectomy changes *versus,* 570–573
　　with paraspinal extension and vertebral osteomyelitis, 477–479
　　　axial short TR images, pre- and postcontrast, 478
　　　CT-guided aspiration biopsy in, 479
　　　disc extension into dorsal paravertebral muscles, 478
　　　displacement of spinal cord in, 477
　　　encroachment on epidural space, 477
　　　gallium scanning and, 479
　　　L1 and L2 loss of height in, 477
　　　L1 end plate destruction in, 477
　　　lumbar thecal sac in, 478
　　　radionuclide scanning and, 479
　　　sagittal short TR image, 477
　　　sagittal short TR image, postcontrast, 477–478
　　postoperative with wound infection and draining sinus tract, 480–482
　　　axial short TR images, 481
　　　butterfly configuration of disc, 480–481
　　　CT-guided aspiration biopsy with culture in, 482
　　　extension of inflammation into intervertebral foraminae, 480–481
　　　inflammation of prevertebral soft tissue component in, 480–481
　　　L5-S1 disc expansion in, 481
　　　parasagittal short TR images, 480–481
　　　sagittal short TR images, 480–481
　　　thecal sac compression in, 480–481
　　posttraumatic with psoas and other abscesses, 470–476
　　　aorta displacement in, 473–474
　　　axial intermediate TR images, 473–474
　　　axial short TR images, 472, 474, 475
　　　cauda equina nerve roots in, 475
　　　CT-guided biopsy in, 475
　　　CT scan, 472, 474
　　　degenerative disc disease *versus,* 475
　　　final plain film, 476
　　　fusion of L3-4 bodies, 476
　　　lateral plain film, 473–474
　　　L3-4 disc projection into vertebral canal, 471, 474
　　　L3 vertebral body end plate in, 470, 474
　　　metastases *versus,* 475
　　　offset of L3 relative to L4 in, 471, 474
　　　paraspinal soft tissue mass, 470, 474
　　　plain film, 470, 474, 475
　　　prevertebral abscess in, 470, 474
　　　psoas muscle abscess, 472, 474, 475
　　　sagittal intermediate TR image, 471, 474
　　　sagittal long TR image, 471, 474
　　　sagittal short TR images, pre- and postcontrast, 470, 474
　　and secondary epidural and paraspinal abscess, 483–486
　　secondary to retropharyngeal abscess, 498–502
　　with soft tissue component and destruction of vertebral body end plate, 467–469
　　　abdominal aortic aneurysm displacement in, 467–468
　　　CT at L3-L4 intervertebral disc, 460, 467–468
　　　CT-guided biopsy in, 468, 469
　　　degenerative changes in interfacet joints in, 467–468
　　　osteophytes at L5, 467–468
　　　plain film, L2-L5, 467–468, 469
　　　psoas muscle evaluation in, 468
　　　soft tissue mass in, 468
　　　spinal sclerosis in, L3-4, 467–468, 469
　　　spinal stenosis in, L3-4, 467–468
　　and vertebral osteomyelitis; bilateral psoas, epidural, paraspinal abscesses, 487–490
　　with vertebral osteomyelitis, L3-4, and spinal stenosis, 781–784

　　anterolisthesis, L3 on 4 and L4 on 5, 782, 784
　　axial short TR image, L3 pre- and postcontrast, 782–783
　　axial short TR images, L3-4, 783
　　cauda equina nerve root in, 782, 784
　　CT-guided biopsy in, 784
　　versus degenerative changes in, 784
　　degenerative changes in, interfacet, 783, 784
　　ligamentum flavum hypertrophy and, 781, 783, 784
　　sagittal long TR image, lumbar, 781
　　sagittal short TR image, lumbar, 781
　　sagittal short TR image, lumbar postcontrast, 782–783
　　spondylolisthesis in, secondary to degenerative changed, 784
　　versus spondylolisthesis, 783
　with vertebral osteomyelitis; psoas and epidural abscesses, lumbar through thoracic spine, 487–490
　　axial short TR image, postcontrast, 488–489
　　cauda equina nerve root compression in, 487, 489
　　fat-suppressed sagittal short TR image, 488–489
　　L4-5 disc space narrowing, 487, 489
　　L4 inferior end plate in, 487, 489
　　L5 superior end plate in, 487, 489
　　lumbar thecal sac compression, 487, 489
　　organisms in, 489–490
　　paraspinal abscesses, 488–489
　　psoas muscle abscesses, 488–489
　　sagittal intermediate TR image, 487–489
　　sagittal short TR image, 487–489
Disc migration, 635
　imaging slices for, 623, 624
Disc(s)
　cervical
　　axial short TR image, C4, 8
　lumbar
　　axial long TR image, 49, 55
　　L3-4, long TR image, 53
　　midsagittal long TR image, standard spin-echo technique, 33
　　sagittal short TR image, 40
　pediatric, 24, 25
　projection into intervertebral foramen
　　parasagittal short TR image, 38
DISH. *See* Diffuse idiopathic skeletal hyperostosis (DISH)
Dislocation
　C1-2 in rheumatoid arthritis, 544–548
　C5 on C6 with nuchal ligament disruption and disc herniation, 302–305
　　axial CT scan, 304
　　axial short TR images, 303–304
　　lateral plain film of cervical spine, 302
　　sagittal intermediate and long TR images, 303–304
　posttraumatic
　　Down's syndrome with C1-2 subluxation *versus,* 824, 825
Distraction of L1-2 interfacet joints
　with compression fracture of L1, 272–274
Dorsal root ganglion
　cervical
　　axial short TR image, 15
　　parasagittal short TR image, 12
　lumbar
　　axial long TR image, 54
　　axial short TR image, 46
　　axial short TR image, pre- and postinfusion, 51
　　coronal short TR image, 36
　　parasagittal short TR image, 37, 38
　　normal short TR image, postinfusion, 14, 15
Dowager's hump, 325
Down's syndrome
　in adolescent, 133–134
　with C1-2 dislocation, congenital heart disease, atrial septal defect, 133–134
　　lateral view of cervical spine, 133
　　sagittal short TR image, 133
　C1-2 dislocation in, 133–134
　C1-2 subluxation in, 823–825
　　axial CT scan, upper cervical spine and foramen magnum, 823–824
　　cervical spinal cord compression and displacement in, 825
　　lateral plain film, upper cervical spine and skull base, 823–824

　　odontoid process projection into foramen magnum, 823–824, 825
　　sagittal long TR image, posterior fossa and upper cervical spine, 823–824
　　sagittal short TR image, posterior fossa and upper cervical spine, 823–824
　　subarachnoid space compromise in, 823–824, 825
Drop metastases
　from cerebral glioblastoma multiforme, 433–438
　from germinoma, 451–454
　from medulloblastoma, 449–450
　with meningeal carcinomatosis
　　glioblastoma multiforme, recurrent cerebral, *versus,* 438
　meningioma *versus*
　　in 57-year-old female, 188
　myxopapillary ependymoma *versus*
　　low thoracic-upper lumbar, 191
　neurofibromatosis type 2 with schwannomas, postoperative changes, tethered cord *versus,* 129
　neurofibromatosis type 2 with schwannomas *versus,* 794
　postlaminectomy adhesive arachnoiditis *versus,* 741
　from recurrent ependymoma
　　axial short TR images, 199–200
　　sagittal short TR images, 198, 200
　from recurrent ependymoma *versus* medulloblastoma, 200
　from recurrent posterior fossa ependymoma, 198–200
　from recurrent posterior fossa medulloblastoma
　　CT scans, postinfusion, 449–450
　　sagittal short TR image, 449–450
　schwannoma *versus,* 177, 183
Dumbbell-shaped tumors, 127, 217–224
Duplication cyst of rectum, sacral myelomeningocele *versus,* 89
Dura
　astrocytoma in, 168, 170
　meningeal metastases in, 861–867
Dural tear, with cerebrospinal fluid leakage, in fracture dislocation of L1-2 spinous processes, 282–283
Dysraphism
　in agenesis and tethered cord, 100–101
　in Chiari II malformation, 78, 79, 80–82
　in neonate, 100–101

E

Encephalomyelitis, postinfectious, multiple sclerosis *versus,* 706
Encephalomyelopathy, postvaccination, 716–718
End plate herniations, of disc, 771–772
End plates, vertebral, cervical, 5
Ependymoma, 137–140
　astrocytoma and neurofibroma of dorsal root ganglion *versus,* 143, 144
　astrocytoma of distal spinal cord *versus,* 233–234
　astrocytoma *versus,* 171
　axial long TR image, 139
　axial short TR image, C3 postcontrast, 138, 139
　at C3, 137, 139, 140
　cavernous angioma of spinal cord *versus,* 837
　dilated Virchow-Robin spaces and, 195–197
　glioma of cervical spinal cord and cerebellum *versus,* 150
　intramedullary
　　in neurofibromatosis type 2, 236, 239, 240
　lumbar
　　with hemorrhagic deposits, 197
　　sagittal short TR images, 195
　　with Virchow-Robin spaces in brain, 196
　metastatic deposits from, 196, 197
　metastatic spread of, 163
　myxopapillary
　　lumbar, 189–191. *See also* Myxopapillary ependymoma
　　with hemorrhage, 192–194
　　schwannoma *versus,* 177
　in neurofibromatosis type 2, 129, 235–240, 241–245
　pilocystic astrocytoma *versus,* 166
　postoperative, C1-7, 161–163
　　axial short TR images, 162–163
　　cystic area in, 161, 163
　　sagittal short TR images, 161, 163

INDEX

recurrent posterior fossa, 198–200
  drop metastasis from, 198–200
sagittal long TR image, 137, 139
sagittal short TR image
  C2-5, 137, 139
  postcontrast, 137, 139
spinal cord
  cavernous angioma of spinal cord with hemorrhage *versus*, 775
  postoperative changes, 161–163
  surgery for, postoperative changes following, 736–738
spinal cord metastasis *versus*, 153
subarachnoid space compromise, 137, 139
with syrinx cavity, 849–852
  axial short TR image, T4, 851–852
  axial short TR image, T10, 851–852
  sagittal long TR image, lower cervical and thoracic spine, 850, 852
  sagittal long TR image, upper thoracic spine, 850, 852
  sagittal short TR image, lower cervical and thoracic spine, 849
  sagittal short TR image, lower cervical/thoracic spine postcontrast, 850, 852
  sagittal short TR image, thoracic spine, 850, 852
  syrinx, C2-T6 and distal end of spinal cord, 850, 851–852
Epidermoid tumor
  post spinal tap, 264
  schwannoma at L3 *versus*, 183
  synovial cyst at left L3-4 interfacet joint *versus*, 672
Epidural abscess, 487–490, 785–789
  cervical disc herniation, at C4-5 level *versus*, 538, 539
  in diabetes mellitus patient, 491, 492, 494, 495, 496, 497
  multilevel anterior and posterior, 491–497
  secondary to retropharyngeal abscess, 498–502
  postoperative disc infection *versus*, 482
  postoperative discitis with wound infection and draining sinus tract *versus*, 482
  secondary to discitis, 483–486
  secondary to retropharyngeal abscess, 498–502
    axial short TR image, midcervical postcontrast, 499, 501
    axial short TR image, upper cervical at C3, 499, 501
    C5-6 disc space narrowing in, 498, 502
    cervical spinal cord compression in, 498, 499, 500–501
    C2-3 to C7 enhancement, 501
    degenerative changes in cervical spine, 498
    parasagittal TR image, postcontrast, 499, 501
    prevertebral soft tissue mass, C2-C7, 498, 499, 501, 502
    sagittal short TR image, postcontrast, 498, 501
    sagittal T1W image of cervical spine, 498
    trachea displacement in, 498
Epidural abscess; paraspinal and psoas muscles abscesses
  axial short TR images
    epidural abscess, 494, 496
    lumbar region, 492, 496
    paraspinal muscles, 494, 496
    postcontrast, cervical spinal cord, 495–496
    precontrast at C2, 494, 496
    psoas muscle, 494, 496
    at T6, 492, 496
  cerebrospinal fluid and, 497
  cervical spinal cord displacement and compression in, 492, 495
  in diabetes mellitus patient with bacteremia, 491–497
  epidural abscess, 491, 492, 495, 496, 497
  laminectomy for, 497
  meninges in, 491
  sagittal short TR images
    lumbar, 491
    lumbar subarachnoid space, 491, 497
    meninges on, 491
    thecal sac in, 491
    thoracic, 492, 495
  soft tissue mass in
    at C3-5 level, 492, 495
    in subarachnoid space obliteration, 492, 495
  subarachnoid space in
    soft tissue obliteration of, 492, 495
  thecal sac in, 491, 495–496

Epidural and prevertebral abscesses, 785–789
  axial long TR image, 786, 788
    prevertebral abscess on, 787, 789
  axial short TR image
    epidural abscess on, 787, 789
    prevertebral abscess on, 787, 789
    spinal cord compression and displacement on, 787, 789
    subarachnoid space obliteration on, 787, 789
  axial short TR images, pre- and postcontrast, 787–788
  sagittal intermediate TR image, 785
    disc space narrowing on, C4-5, C5-6, C6-7, 785, 789
    spinal cord edema on, 785, 789
  sagittal long TR image, cervical, 785, 786, 788
  sagittal short TR image, postcontrast
    abscess cavity at C5-6, 785, 789
Epidural catheter placement
  axial short TR images
    lumbar region, 310–311
    thecal sac at kidney level, 309, 311
  epidural hematoma; blood in thecal sac, air in vertebral canal, 308–312
  sagittal short TR image
    air in vertebral canal, 311–312
    lower thoracic and lumbar region, 308, 311
    osteophytes in lumbar region, 308, 311
    thoracic region, 309, 311
Epidural fat
  in Chiari I malformation with focal syrinx, 72
  in Chiari II malformation
  in neonate, 78
  lumbar
    axial short TR image, 45
    midsagittal long TR image, standard spin-echo technique, 33
    midsagittal short TR image, 30, 34
Epidural hematoma, 742–743
  cause unknown, 799–801
    axial short TR image, lumbar, 799–800
    axial short TR image, spine, 800–801
    hemorrhage in, 799–800, 801
    osteophyge in, L2-3, 800–801
    sagittal short TR image, lumbar, 799–800
    sagittal short TR image, spine with reformatting technique, 800–801
    spinal cord compression, T11-L3 799–800, 801
    subarachnoid space obliteration, T11-L3, 799–800, 801
    thecal sac compression in, 799–800, 801
  epidural lipomatosis *versus*, 750, 751
  in hangman's fracture, 297
  lumbar region, 744–746
    axial CT postinfusion, 744
    marrow of vertebral bodies in, 744–745, 746
    sagittal long TR image, 744–745
    sagittal short TR image, 744–745
    thecal sac compression in, 744, 745
  methemoglobin phase in, 306, 311
  in multiple myeloma, 407–409
  with pleural effusions
    in multiple myeloma, 407–409
  post epidural block, 306–307
    axial short TR image, 306–307
    sagittal long TR image, lumbar, 306–307
    sagittal short TR image, lumbar, 306–307
  post epidural catheter placement, 309, 311, 312
  post spinal anesthesia, 742–743
    axial short TR image, L5, 742–743
    displacement of dura in, 742, 743
    sagittal long TR image, 742
    sagittal short TR image, lumbar, 742
  small, 306–307
  spontaneous secondary to coumadin therapy, lumbar, 313–316, 317–319, 746
    axial short TR image, L2, 314–315
    axial short TR image, L1 level, 315
    sagittal short TR image, 313
    sagittal short TR image with straightening algorithm, 314–315
    spinal canal compromise in, 316
    thecal sac compression in, 314–315
  spontaneous secondary to coumadin therapy, midthoracic, 317–319
    axial short TR image at T5, 317–318
    epidural fat in, 318

sagittal short TR images, 317–318
subarachnoid space compression in, 318
thoracic
  with blood in thecal sac; air in vertebral canal, 308–312
Epidural lipoma, epidural hematoma *versus*, 743
Epidural lipomatosis, 750–751
  axial short TR image, 750
  clinical history in, 750
  disc bulging in, multiple, 750
  idiopathic, causes of, 751
  sagittal short TR image, 750
  thecal sac compression in, 750
Epidural metastases
  in lung cancer, 386–388
  with T11 and L4 vertebral metastases, 845–848
Epidural venous plexus
  cervical
    normal, 10
  disc fragment, recurrent migratory post lumbar laminectomy *versus*, 644
  lumbar
    midsagittal short TR image, 31
Esophagus
  axial short TR image, 15
  cancer of, postradiation changes and, 725–727
Ewing's sarcoma
  metastatic
    bone *versus* soft tissue component in, 370
    compression fracture, T8, 369
    myelography in, 370
    sagittal short TR images, 369–370
    soft tissue epidural mass, T2, 369–370
    spinal cord compression at T2, T8, 369–370
    spinous process expansion, T2, 369
  multiple myeloma with infiltration of vertebral body marrow and soft tissue mass *versus*, 406

F

Facets, bilateral perched, 300–301
Fall from sitting position, 269–271
Fast-spin echo technique, rapid acquisition with relaxation enhancement in, 62
Fat
  bone marrow
    postradiation, 339
  as contrast agent, 356
  at end of clivus, 13
  thoracic, 20
Fat saturation technique
  use of cervical, 4
  MR imaging of brachial plexus, 361
Fat-suppression short TR images, 337
Filum terminale
  axial CT image postmyelogram, 56
  midsagittal long TR image
    in distal end of thecal sac, 32
Filum terminale lipoma
  sacral agenesis with, 93–96
  tethered cord with, 104–106
Flexion injury
  hangman's fracture in, 292–297
  perched facets from, bilateral, 300–301
Foramen magnum
  in Chiari II malformation, 80–82
  in Chiari malformation
    axial short TR image, 68–69
    high signal intensity fat area and, 9
    midsagittal short TR image, 9
    sagittal long TR image, 13
    sagittal short TR image, 5, 10
Foramen of Magendie, in pilocytic astrocytoma, 164, 166
Foramina transversarium
  cervical
    coronal long TR image, 7
    parasagittal short TR image, 11
    vertebral artery in, 11
Fracture dislocation
  C4 on C5 with scoliosis and posttraumatic syrinx cavity, 289–291
    coronal short TR image, 290–291
    sagittal midline reconstruction from CT scan, 290–291
    sagittal short TR images, 289–290

Fracture dislocation (*continued*)
  hangman's C2 on C3 with disc herniation, 292–297
    axial CT scans, 293, 296
    axial short TR images, 295–296
    lateral cervical plain film, 292, 296
    parasagittal long TR image, 294, 296
    sagittal long TR image, 294, 296
    sagittal midline reconstruction from CT scan, 292, 296
    sagittal short TR image, 294, 296
    spinal cord compression in, 294, 296, 297
    subarachnoid space compression in, 295–296
  of L1-2 spinous processes
    with dural tear and cerebrospinal fluid leakage, 282–283
  T6-7 with cord contusion and paraspinal hematoma, 276–281
    anteroposterior plain film, thoracic, 276, 279
    axial CT scan at T6, 277, 280
    axial CT scan at T7, 278, 280
    axial short TR images at T7 level, 278, 280
    compression deformity, T6/T7 vertebral bodies, 276, 277, 279
    hematoma in, 277, 280
    pleural effusions in, 277, 280
    retropulsion, vertebral bodies into cerebral canal, 276, 277, 279
    sagittal long TR image, 277, 279
    sagittal short TR image, 276, 279
    syrinx cavity development in, 280
Fractures. *See also* Comminuted fracture; Compression fractures; Odontoid fracture(s)
  pathologic
    in metastatic disease, 397–398
    in osteoblastic disease, 417–420
Fusion
  C4-5, osteophyte formation with subarachnoid space compromise and myelomalacia, 567–569
  C5-6 and C6-7 levels
    postoperative changes with, 563–566
    metallic plate and fixating screws in, 838–841

G

Ganglioglioma, ependymoma with syrinx cavity *versus*, 852
Gastrointestinal tumors, osteoblastic and osteolytic metastases *versus*, prostatic, 803
Germinoma
  with drop metastases and spinal meningeal carcinomatosis, 451–454
    axial intermediate TR image, pineal gland, 453–454
    axial long TR image, pineal gland, 453–454
    axial short TR image, brain, postcontrast, 452, 454
    brain in, 451, 452, 453, 454
    correlation with cerebrospinal fluid analysis, 454
    hydrocephalus in, obstructive, 452, 454
    pineal gland level in, 452, 453, 454
    sagittal short TR image, brain, postcontrast, 452, 454
    sagittal short TR image, distal end of spinal cord, 451, 454
    sagittal short TR image, postcontrast, 451, 454
    soft tissue surrounding spinal cord, 451, 454
    subarachnoid space obliteration in, 451, 454
  potential metastasis to suprasellar cistern, 454
Glioblastoma multiforme
  cerebral recurrent with drop metastases and meningeal carcinomatosis, 433–438
    axial short TR image, lumbar, 433, 437
    basal ganglia in, 434, 437
    brain, 434, 437
    brain imaging in, 437–438
    cauda equina nerve roots in, 433, 435, 437
    from central nervous system or other primary, 438
    coronal short TR image, brain, 434, 437
    distal thecal sac in, 435, 436–437
    edema in, 434, 437
    importance of postinfusion scan, 438
    left frontal lobe in, 434, 437
    L5-S1 intervertebral disc herniation in, 433, 436–437
    lumbar thecal sac in, 435, 437
    in pediatric patient, primitive neuroectodermal tumor comparison with, 438

porencephaly in, postoperative, 434, 437
sagittal long TR image, lumbar, 436–437
sagittal short TR images, lumbar, 433, 435, 437
Glioma
  of cervical spinal cord and cerebellum, 149–150
    sagittal T1W image, postcontrast, 149–150
    sagittal T1W image C2-6, 149–150
  in child, 149–150
Gluteal muscles, postpolio, 766
Gradient-echo images, magnetic susceptibility of, 346
Granulocytic sarcoma. *See* Chloroma (granulocytic sarcoma)
Guillain-Barré syndrome, cytomegalovirus CT brain scan comparison with, 521

H

Hangman's fracture. *See also under* Fracture dislocation
  C2 on C3 with disc herniation, 292–297
  definition of, 297
Headache, in germinoma with drop metastases and spinal meningeal carcinomatosis, 451–454
Hemangioblastoma
  cerebellar
    axial short TR image, 258–259
    lesion-associated, 259
  cerebral, 857–860
  of cervical spinal cord
    sagittal short TR image, 258–259
    glioma of cervical spinal cord and cerebellum *versus*, 150
  spinal, 857–860
    in von Hippel-Lindau disease, 258–259
  in von Hippel-Lindau disease
    cerebellar, 599–601
    spinal cord, 258–259, 599–601
Hemangioma, in T11 vertebral body, 269, 271
Hematoma. *See also* Epidural hematoma
  chloroma *versus*, 379
  lipoma, L2 level with tethered spinal cord and diastematomyelia *versus*, 821, 822
  L2-3 midline disc herniation with sequestered fragment L4-5 and hemorrhage *versus*, 654
  MR *versus* CT scanning for, 280
  paraspinal
    in fracture dislocation with cord contusion, 276–281
    midlumbar bilateral, 310–311, 312
    with T6 and T7 fractures, 277, 280
  posttraumatic
    epidural hematoma *versus*, 801
  soft tissue
    with cervical spinal cord injury, 305
  spinal cord
    with L1 compression fracture, 284–285
Hematopoiesis
  extramedullary, 752–755
    axial short TR image, postcontrast, 753–754
    characterization of, 755
    clinical history and, 755
    conditions associated with, 755
    coronal short TR images, pre- and postcontrast, 752, 753–754
    flow void areas in, 752, 753–754
    marrow in lumbar region, 754, 755
    sagittal long TR image, 754
    sagittal short TR image, lumbar, 754
    spondylolisthesis in, L5-S1, 754
Hemicords
  in diastematomyelia, 115, 116–117, 121, 123–124
  diplomyelia *versus*, 117
Hemophilia, spontaneous epidural hematoma *versus*, 319
Hemorrhage. *See also* Blood
  with hemangioblastoma, 259
  posttraumatic
    spinal cord arteriovenous malformation with subarachnoid hemorrhage *versus*, 613
  of schwannoma, 177
  spontaneous epidural hematoma *versus*, 319
  subacute
    lipoma *versus*, 96
Hemorrhagic infarct, eighth cranial nerve, bilateral acoustic/multiple schwannomas *versus*, 132
Hemorrhagic tumor, spinal cord arteriovenous malformation with subarachnoid hemorrhage *versus*, 613

Hemosiderin, 311
Hemosiderin deposition
  with cavernous angioma, 837
  with hemangioblastoma, 259
Hemothoraces, with fracture dislocation of T6-7, 279–280
Hepatitis B vaccination, transverse myelopathy following, 712–715, 716–718
Hilar lymphadenopathy, postradiation changes and, 728–730
Horseshoe kidney, 102–103
Hydromyelia, in Chiari malformation, 70
Hyperostosis, diffuse idiopathic skeletal, 581–583

I

Idiopathic transverse myelopathy
  multiple sclerosis *versus*, 702
  transverse myelopathy postimmunization *versus*, 715
Iliac crest, chordoma involving, 831–833
Imaging sequences
  axial gradient-echo, 29
  axial short and long TR, 29
  cervical
    fat-saturated, 4
  sagittal short and long TR, 29
Imperforate anus, sacral agenesis with filum terminale lipoma in, 93–96
Infant
  coccygeal agenesis in, 90–92
  M. tuberculosis meningitis with pneumonitis in
    cerebrospinal fluid analysis and, 508
    meninges in, 507–508
    sagittal short TR images, 507–508
    subarachnoid space below C5 in, 507–508
    vertebral body end plates in, 507–508
  meningomyelocele in, 90–92
  pneumonitis and meningitis in, 507–508
  sacral teratoma in, 260–262
    calcification in, 260, 261
    sagittal T1W image, 260–261
    sagittal T2W image, 261
    thecal sac in, lumbar, 260–261
  tethered cord in, 90–92
Infarct
  bone marrow, 756–759
  hemorrhagic, cranial nerve, 132
  multiple sclerosis *versus*, 791, 792
Inferior vena cava flow void, axial short TR image, 46
Inflammatory disease
  lung cancer with bony and epidural metastases *versus*, 388
  metastatic breast cancer with adenopathy *versus*, 359
Inflammatory meningitis, bacterial, meningeal carcinomatosis *versus*, 432
Inflammatory process
  breast cancer metastatic to C2 vertebral body with cord compression *versus*, 385
  drop metastases from recurrent posterior fossa medulloblastoma *versus*, 450
  Mycobacterium tuberculosis versus sarcoidosis, 515
  neurofibromatosis type 1 with plexiform neurofibromas in cervical spine *versus*, 816, 817
  neurofibromatosis type 2 with schwannomas *versus*, 794
Interfacet joint fluid, axial long TR image, 55
Interfacet joint(s)
  cervical
    parasagittal short TR image, 12
  degenerative changes in lumbar
    axial long TR image, 54
  lumbar
    axial short TR image, 46
  thoracic and lumbar
    Mycobacterium tuberculosis in, 512–515
Intervertebral discs. *See* Disc(s)
Intervertebral foramen
  lumbar
    parasagittal short TR image, 37, 38
    in neurofibromatosis type 1 with multiple plexiform and dumbbell-shaped tumors
      cervical, 219, 223
    in neurofibromatosis type 1 with multiple plexiform neurofibromas

INDEX

cervical, 212, 213, 215, 216
   lumbar, 214, 215
   parasagittal short TR image, 11
   T5-6 and T6-7
   renal cell cancer metastasis to, 372
Intramedullary enhancing lesions, neurofibromatosis type 1 with multiple plexiform neurofibromas *versus*, 216
Intramedullary infection, transverse myelopathy *versus*, 723, 724
Intramedullary inflammatory process, spinal cord ischemia with areas of enhancement *versus*, 608
Intramedullary metastases, transverse myelitis *versus*, 711
Intramedullary metastatic deposit, postradiation changes in spinal cord and vertebral bodies *versus*, 726, 727
Intramedullary tumor, cervical, imaging sequences in, 3
Intravenous drug abuse, discitis in, 483–486, 487–490

J

Jugular vein
   flow void, 250–251
   normal short TR image, postinfusion, 14

K

Kidney
   coronal short TR image, 36
   horseshoe
      in sacral agenesis with tethered cord, 102–103
   lesions in
      in sacral agenesis, 96
Klippel-Feil anomaly, 549–552
   with Chiari I malformation, tethered cord, lipoma, sacral agenesis, 112–114
      lipoma and, 112
      sacral agenesis and, 112
      sagittal intermediate TR image, T8, 113
      sagittal short TR image, 112
         fusion of T1-T2 and T6-T7, 112–113
      sagittal short TR image, lumbar, 113
   Chiari I malformation-associated, 112–114
   description of, 551
Kyphosis
   dorsal
      with osteoporotic compression fractures, 325
   L3-4 level
      in discitis with epidural and paraspinal abscesses, 483
   thoracic
      in adenocarcinoma, metastatic uterine, 353–355
      normal, 20
      secondary to osteoporosis, 320
   T4 level
      in metastatic breast cancer, 360–361

L

Lamina, cervical, axial short TR image, 15
Laminectomy
   complete bilateral with discectomy
      recurrent herniated disc fragment following, 637–639
   indication of previous
      in chordoma, recurrent postoperative, 250–251
   lumbar post operative
      recurrent herniated disc migration behind L5 vertebral body, 640–644
   postoperative adhesive arachnoiditis and, 739–741
   postoperative changes with, 182–183, 736, 804–805
   postsurgical clips and, cervical and thoracic, 857, 859–860
   synovial cyst following, 670–672
Laryngeal ventricle, sagittal short TR image, 10
Lateral recess
   L4-5, stenosis of, 677–678
   lumbar articulating facet-vertebral body
      axial long TR image, 50
Leiomyosarcoma
   rectal
      sacral myelomeningocele *versus*, 89
   spinal cord metastasis from, 151–153

Leptomeningeal carcinomatosis, 429–432, 853–856
Leukemia. *See also* Acute lymphocytic leukemia; Acute myelogenous leukemia
   multiple myeloma with marrow involvement *versus*, 394
Leukemic infiltrate
   in bone marrow
      with bony calvarium metastases, 865, 866, 867
      with dural meningeal metastases, 864, 866, 867
      with granulocytic sarcoma (chloroma) of neck; dural meningeal metastases
         axial short TR images, cervical, 862, 866, 867
         axial short TR images, upper thoracic, 863, 866
         coronal short TR image, brain postcontrast, 864, 866
         mass lateral to vertebral column in, 862, 863, 866, 867
         radionuclide scan in, 867
         sagittal intermediate TR images, cervical, 862, 866
         sagittal short TR images, cervical, 861
         soft tissue mass in, T3-4, 861, 867
         subarachnoid space compromise in, 862, 863, 866, 867
      with granulocytic sarcoma (chloroma) of neck; dural meningeal metastases; bony calvarium metastases, 861–867
      and leptomeningeal carcinomatosis, 853–856
         axial short TR image, thoracic postcontrast, 855
         cauda equina nerve roots in, 854–855, 856
         clinical history in, 856
         distal spinal cord in, 856
         marrow of vertebral bodies in, 853, 855
         pleural effusions in, bilateral, 856
         sagittal fat suppression image, lumbar, for meningeal carcinomatosis, 854–855, 856
         sagittal intermediate TR image, lumbar spine, 853
         sagittal long TR image, lumbar spine, 854–855
         sagittal long TR image, thoracic, 854–855
         sagittal long TR image, thoracic postcontrast, 854–855
         sagittal short TR image, lumbar spine, 853
      with metastases in thecal sac and meningeal carcinomatosis, 443–446
   in bone marrow with bony calvarium metastases
      axial intermediate/long TR images, brain, 863, 866
      axial short TR image, bony calvarium, 865, 866
      axial short TR image, brain postcontrast, 864, 866
   throughout visualized marrow
      axial long TR image, 444–445
      cauda equina nerve roots in, 445, 446
      with fracture L1 vertebral body, and metastases in thecal sac, meningeal carcinomatosis, 443–446
      sagittal and parasagittal long TR images, 443–444, 445
      sagittal short TR image, 443, 445
      sagittal short TR image, postcontrast, 445
   in vertebral body marrow
      and meningeal carcinomatosis, 455–457
   in vertebral column marrow, 861–867
Lhermitte's sign, in Chiari malformation, 70
Ligamentum flavum
   axial short TR image, 46
   lumbar disc bulge and, L4-5 with lateral recess stenosis, 677–678
Ligamentum flavum hypertrophy
   characterization of, 675–676
   in discitis with vertebral osteomyelitis, L3-4, and spinal stenosis, 781, 783, 784
   in lumbar disc herniation
      L2-3 midline with fragment sequestered at L4-5, 652, 653, 654
   spinal stenosis with, 673, 675, 676
   and vacuum degenerative changes of lumbar disc, 679–680
Lipoma. *See also* Epidural lipoma
   caudal regression syndrome with tethered cord and vertebral anomalies *versus*, 99
   epidural hematoma *versus*, 801
   of filum terminale
      sacral agenesis with, 93–96
      tethered cord with, 104–106
   L2 level with tethered cord and diastematomyelia, 818–822
      axial fat saturation image, L3, 820–821

axial long TR image, L3, 820–821
axial short TR image, L2, 819, 821
chemical shift artifact in, 820, 822
clinical history in, 816
danger of myelography in, 822
dysraphism in, 822
lipoma, L2, 818, 819, 821
midsagittal long TR image
parasagittal long TR image, 819, 821
sagittal short TR image, lumbar, 818
spinous processes in, incomplete midlumbar, 822
tethered spinal cord, 820, 821–822
tethered cord with, 109–111
Lumbar disc
   axial short TR image, 45
   conspicuity of
      long *versus* short TR images in, 628
   migration of
      L-2 to lateral recess, 646
      and sequestration at L4-5, 632–636
Lumbar disc bulge
   L4-5 with lateral recess stenosis on right, 677–678
      axial CT scans at L4-5 postmyelogram with bone window width technique, 677–678
      intervertebral foraminal stenosis, 678
      ligamentum flavum prominence in, 677–678
      osteophyte in, 677–678
Lumbar disc herniation
   L2-3 with disc fragment migration, 645–646
      axial short TR image, L2-3, 645–646
      sagittal long TR image, 645–646
   L2-3 midline with fragment sequestration at L4-5, 651–654
      axial long TR image, L4 midbody, 652–653
      axial short TR image, L2-3, 653
      cauda equina nerve roots within thecal sac, 652–653
      disc prominence at L2-3, L4-5, 652
      hemorrhage along dorsal aspect in, 651, 652–653, 654
      left parasagittal short TR image, 652–653
      ligamentum flavum hypertrophy in, 652, 653, 654
      right parasagittal short TR image, 651
      sagittal intermediate TR image, 652–653
      sagittal short TR image, 651
      soft tissue mass encroachment on thecal sac, 652–653
      spinal stenosis in, 652–653, 654
      superior extrusion of nucleus pulposus in, 654
      thecal sac compression in, 652–653, 654
   L2-3 migration to lateral recess, 646
   L4-5
      axial short TR images, 623–624
      epidural fat obliteration in, 623–624
      evaluation with multi-angle images, 623, 624
      extrusion and on sagittal long TR image, 623–624
      nerve root compression in, 648–649, 650
      nerve root encroachment in, 623–624
      posterior displacement of nerve root in, 648–649, 650
      sagittal short TR image in, 622
      thecal sac compression in, 646, 648, 649, 650
      thecal sac displacement/compression in, 623–624
   L4-5 with disc degeneration at L3-4 and L5-S1, 619–621
      avulsion fracture in, 620–621
      axial short TR images, 620–621
      CT for avulsion fracture in, 621
      dorsal root ganglion in intervertebral foramen, 620–621
      obliteration of subarachnoid space in, 619
      sagittal long TR image, 619
      sagittal short TR image, 619
      thecal sac compression in, 620–621
   L4-5, disc migration and sequestration in, 632–636
      axial short TR images at L2, 634–635
      axial short TR images at L5, 633, 635
      Batson's plexus enhancement in, 633, 635
      cauda equina nerve root enhancement and, 634–635, 636
      epidural venous plexus in, 633, 635
   L4-5, left lateral, with encroachment on intervertebral foramen, 647–650
      axial short TR images, 648, 649, 650
      clinical evaluation in, 650
      conjoined nerve roots in, 647, 650

Lumbar disc herniation (*continued*)
   dorsal root ganglion in, 649–650
   fat obliteration in, 648–649
   left parasagittal short TR image, at intervertebral foramen, 647, 648, 649
   MR imaging *versus* myelography in, 650
   obliteration of foramen in, 648–649
   sagittal short TR image, 647, 649
  L5-S1 disc prominence in, 632
   midsagittal short TR image, 633, 635
   nerve root sleeve obliteration at L5, 633, 635
   parasagittal short TR image, postcontrast, 633, 635
   sagittal long TR image, 632
   sagittal short TR image, 632
   soft tissue mass behind L5, 632, 633, 635
   thecal sac obliteration at L5, 633, 635
  L5-S1, lateral, 625–628
   axial short TR images, 627
   cauda equina nerve root displacement in, 627, 628
   with disc degeneration, 628
   epidural fat obliteration in, 627
   parasagittal long TR image, 626–627
   retrolisthesis and, 625
   sagittal long TR image, 625
   sagittal short TR image, 625
   vacuum degenerative change *versus* calcification in, 625
  L5-S1 and L4-5
   axial short TR image, L5-S1, 630–631
   axial short TR images, 630–631
   commonality of, 631
   compression of nerve root sleeve in, 630–631
   determination of laterality in, 631
   epidural fat and, 631
   fast spin echo technique *versus* long TR images for, 631
   left parasagittal long TR image, fast spin echo technique, 630–631
   midsagittal long TR image, fast spin echo technique, 630–631
   nerve root displacement in, 630–631
   parasagittal short TR images, left/right, 629
   soft tissue mass at L5-S1, 630–631
   thecal sac effacement in, 631
Lumbar disc migration and sequestration L4-5, 632–636
Lumbar spine
  chordoma involving, 831–833
  compression fractures, 272–275
  helical CT scanning of, 624
  infant
   axial short TR image, 91–92
   long TR image, 90, 92
   sagittal short TR image, 90
  lymph node enlargement
   sagittal short TR image, 42
  normal anatomy, 29–64
   axial computed tomography, 56–58
   axial long TR images, 50, 54–55
   axial short TR images, 45–49
    pre- and postinfusion, 44, 51, 60
   coronal short TR images, 35–36
   long TR images, 52–53
   midsagittal long TR images, 32–33
   midsagittal short TR images, 30–31
   MR myelography, 61
   parasagittal long TR images, 59
   parasagittal short TR image, 58
   parasagittal short TR images, 37–39, 58
   pediatric, 40–41
   sagittal intermediate signal intensity, 43
   sagittal long TR images, 41
   sagittal short TR images, 40, 42–44
  postoperative changes in
   secondary to laminectomy, 183
  Tarlov cysts, 58–61
Lumbar vertebrae
  hypoplastic
   in neonate, 100
  renal cell cancer metastasis to, 371–376
Lumbar vertebral canal, in Chiari II malformation, 77–78
Lung cancer
  with bony and epidural metastases and cord compression, 386–388
   axial short TR image, 387–388

axial short TR image, upper lumbar, 387–388
evaluation of epidural fat and cerebrospinal fluid, 388
marrow of vertebral bodies in, 386, 388
pleural effusion in, 387–388
sagittal long TR image of thoracic spine, 386, 388
sagittal short TR image of thoracic spine, 386, 388
thoracic spinal cord compression in, 387–388
vertebral pedicle involvement in, 387–388
  metastatic with lung nodules on chest CT, 362–366
   axial short TR images, 363, 364, 365
   bone destruction in, 364, 365
   chest CT *versus* plain film in, 366
   CT scan with CT-guided biopsy, 364–365
   C3 vertebral body marrow and height in, 363, 365
   pedicle expansion into thecal sac in, 363, 365
   posteroanterior and lateral plain films, 362, 365
   sagittal short TR images, 363, 365
   soft tissue mass in, 364–365
   spinal cord displacement in, 363, 365
Lymph node(s)
  enlarged
   secondary to non-Hodgkin's lymphoma, 347–349
  lumbar, enlarged
   sagittal short TR image, 42
  paratracheal
   in metastatic renal cell cancer, 371–376
  prevertebral lumbar
   axial short TR images, pre- and postcontrast, 44
Lymphoma
  leukemic infiltrate in bone marrow
   with granulocytic sarcoma (chloroma) of neck; dural meningeal metastases; bony calvarium metastases *versus*, 867
  lumbar spine in
   sagittal short TR image, 42
  meningeal carcinomatosis *versus*, 432
  multiple myeloma with marrow involvement *versus*, 394
  versus vertebral metastases secondary to non-Hodgkin's lymphoma, 349

M

Magnetic resonance imaging (MRI), contrast material for, 3
Magnetic resonance (MR) myelography
  adjunctive to MR and CT scanning, 682
  application of, 682
  description of, 682
  fast spin-echo, 62
  rapid aquisition with relaxation enhancement, 62
  three-dimensional
   of lumbar spine, 61
   versus myelography, 62
  three-dimensional gradient echo-pulse, 62
Magnetic resonance (MR) study
  lumbar spine
   fast *versus* standard spin-echo technique, 32
   standard spin-echo, 33
Magnetic susceptibility artifact
  in Chiari I malformation with postoperative changes in posterior fossa, syrinx cavity, 811, 812
  in chordoma, recurrent postoperative, 252
  in disc fragment, recurrent migratory post lumbar laminectomy, 643, 644
  in gradient echo image
   in cavernous angioma, 837
  from metallic implants, 345–346
  with metallic fusion plate and fixating screws post discectomy C5-6, C6-7, 838, 839, 840, 841
  postlaminectomy
   in von Hippel-Lindau syndrome with multiple spinal and cerebral hemangioblastomas, 857, 859, 860
Marrow
  edema of
   with disc fragment, 639
  infarction of
   in breast cancer, 461–462
   in sickle cell anemia, 756–757
  multiple myeloma involvement of, 392–394
  normal, signal intensity in *versus* intervertebral disc, 457

Medulla
  in metastatic colon carcinoma, 202, 204
  in pilocytic astrocytoma
   cystic lesion in, 155, 158
   expansion of, 164, 166
Medulloblastoma
  in child
   diffuse osteoblastic metastases in, 423
  colon cancer metastatic to subarachnoid space *versus*, 448
  with drop metastases
   M. tuberculosis meningitis with pneumonitis *versus*, 507–508
  metastatic
   to subarachnoid space, 450
  posterior fossa with drop metastases, 449–450
  recurrent posterior fossa with multiple drop metastases, 449–450
Melanoma, breast cancer, metastatic with osteoblastic metastases, epidural component and spinal cord compression *versus*, 413
Meningeal carcinomatosis
  breast cancer, metastatic with osteoblastic metastases, epidural component and spinal cord compression *versus*, 413
  cerebral, 461–463
   secondary to breast cancer, 433–438
  from cerebral glioblastoma multiforme with drop metastases, 429–432
  contrast enhancement in, 29
  cytomegalovirus radiculitis *versus*, 521
  from diffuse bone metastases, 439–442
  epidural abscess *versus*, 496
  imaging of, contrast enhanced, 3
  from leukemic infiltrate, 443–446
  in vertebral body marrow, 455–457
  M. tuberculosis meningitis with pneumonitis *versus*, 508
  meningitis postcraniotomy with arachnoid adhesions *versus*, 506
  Mycobacterium tuberculosis without sarcoidosis *versus*, 511
  postlaminectomy adhesive arachnoiditis *versus*, 741
  postradiation change in non-Hodgkin's lymphoma *versus*, 732
  sarcoidosis of central nervous system *versus*, 518
  secondary to breast cancer, 429–431, 433–438
   axial short TR images, 430, 432
   cauda equina nerve roots in, 429, 430, 432
   cerebral meninges in, 431–432
   coronal short TR images of brain, 431–432
   metastatic deposit in L4 vertebra, 429, 432
   primary tumor search in, 432
   primary tumor types in, 432
   sagittal short TR images, 429, 432
   spinal and cervical leptomeninges in, 432
  spinal
   from drop metastases, 451–454
   secondary to breast cancer, 433–438
Meningeal metastases, dural, 861–867
Meningioma(s)
  metastatic colon carcinoma *versus*, 205
  in neurofibromatosis type 2, 129, 235–240, 241–245
  schwannoma *versus*, 179
  spinal
   in neurofibromatosis type 2, 238, 239, 240
  T8-9 disc herniation with calcification in adenocarcinoma patient *versus*, 594
  T6-7 disc herniation with calcification *versus*, 592
  thoracic
   axial short TR image postcontrast, 184–185
   sagittal short TR images, 184–185
   spinal cord compression with, 185
  thoracic disc herniation *versus*, T6-7, 590
  in 57-year-old female, 186–188
   axial CT scan, 186, 188
   axial postmyelogram CT scan, 187–188
   lateral view of myelogram, 186, 188
   sagittal reconstruction view of postmyelogram CT scan, 187–188
Meningitis, 491–497
  bone metastases and spinal meningeal carcinomatosis *versus*, 441
  chemical with arachnoid adhesions, 503–506

INDEX

epidural abscess *versus*, 496, 497
infective
  glioblastoma multiforme, recurrent cerebral with meningeal carcinomatosis *versus*, 438
inflammatory, 432
M. tuberculosis with pneumonitis, 507–508
postcraniotomy with arachnoid adhesions, 503–506, 504–506
  axial short TR image, L4, 505–506
  axial short TR image, T9, 504, 506
  cauda equina nerve roots in, 504, 505–506
  cerebrospinal fluid culture in, 506
  meninges of brain in, 503, 505–506
  sagittal short TR images, lower thoracic and upper lumbar, 504, 506
  syrinx cavity in, 504, 506
Meningocele
  anterosacral
    MR imaging *versus* myelography of, 89
  in Chiari II malformation
    in neonate, 78, 79
  occipital
    in Chiari III malformation, 87
Meningoencephalocele, in Chiari III malformation, 87
Meningomyelocele
  in Chiari II malformation, 77–79
    in neonate, 78, 79
  congenital, 90–92
  in infant, 90–92
  tethered cord, coccygeal agenesis and, 90–92
Metallic fusion plate and fixating screws
  cervical spine post discectomy C5-6, C6-7, 838–841
    axial gradient echo image, C6, 840
    axial short TR images, C6 pre- and postcontrast, 839–840, 841
    comparison with plain film, 840
    magnetic susceptibility artifact in, 838, 839, 840, 841
    sagittal intermediate TR image, cervical spine, 838, 841
    sagittal long TR image, cervical spine, 839–840, 841
    sagittal short TR image, cervical spine, 838
  in C5, 6, and 7 vertebral bodies
    and metastases to vertebral bodies and spinous processes, 344–346
    MR imaging effect on, 346
    postsurgical changes in, 344–346
Metastasis(es)
  accuracy of MR imaging and, 337
  from another primary
    leukemic infiltrate in bone marrow and leptomeningeal carcinomatosis *versus*, 855, 856
  cancers similar to, 356
  diffuse
    neurofibromatosis type 1 with plexiform neurofibromas in cervical spine *versus*, 816, 817
    with pathologic fractures post breast cancer treatment, 842–844
  diffuse bony
    with fractures of T10, L1, L2, 842–844
  diffuse vertebral body with compression fracture at T6, 397–398
    clinical history in, 398
    compression fracture of T6, 397
    radionuclide bone scan and, 398
    sagittal reconstruction image, thoracic spine, 397–398
    sagittal short TR images, 397
    soft tissue component extension into T6 vertebral canal, 397
  at end of thecal sac, 443–445
  epidural
    lung, 386–388
    with vertebral, T11 and L4, 845–848
  hemorrhagic
    cavernous angioma of spinal cord with hemorrhage *versus*, 775
  meningeal dural, 861–867
  Mycobacterium tuberculosis versus sarcoidosis, 515
  postradiation changes, 338–339
  T11 and L4 vertebral bodies with epidural metastases, 845–848
    axial short TR images, T11 midbody pre- and postcontrast, 847

axial short TR images, T11 pre- and postcontrast, 846–847
epidural encroachment on thecal sac, T12-L1, 847–848
osteophyte formation in, 847–848
sagittal long TR image, 845
sagittal short TR image, L4, 845
sagittal short TR image, postcontrast, 845–846
sagittal short TR image, postcontrast with fat suppression technique, 845–846, 847
thecal sac at L4, 847–848
von Hippel-Lindau disease with cerebellar and spinal hemangioblastomas *versus*, 599–601
Metastatic deposit(s)
  chordomas with postoperative changes *versus*, 251
  dermoid tumor *versus*, 264
  neurofibromatosis type 2 *versus*, 230–232
  osteoblastic and osteolytic, 461–463
  signal intensity of marrow *versus* tumor, 337
Metastatic disease. See also Osteoblastic metastatic disease; Osteolytic and osteoblastic metastases
  breast or prostate
    multiple myeloma *versus*, 409, 416
  chordoma: distal lumbar spine, iliac crest, sacrum, coccyx *versus*, 832, 833
  colon carcinoma metastasis *versus*, 368
  compression fracture, 321, 323
  discitis with vertebral osteomyelitis, L3-4, and spinal stenosis *versus*, 781
  L2-3 midline disc herniation with sequestered fragment at L4-5 *versus*, 654
  lung cancer with bony and epidural metastases *versus*, 388
  multiple sclerosis *versus*, 692, 693
  versus osteogenic carcinoma, 337
  from primary tumor, 205
  thyroid
    versus renal cell carcinoma, 382
  traumatic compression fracture *versus*, 271
  versus vertebral metastases secondary to non-Hodgkin's lymphoma, 349
Methemoglobin, 311, 317, 319
MISME. See Multiple inherited schwannoma, meningioma, ependymoma (MISME); Neurofibromatosis type 2
Motorcycle accident, fracture dislocation T6-7, with cord contusion and paraspinal hematoma, 276–281
Motor vehicle accident
  anterolisthesis of C4 on C5 with herniated disc, 286–288
  compression fracture of L1 with spinal cord hematoma, 284–285
  ejection at high speed, 282–283
  flexion injury with fracture dislocation
    axial short TR image, lower thoracic/lumbar, 282–283
    dural tear with cerebrospinal fluid/blood leakage, 282–283
    L1-2 spinous processes, 282–283
    sagittal long TR image lower, thoracic/lumbar, 282–283
    sagittal short TR image, lower thoracic/lumbar, 282–283
Multiple inherited schwannoma, meningioma, ependymoma (MISME), 239, 794–795. See also Neurofibromatosis type 2
Multiple myeloma, 395–396
  versus amyloidosis, 391
  amyloidosis in, 759
  axial short TR image
    thoracic spinal cord compression in, 403
  with bony involvement and cord compression from soft tissue mass, 402–406
    axial short TR images, pre- and postcontrast, 405–406
    fat infiltration of paraspinous muscles, 405–406
    parasagittal short TR image, postcontrast, 405–406
  breast cancer with osteoblastic and osteolytic deposits throughout bone; cerebral carcinomatosis *versus*, 463
  calvarium destruction in, 390, 391
  characterization of, 391
  with compression fractures
    at T12, L1, L2, L3, L4, L5, 392, 393–394

CT scan in, 396
  with bone window widths, 390
description of, 403
with diffuse marrow involvement and multiple compression fractures, 392–394
epidural hematoma and pleural effusions in, 407–409
  axial long TR image, lumbar, 408–409
  axial short TR, 408–409
  axial short TR image, 408–409
  axial short TR image, lumbar, 408–409
  compression fracture in, 408–409
  epidural fat and, 407, 409
  epidural hematoma, 407, 409
  pleural effusions, 408–409
  sagittal short TR image, cervical and upper thoracic, 407, 409
  spinal cord displacement and compression in, 407, 409
with infiltration of vertebral body and soft tissue mass
  compression fractures in, 408–409
with infiltration of vertebral body marrow with soft tissue mass, 404–406
  compression fracture of L5 vertebral body, 404
  degenerative changes at multiple levels, 404
  extension into dorsal paraspinal muscles, 406
  marrow of vertebral bodies and, 404
  osteophytes in, 404
  sagittal short TR images, 404
  soft tissue tumor, L3 level, 404, 405–406
with involvement of spine and bony calvarium, 389–391
  anteroposterior plain film of spine, 389–390, 391
  bone destruction in bony calvarium, 390, 391
  CT brain scan postinfusion, 390
  CT scan with bone window width, 390
  degenerative changes with osteophytes at C5, C6, C7, 389–390
  expansion of frontal bone, 390
  marrow of vertebral bodies, 389–390
  pedicle at L3 level, 389–390
  radionuclide bone scan correlation with, 391
leukemic infiltrate in marrow
  with granulocytic sarcoma (chloroma) of neck; dural meningeal metastases; bony calvarium metastases *versus*, 867
leukemic infiltrate in marrow and leptomeningeal carcinomatosis *versus*, 855, 856
with marrow involvement and compression fractures, 392–394
  axial short TR image, 395–396
  clinical considerations in, 396
  compression fractures, L1 and L4 vertebral body, 395
  with disc protrusion, lumbar, 395
  marrow involvement, 395, 396
  sagittal short TR image, 395
  sagittal short TR image, postcontrast, 393–394
  sagittal short TR image, thoracic, 392, 393–394
  subarachnoid space compression in, 395–396
  transverse process in, lumbar, 395–396
metastases to vertebral bodies with compression fracture *versus*, 398
metastases *versus*, 344–346
metastatic lung cancer *versus*, 366
metastatic osteoblastic prostate carcinoma *versus*, 416
osteoblastic and osteolytic metastases *versus*, prostatic, 803
osteoblastic metastatic prostate cancer *versus*, 352
osteolytic and osteoblastic metastases *versus*, diffuse, 797, 798
pleural effusions in, bilateral bloody, 408–409
postsurgical changes with metallic implants and metastases *versus*, 346
with rapid progression, 399–401
  axial short TR images, L4 pre- and postcontrast, 401
  compression fractures at L1, L4, L5, 399–400
  marrow of vertebral bodies in, 400–401
  paraspinal mass in, 401
  pedicle expansion in, 400–401
  retropulsion of L1 component into vertebral canal, 399–400
  sagittal long TR image, 400–401

Multiple myeloma (*continued*)
  sagittal short TR images, 399–400
  spinal cord displacement in, 399–400
  renal cell cancer metastatic to lung and thoracic/lumbar vertebrae *versus,* 375
  sagittal long TR image
    lower cervical and upper thoracic spine, 402
  sagittal short TR image
    degenerative changes in cervical spine, 402
    epidural mass on, 402
    thoracic spinal cord displacement, 402
  sagittal short TR image postcontrast, 402–403
    thoracic spinal cord compression on, 402–403
  schwannoma in, 180–181
  spinal cord compression
    from soft tissue component, 394
    with thoracic vertebral body marrow involvement, 393–394
  unusual presentation of, 845–848
  with vertebral body marrow infiltration and soft tissue mass, 404–406
Multiple myeloma, Polyneuropathy, Organomegaly, Endocrinopathy, Myeloma, Skin changes (POEMS)
  osteoblastic metastatic prostate cancer *versus,* 352
Multiple sclerosis
  blurred vision in, 707, 708
  of brain, 689–693, 790–792
  brain and spinal cord, 689–693, 694–698
    in adolescent, 694–698, 790–792
    arcuate fibers in, 696, 697, 698
    axial FLAIR image, brain, 697
    axial long TR image, brain, 695, 697, 698
    axial long TR image, brain at lateral ventricles, 691–692, 790, 791
    axial long TR image, central spinal cord, 695, 697, 698
    axial long TR image, upper cervical spinal cord, 790–791
    axial short TR image, brain, 696–697
    axial short TR image, brain pre- and postcontrast, 691–692
    axial short TR image, postcontrast C4, 690, 692
    cerebrospinal fluid analysis in, 692, 792
    cervical cord findings in, 692–693
    corpus callosum in, 695, 697, 698, 790, 792
    edema in, spinal cord, 699, 701, 702
    frontal horn of lateral ventricle in, 700–701, 702
    periventricular areas of brain in, 692
    plaque in spinal cord in, 790, 792
    preventricular area in, 697
    sagittal long TR image, 694, 697
    sagittal short TR image, postcontrast C4, 690, 692
    sagittal short TR image, thoracic spinal cord, 694
    subarachnoid fluid in, 694, 697
  cerebrospinal fluid analysis in, 702, 706
  cervical spinal cord in
    imaging sequences in, 3
  MR imaging of brain in, 702
  postradiation changes in spinal cord and vertebral bodies *versus,* 726, 727
  postradiation changes with spinal cord enhancement *versus,* 729, 730
  probable, 697–702, 699–702
    axial intermediate TR image, 700–701
    axial long TR image, 700–701
    sagittal long TR image, C1 through C7, 699, 701
    sagittal short TR image, cervical spine, 699, 701
    sagittal short TR images, mid- and upper cervical, 700–701
  sex difference in, 702, 706
  spinal cord, 689–693, 694–698, 703–706, 707–708, 790–792
    axial short TR image, 705, 706
    axial short TR images, C2-3 pre- and postcontrast, 704–705, 706
    sagittal intermediate TR image, cervical, 707–708
    sagittal long TR image, C2-3 postcontrast, 704–705, 706
    sagittal short TR images, C2-3 and C5-6 postcontrast, 703, 705, 706
    sagittal short TR images, cervical pre- and postcontrast, 707–708
  spinal cord findings in, 692
  transverse myelitis *versus,* 711
  transverse myelopathy *versus,* 715
  white matter in, 697, 698

Mycobacterium avium intracellulare
  inflammatory process of
    metastatic breast *versus,* 385
  Mycobacterium tuberculosis without sarcoidosis *versus,* 509–511
Mycobacterium species
  in discitis, 475, 479, 489–490
Mycobacterium tuberculosis
  in discitis, 485
  in infant
    pneumonitis and meningitis with, 507–508
  inflammatory process of, 385
  in interfacet joints, thoracic and lumbar, 512–515
    axial short TR images, pre- and postcontrast, 513, 515
    cerebrospinal fluid analysis in, 515
    correlation with neuroradiologic imaging, 515
    CT-guided needle aspiration with culture in, 515
    parasagittal short TR image, lumbar paraspinal area, 513, 515
    parasagittal short TR image, postcontrast, 514–515
    radionuclide bone scan in, 515
    sagittal short TR images, 513, 515
    temporal bone involvement and, 515
  meningitis and, 506
  pneumonitis and meningitis with, 507–508
  sarcoidosis of central nervous system *versus,* 518
  transverse myelopathy *versus,* 724
  without sarcoidosis, 509–511
    axial short TR image, 510–511
    cervical spinal cord compression in, 510–511
    cervical spinal cord widening in, 509
    leptomeninges surrounding cervical spinal cord, 510–511
    medulla narrowed at craniocervical junction, 509
    sagittal long TR image, 510–511
    sagittal short TR image, 509–511
    sagittal short TR image, postcontrast, 510–511
    subarachnoid space in, 510–511
    upper cervical cord to C2 in, 510–511
Myelitis
  transverse. *See also* Transverse myelopathy (myelitis)
    postimmunization, 712–715
    secondary to multiple sclerosis, 719–721
    of unknown cause, 709–711, 722–724
Myelofibrosis, breast cancer with osteoblastic and osteolytic deposits throughout bone; cerebral carcinomatosis *versus,* 463
  osteolytic and osteoblastic metastases *versus,* diffuse, 797, 798
  sickle cell anemia with multiple bone infarcts *versus,* 757
Myelography
  in metastatic Ewing's sarcoma spinal cord compression
    cervical or lumbar tap and, 370
  versus MR imaging
    in renal cell cancer metastatic to lung and thoracic/lumbar vertebrae, 376
  MR scanning *versus*
    for meningioma, 185
  in osteoblastic metastatic prostate cancer, 352
  for postsurgical changes with metallic plate and screws, 346
Myelography with postmyelogram CT scan, *versus* MRI, for cervical disc herniation, 534, 536, 539
Myelomalacia
  from C5-6 disc herniation, 574–578
  from degeneration with osteophyte formation and trauma, 540–543
  degenerative changes with osteophyte formation *versus,* 543
  post C4-5 fusion and osteophyte formation, 567–569
Myelomeningocele
  anterior sacral, 88–89
    sagittal long TR image, 88
    sagittal short TR image, lower lumbar, 88
    thecal sac extension in, 88
  Chiari II malformation and, 77–79, 80–82
  sacral
    anterior, 88–89
    CT scanning in, 89
    tethered cord and lipoma with, 109–111
Myxopapillary ependymoma
  dermoid tumor *versus,* 264
  lower thoracic-upper lumbar, 189–191

axial short TR images postcontrast, 190
sagittal short TR images postcontrast, 189
lumbar
  axial short TR images, 193–194
  with hemorrhagic areas, 192–194
  sagittal short TR images, 192
metastases from, 194

N

Neonate
  sacral agenesis with filum terminale lipoma in, 93–96
    axial short TR image, 94–95
    Chiari III malformation
      with occipital meningocele/meningoencephalocele, 87
      sagittal short TR image of skull, 86
    Chiari II malformation with meningomyelocele, sacral agenesis, 77–79
    long TR image, 94–95
    sagittal intermediate TR image, 93, 95
    sagittal short TR image, 93, 95
    short TR image, at intervertebral disc of L4-5, 95
  sacral and coccygeal agenesis, sinus tract, spinal dysraphism, tethered cord in, 100–101
  tethered cord, sacral agenesis, horseshoe, pelvic kidney in, 102–103
Nerve, lumbar, coronal short TR image, 36
Nerve roots, L3-4, long TR image, 53
Neural foramen, axial short TR image, 60
Neuroblastoma, diffuse osteoblastic metastases in, 423
Neurofibroma, 141–144. *See also* Plexiform neurofibroma
  of dorsal root ganglion bilaterally, 141–144
  drop metastasis *versus,* 200
  dumbbell appearance of
    enlarged lymph nodes *versus,* 349
  L2-3 disc herniation with fragment migration *versus,* 646
  schwannoma *versus,* 177, 179
  Tarlov cyst *versus,* 61
Neurofibromatosis
  with bilateral acoustic schwannomas, meningiomas, and spinal cord ependymomas, 241–245
    axial short TR image, 242, 244
    coronal short TR images, 244–245
    magnetic susceptibility artifact, 241
    parasagittal short TR image, 242, 244
    sagittal long TR image, 242, 244
    sagittal T1W images, 241, 244
  bilateral acoustic schwannomas in, 242, 244, 245
  central. *See* Neurofibromatosis type 2
  meningiomas in, 242, 244
  peripheral form. *See* Neurofibromatosis type 1
Neurofibromatosis type 1, 239
  astrocytoma in, 141–144. *See also* Astrocytoma, with neurofibroma
  astrocytoma of distal spinal cord *versus,* 233–234
  axial postcontrast image, midhumerus, 126–127
  congenital, 125–127
    plexiform neurofibroma in, 125, 127
  coronal short TR image, chest and thoracic spine, 125, 127
  long TR image, 126–127
  with multiple plexiform neurofibromas, 211–216, 225–229
    in adolescent patient, 225–229
    at all levels, 225–229
    axial image, upper lumbar region, 227, 229
    brachial plexus in, 213, 215
    spinal canal soft tissue masses in, 225, 228
  with multiple plexiform neurofibromas and dumbbell-shaped tumors, 217–224
    anterior scalenus muscle, 218, 223
    carotid artery flow void, thoracic inlet, 219, 223
    cervical region, 217, 218, 219, 223, 224
    globes of orbit and, 222, 224
    intervertebral foramina in, cervical, 219, 223
    left subclavian vein flow void in, thoracic inlet, 219, 223
    lumbar region, 220, 221, 222, 223–224
    right subclavian vein flow void, thoracic inlet, 219, 223
    spinal cord compression in, 220, 221, 223
    spinal cord displacement in, 220, 223

supraclavicular region in, 217, 223
trachea in, 219, 223
with multiple spinal neurofibromata and plexiform neurofibroma
on right brachial plexus, 125
with plexiform neurofibromas, cervical spine, 813–817
axial long TR image, C4-5, 814, 816
axial short TR image, C4-5, pre- and postcontrast, 815–816
bilateral, 814, 815, 816, 817
brachial plexus nerve roots in, 814, 816
cervical spinal cord expansion in, 813, 816
coronal short TR image, cervical postcontrast, 815–816
coronal short TR image, cervical spine postcontrast, 815–816
coronal short TR image, vertebral artery postcontrast, 815–816
mass at C1-2 level, 813, 816
midsagittal short TR image, postinfusion, 813
parasagittal short TR image, postinfusion, 814, 816
sagittal short TR image, 813
spinal cord compression in, 815–816, 817
with plexiform neurofibromata in cervical spine, 813–817
short TR image, supraclavicular, 125, 127
Neurofibromatosis type 2
astrocytoma in, 167–171
axial short TR image
pre- and postcontrast, 130–131
with bilateral acoustic schwannomas, 241–245
with cerebral meningiomas and acoustic schwannomas, 238, 239
characterization of, 132
definition of, 129
description of, 239
with meningiomas and ependymomas, 241–245
with multiple schwannomas, 793–794
with plexiform neurofibromas, 230–232
with plexiform neurofibromas in intervertebral foramina, sternocleidomastoid muscle, intradural space
axial short TR images, C5, 231–232
cervical and thoracic, 230–232
sagittal short TR images, 230, 232
sagittal short TR image
lumbar, postcontrast, 131
sagittal T1W image
falx cerebri on, 238–239
with schwannomas, 794–795
with schwannomas, lumbar spine
cauda equina nerve roots in, 793–794
cerebrospinal fluid analysis in, 794
clinical history and, 794
disc herniation in, L4-5, 793, 794
retrolisthesis in, L5 on S1, 793, 794
sagittal images, 793–794
with schwannomas, postoperative changes, tethered cord, 128–129
spinal cord tethering in, postoperative, 128–129
with spinal schwannoma, meningioma, and ependymoma, 235–240
axial T1W image, cauda equina region, 238–239
sagittal T1W image of cervical and thoracic spine, 235, 236, 237, 239
sagittal T1W image of thoracic and upper lumbar subarachnoid space, 236, 237, 239
Non-Hodgkin's lymphoma
postradiation change in, 731–732
vertebral metastases and lymph node enlargement in, 347—349
abdominal aorta flow void and, 347, 349
axial short TR image, 348–349
epidural enhancement, 348–349
marrow in L3 and L4 vertebral bodies, 348–349
parasagittal short TR image, 347–348, 349
sagittal short TR image, lumbar, 347, 349
sagittal short TR images, 347, 349
soft tissue masses, 348–349
thecal sac in, 347–348
Nucleus pulposus, lumbar disc, axial long TR image, 49

O

Ochronosis (alkaptonuria)
calcified T6-7 herniated disc versus, 598
characterization of, 598
intervertebral disc calcification in, 598

Odontoid fracture(s)
medicolegal problems and, 299
old, 298–299
posttraumatic, 298–299
type I, 299
type II, 298–299
sagittal long TR image, 298–299
sagittal short TR image, 298–299
type III, 299
Odontoid process, 5
coronal long TR image, 7
degenerative changes in, 249, 251
in Down's syndrome
dislocation of, 133–134
subluxation of, 133–134
midsagittal short TR image, 9
sagittal long TR image, 6
sagittal short TR image, 5
Optic neuritis
multiple sclerosis and, probable, 699–702
and transverse myelopathy secondary to multiple sclerosis, 719–721
Osteoarthritis, amyloidosis in, 759
Osteoblastic and osteolytic metastases
from prostate cancer
axial CT scan, T11, 802–803
lateral plain film, thoracolumbar spine, 802–803
sclerosis, T11 vertebral body, 802–803
Osteoblastic metastatic deposits
breast cancer metastatic to vertebral body marrow and spinal epidural space versus, 460
diffuse, 460–463
in prostate cancer, 350–352
cervical and upper thoracic, 350–351
lumbar, 350–351
sagittal short TR images, 350–351
sagittal short TR images post scoliosis correction program, 350–351
scoliosis in, 350–351
Osteoblastic metastatic disease
in breast cancer, 410–411, 412–413
MR image correlation with plain film, 411
osteoblastic metastatic prostate cancer versus, 352
diffuse
in prostate cancer, 350–351, 795–798
from primary osteogenic sarcoma, 421–423
with multiple pathologic fractures, 417–420
in primary osteogenic carcinoma, 421–423
axial short TR images, 422–423
compression fractures of L1, L3, L4 vertebral bodies, 421
L5 vertebral body encroachment on subarachnoid space, 421
radionuclide scanning in, 423
retropulsion of vertebral body into vertebral canal, 422–423
sagittal long TR image, lumbar region, 422–423
sagittal short TR images, 421
from prostate cancer, 340–343, 350–352, 414–416, 802–803
response to long TR sequences, 337
with soft tissue component in lower cervical region, 417–420
Osteochondroma
T6-7 disc herniation with calcification versus, 592
T8-9 disc herniation with calcification in adenocarcinoma patient versus, 594
Osteogenic carcinoma, metastatic breast cancer versus, 337
Osteolytic and osteoblastic metastases
diffuse, 795–798
axial short TR images, pre- and postcontrast, 796–797
bone biopsy in, 797
coronal image in, 797
disc reversal sign in, 795, 797
marrow of vertebral bodies in, 795, 796, 797
radionuclide bone scan in, 797
sagittal long TR image, lumbar, 795
sagittal short TR image, lumbar, 795
sagittal short TR image, lumbar postcontrast, 796–797
spinal processes in, 795, 797
Osteolytic metastases
breast cancer metastases in vertebral body marrow and spinal epidural space versus, 460

conversion to osteoblastic deposits, 420
diffuse, 461–463, 795–798
response to long TR sequences, 337
Osteomyelitis
C5 and C6 levels and retropharyngeal abscess, 498, 501, 502
discitis and, 570–573
epidural abscess versus, 502
at L3-4 and spinal stenosis, 781–784
vertebral, 487–490
discitis with, 477–479
Osteophytes
diffuse idiopathic skeletal hyperostosis versus, 580–582
end plates, C5 and C6, 9
formation and chordoma, 249, 251
formation of and myelomalacia, 540–543
at L2-3 level, 338–339
post C4-5 fusion, 567–569
Osteoporosis
compression fractures in
kyphosis with, 320, 325
L3, L4, L5, 182–183
thoracic, 320–325
in lumbar spine
synovial cyst and, 666, 669
traumatic compression fracture versus, 271

P

Paget's disease
characterization of, 674–675, 676
at L5, S1, S2, sacral alae and iliac crests, incidental, 675, 676
of lumbar spine, sacral alae, and iliac crests, 673–676
plain film in, 676
radionuclide bone scanning in, 675
Pantopaque®. See Retained Pantopaque
Paraneoplastic syndrome
postradiation changes in spinal cord and vertebral bodies versus, 727
transverse myelitis versus, 711
Paraplegia, in cavernous angioma of spinal cord with hemorrhage, 773–775
Paraspinal mass, postradiation changes versus, 339
Paraspinal muscles
abscess of, 491–497
in diabetes mellitus patient, 493, 494, 496
secondary to discitis, 483–486
postpolio, 766
Pathologic fractures
in metastatic disease
from breast cancer, 842–844
vertebral body, 397–398
in osteoblastic disease, 417–420
Pedicle, lumbar, coronal short TR image, 36
Pelvis, in neurofibromatosis type 1 with plexiform neurofibromas, axial long TR image, 226, 229
Perched facets
from acute neck flexion injury, 300–301
compression of nerve rootlets in, 301
C4 on C5 subluxation, 300
lateral plain film, 300
treatment of, 301
bow tie appearance of, 301
Pilocytic astrocytoma, 145–148, 154–160
in adolescent, 164–166
axial short TR image
postcontrast, 147–148
at tumor midportion, 147–148
axial short TR image, C2, odontoid tip, 157–158
axial short TR image, C1 postcontrast, 157–158
C1-3
axial short TR image, tip of odontoid, 157–158
cystic lesion in medulla, 155, 158
cystic portion of tumor, 159
parasagittal long TR image, 155, 158
sagittal long TR image, C1-T1, 155, 158
sagittal short TR images, 155, 158
spinal cord enlargement, 156, 158
subarachnoid space obliteration in, 156, 157, 158
cervical spinal cord in, 164–166
characterization of, 144
glioma of cervical spinal cord and cerebellum versus, 150

Spinal cord compression (*continued*)
  MR imaging *versus* other methods for, 376
  in multiple myeloma with soft tissue mass, 402–403
  at T2 in Ewing's sarcoma, 369–370
  in uterine adenocarcinoma, metastatic, 353–356
Spinal cord edema
  with epidural and prevertebral abscesses, 785, 789
  with traumatic compression fracture, 271
Spinal cord infarction
  acute disseminated encephalomyelopathy *versus*, 718
  astrocytoma of distal spinal cord *versus*, 233–234
  transverse myelopathy *versus*, 715, 723, 724
Spinal cord ischemia, 607–609
  postradiation changes in spinal cord and vertebral bodies *versus*, 726, 727
  in spinal cord arteriovenous malformation, 610–614
Spinal cord lipoma, 747–749
  axial short TR image, 748
  congenital, 749
  degenerative changes and, incidental, 747
  osteophytes with, 747
  post laminectomy, 747
  sagittal long TR image, 747–748
  sagittal short TR image, 747
Spinal cord metastasis
  ependymoma *versus*, 140
  from leiomyosarcoma, 151–153
    axial long TR image, 152–153
    axial short TR image, pre- and postcontrast, 152–153
    sagittal short TR images, 151, 153
Spinal cord tumor(s)
  chordoma, 248–257
  dermoid, 263–264
  hemangioblastoma, multiple
    in von Hippel-Lindau disease, 258–259
  intradural, 175–205
  intramedullary, 137–171
  multiple sclerosis *versus*, 692, 708
  neurofibromatosis, 211–245
  postoperative changes post discectomy with spinal fusion *versus*, 580
  primary
    acute disseminated encephalomyelopathy *versus*, 718
  sacral teratoma, 260–262
  spinal cord ischemia with areas of enhancement *versus*, 608, 609
  spinal cord lipoma *versus*, 748, 749
  transverse myelitis *versus*, 711
  transverse myelopathy secondary multiple sclerosis *versus*, 721
Spinal laminar line, 5
Spinal stenosis, 677–678
  with cervical spinal cord injury, 305
  C5 from anterolisthesis C4 on C5, 291
  evaluation of lumbar
    CT of lumbar and lower thoracic vertebral canal in, 680
    MR imaging for spondylolisthesis in, 680
  helical CT scanning in, 624
  L3-4 from osteomyelitis, 781–784
  L3-4 secondary to ligamentum flavum hypertrophy/encroachment on vertebral canal, 673–676
    axial short TR images, L5 and S1 vertebral bodies, 674–675
    axial short TR images, L5 vertebral body
    Paget's disease at L5, S1, S2, incidental, 673, 675
    Paget's disease in, incidental, 673, 675
    sagittal long TR image, 673, 675
    sagittal short TR image, 673, 675
  L4-5 and L3-4 with bulging discs at L3-4, L4-5, L5-S1, 681–682
    encroachment on subarachnoid space, 681–682
    encroachment on thecal sac with, 681–682
    ligamentum flavum hypertrophy in, 681–682
    posteroanterior short TR image of MR myelogram, 681–682
    sagittal short TR image with MR myelography, 681–682
  lateral recess, 677–678
  with vacuum degenerative changes of lumbar disc, 679–680
    axial CT scan with tissue bone width technique, 679–680
    axial CT scan with tissue window width technique, 679–680
    cystic degenerative change in, 679–680
    interfacet joint narrowing in, 679–680
    ligamentum flavum hypertrophy in, 679–680
Spinous processes
  cervical
    metastases to, 344–346
    sagittal short TR image, 10
  L5
    midsagittal short TR image, 34
  lumbar
    axial short TR image, 46
    normal short TR image, postinfusion, 14
    sagittal long TR image, 6
  thoracic
    normal, 20
Spondylolisthesis
  anterior
    secondary to degenerative changes, 182–183
  grade 1, 655–658
  grade 4, 662–665
  L2 on L3, 181
  secondary to bilateral spondylolysis, 655–658, 659–661
Spondylolisthesis, grade 1
  interfacet joint changes and, 658
  secondary to bilateral spondylosis at L4-5, 655–658
    axial short TR image, L3-4, 656–657
    axial short TR image, L4-5, 657
    parasagittal short TR image, 656–657, 658
    pars interarticularis interruption in, 656, 657, 658
    pseudobulge encroachment on intervertebral foramen, 656, 657
    sagittal long TR image, 655, 658
    sagittal short TR image, 655, 658
    spondylolysis in, 657, 658
Spondylolisthesis, grade 4, 662–665
  axial short TR image
    L4 level, 664
    L5 vertebral body, 663–664, 665
    S1 superior end plate, 663–664, 665
  epidural fat in, 662, 663–664, 665
  epidural space enlargement in, 662, 663–664
  nerves at L4 level, stretched, 664, 665
  pseudobulging disc, 662, 663, 664, 665
  sagittal long TR image, 662, 664
  sagittal short TR image, 662
  spinal stenosis in, 662, 664, 665
Spondylolysis
  bilateral, L4-5 level, 655–658
  bilateral and grade 1 spondylolisthesis, 659–660
    axial short TR image at interface joint, 660, 661
    axial short TR image at pars defect, 660
    disc prominence in, L5-S1, 659, 661
    displacement of L5 on S1 in, 659
    epidural space enlargement in, 659, 661
    parasagittal short TR image at interfacet joints, 659–660, 661
    pars interarticularis interruption at L5, 659–660, 661
    pseudobulging disc in, L4-5 i, 659, 661
    sagittal short TR image, 659, 661
    sclerosis in, 660
  definition of, 580
  postoperative changes post discectomy with spinal fusion *versus*, 580
Sternocleidomastoid muscle
  plexiform neurofibromas in, 230–232
  soft tissue masses
    in neurofibromatosis type 2, 231–232
Subarachnoid space, colon cancer metastasis to, 447–448
Subclavian veins, right and left, in neurofibromatosis type 1, 219, 223
Subluxation
  C1-2 in Down's syndrome, 823–825
  C2 on C3, 294, 296
  C4 on C5, 300
  C5 on C6, 304
  postsurgical, 344–345
Synovial cyst, 666–669
  calcification of, 672
  characterization of, 669
  versus herniated discs, 672
  interfacet degenerative changes with, 669
  at L3-4 interfacet joint, 670–672
    anterolisthesis in, anterior, 670
    axial short TR image, L3-4, 671–672
    axial short TR image, vertebral pedicle at L4, 671–672
    bulging discs, T12-L1, L1-2, L2-3, 670, 672
    cauda equina nerve roots displacement in, 670, 672
    disc space narrowing in, L5-S1, 670
    epidural fat obliteration in, 670
    irregularity of inferior articulating facet in, 671–672
    osteophytes in, 670
    retrolisthesis, L2 on L3 and L1 on L2, 670
    sagittal long TR image, 670, 672
    sagittal short TR image, 670
    thecal sac displacement/compression in, 671–672
    thecal sac obliteration in, 670, 672
  lumbar spine
    anterolisthesis of L4 in, 666, 669
    axial long TR image, 668
    axial short TR image, 667–668
    midsagittal long TR image, 666
    osteoporosis in, 666, 669
    parasagittal long TR image, 667–668
    sagittal short TR image, 666
    thecal sac displacement and compression in, 667–668
  spinal stenosis and, 672
Syringohydromyelia
  in Chiari I malformation, 79, 85
  in Chiari III malformation, 87
Syringomyelia, diastematomyelia-associated, 118
Syrinx cavity, 810–812
  benign
    pilocytic astrocytoma *versus*, 146, 148
  C4
    in fracture dislocation of C4 on C5, 289–291
  cervical, 579–580
    in Chiari III malformation, 86
    evaluation of, 76
    imaging sequences in, 4
    in Chiari I malformation, 71
    in Chiari malformation, 83–85
    in child, 104–106
  decompression of, cervical
    postoperative follow-up, 83–85
  diastematomyelia-associated, 122–124
  distal cord
    tethered cord with filum terminale lipoma with, 104–106
  evaluation for
    in Chiari I malformation, 70
  multiple sclerosis *versus*, 702, 706
  posttraumatic
    spinal cord ependymoma removal *versus*, 164
  response to shunt tube placement
    MR evaluation of, 85
  thoracic
    axial short TR image, 75–76
    sagittal long TR image, 74–75
    sagittal short TR image, 74–75
  thoracic-lumbar
    in Chiari II malformation, 77–78
  traumatic injury and, 280

T

Tarlov cysts
  definition of, 61
Teratoma
  description of, 262
  malignant potential of, 262
  sacral, 260–262
    caudal regression syndrome with tethered cord and vertebral anomalies *versus*, 99
    in infant, 260–262
    sacral agenesis with filum lipoma *versus*, 96
    sacral myelomeningocele *versus*, 89
Tethered cord
  in agenesis and spinal dysraphism, 100–101
  in Chiari II malformation, 80–82
  in neonate, 78, 79
  congenital, 90–92, 100–101
    with filum terminale lipoma, syrinx of distal cord, expanded lumbar canal, 104–106
    lipoma, myelomeningocele and, 109–111
    sinus tract, 107–108
  in infant, 90–92

INDEX

with lipoma
  at L2, 818–822
  and myelomeningocele, 109–111
lower thoracic and upper lumbar
  in neurofibromatosis type 2, 128, 129
meningomyelocele, coccygeal agenesis and, 90–92
in neonate, 100–101, 103
postlaminectomy, 163
postoperative, 768–770
post pilocytic astrocytoma removal, 160
sacral agenesis, horseshoe kidney and, 102–103
secondary to surgery, 129
sinus tract, 107–108
T12-L1
  post laminectomy, 804–805
Tethered cord, lipoma, myelomeningocele
  in infant
    parasagittal image, left side, 110–111
    parasagittal image, right side, 109–110
    sagittal intermediate signal intensity image, 110–111
    sagittal short TR image, 109–110
Tethered cord, sacral agenesis, horseshoe pelvic kidney
  neonatal
    sagittal short TR image, 103
Tethered cord and sinus tract
  in infant, 107–108
    sagittal short TR image, 107
Tethered cord with filum terminale lipoma, syrinx of distal cord, expanded lumbar vertebral canal, 104–106
  axial short TR image, 104, 106
  chemical shift artifact in, 106
  in child, 104–106
  sagittal long TR image, 106
  sagittal short TR image, 104, 106
  vertebral canal expansion in, 105–106
Thecal sac
  long TR image of, 52
  lumbar
    axial CT images, 56, 57
    MR myelogram, three-dimensional, 61
    parasagittal long TR image, 59
  metastasis to
    in acute myelogenous leukemia, 443–445
    from leukemic infiltrate, 443–446
  termination of
    midsagittal short TR image, 34
  thoracic
    blood in, 308–312
Thoracic disc herniation
  T6-7, 587–590
    axial short TR images, T5-6 and T6-7, 588, 589
    calcification of, 590
    CT scanning for calcification in, 590
    kyphosis and, 587–588, 590
    midsagittal long TR image, 587–588
    midsagittal short TR image, 587–588
    mushroom-shaped mass in, 587–588, 589
    parasagittal long TR image, 588–589
    spinal cord compression in, 589
    spinal cord displacement in, 587–588, 589
  T6-7 with calcification, 591–592
    axial CT scan below T6-7, 591–592
    axial CT scan postmyelogram using bone width technique, 591–592
    axial CT scan postmyelogram using soft tissue window widths, 591–592
  T6-7 with compromise of vertebral canal, 595–598
    in adolescent, 595–598
    axial CT scan at superior end plate of T7, 595, 597
    axial CT scan using bone window widths, 595, 597
    axial CT scan using bone window widths at T7-8, 596–597
    axial CT slice, 595, 597
    calcification of disc in, 595, 596, 597, 598
    left parasagittal reconstruction of spine with bone window widths, 597–598
    midsagittal reconstruction image using bone window widths, 596–597
    vertebral canal compromise in, 595, 596, 597
  T8-9 with calcification in adenocarcinoma patient, 593–594
    axial CT image, T8-9, 593–594
    axial CT image with bone window technique, 593–594

nucleus pulposus displacement in, 594
pleural effusions in, 594
spinal cord displacement and compression in, 593–594
Thoracic spinal cord
  astrocytoma in, 168, 170
  hemangioblastomas in, 599–601
  ischemia and presumed infarction in, 602–606
  midsagittal short TR image
    at L1 vertebral body, 32
  multiple sclerosis in, 694
Thoracic spinal cord infarction, post aortic aneurysm repair, 602–606
Thoracic spinal cord ischemia
  with areas of enhancement, 607–608
    hemangioma in T9 vertebral body, 608, 609
    incidental disc protrusion at L3-4 and L5-S1, 608
    within lumbar vertebral bodies, 608
    sagittal long TR image, 607
    sagittal long TR image at conus medullaris, 608
    sagittal short TR image, postcontrast, 607
    sagittal short TR image at conus medullaris, 608
    spinal cord enlargement in, 607
  infarction from, 606
  transient in elderly patient, 605–606
Thoracic spinal cord ischemia and infarction
  axial short TR image, 604–605
    postcontrast, 604–605
  left parasagittal long TR image, 603, 605
  left parasagittal short TR image, 603–604
  paraspinal fluid collection in, 604–605, 606
  pleural effusion in, 604–605, 606
  post aortic aneurysm repair, 602–606
  sagittal long TR image, 603–604
  sagittal short TR images
    postcontrast, 602, 604
    precontrast, 602
  signal intensity variation in
    secondary to flow-related, 603, 605, 606
  signal intensity within vertebral bodies
    secondary to osteoporosis, 606
  subarachnoid space obliteration in, 602
  thoracic aorta in
    enlargement of, 603–604, 605
    narrowing of lower, 603, 605
Thoracic spine
  distal
    in Chiari I malformation with focal syrinx, 72
  normal anatomy, 17–25, 19–25
    axial images, 19
    axial long TR image, 23
    contrast enhancement of, 19
    imaging of, 19
    pediatric, 24, 25
    sagittal long TR image, 21, 22, 25
    sagittal short TR image, 20, 24
Thoracic vertebrae
  renal cell cancer metastasis to, 371–376
Tonsillar ectopia
  defined, 70
  sagittal short TR image, 10
Trachea, in neurofibromatosis type 1, 219, 223
Transverse ligaments
  cervical
    sagittal long TR image, 13
Transverse myelitis. See Transverse myelopathy (myelitis)
Transverse myelopathy (myelitis). See also Acute disseminated encephalomyelopathy (ADEM)
  acute disseminated encephalomyelopathy versus, 718
  causes of, 721, 723
  cause unknown, 722–724
    in adolescent, 722–724
    correlation of imaging with clinical history, 724
    sagittal long TR images, cervical and upper thoracic, 722–723
    sagittal short TR image, thoracic postcontrast, 722
  idiopathic
    transverse myelopathy secondary multiple sclerosis versus, 721
  post hepatitis B vaccination, 712–715
  postimmunization, 712–715
    axial long TR image, 713–714
    axial short TR image, postcontrast, 714
    clinical course of, 715

    sagittal long TR image, medulla through C5-6, 712, 714
    sagittal short TR image, C2 through C5, 712, 714
    sagittal short TR image, lower medulla through C3-4 postcontrast, 713–714
  postradiation changes in spinal cord and vertebral bodies versus, 726
  secondary to multiple sclerosis, 719–721
    axial short TR images, thoracic spinal cord, 720–721
    brain imaging correlation with spinal imaging in, 721
    cerebral cortex defect in, 720–721
    clinical history in, 721
    corpus callosum defect in, 720–721
    optic neuritis in, 721
    sagittal short TR image, brain, 720–721
    sagittal short TR images, thoracic spinal cord, 719
  spinal cord ischemia with areas of enhancement versus, 608, 609
  thoracic spinal cord ischemia and infarction versus, 605
  of unknown cause, 709–711
    axial short TR image, postcontrast, 710
    cervical spinal cord edema in, 709
    sagittal short TR image, thoracic postcontrast, 710
    sagittal short TR images, pre- and postcontrast, 709
Trauma
  anterolisthesis of C4 on C5
    with herniated disc at C4-5 level, 286–288
  compression fracture in
    with cord edema, 269–271
    L1, 272–275
    L1 with distraction of interfacet joints, 272–275
    L1 with spinal cord hematoma, 284–285
    multiple, 322–323
    osteoporosis-related, 324–325
    T4 and T12, osteoporosis-related, 320–321
  dislocation of C5 on C6 in
    with nuchal ligament disruption and herniation of C5-C6 disc, 302–305
  epidural hematoma in, 306–307
    with blood in thecal sac, air in vertebral canal, 308–312
    in midthoracic region, Coumadinrelated, 317–319
    spontaneous, 313–316
  flexion in
    with fracture dislocation L1-2, 282–283
  fracture dislocation in
    C4 on C5, scoliosis and posttraumatic syrinx cavity associated with, 289–291
    C2 on C3 with herniated disc, 292–297
    L1-2, 282–283
    T6-7 with cord contusion and paraspinal hematoma, 276–281
  odontoid fractures in, 298–299
  perched facets from
    bilateral, 300–301
Tumor(s)
  cervical
    cervical disc herniation, C5-6 level, right side versus, 530
    imaging sequences and contrast material in, 3
  spinal cord
    contrast enhancement in, 29

U

Uncinate process
  cervical
    axial short TR image, 14
    coronal long TR image, 7
  cervical, C4
    axial short TR image, 8
  normal short TR image, postinfusion, 14

V

Vagus nerve, neurofibroma of, 212, 216
Vascular insult, Chiari I malformation with focal syrinx versus, 70
Vasculitis, multiple sclerosis versus, 791, 792
Venous plexus, cervical vertebral body, sagittal short TR image, 10

Venous plexus flow void
   coronal short TR image, 36
Ventriculitis, cerebral, cytomegalovirus radiculitis *versus,* 521
Vertebral anomalies, diastematomyelia *versus,* 121
Vertebral arteries
   cervical, 7
   in foramen transversarium, 11
Vertebral body
   cervical, 7
   dorsal root ganglion, L5
     long TR image of, 52
   endplates of lumbar
     sagittal intermediate intensity image, 43
   L1
     axial short TR image, 60
     spinal cord termination at, 35
   lumbar
     parasagittal short TR image, 39
     sagittal long TR image, 41
   midsagittal short TR image, L4 and L5, 31
   normal pediatric
     sagittal short TR image, 24
   postradiation changes in, 725–727
Vertebral body height
   lumbar
     midsagittal short TR image, 30
     sagittal short TR image, 42
Vertebral canal
   in Chiari I malformation with focal syrinx, 72
expansion of
   in pilocystic astrocytoma, 164, 166
tissue in from spinal tap
   synovial cyst at left L3-4 interfacet joint *versus,* 672
Vertebral metastases. *See also under* Non-Hodgkin's lymphoma
   and lymph node enlargement, 347–349
Vertebral pedicle
   lumbar
     axial CT image postmyelogram, 56
     axial short TR image, 47
     axial short TR image, postcontrast, 48
   in metastatic disease, 337
Virchow-Robin spaces
   axial short TR image of brain, 196
   dilated, 195–197
Von Hippel-Lindau disease
   with cerebellar and spinal hemangioblastomas, 599–601
   in adolescent patient, 599–601
   axial short TR image, T7, 600–601
   cerebellar, 600–601
   coronal short TR image, brain, 600–601
   sagittal short TR image, postcontrast, 599
   spinal cord displacement in, 599
   subarachnoid space lesions in, 599, 600–601
hemangioblastoma in, 599–601
   multiple, 258–259
   spinal and cerebral, 857–860
   spinal cord, 258–259
   typical findings in, 601
Von Hippel-Lindau syndrome
   with multiple spinal and cerebral hemangioblastomas, 857–860
   magnetic susceptibility artifact in, 857, 859, 860
   parasagittal short TR image, brain postcontrast, 859
   parasagittal short TR image, cervical spine, 857
   post laminectomy clips in, cervical and thoracic, 857, 859–860
   postoperative changes in, from occipital craniectomy, 860
   sagittal short TR image, brain postcontrast, 858–859
   sagittal short TR image, cervical spine, 857
   sagittal short TR image, thoracic spine, 858–859
Von Recklinghausen's disease. *See* Neurofibromatosis, type 1

W

Wallerian degeneration
   spinal cord ependymoma removal *versus,* 164
Whiplash injury
   degenerative changes with osteophyte formation post-trauma, 541–543